Military Medicine in Iraq and Afghanistan

A Comprehensive Review

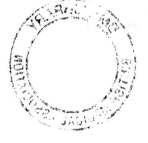

Military Medicine in Iraq and Afghanistan

A Comprehensive Review

Edited by

Ian Greaves
United Kingdom Defence Medical Services
and
James Cook University Hospital
Middlesbrough, United Kingdom

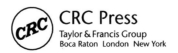

CRC Press
Taylor & Francis Group
Boca Raton London New York

CRC Press is an imprint of the
Taylor & Francis Group, an **informa** business

CRC Press
Taylor & Francis Group
6000 Broken Sound Parkway NW, Suite 300
Boca Raton, FL 33487-2742

© 2019 by Taylor & Francis Group, LLC
CRC Press is an imprint of Taylor & Francis Group, an Informa business

No claim to original U.S. Government works

Printed on acid-free paper

International Standard Book Number-13: 978-1-138-55423-8 (Hardback)
International Standard Book Number-13: 978-0-8153-7759-7 (Paperback)

**Visit the Taylor & Francis Web site at
http://www.taylorandfrancis.com**

**and the CRC Press Web site at
http://www.crcpress.com**

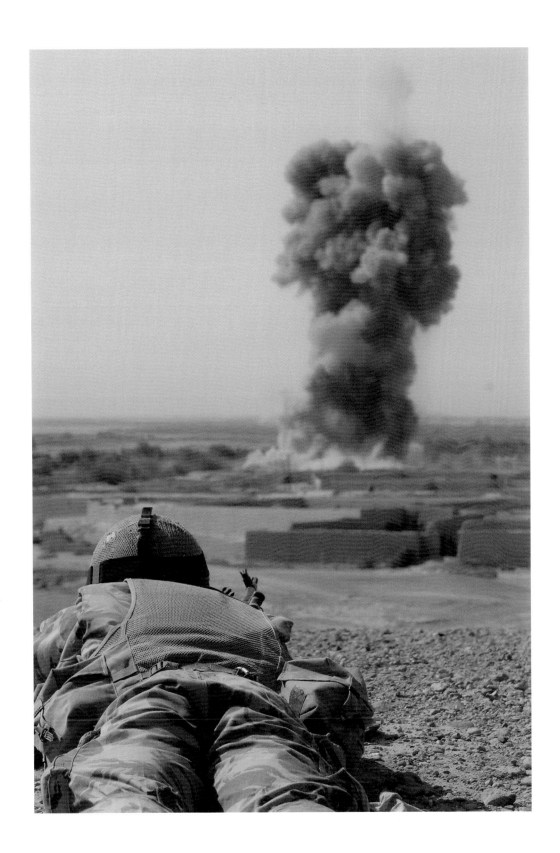

Contents

Preface

A LASTING LEGACY?

The concept of regular advances in care for the military casualty arising from combat experience and forming steps in a continuous process of improvement in clinical care is an attractive one but is an aspiration that more often than not fails to happen. The period between conflicts is often associated with loss of corporate knowledge as individuals retire and as the political imperative to maintain support (and indeed interest) in the Defence Medical Services fades. This is a phenomenon affecting not only the United Kingdom but also the majority of nations.

Unsurprisingly, therefore, most conflicts start with limited medical capability. There is thus an inevitable need as each conflict progresses for rapid development in the delivery of clinical care to ensure that the wounded and ill are looked after, and mortality and morbidity are reduced where possible.

Experience shows that from the Crimean War onwards, advances in treatment have occurred during conflict, yet there has been relative failure to consolidate this knowledge with the coming of peace. The phenomenon is well accepted by most North Atlantic Treaty Organisation forces, but medical delivery during periods of peace, or more specifically when casualties are not being taken, is seen as too expensive by the higher commands of most nations and indeed by their political leaders. It is this perpetual fluctuation in patient management that we must try to avoid whilst remaining fiscally prudent and politically realistic.

In the 1990s, there were enormous reductions in military medicine. Some were sensible and necessary, but others reduced overall care pathways and degraded clinical capability. It took until 2006 to achieve real improvement, and the resulting advances in regimes and research innovations described in this book demonstrated a capacity for forward thinking and an ability to learn from experience that has been of great benefit nationally and internationally, in military and civilian practice alike. By 2014, however, the reduction in visible warfare in Iraq and Afghanistan, and the consequent decline in casualty numbers, led to overall reductions in military numbers and problems with financial management across Defence. The supply of medical capabilities inevitably came once more under review, with finances being under especially close scrutiny.

It is therefore important that the readers of this book are aware that although many of the developments have now found their place in contemporary civilian practice, the ability of the DMS to respond in the same way in the future is inevitably a function of political support, military commitment and financial policy. Nothing can be taken for granted.

What is clear is that effective interaction between primary healthcare, secondary healthcare, nursing, mental healthcare and rehabilitation ensures the continuance of the best care pathways, reduces inappropriate investigation, prevents duplication of effort and consequently facilitates effective care, allowing, where possible, a successful return to active duty. Consequently, the cost is reduced. The option to see a reduction in medical care as part of the 'peace dividend' will, in the longer term, be counterproductive and, perhaps counter-intuitively, expensive. Working together as multidisciplinary teams, focusing research profiles and always remembering that the patient is at the heart of all we do require commitment from clinicians, commanders and politicians alike.

Alasdair Walker, CB, OBE, QHS
Surgeon General 2015–2017

Martin Bricknell, OStJ, QHP
Surgeon General 2017–

Dedicated to the memory of

All those, including the four members of The Royal Army Medical Corps, who gave their lives in Iraq and Afghanistan

In Arduis Fidelis

Role of honour

Sergeant John Nightingale, Royal Logistic
Corps, aged 32

Corporal Ian Plank, Royal Marines, aged 31

Gunner Duncan Pritchard, 16 Squadron RAF
Regiment, aged 22

Corporal Dewi Pritchard, Royal Military
Police, aged 35

Sergeant Steven Roberts, 2nd Royal Tank
Regiment, aged 33

Operator Mechanic (Communications) Ian
Seymour, 148 Commando Battery Royal
Artillery, aged 29 years

Lance Corporal Karl Shearer, Household
Cavalry Regiment

Corporal David Shepherd, Royal Air Force
Police, aged 34

Private Jason Smith, 52nd Lowland Regiment
(Volunteers) attached to 1st King's Own
Scottish Borderers, aged 32

Lance Corporal Barry Stephen, 1st Battalion
The Black Watch, aged 31

Warrant Officer Second Class Mark Stratford,
Royal Marines, aged 39

Private Ryan Lloyd Thomas, The Royal
Regiment of Wales, aged 18

Major Matthew Titchener, Royal Military
Police, aged 32

Fusilier Kelan Turrington, Royal Regiment of
Fusiliers, aged 18

Lieutenant Alexander Tweedie, Household
Cavalry Regiment, aged 25

Company Sergeant Major Colin Wall, Royal
Military Police, aged 34

Major Jason Ward, Royal Marines, UK
Landing Force Support Group, aged 34

Lieutenant Philip, West Royal Navy, 849 Naval
Air Squadron, aged 32

Flight Lieutenant David Rhys Williams, Royal
Air Force, 9 Squadron

Lieutenant James Williams, Royal Navy, 849
Naval Air Squadron, aged 28

Lieutenant Andrew Wilson, Royal Navy, 849
Naval Air Squadron, aged 36

2004

Sergeant Paul Connolly, Royal Electrical &
Mechanical Engineers, aged 33

Lance Corporal Andrew Craw, Argyll &
Sutherland Highlanders, aged 21

Fusilier Gordon Gentle, Royal Highland
Fusiliers, aged 19

Flight Lieutenant Kristian Gover, 33 Squadron
RAF, aged 30

Sergeant Stuart Robert Tennant Gray, 1st
Battalion The Black Watch, aged 31

Corporal Richard Ivell, Royal Electrical &
Mechanical Engineers, aged 29

Fusilier Stephen Jones, The Royal Welch
Fusiliers, aged 22

Gunner David Lawrence, Royal Artillery,
aged 25

Private Paul Lowe, 1st Battalion The Black
Watch, aged 19

Private Scott McArdle, 1st Battalion The Black
Watch, aged 22

Private Kevin McHale, The Black Watch,
aged 27

Private Lee O'Callaghan, Princess of Wales'
Royal Regiment, aged 20

Chief Petty Officer Simon Roger Owen, HMS
CHATHAM, aged 38

Sergeant Norman Patterson, Cheshire
Regiment, aged 28

Private Christopher Rayment, Princess of
Wales' Royal Regiment, aged 22

Staff Sergeant Denise Michelle Rose, Royal
Military Police, aged 34

Major James Stenner, Welsh Guards, aged 30

Corporal Marc Taylor, Royal Electrical &
Mechanical Engineers, aged 27

Lance Corporal Paul Thomas, The Light
Infantry, aged 29

Sapper Robert Thomson, Royal Engineers,
aged 22

Private Pita Tukutukuwaqa, The Black Watch,
aged 27

Rifleman Vincent Windsor, Royal Green
Jackets, aged 23

2005

Major Matthew Bacon, Intelligence Corps,
aged 34

Lance Corporal Alan Brackenbury, The King's
Royal Hussars, aged 21

Chief Technician Richard Brown, RAF
Lyneham, aged 40

Private Mark Dobson, Tyne-Tees Regiment,
aged 41

Signaller Paul William Didsbury, 21st Signal Regiment (Air Support), aged 18

Flight Sergeant Mark Gibson, 47 Squadron, RAF Lyneham, aged 34

Private Phillip Hewett, 1st Battalion Staffordshire Regiment, aged 21

Sergeant Chris Hickey, 1st Battalion the Coldstream Guards, aged 30

Sergeant John Jones, 1st Battalion The Royal Regiment of Fusiliers, aged 31

Lance Corporal Steven Jones, Royal Signals, aged 25

Fusilier Stephen Robert Manning, Royal Regiment of Fusiliers, aged 22

Squadron Leader Patrick Marshall, Royal Air Force, Headquarters Strike Command, aged 39

Captain Ken Masters, Royal Military Police, aged 40

Fusilier Donal Anthony Meade, Royal Regiment of Fusiliers, aged 20

Master Air Engineer Gary Nicholson, 47 Squadron, RAF Lyneham, aged 42

Sergeant Robert O'Connor, RAF Lyneham, aged 38

Flight Lieutenant Paul Pardoel, 47 Squadron, RAF Lyneham, aged 35

Second Lieutenant Richard Shearer, 1st Battalion Staffordshire Regiment, aged 26

Flight Lieutenant Andrew Smith, 47 Squadron, RAF Lyneham, aged 25

Private Leon Spicer, 1st Battalion Staffordshire Regiment, aged 26

Flight Lieutenant David Stead, 47 Squadron, RAF Lyneham, aged 35

Guardsman Anthony John Wakefield, 1st Battalion, The Coldstream Guards, aged 24

Corporal David Williams, RAF Lyneham, aged 37

2006

Lance Corporal Dennis Brady, Royal Army Medical Corps, aged 37

Lieutenant Commander Darren Chapman Royal Navy, 847 Naval Air Squadron, aged 40

Marine Paul Collins, 847 Naval Air Squadron, aged 21

Corporal Matthew Cornish, 1 Light Infantry, aged 29

Corporal John Johnston Cosby, 1st Battalion The Devonshire and Dorset Light Infantry, aged 28

Wing Commander John Coxen, RAF Benson, aged 46

Captain David Dobson, Army Air Corps, aged 27

Lance Corporal Allan Douglas, 1st Battalion, The Highlanders, aged 22

Staff Sergeant Sharron Elliott, Intelligence Corps, aged 34

Private Lee Ellis, 2nd Battalion, The Parachute Regiment, aged 23

Lance Corporal Paul Farrelly, Queen's Dragoon Guards, aged 27

Private Marc Ferns, The Black Watch, aged 21

Kingsman Jamie Hancock, 2nd Battalion, The Duke of Lancaster's Regiment, aged 19

Sergeant Graham Hesketh, 2nd Battalion, The Duke of Lancaster's Regiment, aged 35

Sergeant Jonathan Hollingsworth CGC, QGM, The Parachute Regiment, aged 35

Captain Richard Holmes, 2nd Battalion, The Parachute Regiment, aged 28

Warrant Officer Class 2 Lee Hopkins, Royal Corps of Signals, aged 35

Marine Jason Hylton, 539 Assault Squadron Royal Marines, aged 33

Private Joseva Lewaicei, 2nd Battalion, The Royal Anglian Regiment, aged 25

Lieutenant Tom Mildinhall, Queen's Dragoon Guards, aged 26

Private Adam Morris, 2nd Battalion, The Royal Anglian Regiment, aged 19

Flight Lieutenant Sarah-Jayne Mulvihill, Royal Air Force, aged 32

Corporal Ben Nowak, 45 Commando Royal Marines, aged 27

Lieutenant Richard Palmer, Royal Scots Dragoon Guards, aged 27

Corporal Gordon Alexander Pritchard, Royal Scots Dragoon Guards, aged 31

Trooper Carl Smith, 9th/12th Royal Lancers (Prince of Wales's), aged 23

Lieutenant Tom Tanswell, 58 (Eyre's) Battery, 12 Regt Royal Artillery, aged 27

Gunner Lee Thornton, 58 (Eyre's) Battery, 12 Regiment Royal Artillery, aged 22

Gunner Samuela Vanua, 58 (Eyre's) Battery, 12 Regiment Royal Artillery, aged 27

Gunner Stephen Robert Wright, 58 (Eyre's) Battery, 12 Regiment Royal Artillery, aged 20

2007

Private Craig Barber, 2nd Battalion The Royal Welsh, aged 20

Major Nick Bateson, Royal Corps of Signals, aged 49

Sergeant John Battersby, Queen's Lancashire Regiment, aged 31

Leading Aircraftman Martin Beard, No. 1 Squadron Royal Air Force Regiment, aged 20

Second Lieutenant Jonathan Carlos Bracho-Cooke, 2nd Battalion, The Duke of Lancaster's Regiment, aged 24

Corporal Jeremy Brookes, 4th Battalion the Rifles, aged 28

Lance Corporal James Cartwright, 2nd Royal Tank Regiment, aged 21

Lance Sergeant Chris Casey, 1st Battalion, Irish Guards, aged 27

Senior Aircraftman Matthew Caulwell, 1 Squadron RAF Regiment, aged 22

Rifleman Daniel Lee Coffey, Second Battalion The Rifles, aged 21

Sergeant Eddie Collins, The Parachute Regiment, aged 33

Private Eleanor Dlugosz, Royal Army Medical Corps, aged 19

Rifleman Paul Donnachie, 2nd Battalion The Rifles, aged 18

Senior Aircraftman Christopher Dunsmore, 504 Squadron Royal Auxiliary Air Force Regiment, aged 29

Corporal Steve Edwards, 2nd Royal Tank Regiment, aged 35

Guardsman Stephen Ferguson, 1st Battalion Scots Guards, aged 31

Corporal Lee Fitzsimmons, Special Air Service, aged 26

Lance Corporal Timothy Darren 'Daz' Flowers, Royal Electrical Mechanical Engineers, aged 25

Lance Corporal Ryan Francis, 2nd Battalion The Royal Welsh, aged 23

Kingsman Alex Green, 2nd Battalion, The Duke of Lancaster's Regiment, aged 21

Major Paul Harding, 4th Battalion, The Rifles, aged 48

Lance Corporal Sarah Holmes, 29 Postal Courier and Movement Regiment, aged 26

Kingsman Alan Joseph Jones, 2nd Battalion, The Duke of Lancaster's Regiment, aged 20

Corporal Paul Joszko, 2nd Battalion, The Royal Welsh, aged 28

Private Scott Kennedy, Black Watch, 3rd Battalion, The Royal Regiment of Scotland, aged 20

Private James Kerr, Black Watch, 3rd Battalion The Royal Regiment of Scotland, aged 20

Corporal Ben Leaning, The Queen's Royal Lancers, aged 24

Rifleman Aaron Lincoln, 2nd Battalion, The Rifles, aged 18

Senior Aircraftman Peter McFerran, 1 Squadron Royal Air Force Regiment, aged 24

Sergeant Mark J. McLaren, 230 Squadron Royal Air Force, aged 27

Corporal Kris O'Neill, Royal Army Medical Corps, aged 27

Colour Sergeant M.L. Powell, The Parachute Regiment, aged 37

Corporal Christopher Read, Royal Military Police, aged 22

Lance Corporal Kirk Redpath, 1st Battalion, Irish Guards aged, 22

Sergeant Wayne Rees, The Queen's Royal Lancers, aged 36

Corporal John Rigby, 4th Battalion, The Rifles, aged 24

Private Luke Daniel Simpson, 1st Battalion, The Yorkshire Regiment, aged 21

Kingsman Adam James Smith, 2nd Battalion The Duke of Lancaster's Regiment, aged 19

Sergeant Mark Stansfield, Royal Logistics Corps, aged 32

Private Michael Tench, 2nd Battalion, The Light Infantry, aged 18

Private Kevin Thompson, Royal Logistic Corps, aged 21

Trooper Kristen Turton, The Queen's Royal Lancers, aged 27

Rifleman Edward Vakabua, 4th Battalion, The
Rifles, aged 23

Corporal Rodney Wilson, 4th Battalion, The
Rifles, aged 30

Kingsman Daniel Wilson, 2nd Battalion,
The Duke of Lancaster's Regiment,
aged 28

Private Johnathon Dany Wysoczan, 1st
Battalion The Staffordshire Regiment,
aged 21

Second Lieutenant Joanna Yorke Dyer, The
Intelligence Corps, aged 24

2008

Sergeant Duane 'Baz' Barwood, 903
Expeditionary Air Wing, Royal Air Force,
aged 41

Colour Sergeant Nicholas Brown, The
Parachute Regiment, aged 34

Corporal Lee Churcher, 20th Armoured
Brigade, Royal Engineers, aged 32

Lance Corporal David Kenneth Wilson, 9
Regiment Army Air Corps, aged 27

2009

Private Ryan Wrathall, 1st Battalion, The
Princess of Wales's Royal Regiment,
aged 21

OPERATIONS IN AFGHANISTAN

2002

Sergeant Robert Busuttil, Royal Logistic Corps,
aged 30

Corporal John Gregory, Royal Logistic Corps,
aged 30

Private Darren John George, Royal Anglian
Regiment, aged 23

2004

Private Jonathan Kitulagoda, Rifle Volunteers,
aged 23

2005

Lance Corporal Steven Sherwood, 1st
Battalion, Royal Gloucestershire,
Berkshire and Wiltshire Light Infantry,
aged 23

2006

Flight Sergeant Gary Wayne Andrews, RAF
Kinloss, aged 48

Sergeant Paul Bartlett, Royal Marines, aged 35

Flight Sergeant Stephen Beattie, RAF Kinloss,
aged 42

Flight Sergeant Gerard Martin Bell, RAF
Kinloss, aged 48

Corporal Bryan James Budd VC, 3rd Battalion,
The Parachute Regiment, aged 29

Lance Corporal Peter Edward Craddock, 1st
Battalion, Royal Gloucestershire, Berkshire
and Wiltshire Regiment, aged 31

Corporal Mark Cridge, 7 Signal Regiment,
aged 25

Private Andrew Barrie Cutts, Royal Logistic
Corps, aged 19

Flight Sergeant Adrian Davies, RAF Kinloss,
aged 49

Corporal Oliver Simon Dicketts, 1st Battalion,
The Parachute Regiment, aged 27

Ranger Anare Draiva, 1 Royal Irish Regiment,
aged 27

Lance Bombardier James Dwyer, Royal
Artillery, aged 22

Captain Alex Eida, Royal Horse Artillery,
aged 29

Lance Corporal Jabron Hashmi, Intelligence
Corps, aged 24

Lance Corporal Jonathan Peter Hetherington,
14 Signal Regiment, aged 22

Private Damien Jackson, 3rd Battalion, The
Parachute Regiment, aged 19

Second Lieutenant Ralph Johnson, Household
Cavalry Regiment, aged 24

Flight Lieutenant Steven Johnson Royal Air
Force, RAF Kinloss, aged 38

Sergeant Benjamin James Knight, RAF
Kinloss, aged 25

Sergeant John Joseph Langton, RAF Kinloss,
aged 29

Lance Corporal Luke McCulloch, 1 Royal Irish
Regiment, aged 21

Flight Lieutenant Leigh Anthony Mitchelmore,
Royal Air Force, RAF Kinloss, aged 28

Lance Corporal Paul Muirhead, 1 Royal Irish
Regiment, aged 29

Flight Lieutenant Gareth Rodney Nicholas,
Royal Air Force, RAF Kinloss, aged 40

Lance Corporal Ross Nicholls, Blues and
Royals, aged 27

Private Craig O'Donnell, The Argyll and
Sutherland Highlanders, 5th Battalion the
Royal Regiment of Scotland, aged 24

Captain David Patton, The Parachute
Regiment, aged 38

Captain Jim Philippson, 7 Parachute Regiment
Royal Horse Artillery, aged 29

Sergeant Gary Paul Quilliam, RAF Kinloss,
aged 42

Private Leigh Reeves, Royal Logistic Corps,
aged 25

Flight Lieutenant Allan James Squires, Royal
Air Force, RAF Kinloss, aged 39

Flight Lieutenant Steven Swarbrick, Royal Air
Force, RAF Kinloss, aged 28

Lance Corporal Sean Tansey, The Life Guards,
aged 26

Corporal Peter Thorpe, Royal Signals, aged 27

Marine Richard J Watson, 42 Commando
Royal Marines, aged 23

Marine Jonathan Wigley, 45 Commando Royal
Marines, aged 21

Marine Joseph David Windall, Royal Marines,
aged 22

Marine Gary Wright, 45 Commando Royal
Marines, aged 22

Corporal Mark William Wright, 3rd Battalion,
The Parachute Regiment, aged 27

2007

Lance Corporal Jake Alderton, 36 Engineer
Regiment, aged 22

Guardsman David Atherton, 1st Battalion,
Grenadier Guards, aged 25

Corporal Darren Bonner, 1st Battalion, The
Royal Anglian Regiment, aged 31

Private Johan Botha, 2nd Battalion, The
Mercian Regiment

Sergeant Craig Brelsford, 2nd Battalion, The
Mercian Regiment, aged 25

Senior Aircraftman Christopher Bridge, 51
Squadron, Royal Air Force Regiment,
aged 20

Lance Bombardier Ross Clark, 29 Commando
Regiment Royal Artillery, aged 25

Marine Thomas Curry, 42 Commando Royal
Marines, aged 21

Lance Corporal George Russell Davey, 1st
Battalion the Royal Anglian Regiment,
aged 23

Guardsman Simon Davison, 1st Battalion
Grenadier Guards, aged 22

Captain Sean Dolan, 1st Battalion, The
Worcestershire and Sherwood Foresters,
aged 40

Guardsman Neil 'Tony' Downes, 1st Battalion
Grenadier Guards, aged 20

Private Ben Ford, 2nd Battalion, The Mercian
Regiment, aged 18

Lance Corporal Mathew Ford, 45 Commando
Royal Marines, aged 30

Private Robert Graham Foster, 1st Battalion,
The Royal Anglian Regiment, aged 19

Corporal Mike Gilyeat, Royal Military Police,
aged 28

Private Chris Gray, A Company, 1st Battalion,
The Royal Anglian Regiment, aged 19

Lance Corporal Alex Hawkins, 1st Battalion,
The Royal Anglian Regiment, aged 22

Guardsman Daryl Hickey, 1st Battalion,
Grenadier Guards, aged 27

Captain David Hicks, 1st Battalion, The Royal
Anglian Regiment, aged 26

Marine Jonathan Holland, 45 Commando
Royal Marines, aged 23

Sergeant Lee Johnson, 2nd Battalion, The
Yorkshire Regiment, aged 33

Lance Corporal Michael Jones, Royal Marines,
aged 26

Sergeant Barry Keen, 14 Signal Regiment, aged 34

Private Aaron James McClure, 1st Battalion,
The Royal Anglian Regiment, aged 19

Captain John McDermid, The Royal Highland
Fusiliers, 2nd Battalion, The Royal
Regiment of Scotland, aged 43

Lance Bombardier Liam McLaughlin, 29
Commando Regiment Royal Artillery,
aged 21

Colour Sergeant Phillip Newman, 4th
Battalion, The Mercian Regiment, aged 36

Guardsman Daniel Probyn, 1st Battalion,
Grenadier Guards, aged 22

Private Tony Rawson, 1st Battalion, The Royal
Anglian Regiment, aged 27

Marine Benjamin Reddy, 42 Commando Royal
Marines, aged 22

Major Alexis Roberts, 1st Battalion, The Royal
Gurkha Rifles, aged 32

Trooper Jack Sadler, The Honourable Artillery
Company, aged 21

Lance Corporal Paul 'Sandy' Sandford,
1st Battalion, The Worcestershire and
Sherwood Foresters, aged 23

WO2 Michael 'Mick' Smith, 29 Commando
Regiment Royal Artillery, aged 39

Marine Scott Summers, 42 Commando Royal
Marines, aged 23

Private John Thrumble, 1st Battalion, The
Royal Anglian Regiment, aged 21

Private Brian Tunnicliffe, 2nd Battalion, The
Mercian Regiment, aged 33

Corporal Ivano Violino, 36 Engineer
Regiment, aged 29

Sergeant Dave Wilkinson, 19 Regiment Royal
Artillery, aged 33

Private Damian Wright, 2nd Battalion, The
Mercian Regiment, aged 23

Drummer Thomas Wright, 1st Battalion, The
Worcestershire and Sherwood Foresters,
aged 21

2008

Trooper Ratu Sakeasi Babakobau, Household
Cavalry Regiment, aged 29

Corporal Jason Stuart Barnes, Royal Electrical
and Mechanical Engineers, aged 25

Lance Corporal James Bateman, 2nd Battalion
The Parachute Regiment, aged 29

Corporal Marc Birch, 45 Commando, Royal
Marines, aged 26

Signaller Wayne Bland, 16 Signal Regiment,
aged 21

Corporal Sarah Bryant, Intelligence Corps,
aged 26

Private Peter Joe Cowton, 2nd Battalion, The
Parachute Regiment, aged 25

Ranger Justin James Cupples, 1st Battalion, The
Royal Irish Regiment, aged 29

Private Nathan Cuthbertson, 2nd Battalion,
The Parachute Regiment, aged 19

Marine Damian Davies, Commando Logistic
Regiment, Royal Marines, aged 27

Corporal Robert Deering, Commando
Logistic Regiment, Royal Marines,
aged 33

Corporal Barry Dempsey, The Royal Highland
Fusiliers, 2nd Battalion, Royal Regiment of
Scotland, aged 29

Private Jeff Doherty, 2nd Battalion, The
Parachute Regiment, aged 20

Marine Neil David Dunstan, 3 Commando
Brigade Royal Marines, aged 32

Colour Sergeant Krishnabahadur Dura, 2nd
Battalion, The Royal Gurkha Rifles,
aged 36

Corporal Liam Elms, 45 Commando Royal
Marines, aged 26

Marine Tony Evans, 42 Commando Royal
Marines, aged 20

Lance Corporal Steven 'Jamie' Fellows, 45
Commando Royal Marines, aged 28

Private Daniel Gamble, 2nd Battalion, The
Parachute Regiment, aged 22

Corporal Darryl Gardiner, Royal Electrical and
Mechanical Engineers, aged 25

Marine Dale Gostick, 3 Troop Armoured
Support Company, Royal Marines, aged 22

Lance Corporal James Johnson, B Company,
5th Battalion, The Royal Regiment of
Scotland, aged 31

Lance Corporal Richard Larkin, Special Air
Service, aged 39

Corporal Damian Stephen Lawrence, 2nd
Battalion The Yorkshire Regiment (Green
Howards), aged 25

Lieutenant Aaron Lewis, 29 Commando
Regiment Royal Artillery, aged 26

Senior Aircraftman Graham Livingstone, 3
Squadron, Royal Air Force Regiment,
aged 23

Marine Alexander Lucas, 45 Commando Royal
Marines, aged 24

Sergeant John Manuel, 45 Commando Royal
Marines, aged 38

Marine David Marsh, 40 Commando Royal
Marines, aged 23

Lance Corporal Nicky Mason, 2nd Battalion,
The Parachute Regiment, aged 26

Sergeant Jonathan Mathews, The Highlanders,
4th Battalion, The Royal Regiment of
Scotland, aged 35

Marine Robert Joseph McKibben, 1 Brigade
Reconnaissance Force, Royal Marines,
aged 32

Trooper James Munday, Household Cavalry
Regiment, aged 21

Private Charles David Murray, 2nd Battalion,
The Parachute Regiment, aged 19

Rifleman Stuart Nash, 1st Battalion, The Rifles,
aged 21

Warrant Officer Class 2 Gary 'Gaz' O'Donnell
GM, 11 Explosive Ordnance Disposal
Regiment Royal Logistic Corps, aged 40

Trooper Robert Pearson, The Queen's Royal
Lancers Regiment, aged 22

Rifleman Yubraj Rai, 2nd Battalion, The Royal
Gurkha Rifles, aged 28

Private Jason Lee Rawstron, 2nd Battalion, The
Parachute Regiment, aged 23

Corporal Sean Robert Reeve, Royal Signals,
aged 28

Lance Corporal Kenneth Michael Rowe, Royal
Army Veterinary Corps, aged 24

Warrant Officer 2nd Class Dan Shirley, Air
Assault Support Regiment, Royal Logistic
Corps, aged 32

Marine Georgie Sparks, 42 Commando Royal
Marines, aged 19

Paul Stout, Special Air Service, aged 31

Senior Aircraftman Gary Thompson, 504
Squadron, Royal Auxiliary Air Force
Regiment, aged 51

James Thompson, serving with the 5th Scottish
Regiment Battle Group

Lieutenant John Thornton, 40 Commando
Royal Marines, aged 22

Lance Corporal Benjamin Whatley, 42
Commando Royal Marines, aged 20

Private Joe John Whittaker, 4th Battalion The
Parachute Regiment, aged 20

Warrant Officer 2nd Class Michael Norman
Williams, 2nd Battalion, The Parachute
Regiment, aged 40

2009

Private Kyle Adams, The Parachute Regiment,
aged 21

Rifleman William Aldridge, 2nd Battalion, The
Rifles, aged 18

Rifleman Philip Allen, 2nd Battalion, The
Rifles, aged 20

Acting Sergeant John Paxton Amer, 1st
Battalion, Coldstream Guards

Fusilier Simon Annis, 2nd Battalion, The Royal
Regiment of Fusiliers

Captain Ben Babington-Browne, 22 Engineer
Regiment, Royal Engineers, aged 27

Rifleman James Backhouse, 2nd Battalion, The
Rifles, aged 18

Rifleman Samuel John Bassett, 4th Battalion,
The Rifles, aged 20

Sergeant Sean Binnie, The Black Watch, 3rd
Battalion, The Royal Regiment of Scotland,
aged 22

Major Sean Birchall, 1st Battalion, Welsh
Guards, aged 33

Corporal Stephen Bolger, The Parachute
Regiment

Corporal Steven Boote, Royal Military Police,
aged 22

Private John Brackpool, 1st Battalion, Welsh
Guards, aged 27

Lance Corporal Richard Brandon, Royal
Electrical and Mechanical Engineers,
aged 24

Rifleman James Stephen Brown, 3rd Battalion,
The Rifles, aged 18

Lance Corporal Tommy Brown, The Parachute
Regiment

Fusilier Louis Carter, 2nd Battalion The Royal
Regiment of Fusiliers

Warrant Officer Class 1 Darren Chant,
1st Battalion, The Grenadier Guards,
aged 40

Lance Corporal David Dennis, The Light
Dragoons, aged 29

Lance Corporal Adam Drane, 1st Battalion,
The Royal Anglian Regiment, aged 23

Kingsman Jason Dunn-Bridgeman, 2nd
Battalion, The Duke of Lancaster's
Regiment, aged 20

Private Gavin Elliott, 2nd Battalion, The
Mercian Regiment, aged 19

Private Kevin Elliott, The Black Watch, 3rd
Battalion, The Royal Regiment of Scotland,
aged 24

Lance Corporal Dane Elson, 1st Battalion,
Welsh Guards, aged 22

Corporal Joseph Etchells, 2nd Battalion, The
Royal Regiment of Fusiliers, aged 22

Lieutenant Mark Evison, 1st Battalion, Welsh
Guards, aged 26

Lance Sergeant Tobie Fasfous, 1st Battalion, Welsh Guards, aged 29

Rifleman Andrew Ian Fentiman, 7th Battalion, The Rifles, aged 23

Lance Corporal James Fullarton, 2nd Battalion, The Royal Regiment of Fusiliers, aged 24

Corporal Tom Gaden, 1st Battalion, The Rifles, aged 24

Rifleman Jamie Gunn, 1st Battalion, The Rifles, aged 21

Captain Mark Hale, 2nd Battalion, The Rifles, aged 42

Trooper Brett Hall, 2nd Royal Tank Regiment, aged 21

Trooper Joshua Hammond, 2nd Royal Tank Regiment, aged 18

Lance Corporal Christopher Harkett, 2nd Battalion, The Royal Welsh, aged 22

Corporal John Harrison, The Parachute Regiment, aged 29

Lance Bombardier Matthew Hatton, 40th Regiment Royal Artillery, aged 23

Lance Corporal James Hill, 1st Battalion, Coldstream Guards, aged 23

Lance Corporal Kieron Hill, 2nd Battalion, The Mercian Regiment, aged 20

Lance Corporal Dale Thomas Hopkins, The Parachute Regiment, aged 23

Bombardier Craig Hopson, 40th Regiment Royal Artillery, aged 24

Corporal Simon Hornby, 2nd Battalion, The Duke of Lancaster's Regiment, aged 29

Corporal Jonathan Horne, 2nd Battalion, The Rifles, aged 28

Rifleman Aidan Howell, 3rd Battalion, The Rifles, aged 19

Sergeant Lee Andrew Houltram, Royal Marines

Rifleman Daniel Hume, 4th Battalion, The Rifles

Private Richard Hunt, 2nd Battalion, The Royal Welsh, aged 21

Guardsman Jamie Janes, 1st Battalion, Grenadier Guards, aged 20

Corporal Dean Thomas John, Royal Electrical and Mechanical Engineers, aged 25

Guardsman Christopher King, 1st Battalion, Coldstream Guards, aged 20

Lance Corporal Stephen 'Schnoz' Kingscott, 1st Battalion, The Rifles, aged 22

Lance Corporal David Leslie Kirkness, 3rd Battalion, The Rifles, aged 24

Marine Michael 'Mick' Laski, 45 Commando, Royal Marines, aged 21

Trooper Phillip Lawrence, Light Dragoons, aged 22

Private Robert Laws, 2nd Battalion, The Mercian Regiment, aged 18

Acting Sergeant Michael Lockett MC, 2nd Battalion, The Mercian Regiment

Craftsman Anthony Lombardi, Royal Electrical and Mechanical Engineers, aged 21

Sergeant Robert David Loughran-Dickson, Royal Military Police, aged 33

Marine Jason Mackie, Armoured Support Group, Royal Marines, aged 21

Marine Travis Mackin, 45 Commando, Royal Marines, aged 22

Guardsman James Major, 1st Battalion, The Grenadier Guards, aged 18

Corporal Loren Owen Christopher Marlton-Thomas, 33 Engineer Regiment, aged 28

Corporal Thomas 'Tam' Mason, The Black Watch, 3rd Battalion, The Royal Regiment of Scotland, aged 27

Serjeant Paul McAleese, 2nd Battalion, The Rifles, aged 29

Acting Serjeant Stuart McGrath, 2nd Battalion, The Rifles, aged 28

Private Robert McLaren, The Black Watch, 3rd Battalion The Royal Regiment of Scotland, aged 20

Lieutenant Paul Mervis, 2nd Battalion, The Rifles, aged 27

Sergeant Stuart 'Gus' Millar, The Black Watch, 3rd Battalion, The Royal Regiment of Scotland, aged 40

Lance Corporal Nigel Moffett, The Light Dragoons, aged 28

Corporal Kevin Mulligan, The Parachute Regiment, aged 26

Rifleman Joe Murphy, 2nd Battalion, The Rifles, aged 18

Corporal Daniel 'Danny' Nield, 1st Battalion, The Rifles, aged 31

Corporal James Oakland, Royal Military
Police, aged 26

Lance Corporal Michael David Pritchard,
Royal Military Police, aged 22

Private James Prosser, 2nd Battalion, The Royal
Welsh, aged 21

Corporal Kumar Pun, The 1st Battalion, The
Royal Gurkha Rifles

Serjeant Chris Reed, 6th Battalion, The Rifles,
aged 25

Lance Corporal Robert Martin Richards,
Armoured Support Group Royal Marines,
aged 24

Acting Corporal Richard 'Robbo' Robinson, 1st
Battalion, The Rifles, aged 21

Lance Corporal Christopher Roney, 3rd
Battalion, The Rifles, aged 23

Sergeant Ben Ross, 3rd Regiment, Royal
Military Police, aged 34

Sapper Jordan Rossi, 38 Engineer Regiment,
Royal Engineers, aged 22

Captain Tom Sawyer, 29 Commando Regiment
Royal Artillery, aged 26

Staff Sergeant Olaf Sean George Schmid GC,
Royal Logistic Corps, aged 30

Corporal Lee Scott, 2nd Royal Tank Regiment,
aged 26

Serjeant Phillip Scott, 3rd Battalion, The Rifles,
aged 30

Rifleman Adrian Sheldon, 2nd Battalion, The
Rifles, aged 20

Captain Daniel Shepherd, Royal Logistic
Corps, aged 28

Rifleman Daniel Simpson, 2nd Battalion, The
Rifles, aged 20

Marine Darren 'Daz' Smith, 45 Commando
Royal Marines, aged 27

Corporal Graeme Stiff, Royal Electrical and
Mechanical Engineers, aged 24

Fusilier Petero 'Pat' Suesue, 2nd Battalion, The
Royal Regiment of Fusiliers, aged 28

Sergeant Matthew Telford, 1st Battalion, The
Grenadier Guards, aged 37

Rifleman Cyrus Thatcher from 2nd Battalion,
The Rifles, aged 19

Lieutenant Colonel Rupert Thorneloe, MBE,
Commanding Officer, 1st Battalion Welsh
Guards

Rifleman Aminiasi Toge, 2nd Battalion, The
Rifles, aged 26

Lance Corporal Paul Upton, 1st Battalion, The
Rifles, aged 31

Warrant Officer Class 2 Sean Upton, 5th
Regiment Royal Artillery, aged 35

Sergeant Simon Valentine, 2nd Battalion, The
Royal Regiment of Fusiliers, aged 29

Sapper David Watson, 33 Engineer Regiment,
Royal Engineers, aged 23

Corporal Nicholas Webster-Smith, Royal
Military Police, aged 24

Trooper Christopher Whiteside, The Light
Dragoons, aged 20

Rifleman Daniel Wild, 2nd Battalion, The
Rifles, aged 19

Private Jason George Williams, 2nd Battalion,
The Mercian Regiment, aged 23

Corporal Danny Winter, 45 Commando, Royal
Marines, aged 28

Acting Corporal Marcin Wojtak, 34 Squadron,
RAF Regiment, aged 24

Private Johnathon Young, 3rd Battalion, The
Yorkshire Regiment, aged 18

2010

Rifleman Peter Aldridge, 4th Battalion, The
Rifles, aged 19

Rifleman Jonathon Allott, 3rd Battalion, The
Rifles, aged 19

Rifleman Carlo Apolis, 4th Battalion, The
Rifles, aged 28

Lance Corporal Jordan Dean Bancroft,
1st Battalion, The Duke of Lancaster's
Regiment, aged 25

Corporal David Barnsdale, 33 Engineer
Regiment, Royal Engineers, aged 24

Major James Joshua Bowman, 1st
Battalion, The Royal Gurkha Rifles, aged 34

Marine Steven James Birdsall, 40 Commando,
Royal Marines, aged 20

Sapper William Bernard Blanchard, 101 (City
of London) Engineer Regiment, Royal
Engineers, aged 39

Lance Corporal Andrew Breeze, 1st Battalion,
The Mercian Regiment, aged 31

Marine Adam Brown, 40 Commando, Royal
Marines, aged 26

Corporal Lee Brownson CGC, 3rd Battalion, The Rifles, aged 30

Fusilier Jonathan Burgess, 1st Battalion, The Royal Welsh, aged 20

Lance Corporal Barry Buxton, 21 Engineer Regiment, Royal Engineers, aged 27

Serjeant Steven Campbell, 3rd Battalion, The Rifles, aged 30

Lance Bombardier Mark Chandler, 3rd Regiment Royal Horse Artillery, aged 32

Lance Corporal Alan Cochran, 1st Battalion, The Mercian Regiment, aged 23

Marine Jonathan David Thomas Crookes, 40 Commando, Royal Marines, aged 26

Lance Corporal Daniel Cooper, 3rd Battalion, The Rifles, aged 22

Corporal Stephen Curley, 40 Commando, Royal Marines, aged 26

Gunner Zak Cusack, 4th Regiment Royal Artillery, aged 20

Lieutenant Douglas Dalzell, 1st Battalion, Coldstream Guards, aged 27

Sergeant Steven William Darbyshire, 40 Commando, Royal Marines, aged 35

Guardsman Christopher Davies, 1st Battalion, Irish Guards, aged 22

Kingsman Sean Dawson, 2nd Battalion, The Duke of Lancaster's Regiment, aged 19

Kingsman Darren Deady, 2nd Battalion, The Duke of Lancaster's Regiment, aged 22

Captain Martin Driver, 1st Battalion, The Royal Anglian Regiment, aged 31

Corporal Steven Thomas Dunn, 216 (Parachute) Signal Squadron, Royal Signals, aged 27

Rifleman Luke Farmer, 3rd Battalion, The Rifles, aged 19

Sapper Darren Foster, 21 Engineer Regiment, Royal Engineers, aged 20

Sergeant Paul Fox, 28 Engineer Regiment, Royal Engineers, aged 34

Bombardier Stephen Raymond Gilbert, 4th Regiment Royal Artillery, aged 36

Corporal Richard Green, 3rd Battalion, The Rifles, aged 23

Lance Sergeant Dave Greenhalgh, 1st Battalion Grenadier Guards, aged 25

Captain Andrew Griffiths, 2nd Battalion, The Duke of Lancaster's Regiment, aged 25

Senior Aircraftman Kinikki 'Griff' Griffiths, 1 Squadron, Royal Air Force Regiment, aged 20

Private James Grigg, 1st Battalion, The Royal Anglian Regiment, aged 20

Sapper Ishwor Gurung, 69 Gurkha Field Squadron, Royal Engineers, aged 21

Rifleman Suraj Gurung, 1st Battalion, The Royal Gurkha Rifles, aged 22

Private Douglas Halliday, 1st Battalion, The Mercian Regiment, aged 20

Lance Corporal Scott Hardy, 1st Battalion, The Royal Anglian Regiment, aged 26

Corporal Christopher Lewis Harrison, 40 Commando, Royal Marines, aged 26

Marine Matthew Harrison, 40 Commando, Royal Marines, aged 23

Marine David Charles Hart, 40 Commando, Royal Marines, aged 23

Private Robert Hayes, 1st Battalion, The Royal Anglian Regiment, aged 19

Lance Corporal Darren Hicks, 1st Battalion, Coldstream Guards, aged 29

Rifleman Daniel Holkham, 3rd Battalion, The Rifles, aged 19

Marine Richard Hollington, 40 Commando, Royal Marines, aged 23

Corporal Harvey Holmes, 1st Battalion, The Mercian Regiment, aged 22

Colour Sergeant Martyn Horton, 1st Battalion, The Mercian Regiment, aged 34

Marine Anthony Dean Hotine, 40 Commando, Royal Marines, aged 21

Private John Howard, 3rd Battalion, The Parachute Regiment, aged 23

Trooper Andrew Martin Howarth, The Queen's Royal Lancers, aged 20

Senior Aircraftman Scott 'Scotty' Hughes, 1 Squadron Royal Air Force Regiment, aged 20

Private Alex Isaac, 1st Battalion, The Mercian Regiment, aged 20

Sergeant Andrew James Jones, Royal Engineers, aged 35

Lance Corporal Tom Keogh, 4th Battalion, The Rifles, aged 24

Rifleman Martin Kinggett, 4th Battalion, The Rifles, aged 19

Corporal Jamie Kirkpatrick, Royal Engineers, aged 32

Rifleman Remand Kulung, 1st Battalion, The Mercian Regiment (Cheshire), aged 27

Trooper James Anthony Leverett, Royal Dragoon Guards, aged 20

Staff Sergeant Brett George Linley, The Royal Logistic Corps, 29 years old

Warrant Officer Class 2 David Markland, 36 Engineer Regiment, Royal Engineers, aged 36

Rifleman Mark Marshall, 6th Battalion, The Rifles, aged 29

Rifleman Liam Maughan, 3rd Battalion, The Rifles, aged 18

Lance Sergeant Dale Alanzo McCallum, 1st Battalion Scots Guards, aged 31

Private Sean McDonald, The Royal Scots Borderers, 1st Battalion, The Royal Regiment of Scotland, aged 26

Sapper Guy Mellors, 36 Engineer Regiment, Royal Engineers, aged 20

Ranger Aaron McCormick, 1st Battalion, The Royal Irish Regiment, aged 22

Private Jonathan Monk, 2nd Battalion, The Princess of Wales's Royal Regiment, aged 25

Sergeant David Thomas Monkhouse, The Royal Dragoon Guards, aged 35

Lance Corporal Stephen Daniel Monkhouse, 1st Battalion Scots Guards, aged 28

Corporal John Moore, The Royal Scots Borderers, 1st Battalion, The Royal Regiment of Scotland, aged 22

Lance Corporal Joseph McFarlane Pool, The Royal Scots Borderers, 1st Battalion, The Royal Regiment of Scotland, aged 26

Corporal Arjun Purja Pun, 1st Battalion, The Royal Gurkha Rifles, aged 33

Lance Corporal David Ramsden, 1st Battalion, The Yorkshire Regiment, aged 26

Sergeant Peter Anthony Rayner, 2nd Battalion, The Duke of Lancaster's Regiment, aged 34

Captain Daniel Read, Royal Logistic Corps, aged 31

Corporal Liam Riley, 3rd Battalion, The Yorkshire Regiment, aged 21

Corporal Taniela Tolevu Rogoiruwai, 1st Battalion, The Duke of Lancaster's Regiment, aged 32

Bombardier Samuel Joseph Robinson, 5th Regiment Royal Artillery, aged 31

Sapper Daryn Roy, 21 Engineer Regiment, Royal Engineers, aged 28

Lieutenant John Charles Sanderson, 1st Battalion, The Mercian Regiment, aged 29

Private Thomas Sephton, 1st Battalion The Mercian Regiment, aged 20

Lance Corporal Graham Shaw, 3rd Battalion, The Yorkshire Regiment, aged 27

Trooper Ashley Smith, Royal Dragoon Guards, aged 21

Sapper Mark Antony Smith, 36 Engineer Regiment, aged 26

Senior Aircraftman Luke Southgate, II Squadron Royal Air Force Regiment, aged 20

Corporal Matthew James Stenton, The Royal Dragoon Guards, aged 23

Corporal Seth Stephens CGC, Royal Marines

Guardsman Michael Sweeney, 1st Battalion Coldstream Guards, aged 19

Kingsman Ponipate Tagitaginimoce, 1st Battalion The Duke of Lancaster's Re

Lance Corporal Michael Taylor, 40 Commando, Royal Marines, aged 30

Marine Scott Gregory Taylor, 40 Commando, Royal Marines, aged 21

Corporal Matthew Thomas, Royal Electrical and Mechanical Engineers

Corporal Stephen Thompson, 1st Battalion, The Rifles, aged 31

Rifleman Mark Turner, 3rd Battalion, The Rifles, aged 21

Lieutenant Neal Turkington, 1st Battalion, The Royal Gurkha Rifles, aged 26

Lance Sergeant David 'Davey' Walker, 1st Battalion Scots Guards, aged 36

Corporal Stephen Walker, 40 Commando, Royal Marines, aged 42

Marine Paul Warren, 40 Commando, Royal Marines, aged 23

Corporal Terry Webster, 1st Battalion, The Mercian Regiment, aged 24

Warrant Officer Class 2 Charles Henry Wood, 23 Pioneer Regiment Royal Logistic Corps, aged 34

Lance Corporal of Horse Jonathan Woodgate, Household Cavalry Regiment, aged 26

2011

Marine Samuel Giles William Alexander MC, 42 Commando, Royal Marines, aged 28

Lieutenant Oliver Richard Augustin, 42 Commando, Royal Marines, aged 23

Warrant Officer Class 2 Colin Beckett, 3rd Battalion The Parachute Regiment, aged 36

Private Martin Simon George Bell, 2nd Battalion The Parachute Regiment, aged 24

Private Gareth Leslie William Bellingham, 3rd Battalion, The Mercian Regiment, aged 22

Sapper Elijah Bond, 35 Engineer Regiment, Royal Engineers, aged 24

Lieutenant David Boyce, The Queen's Dragoon Guards, aged 25

Lance Sergeant Mark Terence Burgan, 1st Battalion Irish Guards, aged 28

Colour Sergeant Alan Cameron, 1st Battalion Scots Guards, aged 42

Lieutenant Daniel John Clack, 1st Battalion The Rifles, aged 24

Major Matthew James Collins, 1st Battalion Irish Guards, aged 38

Ranger David Dalzell, 1st Battalion, The Royal Irish Regiment, aged 20

Squadron Leader Anthony Downing, Royal Air Force, RAF Kinloss, aged 34

Lance Corporal Peter Eustace, 2nd Battalion, The Rifles, aged 25

Colour Serjeant Kevin Charles Fortuna, 1st Battalion, The Rifles, aged 36

Lance Corporal Martin Joseph Gill, 42 Commando, Royal Marines, aged 22

Private Matthew James Sean Haseldin, 2nd Battalion, The Mercian Regiment, aged 21

Captain Lisa Jade Head, Royal Logistic Corps, aged 29

Private Lewis Hendry, 3rd Battalion, The Parachute Regiment, aged 20

Private Dean Hutchinson, The Royal Logistic Corps, aged 23

Captain Tom Jennings, Royal Marines, aged 29

Private John King, 1st Battalion, The Yorkshire Regiment, aged 19

Private Thomas Christopher Lake, 1st Battalion, The Princess of Wales's Royal Regiment, aged 29

Rifleman Martin Jon Lamb, 1st Battalion, The Rifles, aged 27

Private Conrad Lewis, 4th Battalion, The Parachute Regiment, aged 22

Lance Corporal Kyle Cleet Marshall, 2nd Battalion, The Parachute Regiment, aged 23

Lance Corporal McKee, 1st Battalion, The Royal Irish Regiment, aged 27

Lance Corporal Jonathan James McKinlay, 1st Battalion, The Rifles, aged 33

Highlander Scott McLaren, The Highlanders, 4th Battalion, The Royal Regiment of Scotland, aged 20

Marine Nigel Dean Mead, 42 Commando, Royal Marines, aged 19

Corporal Lloyd Newell, The Parachute Regiment

Corporal Mark Anthony Palin, 1st Battalion, The Rifles, aged 32

Corporal Michael John Pike, The Highlanders, 4th Battalion, The Royal Regiment of Scotland, aged 26

Private Daniel Steven Prior, 2nd Battalion, The Parachute Regiment, aged 27

Rifleman Vijay Rai, 2nd Battalion, The Royal Gurkha Rifles, aged 21

Lance Corporal Richard Scanlon, 1st The Queen's Dragoon Guards, aged 31

Rifleman Sheldon Lee Jordan Steel, 5th Battalion, The Rifles, aged 20

Lance Corporal Liam Richard Tasker, Royal Army Veterinary Corps, aged 26

Private Matthew Thornton, 4th Battalion, The Yorkshire Regiment, aged 28

Private Joseva Saqanagonedau Vatubua, 5th Battalion, The Royal Regiment of Scotland, aged 24

Lance Corporal Paul Watkins, 9th/12th Royal Lancers, aged 24

Sergeant Barry John Weston, 42 Commando, Royal Marines, aged 40

Private Robert Wood, 17 Port and Maritime Regiment Royal Logistic Corps, aged 28

Marine James Robert Wright, 42 Commando, Royal Marines, aged 22

2012

Lance Corporal James Ashworth VC, 1st Battalion, Grenadier Guards, aged 23

Captain Walter Barrie, 1st Battalion, Royal Regiment of Scotland, aged 41

Captain Rupert William Michael Bowers, 2nd Battalion, The Mercian Regiment, aged 24

Lieutenant Andrew Robert Chesterman, 3rd Battalion, The Rifles, aged 26

Sergeant Nigel Coupe, 1st Battalion, The Duke of Lancaster's Regiment, aged 33

Sergeant Lee Paul Davidson, The Light Dragoons, aged 32

Lance Corporal Lee Thomas Davies, 1st Battalion, Welsh Guards, aged 27

Corporal Channing Day, Royal Army Medical Corps, aged 25

Lieutenant Edward Drummond-Baxter, 1st Battalion, Royal Gurkha Rifles, aged 29

Lance Corporal Michael Foley, Adjutant General's Corps, aged 25

Private Anthony Frampton, 3rd Battalion, The Yorkshire Regiment, aged 20

Lance Corporal Duane Groom, 1st Battalion Grenadier Guards, aged 32

Lance Corporal Gajbahadur Gurung, Royal Gurkha Rifles, aged 26

Corporal Alex Guy, 1st Battalion, The Royal Anglian Regiment, aged 37

Corporal Jake Hartley, 3rd Battalion, The Yorkshire Regiment, aged 20

Captain Stephen James Healey, 1st Battalion, The Royal Welsh, aged 29

Private Christopher Kershaw, 3rd Battalion, The Yorkshire Regiment, aged 19

Lance Corporal Siddhanta Kunwar, 1st Battalion The Royal Gurkha Rifles, aged 28

Sergeant Jonathan Eric Kups, Royal Electrical and Mechanical Engineers, aged 38

Rifleman Sachin Limbu, 1st Battalion, The Royal Gurkha Rifles, aged 23

Captain Carl Manley, Royal Marines, aged 41

Corporal Brent John McCarthy, RAF Brize Norton, aged 25

Corporal David O'Connor, 40 Commando Royal Marines, aged 27

Warrant Officer Class 2 Leonard Perran Thomas, Royal Corps of Signals, aged 44

Sapper Connor Ray, Royal Engineers, aged 21

Corporal Andrew Steven Roberts, 23 Pioneer Regiment, The Royal Logistic Corps, aged 32

Guardsman Craig Andrew Roderick, 1st Battalion, Welsh Guards, aged 22

Guardsman Michael Roland, 1st Battalion, Grenadier Guards, aged 22

Signaller Ian Gerard Sartorius-Jones, Royal Corps of Signals, aged 21

Guardsman Jamie Shadrake, 1st Battalion, Grenadier Guards, aged 20

Private Ratu Manasa Silibaravi, Royal Logistic Corps, aged 32

Lance Corporal Matthew David Smith, Royal Engineers, aged 26

Corporal Jack Leslie Stanley, The Queen's Royal Hussars, aged 26

Private Gregg Thomas Stone, 3rd Battalion The Yorkshire Regiment, aged 20

Sergeant Luke Taylor, Royal Marines, aged 33

Corporal Michael John Thacker, 1st Battalion The Royal Welsh, aged 27

Sergeant Gareth Thursby, 3rd Battalion, The Yorkshire Regiment, aged 29

Senior Aircraftman Ryan Tomlin, 2 Squadron RAF Regiment, aged 21

Captain James Anthony Townley, Corps of Royal Engineers, aged 29

Guardsman Apete Saunikalou Ratumaiyale Tuisovurua, 1st Battalion Welsh Guards, aged 28

Private Daniel Wade, 3rd Battalion, The Yorkshire Regiment, aged 20

Guardsman Karl Whittle, 1st Battalion, Grenadier Guards, aged 22

Private Daniel Wilford, 3rd Battalion, The Yorkshire Regiment, aged 21

Private Thomas Wroe, 3rd Battalion, The Yorkshire Regiment, aged 18

2013

Lance Corporal James Brynin, The Intelligence Corps, aged 22

Warrant Officer Class 2 Ian Fisher, 3rd Battalion, The Mercian Regiment, aged 42

Fusilier Samuel Flint, 2nd Battalion, The Royal Regiment of Scotland, aged 21

Private Robert Murray Hetherington, 2nd Battalion, The Royal Regiment of Scotland

Captain Richard Holloway, Royal Engineers, aged 29

Corporal William Thomas Savage, 2nd Battalion, The Royal Regiment of Scotland, aged 30

Kingsman David Robert Shaw, 1st Battalion, The Duke of Lancaster's Regiment, aged 23

Sapper Richard Reginald Walker, Royal Engineers, aged 23

Lance Corporal Jamie Webb, 1st Battalion, The Mercian Regiment, aged 24

2014

Flight Lieutenant Rakesh Chauhan, Royal Air Force, RAF Odiham, aged 29

Captain Thomas Clarke, Army Air Corps, aged 30

Warrant Officer Class 2 Spencer Faulkner, Army Air Corps, aged 38

Sapper Adam Moralee, 32 Engineer Regiment, Royal Engineers, aged 23

Lance Corporal Oliver Thomas, Intelligence Corps, aged 26

Corporal James Walters, Army Air Corps, aged 36

2015

Lance Corporal Michael Campbell, 3rd Battalion Royal Welsh Regiment, aged 32

Flight Lieutenant Geraint Roberts, Royal Air Force, RAF Benson, aged 44

Flight Lieutenant Alan Scott, Royal Air Force, RAF Benson, aged 32

Disclaimer

The views and opinions expressed are those of the authors alone and should not be taken to represent those of Her Majesty's Government, Ministry of Defence, Her Majesty's Armed Forces or any government agency.

Note on Royalties

All the royalties from the sale of this book will be donated to military medical charities.

Introduction

This book is a detailed review of the experiences of the *United Kingdom Defence Medical Services* on deployment in Iraq (the *Second Gulf War – Operation Telic*) and Afghanistan (*Operation Herrick*). Individual chapters discuss the challenges, failures and achievements of clinicians, planners, researchers and commanders in delivering effective care to deploying, deployed and returning personnel.

It is undoubtedly in the field of trauma that the improvements in patient care are best known; however, the profile of the improvements in trauma care that have arisen from recent campaigns may overshadow what has happened in other fields of clinical endeavour. It is important that these contributions by other specialties are not forgotten. Aside from trauma, most other specialties have also seen very significant developments, particularly transfusion medicine, rehabilitation and mental health, and it is often the key role of other lower profile specialties in preserving the fighting strength, which has allowed the deployment of an effective fighting force: this is particularly true of internal medicine, primary care and blast protection. The care provided for casualties on both campaigns has been a joint effort of clinicians, scientists, logisticians and commanders, empowered at least in part by the public profile of injury and mortality rates. Equally, we do not want to 'oversell' the medical achievements of these campaigns, and we have tried to offer a broad approach that recognises both the advances and the challenges of deployed care across the whole clinical spectrum.

This book both answers and asks questions. It begins with a history of the recent conflicts in *Iraq* and *Afghanistan* in which challenging questions are asked. Perhaps, these wars are too close to be considered in an entirely rational and impartial way, but it does seem to me as if some degree of consensus is emerging, and if both these conflicts are now seen in the light of subsequent events, 'dodgy dossiers', public enquiries and an uncertain shape of future Defence capability, this does not detract even in the slightest from the commitment, courage and bloody-minded persistence, not to mention the humour, of the members of Her Majesty's Armed Forces of all kinds from pilots to logisticians, engineers to infantry. Such is the quality of the British serviceman or woman.

Chapters 3 and 4 deal with the pre-hospital and emergency department management of the severely wounded, discussing the challenges of the deployed environment and the changes in practice and organisation that have resulted from our experience, many of which are now reflected in practice within the National Health Service. Chapters 5 to 7 discuss the subjects of anaesthesia, pain management, intensive care medicine and aeromedical evacuation, all elements vital to providing the best experience for patients. Chapters 8 to 11 consider the management on deployment and in the United Kingdom of complex and life-changing injuries. Routine and emergency medical problems are also considered (Chapter 12), and the essential but often overlooked support services, most importantly imaging and blood transfusion, which have transformed military and now civilian trauma practice are also discussed.

One of the most controversial areas following these campaigns has been the subject of mental health; this is discussed in detail in Chapter 15, which offers a summary of the mental health consequences of service in the Armed Forces in general and, more specifically, of deployment. As such, it provides answers to many of the questions that have generated much heat, and little light, in this area in recent years. Similarly, HM Forces, including the Defence Medical Services, have been criticised over the management of detainees and prisoners: as a result, this book would be incomplete without appropriate reflections on this subject (Chapter 20). Primary care and the care of children are also considered, as is, importantly, rehabilitation, where the United Kingdom has achieved an International reputation as a result of the work of the *Defence Medical Rehabilitation Services*. The vital role of the Royal Navy at sea is also considered, not forgetting the many Navy and Royal Marines personnel who served, and lost their lives, on land alongside their colleagues from the other services.

Whilst the aim of the contributors and the editor of this book is to capture the advances that have followed deployed experience, this book is not in any way intended to be self-regarding. There were problems, not all of which have been overcome; not everyone got everything right every time and mistakes were made. Whilst no criticism is made of individuals, where necessary, system failures are discussed, in the hope that they can be remedied sooner rather than later and that appropriate lessons will be learned. Nevertheless, it must be remembered that Armed Forces on deployment are carrying out complex tasks, in a hostile and distant environment and within a complex organisation.

Medically, one of the most important results of the campaigns described in this volume is the enormous amount of material that has been published in book form and as papers in learned journals by members of the Defence Medical Services and their academic colleagues. A list of books and over 1000 papers is included as Appendix D arranged by subject. Executive summaries of the *Audit Commission* and *Care Quality Commission* reports into deployed medical care may be found in Appendices E and F.

Attitudes to the *Defence Medical Services* change when combat stops. History suggests that organisational decline inevitably follows the achievements of clinicians in wars as those clinicians retire or leave the service, their duty done. Institutional memory is short and easily forgotten: this is one of the reasons for this volume. These lessons will inevitably have to be relearned, at least in part, next time, and this learning may come at a significant cost. Over the achievements of clinicians from team medic to hospital specialist hovers the experience that such services are less regarded and hence less supported and funded in times of peace: time will tell.

The considerable cost in terms of death and disability has left a legacy of effects that will last for many years. No apology is made, therefore, for including the role of honour of the men and women who were killed or died on these two campaigns. The book is dedicated to them in recognition and gratitude for their sacrifice.

I am immensely grateful to the trustees of the Royal Army Medical Corps Charities for the substantial donation, which has made the publication of this book possible in its current form.

It has been a privilege to edit and contribute to this book. I hope that it will lead to a greater awareness, inside and outside the Armed Forces, of the efforts made to improve health and save life by clinicians of all kinds and all those who support them, and that my colleagues, past and present, feel that that this volume does them justice.

Colonel Ian Greaves
Editor

Contributors

Dominic Aldington BSc(Hons) MBBS FRCA FFPMRCA RAMC (Rtd)
Hampshire Hospitals Foundation Trust, Hampshire, United Kingdom

Andy Barlow MBChB DFRSH MAcadMEd RAMC
Academic Department of Military General Practice, Royal Centre for Defence Medicine, Birmingham, United Kingdom

Jodie Blackadder-Weinstein MBChB BSc MRCGP FSRH RAF
Academic Department of Military General Practice, Royal Centre for Defence Medicine, Birmingham, United Kingdom

Sebastian Bourn FRCA RN
Institute of Naval Medicine, Alverstoke, United Kingdom

Johno Breeze PhD FRCS MFDS RAMC
Queen Elizabeth Hospital Birmingham, Academic Department of Military Surgery and Trauma, Royal Centre for Defence Medicine, Birmingham, United Kingdom

Dan Connor BMedSci BM BS FRCA
Queen Alexandra Hospital, Portsmouth, United Kingdom

Nicholas Dodds RN
Institute of Naval Medicine, Alverstoke, United Kingdom

Heidi Doughty OBE OStJ TD MBA FRCP FRCPath L/RAMC
NHS Blood and Transplant, Birmingham, United Kingdom

John Etherington CBE FRCP L/RAMC
Defence Medical Rehabilitation Centre, Headley Court Epsom, United Kingdom

Iain Gibb FRCS FRCR Ed L/RAMC
Portsmouth Hospitals Trust, Portsmouth, United Kingdom

Natalie Glover BSc MBBCh FRCA DRTM RAF
Royal Gwent Hospital, Newport, University Hospital of Wales, Cardiff, Wales, United Kingdom

Lorraine Greasley QGM FRCEM L/RAMC
John Radcliffe Hospital, Oxford, United Kingdom

Ian Greaves OStJ FRCEM FRCP FRCSEd FIMC FASI FRSA DTM&H DMCC DipMedEd L/RAMC
James Cook University Hospital, Middlesbrough, United Kingdom and Royal Centre for Defence Medicine, Birmingham, United Kingdom

Ian Gurney BMedSci BM BS DipMedTox FRCEM RAMC
Defence Medical Services and Plymouth Hospitals NHS Trust, Plymouth, Devon, United Kingdom and Royal Centre for Defence Medicine, Birmingham, United Kingdom

Richard Heames FRCA RN
Southampton Hospital NHS Trust, Southampton, United Kingdom

Simon Horne BA BM BCh DIMC DCH DMCC DHA FRCS(Ed) A&E FRCEM RAMC
Derriford Hospital, Plymouth, United Kingdom and Royal Centre for Defence Medicine, Birmingham, United Kingdom

Elspeth Hulse MB ChB FRCA Dip Med Tox PhD RN
Royal Infirmary of Edinburgh, Edinburgh, United Kingdom and Department of Military Anaesthesia and Critical Care Medicine, Royal Centre for Defence Medicine, Birmingham, United Kingdom

Paul Hunt MD FRCEM FFICM DIMC RAMC
James Cook University Hospital, Middlesbrough, United Kingdom and Royal Centre for Defence Medicine, Birmingham, United Kingdom

Clinton Jones BSc MBChB FRCA DiplMC Dip RTM RAMC
Aintree University Hospital NHS Foundation Trust, Liverpool, United Kingdom

Norman Jones MBE ARRC RGN RMN BSc(Hons) MSc PhD QARANC
Academic Department Military Mental Health Kings College, London, United Kingdom

Mansoor Ali Khan PhD FRCS FEBS FACS RN
St Mary's Hospital, London, United Kingdom and Royal Centre for Defence Medicine, Birmingham, United Kingdom

Emrys Kirkman OBE PhD
Defence Scientific and Technical Laboratories, Porton Down, United Kingdom

Eluned Lewis BSc(Hons) MSc PhD FIMMM
Engineering Group, D S&EQT MOD Abbey Wood, Bristol, United Kingdom

Niall Martin MBBS MD MSc DMCC AKC FRCS(Plast)
St Andrew's Burn Service, Broomfield Hospital Chelmsford, Chelmsford, United Kingdom and Department of Military Surgery and Trauma, Birmingham, United Kingdom and Queen Mary University of London, London, United Kingdom

Jonathan Matthews MBBCh MFSEM(UK) FRCSEd(Tr&Orth) RN
Royal Cornwall Hospitals Trust, Cornwall, United Kingdom

Simon J. Mercer MB ChB MAcadMEd FHEA FCollT FRCA MMEd RN (Rtd)
Aintree University Hospitals NHS Foundation Trust Liverpool, United Kingdom

Paul Moor BMedSci BM BS FRCA RAMC
Derriford Hospital, Plymouth, United Kingdom

Sue Pope RAMC
Defence Medical Rehabilitation Centre Headley Court, Epsom United Kingdom

Ross Moy FRCEM RAMC
John Radcliffe Hospital, Oxford, United Kingdom

Arul Ramasamy PhD RAMC
Imperial College, London, United Kingdom

Paul Reavley MBChB FRCEM FRCSEd (A&E) MRCGP Dip Med Tox RAMC
Bristol Royal Infirmary and Bristol Royal Hospital for Children, Bristol, United Kingdom and formerly Defence Medical Services UK, Lichfield, United Kingdom and Royal Centre for Defence Medicine, Birmingham, United Kingdom

Rory Rickard PhD FRCS RN
Derriford Hospital, Plymouth, United Kingdom and Royal Centre for Defence Medicine, Birmingham, United Kingdom

Matthew Roberts MA BM BCh DMCC FRCA
University of Colorado, Denver, Colorado and Denver Health Medical Center, Denver, Colorado

Rob Russell FRCP FRCEM MIHM DiplMC RCSEd L/RAMC
Headquarters Surgeon General's Department DMS Whittington, Staffordshire, United Kingdom

Jason E. Smith MBBS MSc MD FRCP FRCEM RN
Derriford Hospital, Plymouth, United Kingdom
and Royal Centre for Defence Medicine,
Birmingham, United Kingdom

Mike Smith MBChB BEng(Hons) PhD FRCGP RAMC
Academic Department of Military General
Practice, Royal Centre for Defence Medicine,
Birmingham, United Kingdom

Sarah Stapley MB ChB FRCS(Eng) FRCS (Tr & Orth) DM RN
Queen Alexandra Hospital, Portsmouth, United
Kingdom and Royal Centre for Defence Medicine,
Birmingham, United Kingdom

Helen L. Surgenor MBChB FRCA RAF
John Radcliffe Hospital, Oxford, United Kingdom

David Vassallo LRCP MRCS DMCC DHMSA FRCS(Ed) MA
L/RAMC
Robertson House, Royal Military Academy
Sandhurst, Camberley, United Kingdom

Sarah Watts MRCVS PhD
Defence Scientific and Technical Laboratories
Porton Down, United Kingdom

Duncan Wilson MB ChB FRCP L/RAMC
Royal Centre for Defence Medicine, Birmingham,
United Kingdom

Rich Withnall MD MA MSc FRCGP FAcadMEd CMgr RAF
Academic Department of Military General
Practice, Royal Centre for Defence Medicine,
Birmingham, United Kingdom

Tom Woolley FRCA MD L/RAMC
Academic Department of Military Anaesthesia
and Critical Care Medicine, Royal Centre for
Defence Medicine and Derriford Hospital,
Plymouth, United Kingdom

Chris Wright MB ChB DIMC FRCEM RAMC
St. Mary's Hospital, Imperial Healthcare NHS
Trust, London, United Kingdom and Royal
Centre for Defence Medicine, Birmingham,
United Kingdom

Military abbreviations

AASG	Air assault surgical group
ADMACC	Academic Department of Military Anaesthesia and Critical Care
ADMEM	Academic Department of Military Emergency Medicine
ADMGP	Academic Department of Military General Practice
ADMM	Academic Department of Military Medicine
ADMMH	Academic Department of Military Mental Health
ADMR	Academic Department of Military Rehabilitation
ADMS	Academic Department of Military Surgery
AE	Aeromedical evacuation
AECC	(i) Aeromedical coordination cell, (ii) Strategic Aeromedical Evacuation Centre
AECO	Aeromedical Evacuation Control Officer
AELO	Aeromedical liaison officer
AEOO	Aeromedical evacuation operations officer
AeVacS	Aeromedical evacuation squadron
AGOMM	Advisory Group on Military Medicine
AME	Airworthy medical equipment
AMS	Army Medical Services
AMSTC	Army Medical Services Training Centre
ANA	Afghanistan National Army
ANP	Afghan National Police
ANSF	Afghan National Security Forces
AO	Area of operations
AOR	Area of responsibility
APOD	Air port of disembarkation

ASCAB	Armed services consultant appointment board
ATACCC	Advanced Technology Applications to Combat Casualty Care (Conference)
BABT	Behind armour blunt trauma
BAR	British Army Review
BARTS	Battlefield Advanced Resuscitation Techniques and Skills
BASICS	British Association of Immediate Care (Schemes)
BATLS	Battlefield Advanced Trauma Life Support
BCD	Battlefield casualty drills
BFA	Battlefield ambulance
BG	Battle Group
BI	Battle injury
BMH	British military hospital
Bn	Battalion
BSN	(camp) Bastion
BST	Blood Supply Team
CA	Clinical advisor: the head of a cadre in a single service, reporting to the DCA who is head of the cadre across Defence.
CAP	Company aid post
CASEVAC	Casualty evacuation
CASH	Combat support hospital (US)
CBA	Combat body armour
CBA-IS	Combat body armour internal security
CBRN	Chemical, biological, radiation and nuclear
CC	Combat casualty
CCAST	Critical care air support team
CCC	Combat casualty care
CCCRP	Combat Casualty Care Research Programme

CCTS	Containerised CT scanner
CDI	Centre for Defence Imaging
CDPath	Centre for Defence Pathology
CDR	Centre for Defence Radiology
CDS	Chief of the Defence Staff (Professional Head of the Armed Forces)
CENTCOM	(US) Central Command
CEPP	Carrier Enabled Power Projection
CFSG	Commando forward surgical group
CGC	Conspicuous Gallantry Cross
CGOs	Clinical Guidelines for Operations
CGS	Chief of the General Staff (Professional Head of the Army)
CJTF	Combined Joint Task Force
CIA	Central Intelligence Agency (US)
C-IED	Counter-IED
CIMIC	Civil-military cooperation
CLIX	Clinical information exploitation (team)
CMAG	Clinical materiel advisory group
CMP	Civilian medical practitioners
CMT	Combat medical technician
CO	Commanding officer
CoAT	Coverage of Armour Tool
COB	Contingency Operating Base
CoC	Chain of Command
COIN	Counter-insurgency
COLPRO	Collective protection (from CBRN threats)
CONDO	Contractor Deployed on Operations
CPAT	Coverage of armour tool
CP	Control/check point
C-Pers	Captured person
CPO	Chief petty officer (Royal Navy)
CPOMA	Chief petty officer medical assistant
CS	Close support
CSH	Combat support hospital
CSMR	Close support medical regiment
CCTS	Containerised CT scanner
CVF	Carrier Vessel Future
DA	Dental assistant
DASA	Defence Analytical Services and Advice
DCA	Defence consultant advisor (Tri-service Clinical head of a specialty)
DCMH	Department of community mental health
DCR	Damage control resuscitation

DEPSIG	Defence Paediatric Special Interest Group
DERA	Defence Evaluation and Research agency
DE&S	Defence Equipment and Support (also DES)
DFC	Distinguished Flying Cross
DfID	Department for International Development
DGAMS	Director General Army Medical Services (obsolete, post dis-established)
DI	Defence Intelligence
DLO	Defence Logistics Organisation
DLOD	Defence Lines of development
DMAPCC	Department of Military Anaesthesia, Pain and Critical Care
DMD	Deployed medical director
DMHS	Defence Mental Health Services
DMICP(D)	Defence Medical Information Capability Programme (Deployed)
DMRC	Defence Military Rehabilitation Centre
DMRE	Defence Medical Research and Exploitation
DMRP	Defence Medical Rehabilitation Programme
DMRT	Deployed medical rehabilitation team
DMS	Defence Medical Services
DMOCG	Defence Medical Operational Clinical Group
DMSTC	(i) Defence Medical Services Transfusion Committee, (ii) Defence Medical Services Training Centre
DNBI	Disease and nonbattle injury
DO	Dental officer
DoD	Department of Defense (US)
DoW	Died of wounds
DPHC	Defence Primary Health Care
DRASH™	Deployable Rapid Assembly Shelter
DS	Dressing station
DSA	Defence specialist adviser
DSAT	Defence Systems Approach to Training
DSF	Director, Special Forces
Dstl [sic]	Defence Scientific and Technical Laboratories
DU	Depleted Uranium
ECBA	Enhanced combat body armour

EFP	Explosively formed projectile	IISS	International Institute for Strategic Studies
EOD	Explosive ordnance disposal		
EP-UBACS	Enhanced protection-under body armour combat shirt	IMAP	Interactive Mapping Analysis Platform
ERI	Exercise rehabilitation instructor	IN	Iraqi Navy
FCO	Foreign and Commonwealth Office	IPT	Integrated project team
FE@R	Force elements at readiness	IRT	Initial/incident response team
FFD	First field dressing	ISAF	International Security Assistance Force
FMCC	Flight movement coordination cell		
FMED	Field Medical Equipment Depot (Obsolete)	ISO	Iso-container
		ISTAR	Intelligence, surveillance, target acquisition and reconnaissance
FMHT	Field mental health team		
FMRT	Field medical rehabilitation team	JAM	Jaish al-Mahdi Militia (Mahdi Army)
FOB	Forward operating base	JADTEU	Joint Air Delivery Test and Evaluation Unit
FRT	Forward rehabilitation team		
FSG	Forward surgical group	JF Log C	Joint Force Logistical Component
FSp	Forward support	JFSp	Joint Force Support (also JFS)
FU	Formed unit	JHF	Joint helicopter force
FwdRT	Forward Rehabilitation Team	JOA	Joint operations area/joint area of operations
GC	George Cross		
GCS	Global Combat Ship	JSP	Joint Service Publication
GDMO	General duties medical officer – a junior doctor usually within five years of qualification who is gaining military experience with a formed unit	JTCCC	Joint Theatre Clinical Case Conference
		JTTR	Joint Theatre Trauma Registry
		KAF	Kandahar Air Field
		KCIA	Kuwait City International Airport
GHB	Golden Hour Box	KCMHR	King's Centre for Military Health Research
GOC	General Officer Commanding		
GS	General support	KIA	Killed in action
GSMR	General support medical regiment	LLCR	Low level capability requirement
GSW	Gunshot wound	LMA	Leading medical assistant (Royal Navy)
HADRO	Humanitarian assistance and disaster relief operations		
		LMA (SM)	Leading medical assistant (submarine) (Royal Navy)
HAS	Helicopter assault force		
HEAS	High-explosive, anti-tank	LN	Local national
HIM	Hospital information manager	LO	Liaison officer
HLCR	High level capability requirement	LOAC	Law of Armed Conflict
HLS	Helicopter landing site	LoC	Lines of communication
HN(S)	Host nation (support)	LSDA	Leading seaman dental assistant
HOSPEX	Hospital exercise	MA	Medical assistant (Royal Navy)
HQ	Headquarters	MA (SM)	Medical assistant (Submarine) (Royal Navy)
HQ AIR	Headquarters Air Command		
IA	Individual augmentee	MACE	Major Trauma Audit for Clinical Effectiveness
ICNO	Infection control nursing officer		
ICU	Intensive care unit (also ITU: intensive therapy unit)	MAPLS	Military Advanced Paediatric Life Support
ID	Infanty division (US)	MASH	Mobile army surgical hospital
IDF	Indirect fire	MATT	Military annual training test
IED	Improvised explosive device	MC	Military Cross

MDHU	Ministry of Defence Hospital Unit (obsolete)		OF2, captain; OF3, major; OF4, Lt colonel; OF5, colonel; OF6, brigadier;
MDSS	Medical and dental sterile supplies		OF7, major general; OF8, Lt general;
Med	Medical		OF9, general. Navy: OF1, midshipman/
MEDCAP	Medical Civic Action Plans		sub-lieutenant; OF2, lieutenant; OF3,
MEDEVAC	Medical evacuation		Lt commander; OF4, commander;
MEDSEM	Medical seminars		OF5, captain; OF6, commodore; OF7,
MEF (US)	Marine Expeditionary Force		rear admiral; OF 8, vice admiral;
MERT (E)	Medical emergency response team (Enhanced)		OF9, admiral. RAF: OF1, pilot officer/ flying officer; OF2, flight lieutenant;
MHA	Military helicopter aircrew		OF3, squadron leader; OF4, wing
MITC	Maritime in transit care		commander; OF5, group captain; OF6,
MiTT	Military Transition Team		air commodore; OF7, air vice marshal;
MLRS	Multiple launch rocket systems		OF8, air marshal; OF9, air chief
MND	Multi-National Division		marshal. OF10 (field marshal, marshal
MO	Medical officer		of the Royal Air Force, admiral of the
MOD	Ministry of Defence		fleet) is no longer used.
MOIC	Medical officer in charge	OMHNE	Operational Mental Health Needs
MOLLE	Modular lightweight load-carrying equipment	OMLT	Evaluation
		OMLT	Operational mentoring and liaison team
MOST	Military Operational Surgical Training Course	OpEDAR	Operational Emergency Department Attendance Register
MSA	Medical Supplies Agency	OPCP	Operational Patient Care Pathway
MSS	Medical Supply Squadron	OR	Non-officer rank grading (NATO)
MST	(i) Mission-specific training, (ii) medical support team		Army: OR 1 and OR 2, Private or equivalent; OR 3, Lance Corporal;
MT	Medical technician (merchant navy equivalent of MA)		OR 4, Corporal; OR 5, No Army equivalent; OR 6, Army Sergeant; OR
MTF	Medical treatment facility		7, Staff or colour sergeant; OR 8, Army
MTP	Modified Terrain Pattern (camouflage material)		Warrant officer class 2; OR 9, Army Warrant officer class 1. Navy: OR 1,
MTSF	Modular Transportable Surgical Facility		No equivalent; OR 2, Able seaman; OR 3, No equivalent; OR 4, Leading
MWC	Maritime Warfare Centre		rate; OR 5, No equivalent; OR 6, Petty
MWD	Military working dog(s)		officer; OR 7, Chief petty officer; OR 8,
NATO	North Atlantic Treaty Organization		No equivalent; OR 9, Warrant officer.
NATS	Navy Afloat Trauma System		RAF: OR 1, Aircraftman; OR 2,
NBI	Non-battle injury		Senior/leading aircraftsman; OR 3,
NCHQ	Naval Command Head Quarters		Lance corporal (RAF Regiment only);
NCO	Non-commissioned officer		OR 4, Corporal; OR 5, No equivalent;
NEO	New entry operation		OR 6, Sergeant; OR 7, Flight
NGO	Non-governmental organisation		Sergeant/Chief technician; OR 8, No
NSE	National Support Element		equivalent; OR 9, Warrant officer.
NTM	Notice to move		
OC	Officer commanding	ORBAT	Order of battle
ODMC	Operational Deployed Medical Capability (project)	ORMHP	Operationally related mental health problem
OF	Officer rank grading (NATO): Army: OF1, 2nd lieutenant/lieutenant (Lt);	PACCSIG	Paediatric Anaesthesia and Critical Care Specialist Interest Group

PAR	Population at risk	ROMD	Regional occupational medicine department
PB	Patrol base	RORT	Role 1 rehabilitation team
PCRF	(i) Primary casualty receiving facility, (ii) primary care rehabilitation facility	RPG	Rocket propelled grenade
PDT	Pre-deployment training	R&R	Rest and recovery/recuperation
PECC	Patient Evacuation Control Cell	RRU	Regional rehabilitation unit
PFA	Parachute field ambulance	RSI	Rapid sequence induction of anaesthesia (now PHEA)
PHP	Personal hearing protection	RUSI	Royal United Services Institute
PIES	Proximity, Immediacy, Expectancy, Simplicity	SAF	Small arms fire
PIHP	Personal interfaced hearing protection	SERE	Survival, evasion, resistance and escape (training)
PJ	Para-rescueman	SGD	Surgeon General's Department
PJHQ	Permanent Joint Head Quarters	SGPL	Surgeon General's policy letter
PJOB	Permanent joint operating base	SIG	Specialist interest group
PO	Petty Officer (Royal Navy)	SIL	Seriously ill
POI	Point of injury	SIRS	Steroids and Immunity from Injury through to Rehabilitation Study
POMA	Petty officer medical assistant		
POSM	Post-operational stress management	SITREP	Situational report
POW	(i) Point of wounding, (ii) prisoner of war	SM	Submarine
		SMO	Senior medical officer
PPA	Principal project area	SNO	Senior nursing officer
PPS	Pelvic protection system	SO	Staff officer The number indicates the seniority of the appointment, the lower the number, the more senior
PRR	Personal role radio		
PRT	Provincial Reconstruction Team		
PRU	Personnel Recovery Unit	SOP	Standard operating procedure
QHP	Honorary Physician to HM Queen Elizabeth II	SOR	Statement of requirement
		Sqn	Squadron
QHS	Honorary Surgeon to HM Queen Elizabeth II	STRATOS	Science and Technology Rapid assistance to Operations
RAF	Royal Air Force	STRATEVAC	Strategic (medical) evacuation
RAMP	Reception arrangements for military patients	SWM	Surface wound mapping
		TA	Territorial Army – obsolete, now the *Reserves*
RAP	Regimental aid post		
RC	Regional Command	TACEVAC	Tactical (medical) evacuation
RCDM	Royal Centre for Defence Medicine	TFH	Taste Force Helmand
RCO	Rehabilitation co-ordination officer	THOR	Trauma Haemostasis and Oxygenation Research Network
RFA	Royal Fleet Auxiliary		
RHH	Royal Hospital Haslar (Portsmouth)	TIC	Troops in contact
RHQ	Regimental headquarters	TIRS	Theatre Intensive Rehabilitation Service
RIP	Relief in place		
RLC	Royal Logistic Corps	TLD	Third location decompression
RM	Royal Marines	TMC	Troop medical centre
RMHP	Reserves Mental Health Programme	TMW	Tactical Medical Wing
RMO	Regimental medical officer	TOA	Transfer of authority
RMP	Royal Military Police	TRiM	Trauma Risk Management
RN	Royal Navy	TSAA	Tri-service anaesthetic apparatus
RNH	Royal Naval Hospital	TTCP	The Technical Cooperation Panel
RNMS	Royal Navy Medical Service	UBACS	Under body armour combat shirt

UNSCR	United Nations Security Council Resolution	VBIED	Vehicle-borne improvised explosive device
UOR	Urgent operational requirement	VC	Victoria Cross
UPS	Uninterruptible power supply	VOIP	Voice over internet protocol
USAF	US Air Force	VSIL	Very seriously ill
USN	US Navy	WHIS	Whole hospital information system
USNMRC	US Navy Medical Research Centre	WI	Wounded in action
USNS	US naval ship	WIA	Wounded in action
(V)	Volunteer, i.e. Reserve unit	WIS	Wounded, injured and sick
		WMIK	Weapon mount installation kit

Medical abbreviations

AABB	American Association of Blood Banks
AAGBI	Association of Anaesthetists of Great Britain and Ireland
AD	Advanced directive
AHP	Allied Health Professional
AIS	Abbreviated Injury Score
ANTS	Anaesthetist's non-technical skills framework
APLS	Advanced Paediatric Life Support
APMS	Adult Psychiatric Morbidity Survey
APRV	Airway pressure release ventilation (mode)
aPTT	Activated partial thromboplastin time
ARDS	Adult respiratory distress syndrome
ARF	Acute renal failure
ASCOT	A Severity Characterisation of Trauma (trauma scoring system)
ATC	Acute trauma coagulopathy
ATD	Adult therapeutic dose
ATLS®	Advanced Trauma Life Support
ATMIST	Handover mnemonic: age, time of injury, mechanism of injury, injuries sustained, signs and symptoms, treatment given
ATR	Standard operating procedure
AUDIT	Alcohol use disorders identification test
BBV	Blood-borne virus
BD	Base deficit
BEA	Blood Establishment Authorisation
BMS	Biomedical scientist
BRLI	Blast-related lung injury
BTC	Barriers to care
CAF	Continuous assurance framework
CBIS	Centre for Blast Injury Studies
CBRN	Chemical biological radiation and nuclear
CBT	Cognitive and behaviour therapy
CCSIG	Critical care special interest group
CCT	Certificate of completion of specialist training
CG	Clinical governance
CISD	Critical incident stress debriefing
CL	Cutaneous Leishmaniasis
CMD	Common mental disorder (symptoms)
CMHN	Community mental health nurse
CNS	Central nervous system
COPD	Chronic obstructive pulmonary disease
CoSHH	Control of Substances Hazardous to Health
COVS	Clinical outcome variability scale
CPD	Continuous professional development
CR	Computed radiography
CRM	Crew resource management
CRPS	Chronic regional pain syndrome
CT	Computed tomography
CTPM	Post-mortem CT imaging
CTU	Clinical Trials Unit
CVC	Central venous catheter
DCR	Damage control resuscitation
DCS	Damage control surgery
DOPTSD	Delayed-onset PTSD
DR	Digital radiography
DTM&H	Diploma in Tropical Medicine and Hygiene
DU	Depleted uranium
ECMO	Extracorporeal membrane oxygenation
ED	Emergency department
EDP	Emergency donor panel
FFP	Fresh frozen plasma
ELISA	Enzyme-linked immunosorbent assay

EM	Emergency medicine	ITU	Intensive therapy unit (also called intensive care unit)
EMDT	Eye movement desensitisation and reprocessing	IVC	Inferior vena cava
ETC	European Trauma Course	LIMS	Laboratory Information Management System
ETCO₂	End-tidal carbon dioxide	LMA	Laryngeal mask airway
FASS	Foot and Ankle Severity Score	LRTI	Lower respiratory tract infection
FAST	Focussed abdominal sonography for trauma	MAST	Military Anti-Shock Trousers
FOI	Fibre optic intubation	MCE	Mass casualty event
FFP	Fresh frozen plasma	MDCT	Multi-detector computed tomography
GA	General anaesthetic	MDSS	Medical device sterilisation services
GCS	Glasgow Coma Scale	MDT	Multi-disciplinary team
G(I)M	General (internal) medicine	MEDSEM	Medical seminars
GMC	General Medical Council	MESS	Mangled Extremity Severity Score
GMI	Graded motor imagery	MHRA	Medicines & Healthcare Products Regulatory Agency
GP	General practitioner		
GRoW	Gradual return to work (programmes)	MIAC	Multi-disciplinary injury assessment clinic
GSW	Gunshot wound		
HBOC	Haemoglobin-based oxygen carrier	MIMMS	Major Incident Medical Management and Support
HCPC	Health & Care Professions Council		
HDU	High-dependency unit	MPK	Microprocessor knee (prothesis)
HEMS	Helicopter Emergency Medical Service	MRI	Magnetic resonance imaging
HIV	Human immunodeficiency virus	mRNA	Mitochrondial ribonucleic acid
HO	Heterotropic ossification	MSA	Medical Supplies Agency (obsolete)
HPA	Health Protection Agency	MSK	Musculo-skeletal
HPMK	Hypothermia Prevention Mitigation Kit™	MRSA	Methicillin resistant *Staphylococcus aureus*
HSD	Hypertonic saline dextran	mTBI	Mild traumatic brain injury
IBS	(i) Intra-operative blood salvage, (ii) Irritable bowel syndrome	MTC	(i) Major trauma centre (ii) Massive transfusion capability
ICD	International Classification & Disease	MTP	Massive transfusion protocol
ICM	Intensive care medicine	MVC	Motor vehicle collision
ICP	Intra-cranial pressure (monitoring)	NBS	National Blood Service (obsolete)
ICRC	International Committee of the Red Cross	NCEPOD	National Confidential Enquiry into Peri-Operative Deaths
ICU	Intensive care unit (also called Intensive therapy unit)	NCTH	Non-compressible torso haemorrhage
		NGO	Non-governmental organisation
IM	Intra-muscular	NHS	National Health Service
INR	International Normalised Ratio – a measure of blood clotting capability; the higher the score, the less effective the clotting process	NHSBT	NHS Blood and Transplant
		NIAA	National Institute of Academic Anaesthesia
		NICE	National Institute Clinical Excellence (now NIHCE)
IO	Intraosseous		
IQR	Interquartile range	NIHCE	National Institute for Heath and Clinical Care Excellence (formerly NICE)
IV	Intra-venous		
IPPV	Intermittent positive pressure ventilation	NIHL	Noise-induced hearing loss
		NIHHL	Noise-induced hidden hearing loss
IS	Information system	NISS	New injury severity score
ISS	Injury Severity Score	OA	Open abdomen

ODP	Operating department practitioner	RIS	Radiology Information System
OOPT	Out of programme training	RLP	Residual limb pain
OPS	Operational performance statement	ROM	Range of movement
OSPE	Objective Structured Practical Examination	ROSC	Return of spontaneous circulation
		ROTEM™	Rotational thrombo-elastometry
OT	Occupational therapy	RRT	Renal replacement therapy
PAC	Pulmonary artery catheter	RSI	Rapid sequence induction (of anaesthesia)
PACS	Patient Archive and Communications System		
		RT	Resuscitative thoracotomy
PAM	Pneumatic acid to mobilization	SI	Shock Index
PAP	Plasmin–antiplasmin	SIG	Specialist interest group
PBLI	Primary blast lung injury	SMART	Specific, measurable, achievable, realistic, and time bound
PCA	Patient controlled analgesia		
PCR	Polymerase chain reaction	SME	Subject matter expert
PPE	Personal protective equipment	SNOM	Selective non-operative management (of abdominal injury)
PD	Psychological debriefing		
PHC	Primary healthcare	STACK	Systolic blood pressure, Temperature, Acidosis, Coagulation and Kit (including blood products used)
PHE	Public Health England		
PHEA	Pre-hospital emergency anaesthesia		
PHEC	(i) Pre-hospital emergency care, (ii) The Pre-Hospital Emergency Medicine Course		
		SWM	Surface wound mapping
		TARN	Trauma Audit and Research Network
		TBI	Traumatic brain injury
PHEM	Pre-hospital emergency medicine	TBSA	Total body surface area
PHPLS	Pre-hospital Paediatric Life Support Course	TCA	Traumatic cardiac arrest
		TEG	Thromboelastography
PICU	Paediatric intensive care unit	TENS	Transcutaneous electrical nerve stimulation
PLP	Phantom limb pain		
POCT	Point-of-care testing	TIA	Transient ischaemic attack
POW	Prisoner of War	TIC	Trauma induced coagulopathy
PPFOM	Pre-prosthetic functional outcome measure	TIVA	Total intravenous anaesthesia
		TNC	Trauma nurse coordinator
pRBC	Packed red blood cells	TNP	Topical negative pressure (dressing)
PT	Prothrombin time	TNPWT	Topical negative pressure wound therapy
PTS	Permanent threshold shift		
PTSD	Post-traumatic stress disorder	TPN	Total parenteral nutrition
QEHB	Queen Elizabeth Hospital Birmingham	TRALI	Transfusion-related acute lung injury
		TRISS	Trauma Revised Injury Severity Score (trauma scoring system)
QoL	Quality of life		
RAMC	Royal Army Medical Corps	TTL	Trauma team leader
RBC	Red blood cells	TTS	Transient threshold shift
RCC	Red cell concentrate	TXA	Tranexamic acid
RCoA	Royal College of Anaesthetists	VAC	Vacuum assisted closure
RCT	Randomised controlled trial	VAP	Ventilator associated pneumonia
R&D	Research and development	vCJD	Variant Creutzfeldt–Jakob disease
REBOA	Rapid endovascular balloon occlusion of aorta	Voc OT	Vocational Occupational Therapist
		VTE	Venous thrombo-embolism
rFVIIa	Recombinant (blood clotting) factor VIIa	WHO	World Health Organisation

A note on operation names

Operation names used by the UK Armed Forces are (usually) single word names chosen at random by a computer specifically so that there is no connection between the name and the nature or aim of the operation, and names do not in themselves become politically sensitive. Names are also required to be appropriate in that they are not frivolous, ethnically or politically sensitive or capable of mis-interpretation. US naming conventions are different, and names such as *Operation Enduring Freedom* (the US name for Operations in Afghanistan) would not be allocated to a UK operation. The main UK operations in Afghanistan constituted *Operation HERRICK* and in Iraq, *Operation TELIC*. By convention, the name of the operation is given in capitals. For ease of reading, I have not followed this convention in the text. Each tranche of *Operations Telic* and *Herrick* was numbered sequentially and almost invariably lasted six months, the length of deployment of most field units. Thus, *Operation Herrick 4* was the fourth six-month period after the beginning of the campaign.

Echelons and levels of clinical care

ECHELONS OF CARE

Role 1 Medical support – is that which is integral to or allocated to a small unit and will include the capabilities for providing first aid, immediate life-saving measures and triage (*NATO definition*).

Role 2 Medical support – is provided at larger unit level, usually of brigade or larger size (or other service equivalent), although it may be provided farther forward, depending upon the operational requirements. In general, it will be prepared to provide evacuation from Role/ Echelon 1 facilities, triage and resuscitation, treatment and holding of patients until they can be returned to duty or evacuated, as well as emergency dental treatment (*NATO definition*).

Role 3 Medical support – is normally provided at division level and above. It includes additional capabilities, such as specialist diagnostic resources, specialist surgical and medical capabilities, preventive medicine, food inspection, dentistry and operational stress management teams when these are not provided at level 2 (*NATO definition*). Role 3 support is usually provided by a field hospital.

Role 4 Medical support – offers definitive care of patients for whom the treatment required is longer than the theatre evacuation policy or for whom the capabilities usually found at Role/ Echelon 3 are inadequate. This would normally comprise specialist surgical and medical procedures, reconstruction, rehabilitation and convalescence. This level of care is usually highly specialised and time-consuming and normally provided in the country of origin. Under very unusual circumstances, this level of care may be established in a theatre of operations (*NATO definition*). UK Role 4 is the Queen Elizabeth Hospital, Birmingham.

Note: (*E*) *enhanced refers to the addition of capability and (A) – afloat, to the maritime capability at the same echelon.*

LEVELS OF CLINICAL CARE

Throughout this book, reference is frequently made to levels of care. In brief, these levels are as follows:

Level 1 – Ward-based care without the need for organ support. However, the patient may need simple interventions such as an intravenous line or oxygen.

Level 2 – High-dependency unit (HDU) care. HDU patients might need support for a single organ (except mechanical ventilation), such as renal replacement therapy, drugs to support heart function (inotropes) or invasive monitoring. The normal staffing rate is one for every two patients.

Level 3 – Intensive care. Patients in the intensive therapy unit are likely to require support for two or more organs or systems or may need ventilation alone. Each patient will have a dedicated nurse, and there is a high level of resident medical cover.

Acknowledgements

First of all, I would like to express my gratitude to the Trustees of the *Royal Army Medical Corps Charity* for a substantial donation in support of this project. I would also like to express my sincere gratitude for the help I have received from Col Cliff Dieppe L/RAMC, Representative Colonel Commandant RAMC, and Maj (Rtd) Marie Ellis, Regimental Secretary RAMC. I am grateful to the former Surgeon General, Surg Vice Adm Alasdair Walker CB OBE for reading the manuscript before submission, and my thanks are also due to Maj. Gen. Martin Bricknell and to Brig Tim Hodgetts CBE for their support. At Surgeon General's Department, Ailsa Keogh has eased the manuscript through the complexities of clearance, for which I am most grateful. My secretary, Mrs Mandy Wright, was as ever a great support.

I am profoundly grateful to all the principle chapter authors for all their hard work in capturing our experience. I hope the final result is as they would wish.

For assistance with illustrations, I am grateful to SSgt Barber, Maj David Cooper RAMC, Dr Mark de Rond, Col Scott Frazer L/RAMC, Dr Robert Fryer, Maj Duncan Gray RAMC, Jason Howe, Lt Col Paul Hunt RAMC, Col Tim Lowes L/RAMC, Surg Cdr Adrian Mellor RN, Lt Col Ross Moy RAMC, Mr Dominic Power, Mr Darren Roberts, Lt Col Derek Saunders and Major Helen Wilson QARANC. Particular thanks are due to Stuart Brown (www.skipperpress.com), Graeme Lothian (http://www.graemelothian.com) and David Rowlands (www.davidrowlands.co.uk), distinguished military artists, for permission to use their paintings.

A particular debt is owed to Col David Vassallo L/RAMC for preparing the deployed forces tables.

On behalf of the principle chapter authors, I would also wish to express my gratitude to Lt Col (Rtd), Dominic Aldington RAMC, Maj Andy Barlow RAMC, Wg Cdr Robin Berry RAF, Wg Cdr Kristina Birch RAF, Sqn Ldr Jodie Blackadder-Weinstein RAF, Col Jon C. Clasper CBE L/RAMC, Surg Cdr D Connor RN, Wg Cdr Ian Ewington RAF, Prof Nicola T. Fear, Surg Cdr David Gay RN, Prof Neil Greenberg, Col Stuart Harrison L/RAMC, Col Jeremy Henning L/RAMC, Surg Cdr S Hutchings RN, Lt Col Andrew Johnston RAMC, Mrs Joan Jones MBE, Lt Col Graham Lawton RAMC, Lt Col S Lewis RAMC, Col Tim Lowes RAMC, Lt Col J McNicholas RAMC (Rtd), Lt Col P Moor RAMC, Lt Col Linda Orr RAMC, Lt Col Harry Pugh, the late Dr Sam Rawlinson OBE, Wg Cdr Robert Scott, Lt Col Mike Smith RAMC, Sqn Ldr Marc Spinks RAF, Lt Cdr T Stevenson, Dr Emma Watkins, Maj Catriona Watson RAMC, Prof Sir Simon Wessely, Surg Cdr Mark Whittaker RN, Col Tom Woolley L/RAMC and Ms Yvonne Yau.

I am grateful to Capt Allan Pang RAMC for assistance with literature searches and to Surg Lt Cdr Sophie Butterworth RN and Major David Hindmarsh RAMC for their painstaking fact checking of the *Role of Honour*. Many thanks are also due to Sq Ldr Natalie Lonsdale and Surg Lt Cdr Butterworth (again) for formatting and correcting the bibliographies. I would like to offer my thanks to Surg Rear Adm (Rtd) Lionel Jarvis CBE for his wise advice and support.

Organisations that have helped with the preparation of the book include the Centre for Defence Pathology (Blood Supply Team), Headquarters Surgeon General, US Armed Services Blood Programme, National Health Service Blood and Transplant and the apheresis nursing leads, Trauma Haemostasis and Oxygenation Research Network and Queen Elizabeth Hospital Birmingham.

At *Taylor & Francis*, Miranda Bromage recognised the value of this project and guided it through acceptance to publication. Relationships with publishers under the strain of deadlines and complex projects are not always plain sailing: this one was, and I'm really grateful to Miranda, Cherry Allen, Amy Rodriguez, Amor Nanas, Kyle Meyer and Gabriel Schenk.

Finally, I would like to thank Julia, Tom and Owen for putting up with the fact that most of the work on this project was done in the evenings and at weekends.

This book has been a coordinated effort by many people: it is almost inevitable that I have missed out someone who has made a significant contribution: to them, I can only offer my sincere thanks and genuine apology.

Ian Greaves

Colour plate acknowledgements

COLOUR PLATE CREDITS

Illustrations marked *editor's collection* have been taken by me or very kindly given to me over the years by clinical colleagues and other photographers. Where the source is known, it is acknowledged with gratitude. If anyone recognises an unacknowledged image, please let me know and a suitable acknowledgement will be made in future editions. I am most grateful to all the individuals and organisations listed below for allowing me to reproduce the following illustrations:

1. *Tented Field Hospital Operation Telic 4*, image courtesy of militaryimages.net
2. *Emergency Department, COB*, editor's photograph
3. *British troops in Basra*. (Courtesy of The Regimental Museum of The Royal Welsh.)
4. *CMTs working on a casualty*, editor's collection
5. and 6. *RAP, Camp Abu Naji* and *CAP, Operation Telic*, by kind permission of Lt Col Paul Hunt RAMC
7. *FOB Musa Qal'eh*, by kind permission of *Maj David Cooper RAMC*
8. Operations in the "Green Zone", editor's collection
9. *A typical Afghan townscape*, editor's collection
10. *Camp Bastion*, Crown copyright
11. *MERT lands*, editor's collection
12. *In-flight resuscitation*, Crown copyright (RAF)
13. *Evacuating an injured casualty*, Crown copyright (RAF)
14. *Entrance to the emergency department*, by kind permission of Lt Col Paul Hunt RAMC
15. *Resuscitation in the ED*, editor's photograph
16. *The operating theatre*, editor's photograph
17. *Improvised traction device*, editor's photograph
18. *Brydon Lines*, editor's photograph
19. *The new Camp Bastion hospital*, editor's photograph
20. The New Camp Bastion hospital, photograph by Cpl Steven Peacock
21. *The main corridor*, editor's collection
22. *Resuscitation in the new facility*, Crown copyright
23. *The Bastion Hospital CT facility*, by kind permission of Col Iain Gibb L/RAMC
24. *A patient being evacuated*, copyright holder not known
25. QEH Birmingham, copyright holder not known
26. *Sandstorm*, editor's collection
27. *Treating a child with the aid of an interpreter*, editor's photograph
28. *Lowering the flag*, Crown copyright
29. *Simon Pegg at Headley Court*, Crown copyright
30. *War Memorial Camp Bastion*, Crown copyright
31. HM Queen Elizabeth II unveils the Iraq and Afghanistan Memorial. Crown copyright.
32. Medical care overview, Crown copyright

TEXT ILLUSTRATION CREDITS

I am also grateful to the owners of the following websites for their kind permission to reproduce a number of the illustrations in the text:

- www.militaryimages.net (Figure 4.1)
- www.tacmedaustralia.com.au (Figure 4.6)
- www.wartimegenitaltrauma.wordpress.com /penile-reconstruction (Figure 10.16)
- http://blogs.discovermagazine.com (Figure 12.1) http://www.usnews.com (Figure 16.5)
- Figure 3.5 is from Wikimedia Commons.

Experience is a jewel, and it had need be so, for it is often purchased at an infinite rate.

Shakespeare

A brief history of *Operations Telic* and *Herrick*

'The first, supreme, the most far-reaching act of judgement that the statesman and commander have to make is to establish…the kind of war on which we are embarking…this is the first strategic question and the most comprehensive'.

Clausewitz[1]

'The key lesson is that we ignore previous experiences of campaigns and those of our allies at our peril'.

3 PARA, Afghanistan, 2007[2]

INTRODUCTION

The momentous attacks of 11 September 2001 were the precipitating causes for both *Operation Telic* and *Operation Herrick*, the British military operations in Iraq and Afghanistan, respectively. This date (universally referred to as *9/11*) saw Osama bin Laden's militant Islamist organisation, *Al Qaeda*, hijack four American airliners and transform them into the largest suicide bombs the World has ever seen. Two of the jets were flown into the Twin Towers of the World Trade Center, New York (Figure 1.1), and a third was deliberately flown into the Pentagon in Washington, DC. The last one crashed into a field in the State of Pennsylvania, after the brave attempts of its passengers to subdue their hijackers diverted them from their intended target, possibly the White House on Capitol Hill. These unprecedented attacks on mainland United States cost almost 3000 lives and were as traumatising to the American psyche as the attack on Pearl Harbor, on that other 'date which will live in infamy', 7 December 1941.

Just as the Pearl Harbor attack precipitated American entry into the Second World War, the 9/11 attacks (albeit by a terrorist organisation rather than an enemy state) led directly to US military intervention in Afghanistan under *Operation Enduring Freedom*. They would also precipitate the subsequent invasion of Iraq (*Operation Iraqi Freedom*) as part of what President George W. Bush declared would be a global 'War on Terror'. The latter campaign was a highly controversial 'War of Choice' against a country that had nothing to do with 9/11,[3] and it ended up, predictably, serving 'as a force multiplier for terrorists like Al Qaeda'.[4] The United Kingdom's invasion of Iraq in support of the United States, under *Operation Telic*, would arguably become 'the most contentious war that the United Kingdom has ever fought'.[5]

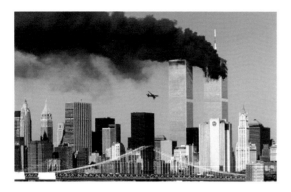

Figure 1.1 The attack on the Twin Towers, 11th September 2001.

THE RESPONSE TO 9/11

Prime Minister Tony Blair's New Labour Government had been elected in 1997 espousing a policy of liberal interventionism and was buoyed by recent military successes in Kosovo (*Operation Agricola*, 1999) and Sierra Leone (*Operation Palliser*, May–June 2000) and a hostage rescue mission (*Operation Barras*, September 2000). The British Government responded immediately in support of the United States after 9/11, wholeheartedly committing troops to strengthen the United Kingdom's 'special relationship' with the United States. This was very much its main policy objective but was never

actually backed with sufficient numbers of troops or with enough resources to accomplish the tasks for which the troops had been offered. This would later be compounded by the severe economic recession of 2008 onwards, which limited the capacity of both the United States and the United Kingdom to commit further resources. There was also increasing pressure, in the United Kingdom especially, to reduce military commitments in two campaigns that appeared to be lasting far longer than envisaged. This failure to commit sufficient resources would ultimately end in strategic defeat in both Iraq and Afghanistan, seriously compromising that very same 'special relationship',[6] although the bravery and dedication of British troops on the ground were never in question.

Afghanistan

Once the Taliban regime in Afghanistan (Figure 1.2) refused to surrender Osama bin Laden and his followers, from 7 October 2001 onwards, British troops rapidly became engaged in a series of operations as part of the US-led coalition supporting the *Northern Alliance* against the Taliban (the Northern Alliance would, in due course, become the *Afghan Interim* and then *Transitional Administration*). It had been over 80 years since British regular troops last set foot on the plains and in the formidable mountains

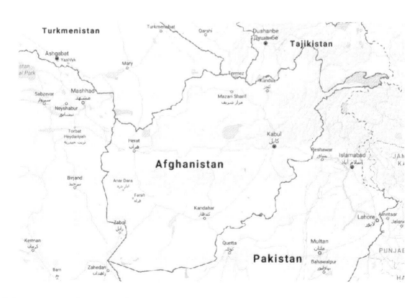

Figure 1.2 Afghanistan and surrounding countries.

and passes of Afghanistan, in the short-lived Third Afghan War of 1919. Their successors were about to relearn some hard lessons.[7,8]

Kabul (the capital) fell on 13 November and Kandahar [the Taliban's spiritual home] on 7 December 2001, with the remnants of the Taliban and Al-Qaeda retreating into the Pashtun heartlands in Waziristan, in northwest Pakistan. Hamid Karzai was then installed in Kabul as interim president and head of the *Afghan Interim Administration*, supported by the *International Security Assistance Force* (ISAF). ISAF had just been created in accordance with the Bonn Conference of December 2001, under the authority of the United Nations (UN) Security Council.[9]

Each of the British operations in this 'Fourth Afghan War' would be allocated its own distinctive codename until late 2004 – *Veritas* (the initial contribution of air crew and Special Forces), *Oracle* (incorporated within *Veritas*), *Fingal* (the UK contribution to ISAF in Kabul from December 2001, including leadership of ISAF for the first six months of its existence) and *Tarrock* (the UK contribution to ISAF operations in Northern Afghanistan).

Shift of focus to Iraq

With the Taliban apparently defeated and with US Special Forces continuing the hunt for Osama bin Laden, the US focus in its 'War on Terror' shifted in 2002 to Saddam Hussein's brutal regime in Iraq and 'unfinished business' from 1991, focussing on the ostensible threat of weapons of mass destruction as a reason to achieve regime change (Figure 1.3). Saddam had seized power in Iraq in 1979, and his forces had invaded Iran in September 1980 and Kuwait in August 1990. He had used chemical weapons in Iran and against his Kurdish subjects. After Kuwait had been liberated in the first Gulf War in 1991, no-fly zones were imposed in northern and southern Iraq (enforced by US and UK aircraft), and the UN Special Commission was set up to monitor Iraq's military arsenals. Increasing obstruction by the Iraqi authorities led to UN weapons inspectors being withdrawn in December 1998.[10]

George W. Bush's election as US president in November 2000 and the 9/11 attacks in 2001 transformed the political scene. From the very first day after 9/11, Bush and his ambitious neo-conservative ideologues, particularly Vice President Dick Cheney and Defense Secretary Donald Rumsfeld, determined to use 9/11 as the excuse for removing Saddam Hussein from power and re-asserting US power in the Middle East, disregarding the fact that Saddam had nothing to do with 9/11.[11] On 12 September 2002, one day after the first anniversary of 9/11, President Bush formally began

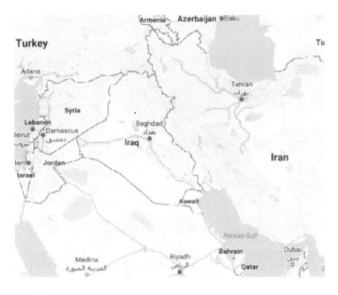

Figure 1.3 Iraq and its neighbours.

arguing the case for a pre-emptive invasion of Iraq in a speech to the UN General Assembly, on the basis that Saddam Hussein's government was violating UN resolutions, primarily on weapons of mass destruction.[12] Just days later, on 24 September, Prime Minister Tony Blair presented his now-discredited 'September Dossier' outlining the apparent threat posed by Iraq through its weapons of mass destruction, for debate in the House of Commons.[13,14]

Concerted US political and military pressure soon led to the UN declaring that it would no longer tolerate Iraq's defiance of international law. *UN Security Council Resolution* (UNSCR) 1441 was unanimously adopted on 8 November 2002, declaring Iraq in material breach of previous resolutions and setting out new procedures for inspections, giving Iraq a final opportunity to comply.[15] Contingent military planning led to a massive build-up of US forces in the Gulf, strengthening diplomatic pressure on Iraq, while building up the momentum for war. UN weapons inspectors were allowed back into Iraq by the end of November, but Iraqi obstruction continued. On 15 February 2003, massive 'Stop the War' protests occurred around the world, with over a million protesting in Britain alone. Regardless of these protests, on 24 February 2003, the United Kingdom, United States and Spain tabled a draft resolution, declaring that Iraq had failed to comply with *Resolution 1441*. It soon became evident that the UN Security Council would not reach consensus on this matter, not the least because the UN Charter and international humanitarian law prohibited pre-emptive military action against another sovereign country. Nonetheless, the United States and the United Kingdom decided to proceed with military action on their own, together with Australia. The world is still dealing with the political and social fallout of this arguably illegal invasion and occupation, and the precedent this 'War of Choice' set for other nations with an eye on the territory of their neighbours.[16]

UK military planning

The United Kingdom's Ministry of Defence (MOD) had to balance the possibility of overt preparations prejudicing the diplomatic process against the need to be ready to take action if the diplomatic process failed. Consequently, enabling activities

for a potential large-scale deployment to the Gulf region only commenced in early December 2002.[17] The favoured option was to enter Iraq from the north through the Kurdish region of Turkey, with the United Kingdom contributing a Brigade's worth of troops, but public pressure forced the moderate Islamic government of Turkey to withdraw its support in December and deny passage through its territory. Planning hurriedly switched to the southern option of invading Iraq through Kuwait and the Gulf, necessitating a significant increase in forces. UK Regular military forces received formal notification around Christmas Day 2002 to prepare for military action and began deploying on 16 January 2003. With regard to reservist personnel, the Secretary of State for Defence announced their first call-out on 7 January 2003, with a larger call-out of selected reservists (mainly medical) on 30 January 2003. The majority of reservists received their compulsory mobilisation orders with less than two weeks' notice, although most were given advance warning.[18] Some Reservists were still flying into theatre as hostilities commenced. The coalition forces invaded Iraq on the night of 20 March 2003, achieving a degree of surprise through the near-simultaneous start of ground and air offensives.

COMBAT OPERATIONS IN IRAQ

Almost a third of the British Army was to deploy to the Gulf within the first six months of *Operation Telic*. This included over 5000 Territorial Army and Regular Reservists, the largest number called up since the Suez crisis in 1956.[19] At the peak of major combat operations in spring 2003, the United Kingdom had a total of 46,000 military personnel deployed in Iraq, including 28,000 on land. Combat operations ceased in May.

The British Army had been configured since the *1998 Defence Review* by the incoming Labour government to be capable of fielding either a divisional force in a full scale crisis or running two concurrent brigade-sized operations (one warfighting for six months, and the other engaged in an enduring non-warfighting operation). Crucially, the two brigade operations could only overlap for six months.[20] These constraints, and a lack of strategic oversight, would bedevil the campaigns in both Iraq and Afghanistan,[21] as force levels were imposed and then applied to the tactical problem, rather than the tactical problem defining the level of forces required.[22] Thus, the stage was set for strategic failure in both campaigns from the beginning.

Whitehall thus initiated moves in May 2003 to rapidly reduce force levels in Iraq by two brigades, aiming to have only 8600 troops in theatre in 2004. This constraint remained despite the deployed forces by then having to cope with a Shi'ite insurgency throughout southern Iraq. Whitehall proceeded with progressive reductions, to 8500 in May 2005 and to 7200 in May 2006. Thereafter, between 2006 and 2009, following deployment into Helmand, the United Kingdom struggled to sustain two brigade-size operations simultaneously in medium-intensity counterinsurgency campaigns in both Iraq and Afghanistan. Forces in Iraq were reduced to 5500 in May 2007,[23] before the United Kingdom withdrew completely in 2009 under the pressure of trying to sustain the operation in Afghanistan.

Following the *1st (UK) Armoured Division's* deployment on *(Operation) Telic 1*, there would be a total of 12 Brigade-sized deployments to Iraq, each of six months' duration, until *Telic 13* brought the operation to a close in May 2009. A total of 179 British Armed Forces personnel or MOD civilians would lose their lives during *Operation Telic*, 136 of them dying as a result of hostile action.[24] Importantly, 'their lives were lost, not wasted – they answered the call of duty undaunted and achieved much against near impossible odds'.[25]

Counterinsurgency in crisis

Despite the fact that the British had greater and more recent experience than their American counterparts in fighting insurgencies, the Army's organisational memory had faded quickly since the peace settlement of 1997 in Northern Ireland, with *counter-insurgency* (COIN) doctrine no longer being taught in the British Military. It had taken the permanent deployment of 13 infantry battalions to Northern Ireland to contain the insurgency there (and even then, with the support of a trusted police force and a deep understanding of local culture), yet in Iraq, the United Kingdom attempted to meet a much more violent insurgency in Basra (three times the size of Belfast) and elsewhere with

only three battalions (and with no support from a corrupt police force or understanding of local tribal culture and language).[26] The military would have to relearn COIN the hard way in both Iraq and Afghanistan.[27]

MEANWHILE, BACK IN AFGHANISTAN...

In January 2003, a resurgent Taliban commenced an insurgency in Afghanistan, infiltrating from Pakistan, the insurgency gathering momentum throughout the summer and setting the pattern for future years. In August 2003, at the request of the UN and the Government of the Islamic Republic of Afghanistan, the North Atlantic Treaty Organization (NATO) took on the leadership of ISAF, initially providing security around Kabul (the British continuing to contribute under *Operation Fingal*), then gradually expanding ISAF's presence by late 2006 to cover the whole country. At its height between February and July 2011, ISAF deployed more than 132,000 troops, with up to 51 NATO and partner nations contributing at various times.[28,29,30]

In April 2004, the United Kingdom deployed a single light infantry battalion (the 1st Battalion The Green Howards), known in theatre as the *Afghan Roulement Infantry Battalion*, to provide security for ISAF in Kabul and in northern Afghanistan, under *Operations Fingal* and *Tarrock*, respectively. In late 2004, the *UK Chief of the Defence Staff* (CDS), seeking to rationalise UK Operational activity in Afghanistan, consolidated the various codenames into one single codename covering all UK contributions within the Joint Area of Operations. This Area was defined as the territory and airspace of Afghanistan. This new operational codename, *Operation Herrick*, came into force on 1 October 2004.[31]

The codenames *Herrick 1–3* were assigned to the three *Afghan Roulement Infantry Battalion* deployments thereafter, namely those of the *1st Battalion The Worcestershire and Sherwood Foresters* (1 October 2004–30 April 2005), the *2nd Battalion The Royal Gurkha Rifles* (29 March–3 October 2005) and the *1st Battalion The Royal Gloucestershire, Berkshire and Wiltshire Light Infantry* (3 October 2005–3 April 2006) (Figure 1.4).[32]

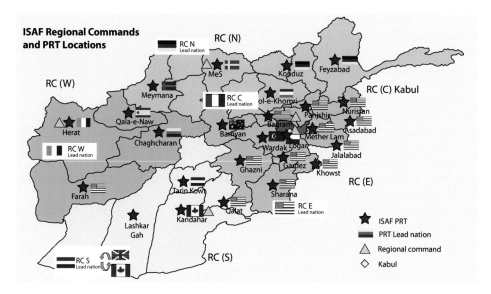

Figure 1.4 ISAF Regional Commands 2006–2010 (summer). The RC (South) Lead Nation rotated between the United Kingdom, Canada and the Netherlands. (From NATO. ISAF placemats archive. 12 January 2009. http://www.nato.int/cps/en/natolive/107995.htm.)

The UK land commitment in Afghanistan changed significantly with *Herrick 4* (April to October 2006), with the deployment of 3300 troops under the command of 16 Air Assault Brigade into Helmand Province as part of the overall ISAF expansion throughout Afghanistan. Thereafter, larger brigade-strength roulements to Helmand (Figure 1.5) occurred every six months until the end of 2014, with the maximum number of British troops in the country reaching 9500 throughout

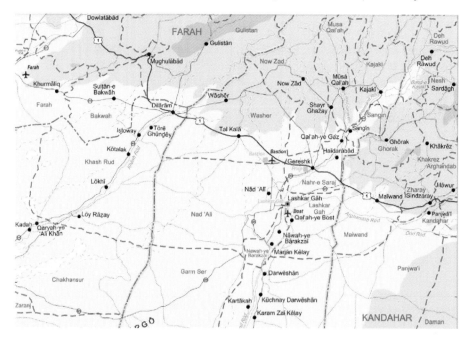

Figure 1.5 Helmand Province, southwest Afghanistan.

2010–2012.[33] The last deployment was *Herrick 20*, formally ending in November 2014, with a small number of troops remaining thereafter, mainly to provide training at the new Afghan National Army (ANA) Officer Academy in Kabul. A total of 453 British servicemen and women would lose their lives during *Operation Herrick*, of whom 405 were directly attributable to hostile action.[34]

For comparison, 722 service personnel died due to hostile action in Northern Ireland between 14 August 1969 and 31 July 2007, while the operation with the largest number of deaths among UK Armed Forces personnel post World War II was Malaya, with 1443 deaths between 16 June 1948 and 31 July 1960.[35]

Thus, the British military commenced the first decade of the twenty-first century with unforeseen operations abroad, in Sierra Leone and then Afghanistan and Iraq. Many individuals and units deployed on multiple occasions to both Iraq and Afghanistan over some 13 years. The crucible of these years of intensive and symbiotic operations resulted in rapid accumulation of individual and collective combat experience and knowledge at all levels throughout the Forces, eventually leading to adaptation and transformation while in conflict as harsh lessons were learned.[36,37] The challenges from the casualty load across both theatres, which actively engaged the whole of the Defence Medical Services, would simultaneously catalyse a revolution in military medical care.

KEY SOURCES FOR *OPERATIONS HERRICK* AND *TELIC*

While no Official Military History has yet been commissioned for *Operation Telic* or *Herrick* (the last such being on the Falklands War, *Operation Corporate*), the UK MOD has conducted several internal studies. The background to the conflict in Iraq and the planning, deployment and combat phases of the operation, together with some early lessons identified, were first described in the MOD report *Operations in Iraq – First Reflections* in July 2003[38] and then updated in *Operation Telic – United Kingdom Military Operations In Iraq* in December 2003.[39] The war-fighting operations (*Telic 1*) were further analysed in *Operations in Iraq – An Analysis from a Land Perspective*,

published in 2005.[40] The analysis of *Operations Telic 2–5*, published in 2006, is available on the Internet,[41] and Brigadier Barry's critical analysis of *Operations Telic 5–13* was released publicly in September 2016.[42,43] Various critical articles were published in the *British Army Review* (*BAR*; the Army's in-house journal), such as the one in 2009 by US Colonel Peter Mansoor, General Petraeus's former chief of staff, who controversially opined that British political and military leaders had abdicated responsibility for protecting the Iraqi people in Basra.[44,45] Most of these *BAR* articles (but not Mansoor's) were collated in a single-volume special report.[46]

The main MOD report on the Afghanistan conflict is the *Operation Herrick Campaign Study*, published internally in 2015. A redacted version has now been released publicly following a Freedom of Information request.[47] The health service support organisational lessons identified by this study, and the actions being taken to implement them, were further examined and published as a definitive record in the *Journal of the Royal Army Medical Corps*.[48]

Every military unit returning from Iraq or Afghanistan submitted a post-operational report, and each unit also documented its experiences in regimental or unit journals, sometimes on YouTube or regimental association websites, and occasionally in books about specific deployments. A few recently published regimental histories describe unit experiences during both campaigns. Select reading lists relating to each campaign are provided later in this volume.

There have been numerous academic papers, not least by the *Royal United Services Institute* (the United Kingdom's pre-eminent military think-tank), which published several papers analysing the United Kingdom's military decision making in Iraq and in Afghanistan.[49,50,51] Several critical books have appeared since the end of *Operation Telic*, commencing with that by defence analyst Richard North in 2009, who laid the blame for Britain's failure in Iraq on the failure by Tony Blair's government to provide the Army with the forces and equipment required.[52] The testimonies of many of the United Kingdom's recently retired senior officers reflecting critically on their experience leading operations in Iraq and Afghanistan were published in 2013 as *British*

Generals in Blair's Wars. This book gives a real sense of how the character of these wars changed even as they were being fought, as well as giving good accounts of operations such as *Operation Sinbad* and *Operation Charge of the Knights*.[53] Three autobiographies by recently retired British generals, who were successively chief of the General Staff from 2003 to 2010, with General Sir David Richards also being promoted to CDS (the most senior serving military officer in the Armed Forces) in 2010–2013, shed further light on both campaigns.[54,55,56] In addition, the *Sunday Times* Defence correspondent, Tim Ripley, published a comprehensive history of the *Operation Telic* campaign as an eBook (2014), later revised and published in paperback (May 2016).[57] An anonymous US librarian has compiled a useful website listing most of the publications relating to US and UK operations in Iraq and Afghanistan.[58] In January 2017, the *International Institute for Strategic Studies* (IISS) published a strategic analysis of both campaigns focussing on the military issues of greatest relevance for the future.[59] In September 2017, Professor Theo Farrell, previously head of the War Studies Department at King's College London, published an authoritative study of Britain's war in Afghanistan, concluding that despite British and American tactical successes, the war was strategically unwinnable after 2002 due to Afghan government corruption and Pakistani support for the Taliban.[60]

The Chilcot report

On 6 July 2016, Sir John Chilcot published his long-awaited *Report of the Iraq Inquiry*, the key document for understanding *Operation Telic*.[61] Three books to date (April 2017), in addition to the IISS study, draw extensively on the Chilcot Report or the Inquiry's proceedings. Former military intelligence officer Frank Ledwidge published a damning critique of the United Kingdom's political and military leadership in 2011 (revised in 2017 after the Chilcot Report lent further credence to his arguments).[62] Major General Christopher Elliott, in his comprehensive study of senior British military leadership and decision making in this period, examined in detail how the mismatch of policy and resources (the ends and the means), and the surprising lack of strategic direction (the ways) connecting

them, seriously affected the two campaigns. Major General Elliott drew extensively on personal interviews with key figures as well as on the Chilcot Inquiry proceedings to inform his analysis (2015).[63] Jeremy Greenstock (UK Ambassador to the UN before the invasion and subsequently Special Envoy for Iraq) was uniquely placed to present the political perspective and describe how Britain's decision to go to war in Iraq fitted into the international context (2016, published after Chilcot).[64]

An Army Reserve surgeon drew on open sources and personal contacts to publish an unofficial medical history, initially just of *Operation Telic 1* on a CD-ROM, but then of the whole of *Operation Telic* as an eBook (2015).[65] The *Journal of the Royal Army Medical Corps* and the *Journal of the Royal Naval Medical Services*, amongst others, documented many medical aspects and lessons from both campaigns.

OPERATION TELIC PHASE BY PHASE

'You are not particularly welcome here. Remember what happened when you were here last time…'[66]

Operation Telic 1 (1st UK Armoured Division, February to June 2003)[67]

PLANNING PHASE

The UK, US and Australian Coalition was under the overall command of US General Tommy Franks, Commander in Chief US Central Command (CENTCOM). General Franks would later describe the US plan for the invasion of Iraq, *Operation Iraqi Freedom*, in his memoir *American Soldier*.[68] In essence, US land forces would invade along two main avenues from the south. Army forces would advance west of the Euphrates River in a long arc that curved from their departure lines in Kuwait to reach Baghdad, while the *1st Marine Expeditionary Force* would follow the road network along the Tigris River further east. Britain would provide one of the five divisions participating in the invasion. The British ground forces would pivot northeast out of Kuwait and isolate Basra, Iraq's second city and the capital of the Shi'a south, forming a protective cordon around the southern oil fields

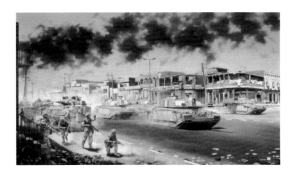

Figure 1.6 Liberation of Basra. (Courtesy of David Rowlands, Military Artist.)

where most of Iraq's oil was produced (Figure 1.6). US, British and Australian Special Forces would control Iraq's western desert, to prevent the launch of long range SCUD missiles against Jordan and Israel. General Franks' objective was to reach Baghdad as soon as possible, bypassing Iraqi forces if necessary, to secure the acquiescence of the Iraqi population and the early collapse of Saddam Hussein's regime, preventing Saddam from using weapons of mass destruction or creating major environmental damage as he had in the 1991 Gulf Conflict.

PREPARATION PHASE

Royal Navy

The British maritime contribution to the Coalition was built on the standing Royal Navy presence in the Gulf. *Naval Task Group 2003*, led by HMS Ark Royal, was expanded into a much larger force totalling some 9000 personnel. It included submarines armed with Tomahawk cruise missiles and a significant amphibious capability with the helicopter carrier *HMS Ocean, Headquarters 3 Commando Brigade Royal Marines, 40 Commando and 42 Commando* (some 4,000 personnel), and hospital facilities in *RFA Argus*. This was the largest amphibious force deployed since the Falklands campaign in 1982.[69]

Land forces

The United Kingdom committed land forces in divisional strength: the *1st (UK) Armoured Division*, which was specially reinforced for this operation. It finally deployed with three brigades executing a mix of light role and armoured tasks, and a logistics brigade: its own *7 Armoured Brigade* (known as the Desert Rats), together with *16 Air Assault Brigade*,

3 Commando Brigade, 102 Logistics Brigade and the *Joint Helicopter Force. 1st (UK) Armoured Division* was under command of the US *1st Marine Expeditionary Force (1 MEF)*, which itself was subordinated to *Combined Force Land Component Command*.* The UK land force deployment would eventually total some 28,000 personnel, the largest such deployment since the First Gulf War.

Air assets

The Royal Air Force (RAF) contributed some 8100 personnel together with 113 fixed wing aircraft to *Operation Telic*; these assets were distributed across eight deployed operating bases in seven countries. In addition, the *Joint Helicopter Command* deployed more than 100 helicopters from all three Services, including Puma and Chinook support helicopters.[70]

INVASION PHASE

On 18 March 2003, the UK Parliament passed a vote by 412 votes to 149 authorising military action against Iraq, and within minutes, Special Forces patrols crossed the border from Jordan into western Iraq on the hunt for Scud missile launchers.[71] *Operation Telic* (the UK contribution to *Operation Iraqi Freedom*) officially began with the issuing of the *Operation Telic Executive Order*, directing military action to commence, on 19 March 2003 (at precisely 06:51 hours Zulu), following the expiry of a US/UK ultimatum to Iraqi President Saddam Hussein, at which stage diplomacy was deemed to have failed. UK Forces, in conjunction with US Forces, were directed to remove the Iraqi Regime. 19 March 2003 was designated *D day*.[72] A 'shock and awe' air offensive commenced immediately, and the invasion of Iraq commenced on the night of 20 March (designated as *G Day*), with one of the earliest actions being an airborne assault by Royal Marines to secure the oil terminals of the Al Faw peninsula and prevent their wanton destruction.

British forces took control of Basra city on 8 April, and US forces formally occupied Baghdad on 9 April. Saddam Hussein's regime had fallen by 14 April 2003, and most of Iraq was taken under

---

* Combined Force Land Component Command would be replaced by Combined Joint Task Force 7 on 14 June 2003 as the operational headquarters for all ground units in the CENTCOM theatre of operations.

coalition control within four weeks. On 1 May, just six weeks after launching the invasion, President Bush declared 'mission accomplished' and the end of major combat operations.[73] Later events would show how premature this was, as well as showing the lack of prior planning for the crucial post-invasion phase (known as *Phase IV* in military parlance – *Phase I* is the battle-planning phase, *Phase II* is the preparatory phase with build-up of materiel and personnel, *Phase III* is the actual battle (or invasion in this instance), and *Phase IV* is the post-conflict phase, which requires prior planning to deal with conflict resolution, security, reconstruction and recovery. Phase IV is crucially dependent on the provision of sufficient numbers of trusted security personnel, particularly police, a factor completely missing in post-invasion Iraq).

As Jeremy Greenstock, former UK Ambassador to the UN and UK Special Envoy for Iraq, said: 'The fundamental error of the Coalition was to have lost control of security almost immediately after the invasion was over. President Bush in effect set the wrong mission for CENTCOM Commander General Tommy Franks: he needed to deliver not just an Iraq without Saddam, but a secure and functioning Iraq without Saddam'.[74]

POST-CONFLICT PHASE

Even while Basra City was being liberated by 7 Armoured Brigade, the abrupt departure of Ba'athist government officials and security personnel was followed immediately (and to some extent unexpectedly) by widespread looting and general lawlessness, with crowds of Iraqi civilians systematically stripping bare recently vacated government buildings as well as police stations, army barracks, schools and commercial premises – and more ominously, abandoned Iraqi Army arms depots and ammunition dumps. The post-conflict political disintegration and violence were not completely unexpected, although they were unplanned for, with clear warnings by the Defence Intelligence Staff, for instance, being ignored, as the Chilcot Report subsequently made clear.[75] Public utilities everywhere simply ground to a halt, with power and water supplies across Basra stopping altogether. Fortunately, British units had taken over the power station and sewage works before they could be attacked, but their personnel were too

few in number to tackle the city-wide looting, and it would be a painfully long time before essential services to this city of a million people could be restored. The city's three major hospitals – the *Az Zubayr Hospital*, the *General Hospital* and the *Teaching Hospital* – remained open and fully functional due to British military protection.

Most of 7 Armoured Brigade's troops would be occupied for weeks to come in mobile patrols and guarding essential services while trying to control this lawlessness, with many military personnel being re-roled into *civil military co-operation* (CIMIC) to help get basic infrastructure, water supplies, health services and local administration back up and running. Not surprisingly, given the lack of clean running water and basic hygiene facilities, and the onset of the debilitating summer heat, serious outbreaks of viral infective gastro-enteritis (diarrhoea and vomiting) began taking a significant toll amongst the troops, with a major outbreak even hitting the main divisional medical facility, *34 Field Hospital*.[76]

Immediately following the end of combat operations (and further highlighting the lack of planning for establishing security in the post-invasion phase), the MOD started to dramatically reduce the 46,000 strong British Force, bringing back *3 Commando Brigade* and *16 Air Assault Brigade* within weeks, leaving *7 Armoured Brigade* to look after southern Iraq. The MOD secured approval from the Treasury to fund the deployment of around 8000 troops to Iraq for a year, in the hope that other countries could be persuaded to send troops to bolster the residual British presence.

Such politically constrained low troop levels (only a small proportion of which translates to 'boots on the ground' in the form of patrolling soldiers) took no account of the actual number of troops really required to ensure a secure post-conflict environment and to meet the obligations of an occupying force under international law. James Quinlivan had calculated exactly these requirements for the influential RAND organisation and had concluded that at least 20 security personnel (soldiers and police combined) per 1000 civilians are required for success in a counterinsurgency environment – which was the ratio that Britain had deployed (troops and police) for the Malayan Emergency in 1952 as well as in Northern

Ireland during the *Troubles*.[77] This ratio would translate to approximately 20,000 troops for Basra City's million-plus population alone, where there was no co-operation by the police. A tranquil environment would have required a tenth of that, still 2000 personnel. It is not surprising that the relatively few British troops left in Basra and elsewhere in Iraq were overwhelmed by the task facing them. The British could never deploy more than a battle group (approximately 500 men) on the streets of Basra at any time. Clausewitz's dictum, quoted at the head of this chapter, applies just as much to the post-conflict phase as to combat operations.

SNATCHING DEFEAT FROM THE JAWS OF VICTORY

The decisive moment came in May 2003, when Paul Bremer, the newly arrived head of the temporary US-led *Coalition Provisional Authority* in Baghdad, issued two highly contentious decrees (*Coalition Provincial Authority Orders 1 and 2*) that would profoundly impact subsequent events in Iraq. On 15 May, he launched a de-Ba'athification policy banning former Ba'ath Party members from public sector employment (ignoring the political reality that every person so employed, including doctors, teachers and civil servants, had been compelled to enrol in the Ba'athist party). Nearly 80,000 people were immediately affected, and chaos ensued as hospitals and schools closed down. The security problem was gravely compounded a week later, on 23 May, when Bremer dissolved the Iraqi Armed Forces (comprising some 385,000 personnel who were sent home unpaid but retaining their weapons) and the Ministry of the Interior (which included the police and other security forces: over 280,000 personnel).[78] This date was the day 'that we snatched defeat from the jaws of victory and created an insurgency' as the decrees made Iraq ungovernable.[79] Bremer also insisted, upon holding elections before handing over power to the Iraqis, a process that would delay the setting up of a new Iraqi government for almost two years, until 2005, over-ruling Jeremy Greenstock's vigorous insistence on a much more rapid transfer of power to the Iraqis in order to give them an early sense of ownership of their liberated country. Bremer's decrees triggered a paradigm shift in public perceptions, as Iraqis now began to look upon Coalition forces no longer as welcome liberators but as occupiers, as well as providing the militias with many thousands of now unemployed but well-armed, experienced and disgruntled recruits to their ranks. Violence soon erupted in Baghdad and the north as the newly freed Shias settled scores with the minority Sunnis, with the Kurds attempting to break away in the north, and the United States, in trying to quell the inter-ethnic violence, only succeeding in uniting the people against the 'invader'.

This paradigm shift in perceptions, as well as the start of the insurgency in the south, was heralded by the tragic events on 24 June 2003, when six members of the *Royal Military Police* (RMP) who were training local police were killed in a riot in Majar al-Kabir in Maysan Province. This followed a search operation elsewhere in the town by members of the *Parachute Regiment*, in an operation interpreted as deeply provocative by the locals. Neither the RMPs nor the Paras knew the other was in town, so the RMP soldiers were left unsupported, in a failure of command and control, and of communications.[80]

Operation Telic 2 (HQ 3rd [UK] Mechanised Division and 19 Mechanised Brigade, July to October 2003)

MULTI-NATIONAL DIVISION (SOUTH-EAST)

The *Headquarters of 3rd (UK) Mechanised Division* took over from its predecessor on 11 July, and in line with plans to internationalise the allied security forces and allow British troops to draw down in numbers, it was renamed *Headquarters Multi-National Division (South-East) – HQ MND(SE)* the next day, taking on responsibility for the four south-eastern provinces of Iraq (Muthanna, Dhi Qar, Maysan and Basrah; Figure 1.7). The first allied contribution was a Danish battle group. The Division's composition would remain predominantly British for the whole of *Operation Telic*, although it would eventually incorporate troops from Australia, the Czech Republic, Denmark, Italy, Japan, Lithuania, New Zealand, Norway, Portugal and Romania at various times. HQ MND(SE) was led by Major General Graeme Lamb as General Officer Commanding MND(SE),

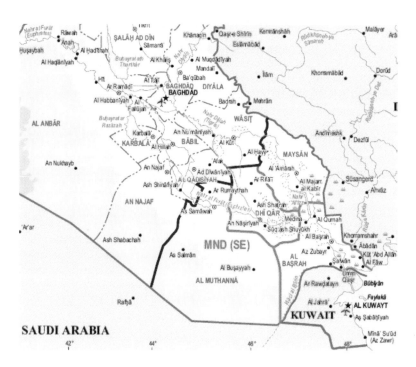

Figure 1.7 MND (SE) and its area of responsibility – Muthanna, Dhi Qar, Maysan and Basrah Provinces.

from July to December 2003.[81] He reported to the US General in charge of CJTF-7, Lieutenant General Sanchez (whose focus would remain on Baghdad), as well as to Lieutenant General John Reith at *Permanent Joint Headquarters* (PJHQ), the UK's strategic HQ overseeing overseas operations.

7 Armoured Brigade in Basra City handed over to 19 Brigade, commanded by Brigadier Bill Moore. The new Brigade, reinforced to six battalion-sized battle groups, was the mainstay of the Division, covering both Basrah and Maysan Provinces. Four of the six battle groups acted as Framework battle groups (also known as Ground Holding battle groups) responsible for distinct areas of operations and were supported by two reconnaissance squadrons of the *Light Dragoons* and a Challenger 2 main battle tank squadron.

The now-9,500 strong British contingent commenced moves to further reduce in number by September 2003, with two of the six battle groups being short-toured, and 19 Brigade headquarters moving out from Basra Palace to Basra International Airport, as a preliminary to merging divisional and brigade headquarters.

However, no sooner had 19 Brigade arrived in theatre than the tempo of operations picked up

considerably, with the security situation deteriorating rapidly as civilians became disenchanted with the slow pace of reconstruction and the lack of electricity and water supplies, especially in the searing summer heat. The rest of the summer saw multiple incidents ranging from intense fire fights to large-scale riots. The newly arrived troops wilted in the heat, with many being admitted to hospital with heat exhaustion. At least two of the 179 British deaths on *Operation Telic* were related to heat stroke. Future troop rotations would occur in April and November specifically to avoid the problem with acclimatisation.

BAHA MOUSA INCIDENT

The defining event of *Operation Telic 2* was the death of Baha Mousa, a local hotel receptionist, while in British custody. On 15 September 2003, soldiers from the *Queen's Lancashire Regiment* (QLR) detained Baha Mousa and nine other civilians and took them to their base for interrogation. For 48 hours, the handcuffed Iraqis were hooded with sandbags, forced into painful stress positions and 'kicked and punched with sustained cruelty'.[82] Baha Mousa died of his injuries, and two others were hospitalised at BMH Shaibah. Baha Mousa's death set in train court martial proceedings against seven soldiers of the QLR, although the result was controversial, with only one soldier being found guilty and imprisoned.

The subsequent Gage Inquiry (2011) into Baha Mousa's death and the torture of the detainees noted that the British Army had been banned since 1972 from using five techniques (hooding, white noise, sleep deprivation, food deprivation and painful stress positions) on prisoners. Unfortunately, the lack of a system for sustaining organisational knowledge within the MOD resulted in such knowledge being lost, with 'no written policy or doctrine banning the practices' at the time of the Iraq War,[83] although this has now been rectified. In separate proceedings, the General Medical Council decided in December 2012 that the QLR's regimental medical officer had failed in his duty of care towards Baha Mousa and the other detainees and removed his name from the Medical Register.[84]

Following the Gage Inquiry, the Army systematically improved its approach to sustaining and retrieving organisational memory through its Historical Branch in Whitehall.[85] The data it gathered, for instance, helped the Al-Sweady Public Inquiry in 2014 dismiss malicious allegations by Phil Shiner's now-discredited Public Interest Lawyers that UK soldiers had mistreated other Iraqis in 2004 during *Operations Telic 3* and *4*.[86] Phil Shiner was 'struck off' the Solicitors' Register on the grounds of professional misconduct in February 2017. It was Phil Shiner who had reported the QLR's Regimental Medical Officer to the General Medical Council.[87]

Telic 3 (20 Armoured Brigade, November 2003 to April 2004)

20 Armoured Brigade took over responsibility for the Iraqi provinces of Basrah and Maysan from 6 November 2003 to 24 April 2004. The Brigade's first two months on *Operation Telic 3* were dominated by low-level counterterrorist battles against fanatical Fedayeen and foreign fighters infiltrating across the long and porous border with Iran and actively supported by Iranian Al Quds forces. Although post-operational reports also mention former Ba'athist Regime loyalists in this context,[88]

the latter generally had enough to contend with without choosing to fight the British. Almost unrecognised at this stage by the British in Basra, although again foretold by the Defence Intelligence Staff, the various Shi'a militias were terrorising and kidnapping local civilians and committing widespread reprisal killings. These Shi'a death gangs were commencing a wholesale programme of ethnic cleansing that would characterise the next two years, torturing and killing Basrawis not of their own persuasion (especially Sunnis, Christians, former Regime loyalists, academics and westernised Iraqis) and setting the conditions for a fundamentalist Shi'a-dominated south.[89]

A UN Security Council Resolution, UNSCR 1511, signed just before the start of *20 Armoured Brigade's* tour, had set the basis for rebuilding Iraq and establishing security.[90] The aim was eventually to transfer authority from the *Coalition Provisional Authority* to an *Iraqi Transitional National Assembly*. The middle two months of *20 Armoured Brigade's* tour were dominated by security sector reform in order to achieve this aim: the building of capacity in the Iraqi Security Forces (especially the paramilitary *Iraqi Civil Defence Corps* and police) and civilian Iraqi institutions. Security sector reform would remain an objective, although sometimes only an aspiration, for the rest of *Operation Telic*.

WORSENING SECURITY SITUATION

Every British battle group from now on became heavily involved in running training programmes for Iraqi personnel, with police recruits being equipped and trained by British forces. However, in the haste to build up the Iraqi Police Service and reverse the disastrous results of Bremer's de-Ba'athification policy, British commanders inadvertently compounded the problem by prioritising quantity over quality. A decision to co-opt large numbers of militia members into the fledgling police force in a bid to win them over and give them a stake in the new government security structure would backfire seriously, as criminal elements purposely infiltrated the police.

The result was that law and order was effectively handed over to the militias, with many of the most serious crimes and murders being committed by rogue police over the next two years.

The worst of the rogue police teams was the ironically named *Serious Crimes Unit*, based in the Jamiat police station in Basra, members of which became more involved in committing serious crimes than investigating them. The *Serious Crime Unit's* death gangs were not just a threat to Basrawis – they were often suspected of colluding in attacks against British troops, and in September 2005, during *Operation Telic 6*, they kidnapped two undercover members of the Special Air Service (see page 17).

The final two months of *Operation Telic 3* were dominated by high-intensity operations against resurgent Shia Militias (notably the *Jaish al-Mahdi* [JAM]) inflamed by events in Baghdad and Fallujah (see below).

MUQTADA AL SADR AND THE *JAM* MILITIA (MAHDI ARMY)

Muqtada al Sadr was an influential and fanatical 29-year-old Shia cleric based in the northern Holy City of Najaf. His father had been murdered by Saddam's military police and he had been under house arrest for most of the 1990s, giving him immense credibility with the Shia underclass.[91] Once Saddam's regime fell, Sadr quickly built up a network of supporters in the Shi'ite city slums of Baghdad and across southern Iraq, particularly in Maysan province, vying for political control of local councils and security institutions, as well as setting up his own militia. This was known as the Mahdi Army or *Jaish al-Mahdi* (JAM), dressed in distinctive black pyjama uniforms. The first JAM units in Basra were established in October 2003, soon beginning low-level attacks against British troops and intimidating civilians working for the occupation forces. The fractious and notoriously unruly Maysan province, where the local population believed they had liberated themselves from Saddam and viewed the British troops as illegitimate occupiers, soon became the epicentre for this unrest. This was compounded by a very weak British presence, with only one battle group of 1000 troops from the *Light Infantry* and *Royal Regiment of Wales* trying to control an area the size of Northern Ireland, without even the backing of a local police force – for comparison, Saddam had to garrison Maysan province with a whole Iraqi Army Corps to keep control.[92] Maysan's capital was Al Amarah, straddling the River Tigris

and strategically located on the main highway (Route 6) between Basra and Baghdad. It was also relatively close to the Iranian border, so it was the first stop for insurgents infiltrating from Iran.

TURNING POINT – FIRST SADR UPRISING

The situation spiralled out of control very rapidly at the beginning of April 2004 following a controversial order by Bremer in Baghdad on 28 March to close down a Sadr-controlled newspaper that he accused of fomenting the growing insurgency against US troops. The lynching of four US contractors in Fallujah three days later led to US Marines storming Fallujah and causing heavy civilian casualties amongst both Sunnis and Shias, with Sadr's top lieutenant being arrested. Within 24 hours, Baghdad's Sadr City and southern Iraq were ablaze as Iraq's Sunni and Shia communities united in outrage against the occupiers, in the 'First Sadr Uprising'.

The sudden escalation of attacks in early April by the JAM in Basra was later described by Major General Graeme Lamb to the Iraq Inquiry as 'like a switch had been flicked'.[93] The troops could no longer safely patrol in the lightly armoured Snatch Land Rovers with dismounted troops wearing berets.

In the south, the strategically located city of Al Amarah (the scene of a fierce battle against the British in June 1915) was the first to be engulfed in riots with the *Light Infantry Battlegroup* coming under heavy and sustained mortar, rocket and small-arms attack. In Basra, the fledgling Iraqi government's council building fell to JAM fighters. Incensed by Al-Jazeera television reports, Bremer demanded that General Sanchez order the British Army to storm the building, but Major General Stewart, in command of MND(SE), refused to risk turning Basra into another Fallujah without an attempt at negotiation. Fortunately, Brigadier Nick Carter managed to persuade the Sadr fighters to hand the building back peacefully to the Iraqi authorities, but General Stewart's refusal to follow Bremer's directive, coupled with serious political concerns in the United Kingdom about intended US actions in Fallujah, caused a major rift in US–UK relations.[94]

ABU GHRAIB SCANDAL

The JAM and other militias, and indeed the Iraqi population in general, were further incensed by the publication of photographs in April 2004 showing US soldiers torturing Iraqi prisoners at Abu Ghraib. The Abu Ghraib scandal caused support in the United Kingdom for British participation in the occupation to drop to a new low, at the same time as the volatility and high intensity of violence necessitated a return to a war-fighting posture by *20 Armoured Brigade*.[95] Heavy attacks on British forces continued throughout April, a new feature being the use of multiple co-ordinated suicide car bomb attacks ('vehicle-borne improvised explosive devices' [*IEDs*]) from 21 April, believed to be Iraqi Sunni in origin, targeting Iraqi police stations and co-located British bases and checkpoints. The drastically worsening security situation in April, exacerbated by the response to the Abu Ghraib scandal, led many of the Iraq Inquiry's witnesses to conclude that the spring of 2004 was the turning point of the campaign.[96]

Operation Telic 4 (1 Mechanised Brigade, May to October 2004)

Faced with continued heavy fighting throughout southern Iraq, the incoming *1 Mechanised Brigade* had to take over bases and responsibilities under fire. Although troop numbers were relatively unchanged, the Brigade effectively doubled the number of armoured infantry companies, replacing the vulnerable Snatch Land Rovers with Warriors, and an infantry battalion by an armoured infantry battalion, as well as deploying Challenger 2 battle tanks from their depot at Shaibah Logistics Base. The Brigade's tour would be highly kinetic.

The *1st Battalion, Princess of Wales's Royal Regiment* (1 PWRR), who took over responsibility for Maysan Province on 18 April, saw intense fighting immediately and almost every day for six months.[97] The two main periods of activity were in April and May during the First Sadr Uprising, and from 2 to 26 August during a second uprising. During this tour, the battalion's main operations were given codenames from the London Underground map, starting with *Operation Pimlico* on 1 May, *Operation Knightsbridge* on 3 May and Operation *Waterloo* on 8 May (undertaken to reassert control over Al Amarah) (Figure 1.8).[98]

The *Battle for Danny Boy* (named after a permanent vehicle checkpoint 6 km south of Al

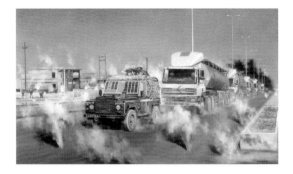

Figure 1.8 'Fighting logistics through' (water convoy under attack in Basra, 8 May 2004). (Courtesy of David Rowlands, Military Artist.)

Amarah, itself named after an Irish traditional tune) occurred on 14 May, when a patrol from the *Argyll & Sutherland Highlanders* was ambushed there by over 200 heavily armed insurgents and had to be rescued by a Warrior group.[99] Over 70 insurgents were killed during the fighting, and several were captured. The bodies of some 20 of the dead were taken back to the nearby British base in Abu Naji for identification purposes. The bodies were returned to senior local officials and relatives the next day, by which time malicious rumours were circulating amongst the Iraqis that the dead had been captured alive and then executed (as had often happened at Abu Naji under Saddam's regime). The bodies were later videotaped at the local hospital morgue and a CD was then circulated in the souks, with uncorroborated accusations of torture and mutilation appearing in the local and international press (already inflamed by revelations of torture at Abu Ghraib). This media backlash against troops who had observed their rules of engagement and responded to a murderous ambush '*with exemplary courage, resolution and professionalism*' was deeply wounding[100] yet taught the British valuable lessons about the management of dead insurgents, whose bodies would subsequently be carefully photographed and left at the scene. The troops involved would eventually be completely exonerated by the Al-Sweady Inquiry in 2014, which '*established beyond doubt that all the most serious allegations, made against the British soldiers involved in the Battle of Danny Boy and its aftermath...have been found to be wholly without foundation and entirely the product of deliberate lies, reckless speculation and ingrained hostility*'.[101]

PRIVATE JOHNSON BEHARRY

During *Operation Telic 4*, the besieged CIMIC House in Al Amarah could only be resupplied by heavily escorted convoys (under *Operation Whitechapel*). Following one of these, Private Johnson Beharry from 1 PWRR was awarded the Victoria Cross for driving his damaged Warrior out of an ambush and saving his comrades' lives and repeating this a month later, on 12 June 2004, despite sustaining life-threatening head injuries from an RPG explosion. The seriously injured Private Beharry was evacuated by IRT Chinook to a civilian hospital in Kuwait for computed tomography scans and initial surgery, before being transferred to the Queen Elizabeth Neuroscience Centre at the University Hospital in Birmingham for definitive surgery and rehabilitation (Figure 1.9).[102]

Following the *Second Sadr Uprising* (2–26 August), the violence in Iraq suddenly subsided, after the Mahdi Army miscalculated and was defeated in a pitched battle against US and Iraqi coalition forces in Najaf. The Shia spiritual leader, Grand Ayatollah Ali al-Sistani, called for a truce, which was agreed, and as a result, relative peace returned for a while.

In the north, the United States had commenced planning for an offensive by 10,000 troops against a pocket of 3000 fanatical Sunni insurgents holding the town of Fallujah. Unless the insurgency there could be quelled, it would threaten the Iraqi elections

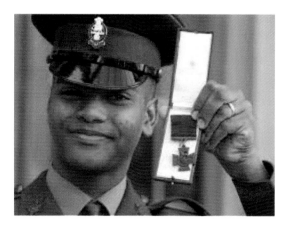

Figure 1.9 Private Johnson Beharry VC, PWRR.

scheduled for 30 January 2005 in accordance with the newly ratified UNSCR 1546.[103] General Casey called for British help, and it was decided that the *Black Watch* (the theatre reinforcement battle group) would defer their roulement home (scheduled for October) and move north in order to join the cordon south of Fallujah, thereby releasing US troops for the planned assault (named *Operation Phantom Fury* by the United States) in the second week of November.

Operation Telic 5 (4 Armoured Brigade, November 2004 to April 2005)

OPERATION BRACKEN

The *Black Watch* mission to Fallujah, codenamed *Operation Bracken*, commenced on 28 October. An advance party flew to Baghdad and a major road convoy left *Shaibah Logistic Base* for the move to *Camp Dogwood*, on the banks of the Euphrates, in the midst of a hostile Sunni population, prior to taking over their area of operation. They faced multiple IEDs and rocket attacks, and on 4 November, the first British fatalities, and the first to suicide bombing in Iraq, were sustained when a suicide bomber killed three *Black Watch* soldiers and an interpreter at a checkpoint, also injuring eight others, and prompting intense political debate back in the United Kingdom.

During their month-long operation, the *Black Watch* effectively blocked and seriously disrupted insurgent activity, culminating in *Operation Tobruk* on 25 November, a battle group-sized mission involving 650 troops in 116 tracked vehicles in the final operation conducted by the *Black Watch* before its impending amalgamation. This all came at a cost – during *Operation Bracken*, the battle group endured three suicide attacks, 25 large IED explosions and daily indirect fire (IDF), a total of 120 serious incidents. In all, five *Black Watch* soldiers and one interpreter were killed and 17 wounded. Four Warriors and one Scimitar light tank were irreparably damaged and two helicopters were damaged by ground fire. The *Black Watch* returned to Scotland in mid-December, in time to hear the defence secretary announce plans to disband one Scottish battalion and amalgamate the other five into a new 'super regiment'.[104]

MND(SE)

The UK Brigade within MND(SE) on *Operation Telic 5*, *4 Armoured Brigade* (normally based in Germany and distinguished by the 'Black Rat' [Jerboa] emblem) took over responsibility for Basrah and Maysan Provinces from 1 November 2004 to 1 May 2005.[105] It arrived in Iraq after the peak of the fighting during the *Second Sadr Uprising* and never faced the levels of violence experienced during *Operation Telic 4*. Nonetheless, the frequency of serious incidents highlighted the potential for a return to major conflict at any time. The unifying purpose behind the Brigade's activities was to realise the political process defined in UNSCR 1546, which had set the scene for democratic elections on 30 January 2005. The first half of the Brigade's tour was therefore dominated by the preparations necessary to ensure the success of these elections. Thereafter, the Brigade's main activities focussed on security sector reform (training and mentoring Iraqi Security Forces) and operating with the Iraqi Security Forces in COIN missions (Joint Security Operations), together with aiding reconstruction.[106]

The January 2005 election, while a success for the democratic process, resulted in the election of politicians and parties implacably opposed to the continued British presence in Iraq, setting in motion events leading to British withdrawals from Maysan and then Basra that would look like retreats under fire.[107] The new governor in Maysan was Adel al Maliki, a former JAM militia commander, and the new Basra governor was Mohammed al-Waili, a leading member of the Fadhilla party, the mouthpiece for Sadr's movement.

Operation Telic 6 (12 Mechanised Brigade, May to October 2005)

Basra had been relatively quiet after the collapse of the *Second Sadr Uprising* in August 2004 and the elections in January 2005. That changed in summer 2005 when the Iranians decided to escalate the conflict by using their militia proxies (both the JAM and more extremist militias, whom the British dubbed 'Special Groups') to attack the British and force their withdrawal from Iraq. The Al-Quds Force of the *Iranian Revolutionary*

Guard provided training in Iran for sniper and rocket teams and began equipping the militias with large numbers of *explosively formed projectile* (EFP) IEDs, which would prove deadly when used against British vehicles. The first confirmed use of Iranian-provided EFP-equipped IEDs was on 29 May, when Lance Corporal Alan Brackenbury of the *King's Royal Hussars* was killed in an IED attack on a Land Rover patrol in Maysan Province.[108] Three more soldiers were killed on patrol in Al Amarah on 16 July, in the first Snatch Land Rover to be penetrated by this new weapon, necessitating all patrols thereafter to be undertaken in Warriors.[109]

JAMIAT INCIDENT

The fragility of the UK's control over Basra in the face of the Iranian-backed militia offensive became evident on 19–20 September 2005 when British troops had to storm the Jamiat Police Station to rescue two British undercover members of the *Special Air Service* who had been kidnapped and held captive by rogue policemen of the *Serious Crimes Unit*. This rescue operation sparked off a major confrontation with rioters and gunmen, during which a *Staffordshire Regiment's* Warrior was firebombed and set alight.[110] The images of the escaping crew made worldwide headlines (Figure 1.10). Fortunately, all five crew members survived, with only one sustaining serious burns, and he made a remarkable recovery.[111]

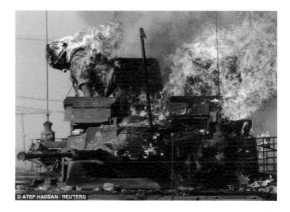

Figure 1.10 Sergeant George Long escaping from burning Warrior, 19 September 2005 – an iconic image from the Iraq campaign.

Operation Telic 7 (7 Armoured Brigade, November 2005 to April 2006)

7 Armoured Brigade arrived in Iraq just weeks after the 'Jamiat incident'. Trust had been eroded, relations with Iraqi civilians and institutions were very strained and practically no security sector reform was taking place in the three provinces of Basra, Maysan and Al Muthanna that came within its remit. Reviving security sector reform and preparations to hand over control of Maysan and Al Muthanna to Provincial Iraqi Control became the focus of initial Brigade activities.

The situation in southern Iraq deteriorated significantly following the terrorist bombing on 22 February 2006 of the Golden Mosque in Samarra (one of the holiest Shi'ite Moslem shrines, 65 km north of Baghdad) in a calculated attempt to ignite a major Sunni-Shi'ite civil war. This was compounded by the escalating anti-Western reaction to the September 2005 publication of the 'Danish cartoons' and revelations in February 2006 in the News of The World of a video showing British soldiers beating Iraqis in Al Amarah in 2003.

Shi'ite militants, particularly in the *Jaish al Mahdi*, openly supported by Iranian al-Quds fighters, increased their activities throughout Iraq, especially in Baghdad and Basra, where they were steadily penetrating the police forces, leading to a surge in sectarian killings. The Jamiat police station in Basra became a de facto JAM interrogation and torture centre, under the control of the thuggish police officer Captain Jaffah.

The Multinational Forces were now facing a determined and increasingly sophisticated IED and IDF campaign, which significantly curtailed conventional operations, although the IED campaign was matched by equally determined counter-IED operations. Captain Kevin Ivison, the ammunition technical officer supporting the *Royal Scots Dragoon Guards* in Al Amarah, would be awarded the George Medal for defusing a secondary device on 28 February 2006 while under sniper fire in the open, although his experiences left him suffering from post-traumatic stress disorder.[112] In April, a co-ordinated rocket attack against Basra Palace during the Queen's Birthday Party organised by the *Foreign and Commonwealth Office* (FCO) led to a withdrawal of FCO and Department for International Development staff. IDF attacks against Multinational Forces had now reached their highest level since March 2003.[113]

Operation Telic 8 (20 Armoured Brigade, May to October 2006)

PRIVATE MICHELLE NORRIS

On 11 June 2006, 19-year-old Private Michelle Norris RAMC, combat medical technician, was attached to C Company 1 PWRR, in Al Amarah. Whilst engaged in a night-time search operation, the Company became embroiled in a heavy fire fight with over 200 insurgents. The warrior that Private Norris was in came under accurate fire and the vehicle commander, Colour Sergeant Page, was shot in the face and very seriously wounded. Private Morris dismounted and climbed onto the top of the vehicle to apply life-saving first aid, disregarding continued sniper fire aimed at her (Figure 1.11). The gunner then dragged her back into the vehicle turret to remove her from the line of fire, and the warrior returned to camp to evacuate the casualty. Private Norris was awarded the Military Cross for her actions, the first female ever to receive this award.[114]

Operation Sinbad

By 2006, the Iraqi police forces had become heavily infiltrated by members of the Iranian-backed

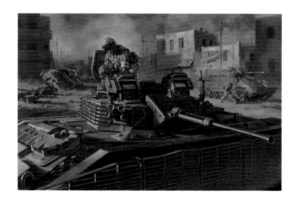

Figure 1.11 Private Michelle Norris MC. (Courtesy of Stuart Brown.)

JAM Army as well as by organised criminals, result-ing in the British effectively having ceded control of Basra to the militias. Major General Richard Shirreff, as the charismatic and energetic new commander of MND(SE) in 2006 July to December, arrived in the-atre determined on a plan, *Operation Salamanca*, to restore security and clean up the police, coupled with intensive reconstruction efforts, aiming to take back Basra City, district by district. British troops would work alongside the Iraqi Army, thereby regaining the initiative and taking the offensive against the Iranian-backed militias. This would allow an acceptable political solution to emerge and also prevent a humiliating strategic defeat for the British. *Operation Salamanca* was rejected by the Iraqi authorities so it was revised as the less ambi-tious *Operation Sinbad*. Coalition commanders in Baghdad supported Sherriff with corps assets (such as surveillance drones) and funds for reconstruc-tion, although an offer to detach a US battalion to Basra was rejected in London.

WITHDRAWAL FROM CAMP ABU NAJI

A pre-requisite for Major General Shirreff's plans was the withdrawal of troops from Camp Abu Naji outside Al-Amarah (where they were under inces-sant heavy indirect fire and regularly sustaining multiple casualties) in order to free them up for *Operation Sinbad*. Shirreff also wanted to avoid the situation that had arisen after the *Queen's Dragoon Guards* had handed over Muthanna Province in July – their base had been looted by civilians four days later. Unfortunately, the withdrawal from Abu Naji did not go smoothly. Intense fighting in the final days also resulted in a Challenger 2 main battle tank being penetrated by an RPG equipped with a tandem charge, this being the first recorded incident of a Challenger 2 being penetrated in this way, and raising the spectre that the militia might now be able to defeat every type of British vehicle. On 24 August, British troops evacuated Camp Abu Naji, leaving it in the hands of Iraqi troops; a few hours later, the guards opened the gates to hundreds of rioters, resulting in the base being looted – this activity being filmed and broadcast live on Arab television channels.[115]

Shirreff launched *Operation Sinbad* between 20 September 2006 and 14 January 2007, in which 1000 British and 2300 Iraqi troops raided Basra police stations in sequence and arrested suspected insurgents and gangsters.[116] The militias responded by using rockets and multiple IEDs, with the UK base at Basra Palace becoming the most rocketed location in the whole of Iraq as the British simply did not have enough assets to suppress all possible firing points. The British troops outfought the Shia militias in many pitched battles as the campaign progressed, leading one local newspaper to describe the British as the 'Lions of Basra'.[117] However, ini-tial successes could not be consolidated due to lack of sufficient resources from London, together with constraints imposed by Iraqi Prime Minister Maliki (who was then reliant on JAM support to keep his weak coalition government in power).[118] The lack of sufficiently trained local Iraqi battal-ions allowed the militias to regroup.

Operation Telic 8 coincided with the deploy-ment of British troops into Helmand Province and the shift of focus of British political and military effort from the ignominious situation in Iraq to Afghanistan.

Operation Telic 9 (19 Light Brigade, November 2006 to April 2007)

The first three months of *Operation Telic 9* were occupied with the ongoing *Operation Sinbad*, although political and military attention in the United Kingdom was distracted by the escalating violence in Helmand, where a full-blown war was now underway. There was one visible outcome from *Operation Sinbad* of great symbolic value – Shirreff was finally given permission to blow up the notorious Jamiat Police Station, which the Royal Engineers did in spectacular fashion on Christmas morning, after British troops released 127 captives, many of whom showed signs of tor-ture and had been expecting to be executed.[119] However, the *Serious Crimes Unit* became fully functional again within months.[120] Basra would remain in the hands of the JAM and its death squads, with Iraqi security forces unable to impose, let alone maintain, the rule of law. This contributed to the conditions that would lead Shirreff's successor into negotiations with JAM during *Operation Telic 9*.[121]

In December 2006, PJHQ in London issued the formal order to begin withdrawing UK troops from Basra city (*Operation Zenith*). On the day that *Operation Sinbad* officially ended, 18 February 2007, Prime Minister Tony Blair announced that 3000 of the 7000 British troops then in Iraq would be withdrawn over the coming months in order to bolster operations in Afghanistan. To quote Ledwidge: '*If any moment can be described as the moment of defeat, this was it*'.[122]

This was in sharp contrast to the political will in America, where, on 23 January 2007, President Bush had announced that an extra five brigades (about 20,000 men) would be deployed to central and northern Iraq in a surge designed to stabilise the country, where the charismatic General David Petraeus had just taken over as *Commander Multi-National Forces Iraq*. Petraeus had a catalytic role in transforming the US Army's approach to COIN and turning their campaign around from slow failure by attrition into manoeuvrist success.[123-124] As Lieutenant General Robin Fry put it, '*The Americans decided they were going to win; the British decided they were going to leave*'.[125]

The political decision to withdraw British troops, and the end of the hamstrung *Operation Sinbad*, coincided with the arrival of Major General Jonathan Shaw (in January 2007) as the new commander of MND(SE). His approach was the opposite of Shirreff's: rather than aiming to achieve security as the essential prerequisite for a political solution, he proposed that security could be achieved only after a political solution had been reached by the Iraqis themselves, and he therefore sought to hand over responsibility as much as possible to the Iraqi security forces. As a first step, he initiated plans to redeploy British troops from their bases in Basra (such as Basra Palace, where they were under daily rocket and mortar attack and resupply was extremely hazardous) to the more easily defensible airport 10 miles away, under *Operation Zenith*. Recognising the reality on the ground of JAM's control over Basra, and assessing that a continued weak British military presence in Basra was counter-productive (attracting over 90% of attacks on security forces), General Shaw negotiated a deal with JAM's Basra commander, Ahmed al-Fartusi, then held captive by the British. Al-Fartusi agreed to renounce violence and allow British troops to withdraw unmolested, in return for a release of JAM prisoners, the last one being al-Fartusi himself. This withdrawal would happen once the British deemed that the local Iraqi *14th Army Division* was sufficiently trained to take over the bases – even though the Iraqi government would still not be strong enough to take over effective control of the city until well into 2008.

Telic 10 (1 Mechanised Brigade, May to October 2007)

Following a temporary ceasefire in July, during which al-Fartusi demonstrated his control over JAM by halting all attacks on coalition forces for three days, the final stage of *Operation Zenith* and the withdrawal from Basra went ahead on 4 September 2007, when the *4th Battalion, The Rifles*, handed over Basra Palace to the Iraqi Army and drove unmolested to Basra Air Station, their route cynically safeguarded by JAM militiamen. The next three months passed peacefully, at least for the British, whose casualty figures dropped significantly (Figure 1.12),[126] but the weakness of the Iraqi Army meant that JAM-led intimidation and terrorisation of the civilian population became rife. As Fairweather said in his book *War of Choice*, the '[British] Faustian bargain undermined the very institutions that the British had gone to Iraq to create…the city was nothing like the peaceful oasis British Defence chiefs were trying to portray to the media*'.[127]

Operation Telic 11 (4 Mechanised Brigade, November 2007 to May 2008)

Al-Fartusi was released on 31 December 2007, and the last JAM prisoners were released on 2 January 2008. Unsurprisingly, the JAM reneged on their deal. On 6 January, the airport base was subjected to the heaviest rocket assault of the war so far, and by 31 January, rocket and mortar attacks on the British were relentless and at their 'pre-accommodation' level.[128] In February, two convoys, cleared in advance by the British with the JAM, were attacked, a charity worker was killed, and journalist Richard Butler was kidnapped by

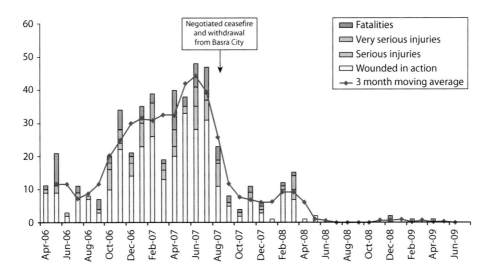

Figure 1.12 British Combat Casualties in Iraq, 2006–2009. (From Casualty Monitor. British Casualties: Iraq. http://www.casualty-monitor.org/p/iraq.html.)

the *Serious Crimes Unit* – he would only be released in April, during the Iraqi-led *Operation Charge of the Knights*.

OPERATION CHARGE OF THE KNIGHTS

For Iraqi Prime Minister Maliki in Baghdad, the continued control by JAM of Iraq's second largest city and its revenues from oil and shipping was an existential threat to his government, not least because the ongoing civil war in Baghdad was being fuelled and financed by the Shi'ite militias in Basra. With his army now reasonably strong and his political position more assured, and with trust in the British having been eroded by their withdrawal from Basra, Maliki planned his own solution. He ordered two additional Iraqi infantry battalions to Basra, then flew to Basra on 24 March and gave his orders to Lieutenant General Mohan, heading the Iraqi 14th Division, who used a plan to retake Basra that had been devised with British Colonels Andrew Bristow and his successor Richard Iron.[129]

The Iraqi Army began operations against the Mahdi Army almost immediately, on 25 March 2008: *Operation Charge of the Knights*, the defining battle for Basra, had begun, using a British-authored plan, but initially not with sufficient resources and without prior consultation with US or UK forces. JAM counterattacked in strength on 27 March

with some 28 simultaneous dawn attacks against army posts across the city, and the newly formed *Iraqi 3rd Brigade* effectively collapsed. Faced with the prospect of defeat, the Iraqi Army redeployed its theatre reserve, the *1st Iraqi Divisional HQ* and the highly experienced *1st Iraqi Brigade*, together with embedded US Marine Corps mentors and trainers, the so-called *Military Transition Teams* (MiTTs), to Basra. Simultaneously, the Coalition despatched its forward Corps HQ and supporting Corps assets, including armed Predator drones and attack helicopters, switching its main effort from Mosul to Basra, in a joint US–UK effort to support the Iraqis, with the British also providing drone surveillance and medical support. Thus enabled, the Iraqi Security Forces launched their decisive attack on 2 April, capturing all their objectives and dramatically regaining the initiative, such that Prime Minister Maliki could order a temporary ceasefire to give a chance for the militias to withdraw peacefully.

Impressed by the professionalism in the US-mentored and -trained *Iraqi 1st Division* compared to the UK-trained but not mentored *14th Division*, Lieutenant General Mohan asked the British to embed trainers within the 14th Division, and 'within 36 hours British forces were back all over Basra, fully embedded into the Iraqi Army' as platoon-sized MiTTs.[130] The offensive phase of

Charge of the Knights ended on 6 May with JAM having been cleared out of Basra by the Iraqi Security Forces, although further operations against JAM in the provinces would continue for several more months. Overall, the decisive victory over JAM was very much an Iraqi victory – and although the Coalition had intervened to help the Iraqis, the circumstances which prompted *Operation Charge of the Knights* still represented a strategic failure for the British in Iraq. As Sir John Chilcot later said, 'It was humiliating that the UK reached a position in which an agreement with a militia group which had been actively targeting UK forces was considered the best option available'.[131]

Operation Telic 12 (7 Armoured Brigade, May to November 2008)

The British military effort, during their remaining year in Basra, concentrated on providing embedded training and operational support to the Iraqi 14th Division in its attempts to provide security for the civilian population. By the end of *Operation Telic 12*, Brigadier Storrie was able to report that the 14th Division was almost fully trained, that the public mood in Basra, in the absence of militia intimidation, was 'upbeat and forward leaning' and that public consent was solid when the British were seen to be operating in support of the Iraqi Security Forces.[132] No UK fatalities occurred during *Operation Telic 12*, the first time during the whole *Telic* campaign.

Operation Telic 13 (20 Armoured Brigade, November 2008 to May 2009)

20 Armoured Brigade returned for its third tour of Iraq to carry out the phased drawdown of UK military capability under *Operation Brockdale* while carrying on with support to the Iraqis under *Operation Telic*. The Divisional Headquarters of MND (South East) and MND (Central) merged into MND (South) under the command of the *US 10th Mountain Division* on 31 March 2009 as US forces replaced the British across Basra Province. Simultaneously, the *Contingency Operating Base* at

Basra airport was formally handed over to the *10th Mountain Division*, with *20 Armoured Brigade* handing over authority to the *2nd Brigade Combat Team* of the US *4th Infantry Division (2/4 ID)* three weeks later, on 20 April.[133] A few British naval assets remained in training roles with the Iraqi navy at Umm Qasr for a little longer, but effectively, *Operation Telic* came to an end in May 2009. The Iraqi parliament did not renew the mandate in July 2009 for these British naval forces to remain in theatre.

The logistic effort involved in withdrawing UK troops and their equipment after six years in Iraq was a massive undertaking. The infrastructure was spread across southeast Iraq and included a bulk fuel installation, a reverse osmosis plant, an ammunition storage point, four purpose-built protective structures and 11 military camps on the *Contingency Operating Base* (COB); 18 outstations; a divisional headquarters; rotary and fixed wing handling and maintenance facilities; and a rendezvous processing point that dealt with hundreds of tons weekly. At the start of *Operation Telic 13*, there were almost 4000 iso-containers on the Contingency Operating Base (COB) alone, over 1000 vehicles and their equipment, 538 tonnes of ammunition and 368 grey and white fleet vehicles. It took six military vessels to remove this equipment capability from Iraq.[134] *Operation Brockdale* and the redeployment of all British troops and equipment via Kuwait would be complete by 31 October 2009.

OPERATIONS IN AFGHANISTAN

2001 Entry into Afghanistan

OPERATION VERITAS (UK)/OPERATION ENDURING FREEDOM (US)

Following 9/11, once the Taliban regime refused to surrender Osama bin Laden and his Al-Qaeda supporters, the United State launched Operation *Enduring Freedom*, supporting the Northern Alliance in their bid to topple the Taliban regime and hunt down Al-Qaeda. The United Kingdom contributed forces under *Operation Veritas*, initially deploying to Bagram airfield in northern Afghanistan before the fall of Kabul and the installation of Hamid Karzai's *Interim Afghan Administration*.

2002–2014 Establishing security

ISAF FOUR-STAGE PLAN

The UN established an ISAF to support Karzai's fragile government, aiming to prevent Afghanistan from again becoming a terrorist haven. The United Kingdom took on leadership of ISAF for its first six months (December 2001 to June 2002), committing its troops under *Operation Fingal*, while the United States shifted its focus to Iraq. NATO took on leadership of ISAF in August 2003, and in October 2003, the *UN Security Council* authorised the expansion of the NATO mission beyond Kabul. NATO and the UN developed a four-stage plan for the country. Under this plan, ISAF would initially provide security in the north, enabling deployment of *Provincial Reconstruction Teams* (PRTs) to develop local infrastructure, then expand security and PRTs to the west, later to the south and east, and eventually to transition all security to Afghan forces. ISAF gradually expanded its remit throughout Afghanistan by late 2006 as up to 51 NATO and partner nations contributed their troops and resources (Figure 1.13).[135]

OPERATION HERRICK PHASE BY PHASE

2003–2006 Return of the Taliban

The Taliban may have lost the opening stages of the war, but they had not accepted defeat, disappearing into the countryside and retreating into the Pashtun heartlands in the *Federally Administered Tribal Area* of northwest Pakistan to regroup. Time was on their side, as it had been on the side of their Mujahideen predecessors against the Soviets. By January 2003, they had begun to infiltrate back into Afghanistan, commencing an insurgency that would sorely challenge ISAF and the fledgling Afghan security forces over the years, as each side strove to achieve dominance throughout the country. Their maintenance of secure bases in the Pashtun heartlands, largely untouchable by either NATO or the Pakistani military, enabled the insurgency to grow steadily, posing a potentially fatal threat to Afghan security. Initially, the Taliban focussed on Kandahar Province, their spiritual home and geographically closest to their strongholds around Quetta in Pakistan, but the arrival of the British in Helmand in 2006 and their actions there generated opportunities for the Taliban, which they exploited – the British had effectively created and then vigorously stirred up a hornets' nest.[136]

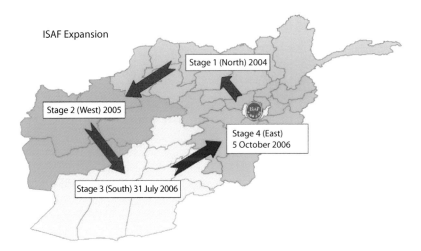

ISAF Expansion

Stage 1 (North) 2004

Stage 2 (West) 2005

Stage 4 (East) 5 October 2006

Stage 3 (South) 31 July 2006

Figure 1.13 ISAF Four-Stage Plan for Provision of Security in Afghanistan. (From NATO. ISAF Placemats. 12 January 2009. http://www.nato.int/isaf/placemats_archive/2009-01-12-ISAF-Placemat.pdf.)

2006 Entry into Helmand

The choice of troops for Britain's initial deployment is best described by Theo Farrell, Professor of War Studies at King's College London: 'This new campaign was a stretch for a small army which had 8,500 troops deployed in Iraq in 2005–2006. The British Army then stood at 101,000, with seven deployable brigades. In addition, the Royal Marines also had a deployable brigade: 3 Commando Brigade. The heavy and medium brigades were all committed to the Iraq campaign. Accordingly the Army's elite light brigade, 16 Air Assault Brigade, was selected to provide the first British task force for Helmand, with 3 Commando Brigade to follow in the second tour. However, the Ministry of Defence (MOD) decided to cap the UK task force at 3,150 troops; in other words, only a half brigade in strength. Its primary job was to protect the Provincial Reconstruction Team (PRT) and to create security in the key ground between and surrounding the provincial capital of Lashkar Gah and the main economic town of Gereshk'.[137]

The first two *Operation Herrick* tours ended up being primarily kinetic in nature, as the British fought to establish themselves in Helmand. The COIN doctrine had been neglected and its hard-learnt lessons had been forgotten by the British Army, no longer forming part of the UK's institutionalised approach.[138] The British Army would have to re-learn COIN the hard way in Afghanistan as they did in Iraq.

OPERATION HERRICK 4 (16 AIR ASSAULT BRIGADE, APRIL TO OCTOBER 2006)

With ISAF expanding its security remit southwards throughout Afghanistan (ISAF Stage 3), the United Kingdom committed its troops to Helmand Province in the southwest. Under the original 'Helmand Plan', outlined previously, the troops would concentrate on protecting the PRT and establish a 'security triangle' around the population centres of *Lashkar Gah* (the provincial capital) and *Gereshk* (the economic centre), enabling good governance and a development programme to be initiated, with the British mainly operating out of the specially constructed *Camp Bastion*.

Under-resourced from the outset due to political constraints, the UK's *3 Para Battle Group*, commanded by Brigadier Ed Butler, deployed in April 2006, only 3150 personnel strong, largely drawn from *16 Air Assault Brigade*. The battle group essentially consisted of a single light infantry battalion (*3rd Battalion, Parachute Regiment*, known as 3 Para, with attached platoons from the *Gurkhas* and *Royal Irish Regiment*, fewer than 600 fighting soldiers in all) with supporting light armour (*Household Cavalry Regiment* with its Combat Vehicle Reconnaissance [Tracked] and Scimitars) and a battery of artillery (*7th Parachute Regiment, Royal Horse Artillery* with 105 mm guns), together with helicopter air support (Apaches, Lynx and Royal Air Force [RAF] Chinooks), and combat service support, including medical assets. The British were ably supported from the start by two attached units of Danes and Estonians (whose vehicles were better suited to the terrain), two nations who would stand squarely beside the British throughout the Helmand campaign.[139]

The deployment was beset by trouble, compounded by the early enforced removal of the then governor of Helmand, Sher Mohammed Akhundzade, a notoriously corrupt warlord heavily involved in the opium trade; in retaliation, he reportedly told his disgruntled 3000-strong militia to join the Taliban against the British. Newly appointed Governor Daoud and President Karzai then put intense diplomatic pressure on Brigadier Butler to also support the government district centres in Musa Qala, Now Zad and Sangin. The result was the discarding of the 'Helmand Plan' and serious over-stretch as British platoons established themselves in the district centres from June onwards, dispersed and vulnerable across a 600 square mile area. The Helmand commitment never really recovered from this fateful decision.[140]

The British platoons inevitably became fixed in place with serious restriction of their freedom of manoeuvre. Their putative 'inkblot' COIN strategy withered on the vine as the Taliban massed to the attack, rapidly besieging the isolated defenders and engaging the platoon houses in prolonged and intense combat. Helicopter resupply and medevac became increasingly dangerous, and artillery, Apache gunships and Harrier jets had to be called in to break up the Taliban attacks, laying waste to the town centres and the very areas that the British had been called in to protect. Thirty-five British soldiers would lose their lives during *Operation Herrick 4*, in a total of 537 contacts ('Troops in Contact' [TICs]) with the Taliban, most of them being killed by small-arms fire, RPGs, and mortars.[141]

Nonetheless, despite the vulnerability of the platoon houses, the Taliban never succeeded in overrunning any outpost and suffered very heavy casualties in their attempts to do so. Their losses would soon force them to change their tactics; by the end of the next *Operation Herrick* roulement, they had switched to besieging the outposts by surrounding them with IEDs, thereby minimising their own losses while significantly increasing those suffered by the British.

OPERATION HERRICK 5 (3 COMMANDO BRIGADE, OCTOBER 2006 TO APRIL 2007)

Learning from the experience of their predecessors, *3 Commando Brigade*, primarily comprising *42* and *45 Commandos Royal Marines*, with elements from the *Royal Regiment of Fusiliers* and others, was reinforced from the outset, deploying with extra assets and manoeuvre capability, including combat Intelligence, surveillance, target aquisition and reconnaisance (ISTAR) assets, to increase situational awareness, and they benefitted in particular from their Viking armoured and tracked personnel carriers. They discarded the *platoon house* strategy in favour of mounting a series of large-scale offensive operations, to seize back the initiative from the Taliban, largely through use of *Mobile Operation Group* patrols, which would 'advance to ambush' and then suppress the Taliban through superior firepower. By the end of their tour, the Royal Marines had largely cleared the Sangin Valley of insurgents and had recorded over 800 TICs, suffering 12 deaths in the process. Most deaths and other casualties were caused by small arms and RPGs, but IEDs were increasingly taking their toll as the Taliban began to switch tactics.

It was during this tour that Apache pilot Captain Tom O'Malley would be awarded the *Distinguished Flying Cross* (DFC) after flying his helicopter into a Taliban compound (Jugroom Fort, near Garmsir) with two Royal Marines strapped to the side to try and save a fatally wounded comrade on 15 January 2007. The pilot of a second Apache, carrying two more Marines, also received the DFC, and the Marines involved were awarded the Military Cross.[142,143] No British serviceman would ever be captured by the Taliban during *Operation Herrick* and no dead soldier would be left behind on the battlefield.

Sangin – the town that cost 100 British lives

If there is one name that epitomises the trials and tribulations of the British deployment into Helmand, and the bravery and fortitude of the individual British soldier when facing almost impossible challenges, it is *Sangin*. This small farming town in the upper Helmand river valley, a cluster of high-walled compounds on the edge of a network of opium fields, was typical of many other villages and towns in Helmand. It had no strategic importance per se, except that it housed a government building symbolising the distant rule of Kabul. British troops first deployed there in Summer 2006 at the request of Governor Daoud and President Karzai, to defend the District Centre. 3 Para's Platoon House endured a bitter siege, with casualty evacuation and resupply by helicopter, supported by air strikes and artillery, which ironically destroyed the town centre and the livelihoods of the people they had been sent to protect. Corporal Bryan Budd would be awarded a posthumous Victoria Cross for his bravery in action during a Taliban ambush there on 20 August 2006. The town was dubbed 'Sangingrad' by the troops during their four years supporting the ANA there, for the ferocity of the fighting and the casualty rates, especially from the networks of IEDs laid in the alleys and fields once the Taliban changed tactics. The *US Marine Corps* took over the district from the Royal Marines on *Operation Herrick 12*, in 2010, to face similar problems. Over 100 British troops died in Sangin, a quarter of the British deaths in Afghanistan, with the ANA sustaining many more fatalities. The Taliban re-entered the district in force and besieged the town once NATO troops withdrew in 2014, and although Afghan forces were supported by US Special Forces and air strikes, the government buildings and town eventually fell to a renewed Taliban onslaught on 22 March 2017.[144]

2007–2009 The Guerrilla War

In the face of increasing Taliban influence, each of the next four *Operation Herrick* brigades would concentrate in their own way on applying core COIN concepts in attempting to bring security to Helmand, trying to win over the local population and contest Taliban authority. Training back in the United Kingdom became much more systematic and COIN centred, as COIN began to be injected 'back into the lifeblood of the British Army'.[145]

OPERATION HERRICK 6 (12 MECHANISED BRIGADE, APRIL TO OCTOBER 2007)

Responsibility for the newly designated Task Force Helmand now fell to *12 Mechanised Brigade*, deploying with two battle groups based on an infantry core (the *Grenadier Guards*, *Royal Anglians* and *Mercians*, later reinforced by the *1st Battalion, Royal Welsh Regiment*, effectively creating four battalion-size manoeuvre elements) supported by light armour (*Light Dragoons*) and artillery (*39 Regiment Royal Artillery*). The *Royal Tank Regiment* deployed with their new six-wheeled armoured Mastiff vehicles ('the Mastiff Group'), thereby providing protected mobility for the infantry and filling a critical capability gap, being much less vulnerable to IEDs (Figure 1.14).

The brigade chose to take on the Taliban in the Green Zone around the Helmand River, particularly between Gereshk and Sangin. A 'clear and hold' policy was initiated in the latter part of *Operation Herrick 6* whereby patrols would turn

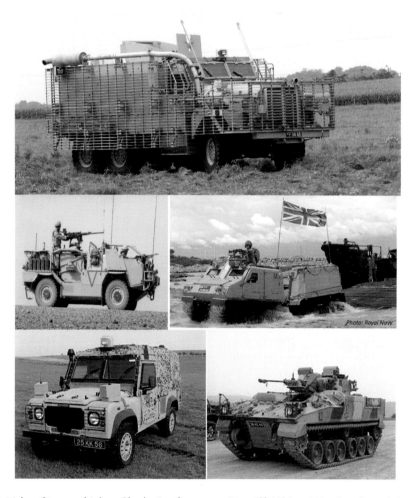

Figure 1.14 British military vehicles: Clockwise from top: Mastiff, Viking, Warrior, Snatch Land Rover and Jackal.

captured compounds into strongpoints and semi-permanent *patrol bases* (PBs), restricting Taliban freedom of movement and exerting 'persistent presence' in contested areas. This marked a shift from the previous modus operandi of repeated clearances of the upper Gereshk and upper Sangin Valleys (described by Brigadier Lorimer as 'mowing the lawn' as the Taliban would invariably return after each clearance) (Figure 1.15).

Political concerns regarding collateral damage and civilian deaths led to more restrictive rules of engagement in July 2007, with *Guidance Card Alpha* (the Armed Forces personal issue card detailing the rules governing engagement with the enemy) limiting the use of deadly force and setting the tone for future deployments, although exemptions could be granted for specific offensive operations. The brigade ended its tour with *Operation Palk Wahel* (*Hammer Blow*), deploying Warrior infantry fighting vehicles ('the Warrior Group') for the first time and pushing the Taliban out of Kajaki and the Upper Gereshk Valley back towards Musa Qala, the only town in Helmand they still controlled (Figure 1.16).

OPERATION HERRICK 7 (52 INFANTRY BRIGADE, OCTOBER 2007 TO APRIL 2008)

The new brigade for Task Force Helmand again had four manoeuvre elements, comprising *40 Commando RM*, *Yorkshire Regiment* (*Green Howards*), *Coldstream Guards* and *Royal Gurkha Rifles*, supported by light armour (*Household Cavalry*) and the *Mastiff* and *Warrior Groups* (*King's Royal Hussars* and *Scots Guards*). 52 Infantry Brigade expanded its predecessor's 'clear

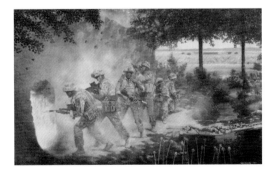

Figure 1.15 'Helmand Vikings', summer 2007 (1st Battalion, The Royal Anglian Regiment). (Courtesy of David Rowlands, Military Artist.)

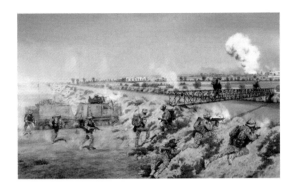

Figure 1.16 The storming of Objective FAN (Zumbelay) during *Operation Palk Wahel*, 19 September 2007. (Courtesy of David Rowlands, Military Artist.)

and hold' policy to one of 'clear, hold and build', actively including reconstruction and development in its plans. Its main offensive success was the recapture of Musa Qala after three days' intensive fighting in early December 2007, during *Operation Mar Karadad* (*Snakebite*), a joint operation involving Afghan, UK, US, and Danish troops.[146]

Operation Herrick 7 saw a massive surge in the Taliban's use of IEDs as the most effective weapon against ISAF. All the British deaths on this tour were due to IEDs or accidents.

HERRICK 8 (16 AIR ASSAULT BRIGADE, APRIL TO OCTOBER 2008)

16 Air Assault Brigade arrived for their second tour in a much stronger configuration, based on five infantry battalions (*3 Para, 1 Royal Irish, 2 Para, Royal Highland Fusiliers* [*2 Scots*] and *Argyll & Sutherland Highlanders* [*5 Scots*]), with a theatre reserve from *2nd Bn, PWRR*, and supported by light armour (*Household Cavalry*), the *Warrior Group* (*The Highlanders* [*4 Scots*]) and the *Viking Group* (*Queen's Royal Lancers*). Each battle group from this tour onwards would either have a geographical area of responsibility (generally Battle Group North around Sangin, North-West around Musa Qala, Central around Gereshk and South around Garmsir), a mentoring (OMLT) role with the Afghans or a theatre reserve role.

Notwithstanding this, *Task Force Helmand* still lacked resources to clear the southern town of Garmsir, so the *US 24th Marine Expeditionary*

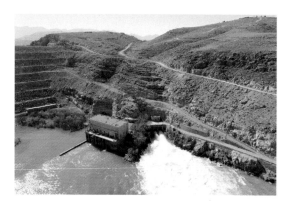

Figure 1.17 Kajaki dam (left) and power station (centre).

Corps deployed to Helmand for this tour, clearing the town and establishing safe PBs before handing responsibility for the area to the British. The tour was also notable for the safe delivery of a new hydroelectric turbine to Kajaki Dam (Figure 1.17), supported by a successful deception operation by the Danes and Special Forces.

OPERATION HERRICK 9 (3 COMMANDO BRIGADE, OCTOBER 2008 TO APRIL 2009)

This was primarily a Navy deployment, under *3 Commando Brigade* on their second tour, led by Brigadier Gordon K. Messenger RM as Commander *Task Force Helmand*. British forces in Helmand were divided into five battle groups, similar to the five of *Operation Herrick 8*, with *Task Force Lashkar Gah* being re-designated as *Battle Group Central-South*. The five battle groups were *Battle Group* (*North West*), covering Musa Qala; *Forward Operating Base* (FOB) Edinburgh, and Now Zad; *Battle Group* (*North*), led by *45 Commando RM*, covering Kajaki, Sangin, FOB Zeebrugger, FOB Inkerman, FOB Robinson, FOB Gibraltar, PB Wishtan, PB Emerald, and PB Tangiers; *Battle Group* (*Centre*), led by the Danish battle group, covering FOB Sandford, FOB Keenan, FOB Price, FOB Armadillo and Gereshk; *Battle Group* (*South*), covering FOB Dwyer, FOB Dehli, Garmsir District Centre, Nawa District Centre, PB Jugroom, PB Hassan Abad, PB Massood and PB Shamshad; and *Battle Group* (*Central-South*), which initially covered PB Argyll, Minerva Lines and Lashkar Gah but expanded in November to include Juno, Shorabak and Bastion. During

this tour, the *United Kingdom National Support Element (Afghanistan) – UK NSE(A) –* was renamed *Joint Force Support (Afghanistan) (JFSp [A])*.

The battle groups were configured around *42* and *45 Commandos*, *The Rifles*, *Royal Gurkha Rifles* and *PWRR*, with a Warrior Group and Viking Group in support. The Danes brought mechanised infantry and Leopard 2 tanks, becoming *Battle Group Centre* around Gereshk. This tour saw the addition of the Jackal mobility vehicle much more suitable for the Helmand terrain and to the equipment scale. Task Force Helmand was now expanding its influence, launching *Operation Sond Chara* (*Red Dagger*) in December to clear Taliban strongholds in Nad Ali and Marjah and prepare the ground for forthcoming incursions into their safe havens in and around the central town of Babaji on *Operation Herrick 10*. The Taliban responded with a dramatic IED offensive in defence of their strongholds – IED finds rose to 40 a week during *Operation Herrick 9*, and most of the 42 British deaths on this tour were due to these weapons.

2009–2011: COIN

A dramatic change in strategy came in May 2009 with the arrival of the new ISAF commander, US General Stanley McChrystal, fresh from leading special operations against the insurgency in Iraq, where the United States had undergone a COIN renaissance, which included deployment of 20,000 extra troops in their 2007 surge. McChrystal's strategic review of the Afghan war persuaded the recently elected US President Barack Obama to deploy a further 35,000 troops to Afghanistan in another surge to overcome the Taliban in key areas and enable the rule of law to prevail. ISAF and the United Kingdom (no longer committed on *Operation Telic*) committed extra troops too, with British personnel in Helmand reaching 9500 by the end of 2009, three times the number with which they had entered the province, and remaining at this peak for two years. The UK Armed Forces formally moved into a campaign footing with the initiation of *Operation Entirety* in 2009, resulting in *Operation Herrick* becoming the institutional main effort.[147] The publication of the new British Army manual 'Countering Insurgency' in October 2009 introduced 10 new

COIN principles into doctrine, training and common use.[148] The British military was successfully transforming in contact.[149]

General McChrystal introduced the policy of 'Courageous Restraint', prohibiting ISAF forces from using air or artillery support against compounds or other civilian structures except in the most extreme circumstances, as well as calling for more targeted operations and ramping up missions by Special Forces. His aim in doing so was to cut civilian casualties to an absolute minimum and thereby undermine Taliban propaganda and recruiting.

OPERATION HERRICK 10 (19 LIGHT BRIGADE, APRIL TO OCTOBER 2009)

19 Light Brigade (nicknamed 'The Black Panthers') took on responsibility for Task Force Helmand on *Operation Herrick 10*, its four battle groups being drawn from the *Welsh Guards, Black Watch (3 Scots), Mercians* and *2 Rifles*. The *2nd Battalion, Welsh Guards* manned the *Warrior Group*, and the *Royal Tank Regiment*, the Vikings, with light armour supplied by the *Light Dragoons*. The *Royal Logistics Corps* manned the upgraded Mastiff 2s.

The tour would be remembered for the casualties sustained during Operation *Panther's Claw* (*Panchai Palang* in Pashtu) from 19 June to 27 July. Some 3000 British, Danish and Estonian troops and 600 Afghan National Security Forces (ANSF) personnel were engaged in this five-week operation, launched to retake the town of Babaji and drive the Taliban out of the crucial area between Lashkar Gah and Gereshk before the forthcoming Afghan elections. It resulted in the heaviest fighting in Helmand since British troops first deployed there in 2006. The Taliban had also buried hundreds of IEDs in the area in advance of this operation. 10 British soldiers lost their lives as a result, including Lt. Col. Rupert Thorneloe, Commanding Officer of *the 1st Battalion, Welsh Guards* and the first British commanding officer to die in battle since the Falklands War. The bloodiest day, and the busiest in the whole campaign for Camp Bastion Hospital, was Friday 10 July, when eight British soldiers were killed and at least 30 British soldiers injured, 15 seriously,[150,151] with a similar number of casualties among Allied troops. This tour resulted in 35 British deaths, 46 seriously wounded and

85 other wounded, with IEDs being the principal killer.

OPERATION HERRICK 11 (11 LIGHT BRIGADE, OCTOBER 2009 TO APRIL 2010)

With over 9000 British troops now committed to Theatre, 11 Light Brigade's deployment was the largest to date, with six infantry battalions (*Grenadier Guards, Coldstream Guards, Rifles, Yorks, Royal Anglians* and *Royal Welsh*) and reinforcements from others (particularly *1 Scots Guards, 1 Scots* [*Royal Scots Borderers*] and *Duke of Lancaster's Regiment*).

With thousands of General McChrystal's surge troops beginning to arrive in theatre, this tour saw the largest joint offensive in the whole of the Helmand campaign, involving 15,000 British, US, Canadian, Danish and Afghan troops, on the months long *Operation Moshtarak* ('Together'). This succeeded in pushing the Taliban from their strongholds in central Helmand (Nad Ali and Lashkar Gah districts and the stronghold of Marjah). For the first time, the ANA took a lead on much of the operation. Almost inevitably, the two operations *Panther's Claw* and *Moshtarak* also resulted in 2009 seeing casualty figures peak for *Operation Herrick*, with 108 British deaths amongst the 9000 troops in theatre, although 2010 would be almost as bloody, with 103 deaths amongst 9500 troops (Figure 1.18).[152,153]

HERRICK 12 (4 MECHANISED BRIGADE, APRIL TO OCTOBER 2010)

4 Mechanised Brigade took over Task Force Helmand for *Operation Herrick 12* with battle groups built around the *Scots Guards, 1 Scots, Mercians, Duke of Lancaster's, 40 Commando Royal Marines, Royal Gurkha Rifles* and *Royal Dragoon Guards*. The brigade's priority was to consolidate the gains from *Operation Moshtarak* in accordance with General McChrystal's vision for secure government. To facilitate this, the US Marine Corps surged into Musa Qala, Sangin, Now Zad and Kajaki, formally taking over control of these areas (and northern and southern Helmand), enabling the British to concentrate on central Helmand. The large *Regional Command (South)* was subdivided in July 2010 into *RC (South West)*, which included Helmand

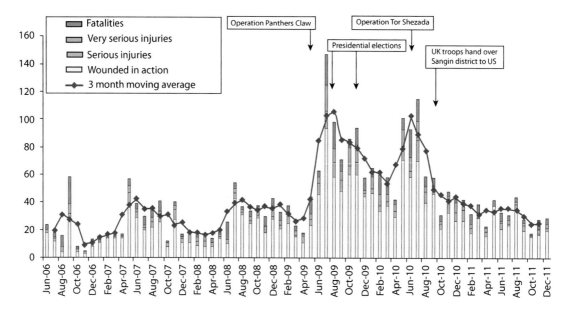

Figure 1.18 British casualties in Afghanistan, 2006–2011. (From Casualty Monitor. British casualties: Afghanistan. http://www.casualty-monitor.org/p/british-casualties-in-afghanistan.html.)

Province, under US command, and a smaller *RC (South)*, with the United Kingdom as lead nation. Sangin was formally handed over to American control in September 2010 (Figure 1.19).[154]

OPERATION HERRICK 13 (16 AIR ASSAULT BRIGADE, OCTOBER 2010 TO APRIL 2011)

16 Air Assault Brigade was the first brigade to return to Afghanistan a third time, in October 2010, its main battle groups being drawn from *2 and 3 Para, 1 Royal Irish, Duke of Lancaster's, Royal Highland Fusiliers (2 Scots), Argyll & Sutherland Highlanders (5 Scots)* and *The Irish Guards*, supported by *The Household Cavalry* and *2nd Royal Tank Regiment*. Strategically, the tour coincided with the NATO summit in Lisbon, on 19 to 20 November, where the member nations met with President Karzai and agreed to gradually withdraw from Afghanistan by 2014, launching a process by which the Afghan government would take leadership for security throughout the country, district by district.[155]

As a result, 16 Air Assault Brigade's focus was on mentoring and developing the ANSF, comprising both ANA and Afghan National Police, in preparation for ISAF Stage 4, with all operations being partnered with the ANA, who would increasingly take the lead on

operations in central Helmand. IEDs still presented the largest threat. However, with more interaction between ISAF mentors and ANA troops, so-called 'Green-on-Blue' or 'Insider' shootings began to occur, with disgruntled Afghan security forces occasionally firing on ISAF troops, jeopardising the trust built up generally between the ANA and their ISAF mentors.

2011–2013: Transition to ANSF

With NATO now firmly committed to withdrawing from Afghanistan in 2014, the stage was set for ISAF Stage 4, transition of responsibility for security in Helmand to the ANSF.

HERRICK 14 (3 COMMANDO BRIGADE, APRIL TO OCTOBER 2011)

3 Commando Brigade took over Task Force Helmand with *42* and *45 Commandos Royal Marine, 1 Rifles, 4 Scots (The Highlanders), Mercians* and *Gurkhas*, supported by *Royal Scots Dragoon Guards* and *Royal Lancers*. The brigade commenced the formal process of transition initiated by the NATO summit, carrying out offensive operations planned and led by the ANA. The focus of most of these operations was on targeting the IED makers.

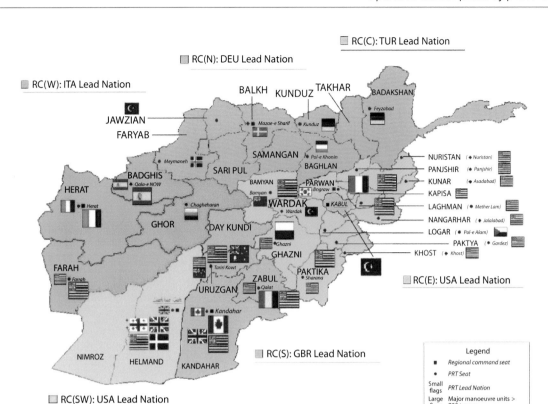

Figure 1.19 ISAF Regional Commands July 2010–2014. (From NATO. Lisbon summit declaration. http://www.nato.int/cps/en/natohq/official_texts_68828.htm.)

In July 2011, responsibility for Lashkar Gah was handed over to Afghan security forces.

UK forces in theatre had now fallen to 6500.[156] British deaths from IEDs simultaneously began to fall dramatically, effectively halving over a year (28 deaths in 2011, compared to 55 in 2010), due to improved counter-IED measures and a reduction in UK operations, and setting the trend for the remaining years.

OPERATION HERRICK 15 (20 ARMOURED BRIGADE, OCTOBER 2011 TO MAY 2012)

20 Armoured Brigade deployed with units from *The Black Watch, 1 Yorks, 2 Rifles, 5 Rifles, 2 Mercians* and *1 PWRR,* supported by *3 Yorks, Queen's Royal Hussars* and *Queen's Dragoon Guards.* The focus remained on developing the effectiveness of the Afghan security forces and maintaining stability in the province. Responsibility for Nad Ali was handed over in November.[157] The main British loss occurred

in March 2012, when a massive IED destroyed a Warrior, killing six soldiers. The medical emergency response team was exceptionally busy during this period (Figure 1.20).

OPERATION HERRICK 16 (12 MECHANISED BRIGADE, MAY TO OCTOBER 2012)

12 Mechanised Brigade deployed with battalions from the *Grenadier Guards, Welsh Guards, 1 Royal Anglians, 3 Rifles, Gurkhas, Yorks* and *Royal Welch Fusiliers,* supported by the *Royal Tank Regiment, Light Dragoons* and *King's Royal Hussars.*[158] It continued the transition process of developing the ANSF, using manoeuvre forces in depth to contest a resurgent threat as ISAF force levels began to drop and setting the conditions for the campaign's final stages. US 'surge' forces throughout Afghanistan were rapidly increasing the rate and scale of their withdrawal and had largely left Helmand by October.[159] Preparations for redeployment of British troops

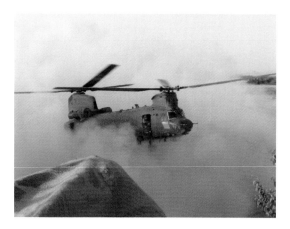

Figure 1.20 Medical emergency response team Chinook in transit to the scene of an incident.

and equipment back to United Kingdom were gathering momentum.[160] IED casualty rates continued to decline.

One notable event in this tour was the courageous action of L/Cpl James Ashworth, 1 Grenadier Guards, who died on 13 June undertaking a grenade attack on a Taliban position, leading to his being awarded a posthumous Victoria Cross (Figure 1.21).[161] This was the second of the three Victoria Crosses to be awarded during the HERRICK campaign. The other two Victoria Crosses were awarded to Corporal

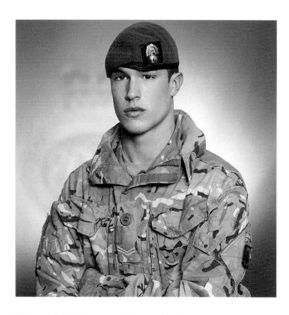

Figure 1.21 James Ashworth VC.

Bryan Budd (posthumously) in 2006 and to Corporal Joshua Leakey in 2013, both soldiers belonging to the Parachute Regiment.

Militarily, the most significant event was the Taliban raid on Camp Bastion on the night of 14 September 2012. Fifteen heavily armed Taliban fighters dressed in US Army uniforms penetrated the base perimeter and launched a co-ordinated attack on the airfield. They killed two US Marines, wounded 17 other personnel, destroyed six US Marine Corps Harrier fighters and severely damaged other aircraft and base infrastructure before 14 of them were killed and the last one captured after a four-hour battle. The loss of the six Harriers represented the largest loss sustained by a US air unit since the Vietnam War. Subsequent investigations revealed that on the night concerned, 12 out of 24 watchtowers had been left unmanned. Two US Marine Corps major generals were held accountable and had to resign their commissions,[162] while the inquiry by the *House of Commons Defence Select Committee* concluded that complacency on the part of the British also played a role in the security lapses.[163,164]

OPERATION HERRICK 17 (4 MECHANISED BRIGADE, OCTOBER 2012 TO APRIL 2013)

4 Mechanised Brigade deployed with *The Scots Guards, 40 Commando Royal Marines, 1 Scots (Royal Scots Borderers), Duke of Lancaster's, 1 Yorks, Gurkhas* and the *Mercians*, supported by *Queen's Royal Lancers* and *Royal Dragoon Guards.*

This tour saw progressive base closures and continuing transition work, with Nad Ali district increasingly handed over to ANSF and offensive operations successfully conducted by the ANA. Unfortunately, six soldiers were killed in 'Green-on-Blue' incidents, and with IED rates continuing to drop due to better counter-IED measures, British fatalities from small-arms fire overtook those from IEDs in 2012 for the first time since 2007.[165] A similar trend was developing across Afghanistan, with significantly more NATO/ISAF fatalities from non-IED causes (180) than from IEDs (132) in 2012.[166]

OPERATION HERRICK 18 (1 MECHANISED BRIGADE, APRIL TO OCTOBER 2013)

Task Force Helmand under *HQ 1 Mechanised Brigade* primarily consisted of the *Irish Guards, 2*

Scots (*Royal Highland Fusiliers*), *Duke of Lancaster's*, *Royal Fusiliers* and *4 Rifles*, as well as the *Royal Tank Regiment* and the *Household Cavalry*. The Brigade had benefitted from the now very sophisticated pre-deployment *Mission Specific Training* programme and a culture of campaign continuity, not the least because it was the third consecutive Brigade to deploy from the 3rd (UK) Division.[167] Transition work with the ANSF continued apace, with the 37 British PBs across central Helmand in April dropping to 12 by October.[168] Task Force Helmand HQ also moved to Camp Bastion after seven years in Lashkar Gah, signalling an important transition statement. The Taliban continued to refine their tactics in the face of the better counter-IED measures, seeking new ways to attack ISAF and undermine the ANSF as ISAF's profile reduced. Specifically, 2013 saw the use of several large suicide vehicle-borne IEDs targeting bases and mobile patrols.[169]

2014: Withdrawal from Theatre

OPERATION HERRICK 19 (7 ARMOURED BRIGADE, OCTOBER 2013 TO JUNE 2014)

7 Armoured Brigade deployed primarily with units drawn from *The Coldstream Guards*, *4 Scots* (*Highlanders*), *Royal Anglians*, *Mercians*, *Royal Welsh*, *Royal Scots Dragoon Guards*, *Queen's Royal Lancers* and *Queen's Own Yeomanry*.[170] Operations were conducted by a manoeuvre battle groups, a new construct for *Operation Herrick*, which was firmly multinational in nature, on this tour comprising a UK Battle Group Headquarters (*4 Scots*) and sub-units from another battalion (*3 Mercian*) together with Estonian and Danish Teams, supporting the ANA. The valuable experiences gained by the manoeuvre battle groups of working tactically alongside allies in coalition operations will be pertinent to future coalition operations.[171] The conclusion of the base closure programme saw *Task Force Helmand* disband on 1 April 2014 and the remaining UK forces placed under command of the US-led HQ Regional Command (South West), formed around the *US Marine Expeditionary Brigade* from the *1st Marine Expeditionary Force*.[172] Units on *Operation Herrick 19* undertook an eight-month tour.

OPERATION HERRICK 20 (20 ARMOURED BRIGADE, JUNE 2014 TO NOVEMBER 2014)

The final Operation Herrick deployment included elements of *1 Armoured Division*, *1 PWRR*, three battalions of *The Rifles*, the *Queen's Dragoon Guards* and the *Queen's Royal Hussars*, operating predominantly from a thinned-out Camp Bastion. The emphasis was on assisting with Afghan election security and on the massive task of redeploying all British equipment back to the United Kingdom. The re-invigorated Taliban exploited the drawdown of UK and US troops by launching a series of concerted large-scale operations in a summer offensive against the ANSF in Sangin, Musa Qala, Now Zad and Kajaki, although the Afghan forces, with some ISAF support, managed to blunt the attacks.[173]

Camp Bastion was officially handed over to the ANA on 27 October 2014 (Figure 1.22),[174] after eight years at the heart of the British military effort in Afghanistan, with the final British troops in Bastion being airlifted to Kandahar in a carefully orchestrated operation.[175] *Operation Herrick* formally ended on 30 November 2014.

NATO formally stood down ISAF and ended combat operations on 28 December 2014. A total of 500 British troops remained in Kabul in a training or force protection role at the newly built *ANA Officer Academy* (informally known as 'Sandhurst in the Sand') under Operation Toral,[176,177] as part

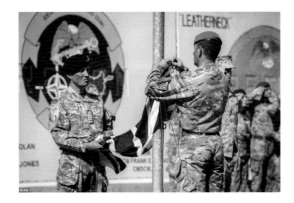

Figure 1.22 Lowering the last Union Flag at Camp Bastion. (From Britain's war in Afghanistan comes to an end after 13 years as flag is lowered over Camp Bastion. Daily Mail, 26 October 2014. http://www.dailymail.co.uk/news/article-2808240/Britain-s-war-Afghanistan-comes-end-13-years-flag-lowered-Camp-Bastion.html.)

of the new NATO-led *Resolute Support Mission* launched on 1 January 2015 to train, advise and assist the Afghan security forces and institutions. Conflict is still ongoing in Afghanistan.

END NOTE

Different sources, even official ones, give slightly different dates for each *Herrick* deployment. The convention used in post-operational reports is to link the start and end of each *Herrick* deployment to the date of *Transfer of Authority* (TOA) between Brigades, usually on the 10 April and 10 October. By contrast, the *Herrick Campaign Study* lists such deployments as May to October or November to April. Moreover, units staggered their arrival and departure dates and some handovers were necessarily prolonged as battle groups took over large areas of responsibility. The dates given in this chapter generally indicate the TOA month.

REFERENCES

1. von Clausewitz, Carl. *On War*. Princeton, NJ: Princeton University Press, 1976. Translated and edited by Professor Sir Michael Howard and Peter Paret.
2. *3 PARA Post-Operational Report, Operation HERRICK 4*. London, 2007.
3. Fairweather J. *A War of Choice: Honour, Hubris and Sacrifice: The British in Iraq*. London: Jonathan Cape, 2011.
4. Edwards A. *Defending the Realm? The Politics of Britain's Small Wars since 1945*. Manchester: Manchester University Press, 2012, p. 238.
5. Hoskins A, Ford M. Flawed, yet authoritative? Organisational memory and the future of official military history after Chilcot. *Br J Mil Hist* 2017;3(2):119–132.
6. Newsinger J. *British Counterinsurgency*. Basingstoke: Palgrave Macmillan, 2015, p. 3.
7. Yorke E. Chasing the Taliban: The Fourth Afghan War. In: *Playing the Great Game – Britain, War and Politics in Afghanistan since 1839*. London: Robert Hale, 2012, pp. 359–425.
8. Barry B. *Harsh Lessons – Iraq, Afghanistan and the Changing Character of War*.

Abingdon: Routledge, for International Institute for Strategic Studies, 2017.
9. NATO. ISAF Mandate. http://www.nato.int /isaf/topics/mandate/ (all internet references in this chapter were still accessible as at 19 April 2017).
10. Introduction. In: *The Fight for Iraq, January– June 2003. The British Army's Role in Liberating a Nation – A Pictorial Account*. London: Ministry of Defence, 2004, pp. 3–4.
11. Newsinger J. America's Wars: Afghanistan and Iraq. In: *British Counterinsurgency*. Basingstoke: Palgrave Macmillan, 2015, pp. 201–206.
12. Statement by President Bush, United Nations General Assembly. 12 September 2002. http://www.un.org/webcast/ga/57 /statements/020912usaE.htm
13. Iraq and Weapons of Mass Destruction – Debate in the House of Commons, 24 September 2002, https://www.theyworkfor you.com/debates/?id=2002-09-24.1.0, and Hansard, 24 September 2002, https://www .publications.parliament.uk/pa/cm200102 /cmhansrd/vo020924/debtext/20924-01 .htm#20924-01_spnew0
14. Chilcot J. *Report of the Iraq Inquiry*. Executive Summary: Weapons of Mass Destruction. London, 16 July 2016, pp. 69–77. http://www.iraqinquiry.org.uk/media /247921/the-report-of-the-iraq-inquiry _executive-summary.pdf
15. United Nations Security Council Resolution 1441 (2002), dated 8 November 2002. http://www.un.org/Depts/unmovic/docu ments/1441.pdf
16. Fairweather J. *A War of Choice: Honour, Hubris and Sacrifice: The British in Iraq*. London: Jonathan Cape, 2011.
17. Ministry of Defence. *Operation Telic – United Kingdom Military Operations In Iraq*. National Audit Office; 11 December 2003. https://www.nao.org.uk/wp-content /uploads/2003/12/030460.pdf
18. House of Commons Select Committee on Defence, Third Report. 16 March 2004. http://www.publications.parliament.uk /pa/cm200304cmselect/cmdfence/57/5709 .htm

19. Jackson M. Foreword. In: *The Fight for Iraq, January–June 2003. The British Army's Role in Liberating a Nation – A Pictorial Account.* London: Ministry of Defence, 2004.

20. House of Commons. *The Strategic Defence Review White Paper.* Published 15 October 1998, p. 24. http://researchbriefings.files .parliament.uk/documents/RP98-91/RP98 -91.pdf

21. Chilcot Report. The Impact of Afghanistan. In: *Executive Summary.* 2016, pp. 99–100, para. 720–732.

22. Maciejewski J. 'Best effort': Operation Sinbad and the Iraq Campaign. In: Bailey J, Iron R, Strachan H (eds.). *British Generals in Blair's Wars.* Farnham: Ashgate, 2013, p. 160.

23. House of Commons Defence Committee. Land operations in Iraq 2007. House of Commons; 3 December 2007. https://www .publications.parliament.uk/pa/cm200708 /cmselect/cmdfence/110/110.pdf

24. Operations in Iraq – British fatalities. https://www.gov.uk/government/fields -of-operation/iraq

25. Nicol M. *Iraq – A Tribute to Britain's Fallen Heroes.* Edinburgh: Mainstream Publishing, 2008, p. 9.

26. Elliott C. *High Command – British Military Leadership in the Iraq and Afghanistan Wars.* London: Hurst & Company, 2015, p. 21.

27. Ucko DH, Egnell R. *Counterinsurgency in Crisis – Britain and the Challenges of Modern Warfare.* New York: Columbia University Press, 2015.

28. North Atlantic Treaty Organisation (NATO). ISAF's mission in Afghanistan (2001–2014). http://www.nato.int/cps/en/natohq/topics _69366.htm

29. NATO. ISAF Mandate. http://www.nato.int /isaf/topics/mandate/

30. NATO. ISAF Placemats Archive, February 2011–July 2011. http://www.nato.int/cps/en /natolive/107995.htm

31. UK operational codenames are randomly chosen by computer. Op HERRICK is named after the poet and song-writer Robert Herrick (1591–1674). http://www.luminarium .org/sevenlit/herrick/herribio.htm

32. NATO. ISAF placemats archive. 12 January 2009. http://www.nato.int/cps/en/natolive /107995.htm

33. NATO. ISAF placemats archive, February 2010–December 2012. http://www.nato.int /cps/en/natolive/107995.htm

34. Op HERRICK casualty and fatality tables. https://www.gov.uk/government /collections/op-herrick-casualty-and-fatality -tables-index

35. https://www.gov.uk/government/uploads /system/uploads/attachment_data/file/512070 /20160331_UK_Armed_Forces_Operational _deaths_post_World_War_II.O.pdf

36. Farrell T, Osinga F, Russell JA (eds.). *Military Adaptation in Afghanistan.* Stanford, CA: Stanford University Press, 2013.

37. Barry B. *Harsh Lessons – Iraq, Afghanistan and the Changing Character of War.* Abingdon: Routledge, for International Institute for Strategic Studies, 2017.

38. Ministry of Defence. *Operations in Iraq – First Reflections.* MOD London; 7 July 2003. Introduction, p. 3. http://www.globalsecu rity.org/military/library/report/2003/iraq 2003operations_ukmod_july03.pdf

39. Ministry of Defence. *Operation Telic – United Kingdom Military Operations in Iraq.* National Audit Office; 11 December 2003. https://www.nao.org.uk/wp-content /uploads/2003/12/030460.pdf

40. Ministry of Defence. AC 71816: *Operations in Iraq – An Analysis from a Land Perspective.* London: MOD, 2005.

41. Ministry of Defence. AC 71844: *Stability Operations in Iraq (Op Telic 2–5). An Analysis from a Land Perspective.* MOD London, 2006. http://download.cable drum.net/wikileaks_archive/file/uk-stbility -operations-in-iraq-2006.pdf

42. Ministry of Defence. AC 71937: *Operations in Iraq, January 2005–May 2009 (Op TELIC 5–13). An Analysis from a Land Perspective.* London: MOD, 29 November 2010, released to the public September 2016. http://operationtelic.co.uk/wp-content /uploads/2014/06/Operations-in-Iraq -REDACTED.pdf

43. Barry B. *The Bitter War to Stabilise Southern Iraq – British Army Report Declassified.* International Institute for Strategic Studies (IISS); 10 October 2016. https://www.iiss.org/iiss%20voices/blogsections/iiss-voices-2016-9143/october-d6b6/the-bitter-war-to-stabilise-southern-iraq—british-army-report-declassified-953d

44. Mansoor P. The British Army and the Lessons of the Iraq War. *British Army Review,* Summer 2009.

45. Ledwidge F. *Losing Small Wars. British Military Failure in Iraq and Afghanistan.* New Haven, CT: Yale University Press, 2011. Revised edition 2017, pp. 254–257.

46. *British Army Review Special Report – Learning 2014, Volume 3: Learning from Conflict – Iraq.* Crown.

47. Lessons Exploitation Centre. *Operation HERRICK Campaign Study.* British Army: Directorate Land Warfare, 2015. https://www.gov.uk/government/uploads/system/uploads/attachment_data/file/492757/20160107115638.pdf

48. Bricknell MCM, Nadin M. Lessons from the organisation of the UK medical services deployed in support of Operation TELIC (Iraq) and Operation HERRICK (Afghanistan). *J R Army Med Corps* 2017; 163(4):273–279.

49. McNamee T (ed.). *War Without Consequences – Iraq's Insurgency and the Spectre of Strategic Defeat. RUSI Essays 2002–2008.* London: RUSI Books, 2008.

50. *The Afghan Papers: Committing Britain to War in Helmand, 2005–06.* Abingdon: Routledge, on behalf of the Royal United Services Institute for Defence and Security Studies, 2011.

51. 'The Afghan Decisions': Four articles by Charles Styles, Josh Arnold-Foster, Matt Cavanagh and Mungo Melvin. *RUSI J* April/May 2012;157(2):40–61.

52. North R. *Ministry of Defeat – The British War in Iraq 2003–2009.* London: Continuum, 2009.

53. Bailey J, Iron R, Strachan H (eds.). *British Generals in Blair's Wars.* Farnham: Ashgate, 2013.

54. Jackson Mike. *Soldier: The Autobiography.* London: Corgi, 2008.

55. Dannatt R. *Leading from the Front.* London: Bantam, 2010.

56. Richards D. *Taking Command.* London: Headline, 2014.

57. Ripley T. *Operation TELIC – The British Campaign in Iraq 2003–2009.* Telic-Herrick Publications, 2016. www.operationtelic.co.uk

58. Books about the Gulf, Iraq, and Afghanistan Wars. http://nostalgia.esmartkid.com/gulfwarbooks.html

59. Barry B. *Harsh Lessons – Iraq, Afghanistan and the Changing Character of War.* Abingdon: Routledge, for International Institute for Strategic Studies, 2017.

60. Farrell T. *Unwinnable – Britain's War in Afghanistan 2001–2014.* London: Bodley Head, 2017.

61. Chilcot J. *Report of the Iraq Inquiry.* London, 16 July 2016. http://www.iraqinquiry.org.uk/

62. Ledwidge F. *Losing Small Wars. British Military Failure in Iraq and Afghanistan.* New Haven, CT: Yale University Press, 2011. Revised edition 2017, pp. 254–257.

63. Elliott C. *High Command – British Military Leadership in the Iraq and Afghanistan Wars.* London: Hurst & Company, 2015.

64. Greenstock J. *Iraq – The Cost of War.* London: William Heinemann, 2016.

65. Rew D. *Blood, Heat + Dust – Operation Telic and the British Medical Deployment to the Gulf 2003–2009.* E-Book; Association of Surgeons of Great Britain & Ireland, 2015. http://www.publications.asgbi.org/bhd_donate/donation_page.html

66. Basrawi clerics to Lieutenant General Sir Peter Wall, summer 2003, reminding him of the Iraq insurgency of 1919–1923 when Britain's attempts to impose an administration upon the tribal sheikhs after driving the Ottomans out of Iraq resulted in the tribes uniting against her (Evidence of Lieutenant General Sir Peter Wall to the Iraq Inquiry, 14 December 2009). Quoted by Ledwidge (2017), p. 17.

67. The dates for the various Op TELIC deployments up to Op TELIC 10 are as released by PJHQ on 24 October 2007 following a Freedom of Information request. http://www.operationtelic.co.uk/documents/mod-telic_dates.pdf. Dates thereafter relate to the Transfer of Authority between Brigades

68. Franks T, McConnell M. *American Soldier*. London: HarperCollins, 2004.

69. Ministry of Defence. *Operations in Iraq – First Reflections*. London, July 2003.

70. Chilcot J. *Report of the Iraq Inquiry*. Volume 7, Section 8 – The Invasion. London, 16 July 2016, pp. 6–7. http://www.iraqinquiry.org.uk/

71. Ripley T. *Operation TELIC – The British Campaign in Iraq 2003–2009*. Telic-Herrick Publications, 2016, p. 77. www.operationtelic.co.uk

72. 16 Close Support Medical Regiment: Operation TELIC – Post Operational Report. dated 1 July 2003.

73. Chilcot J. *Report of the Iraq Inquiry*. Volume 7, Section 8 – The Invasion. London, 16 July 2016, p. 8. http://www.iraqinquiry.org.uk/

74. Greenstock J. *Iraq – The Cost of War*. London: Heinemann, 2016, p. 418.

75. DIS. *Red Team Report on Retaining Support of the Iraq People*. In: Chilcot J. *Report of the Iraq Inquiry*. Section 6.5, paras 570–609, and 855ff. http://www.iraqinquiry.org.uk/. (Discussed in Ledwidge, 2017, pp. 21–25.)

76. *Operations in Iraq – An Analysis from a Land Perspective*. London: MOD, 2003, pp. 5–9.

77. Quinlivan JT. Force requirements in stability operations. *Parameters* 1995;Winter:59–69. http://ssi.armywarcollege.edu/pubs/parameters/Articles/1995/quinliv.htm. Updated in: Quinlivan JT. Burden of victory: the painful arithmetic of stability operations. *Rand Review* 2003;Summer. www.rand.org/publications/randreview/issues/summer2003/burden.html. (Also discussed in Ledwidge, 2017, pp. 142–145).

78. Newsinger J. America's Wars: Afghanistan and Iraq. In: *British Counterinsurgency*. 2nd ed. Basingstoke: Palgrave Macmillan, 2015, pp. 216–217.

79. Ricks T. *Fiasco: The American Military Adventure in Iraq*. London: Allen & Lane, 2006, pp. 161–163.

80. Nicol M. *Last Round*. London: Weidenfeld & Nicolson, 2005.

81. Chilcot J. *Report of the Iraq Inquiry*. Section 9.2. 23 May–June 2004. London, 16 July 2016, p. 240. http://www.iraqinquiry.org.uk/

82. Williams AT. *A Very British Killing – The Death of Baha Mousa*. London: Jonathan Cape, 2012.

83. Gage W. The Report of the Baha Mousa Inquiry. 2011. https://www.gov.uk/government/uploads/system/uploads/attachment_data/file/279190/1452_i.pdf (accessed 23 March 2017).

84. Cobain I. Baha Mousa doctor Derek Keilloh struck off after 'repeated dishonesty.' *The Guardian*. 21 December 2012. https://www.theguardian.com/world/2012/dec/21/baha-mousa-doctor-struck-off (accessed 2 April 2017).

85. Hoskins A, Ford M. Flawed, yet Authoritative? Organisational memory and the future of official military history after Chilcot. *Br J Mil Hist* February 2017;3(2): 119–132.

86. Forbes T. The Report of Al Sweady Inquiry. December 2014. https://www.gov.uk/government/uploads/system/uploads/attachment_data/file/388292/Volume_1_Al_Sweady_Inquiry.pdf

87. Justice for Dr Derek Keilloh – What actually happened? http://www.justice4drkeilloh.org.uk/

88. 20 Armoured Brigade Post Operational Report – Operation Telic 3, dated 4 July 2004.

89. Ledwidge F. *Losing Small Wars. British Military Failure in Iraq and Afghanistan*. New Haven, CT: Yale University Press, 2011. Revised edition 2017, pp. 28–32.

90. United Nations Security Council Resolution 1511. 16 October 2003. https://documents-dds-ny.un.org/doc/UNDOC/GEN/N03/563/91/PDF/N0356391.pdf?OpenElement

91. Ripley T. *Operation TELIC – The British Campaign in Iraq 2003–2009*. Telic-Herrick Publications, 2016, pp. 190, 196–208. www.operationtelic.co.uk

92. Deployment of pre-war Iraqi forces: GlobalSecurity.org. '1 Corps.' http://www.globalsecurity.org/military/world/iraq/1corps.htm

93. Chilcot J. *Report of the Iraq Inquiry.* Executive Summary. London, 16 July 2016, p. 96. http://www.iraqinquiry.org.uk/

94. Ripley T. *Operation TELIC – The British Campaign in Iraq 2003–2009.* Telic-Herrick Publications, 2016, pp. 200–203 (including referenced interviews with General Stewart). www.operationtelic.co.uk

95. 20 Armoured Brigade Post Operational Report – Operation TELIC 3, dated 4 July 2004.

96. Chilcot J. *Report of the Iraq Inquiry.* Executive Summary. The Turning Point. London, 16 July 2016, p. 96, para 701. http://www.iraqinquiry.org.uk/

97. Mills D. *Sniper One.* London: Michael Joseph, 2007. (An account of the 1 PWRR Battlegroup under siege for six months at CIMIC House, Al Amarah.)

98. Holmes R. The first uprising: from Pimlico to Whitechapel. In: Rchard H. *Dusty Warriors.* London: HarperPerennial, 2007, Chapter 5, Round One, pp. 185–226.

99. Holmes R. The battle for Danny Boy. In: Rchard H. *Dusty Warriors.* London: Harper Perennial, 2007, Chapter 5, Round One, pp. 226–246.

100. Al-Sweady inquiry report. Conclusion, para 5.202. https://www.gov.uk/government/publications/al-sweady-inquiry-report

101. Al-Sweady inquiry report. Conclusion, para 5.201. https://www.gov.uk/government/publications/al-sweady-inquiry-report

102. Beharry J. *Barefoot Soldier – A Story of Extreme Valour.* London: Sphere, 2006.

103. United Nations Security Council. Press Release, 8 June 2004. https://www.un.org/press/en/2004/sc8117.doc.htm

104. Ripley T. *Operation TELIC – The British Campaign in Iraq 2003–2009.* Telic-Herrick Publications, 2016, pp. 231–238.

105. 4 Armoured Brigade would become 4 Mechanised Brigade in 2007 on leaving 1 (UK) Armoured Division in Germany and being assigned to 3 (UK) Mechanised Division in the UK.

106. 4 Armoured Brigade Post Operational Report – Operation TELIC 5, dated 29 July 2005.

107. Ripley T. *Operation TELIC – The British Campaign in Iraq 2003–2009.* Telic-Herrick Publications, 2016, p. 259. www.operationtelic.co.uk

108. Nicol M. *Iraq – A Tribute to Britain's Fallen Heroes.* Edinburgh: Mainstream Publishing, 2008, pp. 150–151.

109. Ripley T. *Operation TELIC – The British Campaign in Iraq 2003–2009.* Telic-Herrick Publications, 2016, pp. 263–265. www.operationtelic.co.uk

110. Ripley T. *Operation TELIC – The British Campaign in Iraq 2003–2009.* Telic-Herrick Publications, 2016, p. 267–268. www.operationtelic.co.uk

111. Narain J. Soldier who faced death in burning tank in Iraq set to run 52 marathons to repay medics who rebuilt him. *Daily Mail Online*, 27 December 2010. http://www.dailymail.co.uk/news/article-1341804/Marathon-Man-The-ordeal-troops-blazing-tank-defining-image-Iraq-Now-running-52-marathons-repay-medic-rebuilt-him.html#ixzz4dHHX0qy8

112. Ivison K. *Red One – A Bomb Disposal Expert on the Front Line.* London: Weidenfeld & Nicolson, 2010.

113. 7 Armoured Brigade Op TELIC 7 Post Operational Report, dated 8 May 2006.

114. Collins D. *In Foreign Fields – Heroes of Iraq and Afghanistan in Their Own Words.* Reading: Monday Books, 2007, pp. 286–297.

115. Ripley T. *Operation TELIC – The British Campaign in Iraq 2003–2009.* Telic-Herrick Publications, 2016, pp. 324–326.

116. The Effects of Op SINBAD 20 September 2006–14 January 2007. MOD, Letter to the Secretary of State, dated 16 February 2007, declassified. http://www.iraqinquiry.org.uk

/media/243581/2007-02-16-minute-beadle-to-banner-the-effect-of-op-sinbad-20-september-2006-to-14-january-2007.pdf

117. Elliott C. *High Command – British Military Leadership in the Iraq and Afghanistan Wars*. London: Hurst & Company, 2015, pp. 117–118.

118. Richard I. Basra 2008: Operation Charge of the Knights. In Bailey J, Iron R, Strachan H (eds.). *British Generals in Blair's Wars*. Farnham: Ashgate, 2013, p. 188.

119. Gardham D. Soldiers destroy Basra's 'rogue' police HQ. *The Telegraph*, 26 December 2006. http://www.telegraph.co.uk/news/worldnews/1537861/Soldiers-destroy-Basras-rogue-police-HQ.html

120. Hughes G. Iraqnophobia – The Dangers of forgetting Operation TELIC. *RUSI J* 2013;157(6):54–60.

121. Chilcot J. *Report of the Iraq Inquiry*. Executive Summary. London, 16 July 2016, p. 106, para 768. http://www.iraqinquiry.org.uk/

122. Ledwidge F. *Losing Small Wars. British Military Failure in Iraq and Afghanistan*. New Haven, CT: Yale University Press, 2011. Revised edition 2017, p. 44.

123. Ricks T. *The Gamble: General David Petraeus and the American Military Adventure in Iraq, 2006–2008*. London: Penguin, 2009.

124. MacKinlay J. A Petraeus doctrine for Whitehall – Review essay. *RUSI J* 2009;154(3):26–29.

125. Fry R. Interview on BBC TV's *Secret Iraq*, October 2010. (Quoted by Ledwidge, 2017, p. 44).

126. Casualty Monitor. British Casualties: Iraq. http://www.casualty-monitor.org/p/iraq.html

127. Fairweather J. *A War of Choice: Honour, Hubris and Sacrifice: The British in Iraq*. London: Jonathan Cape, 2011, p. 328.

128. Ledwidge F. *Losing Small Wars. British Military Failure in Iraq and Afghanistan*. New Haven, CT: Yale University Press, 2011. Revised edition 2017, p. 52.

129. Iron R. Basra 2008: Operation charge of the knights. In: Bailey J, Iron R, Strachan H (eds.). *British Generals in Blair's Wars*. Farnham: Ashgate, 2013, pp. 187–199.

130. Iron R. Basra 2008: Operation charge of the knights. In: Bailey J, Iron R, Strachan H (eds.). *British Generals in Blair's Wars*. Farnham: Ashgate, 2013, pp. 187–199.

131. Sir John Chilcot's public statement, 6 July 2016.

132. OP TELIC 12: HQ 7th Armoured Brigade Post Operational Report. 15 December 2008.

133. 20th Armoured Brigade Op Telic 13 Post Operational Report. 6 July 2009.

134. 20th Armoured Brigade Op Telic 13 Post Operational Report. 6 July 2009.

135. NATO. ISAF Placemats. 12 January 2009. http://www.nato.int/isaf/placemats_archive/2009-01-12-ISAF-Placemat.pdf

136. Elliott C. *High Command – British Military Leadership in the Iraq and Afghanistan Wars*. London: Hurst & Company, 2015, p. 158.

137. Farrell T. Improving in war: Military adaptation and the British in Helmand Province, Afghanistan, 2006–2009. *J Strateg Stud* 2010;33(4):567–594.

138. Alderson A. Counter-insurgency: Learn and adapt? Can we do better? *Br Army Rev* 2007(summer):16–21.

139. Jakobsen PV, Thruelsen PD. Clear, hold, train: Denmark's military operations in Helmand 2006–2010. *Danish Foreign Policy Yearbook* 2011:78–105.

140. Newsinger J. America's Wars: Afghanistan and Iraq. In: *British Counterinsurgency*. 2nd ed. Basingstoke: Palgrave Macmillan, 2015, pp. 231–232.

141. Neville L. *The British Army in Afghanistan 2006–14. Task Force Helmand*. Oxford: Osprey Publishing, 2015, pp. 9–24.

142. Marines in rescue bid for comrade. *The Independent*, 17 January 2007.

143. Pryne M. Hero Apache pilot awarded the Distinguished Flying Cross to sell gallantry medals. *The Daily Telegraph*, 1 July 2014. http://www.telegraph.co.uk/news/uknews

/defence/10938151/Hero-Apache-pilot
-awarded-the-Distinguished-Flying-Cross
-to-sell-gallantry-medals.html

144. Tomlinson H, Yaqubi A. Taliban capture
town that cost 100 British lives. *The Times*,
24 March 2017, p. 17.

145. Alderson A. Too busy to learn: Personal
observations on British campaigns in
Iraq and Afghanistan. In: Bailey J, Irons
R, Strachan H (eds.). *British Generals in
Blair's Wars*. Farnham: Ashgate, 2013,
pp. 281–296.

146. Grey S. *Operation Snakebite: The Explosive
True Story of an Afghan Desert Siege*.
London: Penguin Books, 2010.

147. Lessons Exploitation Centre. *Operation
HERRICK Campaign Study*. London: British
Army, Directorate Land Warfare, 2015,
p.iii.

148. *British Army Field Manual, Vol 1, Part 10,
Countering Insurgency*. London: HMSO,
October 2009.

149. Farrell T. Improving in war: Military adaptation and the British in Helmand Province,
Afghanistan, 2006–2009. *J Strateg Stud*
2010;33(4):567–594.

150. UK hospital in Afghanistan copes with
bloodiest day. *Reuters*, 12 July 2009.

151. Camp Bastion's advanced field hospital has
experienced its bloodiest week for British
troops since operations began in Helmand
with wards nearly at full capacity. *The Daily
Telegraph*, 13 July 2009.

152. Afghanistan casualty and fatality tables
(number of Afghanistan UK military and
civilian casualties 7 October 2001 to 31
December 2014). https://www.gov.uk
/government/uploads/system/uploads
/attachment_data/file/394808/20150114
_ENCLOSURE1_British_casualties_in
_Afghanistan_7_Oct_01_to_31_Dec_14.pdf

153. Casualty Monitor. British casualties:
Afghanistan. http://www.casualty-monitor
.org/p/british-casualties-in-afghanistan
.html

154. NATO. Lisbon summit declaration. http:
//www.nato.int/cps/en/natohq/official
_texts_68828.htm

155. 3 Commando Brigade take command of
Task Force Helmand. MOD Announcement,
11 April 2011. https://www.gov.uk/govern
ment/news/3-commando-brigade-take
-command-of-task-force-helmand

156. Neville L. *The British Army in Afghanistan
2006 – 14. Task Force Helmand*. Oxford:
Osprey Publishing, 2015, p. 46.

157. NATO. ISAF Placemats Archive. 6 August
2010. http://www.nato.int/cps/en/natol
ive/107995.htm

158. 12th Mechanised Brigade to replace 20th
Armoured Brigade in Helmand. MOD
Announcement, 9 February 2012. https:
//www.gov.uk/government/news/12th
-mechanized-brigade-to-replace-20th
-armoured-brigade-in-helmand

159. NATO. ISAF Placemats Archive. 8 October
2012. http://www.nato.int/isaf/placemats
_archive/2012-10-08-ISAF-Placemat.pdf

160. Joint Force Support (Afghanistan) (JFSP(A))
13: Post Operational Report, dated 15 July
2012.

161. http://www.victoriacross.org.uk/bbashwor
.htm

162. Ledwidge F. *Losing Small Wars. British
Military Failure in Iraq and Afghanistan*.
New Haven, CT: Yale University Press, 2011.
Revised edition 2017, pp. 128–129.

163. House of Commons Defence Committee.
Afghanistan – Camp Bastion Attack. House
of Commons, 16 April 2014. https://www
.publications.parliament.uk/pa/cm201314
/cmselect/cmdfence/830/830.pdf

164. House of Commons Defence Committee.
Afghanistan – Camp Bastion Attack:
Government response to the committee's
Thirteenth Report of Session 2013–14.
House of Commons, 7 July 2014. https:
//www.publications.parliament.uk/pa
/cm201415/cmselect/cmdfence/526/526.pdf

165. Neville L. *The British Army in Afghanistan
2006–14. Task Force Helmand*. Oxford:
Osprey Publishing, 2015, p. 48.

166. Afghanistan War NATO/ISAF Coalition
Military Deaths caused by IEDs – Status as
of end of 2014. http://stats.areppim.com
/stats/stats_afghanwar_ied.htm

167. Task Force Helmand Op HERRICK 18 Post-Operational Report.

168. Neville L. *The British Army in Afghanistan 2006–14. Task Force Helmand*. Oxford: Osprey Publishing, 2015, p. 48

169. Task Force Helmand Op HERRICK 18 Post-Operational Report. 2013.

170. Neville L. *The British Army in Afghanistan 2006–14. Task Force Helmand*. Oxford: Osprey Publishing, 2015, p. 49–50.

171. Sandford R. Coalition operations: The Manoeuvre Battlegroup Op HERRICK 19. *BAR Special Report – Learning from Afghanistan* 2016;4.2.

172. Operation HERRICK 19: Task Force Helmand Post Operation Report, dated 12 June 2014.

173. Neville L. *The British Army in Afghanistan 2006–14. Task Force Helmand*. Oxford: Osprey Publishing, 2015, p. 50.

174. Britain's war in Afghanistan comes to an end after 13 years as flag is lowered over Camp Bastion. *Daily Mail*, 26 October 2014. http://www.dailymail.co.uk/news/article-2808240/Britain-s-war-Afghanistan-comes-end-13-years-flag-lowered-Camp-Bastion.html

175. Last British soldiers leave Camp Bastion as war in Afghanistan ends. *The Telegraph*, 27 October 2014. http://www.telegraph.co.uk/news/worldnews/asia/afghanistan/11189479/Last-British-soldiers-leave-Camp-Bastion-as-war-in-Afghanistan-ends.html

176. Op TORAL: Sandhurst in the Sands. *YouTube video*, 18 June 2015. https://www.youtube.com/watch?v=1bhAv136ml0

177. NATO. RSM Placemats Archive, May 2015. http://www.nato.int/nato_static_fl2014/assets/pdf/pdf_2015_05/20150508_1505-RSM-Placemat.pdf

2

Organisation of the medical services in Iraq and Afghanistan

'And that's what saved my life, putting that tourniquet on so high up and so effectively'.

Lance Corporal Rory Mackenzie, Royal Army Medical Corps (RAMC), Combat Medical Technician

'If anything positive can be said of war, it would be that it serves as a catalyst for rapid improvements in medical understanding and care'.[1]

INTRODUCTION

As far as military medicine is concerned, the twenty-first century effectively started on 9/11. The subsequent 13 years of intensive operations resulted in rapid accumulation of combat experience, and dissemination of knowledge and best practice, throughout the Defence Medical Services (DMS). Many highly motivated individuals worked together to bring about a military medical revolution that transformed the delivery of care from point of injury on the battlefield (Role 1) through to definitive care and rehabilitation in the United Kingdom (Role 4).[2,3] Many casualties were saved as a result, including Lance Corporal Rory Mackenzie RAMC, quoted earlier, with progressive improvement in survival rates and unprecedented numbers of 'unexpected survivors'.[4] Equivalent efforts were made in trying to heal the hidden effects of wounding.[5]

The revolutionary concepts that influenced combat casualty care from point of wounding or illness through to the home base evolved throughout *Operation Telic* and *Operation Herrick*. By the time *Operation Herrick* ended in 2014, they had formally been incorporated into doctrine and training to ensure they endure. Patients were supported by seven interconnected capabilities of care, encapsulated as the *Operational Patient Care Pathway*[6–8] (Figures 2.1–2.3). Moreover, ensuring wider international dissemination of best medical practice, this UK national medical doctrine has now been merged with North Atlantic Treaty Organization (NATO) medical doctrine as a single publication.[9]

These new concepts and the key medical lessons learned at each level of care during this revolution in military medical care are detailed separately in this book. The key organisational lessons were captured in the Herrick Campaign Study and the main themes were further analysed in the *Journal of the RAMC*.[10,11] This chapter sets the historical context for these concepts and lessons, within their supporting organisational framework, for *Operation Telic* and then for *Operation Herrick*.

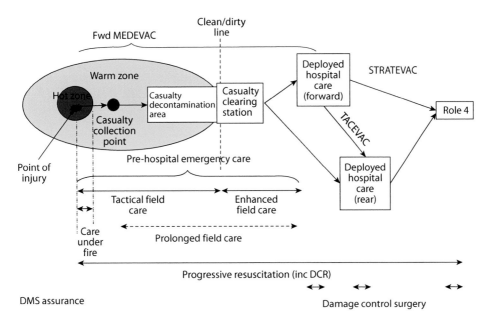

Figure 2.1 The Operational Patient Care Pathway.

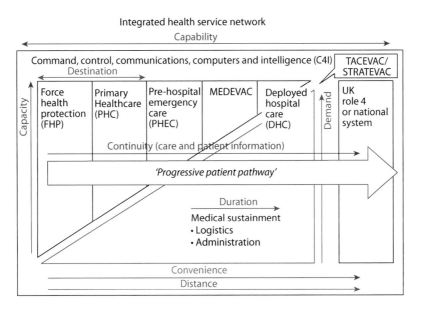

Figure 2.2 Interconnected seven capabilities of care. (From Operation Herrick 19 – Close Support Medical Regiment – Post Operational Observations, dated 28 May 2014.)

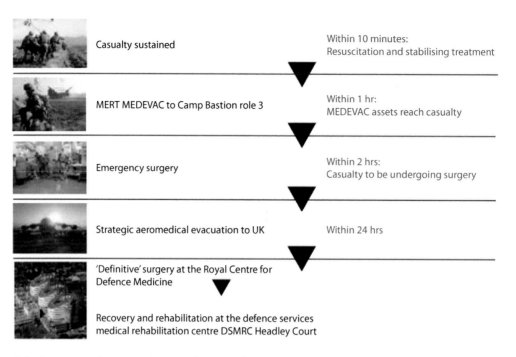

	Casualty sustained	Within 10 minutes: Resuscitation and stabilising treatment
	MERT MEDEVAC to Camp Bastion role 3	Within 1 hr: MEDEVAC assets reach casualty
	Emergency surgery	Within 2 hrs: Casualty to be undergoing surgery
	Strategic aeromedical evacuation to UK	Within 24 hrs
	'Definitive' surgery at the Royal Centre for Defence Medicine	

Recovery and rehabilitation at the defence services medical rehabilitation centre DSMRC Headley Court

Figure 2.3 Operational Patient Care Pathway and clinical timelines on *Operation Herrick* (Herrick campaign study).

OPERATION TELIC – PREPARING FOR THE INVASION

Strategic medical plan

The political direction to prepare to invade Iraq should it fail to comply with UN Security Council Resolution 1441 was given in November 2002.[12] Military planners then had to consider various options for accomplishing this and ensuring that they would have sufficient resources for the purpose. Concurrently, appropriate strategic and operational-level medical estimates were conducted to ensure that each contingency plan could be supported medically. A strategic medical estimate (determining the number and type of casualties expected, and when and where they would occur) was therefore undertaken, while joint operational-level medical planning (to determine the resources required) was conducted by Permanent Joint Headquarters (PJHQ), in association with Front Line Commands, and tested with principal tactical medical commanders and Defence Consultant Advisors.

The favoured military option of entering Iraq from the north had to be abandoned in December when the Turkish government withdrew its support, so planning switched hurriedly to the southern option of entering Iraq through Kuwait. The United Kingdom increased its commitment from *7 Armoured Brigade* alone by adding *3 Commando Brigade* and *16 Air Assault Brig*ade, each with its integral close medical support assets, to the Order of Battle (ORBAT), under *1st (UK) Armoured Division*.

Clinical 1–2–4 timelines

British military medical doctrine of the time dictated that seriously injured casualties should receive skilled resuscitation within one hour of injury, receive damage control surgery if necessary within two hours, receive surgery for head injuries within four hours and receive surgery for other injuries within six hours.[13] This concept of one-, two- and four-hour clinical timelines underpinned all medical planning.

Force health protection

In addition to preparations for the environmental challenges posed by the deserts of Kuwait and

Iraq, the perceived threat of biological and chemical warfare underpinned force protection measures (vaccinations, nerve agent antidotes, personal [PPE] and collective protective equipment [COLPRO] and training). Anthrax, for instance, had made its debut as a weapon of terrorism as recently as October 2001, when 21 people in the United States had contracted this disease from spores sent in the mail.[14] Vaccination against anthrax was offered to service personnel deploying on *Operation Telic*.

MEDICAL ORBAT

Capability and capacity

The medical ORBAT had to ensure sufficient capability to support all three brigades in meeting the 1–2–4 clinical timelines. The demand on precious resources was to be judiciously managed (and the deployed bed capacity kept at the truly necessary minimum) through efficient aeromedical evacuation and the provision of a strong reserve. The final UK operational medical plan for *Operation Telic* determined that in addition to integral single Service Role 1 and Role 2 support, Role 3 support would be required as follows.

ROYAL NAVY

The Royal Navy would provide a 100-bed *primary casualty receiving facility* (PCRF), provided on board *Royal Fleet Auxiliary (RFA) Argus*. This was not a designated hospital ship as she carried weapons systems and had other military roles, so she could be positioned much closer to the battlespace, allowing more rapid transfer of patients to definitive care.[15]

ARMY

The Army provided two 200-bed field hospitals (with another 200-bed field hospital providing the strategic medical reserve). In due course, unforeseeable delays in deploying the equipment for the first 200-bed hospital would necessitate the airborne deployment of a 25-bed field hospital to provide Role 3 capability for the build-up phase in Kuwait, until a full 200-bed capability could be established.

ROYAL AIR FORCE

Strategic aeromedical evacuation to the United Kingdom would be through a casualty staging flight operating out of Kuwait International Airport. The Princess Mary's Hospital, at Royal Air Force (RAF) Akrotiri, Cyprus, would have an embedded *Critical Care Air Support Team* (CCAST) and be augmented to 90 beds to support aeromedical evacuation, also providing a surge capability in the event of a major casualty incident in the Area of Operations.[16]

OPERATION TELIC 1 (1ST [UK] ARMOURED DIVISION FEBRUARY TO JUNE 2003)

Command and control

While the medical command of the maritime and air components of the UK Forces was straightforward, the land forces under *1st (UK) Armoured Division* were divided into a Lines of Communication Component (essentially the forward troops of *7 Armoured Brigade*, *16 Air Assault Brigade* and *3 Commando Brigade*) and a Joint Force Logistic Component (the support troops of *102 Logistic Brigade*), each with its own medical commander (commander medical, referred to as commander med), a situation that had the potential for friction in overlapping areas of operation.

Medical logistics

84 MEDICAL SUPPLY SQUADRON

Logistics underpins all medical care. The unit responsible for supplying deployed land medical assets with their specialist medical operational materiel during the whole of *Operation Telic* was *84 Medical Supply Squadron (84 MSS)*, still an RAMC unit during *Operation Telic 1* but under the command of *9 Supply Regiment Royal Logistic Corps* (RLC), with over 50% of its personnel being drawn from the RLC. *84 MSS* was formed on 1 April 2001 as a result of the 1998 Strategic Defence Review, succeeding the RAMC's eponymous *Field Medical Equipment Depot* (84 FMED), which had supported the Army Medical Services since its formation in 1986, particularly during the First Gulf War (*Operation Granby* 1990–1991) and the Balkan conflicts. *84 MSS* would formally disband as an RAMC unit and migrate to the RLC in April 2005. In March 2006, the squadron also deployed to Afghanistan on *Operation Herrick*, remaining there until October 2014, thereby earning the unique distinction of being the only unit in the Armed Forces to be permanently deployed simultaneously in both theatres for practically the whole of these two campaigns.

84 MSS was key to the operational-level medical mission, but at the time of *Operation Telic 1*, it was under-resourced in terms of transport, communications and specialist storage facilities. It also deployed relatively late into theatre considering its crucial role in meeting unit demands and distributing urgent operational requirements, a situation not helped by the fact that none of the 43 augmentees for its rear troop had any medical logistics experience. In the early stages of *Operation Telic*, this impacted on the efficiency of the whole of the *UK Medical Group*.

The importance of the need to develop and resource *84 MSS* properly in order to ensure a robust, effective and efficient medical logistic chain was a key lesson from the early stages of *Operation Telic*.[17] This was recognised and addressed by the RLC for the rest of *Operations Telic* and *Herrick* – the enduring proof of the RLC's success in this endeavour being the *European Supply Chain Excellence Award* won by the squadron for its sterling performance during *Operation Gritrock* in late 2014.[18]

Pre-hospital emergency care and primary healthcare: Role 1 and Role 2 support

Role 1 support forward was provided by *3 Commando Brigade Royal Marines*, *1 Close Support Medical Regiment* (1 CSMR) and *16 CSMR*, with attached surgical teams providing integral Role 2 support. *5 General Support Medical Regiment* (5 GSMR) would evacuate casualties from the close support (CS) regiments to hospital. *4 GSMR* provided Role 1 support on the lines of communication, evacuating casualties from hospital to the point of departure from theatre. Unlike their CS counterparts, neither of the GSMRs had attached surgical capability because of their proximity to hospital level care.

3 COMMANDO BRIGADE ROYAL MARINES

The medical assistants and doctors of *40* and *42 Commando* and the *Commando Logistic Regiment* provided Role 1 support to *3 Commando Brigade RM* during the assault on Al Faw peninsula on 20 March. Role 2 support was provided by the *Commando Forward Surgical Group* with its two surgical teams, eventually locating on the Al Faw peninsula.

1 CLOSE SUPPORT MEDICAL REGIMENT

1 CSMR, reinforced by personnel from some 40 units representing all three Services, deployed in February 2003 in support of *7 Armoured Brigade* (the Desert Rats), eventually crossing into Iraq on 22 March. It assumed a proven structure similar to that of its predecessor armoured division field ambulances, namely one forward squadron and two dressing stations (DSs) (Figure 2.4).[19]

The forward squadron had four troops each attached to a battlegroup, with A Troop in support of *Royal Scots Dragoon Guards*, B Troop in support of *2nd Royal Tank Regiment*, C Troop in support of *1st Battalion, The Royal Regiment of Fusiliers* and D Troop in support of *1st Battalion, The Black Watch*. The regimental medical officers intrinsic to each of these four battlegroups were junior and inexperienced and were therefore reinforced by a more senior medical officer from the supporting medical troop.

Each of the two DSs (DS 1A and DS 1B) had four resuscitation bays and a surgical team providing Role 2 support. DS 1A was formed from the unit's

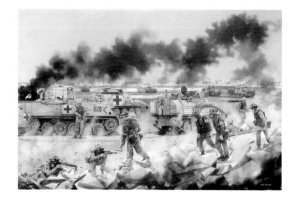

Figure 2.4 'The Sergeant Major's Packet', 28 March 2003: *1 CSMR* recovering the injured during the attack on the Ba'ath Party headquarters in Az Zubayr. (Courtesy of David Rowlands, Military Artist.)

A (29) Close Support Medical Squadron. DS 1B was provided as a formed sub-unit from *3 CSMR*, which was twinned with 1 CSMR. DS 1B would receive the bulk of casualties (including injured children) due to *7 Armoured Brigade* wishing to retain DS 1A (with its COLPRO capability) on wheels in order to move it to any location suffering a chemical warfare strike – the main perceived threat. Several of the unit's armoured and battlefield ambulances (BFAs) were hit by small-arms fire (SAF), one having a lucky escape when a rocket-propelled grenade failed to detonate on impact.[20] DS 1A moved in early April to Basra International Airport to cover the entry into Basra and to act as a diarrhoea and vomiting ward to relieve the load on *34 Field Hospital* at Shaibah. Infective gastroenteritis, exacerbated by field conditions and the heat, afflicted many troops on *Operation Telic*, particularly those advancing into areas recently vacated by Iraqi forces whose standards of environmental hygiene were severely lacking. Divisional environmental health teams were kept extremely busy, supporting individuals and units with field hygiene measures, but nonetheless, there was a continual background incidence of diarrhoea and vomiting, at times seriously impacting upon operational effectiveness. After hostilities officially ended for British coalition forces on 10 April, DS 1A moved on 13 April into the presidential palace at Basra to establish a primary healthcare facility.

A Joint *Divisional Medical Regiment* was then established from elements of *1 CSMR* and *5 GSMR* as a basis for future roulements. This included provision for the Role 2+ (equivalent to Role 2 Enhanced) facility established by *16 CSMR* at Al Amarah in Maysan Province, which was taken over by DS 1A. This facility was three hours' drive north of *34 Field Hospital's* location at Shaibah and so was particularly necessary on no-fly days when support helicopters were grounded by environmental conditions.

16 CLOSE SUPPORT MEDICAL REGIMENT

16 CSMR, together with the rest of *16 Air Assault Brigade*, received official notification on 20 December 2002 of their deployment to Kuwait on *Operation Telic*, with *16 Air Assault Brigade* being tasked with supporting the seizure of the Iraqi Rumallah oilfields. The regimental command group began

deploying on 31 January 2003, with the majority of the 286 personnel who deployed with the regiment (including reserves mainly drawn from *144 Parachute Medical Squadron [V]*, the Regiment's Territorial Army [TA] Squadron) arriving in theatre by 28 February.

16 CSMR initially deployed to concentration area *Eagle* in Kuwait before crossing into Iraq at the start of hostilities. Meanwhile, Medical Troop deployed in support of UK Special Forces. On crossing the border, *19* and *23 Air Assault Medical Squadrons* leapfrogged each other following the Brigade's rapid advance through the oilfields before reaching their final locations around Al-Amarah, where two separate bedding-down facilities had to be established to cope with the large numbers of gastroenteritis cases then being suffered by the Brigade.[21]

The unit's surgical capability was based around two *air assault surgical groups* (AASGs) providing Role 2+ support: 19 Squadron AASG, initially grouped with *3 PARA Battlegroup*, and 23 Squadron AASG. Each AASG had a resuscitation team led by an emergency medicine physician, with anaesthetic support. There were two field surgical teams (comprising one general surgeon, one orthopaedic surgeon, two anaesthetists and eight operating department practitioners) providing an optimal skill mix for performing damage control surgery, backed up by a post-operative intensive and high-dependency care area for up to four patients. During *Operation Telic*, a maximum of three intensive care unit (ICU) patients could be held simultaneously. Additional areas included a lower-dependency ward and laboratory, radiology, psychiatry, chaplaincy and physiotherapy services.

Both AASGs treated many casualties, including Iraqi prisoners of war during the offensive operations of 20 March to 10 April, as well as dealing with several multi-casualty incidents involving critically ill patients, demonstrating the utility of this template for a generic light Role 2+ facility.[22] The AASG depended heavily on a robust evacuation system. This was provided largely by the Regiment's own BFAs in the absence of dedicated UK CASEVAC helicopters, with UK support helicopters being in short supply. The United States did, however, provide several dedicated Blackhawk CASEVAC helicopters in support of *1st (UK) Armoured Division* during warfighting operations.

The unit redeployed to Maysan Province once offensive operations ceased, setting up a surgical Role 2+ facility at Al Amarah. In total, the unit treated 2752 patients on *Operation Telic 1* broadly categorised as 18 priority one, 64 priority two, 2686 priority three (walking casualties), 31 surgical cases and 10 ventilated transfers.[23]

4 GENERAL SUPPORT MEDICAL REGIMENT

4 GSMR, together with *22 Field Hospital* and *33 Field Hospital*, all normally part of *101 Logistic Brigade*, deployed to Kuwait to provide integral medical support to *102 Logistic Brigade* instead, in its role as *Joint Force Logistic Component* (JFLogC). *E (13) Squadron* deployed to the Forward Concentration Area at Camp Coyote to cover the integration training of the arriving troops of *1st (UK) Armoured Division*, while the Regimental Headquarter (RHQ) and Headquarters (HQ) Squadron initially set up at the Rear Support Area at Camp Fox. *A (11) Medical Squadron*, initially co-located at Camp Fox, provided area medical support (primary care) from Kuwait International Airport (the Air Port of Disembarkation [APOD]) up the main supply routes to Camp Coyote.

Just prior to D Day, Tactical HQ and A Squadron moved to Camp Coyote. A Squadron handed over the area medical support in the south to the US Army in order to take on the ground tactical medical evacuation (TACEVAC) role, taking patients from *202 Field Hospital (V)* in Camp Coyote to the RAF's Air Staging Unit at Kuwait International Airport. This necessitated the hiring of several 25-seater coaches for ambulatory patients as the regiment had only deployed with BFAs.

E Squadron split its assets, with medical teams supporting internally displaced persons aid distribution points while a troop provided area medical support to *17 Port and Maritime Regiment RLC* and *23 Pioneer Regiment RLC*, at the main Iraqi port of Um Qasr (whose reputation earned this duty the nickname *Operation Certain Death*). The rest of *E Squadron* then moved forward to Um Qasr along with HQ 102 Logistic Brigade, which had split in two to facilitate the Logistic Brigade, moving forward in direct support of the advancing fighting brigades of *1st (UK) Armoured Division*, leaving half its staff behind to run HQ JFLogC in Camp Arifjan in Kuwait. E Squadron also projected its ambulance

troop north to support *34 Field Hospital* in Shaibah, thereby providing a northern hospital evacuation loop down to *202 Field Hospital* in Camp Coyote.

The rest of the Regiment stayed at Camp Coyote, with A Squadron continuing to provide area medical support and ground TACEVAC for the southern hospital evacuation loop to the APOD. One BFA was despatched to provide medical cover for the team moving north to re-open the UK Embassy in Baghdad, earning the regiment the distinction of being the only British medical unit to reach Baghdad on *Operation Telic 1*, evidenced by a photograph in the Corps Magazine of the BFA crew in front of the *Swords of Qadisiyah*.[24]

The RHQ, HQ Squadron and A Squadron returned to the United Kingdom in May. E Squadron, reinforced with emergency department staff from *202 Field Hospital (V)* in anticipation of the inevitable heat casualties among un-acclimatised incoming troops, remained behind in Camp Coyote until July to provide medical support during the reception, staging, onward movement and integration of troops arriving for *Operation Telic 2*. The regiment's two TA medical squadrons, namely the Maidstone-based *220 (Home Counties)* and the *Leicester-based 222 (East Midlands)*, combined forces to deploy as an aptly named 22 Medical Squadron to form the CS Squadron on *Operation Telic 2*.

5 GENERAL SUPPORT MEDICAL REGIMENT

5 GSMR (like *4 GSMR*) was a wheeled unit rather than an armoured one, that is, one with vehicles that did not have armour protection. Nonetheless, unlike *4 GSMR*, it retained a CS Squadron (A Squadron), based on the old field ambulance structure of DS and medical sections, to provide the manoeuvre reserve for the divisional commander medical to support the operations of the forward fighting Brigades, while B Squadron normally provided area medical support (primary care) in the divisional rear area. Its evacuation function also differed from its sister regiment in that it evacuated casualties from the forward squadrons of the CS medical regiments to the deployed field hospitals.

For *Operation Telic*, it was decided that A Squadron would not provide a manoeuvre capability and that the Reservist B Squadron would not be deploying. A Squadron was therefore re-organised to provide area medical support while retaining the ability to reform the CS Squadron as necessary. To maintain flexibility, Troop HQs were deployed forwards with some ambulances for immediate response to incidents, with the rest of the BFAs in reserve. An Ambulance Control Cell was embedded in Divisional HQ, while A Squadron's HQ stayed on the ground as a focus for the reserve.

The last of the unit's personnel and equipment arrived in theatre barely 48 hours before the start of the land campaign, deploying forwards to support the Brigades. The Regiment was tasked with providing area medical support in the divisional rear area, including the Corps' prisoner of war holding facility, evacuation of battle casualties in the rear area directly to *202 Field Hospital (V)*, evacuation of casualties from the forward Squadrons of the CS medical regiments and the *Commando Medical Squadron* to *34* and *202 Field Hospitals* and provision of infrastructure support to divisional psychiatric and environmental health assets. *5 GSMR* also became responsible for managing the divisional medical radio communication net for the whole of the Medical Group, as well as providing specialist Medical Logistic staff to the Medical Branch of *1st (UK) Armoured Division*.

As the fighting brigades moved forward into Iraq, RHQ and D Squadron initially moved forward near the border town of Safwan. Once Basra was secured, they moved to Shaibah airfield to provide support to *4 GSMR* in moving casualties from *34 Field Hospital* to an ambulance exchange point just within the Kuwaiti border. E Squadron remained with the fighting brigades throughout, with its BFAs variously approaching Basra from the Al Faw peninsula in support of *3 Commando Brigade*, entering Basra with *7 Armoured Brigade*, moving as far north as Al Amarah with *16 Air Assault Brigade* and running the gauntlet of the border crossing point at Safwan. During the campaign, *5 GSMR* saw and treated some 1500 patients (including enemy prisoners of war) and evacuated some 900 casualties (allied and enemy military and Iraqi civilians).[25]

Deployed hospital care – Role 3 support (forward and rear) on Operation Telic 1

RFA Argus (with the sole computed tomography [CT] scanner for British troops) provided Role 3 support afloat (the maritime term being Echelon 3), while Role 3 support ashore was provided by *22, 33, 34* and *202 Field Hospitals*.[26]

RFA ARGUS (PCRF)

RFA Argus deployed on 15 January 2003 and was operational as a 100-bed PCRF in the North Arabian Gulf by mid-February, where she would potentially be well positioned to receive casualties from land operations. In practice, the lack of dedicated CASEVAC helicopters militated against this. She was designated as a Force asset and available for Coalition casualties, although her primary role would be in support of *3 Commando Brigade's* assault on the Al Faw peninsula and providing Echelon 3 support to maritime operations.[27]

From H Hour on 21 March until being stood down on 9 April, the PCRF treated four UK battle casualties, one US battle casualty, 25 prisoners of war, eight displaced persons, 29 non-battle casualties, 50 disease & non-battle injury (DNBI) patients, 374 dental patients, and 138 physiotherapy patients. Sixty-six surgical procedures were conducted, 25% of patients needed CT scanning and 34% of patients were admitted to the intensive care unit. No deaths occurred at the PCRF.[28]

The inability to transfer critically ill and unstable patients from medical units ashore to *RFA Argus* for CT scanning during the warfighting phase underscored the clinical necessity for field hospitals to be provided with their own CT scanner, a deficiency finally rectified in March 2005.[29]

22 FIELD HOSPITAL

22 Field Hospital, then based at Thornhill Barracks, Aldershot, was not originally designated to deploy on *Operation Telic* as it had been extended in role to cover Balkan operations so that *34 Field Hospital* could deploy. However, the planned deployment of *33 Field Hospital's* equipment on 28 January 2003 was delayed at Marchwood Military Port by Greenpeace protestors, so *22 Field Hospital* was urgently tasked by PJHQ to provide an early Role 3 capability in Kuwait during the force generation phase until a 200-bed hospital could be established. The facility was to be supported by robust tactical evacuation and to observe a strictly limited holding policy.

The unit deployed an air-portable 25-bed-capability hospital troop to Camp Coyote (the divisional concentration area, in Kuwait) on 10 February 2003, with less than 10 days' planning and preparation. The unit's equipment, packed into nine standard ISO containers and two Reefers (refrigerated containers), was carried on board a chartered Ukrainian Antonov aircraft. The hospital troop comprised 55 personnel in all (25 cadre staff to provide the command and logistic elements, together with 30 clinical personnel previously nominated to deploy with *33 Field Hospital*). The unit declared full operating capability on 12 February, within three days of arrival in theatre, in effect providing what would now be termed a *Role 2 Enhanced* capability.

Its 25-bed capability was deemed sufficient to support the initial population at risk (PAR) of 3,500 personnel; however, the PAR rose to 23,812 during the three weeks that this hospital was open (its planned period of operating had to be extended until 6 March 2003), before it could be relieved by *33 Field Hospital* once all that hospital's equipment and clinical modules arrived in theatre. During this time, it treated over 600 patients and had over 240 admissions, reaching a peak of 74 inpatients on one day.

This was the second time in just over 12 months that a 25-bed Role 2 Enhanced UK facility had been deployed by air to support operations, although no formal doctrine yet existed for this concept. The previous occasion had been the deployment of a hospital troop by *34 Field Hospital* to Bagram airport, northern Afghanistan, on *Operation Fingal*, from 23 December 2001 to May 2002.[30] Both deployments highlighted the need to formalise this useful air deployable capability. After *33 Field Hospital* had conducted a relief in place (RIP) and handed over to *202 Field Hospital (V)* on 17 March, *22 Field Hospital's* staff and equipment were subsumed into *33 Field Hospital* to become the theatre medical reserve at Camp Coyote, before returning to Aldershot once the reserve was stood down.[31,32]

33 FIELD HOSPITAL

33 Field Hospital, based at Fort Blockhouse, Gosport, commenced internal preparations for deployment in October 2002, before receiving the formal force generation order on 6 January 2003 to prepare to deploy a 200-bed and seven surgical

team capability on *Operation Telic*, with some 400 plus clinical personnel being drawn from a wide variety of other units. The hospital was to be sited within the tactical assembly area (Camp Coyote) to deal with DNBI patients and then provide Role 3 support during the advance into Iraq.

Prior preparation and planning for medical force protection had resulted in the cadre staff already being almost 100% vaccinated as necessary – the augmentees were not as well prepared by their parent units, a lesson identified for the future. *33 Field Hospital* was placed under the operational command of *102 Logistic Brigade* (deploying from Germany) rather than its parent *101 Logistic Brigade*, which presented a peculiar set of logistic and administrative challenges. The blockade of Marchwood Maritime Port on 28 January by the Greenpeace vessel Rainbow Warrior then caused significant delays in shipping the unit's 86 ISO containers' worth of equipment and necessitated the urgent interim deployment of a hospital troop from *22 Field Hospital*.

The unit's equipment eventually arrived in Camp Coyote in Kuwait by 20 February, and an impressively large 200-bed tented Hospital complex, including a 50-bed COLPRO element erected solely by the two attached military bands, was established within three days. The hospital declared full operating capability on 6 March (Figure 2.5). The unit's reassuring presence provided a significant confidence booster to deployed troops regarding their medical support.[33]

Between taking over from *22 Field Hospital* on 6 March and handing over command on 17 March,

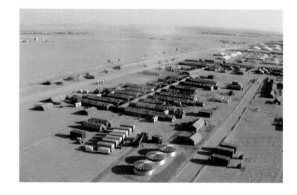

Figure 2.5 *33 Field Hospital* at Camp Coyote, Kuwait.

33 Field Hospital admitted over 360 patients, including minor orthopaedic and general surgery cases, a small amount of trauma and a significant number suffering from medical conditions.[34] On 17 March, three days before the warfighting phase commenced, *33 Field Hospital* handed over the 200-bed complex to *202 Field Hospital (V)*, thereafter forming the theatre medical reserve before returning to the United Kingdom on 10 April in preparation for redeployment on *Operation Telic 2*.

34 FIELD HOSPITAL

34 Field Hospital, based at Strensall near York, commenced preparation for *Operation Telic* in late 2002, finally receiving its force generation order in early February 2003. It deployed its equipment by sea on 14 February, and its personnel from 16 February onwards. It would play a key part in all four phases of *Operation Telic 1*: preparation, shaping the battlespace, ground operations and post-conflict resolution.

The medical plan required *34 Field Hospital* to be held on wheels (that is ready to move) at a tactical assembly area ready to be deployed forward into Iraq at the earliest opportunity in support of combat operations. It initially set up a 25-bed facility just within the Kuwaiti border, before deploying in stages into Iraq from G Day +4 to G Day +7 to establish a robust 200-bed facility on 26 March at its final destination (Shaibah Airfield, some 4 km west of Az Zubayr and 13 km south of Basra, the site of RAF Shaibah in the Second World War and now designated to become a Logistic Base). *7 Armoured Brigade* was still fiercely contesting the area as *34 Field Hospital* deployed to Shaibah, with the airfield being hit repeatedly by indirect fire (IDF) during the building of the hospital, and with *34 Field Hospital* actually deploying forward of *1 CSMR* and its integral Role 2 surgical teams in order to best deliver critical Role 3 medical support during the warfighting. Casualties were delivered directly by armoured ambulances from Role 1 to Role 3, largely negating the need for damage control surgery at Role 2.

By the time *34 Field Hospital* handed over its Role 3 commitment at Shaibah to *202 Field Hospital (V)* on 16 May 2003, it had treated 3500 patients, admitted 2100 of these and carried out 420 surgical operations. Its busiest period was between 27 March and 12 April, with its bed occupancy averaging 185. Most admissions during this period were victims of a large outbreak of gastroenteritis, which seriously affected many units, including the hospital itself, whose own staff accounted for a third of the admissions, largely as a result of the premature introduction of locally sourced fresh rations (including salads and fruit) before rigorous environmental health measures could be fully implemented.[35]

The hospital also treated numerous injured civilians, but it was the large number of paediatric casualties, and the lack of basic paediatric equipment, that created the most angst, especially as requests for paediatric equipment had been repeatedly staffed before and during the warfighting phase but had been consistently rejected or demands diluted.[36] A similar situation would be faced by *202 Field Hospital (V)*.

202 (MIDLANDS) FIELD HOSPITAL RAMC (VOLUNTEERS)

202 Field Hospital (V), based in Birmingham, had been the lead TA field hospital within *2 Medical Brigade* since April 2001, transitioning to high readiness (R5, ready for mobilisation at five days' notice) following recommendations in the recent Strategic Defence Review. It had increased its capability from 100 beds in November 2001 to 200 beds by November 2002. It had also been validated early at full operational capability on *Exercise Log Viper* in September 2002, thereby becoming the only TA hospital with this capability at R5. This had a direct bearing on the decision to mobilise this hospital for *Operation Telic*.[37] Following a protracted period of informal warning orders and false starts between August 2002 and February 2003, *202 Field Hospital (V)* personnel were compulsorily mobilised in early March and deployed to Kuwait in time to conduct an RIP with *33 Field Hospital* in Camp Coyote on 17 March. This deployment necessitated augmentation by individuals from 18 other units to achieve its full warfighting establishment of 566 personnel.

It was originally envisaged that *202 Field Hospital (V)* would primarily receive UK and Coalition casualties, with *34 Field Hospital* being designated as the receiving unit for Iraqi prisoners of war. In the event, *202 Field Hospital (V)* received Iraqi prisoners of war as well as wounded Iraqi civilians. These included a significant proportion of burns as well as paediatric casualties for whom the hospital was neither equipped nor formally staffed. The fortuitous presence of a consultant paediatrician deployed as a physician, and an ingenious anaesthetist, made a considerable difference, but it served to highlight the need to prepare adequately for such casualties.[38]

In addition to its integral clinical capability, *202 Field Hospital* was reinforced by the theatre burns, maxillo-facial and neurosurgical teams during the warfighting. This concentration (a concept proven in the First World War) produced economy of effort, with the burns team seeing the equivalent of a year's peacetime work within a month, although the neurosurgical team was hampered by the lack of a CT scanner as well as delayed arrival of its instruments.[39]

During the warfighting phase between 19 March and 21 April, some 1366 patients were admitted to the hospital, with 63 requiring intensive care. A further 1000 patients were treated by the emergency department but not admitted. The operating department treated over 160 patients, 23 being children. The specialist burns unit treated over 60 cases.[40]

Once the warfighting phase had ended, the hospital at Camp Coyote was drawn down and *202 Field Hospital* redeployed to Shaibah Logistics Base to conduct their second relief in place, on 16 May 2003, taking over the temporary tented facility established by *34 Field Hospital*. They then constructed a more environmentally robust, although still tented, hospital alongside this – a facility that would become known as *British Military Hospital (BMH) Shaibah* (Figure 2.6).

202 Field Hospital returned to the United Kingdom in July 2003 on being relieved by *33 Field Hospital*. Some of its experience was documented in two articles in the *Journal of the RAMC*.[41,42] The unit's major contribution to *Operation Telic* was recorded in an e-book initially covering only *Operation Telic 1* but later revised to form a comprehensive although unofficial medical history of the whole *Telic* campaign.[43,44] *202 Field Hospital* featured prominently in a book commemorating 100 years of the Territorials,[45] and a recently published unit history also covers *Operation Telic*.[46]

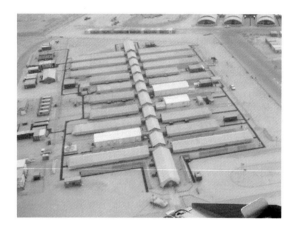

Figure 2.6 British Military Hospital Shaibah.

PRE-HOSPITAL EMERGENCY CARE, PRIMARY HEALTHCARE AND DEPLOYED HOSPITAL CARE: UK MEDICAL GROUP *OPERATION TELIC 2–13*

As this chapter does not purport to be a comprehensive medical history of *Operation Telic* or *Operation Herrick*, only salient points or major organisational changes are noted here. The reader should refer to Chapter 1 for greater situational awareness as operational activity invariably affected the clinical tempo and the way medical assets were organised.

Operation Telic 2 *(July to October 2003)*

UK MEDICAL GROUP

Following the drawdown of combat and medical forces in theatre at the end of *Operation Telic 1*, and the formation of *Multinational Division (Southeast)*, MND(SE), on 12 July, at the start of *Operation Telic 2*, a UK Medical Group was formed on 28 August 2003. This brought all medical assets under a single RHQ. The *UK Medical Group* (with its support, CS and hospital squadrons) provided Role 1 to Role 3 medical support to both UK and multinational forces within the MND(SE) area of operations.

In *Operation Telic 2*, the RHQ, Hospital Squadron and Support Squadron were provided by *33 Field*

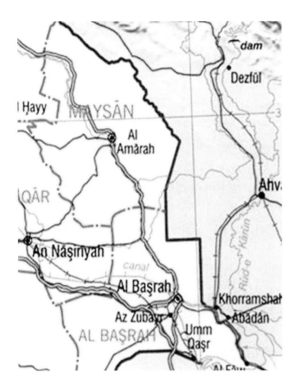

Figure 2.7 Area of responsibility, UK Medical Group.

Hospital (which had taken over BMH Shaibah on 24 July as well as the Role 2+ detachment at Al Amarah).

The CS Medical Squadron (largely provided by *22 Medical Squadron* from *4 GSMR*) had its squadron HQ at Basra Palace, but its evacuation and patient transfer capability was dispersed across Al Basrah and Maysan Provinces.[47] The latter province was the size of Northern Ireland; its long border with Iran allowed free passage of insurgents, and its principal city, Al Amarah, was 200 km north of Basra (Figure 2.7).

COMMAND AND CONTROL

Before the formation of the *UK Medical Group*, the command structure was clear: *33 Field Hospital* was under operational command of *Joint Force Logistic Component*, soon to become *HQ National Support Element*. On formation of the *UK Medical Group*, the commanding officer (CO) of the lead unit supplying the RHQ (initially *33 Field Hospital*, in future either the deploying medical regiment or the field hospital) became *de facto* CO of the *UK*

Medical Group. The *UK Medical Group* became responsible both to HQ MND(SE) and to HQ NSE: it was under the tactical command of HQ MND(SE) and operational control of HQ NSE. Simultaneously, a commander medical, with his own staff branch, was appointed in an advisory role (as Force Medical Advisor) within divisional HQ at MND(SE).

The new command structure unfortunately led to confusion. A workable solution evolved whereby clearly national business (such as UK personnel requiring aeromed) became directed to and from NSE, whereas multinational business (for example Iraqi hospital liaison or coalition forces patient tracking) became the responsibility of MND(SE).[48]

The existence of a commander medical as well as a CO *UK Medical Group* would occasionally create additional friction on future tours, especially if a particular commander medical 'thought that he was [in command]'.[49] This was rectified on *Operation Telic 11*, when the two roles were combined simultaneously with the integration of the separate brigade and divisional HQs into a single HQ.

There was similar confusion and friction on *Operation Herrick 10* and *11*, until the restructuring of RC (South) on *Operation Herrick 12* combined both roles under commander medical. The confusing medical command status on the early *Operation Telic* tours emphasises the necessity for clarity in command structures. During their tour on *Operation Telic 2*, *33 Field Hospital* treated about 1700 patients and performed over 170 surgical operations.

Operation Telic 3 (November 2003 to April 2004)

Operations in Iraq during *Operation Telic 3* proved very demanding particularly for the CS medical squadron, stretched thin on the ground. The first two months of the campaign were dominated by the counterterrorist battle against fanatical Fedayeen and foreign fighters. Success in this battle produced a temporary mid-tour lull in clinical activity as *20 Armoured Brigade* focussed on building capacity in the Iraqi Security Forces (ISF) and wider Iraqi institutions. The final month was dominated by a sudden surge in combat casualties during the First Sadr Uprising, which saw the first use by insurgents of multiple co-ordinated suicide car bomb attacks, together with 122-mm rocket attacks against all British bases.

Operation Telic 4 *(May to October 2004)*

The *UK Medical Group* was heavily involved in caring for casualties during both the First Sadr Uprising (April to May) and the Second Sadr Uprising (2 to 26 August). A Role 2 (-) DS was deployed at the end of October on *Operation Bracken*, the *Black Watch* mission to Fallujah in support of a US offensive against fanatical Sunni insurgents holding the town. This DS would see serious action on 4 November when a suicide bomber caused multiple casualties, including the first death to suicide bombing amongst UK troops.

Operation Telic 5 *(November 2004 to April 2005)*

The *UK Medical Group* on *Operation Telic 5*, whose cadre hospital and medical regiment staff deployed for six months, was supplemented by Regular and Reservist augmentees from 72 different units with 22 different cap badges, typically serving between four and six weeks (consultants in the Regulars) and three months (Reservists).[50] This mixture and the frequent turnover of clinical staff was typical of other *Operation Telic* (and eventually *Operation Herrick*) tours and presented a continual and considerable challenge both in bringing personnel together for pre-deployment training and in managing the clinical churn during deployment. It did, however, have the considerable benefit of rapidly disseminating combat experience and knowledge of best practice widely across the DMS, and as personnel began to return for repeated tours, the learning curve was reduced. The strength of the whole *UK Medical Group* on *Operation Telic 5* was 330 personnel.

UK MEDICAL GROUP COMPOSITION

The RHQ and support squadron, the HQs of both the hospital and CS squadrons, and the hospital squadron were now all co-located at Shaibah Logistics Base. Role 1 assets were based at Al Amarah, Basra City and Shaibah. The Role 2+

facility at Al Amarah and an Emergency Medicine (EM) ward at Shatt Al Arab Hotel in Basra completed the *UK Medical Group*.

NEW HOSPITAL BUILD & CT SCANNER

During the early stages of *Operation Telic 5*, the new tented field hospital structure was completed at Shaibah, although the move into it had to be delayed. A state-of-the-art multi-slice CT scanner, with a teleradiology link to the *Centre for Defence Imaging* at Royal Hospital Haslar, was installed at the new hospital, being commissioned on 4 March 2005. This was the first time a British field hospital had been equipped with CT capability.[51]

CLINICAL TEMPO

Perhaps the most portentous incident during this tour occurred on 20 January 2005, when a suicide bomber detonated his vehicle-borne improvised explosive device (IED) at the main gate of Shaibah Logistics Base, resulting in eight UK casualties (of whom four were evacuated to the United Kingdom) and 12 Iraqi civilian casualties, including one fatality. In March 2005, the increasing threat to soldiers 'outside the wire' resulted in three Saxon ambulances arriving in theatre to begin replacing the vulnerable soft-skinned BFAs previously used by the CS Squadron. By the end of the tour, the *UK Medical Group* had treated 6467 primary healthcare patients, admitted 1069 patients to Role 3, performed over 80 surgical procedures and evacuated 219 patients out of theatre.

Operation Telic 6 *(May to October 2005)*

During this deployment, the *UK Medical Group* was involved in numerous battlegroup and brigade operations as the Iranians escalated the conflict through their militia proxies in Iraq. The presence of a medical support officer as an embedded liaison officer at Brigade HQ ensured that medical advice was always readily available and that medical planning was instituted at an early phase. The new tented (Tier 1) field hospital continued to undergo development with the addition of several Portakabin (Tier 2) buildings.

The turbulence caused by the frequent rotation of consultant clinical staff, usually deploying for only four to six weeks, caused increasing concern during this period of heightened activity. This rapid turnover had most impact on the efficiency of the critical role of clinical director, with seven personnel filling this role over this particular six-month tour. This issue, which seriously impacted all the *Operation Telic* and early *Operation Herrick* tours, would eventually lead to the creation of the standalone appointment of the deployed medical director (DMD) at Camp Bastion, from April 2009 (*Operation Herrick 10*) onwards.[52]

CLINICAL TEMPO

By the end of *Operation Telic 6*, the *UK Medical Group* had treated 6886 primary healthcare patients, admitted 801 patients to Role 3, performed over 168 surgical procedures and evacuated 269 patients out of theatre.[53]

Operation Telic 7 *(November 2005 to April 2006)*

COMMAND STATUS

During *Operation Telic 7*, the *UK Medical Group* command status changed from operational control by UK NSE to operational control by MND(SE). This formalised what had been occurring and lessened scope for confusion, creating a more efficient structure.

FORCE PROTECTION

The increasingly sophisticated IED and IDF campaign against coalition troops and the inadequate protection provided against these by BFAs led to the urgent request for new wheeled armoured ambulances, with nine more upgraded Saxon ambulances being issued as an interim measure. As the Saxons had limited utility in close urban areas, combat medical technicians were deployed inside Warriors for patrols within Basra.

Operation Telic 8 *(May to October 2006)*

RHQ & SUPPORT SQUADRON

These were provided by *22 Field Hospital* (which concurrently provided a hospital squadron to support the deployment of *16 Air Assault Brigade*

into Afghanistan on *Operation Herrick 4*). The *UK Medical Group* deployed straight into theatre in Iraq from pre-deployment HOSPEX training at the *AMS Training Centre* (AMSTC) in York to maintain the operational tempo and focus. This proved invaluable as, immediately upon taking over in theatre, both the CS squadron and the hospital squadron were faced with casualties from a crashed Lynx and an IED attack upon Multi-National Force troops. This set the scene for the rest of the tour as insurgent activity steadily increased, resulting in more casualties from IEDs and from complex direct and indirect fire attacks within the urban environments of Basra City and Al Amarah.

MND(SE) had recognised the difficulty of trying to control Basra City with one Battle Group HQ by instead dividing responsibility for the city in two, with the creation of *Basra City North BG* and *Basra City South BG*. Medical support was accordingly split, initially with a regimental aid post at Basra Palace supporting *Basra City South BG* and a larger medical troop at the Shatt Al Arab Hotel supporting *Basra City North BG*. The imbalance was eventually addressed by the incremental creation of a medical troop capability at Basra Palace, with relocation of staff when the Shaibah Logistic Base Primary Healthcare Medical Facility was closed in December 2006.

The closure of Camp Abu Naji in Maysan Province in August 2006 resulted in the medical troop at Maysan being drawn down and reinvested to form a Divisional Medical Reserve. Concurrently, the *UK Medical Group* was able to deploy two crewed BFAs and an emergency nurse to support the Maysan Battle Group on desert and border operations. The freeing up of medical manpower also allowed the *UK Medical Group* to take on medical support to the *Divisional Temporary Detention Facility* and assure healthcare delivery there.[54]

As a result of this rebalancing, the *UK Medical Group* was now better placed to provide medical support to deliberate security operations in Basra City. During *Operation Sinbad* (the major combined Coalition and Iraqi Army operation against the death squads, militias and rogue police, 20 September 2006 to 14 January 2007),[55] the CS squadron flexed the *Divisional Medical Reserve* between the two medical troops supporting Basra City North and South battlegroups.

Each battlegroup had a full complement of team medics (with combat medical technicians deployed as dismounts in Warriors, backed up by Saxon Ambulances and evacuation by helicopter).

In the meantime, the *UK Medical Group* was also preparing to move the Hospital Squadron from BMH Shaibah to a new Tier 2 location nearing completion by the *Royal Engineers* at the *Contingency Operating Base* (COB) at Basra Air Station, the *Royal Engineers* by now being adept at field hospital construction.[56]

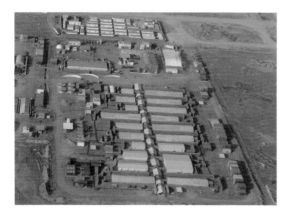

Figure 2.8 BMH Basra, the Tier 2 Hospital location at COB, Basra Air Station (note the concrete blast walls around hospital departments for protection against IDF).

Operation Telic 9 (November 2006 to April 2007)

MOVE TO THE COB

The first half of the tour was marked by the successful move (*Operation Revenant*) of the *UK Medical Group* from Horsley Lines at Shaibah Logistics Base to its new location at the COB, in the first week of January 2007 (Figures 2.8 and 2.9).

The *UK Medical Group* would remain at the COB for the rest of *Operation Telic*. This tour witnessed a substantial increase in the tempo of hostile action (with many casualties from IEDs, IDF and SAF (Figures 2.10–2.12), including injuries and two deaths from within the ranks of the CS medical squadron.[57,58]

Lance Corporal Rory Mackenzie RAMC combat medical technician, whose personal account opened this chapter, sustained a traumatic above-knee amputation of his right leg due to an IED blast under his Warrior on 21 January 2007 – his life was saved by the rapid application of a tourniquet.[59] Corporal Kris O'Neil RAMC and Private Eleanor Dlugosz RAMC, combat medical technicians from *3 CSMR*, together with three other soldiers from *2nd Battalion Duke of Lancaster's Regiment Battle Group*, were killed on patrol in Basra on 5 April 2007 when another IED destroyed their Warrior.

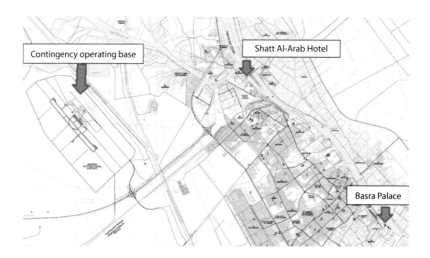

Figure 2.9 British bases in Basra.

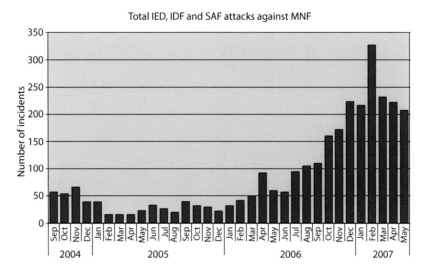

Figure 2.10 Increased tempo of Hostile Action experienced on *Operation Telic 9*. (From Operation TELIC 9 – UK Medical Group Post Operational Report, dated 25 June 2007.)

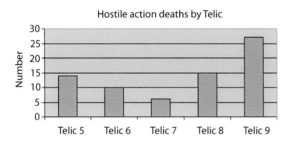

Figure 2.11 UK fatalities from hostile action on *Operation Telic 5–9*.

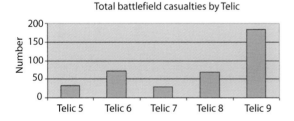

Figure 2.12 UK battlefield casualties on *Operation Telic 5–9*.

Operation Telic 10 *(May to October 2007)*

From a medical support perspective, *Operation Telic 10* can be considered in two phases based solely on the UK military casualty load from hostile action, the dividing line being the temporary ceasefire negotiated with al-Fartusi's *Jaish al-Mahdi* (JAM) militia in July. The tour began with the difficult challenge of conducting the relief in place of a force in contact, with the exceptionally high tempo carrying on from *Operation Telic 9*. The first two months alone saw more casualties received at the Role 2 (Enhanced) Hospital (now BMH Basra) than during the whole of *Operation Telic 8*, with IDF attacks causing practically as many casualties as IEDs. Frequent strategic aeromedical evacuation flights (running, on average, twice a week for the first three months, thereafter weekly) enabled this casualty load to be accommodated, particularly in ICU. The hospital itself was not immune from IDF, with four 122-mm rockets exploding on or immediately around it in July and August (Figure 2.13).[60]

The dangers faced during ground evacuation in Basra meant that CASEVAC from the scene of wounding had hitherto been largely by helicopter, although this became riskier as the surface to air threat increased and safe helicopter landing sites reduced in number with the British withdrawing from the city centre. The arrival of twelve Bulldog armoured ambulances in theatre during *Operation Telic 10* transformed the provision of battlefield treatment and evacuation.

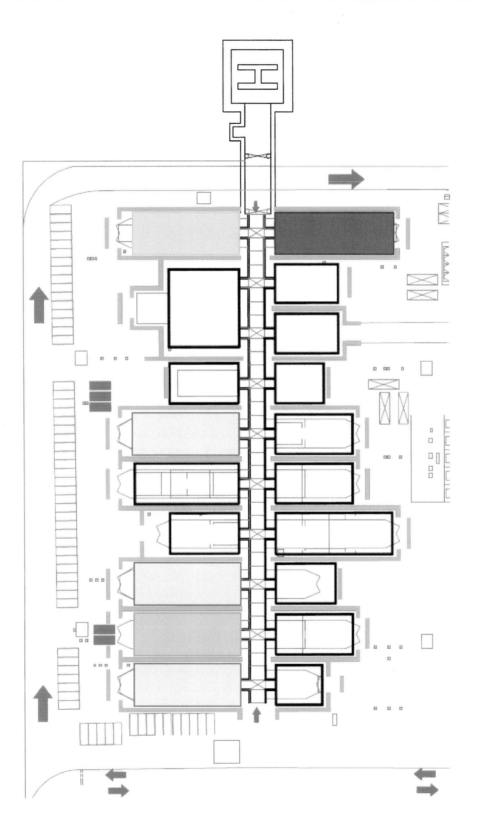

Figure 2.13 Floor plan of COB Hospital on *Operation Telic 11*, showing blast walls between tented departments. Compare with Figure 2.8 (aerial photo, *Operation Telic 9*). The emergency department resuscitation room is in red, the minor injuries area in yellow and operating theatres are in the square block adjacent to minor injuries. The wards are in blue, and physiotherapy, in green. The pathology laboratory is next to the operating theatres. ICU and X-ray are across the corridor opposite the operating theatres. Other elements include welfare, management, pharmacy and the evacuation cell.

Operation Telic 11 *(November 2007 to April 2008)*

COMMAND STATUS

The HQ structure on *Operation Telic 11* moved from separate Brigade and Divisional constructs to an integrated HQ in January 2008. The CO *UK Medical Group* (on *Operation Telic 11* the CO of 1 CSMR) was simultaneously appointed as Commander Medical, which assisted in easing the transition to the integrated HQ.

HOSPITAL SQUADRON

Unusually, on this tour, *1 CSMR* was tasked to provide the hospital squadron for BMH Basra rather than this being supplied by either a regular or reservist field hospital. This necessitated the re-roling of one of its own CS Squadrons (D Squadron) to form the hospital squadron nucleus. There was initial trepidation at this tasking, particularly due to lack of familiarity with running the *Hospital Management Cell*. However, early engagement with AMSTC had allowed a planned programme of relevant pre-deployment courses and training, including exposure to several HOSPEXs. The experiment succeeded in its aim, with the Hospital Squadron and particularly the hospital management cell coping efficiently with the flow of casualties during three major medical incidents in just over two days, with the result that it was repeated for *Operation Telic 12* (when *3 CSMR* would provide the Hospital Squadron).

FORCE PROTECTION

In response to the increased threat of IEDs, the new Mastiff Protected Mobility Ambulance was deployed in February 2008, providing an impressively higher level of protection than the older Saxons and FV432s it replaced. Mastiff also provided an excellent treatment platform forward, enabling greater flexibility in medical planning, particularly valued during *Operation Charge of the Knights*.

OPERATION CHARGE OF THE KNIGHTS

'There are 15 casualties arriving via IRT in one minute, unknown triage category'.

Message received at BMH Basra signalling the third trauma call of the shift, and the third major medical incident in three days, during the Battle for Basra (*Operation Charge of the Knights*, March–April 2008).[61]

Al-Fartusi's JAM militia had renewed their rocket attacks against the British in January 2008, as well as reinforcing their hold over Basra City and channelling funds and fuel to the ongoing civil war in Baghdad. Faced with this serious threat to his government, the now emboldened Iraqi Prime Minister Maliki launched *Operation Charge of the Knights* on 25 March to retake Basra City, initially with Iraqi forces alone but soon reinforced by US and UK assets, including provision of medical support. The *UK Medical Group* focus switched overnight from supporting coalition forces in a defensive posture at the COB to supporting combined operations with the ISF, inevitably leading to the admission of large numbers of ISF and civilian casualties with the attendant challenges. The peak of activity was in the first week, with the hospital dealing with three major medical incidents within three days (Figure 2.14).

The successful outcome of *Operation Charge of the Knights* resulted in freedom of manoeuvre and movement throughout Basra City and the Province being restored to the level of safety achieved at the end of *Operation Telic 1* in 2003. The number of British casualties fell to their lowest level yet and remained equally low hereafter.[62]

Operation Telic 12 *(May to October 2008)*

COMMAND STATUS

The command structure introduced on the previous *Operation Telic* tour (with the CO of the *UK Medical Group* taking on the role of Commander Medical) had worked well, so it was retained for this tour. Similarly, *3 CSMR*, deployed on this tour,

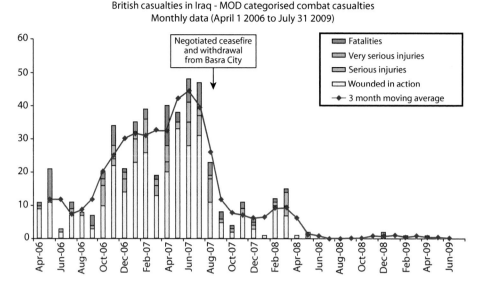

Figure 2.14 British Combat Casualties in Iraq, 2006–2009. (From Casualty Monitor. British Casualties: Iraq. http://www.casualty-monitor.org/p/iraq.html.)

was tasked with providing the Hospital Squadron in addition to RHQ and CS Squadron. *Operation Telic 12* marked the turning point in the campaign as the emphasis changed to mentoring and embedded training with the ISF. No UK personnel died or were injured as a result of enemy action on this tour, for the first time on *Operation Telic* (Figure 2.14).

Operation Telic 13 *(November 2008 to May 2009)*

The focus on this tour was the phased withdrawal of British troops from Iraq under *Operation Brockdale* and the transition to US Forces. The maintenance of effective and appropriate medical support during this dynamic period of transition presented planning and logistic challenges, with the Med Group (led by *22 Field Hospital*) moving from an enduring to a more expeditionary footing. Fortunately, the greatly improved performance of the Iraqi Army meant less insurgent activity and, therefore, significantly fewer casualties.

The Role 2 Enhanced hospital reconfigured internally to a reduced 2/2/2/10 capacity (two emergency bays, two operating theatres, two ICU beds and 10 intermediate care beds) while absorbing and successfully integrating US medical teams (*2/4*

BCT 'Charlie' Med Company and *274 Field Surgical Team*) prior to transfer of authority.

The CS medical squadron, from *1 Medical Regiment*, with its now battle-proven Bulldog and Mastiff ambulances, continued to provide close and local area support to a variety of enduring and framework operations until final departure from theatre.

Overall, the concept of a unified *UK Medical Group* based on a single RHQ, with prehospital and deployed hospital care battlegrouped into different squadrons, worked well on *Operation Telic*, providing the flexibility and co-ordination to support a variety of operations and providing the whole spectrum of care from point of wounding to surgery and evacuation from theatre under one command.[63]

OPERATION HERRICK

Command and control

The medical command chain on *Operation Herrick 4–20* evolved as the campaign progressed. From *Operation Herrick 4 to 9*, the *UK Joint Force Medical Group* had its own CO – *Comd UK JF Med Gp* – who would usually be the CO of the deploying medical regiment. The Medical Group generally comprised an RHQ located at Camp Bastion, one or two

CS medical squadrons providing Role 1 support throughout Helmand Province, a Role 2 (later Role 3) hospital squadron at Camp Bastion and a support squadron providing logistic support. Each squadron initially had its own squadron commander (an officer commanding), before the increasing size of the Role 3 Hospital merited it becoming a distinct unit with its own CO from *Operation Herrick 10* onwards.

The introduction of a divisional-level commander medical – Commander Medical JFSp(A), referred to as Commander Med – in a medical advisory role for *Operation Herrick 10 and 11* blurred the command boundaries with the Comd UK JF Med Gp, causing some confusion, similar to what had happened on *Operation Telic*. This was resolved when the two roles were amalgamated from *Operation Herrick 12* to *19*, as Comd Med JFSP(A), with operational control over the whole Medical Group. This coincided with the CS medical squadron being upgraded to a (theatre) CS medical regiment, commanded by the CO of the deploying CS medical regiment.

Operation Herrick 1–3 (*Afghan Roulement Infantry Battalions, October 2004 to April 2006*)

The three successive Afghan Roulement Infantry Battalions from 1 October 2004 onwards deployed to Kabul and northern Afghanistan with integral Role 1 medical support and, importantly, environmental health technicians. They were supported by an ISAF Role 3 hospital in Kabul.

2006: ENTRY INTO HELMAND

ISAF now began Stage 3 of its plan for security in Afghanistan, expanding into the southwest, with the United Kingdom initially committing 3150 troops, half a brigade, into Helmand Province. The next two Operation Herrick tours became very kinetic.

Operation Herrick 4 (16 Air Assault Brigade, *April to October 2006*)

FRONTLINE MEDICAL SUPPORT – TEAM MEDICS

'My friends from the Regiment all rushed in, even though it was a suspected minefield. They worked to give me first aid on the ground. A young team medic put a surgical airway into my trachea (to help my breathing), which was something that he'd never done before. There is no question that saved my life'.[64]

Lance Bombardier Ben Parkinson MBE. Injured in Afghanistan, aged 22

Pre-deployment training for *16 Air Assault Brigade* aimed to ensure that every fourth soldier within the frontline infantry would be trained to team medic level and thus theoretically be capable of providing immediate medical support for the first 15 minutes after injury, after which they would be supplemented by combat medical technicians from the CSMR.

ROLE 1 SUPPORT – *16 CSMR*

More specialised frontline medical support on *Operation Herrick 4* was provided by *16 CSMR*. The unit deployed with its RHQ and two of its squadrons: *23 Air Assault Medical Squadron* and *181 Air Assault Medical Support Squadron* (Figure 2.15).[65]

The regiment established a primary healthcare facility and a dental clinic at Camp Bastion, together with primary healthcare facilities at the Provincial Reconstruction Team base at Lashkar Gar and Combat Outpost Price near Gereshk, and a further dental clinic in the Multinational Role 3 facility in Kandahar. These four facilities complemented the already established UK Medical Role 1 nodes at Kandahar and Camp Souter, Kabul. The course of operations subsequently required the establishment of a number of additional combat outposts, platoon houses and bases within district centres. Each location was provided with its own medical node (generally one or more combat medical technicians). These were established at Combat Outpost Robinson, the district centres in Musa Qal'eh, Now Zad, Sangin and the Kajaki dam complex.

It was at Kajaki Dam on 6 September 2006 that L/Cpl Paul ('Tug') Hartley RAMC, combat medical technician with *23 Air Assault Medical Squadron*, became the first member of the Army Medical Services to be awarded a gallantry award (the George Medal) during *Operation Herrick* for

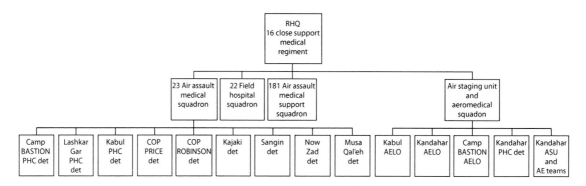

Figure 2.15 Schematic composition of *Operation Herrick UK Joint Force Medical Group*. COP, combat outpost; PHC primary healthcare; AELO, aeromedical evacuation liaison officer; det., detachment; ASU, air staging unit; AE, aeromedical evacuation. (From OP HERRICK 4 – Joint Force Medical Group Post Operational Report, dated 10 October 2006.)

going to the aid of wounded paratroopers trapped in a minefield, at great personal risk, and caring for them while injured himself for the six hours before they could be winched to safety by US Blackhawks. The events that day at Kajaki Dam would later be re-enacted for a British Academy of Film and Television Arts-nominated film which unexpectedly also helped the survivors overcome the effects of post-traumatic stress disorder.[66] Coincidentally, the previous RAMC George Medal recipient, Cpl Colin Lowes, had also deliberately entered a minefield to attend a seriously wounded soldier during the Korean conflict 54 years previously.[67]

PRE-HOSPITAL EMERGENCY CARE – THE MEDICAL EMERGENCY RESPONSE TEAM

As the danger of IEDs largely precluded road evacuation, the pivotal link between casualties on the battlefields of Helmand and the hospital at Camp Bastion was the iconic helicopter-borne medical emergency response team (MERT). Fortunately, air superiority was not contested, although helicopter landing sites most definitely were.

The MERT was a revolutionary concept initially developed by *16 CSMR*, taking the most experienced healthcare professionals (a consultant in emergency medicine or anaesthesia, a nurse and two paramedics) directly to the most critically wounded on the battlefield. It had its precedents in the helicopter-borne IRTs of the 1990s, which carried an anaesthetist and operating department practitioner to the scene of injury.[68]

MERT was introduced on *Operation Herrick 4* in 2006, utilising the skills of clinicians already deployed to Bastion and the RAF's sturdy and spacious CH-47 Chinook helicopter.[69] From 2007, in-flight advanced resuscitation included blood transfusion, a critical life-saving innovation.[70] Anaesthetists or emergency physicians were deployed specifically for the MERT from 2008 onwards.[71]

The MERT was preferentially tasked with evacuating the most severely injured casualties. The wisdom of this intuitive measure was borne out when the outcomes of casualties retrieved by MERT were compared with those retrieved by the smaller US Army Dustoff and US Air Force (USAF) Pedro helicopters (which carried only paramedics).[72,73] The physician-led MERT capability transported a higher percentage of severely injured casualties, while achieving greater than predicted survival. Many hundreds of casualties would be successfully evacuated from the battlefields of Helmand by the MERT, almost always at great personal risk to the medics and RAF crews on board, fortunately without their Chinook ever being shot down, despite being the most-targeted aircraft in Afghanistan.[74,75]

DEPLOYED HOSPITAL CARE – BASTION ROLE 3 ENHANCED (UK) HOSPITAL

22 Field Hospital deployed its Hospital Squadron to Camp Bastion in April 2006 to set up a tented (Tier 1) 25-bed facility, the BSN Role 2 Enhanced (UK) hospital. This was expandable to 50 beds, which were manned by 86 Tri-Service staff. This was concurrent with *22 Field Hospital's* RHQ and Support Squadron also deploying to Iraq for six months, so for the duration of its time on *Operation Herrick*, the hospital squadron was placed under the command of *16 CSMR*. Camp Bastion Hospital would eventually develop to become a powerhouse of medical innovation, reputedly the best trauma hospital in the world, and certainly the busiest in Afghanistan, during the relatively short time of its existence.[76–78] Additional support was provided by RAF primary healthcare staff in an Air Staging Unit and by an RAF Aeromedical Squadron. Individual augmentees (IAs) from the Defence Medical Education & Training Agency and the Defence Dental Services completed the medical ORBAT of 274 personnel.[79]

TACTICAL AND STRATEGIC AEROMEDICAL EVACUATION

The ability to move patients to definitive care elsewhere in Afghanistan (TACEVAC) or to Role 4 in the United Kingdom (STRATEVAC) was critical to keeping Bastion Hospital available to receive further casualties. The *aeromedical evacuation liaison officer* in Bastion played a key role in liaising with the United Kingdom and with civilian and military medical treatment facilities in theatre for transfer of critically ill patients. The CCAST based at Bastion, or UK-based teams, would then provide mobile intensive care capability to safely carry out the transfers.

Operation Herrick 5 (3 Commando Brigade, *October 2006 to March 2007*)

Frontline medical support to *3 Commando Brigade* on *Operation Herrick 5* was provided by the RHQ and CS Squadron formed on the medical squadron of the *Commando Logistics Regiment*. The hospital squadron (manning the BSN Role 2 Enhanced Hospital) was also formed on the medical squadron of the *Commando Logistics Regiment*, with IAs from the Royal Navy, Army and RAF units. It was at the very end of this tour, on 30 March 2007, that the first *Joint Theatre Clinical Case Conference* was held, creating a structure for prompt clinical

feedback on the management of seriously injured UK Service personnel.[80] Clinical governance strongly underpinned all clinical care.

2007 to 2009: The Guerilla War

Operation Herrick had now evolved into a classic counter-insurgency (COIN) campaign. Each of the next four Herrick brigades would apply COIN concepts in a series of deliberate offensive operations, often in complex terrain, initially focussing on 'clear and hold'. Following each operation, small detachments would be established in a series of forward operating bases (FOBs) or patrol bases from which ground could be secured or dominated, to dislocate the insurgents from the populace and theoretically allow reconstruction and development (security sector reform) to take place.

MEDICAL SUPPORT TO COIN OPERATIONS

The spectrum of operations in this complex operating environment required highly agile and quickly available medical support, with medics attached to practically every base and patrol. The highly dispersed nature of the operations meant that there was often no focus on the traditional subunit/ unit aid post, with a strong reliance on team medics supplemented by combat medical technicians before helicopter evacuation could take place.[81] Team medics were highly successful, but they were trained and equipped to provide support only for the first 15–20 minutes after injury, leaving a critical gap in medical support before the MERT arrived. To mitigate this risk, it was often necessary to group combat medical technicians within combat logistic patrols and convoys.

Despite the high-intensity COIN operations, the relatively low battle casualty rates compared to warfighting (with isolated incidents averaging two or three casualties) created the expectancy that every casualty would receive the very best care possible, with the MERT being deployed in practically every instance. Whilst highly capable, it took time for the MERT to arrive at the scene, hence the need for effective emergency medical support on the ground. The main threats to coalition forces at this stage in the campaign were SAF, rocket propelled grenades, recoil-less rifles, mine-strikes and IEDs, including suicide IEDs.

Operation Herrick 6 (12 Mechanised Brigade, *April to October 2007*)

Operation Herrick 6 saw *12 Mechanised Brigade* take over responsibility for what was now called *Task Force Helmand*. Frontline medical support was provided by the Med Group, now comprising some 300 personnel from over 35 different units, commanded by *4 GSMR*.[82] Half of the Med Group (the RHQ and CS Medical Squadron) was formed on *4 GSMR*. There were two small Role 1 detachments at Kandahar (one of which was the aeromedical hub mainly consisting of RAF personnel) and a team based with the British contingent at Kabul. The other half consisted of the Bastion Role 2 (Enhanced) Hospital, based on two TA hospitals in succession: *212 (Sheffield) Field Hospital (Volunteers)* and *208 (Liverpool) Field Hospital (Volunteers)*, each supplying about 80 personnel.

Operation Herrick 7 (52 Infantry Brigade, *October 2007 to April 2008*)

5 GSMR (the predecessor of *5 Armoured Medical Regiment*), from Preston, provided the core of the Med Group. The unit deployed its RHQ, a Regular CS Squadron, a Regular support squadron and elements of the unit's two TA squadrons from Hull and Chorley to provide frontline medical support. The Bastion Role 2 (Enhanced) Hospital was again based on two TA hospitals in succession: *201 (Northern) Field Hospital (Volunteers)* and *243 (The Wessex) Field Hospital (Volunteers)*.

The campaign in Helmand was still evolving, with a steady increase in the number of FOBs, each requiring a medical contingent. This created its own challenge for the CS medical regiment, as the number of medics deployed in support of ground troops on combat patrols was constantly changing, with new tasks pulling on scarce resources. The convoy logistic patrols also became more regular and bigger, thus requiring greater medical support than originally envisaged.[83]

THE MOVE FROM ROLE 2 (ENHANCED) TO ROLE 3 (UK) BASTION HOSPITAL

The major development during *Operation Herrick 7* was the move of Bastion Hospital from the original Tier 1 tented accommodation into purpose-built semi-permanent Tier 2 accommodation in February 2008 (at the start of *Operation Herrick 7B*). *243 Field Hospital* had been in Theatre for just over two weeks when the move to the new facility was achieved.[84] It was at this new Tier 2 hospital, during *Operation Herrick 7B*, that the life-saving process of 'Right Turn Resuscitation', by which critically injured casualties were received by the trauma team within the operating theatre rather than in the emergency department, was introduced.[85] The term has become synonymous with the aggressive and successful damage control resuscitation policy adopted at Bastion and is being increasingly adopted worldwide.

BUILDING BASTION HOSPITAL – TENTS TO PORTAKABIN (TIER 1 TO TIER 2)

'Never again should a project of this magnitude and importance be undertaken without the employment of a dedicated Project Officer from inception to completion'.

Commander Medical (Operation Herrick 7)[86]

In the context of a book dedicated to the medical lessons from Iraq and Afghanistan, it is pertinent to reflect on the key lessons identified during design and construction of the UK's Role 3 medical facility in Afghanistan, Camp Bastion Hospital, as construction issues impinged significantly on the level of care that could be provided. The British Army categorises buildings into three types: Tier 1, Tier 2 and Tier 3. Tier 1 structures are tents and therefore temporary. Such structures are ideal for insertion operations such as entry into Helmand in April 2006, if no pre-existing building can be converted. The original Bastion hospital set up by *22 Field Hospital* was such a tented structure built to a standard pattern, with separate tents for the emergency department, operating theatres, intensive care unit, laboratory, X-ray department, wards and command areas, with inter-communicating corridors. If an operation is expected to last a year or more, then measures are taken to construct a more permanent replacement.

Tier 2 structures are also temporary, but more durable than tents, usually in the form of a

Portakabin-type unit erected from flat pack assembly, either used individually or in a formation. Tier 3 structures are permanent buildings. If an operation is expected to last for several years, or if the facility is eventually to be handed over to the host nation, the Tier 3 option is the most cost-effective even if it might take longer to construct. UK regulations for hospital design are applicable to both Tier 2 and Tier 3 structures but can be better met in Tier 3 structures.

TIER 2 BUILD

By September 2006, within weeks of troops arriving in Helmand for what promised to be a long-term commitment, a contractor was engaged to build a Tier 2 semi-permanent hospital alongside the initial tented facility, to be ready by April 2007. Staff and patients would then move across to the new build, leaving the tented facility in situ for use in emergency, as a resilience hospital. It was also decided to dismantle the now-surplus Tier 2 Portakabin hospital in the British base in Basra, which had been built by the same contractor, and transport its components to Bastion for incorporation in the new build or in the resilience hospital. However, by the time that hospital was dismantled and actually arrived in Bastion (towards the end of 2010), it was so damaged that none of the Basra hospital could be re-used.

In the meantime, the construction of the Tier 2 Bastion hospital had gone ahead, but frustratingly, it had been so ill-managed and beset with so many design flaws and problems that construction practically ceased in 2007. The Royal Engineers were belatedly engaged to bail out the contractor and complete the construction of the hospital through their specialist unit, *170 (Infrastructure Support) Engineer Group*, which happened to have a reservist architect experienced in hospital design.

The Tier 2 hospital eventually opened in February 2008, 10 months later than scheduled, and after clinical care had been carried out in tents for almost two years, through the extremes of an extra summer and winter season. *243 Field Hospital*, just commencing their *Operation Herrick 7B* tour (January to April 2008), closed down the tented hospital and were the first unit to man the new hospital.

The new hospital was designed to care primarily for trauma patients. It had an emergency department with nine resuscitation bays, leading directly into an adjacent operating theatre (the Bastion Right Turn) large enough to support two concurrently working operating tables (later expanded to four). It had an adjacent ICU with four beds. Two intermediate care wards (named Wards One and Two) provided capacity for some 35 patients, and there were two isolation rooms with a single bed in each. A reception and administration area, a pathology laboratory with a large blood bank and an X-ray department with CT scanner (which crucially was adjacent to the emergency department and would eventually be replaced by two higher specification models) completed the setup.[87]

Unfortunately, the lack of development planning in the critical early stages meant that services could not expand sensibly to extend the hospital as required, as became very evident during the increasing tempo of combat operations from 2008 to 2010. Extra ward tents would eventually be erected behind the hospital, to be replaced in their turn by more permanent constructions, while whole departments would be moved around within the hospital in order to create more clinical capacity. Thus, the ICU moved in early 2009 to the larger Ward One area and expanded to 12 beds, being replaced in situ by pathology. The result was a cramped and seemingly disjointed hospital with potentially serious infection prevention and control issues.

Notwithstanding these infrastructure issues and the effort involved in mitigating them to prevent clinical care being interrupted, the new Tier 2 'Role 2 Enhanced Treatment Facility' still represented a huge leap forward in capability. Being temperature controlled and weather protected, it created a much better working environment, minimising the problems associated with the heat, cold and dust of Helmand Province.

The lessons highlighted during the saga of the Tier 2 build (particularly the need for a dedicated and experienced project manager who could see such a project through from start to finish and critically ensure its design was fit for purpose and expansion) were fully documented in post-operational reports.[88] They were further elaborated in an article in the *Royal Engineers Journal*, which should be mandatory reading for medical planners.[89]

Bastion Hospital, in its Tier 2 enhanced capability configuration, was rapidly re-designated as a Role 3 hospital. The only other Role 3 hospitals then in Afghanistan were at Bagram and Kandahar Air Field. Bastion was always busier than either of these and its workload would equal that of the other two combined. It would become renowned during the short period of its busy existence as probably the world's best trauma hospital for the quality of care delivered. The unprecedented numbers of 'unexpected survivors' were its hallmark.

It pays to reflect that, if only there had been effective project management throughout Bastion hospital's construction, this world class Role 3 capability could have been delivered much more quickly and on time, more efficiently and effectively, within a properly designed building (even if still Tier 2), to an even higher standard of excellence.

Operation Herrick 8 (16 Air Assault Brigade, *April to October 2008*)

16 Air Assault Brigade returned to Afghanistan on *Operation Herrick 8* to take command of Task Force Helmand. Frontline medical support was provided by the CS medical regiment formed on *16 Medical Regiment*, and the BSN Role 3 (UK) hospital was based on two TA hospitals in succession: *203 (Welsh) Field Hospital (V)* and *204 (Northern Irish) Field Hospital (V)* (Figure 2.16).

The Med Group on *Operation Herrick 8* consisted of two CS medical squadrons, the hospital squadron and the support squadron. Augmentation came from all three services, both regular and reserve, from 57 provider units, from personnel ranked from private to brigadier and from civilian nurses and welfare workers. The CS squadrons supported battlegroups in northern and southern Helmand. Medical liaison officers linked the units directly to the Med Group to provide situational awareness and to support battlegroup planning. Some 120 medical officers, combat medical technicians and nurses were attached to forward units to support patrolling and static medical centres.

During *Operation Herrick 8 the* Med Group saw an unprecedented number of casualties. The MERT launched 343 times for 976 casualties; the hospital admitted 1049 patients; there were over 11,000 primary healthcare presentations; and over 42,000 individual medical stores demands were made to sustain the medical effort.[90]

MULTINATIONAL COLLABORATION – THE ESTONIAN CONTINGENT AT BASTION

A small but valued contingent from the Medical Service of the Estonian Defence Force, both Regulars and Reservists, was integrated into Bastion Hospital from April 2008 onwards.[91] The Estonians not only contributed to the care of the wounded at Bastion but also took medical lessons from the battlefield back home to revolutionise Estonia's civilian trauma service. Estonia had no national defence force under Soviet occupation from 1940 to 1991. On gaining independence at the end of the Cold War, it had to build up its Defence Force, including its Medical Service, from scratch. Estonia joined NATO in 2004, participated in Balkan peacekeeping missions and from 2005 to 2014 deployed its combat forces to Iraq and Afghanistan, where

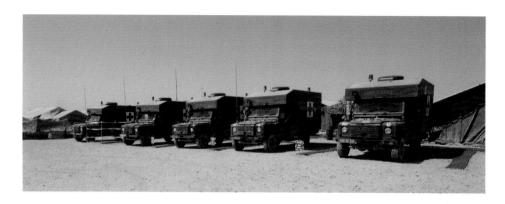

Figure 2.16 Ambulance Troop, Camp Bastion, *Operation Herrick 8.*

it participated in ISAF combat operations alongside UK units in Helmand from 2006 onwards. Estonian casualties entered the British patient care pathway, undergoing resuscitation at Bastion before aeromedical evacuation to Role 4 care in Birmingham and repatriation.

In 2006 and 2007, Estonia began negotiating with the UK Ministry of Defence (MOD) to send a full surgical team to Helmand. Estonian candidates for deployment began attending Battlefield Advanced Trauma Life Support courses in Holland. The turning point came when two reservist civilian surgeons attended the April 2008 annual meeting of the *British Military Surgical Society*. They then participated in the *Principles of War Surgery* course in Birmingham and HOSPEX training in Strensall, where they were validated for deployment. The first Estonian surgeon to deploy was rapidly assimilated fully into clinical practice at Bastion, setting the precedent. Other tours followed.

Operation Herrick 9 (3 Command Brigade, *October 2008 to April 2009*)

As on *Operation Herrick 5*, this was primarily a Navy deployment. Frontline medical support to *3 Commando Brigade* on *Operation Herrick 9* was provided by the RHQ and CS squadron formed on the medical squadron of the *Commando Logistics Regiment*. The hospital squadron was also formed on the medical squadron of the *Commando Logistics Regiment*, with IAs from Royal Navy, Army and RAF units. Rotational thrombo-elastometry was introduced to UK military medical practice during this tour, when a feasibility study carried out at Bastion Hospital between January and March 2009 showed its utility in the management of patients requiring massive transfusion. This was fortuitously just in time for the flood of casualties during the next tour.[92] MA Kate Nesbitt, a medic attached to *1st Battalion the Rifles*, became the first Royal Navy female, and the second female in the Armed Forces, to be awarded the Military Cross for saving a casualty's life under fire.[93]

2009–2011: COIN RENAISSANCE

The Herrick Campaign was revitalised with the arrival in theatre of the new ISAF Commander, US General Stanley McChrystal, in May 2009, and the resulting surge of US troops, with UK troops also increasing greatly in number. This was accompanied by a commensurate increase in medical capability, particularly at Bastion, and a US Role 2 (Enhanced) hospital being established in southern Helmand, at FOB Dwyer.

Operation Herrick 10 (Light Brigade, *April to October 2009*)

The main challenge faced by the DMS on *Operation Herrick 10* was planning for, and coping with, the casualty surges experienced during *Operation Panther's Claw* ('Panchai Palang' in Pashtu), the name reflecting *19 Light Brigade's* nickname, 'The Black Panthers'. This five-week operation, 19 June–25 July 2009, aimed to assert control over and secure the belt of tribal land around the main road leading north from Lashkar Gar (the provincial capital) to Gereshk (the commercial hub) in central Helmand, including the town of Babaji, an area that until then had been firmly in the hands over Taliban insurgents.[94] The intention was to clear the Taliban from this region in time for the 80,000 inhabitants to participate freely in planned presidential elections in the August.

The core of the Med Group was formed from *2 Medical Regiment*, from Hohne, Germany. The unit deployed to theatre with its two squadrons amalgamated into one large CS squadron, its RHQ, its support squadron (providing the G4 [logistics] support) and a G1 (personnel) cell. The Regiment was reinforced with IAs from *4 Medical Regiment* and *225 Medical Regiment (Volunteers)*. Combat medical technicians from the regiment were attached to infantry platoons throughout Helmand in preparation for *Operation Panther's Claw*. Coincident with the US surge into Afghanistan, the US Secretary of State for Defence mandated that all medevac missions be completed within 60 minutes. This resulted in USAF HH-60 Pave Hawk helicopters (Callsign 'Pedro'), manned by two paramedics, being forward located at Camp Bastion, where they supplemented British medevac missions by the RAF Chinook with MERT. Even so, the US Department of Defense openly acknowledged that MERT was the option of choice for evacuation of critically wounded personnel.[95] The US policy was reinforced by the simultaneous publication in early 2009 of an authoritative review by the UK's Academic Department of Military Surgery and Trauma at Royal Centre for Defence Medicine (RCDM) that unequivocally recommended that, to prevent avoidable deaths, there must be an upper limit of two hours from wounding to surgical haemorrhage control for all casualties.[96] These directions shaped preparations to manage casualties during *Operation Panther's Claw*.

Role 3 Support Bastion Hospital was based on *202 Field Hospital (Volunteers)* for *Operation Herrick 10A* (April to July, the period encompassing *Panther's Claw*) and a Danish Reserves Field Hospital for *Operation Herrick 10B* (August to October).

DEPLOYED MEDICAL DIRECTOR

The introduction of the DMD role within the military medical machine during *Operation Herrick 10*, just in time to plan for the frenetic clinical activity that would characterise *Operation Panther's Claw*, exemplifies the importance of leadership skills and operational experience in promoting transformation.

Until early 2009, the senior doctor in British field hospitals doubled up as clinical director. This led to situations where a surgeon or anaesthetist, despite acting as clinical director, would be fully occupied in theatre and unable to deal with other crises. This had not presented an issue in the short periods of clinical activity during *Operation Granby* and up to the opening phase of *Operation Telic* (2003). It was a different matter once the pace and complexity of clinical activity accelerated in Afghanistan, with the change from ballistic to blast injury, when the Taliban adapted by using IEDs with telling effect.

By 2009, many developments in combat casualty care in Afghanistan had come together. The advances in pre-hospital medicine and damage control resuscitation, the rapid evacuation of large numbers of massively wounded personnel to and from Bastion Hospital, the multinational working environment, the inter-disciplinary challenges of clinical innovations, clinical governance issues and the high-intensity workload with its clinical dilemmas and ethical issues had created extremely challenging conditions. These were too complex for individual clinical directors distracted by still

having to care personally for critically ill casualties, especially if they were unfamiliar with new concepts and processes.

These conditions, and operational feedback, led to the concept of the DMD. This person, an experienced clinician, would be formally appointed in a leadership role, without direct clinical responsibilities, working in a triumvirate alongside the CO and senior nursing officer (SNO), with direct managerial responsibility for clinical activity across the hospital and deploying for a minimum of three months.

The first DMD deployed in April 2009. The first two DMDs were experienced military academics; thereafter, a robust selection process was introduced together with structured pre-deployment training, two intensive hospital validation exercises (HOSPEX) at Strensall and finally a week-long handover in theatre.[97] The DMD role has proven invaluable in managing the complex ethical challenges faced on deployment, not the least those related to working with limited resources, with clinicians from other countries and the indigenous health system, upholding the medical rules of eligibility and caring for children in an austere environment.[98]

MULTINATIONAL COLLABORATION – THE US CONTINGENT AT BASTION

Bastion Hospital was augmented from May 2009 by 48 US military medical staff commencing a six-month deployment, arriving as part of President Obama's 'Surge' of 21,000 US Marines into Afghanistan and also in time for *Operation Panther's Claw*. This group was the first of 11 six-month contingents of US medical personnel to be integrated into Bastion Hospital.[99]

The US contingent consisted of IAs drawn from many units and commands across the world (including Navy, Army, Marine Corps and Air Force). On some rotations, they provided up to half the Bastion clinical staff, as well as providing crucial continuity and gaining valuable experience over their six-month tours, compared to the six weeks to three months of many of the UK clinical staff. The head of the US contingent filled the role of deputy DMD until the roles were separated during *Operation Herrick 16*. The overall result of this multinational collaboration was very positive, despite occasional friction (the inevitable consequence of human interaction, especially across different cultures), with a great esprit de corps boding well for UK–US co-operation in future operations.

PREPARING FOR OPERATION PANTHERS CLAW

Bastion Hospital's capability was significantly increased, and extra staff were mobilised, in preparation for *Operation Panther's Claw*: the emergency department increased from 8 bays to 10; the operating theatres increased from two tables to three (surging to four); the ICU increased from four beds to eight, with a surge capability of 10; and the wards increased from 26 to 28 beds, with a surge capability of 50 beds. A consultant radiologist was deployed to Bastion as part of the US contingent, setting a precedent for future tours.[100] As neurosurgical and maxillofacial facilities (including British teams) were now located at Kandahar, head-injured casualties would preferentially be flown there directly from the battlefield.

'THE BLOODIEST DAY'

On Friday 10 July 2009, during the height of *Operation Panther's Claw*, British battlefield casualties reached the highest number in a single day since the Falklands conflict of 1982, let alone for the whole of the *Operation Telic* or *Operation Herrick* campaigns.

Eight British servicemen were killed in action that day, all by IEDs, and 30 were wounded, 15 seriously, with similar numbers among Allied troops, and Bastion Hospital bore the brunt of the action.[101] The month of July also saw the highest number of British fatalities and very seriously and seriously injured casualties on *Operation Herrick* (see Figure 2.17).[102] It was the defining month for the DMS in Afghanistan.

DANISH HOSPITAL SQUADRON, *OPERATION HERRICK 10B*

In the meantime, the Danes had been preparing to deploy to Bastion. Denmark had contributed its Leopard tanks to *Operation Panther's Claw*; now it was its turn to contribute to the medical mission. It had been agreed by the respective ministries of defence that the Danes would deploy their sole reserve field hospital as a hospital squadron to Bastion from August to October 2009. Preparation for this unique multinational collaboration had involved intensive individual and collective training – the Hospital Squadron for *Operation Herrick 10B* would be half Danish and a quarter each British and American. The CO was Danish, assisted by a British DMD, who had learned Danish in preparation for this deployment (Figure 2.18).

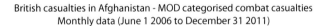

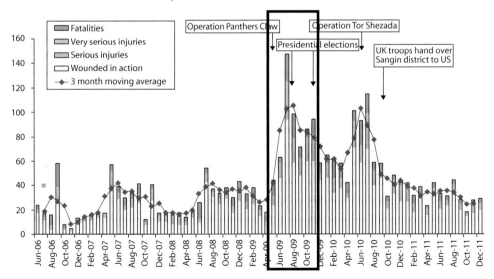

Figure 2.17 British casualties in Afghanistan, 2006–2011. (*Operation Herrick 10* tempo highlighted). (From Casualty Monitor. British Casualties: Afghanistan http://www.casualty-monitor.org/p/british-casualties-in-afghanistan.html.)

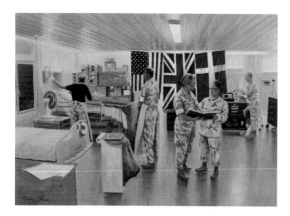

Figure 2.18 Bastion Hospital ICU – a testimony to multinational cooperation. (Courtesy of Graeme Lothian.)

The Danish three-month deployment, following hard on the heels of *Operation Panther's Claw*, turned out to be the most intense period of activity to date at Bastion. Records were broken for the number of surgical procedures, CT scans performed per day, laboratory investigations processed, units of blood transfused and activations of the platelet apheresis and emergency blood donation panels.[103]

Operation Herrick 10 was the most kinetic of all the *Operation Herrick* tours, with 498 Troops in Contact recorded, 35 deaths, 46 seriously wounded and 85 other wounded.[104,105] IEDs were the principal killers and the cause of complex polytrauma in survivors; there were 426 recorded IED incidents, with 84 detonating against or in close proximity to dismounted UK patrols. Smaller Danish medical contingents would continue to deploy to Bastion in variable numbers for much of the rest of the *Operation Herrick* campaign.

Operation Herrick 11 (11 Light Brigade, *October 2009 to April 2010*)

REGIONAL COMMAND (SOUTH)

The start of *Operation Herrick 11* coincided with the United Kingdom taking on leadership of Regional Command (South) in Kandahar from 1 November 2009 to 1 November 2010. RC(South) was one of the five ISAF Regional Commands in Afghanistan in 2009 – a sixth, RC(South West), would be created in July 2010, with Task Force Helmand being transferred to its command (Figure 2.19).

The collective experiences of the multinational medical branch at HQ RC(S) in organising medical support to all regional military operations during this time, including the detailed medical planning for *Operation Moshtarak*,[106] were collated in a special supplement of the *Journal of the RAMC*.[107] This supplement provides an invaluable repository of organisational lessons for medical personnel in leadership roles at HQ.

HQ JFSp(A) had recently moved from Kandahar to Camp Bastion, making it much easier for the incoming commander medical to balance taking on command over the Bastion-based Med Group with working in HQ (the new Command & Control [C2] structure would be formalised at the start of *Operation Herrick 12*). The most significant result of the move from Kandahar was that the HQ, now co-located with its units, could clearly take on command over the Med Group, not just be a coordinating HQ. It could therefore focus its efforts more effectively in direct support of *Task Force Helmand* – just in time to prepare for *Operation Moshtarak*.

UK JOINT FORCE MEDICAL GROUP

Operation Herrick 11 was unique in having a regular field hospital (*33 Field Hospital*) providing the CS Squadron as well as leading the Med Group. *256 (City of London) Field Hospital (Volunteers)* provided the hospital squadron on *Operation Herrick 11A* (October 2009 to January 2010), and *205 (Scottish) Field Hospital (Volunteers)*, on *Operation Herrick 11B* (January to April 2010).

The high tempo of operations seen on *Operation Herrick 10* continued into the first half of this tour, with 180 trauma calls in the first six weeks, thankfully followed by some seasonal reduction. The case mix was dominated by traumatic amputations with extensive bilateral and lower limb disruption secondary to IEDs. One unexpected survivor of such critical injuries underwent transfusion in theatre of an unprecedented 274 units of blood and blood products.[108] This was a tribute to the success of the aggressive damage control resuscitation and massive transfusion policy adopted at Bastion and the organisational support behind it.[109]

There were three main medical organisational challenges during this tour. The first challenge was planning for and providing medical support to

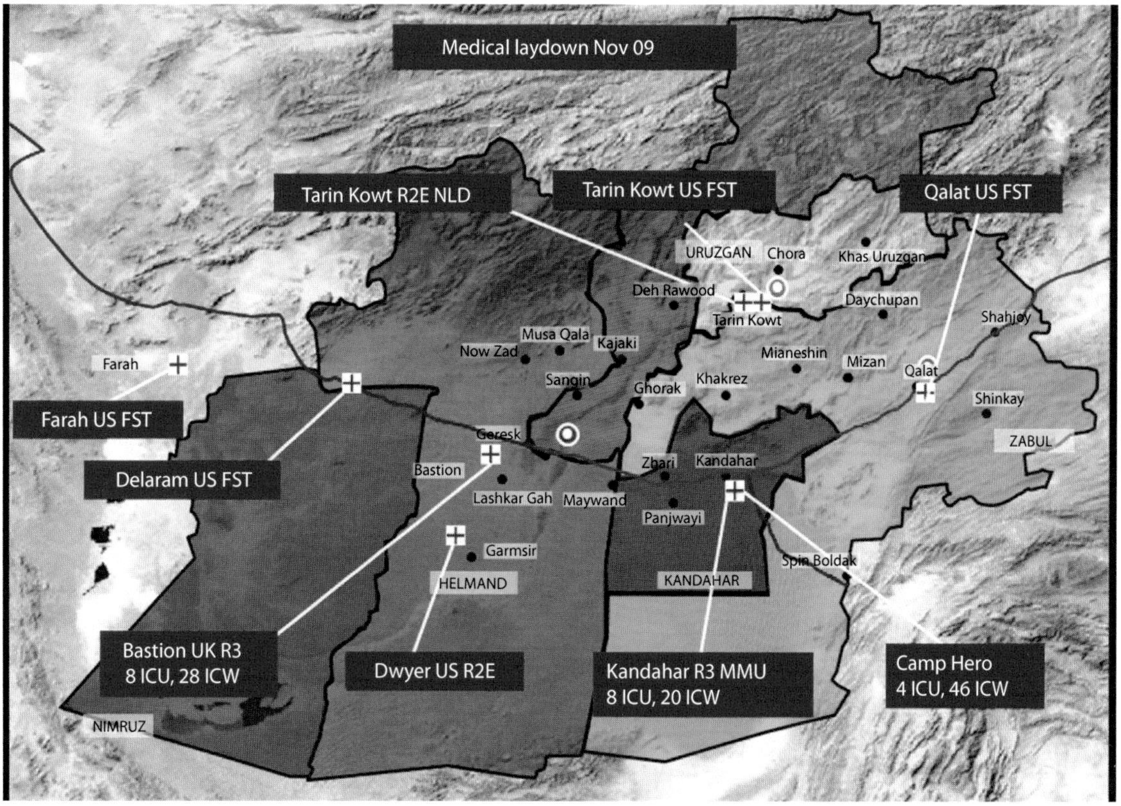

Figure 2.19 ISAF Role 2 & 3 Medical Treatment Facilities in RC (South), November 2009. The relative number of intensive care unit and intermediate care ward beds is shown for the Role 3 hospitals at Bastion and Kandahar, three months before *Operation Moshtarak*.

Operation Moshtarak (the clearance of Nad-e Ali and Lashkar Gah districts by Task Force Helmand, and of Marjah by the US Marines' Task Force Leatherneck).

OPERATION MOSHTARAK

This was the largest joint offensive in the whole *Operation Herrick* campaign. As an RC (S) operation, medical planning for this involved Chief Medical HQ RC(S), Deputy Assistant Chief of Staff Medical at PJHQ and Commander Medical JFSp(A), as well as the COs (and DMD) of the two medical units at Bastion. Planning revolved around the casualty estimate and then increasing the medical support and capacity to meet the expected casualty load over the duration of the operation. The critical capacity was Role 3 ICU availability.

For the Role 3 (UK) Hospital at Bastion, planning involved an increase in capacity of both ICU and the intermediate care cadres and deployment of the third standby MERT and the strategic CCAST from the United Kingdom. Maximum use was made of the newly collocated USAF Casualty Aeromedical Staging Facility to facilitate access to USAF aeromedical capacity and to evacuate as many patients as possible before D Day (12 February 2010). The result was that, despite over 50 battle casualty admissions on D Day (mainly Afghan nationals with gunshot wounds), Bastion Hospital was almost clear of patients for the second day of the operation, enabling both taskforces to continue their momentum.[110]

TWO UNITS

The second challenge was the formation within the Med Group of two formal units, rather than squadrons, by the end of *Operation Herrick 11*: the new (theatre) CSMR and the Camp Bastion Role

3 (UK) Hospital, each with its own CO but sharing an operations room (Ops Room) and support squadron. This enabled the commander of the Med Group to focus on engaging with Task Force Helmand rather than being fixed upon hospital activities.

ICELANDIC ASH CLOUD

The final organisational challenge was managing the disruption to strategic aeromedical evacuation and resupply caused by the Icelandic volcanic eruption in April 2010. This eruption sent a huge ash cloud over the northern Atlantic and Europe, causing a sudden and unexpected halt to the strategic aeromedical evacuation of casualties from Afghanistan, as well as halting the resupply of consumables such as blood and blood products, vital for the massive transfusion protocols used at Bastion. Various contingency plans were developed, exploring the options of evacuating patients to southern Europe, Cyprus and the Middle East, with a few UK patients actually being evacuated via Bagram through the US system before the air bridge re-opened. Blood stocks fortunately never became an issue, as the departure of the outgoing *205 Field Hospital (V)* was also delayed by the ash cloud, so there were plenty of volunteers for the emergency blood donor panel.

Operation Herrick 12 (4 Mechanised Brigade, *April to October 2010*)

REGIONAL COMMAND AND CONTROL

The medical support in RC(S) had its hub at the strategic aeromedical centre at Kandahar. At its peak in the summer of 2010, before the creation of RC(SW) in July, HQ RC(S) oversaw the function of three Role 3 and three Role 2 Enhanced hospitals, eight designated helicopter medical evacuation task lines and five types of medical evacuation aeroplanes. During the tour, the medical staff managed the forward medical evacuation of 8036 casualties compared with 5994 for 2009.[111]

UK JOINT FORCE MEDICAL GROUP

The Med Group was now formally divided into a CS medical regiment (provided by *3 Medical Regiment*) and the Bastion Role 3 (UK) Hospital (its core being *34 Field Hospital*), both under functional command of Comd Med JFSp(A), with the previously separate role of Comd UK JF Med Gp being subsumed into this position. At a stroke, this abolished the potential for friction and confusion at senior command level.

FORCE PROTECTION (ROLE 1 ARMOURED AMBULANCE SUPPORT)

Although the Mastiff Protected Mobility Vehicles operated well in Iraq, a smaller, more manoeuvrable platform was required for the tighter confines of Afghanistan's villages. Four of the new Ridgeback protected BFAs were deployed to Helmand in April 2010.[112]

Operation Herrick 13 (16 Air Assault Brigade, *October 2010 to April 2011*)

The focus for *16 Air Assault Brigade*, the first to return for a third tour, was on mentoring and developing the Afghan National Security Forces (ANSF) in preparation for ISAF Stage 4. The Med Group aligned itself to this at both Role 1 and Role 3.

TEAM MEDICS

Having faced the reality of combat in two previous tours, and seen how prompt action by team medics repeatedly saved lives before qualified medics could arrive at the scene, every second soldier within the Brigade was now trained to team medic level, with the medics from the Med Group refreshing and enhancing this training at every opportunity. A key recommendation from this tour, worth repeating, was that all soldiers deploying forward should be trained to team medic level and that all combat medical technicians should be taught to team medic instructor level during their Phase 2 training.

ROLE 1

Operation Herrick 13 was the first tour that the CS medical regiment (*16 Medical Regiment* in this case) was split into three sub-units with very different roles: A, B and Support Squadrons. A Squadron focused on the delivery of primary and pre-hospital emergency care to Task Force Helmand (with its medics completing 10,102 patrols by the end of tour), while B Squadron focused on primary care to entitled personnel (including detainees) within the main operating bases and on partnering and mentoring the ANSF. The Support Squadron supported both the Role 1 and Role 3 units. The CS medical regiment provided direct medical support to 78 of the 104 task force locations during this tour.[113] An idea of relative workload (for British patients alone) can be gained by considering that the CS medical regiment treated 371 battle casualties and 22,550 DNBI casualties in these six months.

2011 TO 2013 TRANSITION TO ANSF

With the formal process of transition to the ANSF now initiated, and preparations for withdrawal gradually gathering momentum, the emphasis for the Med Group on the next *Operation Herrick* tours would increasingly be on developing the medical capability of the ANSF while supporting operations.

Operation Herrick 14 (3 Commando Brigade, *April to October 2011*)

The composition of the Royal Navy-led Med Group was similar to that on *Operation Herrick 5* and *9*, with IAs drawn from across the Naval Services (Royal Navy, Royal Marine Band Service and Royal Marines), as well as significant proportions of Army and RAF personnel. Lessons had been learned from previous tours, a key success in the preparation for this tour being the formation of the CS medical regiment skeleton RHQ at Navy Command HQ nine months before deployment and its co-location with the *Operation Herrick 14* hospital regiment command team. Role 1 medical support was provided to 4 Main Operating Bases and 77 forward locations, with the medics deployed forward completing over 10,500 patrols.[114]

Operation Herrick 15 (20 Armoured Brigade, *October 2011 to April 2012*)

'The call came through on the radio: one casualty, both legs amputated'.

Captain Tom Blankenstein, Regimental Medical Officer, Operation Herrick 15.

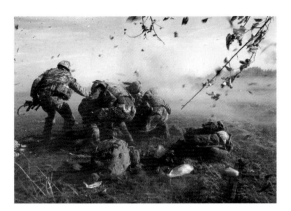

Figure 2.20 Pre-hospital emergency care, *Operation Herrick 15.*

An IED explosion in the early hours of Armistice Day (11/11/11) resulted in a British soldier of the *1st Battalion the Princess of Wales's Royal Regiment* losing both legs – but not his life. This was thanks to the patrol's combat medical technician (from *1 Medical Regiment*) who promptly applied tourniquets and a pelvic binder and gave morphine.[115] The moment when the Chinook carrying the MERT came in to evacuate, the casualty was captured by photographer Jason Howe in an award-winning photograph (Figure 2.20).[116]

This tour saw the fourth, and very successful, iteration of the integrated ops room concept for the Med Gp, with sharing of staff functions below 2nd in Command (2IC) level between the CS medical regiment (*1 Medical Regiment*) and the hospital. The UK Med Gp BSN Role 3 Hospital was commanded by *208 (Liverpool) Field Hospital (Volunteers)* on *Operation Herrick 15A* (October 2011 to Jan 2012) and by *201 (Northern) Field Hospital (Volunteers)* on *Operation Herrick 15B* (January to April 2012).

COMMAND AND CONTROL

The hospital command structure in place by now had proven to be the most efficient at meeting the disparate challenges at Bastion: command rested with the 'triumvirate' of CO, DMD and SNO, interlinked with the 2IC, who also provided the chief of staff function, with a second layer at departmental level. To facilitate this, during *Operation Herrick 15A*, the CO shared an office with the DMD (adjacent to that of the CO of the medical regiment); 2IC shared with the regimental sergeant major (RSM) (also adjacent to medical regiment adjutant and RSM); and the SNO was co-located with hospital reception and the senior wardmaster within the hospital. The rest of the Med Gp HQ and the Ops Room were immediately at hand, allowing instant communication as required.

HOSPITAL STAFFING

To give an idea of the typical composition of Bastion Hospital, the following personnel deployed there on *Operation Herrick 15A*: 58 from 208 Fd Hosp (V), 17 IAs from *2 Medical Brigade*, 77 Regular IAs and 87 US personnel from the 10th Combat Support Hospital (CSH), with the rest of 10th CSH manning the US Role 2/3 facility at FOB Dwyer. Also deployed were six Danes (providing a fifth surgical team in addition to the two US and two UK teams), two civilian Defence Medical Welfare Services staff and five civilian CONDO nurses (contractors deployed on operations; with specialist skills in emergency or intensive care). US/UK interoperability was enhanced by combined training before deployment, particularly at the series of HOSPEX Validation Exercises at AMSTC as well as in Germany, and also by sharing of command responsibilities on deployment.

CAPABILITY

The main areas of capability development during on *Operation Herrick 15A* were the expansion of ICU beds from 14 to 16 beds and the opening of a new 40-bed ward (Ward 3). The tented resilience hospital was drawn down and closed during this tour in preparation for withdrawal.

ANSF MENTORING

The Afghan National Army (ANA) 215 Corps had a troop medical centre (TMC) at Camp Shorabak, adjacent to Camp Bastion. This was a modern hard build with a 20-bed ward facility, two resuscitation bays and a primary healthcare facility, with embedded Danish and US mentors. Bastion's DMD attended bi-weekly ward rounds with the ANA corps surgeon, and regular 'train the trainer' sessions were conducted at both the TMC and at Bastion. These would steadily enhance the capability of the TMC to treat casualties and facilitate the transfer of ANSF and Afghan civilian casualties into the local health system (to

Kabul National Military Hospital and Kandahar Regional Military Hospital for ANSF casualties, and Bost for civilians).

Operation Herrick 16 (12 Mechanised Brigade, *April to October 2012*)

'The medical support to TFH is simply outstanding. Rapid air medevac from point of wounding to the world-class trauma facility at Bastion Role 3 has increased survival rates significantly; the effect of this on the moral component of fighting power cannot be underestimated'.[117]

The average time for a Category A casualty to reach Bastion from point of wounding was 39 minutes on *Operation Herrick 16*, well within the 'Golden Hour'. Role 1 support was provided by *4 Medical Regiment*, with *22 Field Hospital* responsible for deployed hospital care.

ATTACK ON CAMP BASTION

The most noteworthy event during *Operation Herrick 16* was the audacious ground attack against Camp Bastion's airfield by 15 Taliban insurgents disguised in a mixture of US Army uniforms and civilian contractor clothing on the night of 14 September 2012. Bastion Hospital was locked down and guarded by hospital staff during the attack, while the wounded and dead (both Allied and Taliban) were brought in. All those who arrived alive, including one critically wounded insurgent, survived (Figure 2.21).

'The whole hospital, all departments and every staff member performed their duties over that 48 hour period without complaint and with the utmost professionalism. Every casualty who arrived at the hospital alive was treated quickly and efficiently and all survived their injuries. The Front of House team performed quickly and efficiently ensuring that all of the wounded were checked and cleared of weapons etc. before moving into the hospital, ensuring that their

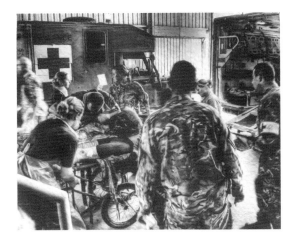

Figure 2.21 Casualties being offloaded at Camp Bastion Hospital, *Operation Herrick* 16.

care and the safety of the staff were not compromised. They also ensured that the dead were looked after with respect and dignity regardless of the side they had chosen to be on'.

WO1(RSM) Andy Game, personal recollection

Operation Herrick 17 (4 Mechanised Brigade, *October 2012 to April 2013*)

ROLE 1 SUPPORT

The new CS medical regiment (formed on *3 Medical Regiment*) continued work on improving ANSF medical capability, shifting focus from partnering to enabling, in line with ISAF strategy, and providing direct support only as a last resort. While helicopter evacuation for the more seriously injured Category A and B casualties remained an ISAF responsibility, over the course of the tour, up to 80% of all ANA casualties would be dealt with by the ANA, with ground evacuation to Shorabak, without recourse to ISAF medical resources.[118]

The key challenge, however, for the CS medical regiment was the medical management of detainees (captured personnel), whose ongoing retention in theatre required a change in philosophy to view this group as a prison population, complete with chronic health needs. This required a complete re-writing of standard operating procedures, with a general practitioner and a primary healthcare nurse being added permanently to the existing establishment of doctors, nurses and medics specifically caring for detainees.[119]

The lead for the Role 3 capability was provided by *243 Field Hospital (Volunteers)* for *Operation Herrick 17A* and *204 Field Hospital (Volunteers)* for *Operation Herrick 17B*. These TA Hospitals, in common with the other TA Hospitals, would later in 2013 be renamed Army Reserve Hospitals and drop the '(Volunteers)' from their title, in accordance with the Future Reserves 2020 plan and a white paper presented to Parliament in July 2013.[120]

The major challenge now taxing medical planners was the absence of an indigenous ANA hospital in Helmand Province, with most major trauma casualties from the *ANA 215 Corps* perforce being admitted to Bastion and now accounting for the majority of inpatients. This represented the key medical risk to successful transition should the ANSF be left without hospital care for their personnel once ISAF forces departed in 2014. A three-stage plan was therefore developed to address this, namely to develop a trauma treatment training centre at the TMC in Shorabak, while constructing a tented Role 2 field hospital in Shorabak, and a 50-bed permanent hospital (to be known as the Regional Military Hospital) to eventually replace that, in advance of Bastion's closure.[121]

Operation Herrick 18 (1 Mechanised Brigade, *April to October 2013*)

ROLE 1 SUPPORT

The CS Medical Regiment (provided by *5 Medical Regiment*) reduced its overall medical footprint in line with overall ISAF reductions whilst maintaining its clinical capability in the face of the Taliban refining their tactics to try and undermine ANSF morale. This was exemplified when the Medical Regiment had to respond to a 55 casualty major medical incident early in the tour.

Whilst there were few ISAF casualties during these six months, an IED strike against a Mastiff on 30 April resulted in another major incident, with three fatalities and six wounded amongst British troops. The summer season also saw a rise in ANSF casualties being received at Bastion. Personnel were therefore reinvested into developing ANA Role 1 medical capability whilst providing additional support to the mentoring project at Shorabak's TMC and the new Role 2 facility.[122]

ROLE 3 SUPPORT

This was led by *33 Field Hospital*, maintaining clinical excellence at Bastion, but now also formally tasked with developing ANSF surgical capability at the ANA Role 2 facility. A concerted all-unit effort resulted in a gratifying total of over 200 surgical procedures (including on Category A, T1 casualties) being performed there by the end of tour, with more than 230 casualties also being transferred directly from Bastion for ongoing care.[123]

2014 Withdrawal from theatre

The last two *Operation Herrick* tours saw the base closure programme completed with transition to the ANSF and final withdrawal from theatre, leaving behind a small training force in Kabul (under *Operation Toral*).

Operation Herrick 19 (7 Armoured Brigade, *October 2013 to April/June 2014*)

ROLE 1 SUPPORT

The CS Medical Regiment on this eight-month-long penultimate tour was provided by *2 Medical Regiment*. With the closure of all bases outside Bastion marking this tour, manoeuvre (CS) medical support 'outside the wire' became limited to the manoeuvre battle group; all area medical support outside Camp Bastion (now designated Joint Operating Base Bastion) now ceased. The exceptions were a Role 1 medical treatment facility at Kandahar Airfield and two in Kabul, namely at Camp Qargha (in a Tier 3 build supporting the new ANA Officer Academy) and Camp Souter (these two would eventually transfer to *Operation Toral*).[124]

ROLE 3 SUPPORT

All ANSF Category B and C casualties were treated by ANSF personnel and, if necessary, admitted to the Role 2 facility at Shorabak from 1 January 2014. In the meantime, the ANSF Regional Military Hospital commenced construction in November 2013 (with a view to completion within two years).

The nucleus for deployed hospital care at Bastion was provided by *203 Field Hospital* on *Operation Herrick 19a* and *202 Field Hospital* on *Operation Herrick 19 B*, each augmented by regulars and other reservists, and a couple of Danish and Estonian personnel. The initial US contingent of 81 personnel had decreased to 53 personnel by the start of *Operation Herrick 19b*, as part of their own withdrawal.

Operation Herrick 20 (20 Armoured Brigade, *April to November 2014*)

'It is my honour to inform you that the Bastion Role 3 Hospital closed at 1000 hrs (L) on the 22nd of September 2014. This has brought to a close an historic era in the story of military medicine'.[125]

Command on *Operation Herrick 20* everted to the pre-*Operation Herrick 10* construct, with a separate commander medical and the CO of the Bastion Role 3 Hospital also commanding the Med Group. The CS medical regiment commenced *Operation Herrick 20* with a much reduced footprint, becoming a medical squadron within the Med Gp. This final Squadron was provided by *30 CS Squadron* from the newly re-organised and renamed *1 Armoured Medical Regiment*. The final field hospital to deploy to Bastion on Operation Herrick was, very fittingly, the regular *34 Field Hospital* – it had also been the first to deploy into Afghanistan after 9/11, setting up a hospital troop at Bagram Airfield on Christmas Eve, 2001, on *Operation Fingal*.

ROLE 4 THE ROYAL CENTRE FOR DEFENCE MEDICINE

The UK's Role 4 during the *Operation Telic* and *Herrick Campaigns* has been the RCDM, a centre for both academic and clinical excellence, at Birmingham, receiving all injured service personnel from overseas. Its genesis following the nadir of the DMS in the late 1990s proves the validity of

Barry Posen's hypothesis in his seminal work on military innovation theory: that an organisation facing defeat can be spurred to innovate.[126]

At the end of the Cold War (1990), there were 19 British military hospitals still in existence across all three Services around the world, and the three Services had their own separate centres of academia and clinical excellence. Drastic restructuring occurred with the post-Cold War peace dividend cuts of the 1994 Defence Cost Studies.[127] DCS 15 (*Front Line First*) resulted in wholesale closure of military hospitals, with the sole survivor in the United Kingdom being the Royal Hospital Haslar, which became tri-service. Military clinicians were dispersed into five small *Ministry of Defence Hospital Units* within National Health Service (NHS) hospitals. Unsurprisingly, many experienced personnel left, and there was a huge drop in morale and corporate knowledge. By 1997, the House of Commons Defence Committee was questioning whether the DMS could even continue to exist and concluded that it would be unable to respond to the demands of a new conflict.[128]

Faced with this existential challenge, the DMS innovated, under the leadership of the remaining cadre of hospital consultants.[129] It was decided to partner military healthcare even closer with the NHS, to close RH Haslar and to open a centre of academic military medicine at a leading university hospital, this becoming the RCDM in Birmingham.[130] The RCDM officially opened on 2 April 2001 at Selly Oak Hospital NHS Trust. The initial problems encountered when injured servicemen began returning from conflict in Iraq and Afghanistan to an NHS without experience in dealing with war wounds were surmounted under combined military and civilian leadership.[131]

In June 2010, RCDM and Selly Oak Hospital relocated to the new Queen Elizabeth Hospital Birmingham.[132] Injured service personnel thereafter would be treated in a dedicated 32-bed trauma and orthopaedic ward within a military environment, whose organisation and ethos are evocatively described in Emily Mayhew's *A Heavy Reckoning*.[133] The Queen Elizabeth Hospital and the RCDM have become the leading trauma hospital in the United Kingdom, and this strong civilian–military partnership is a role model for co-operation, co-ordination and achievement.[134–136] The care casualties received

at RCDM prepared them well for rehabilitation at the next stage on their road to recovery, the Defence Medical Rehabilitation Centre (DMRC) at Headley Court.

ROLE 4 HEADLEY COURT

'They have served their country, buried their mates, cheated death itself and now rise above the hurt their enemies thought they had inflicted on them'.

General the Lord Dannatt, Chief of the General Staff 2006–2009[137]

General the Lord Dannatt was here paying testimony to wounded service personnel who had journeyed to recovery through the DMRC at Headley Court, Surrey. Headley Court was established in 1946 in the aftermath of the Second World War but re-entered the nation's consciousness during the Iraq and Afghanistan Campaigns largely through the fund-raising efforts of the charity Help for Heroes, newly established on 1 October 2007, which actively raised funds for Headley Court. The Headley motto is *Per Mutua*, for the joint effort needed from medics and patients to 'break the shackles' of injury.[138]

Casualties entered Headley once they left the acute care environment of RCDM, in order to mobilise and return to fitness and work as far as possible. Headley has been transformed completely in response to receiving large numbers of complex polytrauma casualties. In 2006, Headley had four beds and no staff and 26 patients throughout the year; the following year, following the UK's deployment to Helmand, there were 10 times the number, even before the casualty surges in Afghanistan of 2009–2010.

That was only the beginning:

'Trying to mobilise somebody with no legs is tricky. To mobilise someone with a fractured pelvis and no legs is even trickier'.

Colonel John Etherington, Director, DMRC[139]

Between 2003 and 2014, in Afghanistan alone, 265 British servicemen sustained 416 amputations – all who survived would eventually pass through Headley.[140] Many would be admitted intermittently over four years or more, undergoing perhaps 25–40 operations, their complex multidisciplinary care being closely co-ordinated with RCDM, where many innovative treatments were being refined to deliver the best functional outcomes. Rehabilitation services simultaneously expanded at Birmingham and at smaller units elsewhere. The key to success was the focus throughout on effective multidisciplinary team working.[141]

The number of new patients has temporarily tailed off with the cessation of *Operations Telic* and *Herrick,* and Headley is to be replaced by a purpose-built facility in Shropshire, but the rehabilitation work continues, often in association with the next centre of excellence, which deals with the mental trauma of injury.

ROLE 4 KING'S COLLEGE AND MENTAL HEALTH

'Seeing someone lose half their body and scream all the way onto the helicopter is traumatic. Seeing someone shot dead is traumatic'.

Captain Johnny Mercer, 29 Commando Regiment Royal Artillery.[142]

Psychiatric battle casualties feature significantly in warfare. The MOD responded to the challenge of mitigating the psychological effects of sending military personnel into danger in Iraq and Afghanistan through the engagement of a novel civilian–military research powerhouse, the *King's Centre for Military Health Research* (KCMHR), as well as initiating the preventive measures of decompression and trauma risk management (TRiM) (see 'Trauma Risk Management' section).[143]

The paradigm shift equivalent to the <C>ABC concept for physically wounded casualties was the formal recognition of 'post traumatic stress disorder' (PTSD) as a distinct entity in 1980.[144] However, PTSD is not the only hallmark of psychological casualty, nor is it the most common.

The First and Second World Wars had shown that the number of psychiatric casualties is related to combat intensity and that effective clinical interventions can be applied.[145] However, prior to *Operation Telic,* the British military had no mechanism for measuring the mental health of their personnel. Two factors then combined in 2003 to bring about a radical change to this situation. Firstly, the impending onset of a second war in Iraq awakened concerns of a repeat of the costly 'Gulf War Syndrome' saga that followed the First Gulf War (1990–1991), when many military personnel developed unexplainable poor physical health.[146] The MOD had then been accused of being slow to react to concerns and could not respond adequately due to poor record keeping.[147] Secondly, the MOD was severely criticised in the 2003 PTSD Class Action for potential negligence in not keeping abreast of modern knowledge regarding the psychological consequences of combat and not ensuring that practice followed doctrine.[148]

King's Centre for Military Health Research

These serious criticisms made the MOD realise that it had to carry out robust mental health surveillance in addition to caring for wounded or ill service personnel. This led to the engagement of the civilian–military collaboration: the KCMHR, at King's College London. KCMHR had carried out extensive research into the 'Gulf War Syndrome',[149] so the MOD commissioned it to proactively monitor the health impact of *Operation Telic,* in collaboration with RCDM's Academic Centre for Defence Mental Health.[150,151] This programme was later expanded to cover conflict in Afghanistan. So far, it has shown that the mental health of deployed British personnel generally remains good, although reservists and medics and those exposed to violent conflict fare worse. Alcohol misuse and depression have proven more significant problems than PTSD,[152] although the increase in PTSD symptoms over time warrants more surveillance and support.[153]

Decompression

Whereas servicemen returning from the Falklands war had time to adjust while travelling by sea, in the early days of conflict in Iraq and Afghanistan, servicemen could be in peril in the morning and have flown home by evening. IAs or reservists returning on their own rather than with formed units, in particular, did not cope well with this sudden change. The British military therefore instituted a system of 'third location decompression' to smooth this transition, enforcing a short stopover in Cyprus to give troops opportunity to swim, sail and relax before finally heading home. It had a positive impact upon alcohol use and mental health for soldiers with a low to moderate degree of combat exposure, and generally troops thought decompression was useful.[154]

Trauma risk management

In the late 1990s, the Royal Marines developed a system of psychological first aid called *trauma risk management*, delivered by trained peers from within their unit rather than by health professionals, which emphasises the normality of emotional reactions to trauma. TRiM was formally adopted as best practice throughout the Armed Forces in 2007 and was widely used in Iraq and Afghanistan.[155] While not designed to prevent or treat PTSD, it positively changes attitudes to mental health, countering its stigma, and certainly appears to benefit both individuals and their unit.[156,157]

There remains, however, no cause for complacency. There is still more to be done, by the MOD, the DMS and the NHS, to mitigate the psychological effects of conflict.

'In 2012, we reached a very unwelcome threshold when, tragically, more soldiers and veterans killed themselves than were killed on operational service in defence of the realm'.

Captain Johnny Mercer, elected MP for Plymouth, 2015[158]

CONCLUSION AND A HISTORICAL PERSPECTIVE

'For all of us here, especially medics, Afghanistan has been the defining operation of our military generation. It has been the catalyst which has catapulted us to the forefront of battlefield trauma care worldwide'.

Final Address: Closure of the Bastion Role 3, 22 September 2014[159]

When the Cold War ended (1989) and the First Gulf War broke out (1990), the three Services had their own separate centres of academia and clinical excellence: the Royal Navy had the Royal Hospital Haslar at Gosport, founded in 1753; the Army Medical Services had the Royal Army Medical College at Millbank, founded in 1906, with clinical expertise concentrated at Queen Elizabeth Hospital, Woolwich; and the Royal Air Force had RAF Wroughton. There were 19 permanent British military hospitals still in existence: 9 in the United Kingdom, 5 in Germany and 1 each in Gibraltar, Cyprus, Hong Kong, Nepal and the Falkland Islands. In addition, there was one full-time regular field hospital (*22 Field Hospital*, augmented by two more in 1996) and 14 TA hospitals. The last time a TA hospital had been mobilised was during the Second World War.

Within one generation, in less than 25 years, by the end of the Afghanistan Campaign and the closure of the operational Camp Bastion Hospital in September 2014, all 19 British military hospitals had ceased to exist or been transferred to civilian use, and several TA hospitals had amalgamated. Secondary care in Germany, Gibraltar, Cyprus and the Falkland Islands has been outsourced to the local civilian healthcare system. The DMS in the United Kingdom are now fully integrated with the NHS, the focal point being the Royal Centre of Defence Medicine within the new Queen Elizabeth Hospital in Birmingham.

The three regular field hospitals have each deployed now on several occasions, and each of the current 10 TA (now Army Reserve) field hospitals has been mobilised and deployed on two or three occasions to Iraq and Afghanistan. Although much has been lost, much more has been gained as the lessons from the battlefield have filtered into the NHS and transformed trauma care worldwide. A revolution in military medical care has occurred, and the DMS has been transformed, arguably for the better. Many casualties who would not previously have survived bear witness to that.

REFERENCES

1. Buckenmaier CI, Mahoney P (eds.). *Combat Anesthesia: The First 24 Hours*. Washington: US Army Medical Department, The Borden Institute, 2015, p. xxiii. http://www.cs.amedd.army.mil/borden/Portlet.aspx?id=4f129d5e-973b-48d9-9fb1-514e6daf90e6

2. Hodgetts T. *A Revolutionary Approach to Improving Combat Casualty Care*. Unpublished Doctoral thesis, City University London, 2012. http://openaccess.city.ac.uk/2040/

3. Vassallo DJ. *Military Medical Revolution: Yes or No? Do the Advances in Military Medicine Since 1990, with Particular Reference to the British Defence Medical Services, Amount to a Revolution in Military Medical Affairs?* Unpublished Dissertation for MA (History of Warfare), King's College London, 2015. Available from the author via djvassallo@aol.com

4. Penn-Barwell J, Roberts SA, Midwinter MJ, Bishop JR. Improved survival in UK combat casualties from Iraq and Afghanistan: 2003–2012. *J Trauma Acute Care Surg* 2015;78(5):1014–1020.

5. King's College London. KCMHR and ADMMH publications. http://www.kcl.ac.uk/kcmhr/pubdb/

6. *Operational Patient Care Pathway*. Ministry of Defence: Joint Service Publication (JSP) 950 Leaflet 1-4-1. 2014. https://www.gov.uk/government/publications/operational-patient-care-pathway

7. Bricknell M. For debate: The Operational Patient Care Pathway. *J R Army Med Corps* 2014;160:164–169.

8. Operation Herrick 19 – Close Support Medical Regiment – Post Operational Observations, dated 28 May 2014.

9. Allied Joint Publication-4.10(B) (NATO Standard, Edition B, Version 1 with UK National Elements, published 28 July 2015). Allied Joint Doctrine for Medical Support, Ministry of Defence: Development, Concepts and Doctrine Centre, Shrivenham: 2015, p. (1)5. https://www.gov.uk/government/uploads/system/uploads/attachment_data/file/454625/20150708-nato_ajp_4_10_uk_secured.pdf

10. Army Directorate Land Warfare. *Operation HERRICK Campaign Study*. MOD, 2015. http://www.gov.uk/government/uploads/system/uploads/attachment_data/file/492757/20160107115638.pdf

11. Bricknell MCM, Nadin M. Lessons from the organisation of the UK medical services deployed in support of Operation TELIC (Iraq) and Operation HERRICK (Afghanistan). *J R Army Med Corps* 2017. Published online first, http://dx.doi.org/10.1136/jramc-2016-000720

12. United Nations Security Council Resolution 1441 (2002). 8 November 2002. http://www.un.org/Depts/unmovic/documents/1441.pdf

13. Army Medical Services Core Doctrine (2000). D/AMD/113/18 dated June 2000 – AMS Core Doctrine Volume 1. Camberley: Army Medical Directorate.

14. Vautier G. Anthrax: A review for the medical officer. *J R Army Med Corps* 2003;149(2): 101–105.

15. Smith JE, Smith SRC, Hill G. The UK maritime Role 3 medical treatment facility: The Primary Casualty Receiving Facility, RFA Argus. *J R Naval Med Serv* 2015;101(1):3–5.

16. Vassallo DJ. *A History of The Princess Mary's Hospital, Royal Air Force Akrotiri 1963–2013 (Limassol: Cyprint, 2012)*. 2nd ed. Kettering: Crest Publications, 2017.

17. Permanent Joint Headquarters: Operation TELIC 1 – Medical Post Operation Report, Para 21, dated 25 September 2003.

18. 84 Medical Supply Squadron wins the ESCEA for Extreme Logistics. Royal Logistic Corps Newsletter, 4 December 2015. http://www.royallogisticcorps.co.uk/84-medical-supply-squadron-wins-the-escea-for-extreme-logistics/

19. David Rowlands, Military Artist. Prints by any of the military artists who have generously allowed their work to be reproduced can be purchased via their websites, details of which are given in the acknowledgements.

20. 1 Close Support Medical Regiment: Interim Post Operational Report and Lessons Learned – OP TELIC. 6 May 2003.

21. 16 Close Support Medical Regiment – Overview. *Royal Army Medical Corps Magazine* 2004;4(1):24.

22. Clasper JC, Jeffrey PA, Mahoney PF. The forward deployment of surgical teams. *Curr Anaesth Crit Care* 2003;14(3):122–125.

23. 16 Close Support Medical Regiment: Operation TELIC – Post Operational Report. 1 July 2003.

24. 4 General Support Medical Regiment. *Royal Army Medical Corps Magazine* 2004; 4(1):18.

25. Information kindly provided by Brigadier Hugh Williamson.

26. Operation TELIC – Post Operation Report: Medical, Volume 1 (of three); Permanent Joint Headquarters, Overview: 1–2. 25 September 2003.

27. Operation TELIC – Post Operation Report: Medical, Volume 1 (of three); Permanent Joint Headquarters, Overview: 4. 25 September 2003.

28. Primary Casualty Receiving Facility RFA *ARGUS* – Post Operational Report Operation TELIC. London: MOD, 25 September 2003.

29. O'Reilly DJ, Kilbey J. Analysis of the initial 100 scans from the first CT scanner deployed by the British armed forces in a land environment. *J R Army Med Corps* 2007;153(3):165–167.

30. Vassallo DJ, Gerlinger T, Maholtz P, Burlingame B, Shepherd A. Combined UK/US Field Hospital management of a major incident arising from a Chinook helicopter crash in Afghanistan, 28 Jan 2002. *J R Army Med Corps* 2003;149:47–52.

31. 22 Field Hospital Deployment OP TELIC – After Action Review, dated 25 May 2003.

32. 22 Field Hospital. *Royal Army Medical Corps Magazine* 2003;3(2):7.

33. 33 Field Hospital – Post Operational Report – OP TELIC, dated 4 June 2003.

34. Annex P, Wards, to: 33 Field Hospital – Post Operational Report – OP TELIC, dated 4 June 2003.

35. Bailey MS, Boos CJ, Vautier G et al. Gastroenteritis outbreak in British Troops, Iraq. *Emerging Infect Dis* 2005;11(10):1625–1628. doi:10.3201/eid1110.050298.

36. 34 Field Hospital – OP TELIC Post Operational Report: Executive Summary, dated 20 June 2003.

37. 202 Field Hospital: Unit Historical Record, 1 April 2002–31 March 2003, Commanding Officer's Comments.

38. 202 Field Hospital POR Lessons Report – Operation TELIC, dated 2 July 2003.

39. Joint Force Logistic Command Medical Post Operation Report 15 April – 30 June 2003. Undated.

40. Green T. *A Jolly Good Show – The Heritage and History of 202 Field Hospital*. Self-published, 2008, p. 247.

41. Roberts MJ, Fox MA, Hamilton-Davies C, Dawson S. The experience of the intensive care unit in a British army field hospital during the 2003 Gulf conflict. *J R Army Med Corps* 2003;149(4):284–290.

42. Kerr G, Clasper JC, Rew DA. Surgical workload from an integrated UK Field Hospital during the 2003 Gulf conflict. *J R Army Med Corps* 2004;150(2):99–106.

43. Rew D. *Blood, Heat + Dust – Operation Telic and the British Medical Deployment to the Gulf in 2003*. Avonworld, 2005, Chapters 10–11. Available as a CD-ROM from the Museum of Military Medicine (formerly the AMS Museum, at Keogh Barracks) and online: http://www.pangrafix.com/bhd/

44. Rew D. *Blood, Heat + Dust – Operation Telic and the British Medical Deployment to the Gulf 2003–2009*. Association of Surgeons of Great Britain & Ireland, 2015. http://www.publications.asgbi.org/bhd_donate/donation_page.html

45. A field hospital in the Second Gulf War. In: Beckett I (ed.). *Territorials – A Century of Service*. Plymouth: DRA Publishing, 2008, pp. 253–254.

46. Green T. *First in, Last Out – 202 Field Hospital On Operations, 2000–2014*. Self-published, 2016.

47. 33 Field Hospital – Op Telic 2 – Post Operation Report, dated 19 November 2003.

48. 33 Field Hospital – Op Telic 2 – Post Operation Report, dated 19 November 2003.

49. Post-operational interview, purposely left anonymous and undated.

50. Post Operational Report – 5 (UK) Medical Group – Operation TELIC 5, dated 25 May 2005.

51. O'Reilly DJ, Kilbey J. Analysis of the initial 100 scans from the first CT scanner deployed by the British armed forces in a land environment. *J R Army Med Corps*, 2007;153(3):165–167.

52. Mahoney PF, Hodgetts TJ, Hicks I. The deployed medical director: Managing the challenges of a complex trauma system. *J R Army Med Corps*, 2011;157(3 Suppl 1):S350–S356.

53. Post Operational Report – 3 Close Support (United Kingdom) Medical Group – Operation TELIC 6, dated 29 November 2005.

54. Operation TELIC 8 – 22 UK Medical Group – Post Operational Report, dated 14 December 2006.

55. The Effects of Op SINBAD 20 September 2006–14 January 2007. MOD, letter to the Secretary of State, 16 February 2007, declassified. http://www.iraqinquiry.org.uk/media/243581/2007-02-16-minute-beadle-to-banner-the-effect-of-op-sinbad-20-september-2006-to-14-january-2007.pdf

56. Merrett SJO. Royal Engineers support to constructing field hospitals. *R Eng J* 2005;119(3):220–225.

57. Operation TELIC 9 – UK Medical Group Post Operational Report, dated 25 June 2007.

58. Operation TELIC 9 – UK Medical Group Post Operational Report, dated 25 June 2007.

59. Froggatt C, Adams B. *Wounded – The Legacy of War*. Germany: Steidl, 2013, pp. 84–89.

60. Operation TELIC 10 – UK Medical Group Post Operational Report, dated 15 November 2007.

61. Message quoted in: Wardley TE. Operation TELIC – A personal View. *J R Naval Med Serv* 2008;94(2):90–91.

62. Casualty Monitor. British Casualties: Iraq. http://www.casualty-monitor.org/p/iraq.html

63. 22 Field Hospital Post Operational Report OP TELIC 13, dated 15 May 2009.

64. Parkinson B. Personal account. In: Froggatt C, Adams B (eds.). *Wounded – The Legacy of War*. Germany: Steidl, 2013, p. 78.

65. OP HERRICK 4 – Joint Force Medical Group Post Operational Report, dated 10 October 2006.

66. Kajaki – The True Story (Kajaki Films Ltd. 2014); Cpl Paul (Tug) Hartley, conversation with author 1 July 2017.

67. Central Chancery of the Orders of Knighthood [Announcement of the award of the George Medal to Cpl Colin Lowes RAMC]. *Army Medical Services Magazine* 1953 (April), p. 36.

68. Vassallo DJ, Graham P, Gupta G, Alempijevic D. "Bomb explosion on the Nis Express" – lessons from a major incident, Kosovo 16 Feb 2001. *J R Army Med Corps* 2005;151:19–29.

69. Davis PR, Rickards AC, Ollerton JE. Determining the composition and benefit of the pre-hospital medical response team in the conflict setting. *J R Army Med Corps* 2007;153(4):269–273.

70. Nicholson RT, Berry R. Pre-hospital trauma care and aero-medical transfer: A military perspective. *Contin Educ Anaesth Crit Care Pain* 2012;12(4):186–189.

71. Pope CD. The medical emergency response team. In: Buckenmaier CI, Mahoney P. (eds.). *Combat Anesthesia: The First 24 Hours*. Washington: US Army Medical Department, The Borden Institute, 2015, pp. 44–46. http://www.cs.amedd.army.mil/borden/Portlet.aspx?id=4f129d5e-973b-48d9-9fb1-514e6daf90e6

72. Apodaca A, Olson C, Bailey J, Butler F, Eastridge B, Kuncir E. Performance improvement evaluation of forward aero-medical evacuation platforms in Operation Enduring Freedom. *J Trauma Acute Care Surg* 2013;75(2 Suppl 2):S157–S163.

73. Morrison JJ, Oh J, DuBose J, O'Reilly D, Russell R, Blackbourne L et al. En-route care capability from point of injury impacts mortality after severe wartime injury. *Ann Surg* 2013;257:330–334.

74. Annett R. *Lifeline in Helmand – RAF Battle-field Mobility in Afghanistan*. Barnsley: Pen & Sword, 2010.

75. British Forces News, 18 November 2015. MERT Saving Lives High in the Sky. http://forces.tv/30067787

76. Vassallo D. A short history of Camp Bastion Hospital: The two hospitals and unit deployments. *J R Army Med Corps* 2015;161:79–83.

77. Vassallo D. A short history of Camp Bastion Hospital: Part 2 – Bastion's catalytic role in advancing combat casualty care. *J R Army Med Corps* 2015;161:160–166.

78. Vassallo D. A short history of Camp Bastion Hospital: Preparing for war, national recognition and Bastion's legacy. *J R Army Med Corps* 2015;161:355–360.

79. OP HERRICK 4 – Joint Force Medical Group Post Operational Report, dated 10 October 2006.

80. Willdridge DJ, Hodgetts TJ, Mahoney PF, Jarvis L. The Joint Theatre Clinical Case Conference (JTCCC): Clinical governance in action. *J R Army Med Corps* 2010;156(2): 79–83.

81. Adapted from: Lt Col Simon Atkinson (Commander UK Medical Group). *Provision of Medical Support in High Intensity COIN Operations*, Annex A to OP HERRICK 6 – UK JF MED GP – Post-Operational Report, dated 21 September 2007.

82. Information from Post-Operational Interviews with Medical Commanders, Land Warfare Centre, conducted by Brigadier (Retd) IA Johnstone OBE, SO1 Post Operational Interviewer, Mission Support Group.

83. Post-Operational Report UK Joint Force Medical Group OP HERRICK 7, dated April 2008.

84. Report on the transition of the Role 2 Enhanced Medical Treatment Facility, Camp Bastion from Tier 1 to Tier 2 Accommodation. Annex F (Annex-F-TierR2E.doc), incorporated within HERRICK 7 Post-Operational Report.

85. Tai NRM, Russell R. Right turn resuscitation: Frequently asked questions. *J R Army Med Corps* 2011; 157(3 Suppl 1):S310–S314.

86. Commander Medical Op HERRICK 7, Post-Operational Report. 1 January 2008.

87. Vassallo D. A short history of Camp Bastion Hospital: The two hospitals and unit deployments. *J R Army Med Corps*, 2015;161(1):79–83.

88. See particularly: Report on the transition of the Role 2 Enhanced Medical Treatment Facility, Camp Bastion from Tier 1 to Tier 2 Accommodation (within Commander Medical Op HERRICK 7 POR).

89. Tarrant JS. Field hospitals – Lessons learnt. *R Eng J* 2012;126:46–55.

90. UK Joint Force Med Group. In: *Operation HERRICK 8, Afghanistan 10 April – 8 October 2008: A Report by 16 Air Assault Brigade*. pp. 29–30 (accessed at the Prince Consort Library, Aldershot, 27 June 2015).

91. Information about the Estonian medical contingent was kindly supplied to the author by Major Tiit Meren.

92. Doran CM, Woolley T, Midwinter MJ. Feasibility of using rotational thrombo-elastometry to assess coagulation status of combat casualties in a deployed setting. *J Trauma Injury Infect Crit Care* 2010;69(Suppl 1):S40–S48.

93. Brown D. Editorial. *J R Naval Med Services* 2009;95(3):123–124.

94. A cruel summer. In: Fairweather J (ed.). *The Good War – Why We Couldn't Win the War or the Peace in Afghanistan*. London: Jonathan Cape, 2014, Chapter 24, pp. 301–318.

95. Committee of Tactical Combat Casualty Care. Tactical evacuation care improvements within the Department of Defense 2011-03. http://www.health.mil/Reference-Center/Reports/2011/08/08

96. Tai NRM, Brooks A, Midwinter M, Clasper JC, Parker PJ. Optimal clinical timelines – A consensus from the Academic Department of Military Surgery and Trauma. *J R Army Med Corps* 2009;155:253–256.

97. Mahoney PF, Hodgetts TJ, Hicks I. The deployed medical director: Managing the challenges of a complex trauma system. *J R Army Med Corps*, 2011;157(3 Suppl 1): S350–S356.

98. Bernthal EM, Draper HJA, Henning J, Kelly JC. 'A band of brothers' – An exploration of the range of medical ethical issues faced by British senior military clinicians on deployment to Afghanistan: A qualitative study. *J R Army Med Corps* 2017;163:199–205.

99. Vassallo D. A short history of Camp Bastion Hospital: Preparing for war, national recognition and Bastion's legacy. *J R Army Med Corps* 2015;161:355–360.

100. Post Operational Report UK Joint Force Medical Group Role 3 Hospital, Op HERRICK 10a, dated 31 July 2009.

101. Graff P. UK hospital in Afghanistan copes with bloodiest day. *Reuters*, 12 July 2009.

102. Casualty Monitor. British Casualties: Afghanistan http://www.casualty-monitor .org/p/british-casualties-in-afghanistan.html

103. Colonel TJ Hodgetts, Deployed Medical Director – DNK/GBR H10B Post-Project Evaluation and Learning Account, dated 5 November 2009.

104. Neville L. *The British Army in Afghanistan 2006 – 14: Task Force Helmand.* Oxford: Osprey, 2015, p. 40.

105. Op HERRICK casualty and fatality tables to 31 December 2014. https://www.gov.uk /government/statistics/op-herrick-casualty -and-fatality-tables-released-in-2014

106. Bricjknell MCM. Medical Lessons from OPERATION MOSHTARAK Phase 2. *J R Army Med Corps* 2011;157(4 Suppl 2) :S463–S467.

107. Managing medical support to operations (special supplement). *J R Army Med Corps* 2011;157(4)(suppl 2):S427–S476.

108. Post Operational Report OP HERRICK 11A, Joint Force Medical Group, Role 3 Hospital Squadron, 256 (City of London) Field Hospital (Volunteers), dated 28 February 2010.

109. Jansen JO, Morrison JJ, Midwinter MJ, Doughty H. Changes in blood transfusion practices in the UK role 3 medical treatment facility in Afghanistan, 2008–2011. *Transfus Med* 2014;24(3):154–161. doi:10.1111/tme .12093. Epub 2013 December 24.

110. Information kindly provided to the author by Brigadier Hugh Williamson.

111. Bricknell MCM. Managing medical support to military operations – The Headquarters Regional Command (South) Experience. *J R Army Med Corps* 2011;157(4 Suppl 2): S428–S429.

112. Army Medical Directorate Lessons Newsletter, Issue 1, June 2010, p. 8.

113. Close Support Medical Regiment Post Operational Report Operation HERRICK 13, dated 2 May 2011.

114. Op HERRICK 14 – Post Operational Tour Report, dated 5 November 2011.

115. Blankenstein T. To make order from chaos. *BMA News* 15 December 2012, p. 10.

116. UK Picture Editors Guild 2012 Photographer of the Year award. www.piced.net/2012 -winners.html

117. Brigadier Doug Chalmers, Commander Task Force Helmand. Quoted from: Op Herrick 16: Task Force Helmand Post Operational Report.

118. Post Operational Tour Report – United Kingdom Medical Group Close Support Medical Regiment Op Herrick 17, dated 25 March 2013.

119. Comd Med Post Operational Report Op Herrick 17/ HQ JFSP(A) 15, dated 25 March 2013.

120. Hammond P. *Reserves in the Future Force 2020: Valuable and Valued.* White Paper presented to the Parliament, July 2013.

121. Comd Med Post Operational Report Op Herrick 17/ HQ JFSP(A) 15, dated 25 March 2013.

122. Operation Herrick 18, 5 Medical Regiment – Post Operational Report, dated 19 September 2013.

123. Operation HERRICK 18, Bastion Role 3 – Post Operational Report, dated 13 October 2013.

124. Operation HERRICK 19, Close Support Medical Regiment – Post Operational Observations, dated 28 May 2014.

125. Communication by Lt Col Jaish Mahan, last CO of Bastion Hospital, to Director General Army Medical Services, 22 September 2014. Reproduced with permission of Lt Col Mahan.

126. Posen BR. *The Sources of Military Doctrine: France, Britain and Germany between the Wars.* Ithaca, NY: Cornell University Press, 1984, p. 47.

127. Raffaelli P. Preface – Military medicine. *Phil Trans Soc B* 2011;366:123.

128. House of Commons Defence Committee. *Seventh Report The Strategic Defence Review: Defence Medical Services – Background*. London: The Stationery Office, 1999.

129. Lillywhite L. The past, present and future of the Defence Medical Services. *J R Army Med Corps* 2009;155 (4):244–245.

130. Jenkins I. The changing world of military health care *J R Naval Med Serv* 2004;90(3): 153–158.

131. Parker C. Foreword. In: Froggatt C, Adams B (eds.). *Wounded – The Legacy of War*. Germany: Steidl, 2013, pp. 10–11.

132. RCDM Birmingham. http://www.raf.mod.uk /PMRAFNS/organisation/rcdmbirmingham .cfm

133. Mayhew E. *A Heavy Reckoning – War, Medicine and Survival in Afghanistan and Beyond*. London: Profile Books, 2017.

134. Evriviades D, Jeffery S, Cubison T, Lawton G, Gill M, Mortiboy D. Shaping the military wound: Issues surrounding the reconstruction of injured servicemen at the Royal Centre for Defence Medicine. *Phil Trans R Soc B* 2011;366:219–230.

135. Hollingsworth AC. The Birmingham Military Trauma Registrar – a personal view. *J R Naval Med Serv* 2012;98(3):21–25.

136. Porter K. Care for the Courageous. *Surgeons News* 2012(June):22–24. http:// www.surgeonsnews.com/back-issues and http://edition.pagesuite-professional.co.uk /Launch.aspx?EID=10d3bfa3-2f03-4d31 -894e-ca35a3ef9a77

137. Dannatt R, Foreword. In: Froggatt C, Adams B (eds.). *Wounded – The Legacy of War*. Germany: Steidl, 2013, pp. 12–13.

138. Ormrod M. *Man Down*. London: Transworld Publishers, 2009, p. 246.

139. Etherington J. The Work of the Defence Medical Rehabilitation Centre, Headley Court – Gresham College Lecture, 24 March 2014. http://www.gresham.ac.uk /lectures-and-events/the-work-of-the -defence-medical-rehabilitation-centre -headley-court

140. Edwards DS, Phillip RD, Bosanquet N, Bull AJ, Clasper JC. What is the magnitude and long-term economic cost of care of the British Military Afghanistan Amputee Cohort? *Clin Orthop Relat Res* 2015;473: 2848–2855.

141. Pope S, Vickerstaff AL, Wareham AP. Lessons learned from early rehabilitation of complex trauma at the Royal Centre for Defence Medicine *J R Army Med Corps* 2017;163:124–131.

142. Mercer J. *We Were Warriors (One Soldier's Story of Brutal Combat)*. London: Sidgwick & Jackson, 2017, p. 199.

143. Greenberg N, Jones E, Jones N, Fear NT, Wessely S. The injured mind in the UK Armed Forces. *Phil Trans R Soc B* 2011;366:261–267.

144. Jones E, Wessely S. A paradigm shift in the conceptualization of psychological trauma in the 20th century. *J Anxiety Disord* 2007; 21:164–175.

145. Jones E, Wessely S. Psychiatric battle casualties: An intra- and interwar comparison. *Br J Psychiatry* 2001;178:242–247.

146. Minshall D. Gulf War Syndrome: a review of current knowledge and understanding. *J R Naval Med Serv* 2014:100(3):252–258.

147. Wessely S. The psychological impact of Operations in Iraq: What has it been, and what can we expect in the future? In: Bailey J, Iron R, Strachan H (eds.). *British Generals in Blair's Wars*. Surrey: Ashgate, 2013, Chapter 17, pp. 201–212.

148. PTSD Class Action. Multiple Claimants v The Ministry of Defence (Part 1) EWHC 1134 (QB). 21 May 2003, Paragraph 5.116. http:// www.bailii.org/ew/cases/EWHC/QB/2003 /1134.html

149. Greenberg N, Wessely S. Gulf War syndrome: An emerging threat or a piece of history? *Emerg Health Threats J* 2008;1,e10. (doi:10.3134/ehtj.08.010)

150. Greenberg N, Jones E, Jones N, Fear NT, Wessely S. The injured mind in the UK Armed Forces. *Phil Trans R Soc B* 2011;366: 261–267.

151. KCMHR and ADMMH publications. http:// www.kcl.ac.uk/kcmhr/pubdb

152. MacManus D, Jones N, Wessely S, Fear NT, Jones E, Greenberg N. The mental health of the UK Armed Forces in the 21st century: Resilience in the face of adversity. *J R Army Med Corps* 2014;160:125–130.

153. Banwell E, Greenberg N, Smith P, Jones N, Fertout M. What happens to the mental health of UK service personnel after they return home from Afghanistan? *J R Army Med Corps* 2016;162:115–119.

154. Jones N, Jones M, Fear NT, Fertout M, Wessely S, Greenberg N. Can mental health and readjustment be improved in UK military personnel by a brief period of structured post-deployment rest (third location decompression)? *Occup Environ Med* 2013; 70(7):439–445.

155. Greenberg N, Langston V, Jones N. Trauma risk management (TRiM) in the UK armed forces. *J R Army Med Corps* 2008;154: 124–127.

156. Greenberg N, Langston V, Everitt B et al. A cluster randomized controlled trial to determine the efficacy of TRiM (Trauma Risk Management) in a military population. *J Trauma Stress* 2010;23:430–436.

157. Wessely S. The psychological impact of Operations in Iraq: what has it been, and what can we expect in the future? In: Bailey J, Iron R, Strachan H (eds.). *British Generals in Blair's Wars*. Surrey: Ashgate, 2013, Chapter 17, pp. 201–212.

158. Mercer J. *We Were Warriors (One Soldier's Story of Brutal Combat)*. London: Sidgwick & Jackson, 2017, p. 323.

159. Mahan JK. Final address: Closure of the Bastion Role 3 on 22 Sep 2014. *J R Naval Med Serv* 2014;100(3):231.

3

Pre-hospital emergency care

INTRODUCTION

War drives progress. The concept of military *pre-hospital emergency care* (PHEC) as an integrated system was developed as a response to the pressures of the conflicts in Iraq and Afghanistan. The system 'developed' rather than 'evolved' because the sharing of ideas across different stages of the patient pathway was key to improving the end-to-end survival of the catastrophically injured combat casualty.[1] Developments were not random, although the implementation of change sometimes appears that way. A requirement constantly to improve performance, coupled with an organisational acceptance of innovation, backed by generous funding, led to striking changes. It can be argued that Iraq and Afghanistan were wars of choice, rather than of necessity. At no time was the UK mainland under direct threat of invasion or widespread destruction. Paradoxically, this creates an even greater pressure to reduce mortality. In order to maintain public support for the ongoing military interventions, the numbers of dead soldiers being repatriated had to be kept as low as reasonably possible: witness the punishing verdicts in the press and in the Courts when military equipment was considered to be defective. PHEC is the first link in the chain of survival, and the first step on casualties' long road to recovery. As we will see, PHEC is arguably the most important step, and certainly the single area of improvement, that has led to the greatest improvement in mortality for our service personnel. Trauma hospitals and rehabilitation units are of little use if the patient does not survive the initial insult. Good epidemiological studies, originally from the US military,

opened the door to the realisation that excellent pre-hospital care could make such a huge difference and ultimately led to the challenging of several long-held medical axioms, the significance of catastrophic external haemorrhage being the most obvious of these. Out of this fell the requirement for techniques to control external haemorrhage, including battlefield tourniquets and haemostatic dressings, as well as the desire to limit damage: for example the dawning recognition that litres of intravenous cold crystalloid fluid were detrimental to the patient.

It is possible to point to the precise moment that the process of transformation of the Defence Medical Services (DMS) was triggered. At 08:46 am on 11 September 2001, Mohammed Atta crashed American Airlines Flight 11 into the North Tower of the World Trade Centre. Ultimately, the attack caused the deaths of 2996 civilians and injured 6000 others. On New Year's Eve 2002, the first regular Army unit entered Afghanistan (2nd Battalion the Parachute Regiment on *Operation Fingal*). The medical team in support (the Regimental Aid Post) carried 'Samway Anchor' tourniquets (but did not know what they were for or how to use them, for the institutional memory had been lost) and bottles of saline (but no way of warming either the patient or the fluids) and they worked in the light of Tilley Lamps. Their understanding of gunshot wounds was limited to a lecture from someone who had seen one once in Northern Ireland, and their concept of blast injuries was non-existent. The desperate desire to save lives was present, but the means, largely, were not. There was no written medical plan of any kind. In October 2014, the last units pulled out of Helmand Province at the resolution

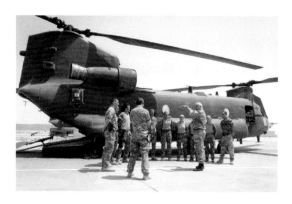

Figure 3.1 General Sir Peter Wall (CGS) visits the Medical Emergency Response Team.

of *Operation Herrick*. These units were supported by a *Medical Emergency Response Team* (MERT): a consultant-led medical team carrying blood products, pre-hospital fluid warmers, chemically heated blankets and the training and confidence to perform pre-hospital procedures such as *pre-hospital emergency anaesthesia* (PHEA) and pre-hospital emergency thoracotomy. Even better, this team was, until the very last moment, intimately linked to the receiving hospital facilities as well as benefitting from an ingrained understanding of the processes that lead to patient death from trauma on the battlefield (Figure 3.1).

DEVELOPMENT OF CIVILIAN PRE-HOSPITAL EMERGENCY MEDICINE IN THE UNITED KINGDOM

The development of military PHEC between 2001 and 2014 coincided with the development of civilian PHEC in the United Kingdom. North American and European models of pre-hospital care began to diverge in the 1990s, with literature in the United States supporting the philosophy of 'scoop and run', whereas European systems tended more towards a 'stay and play' approach.[2] In other words, US pre-hospital clinicians prioritised removal of the casualty from the scene to hospital care, whereas in the United Kingdom, medical lifesaving interventions *at scene* took priority. This difference was exacerbated by the relative differences in funding of healthcare in North America compared to Europe. Private healthcare does not lend itself to physicians

deploying forward of hospital facilities, whereas in a nationally funded healthcare system, physician–paramedic models of care are more likely to be found. Nevertheless, in the United Kingdom, engagement of physicians in pre-hospital care was patchy to say the least and largely dependent on the drive of committed individuals. This difference in civilian models of care is reflected within the relevant militaries – with US military physicians rarely working in the pre-hospital arena.

In the United Kingdom, a few pioneers of civilian pre-hospital care, such as Sir Keith Porter in the Midlands (founder of the *West Midlands Central Accident, Resuscitation and Emergency* Team), and Dr. Alastair Wilson (founder of *London's Air Ambulance*), had driven the development of higher level pre-hospital care teams, led by specially trained physicians, performing physician-only interventions such as *rapid sequence induction of anaesthesia* (RSI; now usually termed *pre-hospital emergency anaesthesia*) and pre-hospital emergent thoracotomy.[3] These and a few other highly organised schemes, usually in rural areas, operated against a background of individual clinicians providing care in their own locale, and often to their own patient population in the case of general practitioners. In many areas there was no provision. The engagement of hospital specialists was limited but the *British Association for Immediate Care* (BASICS) and, later, the *Faculty of Pre-Hospital Care* at the Royal College of Surgeons of Edinburgh, offered education, guidance on clinical and training matters and eventually both a *Diploma* and *Fellowship in Immediate Medical Care* (the preferred term at that time). For a period of time, pre-hospital care was considered 'the Wild-West of Medicine' (as described by Dr. Rod Mackenzie) and was perceived as an area of practice largely confined to rural general practitioners and 'enthusiasts' with all the implied negative connotations that that term can attract. In addition, lack of a sizeable evidence base frequently led hospital-based clinicians to question whether pre-hospital interventions had any value at all. Despite all these challenges, there was a definite trend towards increased engagement of physicians in pre-hospital care, and increasingly towards the involvement of hospital clinicians, particularly emergency physicians and anaesthetists. The inclusion of a physician as part of the standard team on air ambulances became increasingly common (although it is not universal even today). It should be noted that the majority of the service provision was offered *pro bono* by clinicians, although a handful of consultants were allocated time in their job plans. Senior military emergency medicine (EM) consultants had been particularly active in the development of the specialty and strong links were established with a number of schemes, particularly in London and the West Midlands.

On 20 July 2011, *pre-hospital emergency medicine* (PHEM) was approved by the *General Medical Council* as a medical sub-specialty of the existing specialties of EM and anaesthesia. The terminology can cause some confusion, but PHEM is the subspecialty practiced by doctors, whereas PHEC refers to the totality of pre-hospital clinical provision, irrespective of who is providing it. The close nature of the community of pre-hospital physicians in the United Kingdom meant that developments on operations happened synergistically with developments at home. In some areas, such as pre-hospital thoracotomy, the civilian practitioners led the way; in other areas, such as pre-hospital administration of blood products, the military drove development.[4,5] As the Iraq and Afghanistan conflicts developed, trainees in both EM and

anaesthesia were encouraged to gain pre-hospital experience, and in 2008, a specific *Tri-Service Lead* post was established for PHEM. This was initially attached to the role of Defence Consultant Advisor (DCA) EM, with the incumbent at the time having had a longstanding engagement in the subspecialty. In 2014, a separate role of DCA PHEM was created. Following the establishment of PHEM as a sub-speciality, clear guidelines were established requiring the completion of a formal PHEM training scheme and regular pre-hospital practice for trainees who intended to provide pre-hospital care as part of their deployed role.

DEVELOPMENT OF MERT

Military medical officers have always supported *immediate response teams* (IRTs). Throughout *Operation Banner*, in Northern Ireland, a medical officer was on stand-by to move by Lynx helicopter from Bessbrook Mill to the scene of an incident, and there are many other examples from deployments and exercises in other parts of the world. During *Operation Telic*, a rotary wing IRT capability was provided across the British *area of responsibility* (AOR) in Southern Iraq using Puma helicopters (Figure 3.2). The medical officers were usually Royal Air Force (RAF)

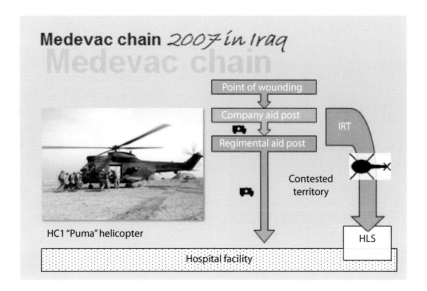

Figure 3.2 Forward MEDEVAC chain in Iraq.

general practitioners from the medical centre at the *air point of disembarkation* and they delivered patients to the Role 2 Field Hospital at Shaibah Logistics Base. On occasion, a consultant in EM was deployed by air from the deployed field hospital. These medical officers were not dedicated to the helicopters; they had primary healthcare duties also. When British Forces first started moving into Afghanistan (New Year's Eve 2001), there was no associated dedicated IRT.

Cover could have been provided by US forces, operating Blackhawk helicopters out of Bagram Airbase, but this was never tested, at least not in the initial phases of the deployment. By the time the task force deployed into the south of the country, setting up *Bastion Logistics Base* in Helmand Province, the CH-47 had become the logistics platform of choice. CH-47 was fast, could be armoured against small-arms fire and could carry up to eight stretchers; in addition, there were almost no restrictions on the amount of medical kit that could be carried. As the fighting intensified, and more casualties began to arrive at the field hospital at Bastion, so medical officers were increasingly used on board the IRT 'cab'.

The concept of using a medical team to provide combat casualty retrieval had never been written into doctrine, but the command chain recognised the requirement and supported *16 Close Support Medical Regiment* in providing this capability. Equipment for the team was initially provided from the field hospital (Figure 3.3).

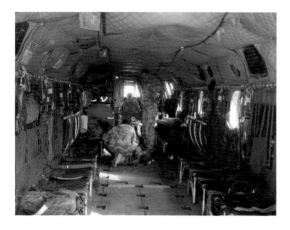

Figure 3.3 Interior of the Chinook (CH47) helicopter with medical equipment loaded.

Team composition

Clinicians continued to support flights to retrieve casualties on an ad hoc basis, with secondary care doctors from EM and anaesthesia taking it in turns to drop what they were doing in the field hospital and fly to locations such as Kajaki Dam, in the north of the province. The use of medical officers in this role was controversial at the time, with some defence consultant advisors reluctant to support the concept.[6] There was an undoubted risk to the MERT airframes with countless incidents of attack from the ground and it was felt to be only a matter of time before a Chinook was shot down The increasing tempo of operations, and increasing casualty load, especially during the summer fighting season, soon overturned objections, and by August 2007, the first *medical officers* were assigned to permanently staff the medical component of the IRT.[7,8] Although at this time, clinical data were not available to support the medically manned MERT, it was apparent that the knowledge that the MERT was available in the event of being injured had a significant effect on morale amongst personnel deployed forwards. Withdrawal of the capability once it was established was never a practical option. One MERT medical officer was added to the deployed manning template from each of anaesthesia and EM, although on occasions later in the campaign, during high-intensity pre-planned operations, an additional MERT medical officer was deployed for limited periods.

This improved the situation for the flight nurses and combat medical technicians who formed the rest of the team, as they could then enjoy continuity from their clinical leads, and team cohesion was improved. Unfortunately, the medical component of the IRT was used far more frequently than the other components, such as Defence Fire and Rescue or working dogs, and gradually the teams became permanently integrated with the helicopters. IRT (Medical) became (Medical) IRT which, spoken aloud, transformed into 'MERT', assumed by all to stand for *medical emergency response team*.

Medical officers on the teams were initially senior trainees; however, in 2011, the Surgeon General stated that injured soldiers would receive consultant-delivered care, and as a result, the

MERT lines were allocated to consultants and more senior, and more experienced, clinicians were deployed on MERT until the end of the campaign.

For most of *Operation Herrick*, there were two MERTs based at Camp Bastion: one led by an EM physician and one by an anaesthetist. Occasionally, one MERT was forward based in support of a particular operation, such as the Brigade of Gurkhas' attack on the Baluchi Valley in Oruzgan Province in November 2007 supported by CH-47 and a MERT based near Tarin Kowt (Figure 3.4).

Other team members included combat medical technicians as well as Army and RAF nurses, although medical support officers, physiotherapists and even an army chaplain flew with the team in the early days. On a number of occasions, individuals flew on the CH47 whose presence could not be justified on clinical grounds, thus exposing individuals to unnecessary risk. One of the first tasks of the Tri-Service lead for PHEM was to ban such activity that exposed individuals to unnecessary and unjustifiable risks. *Operating department practitioners* were trialled for a period of time but were dropped in favour of a paramedic supported system.[9] This optimal team composition of doctor, nurse and two paramedics was adopted for the remainder of *Operation Herrick* (Table 3.1). As a result, the RAF developed a paramedic cadre.

Table 3.1 Optimal composition of an MERT

Clinician	Role
Consultant qualified in PHEM	Clinical leadership, decision making and clinical interventions including PHEA
Flight nurse	Clinical support and communications
Paramedic 1	Clinical support including blood component transfusion
Paramedic 2	Triage, loading plan and control of catastrophic external haemorrhage

Unfortunately, in order to ensure appropriate remuneration, most paramedics were promoted to senior non-commissioned officer rank and, as a consequence, posted into largely administrative roles. As a consequence, in many cases, the only clinical experience paramedics regularly received was on deployed operations. This situation remains only partially resolved, and the situation for paramedics remains radically different from that of nurses and doctors (the other MERT members), who remain in a primarily clinical role when not deployed on operations.

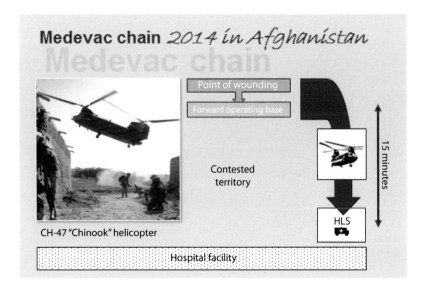

Figure 3.4 Forward medevac chain in Afghanistan.

There were a number of other issues that had to be addressed in order to deliver a clinical capability with effective governance structures: equipment scaling had to be determined, defined and acquired, and standard operating procedures (SOPs) needed to be put in place and governance systems established. Almost inevitably, due to the initial ad hoc development of MERT as an enhanced IRT capability, there was an equipment shortfall which was partially filled, to begin with, using equipment from the hospital. Introduction into theatre by clinicians of individual items of kit was also an issue (discussed further in Chapter 23). As a result, a MERT module was established under the authority of the PHEM and EM equipment committee chaired by DCA EM. This body reviewed all requests for inclusion in the MERT modules and was also responsible for identifying possible new equipment and replacements for obsolete kit. Items not specified in the module were not permitted, except as part of an endorsed trial. DCA EM led a multidisciplinary MERT governance visit to theatre at least once every year for the reminder of *Operation Herrick*.

Two sets of SOPs were established, one administrative (dealing with drug checks, record keeping etc.) and the other clinical. Clinicians were required to follow the protocols given in the SOPs unless there was a very good reason for not doing so, and in the event of this not being the case, such action would potentially be at the clinician's own risk. To some extent, governance issues for MERT were identified at the weekly trauma conference; they could also be picked up separately and forwarded to the Tri-Service Lead, but as Herrick developed, a monthly review of all patient report forms was undertaken by a team headed by the Tri-Service Lead. This process looked particularly at systemic issues or failures, but it also identified idiosyncrasies of practice by individuals.

Working with the Americans

By 2012, more US forces were moving into the area, and MERT began working alongside US Air Force (USAF) *Pedro* parajumpers (based at Camp Bastion), as well as US Army *Dustoff* casualty evacuation helicopters (based at Kandahar Airfield). Relations were initially difficult: the USAF did not suffer from the command and control difficulties faced by MERT, (which often had to wait for launch authority to be granted by the complex North Atlantic Treaty Organization (NATO) command structure) with the result that they would arrive on scene first. There was an almost inevitable tension between, on the one hand, MERTs' perceptions of themselves as a highly skilled resuscitation capability and the US crews as slightly *gung ho* practitioners of scoop and run and, on the other hand, the US perception of MERT as being, on occasion, reluctant to go to the aid of personnel when *their* personnel were happy to be deployed (Figure 3.5).

In fact, on occasion, there *was* some reluctance to deploy MERT, but this was invariably a command decision, not a medical one, and there is no doubt that different rules had to govern the deployment of an asset carrying not only aircrew but also a MERT and force protection element. In the eyes of MERT, *Pedro* and *Dustoff* were militarily highly skilled but less effective medically; the converse view was held by some of the US personnel. In reality, the capabilities were different, and both were necessary and needed. Clinicians in the hospital made every effort to include *Pedro* and *Dustoff* personnel in the medical community, but some reluctance to attend clinical governance meetings, for example, remained.

Nevertheless, relationships did improve, and the relative strengths and weaknesses of each platform came to be appreciated. The Pavehawk helicopters could launch faster than the CH-47 and they had plenty of experience in combat casualty retrieval, for instance having well-developed

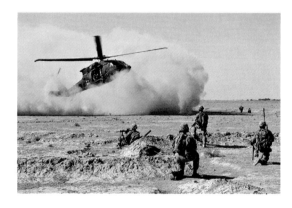

Figure 3.5 Dustoff lands-on.

tactics for managing aviation crash sites. They could sometimes get to casualties that the CH-47 could not reach. MERT, on the other hand, had a greater capacity and a higher medical capability,[10] which were eventually acknowledged by the USAF. The concept of a *Patient Evacuation Control Cell* developed, staffed by US and UK personnel with an understanding of the relative capabilities of MERT, *Pedro* and *Dustoff* and able to assign resources appropriately: truly 'intelligent tasking'. Weekly *pre-hospital care clinical case conferences* were held, where frictions and clinical complaints could be resolved. These were eventually chaired by the deployed medical director for the Field hospital. In late 2014, Camp Bastion was drawing down and the hospital closed its doors. MERT covered the withdrawal of forces, finally moving itself and its logistic supplies to Kandahar, before heading home.

DATA

There are numerous epidemiological studies referencing deaths in combat. The issue with many studies is that the data sets use different terms – they are not homogenous (Figure 3.6).

Fighting in Helmand Province in particular was intense, with a fatality rate of 19/1000/year (nearly four times the US rate of 5/1000/year in Iraq).[11] Fatalities can usefully be divided into those who died before any kind of medical help was offered, those *killed in action*, and those who died subsequent to receiving medical help. Confusion arises from the term *died of wounds* because this means 'after receiving medical help', which may mean following arrival at a medical facility or simply subsequent to receiving medical care of any kind. This distinction becomes more blurred with the development of PHEC and the fact that hospital resources were increasingly pushed forwards into the battlespace. With US and UK soldiers being killed, and many more suffering life-changing injuries, the respective medical services started analysing the data closely and, indeed, collaboratively. It was quickly realised that the pre-hospital phase of the patient pathway was key: 87.3% of all injury mortality occurred in the pre-hospital environment. Of the pre-hospital deaths, 75.7% (n = 3040) were classified as *non-survivable* and 24.3% (n = 976) were deemed *potentially survivable* (PS).[12] A further review of the potential survivors revealed that haemorrhage from major trauma was the predominant mechanism of death in 230 of 287 (80%) PS cases.[13] The majority of deaths occurred within the first 10 minutes of wounding. Consequently, PHEC is the clinical arena that offers the potential

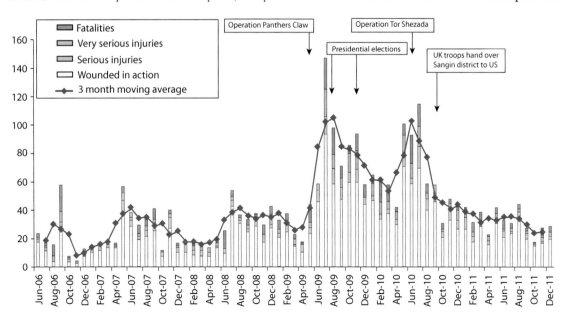

Figure 3.6 British casualties in Afghanistan, June 2006–December 2011.

for the single biggest improvement in mortality. These data also disproved the longstanding belief that trauma deaths were tri-modal in nature, instead describing a $1/x$ asymptotic pattern.

Casualties on the battlefield need battlefield first aid, and they need it immediately.[14] They also need more advanced interventions: waiting for arrival at hospital before these are commenced was no longer acceptable practice. The recognition of this fact required a change in medical 'first principles'.[15] Battlefield casualty drills (BCDs) were rigorously and regularly taught and re-emphasised before and on deployment into theatre. The injury rates from both campaigns meant that deploying personnel became aware, for the first time in a generation, of the importance of basic life-saving skills. The clinical emphasis was changed to place control of life-threatening bleeding as the first priority, and appropriate equipment, including dressings and tourniquets, was issued. One in four deployed personnel was trained as a *team medic* with a level of skills that was still basic but higher than that taught to all personnel as part of the buddy–buddy battlefield first aid-drills system. Thus, battlefield casualties were immediately treated using tourniquets and dressings in order to prevent blood loss, preventing immediate death from exsanguination. Streamlined communications (the '9-liner + ATMIST'; Tables 3.2 and 3.9) ensured that appropriate resources were despatched to the scene. Emergency department level care then arrived on the back of the Chinook.

MERT was credited with further contributing to a hitherto unprecedented improvement in battlefield casualty survival; however, the extent of this was appreciated only when retrospective analyses of the data were made. Having the US and UK capabilities managing the same *population at risk*, across the same AOR, made for an inadvertent un-randomised, un-controlled trial of the respective platforms.

MERT data

Both the United States and the United Kingdom maintain a registry of trauma patients treated on operations: the Joint Theatre Trauma Registry, which contains a wealth of data pertaining to the most severely injured patients treated during the

Table 3.2 NATO '9-liner'

Line 1: Location of the pick-up site
Line 2: Radiofrequency, call sign and suffix
Line 3: Number of patients of precedence:
  A – Urgent;
  B – Urgent surgical;
  C – Priority;
  D – Routine;
  E – Convenience.
Line 4: Special equipment required:
  A – None;
  B – Hoist;
  C – Extraction equipment;
  D – Ventilator.
Line 5: Number of patients:
  A – Litter;
  B – Ambulatory.
Line 6: Security at pick-up site (in peacetime – number of wounds, injuries, and illnesses)
  A – No enemy troops in area;
  B – Possible enemy troops in area (approach with caution);
  C – Enemy troops in area (approach with caution);
  D – Enemy troops in area (armed escort required).
Line 7: Method of pick-up site marking:
  A – Panel;
  B – Pyrotechnic signal;
  C – Smoke signal;
  D – None;
  E – Other.
Line 8: Patient nationality and status:
  A – Coalition military;
  B – Coalition civilian;
  C – Non coalition military;
  D – Non coalition civilian;
  E – EPW
Line 9: NBC contamination (in peacetime – terrain description of pick-up site):
  N – Nuclear;
  B – Biological;
  C – Chemical.

Telic and *Herrick* campaigns. Thus, comparison of the US and the UK systems (i.e. MERT versus *Pedro* and *Dustoff*) can be made.[16] Perhaps unsurprisingly, the MERT platform, with plenty of space and a dedicated four-person medical team proving advanced resuscitation, performs better than the smaller US platforms in terms of patient survival. It is important to remember in considering these data that there were undoubtedly situations in which evacuation by MERT was not possible and lighter platforms offered the only chance of evacuation. Analysis of battlefield data must always be considered in the light of practicalities mandated by the tactical situation. However, a conservative estimate of the difference in survival is that being retrieved by MERT reduced patient mortality by 6% (a statistically significant difference with a *p* value of 0.035)[17] and that this difference was not solely because of a difference in tasking.[18] Only 35% of patients carried by MERT were UK servicemen, the rest being coalition allies and Afghan military, police and civilians; 7.3% of MERT patients were children.[19]

CH-47 Chinook

The advantages of using helicopters rather than ground ambulances to move patients are numerous. They include speed,[20] the ability to cross rough terrain and contested territory and improved comfort for the patient. Civilian air ambulances are normally constrained by their small size and are limited in the number of team members and amount of medical equipment that can be carried. The CH-47 does not suffer from these limitations – its payloads are measured in tonnes rather than kilograms (Figure 3.7). The standby location of the on-duty team was always debated: it would oscillate between the field hospital (therefore

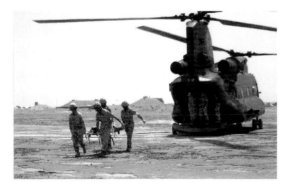

Figure 3.7 Chinook (CH-47) unloading a casualty.

with good links to the receiving facility) and the flight-line (with easy access to the helicopters and making interaction with the flight crew easier, but leading to loss of contact with the hospital). The four-person medical team was usually supported by an eight-man *force protection team*. These were initially Regular Army infantry, then reservist Infantry and eventually members of the RAF Regiment. Force protection provided close protection to the aircraft, establishing a perimeter on landing and searching casualties and any civilians prior to emplaning. The MERT Cab itself was usually accompanied by a pair of Apache gunships. By definition, MERT would be flying to the most dangerous part of the AOR, at that moment, and the scene assessment and firepower brought by the attack helicopters were intended to win the fire-fight and ensure the safety of the landing zone. Most missions were uncontested, although, occasionally, Taliban fighters would find ways around ground defences, for example bringing in indirect fire onto the landing zone outside Now Zad *Forward Operating Base* or suddenly appearing from concealed fox-holes in the 'Green Zone' along the Helmand River. The helicopter was a prize target for the insurgency and was hit by small-arms fire; however, no fatalities were ever sustained on board the cab. Due to the limited numbers of airframes available in theatre, at no time was a CH-47 available for dedicated MERT duties,

MERT interventions

A well-drilled MERT could load a patient; perform a rapid assessment of their injuries; apply measures to stop catastrophic haemorrhage, including packing of junctional wounds and applying a pelvic binder; intubate and ventilate the patient; administer units of red blood cells and fresh frozen plasma at 38°C via intra-osseous (IO) access; and package the patient in warming blankets, all within 10 minutes of first receiving the patient (Figure 3.8). As well as facilitating the aggressive resuscitation of the patient, having a senior clinician on board allowed for rapid and confident high-level decision making.[21,22] During operations in Helmand, this was principally about selecting head-injured patients who would survive the longer trip to Kandahar and benefit from the attentions of the

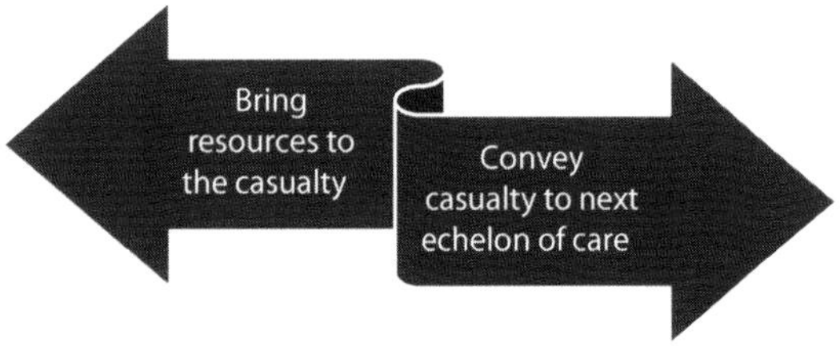

Figure 3.8 Functions of aviation in supporting PHEC.

neurosurgeon based there. Camp Bastion, being ostensibly a Role 2 hospital, only infrequently had a neurosurgical capability.

Possibly the most significant intervention, after control of catastrophic haemorrhage, was the ability to administer blood products. Units of red blood cells were carried from 2008, with (defrosted) fresh frozen plasma from 2010. Some studies credit this intervention with halving mortality, although unpicking the different interventions is difficult.[23] Use of blood products is now well established at this echelon, and it should be remembered that conventional transfusion practice standards, insisted upon by the UK Blood Transfusion Service, were maintained at all times.[24] The difficulty was in ensuring that blood products were maintained at the correct temperature once released from the blood bank. Ordinary beer-coolers or ice-boxes were inadequate and would fail temperature monitoring tests. The breakthrough came with *Golden Hour Boxes* manufactured by Minnesota Thermal Sciences, which use 'phase change technology' to keep the contents at a precise temperature for up to five days. This, along with careful documentation, gave the blood transfusion experts the confidence to release blood products from the laboratory to be used in the pre-hospital arena.[25] This experience was brought back to the United Kingdom, with London's Air Ambulance adopting Golden Hour Boxes and military protocols from March 2012 – a very good example of military medical development influencing civilian practice. Aside from the effects of pre-hospital blood transfusion, the provision of adequate supplies of blood products in theatre was an astonishing logistic achievement, which has not received the recognition it deserves.

PHEA was required for pain management when ketamine sedation was inadequate and to facilitate any painful interventions required, such as packing a pelvic wound or performing thoracostomies.[26] In the early years of MERT, clinician confidence at performing PHEA varied, but as more military clinicians were trained in the technique by civilian air ambulances back in the United Kingdom, the indications for performing anaesthesia on the back of a moving helicopter became better understood and were captured in successive iterations of SOPs.[27] Intubating patients was controversial, but in general, this was performed safely and effectively (Table 3.3).

Some interventions were quickly discarded: while IO access, both sternal and peripheral, proved to be reliable and effective, central venous access was quickly determined to be too dangerous, risking intrathoracic and mediastinal administration of blood products. Pre-hospital emergency thoracotomy remained controversial,[31] although happily, the issuing of larger-size body-armour chest plates reduced the incidence of thoracic injury. The MERT concept reconciles the two competing philosophies of pre-hospital care: 'stay and play' (perform interventions and packaging at scene, but risk delaying surgery

Table 3.3 Intubation success rates on MERT

	Civilian UK emergency department[28]	London HEMS[29]	MERT[30]
Grade I or II view	92.0%	81.0%	96.0%
First attempt success	87.7%	87.5%	94.4%
First or second attempt success		97.8%	98.8%

in hospital) and 'scoop and run' (the North American concept that time to surgery trumps all other concerns). MERT is best described as 'scoop and play'.

TRAINING

Training courses developed rapidly in response to the *Telic* and *Herrick* campaigns. Three-month deployments for clinicians and six-month deployments for non-clinicians meant that personnel were rotating frequently between the UK and the operational areas. Changes to medical 'tactics', for example how to apply a tourniquet, were soon fed back to the training courses at home. The main courses that developed over this period were *Mandatory Annual Training Test 3 (Battlefield Casualty Drills), Team Medic training, Battlefield Advanced Trauma Life Support* (BATLS), and the *Rotary Wing Familiarisation Course*, which became the *MERT Course*. Without strict definitions for terms such as 'first aid' or 'medic', there is a risk of confusion. The *National Health Service Skills for Health* structure can usefully be applied at this point, in order to explain the different levels of PHEC training (Table 3.4). It should be remembered that, as previously stated, PHEM refers to doctors and the General Medical Council recognised sub-speciality, whereas PHEC refers to the entire end-to-end system of emergency healthcare, incorporating non-vocational providers ('first-aiders') all the way through to specialist PHEM physicians.

Table 3.5 Individual issue battlefield first aid items issued by the end of *Operation Herrick*

First field dressing	×2
Combat Application Tourniquet	×2
Morphine auto-injector (10 mg)	×2
BCDs aide-memoire	×1

Level 1: Care under fire and BCDs

In a combat environment, in order to begin performing first aid (Table 3.5), the fire-fight must first be won. This can be considered an extension of the principle of first aid that dangers should be removed and that, above all, the rescuers should not become casualties themselves. Most importantly, this means that unless the tactical situation has improved dramatically, the casualty may have to be moved to a place of relative safety (behind 'cover') before treatment may begin. There is then a requirement to apply life-saving first aid, termed 'care under fire'. Principally, this involves the application of tourniquets to limbs and dressings, including haemostatic dressings, to areas of external bleeding not amenable to tourniquet application. The British Army has long recognised that many individuals do not respond well under the pressure of combat. Long before any concepts such as *crew resource management* or *bandwidth* were shared outside of the aviation industry, the Army knew that soldiers had to be drilled in order to function effectively under fire. Battlefield first aid is no different, and so winning the fire-fight, quick

Table 3.4 DMS levels of PHEC

Level 8	Consultant in PHEM with FIMC	Medical officers providing Specialist PHEM
Level 7	Registrar training in PHEM	
Level 6	Level 5 + two years experience + DIMC	Vocational providers
Level 5	Any doctor, nurse, paramedic	
Level 4	Combat Medical Technicians Class 1	
Level 3	Advanced team medic	Non-vocational providers
Level 2	Team medic, Remote team medic	
Level 1	MATT3, Basic first aid	

Note: DIMC, Diploma in Immediate Medical Care from the Royal College of Surgeons of Edinburgh; FIMC, Fellowship in Immediate Medical Care from the Royal College of Surgeons of Edinburgh.

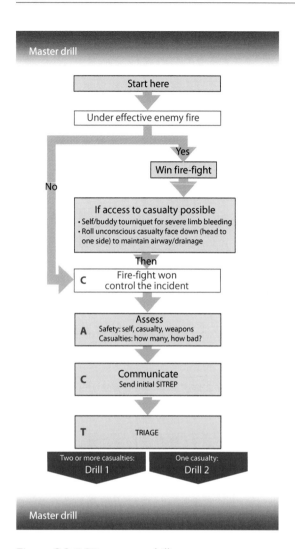

Figure 3.9 BCDs: master drill.

Table 3.6 Contents of the *Operational Team Medic Pouch*

Triangular bandages	x 4
First field dressing	x 6
Haemostatic dressing (Celox)	x 4
Chest seal	x 2
Disposable suction device	x 1
Plastic gloves (pairs)	x 4
Skin-marking pen or pencil	x 1
Shears for cutting clothing	x 1
Combat Application Tourniquet	x 4
Triage labels (pack)	x 1

assessment of a patient and the application of tourniquets and dressings have been turned into BCDs. The Master Drill is shown in Figure 3.9. BCDs are taught annually. The aim is that these simple drills will be as instinctive for the combat soldiers as those that govern their actions in taking on and overcoming the enemy. The number of medical items issued to each individual soldier grew during the *Telic* and *Herrick* campaigns in response to the increase in intensity of fighting. However, there was always an awareness of the potential for degrading combat performance by overloading soldiers, as well as some concern regarding the effect of these *momento mori* or at least reminders of the possibility of injury and death if provision was overdone.

Level 2: Team medic training

UK and US Special Forces have long recognised the benefit of additional training in battlefield first aid. Their concept of 'patrol skills' means that each member of a team has a primary skill and at least one secondary skill, with every fourth soldier receiving additional medical training. This concept has been adopted by conventional forces, although limitations in time and money mean that team medic training is only three and a half days in duration. The concept at this level is to *train-the-trainer*. Once a number of *team medic trainers* returned to their unit, training tended to progress exponentially.

With an original target of one in four soldiers being trained to team medic standard, some units, particularly those front-line infantry units returning to operations after sustaining casualties on previous tours, improved on this, eventually achieving ratios of 1:2 or even better.

Team medics are equipped with the operational *Team Medic Module*, which contains extra items not issued for individual issue (Table 3.6). This module is the most basic of a series of deployable medical modules under the authority, during *Operation Herrick* of DCA EM and now of DCA Pre-Hospital Care.

This equipment is designed to supplement and to augment that issued to individual personnel.

Level 3: Advanced team medic training

Some specialist military teams, such as 16 *Air Assault Brigade Pathfinders* or *Royal Artillery Forward Observation* teams, deploy 'at reach' to high-threat environments, without necessarily being supported by cap-badged DMS personnel. These teams arguably require additional medical training, over and above that of team medic standard. However, this level of training is seldom provided for conventional forces who may lack the time and funding required to achieve it.

Level 4 and 5: BATLS Course

Here, we consider the training for vocational providers: doctors, nurses, paramedics and medics. At the beginning of *Operation Telic*, British Army BATLS and *Battlefield Advanced Resuscitation Techniques and Skills* (BARTS) were well-established courses that had been drifting apart from civilian *Advanced Trauma Life Support* (ATLS) for a number of years, the underlying drivers being the different aetiologies of trauma found in the civilian as opposed to the military arena and the different priorities required in the management of casualties.[32] Both courses were established at the time of the First Gulf War when BATLS itself was accredited by the ATLS organisation, backed by the Royal College of Surgeons, and had equivalence for medical training purposes. Due to the increasing divergence between the courses, this ceased to be the case. BARTS training had, in addition, been

folded into BATLS. The original BATLS Course was aimed at military medical officers but quickly expanded to include nurses and combat medical technicians, rightly adopting a whole-team approach, although the material was often poorly tailored to individual groups of attendees. More recently, recognising the inherent differences between pre-hospital care and in-hospital care, the course has dropped much of the in-hospital content. Blood gases and reviews of plain-film radiographs have been replaced by triage tools and skills such as supra-glottic airway insertion and needle thoracocentesis. The focus of in-hospital team training has become the *Military Operational Surgical Training Course* rather than BATLS. The course content was continually updated throughout the campaigns, adding techniques such as IO access, as the equipment became available.

Level 7 and 8: MERT Course

The first medical officers to attend the dedicated *Rotary Wing Familiarisation Course* did so in early 2007. Medical officers and nursing officers returning from the conflict in Helmand Province quickly rebuilt the course, re-branding it the *MERT Course*. This training is held four times a year and is administered by *Tactical Medical Wing* of the Royal Air Force. During *Operation Herrick*, a rigorous pass/fail element was introduced into these courses: candidates who failed the course could be, and were, prevented from deploying. This course teaches and assesses an individual's ability to apply BATLS concepts and damage control

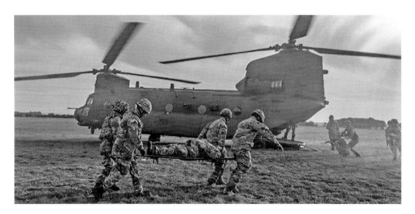

Figure 3.10 A team loads a casualty during the MERT Course.

Table 3.7 Examples of equipment issues for MERT during *Operation Herrick*

Equipment issue	Mitigation
Battery failure in the cold	Batteries kept in accommodation or in sleeping bags
Intubating bougies become overly flexible in the heat	Bougies kept cool inside 'Golden Hour' boxes
Stylets sticking inside endotracheal tubes	Stylets abandoned as a method of assisting intubation
Monitoring failure during missions	Regular equipment checks, and multiple redundancy with spare electromedical items
Pieces of paper lost in the down-draft	Write on the patient's skin
Frequent equipment failures, such as endotracheal tube breakages and anaesthetic circuit breakages	Regular equipment checks and multiple redundancy with plenty of spares carried

resuscitation in a high-tempo operational environment and their ability to function within a small team working with rotary-wing aviation assets, particularly CH-47 (Chinook) aircraft Figure 3.10). In May 2012, a MERT mission resulted in an unrecognised oesophageal intubation, with devastating consequences for the patient. Immediately, attention rightly focussed on the training of the individuals on the team, and further efforts were made to improve the standards of training on the MERT Course and to emphasise the importance of team working. As ever, in modern medicine, interventions have the potential to do great harm, as well as good. Most of the MERT instructors have completed multiple operational tours on MERT, and there is a high ratio of instructors to candidates. Candidates are formed into teams, usually consisting of a medical officer, a flight nurse and two paramedics (mirroring the deployed team structure), and they are put through numerous moulages, both formative and summative, culminating with summative moulages aboard a CH-47 flying tactically. The course currently provides a focus for Level 8 PHEM activity within the military and benefits from instructors and candidates from all three Services. With the end of *Operation Herrick*, and a return to contingency operations, the course has re-focussed yet again, requiring the teams to be flexible in their mindset, accepting the resources they have available, which may

involve smaller airframes or even ground transfer of patients.

On operational deployment, a MERT is equipped with the MERT Module, which contains two monitors, a ventilator, suction devices, warming equipment and enough consumables to manage multiple casualties over multiple missions, without needing to resupply. Equipment issues faced by the MERT during the HERRICK campaign were largely down to the extremes of the environment; examples are given in Table 3.7.

SPECIFIC EQUIPMENT

Control of catastrophic external haemorrhage <C>

The medical mindset had to be re-set. So the paradigm of Airway, Breathing and Circulation (ABC) priorities was changed to Control of Catastrophic

Table 3.8 MARCH

M	Massive haemorrhage control
A	Airway
R	Respirations
C	Circulation
H	Head/hypothermia

(External) Haemorrhage first, followed by Airway, Breathing and Circulation (<C>ABC).[15] Interestingly, the world of special forces had long adopted this mantra, preferring to use the MARCH algorithm (Table 3.8) instead of ABC.

In fact, given the provision of tourniquets and haemostatic dressings, it should be possible to prevent almost all deaths from external exsanguination. This leads to the new, and more satisfying, mantra of 'no patient should be allowed to die from external haemorrhage'.

Battlefield tourniquet master class

'*The tourniquet, if used properly, is perhaps the leading lifesaving device available to soldiers in the field*'.[33] Every member of HM Forces deploying on operations is now required to be competent in the use of an emergency battlefield tourniquet. Despite the clear clinical benefits of battlefield tourniquets, some military clinicians initially resisted their introduction.[34] The debate was soon won[35] and evidence of safety and efficacy soon followed. No limb has been lost solely due to the application of a tourniquet,[36] and by 2008, it was recognised that up to 57% of deaths may have been prevented by earlier tourniquet use.[37]

Although tourniquets may be improvised, provided they are properly applied with adequate force, this should now only be required in exceptional circumstances. It is recognised that in some cases, a single tourniquet may not be sufficient to control bleeding, and for this reason, *team medics* carry supplies of tourniquets so that the injured soldier's buddy is not left without. The amount of force required to control haemorrhage is directly proportional to the diameter of the limb, and the danger of inadequate tightening is that of achieving a pressure less than systolic but higher than venous pressure. This may have the paradoxical effect of increasing bleeding from the limb by allowing arterial inflow but restricting venous outflow from the extremity. Commercially produced tourniquets are more efficacious than improvised ones,[38] with the Combat Application Tourniquet (C-A-T™) selected for issue to combat troops due to its ability to be applied one-handed.

Lessons learned from reviews of tourniquet use on the battlefield

Techniques for the correct and effective use of a tourniquet matured during the conflict, and changes were fed back very rapidly through pre-deployment training or refresher training immediately after arrival in theatre. The decision to apply a tourniquet had to be made rapidly and instinctively; a tourniquet can always be removed. Experience proved that arterial spasm and/or reduced blood pressure might result in a relative absence of bleeding from a traumatic amputation: personnel were still taught to apply a tourniquet. Catastrophic haemorrhage was possible as spasm reduced or resuscitation raised the blood pressure.

Troops were taught to apply a tourniquet directly to the skin 2–3 inches above the injury unless blast injury had caused internal damage to the limb and more proximal application was warranted. The tourniquet was to be placed with the windlass-rod and windlass-clip uppermost in order to avoid pressure sores underneath the patient and the tourniquet was tightened until bleeding was controlled. Failure to control bleeding with a single tourniquet was an indication for applying a second tourniquet side by side with the first, especially when applying them to the thigh area.[39] Troops were warned that a correctly applied tourniquet is very painful and that the patient might sometimes resist application or even try to remove the device. Analgesia was therefore mandatory.

On occasion, experience showed that bleeding from medullary bone ends occurred if the tourniquet was applied below the level of the nutrient (perforating) artery; this could be controlled with a large stump-dressing. After approximately 15 minutes, the tourniquet was to be re-checked. Bleeding from the part of the limb distal to the tourniquet, as well as blood soaking into the fabric of the tourniquet, might mean that extra tightening was required. Only when haemorrhage control was achieved were dressings and splints to be applied.

Use of a tourniquet to control catastrophic haemorrhage mandates categorising the patient as a T1 priority for evacuation. Whoever has applied the tourniquet must ensure that a face-to-face handover is made with the next level of care and that verbal confirmation of the presence of a tourniquet, including the time of application, is made.

First field dressing

The venerable *First Field Dressing* was first issued to troops in World War I. The fallacy of the traditional First Field Dressing was that it was designed 'to soak up to a litre of blood'. Should the first dressing become saturated, then a second was applied over the top. In effect, this had the potential to produce a wick. Of course, the blood is actually better inside the patient than inside the dressing. The modern First Field Dressing incorporates an elasticated bandage, with which firm pressure is applied over the wound. This has the effect of restricting capillary-bed and venous bleeding. The current dressing was selected after a review by senior emergency clinicians of a wide range of commercially available options. Whilst not usually considered as an active haemostatic, cotton-gauze padding contains cellulose, which activates the extrinsic clotting pathway. The modern dressing is lighter, vacuum packed and gamma-irradiated for sterility. The waterproof packaging may also be used as a temporary improvised chest-seal.

The range of dressings available in the current series of pre-hospital modules also allows effective management of capillary-bed bleeding, low-volume venous bleeding and medullary bleeding from fractured bone-ends as well as reducing the risks of infection of an injury by shortening the time available for colonisation by pathogenic bacteria and fungi and preventing flies and dust from landing on an open wound. In the case of burns, dressing the burn wound significantly improves pain control by reducing air flow across the burned surface, and the importance in psychological terms of covering a mutilating wound, so the shocked casualty cannot see it, should not be forgotten. The first field dressing also allows absorption of exudate from a wound, particularly in prolonged field care situations. This promotes wound healing and helps reduce infection by reducing the volume of available fluid that provides a medium for bacteria.

Allowing gas exchange also prevents growth of anaerobic pathogens (causing infection such as gas gangrene).

Junctional bleeding

The neck, axilla and groin are the junctional areas of the body. Haemorrhage is the predominant mechanism in 80% of cases of preventable death on the battlefield. Of these cases, the major body regions where bleeding accounted for mortality were torso (48%), extremity (31%) and junctional (neck, axilla and groin) (21%). Haemostatic dressings and junctional tourniquets were developed specifically to prevent deaths as a result of bleeding from areas of the body not amenable to tourniquet application.

Haemostatic dressings

First-generation haemostatic dressings included *Quikclot Granules™* and *Hemcon Gauze™*. Unfortunately *Quikclot™* granules work via an exothermic reaction and occasionally caused significant burns to the surrounding tissues. The *Hemcon™* dressing was a small, rigid patch that did not fit inside all wounds. Second-generation dressings were soon developed. Following a review of the available evidence at the time, *Celox™* gauze was chosen as the haemostatic dressing for the British Armed Forces. Celox™ modern haemostatic dressings aim to reliably stop 100% of catastrophic external bleeds within 60 seconds. The active ingredient is chitosan, a natural polymer extracted from shrimp shells and highly purified. *Celox™* is considered to be highly effective.[40–42]

IO access

IO needles are discussed in more detail elsewhere, but it is worth commenting here that improvements in technology and the portability of equipment (particularly the EZIO® and FAST1 IO® devices) led to the introduction of forward IO use in military patients on deployed operations.[43] The ease of insertion of these devices made them an essential component in achieving intravenous access in severely shocked patients, especially those who had very often lost one or more limbs. The largest published series of the use of IO access has been described by the UK DMS.[44] Overall success rates of insertion have been found to be excellent, with one series describing successful insertion and use in 85% of cases[45] and others suggesting successful insertion in 90–96% of cases.[44] A case series of PHEA via the IO route has also been published.[46] Complications of IO access are rare but may include infection and retained needle parts.[47]

Communications

In warfare, effective communications are essential, and never more so than when casualties have been sustained. Without a correctly formatted NATO 9-line request (Table 3.2), MERT would not launch. Eventually, the system evolved to the point where MERT clinicians could watch a 9-liner 'drop' (being entered onto the J-CHAT text-based communications system) and anticipate the order to launch. The addition of ATMIST (Table 3.9) improved the quality of the available medical information. The situation on the ground had usually evolved and was seldom 'as given', so the flight nurse would update the receiving hospital with an assessment of the casualties. Often, the poor range of the CH-47 radios meant that information had to be relayed from clinician, to flight crew, to the accompanying Apaches, to Joint Force Helicopter operations, to the Medical Regiment operations cell at Camp Bastion. Unsurprisingly, messages were frequently confused or lost altogether, although if all else failed, the hospital was usually alerted by the sound of the helicopter. The requirement to re-stock with blood products after a mission was key to the continued effectiveness of MERT, and so the message always had to be passed that blood re-supply was required, because the lab required time to defrost the fresh frozen plasma.

Table 3.9 ATMIST clinical addendum to the 9-liner

A	Age of the patient
T	Time of injury
M	Mechanism of injury
I	Injuries sustained or suspected
S	Signs and symptoms
T	Treatment given

Hence, the code-phrase 'Operation Vampire' was adopted. This term was instantly recognisable and seemed successful in making its way through the complexities of the communications network to the laboratory. It was also used by the emergency department as a marker of the severity of the incoming casualties.

HANDOVER

Handover of the patient to the receiving facility is a key component of effective care. First, patients (and escorts) had to be 'sanitised', to ensure that they were not carrying munitions that could endanger the receiving facility or compromise the status of the hospital under the Geneva Convention. There was an ongoing fear that an enemy casualty or member of the Afghan National Security Forces would enter the hospital carrying a loaded weapon or some form of self-detonatable explosive device. Equally, a UK or other coalition casualty might be carrying a weapon with the smaller but still present risk of a firearms accident. Only once the patient had been thoroughly checked were they allowed into the emergency department, even if they are critically ill. A well-disciplined trauma team would then concentrate on the handover being given by the MERT clinician. In this situation, clinicians are unlikely to be able to remember more than a handful of pieces of information: handovers must therefore be short, in the region of 30 seconds, relevant and succinct. The ATMIST structure (Table 3.9) was used as a template for handover throughout operations in Iraq and Afghanistan. Further details can be given to the *trauma team leader* and to the anaesthetic team once the initial primary survey is complete. Documentation had then to be completed immediately, lest another mission be called and the information lost. The quality of record keeping by pre-hospital teams was a persistent issue during *Operation Herrick*, and eventually, the task became a mandatory role for the leader of the MERT. The correct balance of information handover gives the receiving team the essential pieces of information to enable immediate life-saving interventions, without leading the team to make incorrect assumptions (including reinforcement bias, whereby a mistake by the pre-hospital team is perpetuated by the in-hospital team). Well-organised systems then enabled the MERT to re-stock from the emergency department before heading off.

CHALLENGES FOR THE FUTURE

The next conflict will be different to the last but will still see injured troops requiring care. The challenge for PHEC is to try and maintain the current high standards during an era of relative peace. Troops should continue to learn BCDs and should still be equipped with the devices that prevent exsanguination. MERT members are still required to maintain the same levels of confidence that they achieved by the end of *Operation Herrick*. Neither should it be forgotten that the MERT concept, although unquestionably effective, was a solution to a specific situation. Throughout *Operation Herrick*, as during *Operation Telic*, coalition forces had air superiority and, hence, control, and the numbers of casualties at any one time were relatively small in historical terms. In addition, medical evacuation is likely also to have to compete for limited airframe availability as well as limited numbers of appropriately qualified personnel. Neither of the first two conditions will necessarily apply in any future conflict, and the shortage of resources and manpower is likely to get worse rather than better. There is a serious risk that MERT will be seen as the panacea for all combat medical situations and stultify genuinely original thinking in this area: a situation in which a search for a problem to which MERT is the solution bodes ill for combat casualty care. For now, the pre-hospital care deployed to Afghanistan demonstrated beyond doubt the value of an integrated and well-regulated system. The sad reality, however, is that the wounds are not yet healed on the last casualties from Afghanistan and yet elements of the DMS are required to justify their continued existence.

CONCLUSION

Eighty-seven per cent of deaths occur pre-hospital and at least one quarter are preventable. The recognition of this fact was the first step in doing something about it. Good levels of funding, coupled with a willingness to change, meant that battlefield first aid could be developed, equipment issued to

troops to prevent exsanguinations and MERTs led by senior clinicians, armed with blood products, put in place to retrieve the most critically wounded patients. That these changes improved outcomes for our patients is clear. Conservative measurements put the improvement in survival at 6%, others closer to 50%. Between October 2001 and July 2015, a total of 454 British personnel died whilst serving on operations in Afghanistan. Had this number been even higher, the likelihood is that public support for the campaign would have dropped considerably. High-quality, effective PHEC does not win wars, but it does prevent us from losing them.

REFERENCES

1. O'Reilly D, König T, Tai N. Field trauma care in the 21st century. *J R Army Med Corps* 2008;154(4):257–264.
2. Demetriades D, Chan L, Cornwell E et al. Paramedic vs private transportation of trauma patients. Effect on outcome. *Arch Surg* 1996;131(2):133–138.
3. Cooke MW. Immediate care: Specialty or pastime? *Injury* 1994;25:347–348.
4. Hodgetts TJ, Mahoney PF. Military pre-hospital care: Why is it different? *J R Army Med Corps* 2009;155(1):4–10.
5. Wood RJ, Jeevaratnam JA, Clasper JC. Aspects of military pre-hospital care. *J Paramed Pract* 2011;3(2):64–69.
6. Calderbank P, Woolley T, Mercer S et al. Doctor on board? What is the optimal skill-mix in military pre-hospital care? *Emerg Med J* 201;28(10):882–883.
7. Clarke JE, Davis PR. Medical evacuation & triage of combat casualties in Helmand Province, Afghanistan: October 2010–April 2011. *Mil Med* 2012;177(11):26.
8. Davis P, Rickards A, Ollerton J. Determining the composition and benefit of the pre-hospital medical response team in the conflict setting. *J R Army Med Corps* 2007;153: 269–273.
9. Thomas A. An overview of the medical emergency response team (MERT) in Afghanistan: A paramedic's perspective. *J Paramed Pract* 2014;6(6):296–302.

10. Kehoe A, Jones A, Marcus S et al. Current controversies in military pre-hospital critical care. *J R Army Med Corps* 2011;157(3 Suppl 1): S305–S309.
11. Bird S, Fairweather C. Military fatality rates (by cause) in Afghanistan and Iraq: A measure of hostilities. *Int J Epidemiol* 2007;36: 841–846.
12. Eastridge BJ, Mabry RL, Sequin P et al. Death on the battlefield (2001–2011): Implications for the future of combat casualty care. *J Trauma* 2012;73:6(Suppl 5):S431–S437.
13. Eastridge BJ, Hardin M, Cantrell J et al. Died of wounds on the battlefield: Causation and implications for improving combat casualty care. *J Trauma* 2011;71:S4–S8.
14. Blackbourne LH, Baer DG, Eastridge BJ et al. Military medical revolution: Deployed hospital and en route care. *J Trauma Acute Care Surg* 2012;73:S378–S387.
15. Hodgetts TJ, Mahoney PF, Russell MQ, Byers M. ABC to <C>ABC: Redefining the military trauma paradigm. *Emerg Med J* 2006;23:745–746.
16. Olson CM Jr, Bailey J, Mabry R et al. Forward aeromedical evacuation: A brief history, lessons learned from the Global War on Terror, and the way forward for US policy. *J Trauma Acute Care Surg* 2013;75:S130–S136.
17. Morrison JJ, Oh J, DuBose JJ et al. En-route care capability from point of injury impacts mortality after severe wartime injury. *Ann Surg* 2013;257(2):330–334.
18. Apodaca AN, Morrison JJ, Spott MA et al. Improvements in the hemodynamic stability of combat casualties during en route care. *Shock* 2013;40:5–10.
19. Walker N, Russell RJ, Hodgetts TJ. British military experience of pre-hospital paediatric trauma in Afghanistan. *J R Army Med Corps* 2010;156(3):150–153.
20. McLeod J, Hodgetts T, Mahoney P. Combat "Category A" calls: Evaluating the pre-hospital timelines in a military trauma system. *J R Army Med Corps* 2007;153(4):266–268.
21. Nicholson Roberts TC, Berry R. Prehospital trauma and aeromedical transfer. A military perspective. *Contin Educ Anaesth Crit Care Pain* 2012;12:186–189.
22. Tai NR, Brooks A, Midwinter M, Clasper JC, Parker PJ. Optimal clinical timelines: A consensus from the academic department of military surgery and trauma. *J R Army Med Corps* 2011;155:253–256.
23. O'Reilly D, Morrison J, Apodaca A et al. Prehospital blood transfusion in the en-route management of severe combat trauma: A matched cohort study. *J Trauma* 2014;77(3):S114–S120.
24. Hervig T, Doughty H, Ness P et al. Pre-hospital use of plasma: The blood bankers' perspective. *Shock* 2014;41(Suppl 1):39–43.
25. O'Reilly DJ, Morrison JJ, Jansen JO et al. Special report: Initial UK experience of prehospital blood transfusion in combat casualties. *J Trauma Acute Care Surg* 2014;77(Suppl 3):S66–S70.
26. Petz LN, Tyner S, Barnard E et al. Prehospital and en route analgesic use in the combat setting: A prospectively designed, multicenter, observational study. *Mil Med* 2015;180(3S):14–18.
27. Haldane A. Advanced airway management – a medical emergency response team perspective. *J R Army Med Corps* 2010;156 (3):159–161.
28. Graham CA, Beard D, Oglesby AJ et al. RSI in Scottish urban emergency departments. *Emerg Med J* 2003;20:3–5.
29. Harris L. Success in physician prehospital rapid sequence intubation: What is the effect of base specialty and length of anaesthetic training? *Emerg Med J* 2011:28; 225–229.
30. Kehoe J, Jones A, Marcus S et al. Current controversies in military prehospital critical care. *J R Army Med Corps* 2011;157(3 Suppl 1): S305–S309.
31. Morrison JJ, Mellor A, Midwinter M, Mahoney PF, Clasper JC. Is pre-hospital thoracotomy necessary in the military environment? *Injury* 2011;42:469–473.
32. Hodgetts T, Mahoney P, Evans G, Brooks A. Battlefield advanced trauma life support (parts 1 to 3). *J R Army Med Corps* 2006;152 (Suppl):4.
33. Mabry RL. Tourniquet use on the battlefield. *Mil Med* 2006;171(5):352–356.

34. Parker PJ, Clasper J. The military tourniquet. *J R Army Med Corps* 153(1):10–12.

35. Hodgetts TJ, Mahoney PF. The military tourniquet: A response. *J R Army Med Corps* 153(1):12–15.

36. Kragh JF, Walters TJ, Baer DG et al. Survival with emergency tourniquet use to stop bleeding in major limb trauma. *Ann Surg* 2009;249(1):1–7.

37. Beekley AC, Sebasta JA, Blackbourne LH et al. Prehospital tourniquet use in Operation Iraqi Freedom: Effect on hemorrhage control and outcomes. *J Trauma* 2008;64:S28–S37.

38. Stewart SK, Khan MA. Improvised tourniquets: Obsolete or obligatory? *J Trauma* 2015;78(1):178–183.

39. Taylor DM, Vater GM, Parker PJ. An evaluation of two tourniquet systems for the control of prehospital lower limb hemorrhage. *J Trauma* 2011;71(3):591–595.

40. Lawton G, Granville-Chapman J, Parker PJ. Novel haemostatic dressings. *J R Army Med Corps* 2009;155(4):309–314.

41. Granville-Chapman J, Jacobs N, Midwinter MJ. Pre-hospital haemostatic dressings: A systematic review. *Injury* 2011;42(5):447–459.

42. Pozza M, Millner WJ. Celox (chitosan) for haemostasis in massive traumatic bleeding: Experience in Afghanistan. *Eur J Emerg Med* 2011;18(1):31–33.

43. Cooper BR, Mahoney PF, Hodgetts TJ et al. Intra-osseous access (EZ-IO®) for resuscitation: UK military combat experience. *J R Army Med Corps* 2007;153(4):314–316.

44. Lewis P, Wright C. Saving the critically injured trauma patient: A retrospective analysis of 1000 uses of intraosseous access. *Emerg Med J* 2015;32(6):463–467.

45. Vassallo J, Horne S, Smith JE. Intraosseous access in the military operational setting. *J R Nav Med Serv* 2014;100(1):34–37.

46. Barnard EBG, Moy RJ, Kehoe A et al. Rapid sequence induction of anaesthesia via the intraosseous route: A prospective observational study. *Emerg Med J* 2015; 32(6):449–452.

47. Taylor DM, Bailey MS. A complication of the use of an intra-osseous needle (letter). *J R Army Med Corps* 2010;156(2):132.

4

Emergency medicine and resuscitation

INTRODUCTION

A decade of conflict has driven significant advances in the practice of military emergency medicine (EM) and resuscitation; in technical and logistical terms, both the specialty and the emergency departments (EDs) in which it is practiced are very different to those deployed on operations before 2001. The clinical culture within which EM practice takes place has also been transformed, recognising the importance of interpersonal skills, the management of human resources as well as physical ones, and the key role of teamwork – both in training and practice. Now is a good time to reflect on how far the specialty has come and how military practice and civilian practice have been synergistic in improving care, especially for the victims of life threatening multi-system trauma.

EM AS A DEPLOYED SPECIALITY

The first deployment of emergency physicians during the period of *Operations Telic* and *Herrick* was to Afghanistan when, in 2001, a single consultant was sent to a Role 2 Facility at *Bagram Airbase* in support of UK troop operations deployed to Afghanistan as part of *Operation Veritas*. This deployment offered challenges to the speciality that were different from those faced in Kosovo on *Operation Agricola* in 1999 and different again from those that followed less than a decade later as operations in Iraq and Afghanistan reached their peak. The deployment to Kosovo in 1999 had been the first in which the relatively new specialty of EM had been deployed by the *Defence Medical Services* (DMS), and establishing a functional deployable

ED had been one of the main aims. In 1999, the DMS EM Cadre consisted of two consultants and five trainees.

The 2001 deployment to Bagram was perhaps most notable for the infamous Bagram Norwalk-like outbreak of May 2002, when 29 British soldiers and staff of a field hospital in Afghanistan developed vomiting, diarrhoea and fever. One patient developed disseminated intravascular coagulation and two required ventilatory support in the hospital's intensive care unit. Nevertheless, this operation helped to consolidate the still relatively new military specialty of EM as an integral part of a deployed UK military capability, emphasising the potential breadth of clinical presentations to a deployed ED. This contrasted starkly with the traditional model (pre-Kosovo) of surgical teams deploying without such a capability.

Emergency physicians were subsequently deployed in Iraq as part of the Role 2 and Role 3 units sent to Kuwait and the Shaibah Airbase in Basrah in early 2003. The initial war-fighting phase of *Operation Telic* saw the EM cadre deployed almost in its entirety with consultants attached to medical regiments in a Role 2 function, whilst at the two Role 3 capabilities straddling the Kuwaiti border, staffing levels were akin to an average National Health Service (NHS) district general hospital at that time. At the peak of offensive operations, the ED of *22 Field Hospital* at Shaibah Airbase was manned by three EM consultants, three EM senior and three EM junior trainees. With time, this level of capability would be reduced, and, for the majority of the enduring *Operation Telic* deployment, a single EM junior trainee supported a single deployed consultant.

The layout of the ED of a standard tented field hospital is invariably based on a simple basic cruciate structure (Figure 4.1). The main hospital entrance is at one end of the complex, leading directly into the reception and waiting area, accommodated in a tent aligned with the central corridor 'spine'. The first pair of tents leading off each side of this corridor contains the resuscitation area on one side and the medical and minor injuries areas on the other. On recent operations, an additional tent has at times been added to the end of the medical area to provide accommodation for casualties with infectious diarrhoea and vomiting as well as access for such casualties to the department without the need for them to pass through the main waiting area. Once treated, potentially infectious casualties would exit the department the way they had entered and then be transferred to a dedicated ward by an outside route, thereby bypassing other patient areas and avoiding the main internal communication routes. Although the later stages of *Operation Herrick* are associated with the new-build 'Tier 2' hospital on hard standing (Figures 4.2–4.4), it must not be forgotten that a tented field hospital will usually be deployed during the entry phase of future land-based operations. Indeed, in the case of *Operation Telic*, the tented hospital configuration was retained for the duration of the campaign.

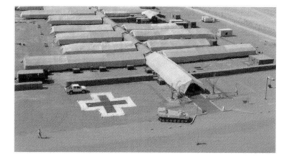

Figure 4.1 Standard tented Role 3 Hospital. The main (ED) entrance is bottom right, with the two elements of the ED on either side of the main spine immediately beyond the ED reception tent. Further wards and departments are positioned at intervals along the corridor with imaging being adjacent to the ED.

Perhaps the greatest advances in resuscitation were made at the Role 3 *medical treatment facility* (MTF) in Camp Bastion, Helmand Province, Afghanistan, between 2006 and 2014. The hospital started out as a modest tented facility (Figure 4.5) but was later developed into a facility with hard standing infrastructure, a 10-bed resuscitation room directly adjacent to a four-table operating theatre and a suite of radiology capability including two computed tomography scanners. It was in this environment that haemostatic resuscitation became a practical reality, damage control resuscitation (DCR) was regularly practised and the term 'right-turn resuscitation' was coined (Figure 4.2).

From a senior clinical delivery perspective, the ED was initially manned by a single UK EM consultant. These consultants were usually individual augmentees deploying away from their role in an NHS hospital to support an established medical unit, but occasionally, the unit deployed with their own cadre EM consultant. The length of the standard operational tour for an emergency physician ranged from 6 to 12 weeks (the tours tending to lengthen as *Operation Herrick* progressed), with a rotation between the regular and reserve consultants resulting in an average deployment cycle of 12–18 months within the EM cadre. However, it should be remembered that the same consultants were initially also rotating through the hospital in Iraq and the period of overlap of the two operations was a significant challenge for the members of what was then still a relatively small cadre. Initially, the deployed EM consultant covered the duties of the *Medical Emergency Response Team* (MERT) doctor, sharing the role with one of the deployed anaesthetists. Later, the MERT clinician became a standalone commitment that was shared between EM and anaesthesia in 2009, eventually evolving to having two clinicians deployed in support of the MERT capability.

EM senior trainees were an integral part of the deployed medical team. They usually deployed for a period of three months, and this period was accredited by the *College of Emergency Medicine* for training (out of programme training) under the supervision of the deployed EM consultant (until late 2013, when the operational tempo decreased to a level below which it was felt that it did not justify recognition for training). Initially, they deployed

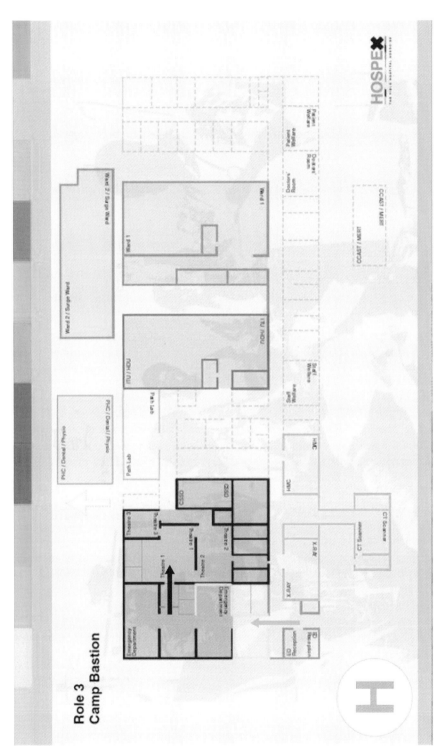

Figure 4.2 Block plan of the Camp Bastion hospital. This is the first stage of the build; subsequent additions would increase the footprint with significantly larger ICU and laboratory facilities. The ED is outlined in red, theatre complex in pink and imaging (bottom) and labs (top) in light blue. The ICU is outlined in purple and the wards in orange. Primary care is on the far right. The original patient entrance was bottom left in the section of the plan marked in grey with the entrance to ED straight ahead (blue arrow). As a consequence, patients taken straight to theatre upon entering the department turned *right* into the operating theatre *right term resus* (red arrow). The term persisted after the entrance was moved to the other end of the department (see Figure 4.4).

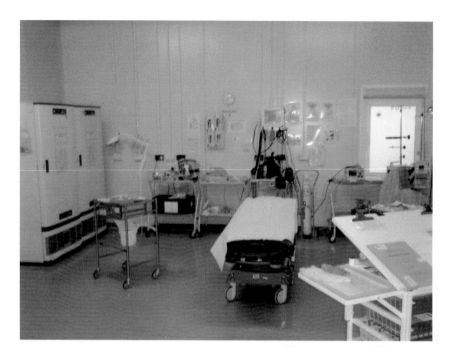

Figure 4.3 One of the ED resuscitation bays in the hardstanding (Tier 2) MTF, Camp Bastion.

at any stage of training, but latterly, the deployment became the realm of the more senior trainees, with the ST4–6 trainees undertaking at least one deployment to *Operation Herrick* during the latter half of their training rotation. In addition to deploying as part of the ED team, many senior trainees also deployed in the MERT clinician role, particularly in the mid to late phase of *Operation Herrick*.

In Afghanistan during 2008, the United States started to contribute medical manpower to the team at Camp Bastion, and the ED went from one to three consultants over the following few months with the addition of US 'attendings'. This allowed a duty roster including a first on-call (where the consultant was resident in the department), a second on-call (available but could be away from the department) and the 'stand-by' third on-call, where the main reason to be called back into the department was in order to help support the response to a multiple casualty incident. In contrast to the relatively short tour lengths of the UK consultants, the US consultants were often deployed for around a year. The multinational makeup of the team persisted until the end of medical operations in Afghanistan in 2014. Despite some pressure

to reduce the disparity between US and UK tour lengths, it was the opinion of Defence Consultant Advisor (DCA) EM and other DCAs that the nature and intensity of the work were resulting in some mental health consequences for deployed clinicians, which, although mild up to that point, could be exacerbated by tours of six months or longer, and thus, plans to lengthen tours were abandoned.

OPERATIONS TELIC AND HERRICK: A NEW CLINICAL CHALLENGE

The main clinical challenge during these operations, and particularly *Operation Herrick*, was the type and severity of the injuries seen, together with the sheer volume of casualties. Situations in which multiple serious injury cases presented simultaneously to the MTF were commonplace, on occasion occurring more than once in a 24-hour period. Not infrequently, the number of cases precipitated a mass casualty or major incident response, when all staff were called back to the hospital from accommodation, rest and dining areas to help manage the influx of patients. In between such incidents, it was fairly normal to experience periods without ED attendances, often extending to several hours, and

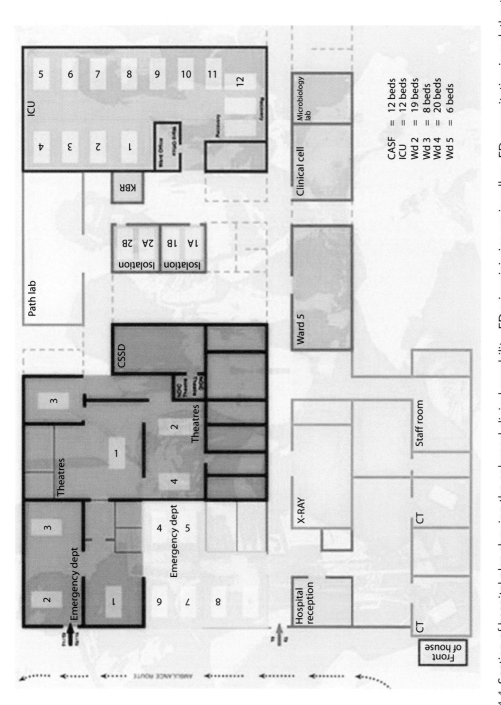

Figure 4.4 Section of hospital plan showing the enlarged clinical capability. ED minor injuries are in red, theatres in pink, imaging and laboratories in blue and ICU in purple. The broken arrows on the left represent the route of ambulances unloading at the ED, and the ambulance entrance is top left marked by a red arrow (patients brought in by this entrance turned *left* into the theatre). The hospital entrance for other patients is marked by a green arrow, bottom left. The main hospital corridor runs across the image from the green arrow.

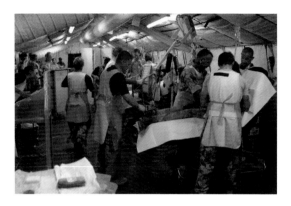

Figure 4.5 First tented field hospital ED at Camp Bastion. The facility on *Operation Telic* was very similar.

the overall numbers of patients seen were generally always well within the capabilities of the deployed ED team. The challenge was not one of total caseload or frequency, as is the usual experience in the NHS setting; it was the extreme severity of some patients' presentations, and frequently having multiple critically injured patients at once.

For all clinicians on their first deployment, the sheer severity of injury in terms of visible tissue damage was something not previously experienced in their NHS practice (Figure 4.6). The severity of injury was overt and affecting, as significant tissue loss and destruction from a blast mechanism were the most common types of injury. This exposure to severely injured patients made major trauma a routine event, and it was this that was the real 'game changer' on deployed operations, leading to new pathways of care and novel treatments through innovation borne of necessity. It inevitably took an emotional toll on staff.

CLINICAL ADVANCES

<C>ABCDE

The paradigm of resuscitation has constantly evolved as lessons from earlier conflicts have been re-learned in the last decade. Through increasing knowledge of the modes of decompensation and cardiac arrest in severely injured battle casualties, the priority in resuscitation has been recognised to be the control of exsanguinating haemorrhage before all else. As a consequence, the sequence of resuscitation, from first aid through to advanced in-hospital resuscitation, has changed from that traditionally taught on trauma resuscitation courses such as the *Advanced Trauma Life Support*® course.[1] *ABC* became *<C>ABC*, where the *<C>* represents control of life-threatening external haemorrhage. This is particularly pertinent on the battlefield in patients with severe extremity trauma, who may benefit from the application of a tourniquet or who have wounds that may benefit from packing with novel haemostatic agents such as Celox. The ethos of DCR incorporates this approach and aims to minimise blood loss from point of injury onwards, maximising tissue oxygenation, retaining clotting function and ultimately optimising

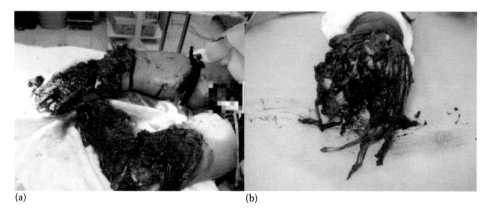

(a)   (b)

Figure 4.6 Blast injuries. (a) Bilateral lower limb amputations. (b) Upper limb amputation showing the avulsive nature of the injuries. Both images demonstrate the massive damage to soft tissue associated with this mechanism of injury.

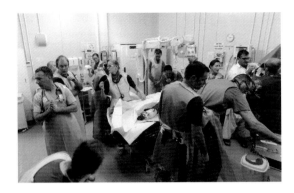

Figure 4.7 Resuscitating the victim of an IED blast. ED, Camp Bastion. Effective raid resuscitation is based on controlled disciplined *parallel* activity.

outcome.[2] *Damage control surgery* (DCS) is an integral part of DCR and, in most cases, is the only way to affect haemorrhage control, particularly in non-compressive torso haemorrhage. The early administration of blood products to manage traumatic coagulopathy is also a key element of DCR (Figure 4.7).

ATMIST

Effective trauma care relies on coordination of pre-hospital and hospital efforts. Many of the advances made in resuscitation involve activation of systems or protocols based on pre-hospital information. This passage of pre-hospital information to the in-hospital environment has been standardised into the *ATMIST format* (Table 4.1), and this has now been incorporated into the standard NATO casualty report, or '9-liner' (page 94).

This format has now been adopted not only across Defence but also within many civilian ambulance services and pre-hospital systems. The passage of critical information such as vital signs allows appropriate preparation (for example activation of a massive haemorrhage protocol) prior to the patient's arrival and is a key enabler for preparation of the ED.[3] Experience on deployment demonstrated the importance of rechecking the correct placement of lines and tubes originally placed in the prehospital environment, the challenging nature of which meant that nothing could be taken for granted.

Table 4.1 ATMIST

A – Age
T – Time of injury
M – Mechanism of injury
I – Injures sustained
S – Vital signs
T – Treatment administered

Intra-osseous access

Intra-osseous (IO) needles have been used in clinical practice since the 1930s and indeed were used during the Second World War but fell out of favour in the 1980s. Until about a decade ago, IO access was usually reserved for paediatric patients in whom intravenous access was not possible or too time-consuming. However, the experience of a decade of critically injured military patients presenting with severe hypovolaemia and the requirement to establish rapid circulatory access while peripherally 'shut-down' necessitated a novel solution. This, in combination with improvements in technology and the reliability of equipment (particularly the *EZ-IO®* and *FAST1®* devices), led to the re-introduction of IO use in military patients on deployed operations.[4] The largest published series of the use of IO access has been described by the UK DMS[5] and includes a description of its use to administer a variety of drugs, along with fluid and blood transfusion. Overall success rates of insertion are good, with one series describing successful insertion and use in 85% of cases[6] and others suggesting successful insertion in 90–96% of cases.[5] A case series of rapid sequence induction of anaesthesia utilising the IO route has also been described.[7] Complications of IO access are rare but may include infection and retained needle parts.[8,9]

TRAUMATIC CARDIAC ARREST AND ED THORACOTOMY

Patients arriving in *traumatic cardiac arrest* (TCA) have, until recently, been thought to have a universally poor chance of survival, with some commentators suggesting intervention to be futile in this patient group. However, recent work looking at outcomes from TCA, particularly in the military population, has shown that the chances of survival following TCA can be as good as for medical causes of cardiac arrest.[10–12] In one study looking at a cohort of military patients, 18 out of 78 patients with TCA survived.[10] In another study looking at a seven-month period in 2009–2010, 14 of 52 patients with TCA had a return of spontaneous circulation, and 4 (8%) survived to discharge.[11]

Further work on outcomes using data from the *Joint Theatre Trauma Registry* (JTTR) suggests that this is reflected over the whole course of the conflicts from 2003 onwards, with an overall survival rate from TCA in this military cohort of 8.7% (Hunt and Smith, unpublished abstract – presented at the *International Conference on Emergency Medicine*, 2016).

Early and aggressive management targeting the reversible causes of hypoxia, tension pneumothorax, hypovolaemia and tamponade is the mainstay of management, and many centres have developed their own protocols for TCA incorporating these features. Resuscitative thoracotomy, traditionally thought to be associated with poor outcomes, was associated with a survival of 21.5%, which increased to 42.3% when the procedure was carried out in the ED.[12] The traditional management of cardiac arrest (instituting chest compressions and the administration of intravenous adrenaline) may not be indicated immediately in all TCA situations.[13] However, further work examining these aspects of resuscitative management is ongoing. Overall, existing dogma regarding the management of TCA has been challenged,[14] and advances during deployed operations have contributed significantly to informing the wider medical community about the management of the most critically injured.

Massive haemorrhage protocols and blood product ratios

It is easy to forget how far resuscitation has advanced over the last decade. In 2003, it was common practice that laboratory test results such as a platelet count or clotting profile were required prior to the release of blood products for transfusion. Resuscitation of hypovolaemic shock was traditionally carried out by administering large (and frequently far too large) volumes of crystalloids.

Much academic ink was spilled in discussing the relative benefits of crystalloids and colloids, not to mention the primacy of Hartmann's solution over normal saline and starches over dextrans. No definitive conclusions were drawn. The development of massive haemorrhage protocols[15] has revolutionised the early management of patients with major trauma, from receiving two litres of warmed crystalloid to receiving as close to whole blood as is possible with component therapy.[16] The cornerstone of haemostatic resuscitation is to target early traumatic coagulopathy as well as to replace oxygen-carrying capacity.

Following early evidence (mainly from retrospective studies looking at combat trauma from US sources) that higher ratios of plasma and platelets may confer a survival benefit, the UK military reviewed its transfusion practices in 2009 and found that 59 patients who underwent massive transfusion received a mean transfusion of 45 units of blood products.[17] There was a high injury burden (median Injury Severity Score, 30), and seven patients in that series received more than 100 transfused units. The overall ratio of units of plasma to packed red blood cells (pRBCs) was 1:1.2, a remarkable achievement of logistics and laboratory efficiency in a deployed setting.

In terms of optimal ratios of blood to other blood products, several retrospective studies have now been overtaken by a large prospective trial – the *PROPPR* study, which randomised civilian trauma patients to receive either 1:1:1 (plasma, platelets and pRBCs) or 1:1:2.[18] Although no overall mortality benefit was found, there were significant differences in early deaths due to bleeding in favour of the higher ratio, supporting as close to 1:1:1 ratios as possible as the initial target. However, all trauma patients are different, and near-patient functional coagulation testing is now employed in the deployed (Role 3) setting, which allows bespoke blood product transfusion depending on the patient's specific requirements.[19] Rotational thromboelastometry (ROTEM™) or thromboelastography (TEG) both allow measurement of clot initiation and function as well as more traditional coagulation parameters. Despite the observed benefit in practice, a recent Cochrane review has suggested that there is not yet enough evidence to support its routine use in guiding trauma resuscitation.[20]

Pharmacological adjuncts to resuscitation

The UK DMS were early adopters of pharmacological adjuncts to the resuscitation of critically hypovolaemic trauma patients, including recombinant activated factor VII (rFVIIa) and tranexamic acid (TXA). Indeed, use of the former resulted in some ill-informed comments by scientists who should have known better regarding alleged use of military personnel for so-called 'drug trials'.

rFVIIa (*Novoseven®*) is a synthetic clotting factor that interacts with tissue factor when administered intravenously; it is licensed in the United Kingdom for the treatment of patients with congenital or acquired haemophilia. After early successes using rFVIIa in the management of trauma patients with haemorrhage,[21,22] several randomised placebo controlled trials have failed to show an improvement in mortality,[23,24] and a meta-analysis concluded that there was no improvement in mortality.[25] Although it was used as an adjunct to massive haemorrhage protocols in the early phases of *Operations Telic* and *Herrick*,[26] it was subsequently withdrawn from use in major haemorrhage within UK DMS protocols.

TXA is an anti-fibrinolytic agent that inhibits plasminogen activation and plasmin activity to prevent breakdown of clot formation. The UK DMS uses TXA as a pharmacological adjunct to the management of massive haemorrhage. This has now been extended to all patients at risk of major haemorrhage, in line with the findings of the CRASH 2 study, which demonstrated a 9% overall reduction in relative risk of mortality and a 15% reduction in death from bleeding in civilian trauma patients with the use of TXA.[27] Current evidence suggests that TXA is less effective, and the risk of adverse effects is greater if the drug is administered after three hours.[28] A retrospective study of the use of TXA in combat trauma patients supported the findings of the CRASH 2 trial and found an absolute risk reduction in mortality of 6.5% in those receiving TXA.[29] TXA is now embedded in both military and civilian management of patients at risk of bleeding.

As UK military trauma patients were being administered very large volumes of pRBC and other blood products, it was noticed that hypocalcaemia was a significant problem particularly in those a massive transfusion.[30] This effect is observed due to the citrate in stored blood forming a complex with serum calcium in vivo. It became necessary to supplement the serum calcium by administering intravenous calcium to patients receiving massive transfusion, and this has now been adopted within the *Clinical Guidelines for Operations*. This has also been mirrored in a civilian setting, where it was found that hypocalcaemia was present after blood transfusion, and the more blood that was transfused, the worse the hypocalcaemia.[31] This is likely to influence practice in civilian trauma systems as well as military systems, and further research is ongoing.

'Right-turn' resuscitation

One of the key elements of DCR is DCS – and a key enabler in facilitating the process was the proximity of the operating theatre to the resuscitation room (see Figures 4.2 and 4.4). In Camp Bastion, the middle phase of *Operation Herrick* saw a hard-standing building replace the tented field hospital. On entry to the resuscitation room within this complex, from the entrance used at that time, a left turn took the patient into the main resuscitation bay, and a right turn took the patient into the operating theatre (Figure 4.2). The term 'right-turn' resuscitation was coined for those patients in whom there was perceived benefit in initiating the resuscitation in the operating theatre, therefore enabling DCS to take place as soon as possible.[32] This enabled the resuscitation team to complete its initial assessment and interventions while the surgical team was initiating DCS. However, the right-turn approach is not without its drawbacks, namely the comparative lack of space, potentially compromised sterility and the greater challenges of performing some investigations in the operating theatre. The concept of over-triage is also a real danger, placing unsalvageable patients in the operating theatre in cases of multiple patients attending simultaneously and consequently tying up valuable and finite theatre resources unnecessarily.

In one study looking at 59 severely injured and shocked patients undergoing surgery, 17 went directly to the operating theatre for resuscitative surgery and the rest spent a mean of 17 pre-operative minutes in the ED. This highlighted the imperative for DCS as part of their resuscitation.[12] The same study found that, with aggressive haemostatic resuscitation, it was possible to normalise physiology during the resuscitation phase even in patients with significant coagulopathy on arrival.[12]

TRAUMA TEAM TRAINING AND HUMAN FACTORS ISSUES

The trauma teams deployed on military operations have been likened to Formula 1 racing pit stop teams and other high-performance groups of individuals who work together towards a complex common goal. In effect, the orchestra of the trauma team is conducted by the team leader, who directs actions to ensure a horizontal approach to resuscitation (while an airway clinician is assessing the airway at the head end, a procedures clinician is gaining intravenous access and obtaining blood for analysis and cross-match, the primary survey clinician is listening to the chest, the radiographer is taking primary survey X-rays and the radiologist is performing focussed abdominal sonography for trauma [FAST]).[33] The use of specific timelines in the resuscitation room to prompt certain actions has also been useful in streamlining processes of care,[33] and such direction may be referred to as 'sign-posting'. Simple measures such as holding a team brief before the patient arrives, providing regular sitreps during the resuscitation and command huddles (where key senior decision-makers come together to agree the management plan) improve the cohesiveness, shared understanding and situational awareness and promote unity of effort of the team.[34,35] These issues are discussed in more detail in Chapter 22. Military emergency physicians developing an understanding of 'human factors' facilitated the evolution of the deployed trauma team from a simple entity delivering ATLS® principles to a highly refined clinical concept in which very senior, very experienced clinicians were provided with a platform to work collaboratively and highly efficiently in solving some genuinely complex clinical challenges. What the notional title afforded the EM consultant of 'team leader' fails to capture is the very 'flattened' hierarchy of the successful military trauma team, where leadership

is distributed amongst the team by virtue of their shared understanding of a shared mental model and shared goals. It is this emphasis on the importance of 'followership' in the team ahead of a more historical 'heroic' model of leadership that supported the outstanding results achieved by these teams. This leadership style can also be referred to as combination of the *transformational* and *transactional* models. In the transformational model, the leader creates a vision to guide through inspiration, executing necessary actions in tandem with team members through a shared belief. The transactional model focuses on supervision, organisation and performance management, which also has its role to play in maximising the effectiveness of the team and promoting best practice, the team members being motivated by the reward of achieving the best possible outcomes.

Training of teams prior to deployment has also been cited as a factor in improved outcomes from major trauma. In contrast to civilian hospital teams, as well as individual training such as the *Battlefield Advanced Trauma Life Support* course, military trauma teams undergo team training prior to deployment and clinical contact, including the *Military Operational Surgical Training* course[36] and a whole hospital exercise (HOSPEX).[37] This ensures that complex interventions, such as the management of TCA or enabling massive transfusion while transferring a patient to the operating theatre, are rehearsed beforehand to allow the choreography and individual technical tasks to be perfected. Another stark contrast with the majority of civilian hospital trauma teams was in the constancy of the composition of the military trauma team, this familiarity and shared experience; inevitably enhancing performance.

TRAINING

In terms of individual training, deployment to a busy operational theatre became a routine part of military EM registrar training. This unique training opportunity afforded EM trainees one-to-one (and at times three-to-one) consultant supervision, a mixed caseload of minor, occupational medical, acute medical and major trauma cases and an invaluable insight into the workings of a deployed military medical facility. Trainees were encouraged to complete a series of workplace-based assessments to incorporate their deployed learning within their standard training portfolios. Dedicated time spent shadowing other members of the deployed team, such as the *deployed medical director*, was provided in order to support trainees in gaining a wider understanding of some of the complex issues at play in managing a deployed MTF.

Many trainees returned from a single *Operation Herrick* training deployment with a logbook of trauma cases that some civilian colleagues would struggle to accumulate in a career of NHS practice. Unsurprisingly, many of those individuals have subsequently taken on senior roles in the development of UK major trauma and pre-hospital networks. When the opportunities for deployment ceased, it became apparent that there was a gap in training between a standard civilian training rotation and what a military EM consultant was expected to deliver in terms of complex trauma management. The end of operations was also expected to lead to a knowledge and practice gap regarding the specific military and clinical competencies required for the deployed environment. This has led to the establishment of a military training fellowship, to be undertaken as part of the military registrar training pathway. The components of this module have been chosen to address the areas where trainees need experience that is not available to them through conventional civilian training in the NHS environment. This fellowship will be undertaken in addition to the standard civilian training programme, to supplement specific military skills such as chemical, biological, radiation and nuclear, trauma team leadership and military staff work. This military module has recently been approved and the first registrars undertaking this module commenced in 2017.

EQUIPMENT ISSUES

The main additions of equipment to the resuscitation room scales were those that facilitated DCR, including diagnostics (i-STAT® measurement of venous blood gas, near patient testing of coagulation with ROTEM™), imaging (mobile X-ray units allowing real-time viewing of plain X-rays) and therapeutics (the Belmont® rapid infuser system

replaced the Level 1® rapid infuser). The equipment contained within military medical modules ensures that the deployed MTF is as well equipped as many civilian health service hospitals. The subject of equipment procurement and supply is covered in more detail in Chapter 23. The ED modules, specifically, were kept under constant review throughout both deployed operations and incremental improvements and new additions made when a capability gap was identified or a significant clinical advance recognised.

OPERATIONAL ANALYSIS (AND RESEARCH)

Operational emergency department attendance record

The *Operational Emergency Department Attendance Register* (OpEDAR) was developed as a clinical tool to inform manning, equipment and training requirements for enduring and new operations. The focus was on the global activity of the ED, not just the military trauma caseload, OpEDAR, collecting data on all attendances, such as minor injury and illness, as well as admission rates. Multivariate quality control models could be applied to OpEDAR to generate dynamic epidemiological statistics, enabling the identification of emerging case clusters to inform doctrine, as well as facilitating deployed commanders in taking appropriate mitigating or preventative action.[38]

In one study, of over 11,000 cases over a three-year period, the hospital's workload was characterised by an increase in explosive and gunshot injuries. The hospital faced a high proportion of attendances for non-battle injury and illness and by patients from the local population. Extrapolation of the data enabled accurate medical planning and pre-deployment training and facilitated preparation for current operations.[39]

Joint theatre trauma registry

Significant advances have been made in the early resuscitation of severely injured patients over the last decade.[40] Much of this has been elucidated and characterised through retrospective analysis of the JTTR. Data on all seriously injured patients (including UK military, coalition forces, detainees and local civilians) treated by the UK DMS on deployed operations are collected by the deployed clinical team and returned to the United Kingdom for validation and entry onto the JTTR. Much of this data collection and stewardship was undertaken by the deployed *trauma nurse coordinators* (TNCs). While TNCs were present in some hospitals in the United Kingdom before this period, the military embraced the role and established it as a core function of the deployed hospital team.

The JTTR was formerly maintained by the *Academic Department of Military Emergency Medicine* (ADMEM) at the *Royal Centre for Defence Medicine* (RCDM) in Birmingham and latterly has been administered by the *Defence Analytical Services and Advice*. Data are prospectively collected from clinical notes, trauma charts and, in the case of death, post-mortem findings. The JTTR holds continuous data on this cohort from 2003, coinciding with the start of hostilities in Iraq. Returns are electronic (where deployed information technology systems allow), with hard copy accompanying UK military patients evacuated to RCDM for definitive care. The default entry criterion for UK JTTR is a casualty who triggers trauma team activation in a deployed field hospital or *Primary Casualty Receiving Facility* afloat. The entry criteria were expanded in 2007 to include all trauma patients returned to RCDM for definitive treatment, irrespective of whether a trauma team response was mandated. All UK Service deaths from trauma are subject to post-mortem examination on repatriation, and a representative from ADMEM attends all examinations and records the detailed findings within JTTR.

In addition to retrospective database analyses, primary laboratory research at Dstl Porton Down underpins the scientific basis for combat casualty care. Much of this work has already influenced practice, including the development of the hybrid haemostatic resuscitation model, assessment of TCA and demonstration of coagulopathy from administration of crystalloid in the pre-hospital phase of management. The Combat Casualty Care Research Programme is covered in detail in Chapter 24.

Ongoing research is underway examining further key elements within the management of TCA and potential uses of blood product substitutes in the management of major trauma.

DISEASE AND NON-BATTLE INJURY

Whilst the severe trauma caseload quite understandably attracted headlines and the majority of research activity, the EDs of *Operations Telic* and *Herrick* saw far greater numbers of disease and non-battle injuries (DNBI) as well as a consistent paediatric caseload (see Chapter 18) throughout more than a decade of activity. In data drawn from *MOD Operational Casualty and Fatality tables*,[41–43] we see that in Iraq, between 2006 and 2009, the percentage of DNBI presentations was 91%, with 9% *wounded in action* (WIA) – 3283 patients compared with 315. From 2006 to 2014, in Afghanistan, the headline percentages were 71% DNBI and 29% WIA, with a ratio of patient numbers of 5255 to 2188. The commonest cause of DNBI presentation was *infectious gastroenteritis*,[44] but these departments saw a huge range of acute minor traumatic and non-traumatic presentations, from sports and environmental injuries, ophthalmology cases through to toxicology and acute neurology, and encompassing all medical specialties in between. Whilst many commentators would describe the blast/amputation complex as the 'signature injury' of these campaigns, it must be acknowledged that the deployed EDs became equally adept at managing any clinical presentation that presented to them. This was especially impressive when considering that, certainly at the start of the campaigns, clinical personnel often worked in austere conditions and with less multidisciplinary resource than they were used to in their customary NHS setting.

PAEDIATRIC EM

Between 2008 and 2012, 766 paediatric patients were registered on the JTTR, with various reports citing paediatric caseloads of between 3% and 18%. What is certain is that from the earliest war-fighting phase of *Operation Telic*[45] to the closing stages of *Operation Herrick*, DMS EM personnel were treating children, with the EM clinicians and nurses frequently the sole repository of regular paediatric experience. Fortunately, the ED modules had been designed to include equipment for the management of children and there was no significant capability gap. EM has therefore played a key role in the development of the *Deployed Paediatric Special Interest Group* and has trained four paediatric EM consultants to work in paediatric major trauma centres with a commitment to maintaining a significant body of paediatric expertise. These specialists in paediatric EM are also mandated to maintain currency in adult practice, and full-time paediatric practice in the NHS is not permitted. It is important to remember that the EM cadre is the only cadre whose members are invariably experienced in the regular assessment and management of children. In addition, the cadre's senior paediatric specialist played a lead role in the development and provision of paediatric training across the DMS.

CONCLUSION

From a clinical specialty still in its infancy in military terms, the Iraq and Afghanistan conflicts drove EM to become a major component of deployed medical capability and a significant contributor to the ongoing research and innovation that arose from that period of operational activity. Lessons learned in Iraq and Afghanistan have helped to shape many of the advances in EM, in particular in the management of severe trauma and pre-hospital care, implemented in civilian practice in recent years. This was a seminal period for military EM in the United Kingdom.

REFERENCES

1. Hodgetts TJ, Mahoney PF, Russell MQ et al. ABC to <C>ABC: Redefining the military trauma paradigm. *Emerg Med J* 2006; 23(10):745–746.
2. Hodgetts TJ, Mahoney PF, Kirkman E. Damage control resuscitation. *J R Army Med Corps* 2007;153(4):299–300.
3. Horne S, Smith JE. Preparation of the resuscitation room and patient reception. *J R Army Med Corps* 2011;157(3 Suppl 1): S267–S272.
4. Cooper BR, Mahoney PF, Hodgetts TJ et al. Intra-osseous access (EZ-IO) for resuscitation: UK military combat experience. *J R Army Med Corps* 2007;153(4):314–316.
5. Lewis P, Wright C. Saving the critically injured trauma patient: A retrospective analysis of 1000 uses of intraosseous access. *Emerg Med J* 2015;32(6):463–467.
6. Vassallo J, Horne S, Smith JE. Intraosseous access in the military operational setting. *J R Nav Med Serv* 2014;100(1):34–37.
7. Barnard EB, Moy RJ, Kehoe AD et al. Rapid sequence induction of anaesthesia via the intraosseous route: A prospective observational study. *Emerg Med J* 2015;32(6): 449–452.
8. Fenton P, Bali N, Sargeant I et al. A complication of the use of an intra-osseous needle. *J R Army Med Corps* 2009;155(2): 110–111.
9. Taylor DM, Bailey MS. A complication of the use of an intra-osseous needle. *J R Army Med Corps* 2010;156(2):132.
10. Russell RJ, Hodgetts TJ, McLeod J et al. The role of trauma scoring in developing trauma clinical governance in the Defence Medical Services. *Philos Trans R Soc Lond B Biol Sci* 2011;366(1562):171–191.
11. Tarmey NT, Park CL, Bartels OJ et al. Outcomes following military traumatic cardiorespiratory arrest: A prospective observational study. *Resuscitation* 2011; 82(9):1194–1197.
12. Morrison JJ, Poon H, Rasmussen TE et al. Resuscitative thoracotomy following wartime injury. *J Trauma* 2013;74(3):825–829.
13. Smith JE, Rickard A, Wise D. Traumatic cardiac arrest. *J R Soc Med* 2015;108(1): 11–16.
14. Smith JE, Le Clerc S, Hunt PA. Challenging the dogma of traumatic cardiac arrest management: A military perspective. *Emerg Med J* 2015;32(12):955–960.
15. Midwinter MJ, Woolley T. Resuscitation and coagulation in the severely injured trauma patient. *Philos Trans R Soc Lond B Biol Sci* 2011;366(1562):192–203.
16. Kirkman E, Watts S, Hodgetts T et al. A proactive approach to the coagulopathy of trauma: The rationale and guidelines for treatment. *J R Army Med Corps* 2007; 153(4):302–306.
17. Allcock EC, Woolley T, Doughty H et al. The clinical outcome of UK military personnel who received a massive transfusion in Afghanistan during 2009. *J R Army Med Corps* 2011;157(4):365–369.

18. Holcomb JB, Tilley BC, Baraniuk S et al. Transfusion of plasma, platelets, and red blood cells in a 1:1:1 vs a 1:1:2 ratio and mortality in patients with severe trauma: The PROPPR randomized clinical trial. *JAMA* 2015;313(5):471–482.

19. Woolley T, Midwinter M, Spencer P et al. Utility of interim ROTEM((R)) values of clot strength, A5 and A10, in predicting final assessment of coagulation status in severely injured battle patients. *Injury* 2013;44(5): 593–599.

20. Hunt H, Stanworth S, Curry N et al. Thrombo-elastography (TEG) and rotational thrombo-elastometry (ROTEM) for trauma induced coagulopathy in adult trauma patients with bleeding. *Cochrane Database Syst Rev* 2015;2:CD010438.

21. Kenet G, Walden R, Eldad A et al. Treatment of traumatic bleeding with recombinant factor VIIa. *Lancet* 1999;354(9193):1879.

22. Rizoli SB, Nascimento B Jr., Osman F et al. Recombinant activated coagulation factor VII and bleeding trauma patients. *J Trauma* 2006;61(6):1419–1425.

23. Boffard KD, Riou B, Warren B et al. Recombinant factor VIIa as adjunctive therapy for bleeding control in severely injured trauma patients: Two parallel randomized, placebo-controlled, double-blind clinical trials. *J Trauma* 2005;59(1):8–15; discussion 15–18.

24. Hauser CJ, Boffard K, Dutton R et al. Results of the CONTROL trial: Efficacy and safety of recombinant activated Factor VII in the management of refractory traumatic hemorrhage. *J Trauma* 2010;69(3):489–500.

25. Yank V, Tuohy CV, Logan AC et al. Systematic review: Benefits and harms of in-hospital use of recombinant factor VIIa for off-label indications. *Ann Intern Med* 2011;154(8): 529–540.

26. Hodgetts TJ, Kirkman E, Mahoney PF et al. UK Defence Medical Services guidance for the use of recombinant factor VIIa (rFVIIa) in the deployed military setting. *J R Army Med Corps* 2007;153(4):307–309.

27. CRASH 2 Trial Collaborators, Shakur H, Roberts I et al. Effects of tranexamic acid on death, vascular occlusive events, and blood transfusion in trauma patients with significant haemorrhage (CRASH-2): A randomised, placebo-controlled trial. *Lancet* 2010;376(9734):23–32.

28. CRASH 2 Collaborators, Roberts I, Shakur H et al. The importance of early treatment with tranexamic acid in bleeding trauma patients: An exploratory analysis of the CRASH-2 randomised controlled trial. *Lancet* 2011;377(9771):1096–1101, 101.e1–101.e12.

29. Morrison JJ, Dubose JJ, Rasmussen TE et al. Military Application of Tranexamic Acid in Trauma Emergency Resuscitation (MATTERs) study. *Arch Surg* 2012;147(2): 113–119.

30. Doughty HA, Woolley T, Thomas GO. Massive transfusion. *J R Army Med Corps* 2011;157(3 Suppl 1):S277–S283.

31. Webster S, Todd S, Redhead J et al. Ionised calcium levels in major trauma patients who received blood in the emergency department. *Emerg Med J* 2016;33(8):569–572.

32. Tai NR, Russell R. Right turn resuscitation: Frequently asked questions. *J R Army Med Corps* 2011;157(3 Suppl 1):S310–S314.

33. Smith JE, Russell RJ, Horne S. Critical decision-making and timelines in the emergency department. *J R Army Med Corps* 2011;157(3 Suppl 1):S273–S276.

34. Arul GS, Pugh HE, Mercer SJ et al. Human factors in decision making in major trauma in Camp Bastion, Afghanistan. *Ann R Coll Surg Engl* 2015;97(4):262–268.

35. Mercer S, Arul GS, Pugh HE. Performance improvement through best practice team management: Human factors in complex trauma. *J R Army Med Corps* 2014;160(2): 105–108.

36. Dubose J, Rodriguez C, Martin M et al. Preparing the surgeon for war: Present practices of US, UK, and Canadian militaries and future directions for the US military. *J Trauma* 2012;73(6 Suppl 5):S423–S430.

37. Davies TJ, Nadin MN, McArthur DJ et al. Hospex 2008. *J R Army Med Corps* 2008; 154(3):195–201.

38. Russell R, Hodgetts T, Ollerton J et al. The Operational Emergency Department Attendance Register (OPEDAR): A new epidemiological tool. *J R Army Med Corps* 2007;153(4):244–250.

39. Stalker A, Ollerton J, Everington S, Russell R, Walker C, White S. A three-year review of emergency department admissions – Op HERRICK 4 to 9. *J R Army Med Corps* 2011; 157(3):213–217.

40. Penn-Barwell JG, Roberts SAG, Midwinter MJ, Bishop JRB. Improved survival in UK combat casualties from Iraq and Afghanistan: 2003–2012. *J Trauma* 2015; 78(5):1014–1020.

41. Operational Casualty and Fatality tables. www.mod.uk.

42. Ministry of Defence. *Treating Illness & Injury Arising on Military Operations*. National Audit Office, 2010.

43. UK Troop Withdrawal from Afghanistan. House of Commons, 2013.

44. Bailey MS, Davies GW, Freshwater DA et al. Medical and DNBI admissions to the UK Role 3 Field Hospital in Iraq during Op TELIC. *J R Army Med Corps* 2016;162:309.

45. Gurney I. Paediatric casualties during Op TELIC. *J R Army Med Corps 2004*;150: 270–272.

5

Anaesthesia and pain management

INTRODUCTION

Improvised explosive devices (IEDs) were responsible for the majority of injuries (more than 75% of those in Iraq)[1] and fatalities (57% in Afghanistan in the period 2001 to 2014)[2] in the combat casualty during the recent conflicts in Iraq and Afghanistan. The poly-trauma caused by IEDs resulted from a combination of *primary effects* (rupture and damage of air-filled/hollow organs), *secondary effects* (penetrating/fragmentation injuries) and *tertiary effects* (injuries created from structural collapse or bodily displacement) of blast. The other effects of blast were rare.[3] The multiple traumatic limb amputations seen during *Operation Herrick* were possibly the result of a combination of primary and tertiary blast forces, although this established hypothesis has now been challenged as a result of recent operational experience (see Chapter 10).[4]

Deaths were primarily caused by haemorrhage at the point of injury. A large (*n* > 4500) US post-mortem study found that nearly all deaths (88%) occurred before reaching a medical facility and that these were due to truncal (67%), junctional (20%) or extremity (14%) haemorrhage.[5] Soldiers exposed to an IED whilst patrolling tended to die of severe lower extremity trauma (48%) and those in vehicles died of severe head (53%) and thoracic (23%) injuries.[6]

The case fatality rate for all UK casualties improved during *Operations Telic* and *Herrick*, reducing from 54% (2003) to 16% (2012).[7] This was largely due to developments in body armour,[1,8] pre-hospital care (for example the use of limb tourniquets and haemostatic agents) and damage control resuscitation (DCR) and surgery (DCS).[9,10] This resulted in severely injured casualties reaching a Role 2/Role 3 facility (*deployed combat support hospital* [CSH]) with a 50% survival probability, measured at a *New Injury Severity Score* of 30 in 2003, but 60 by 2012.[7]

The resuscitation peri- and intra-operative anaesthetic management received at Role 2 or 3 facilities was vital in restoring normal thermal and coagulation parameters with an acceptable haemodynamic status for the injury concerned. This was achieved through the targeted use of fluids and blood products, which also assisted the clearance of oxygen debt and metabolic acidosis and the resolution of coagulopathy.[9] Achieving these physiological goals was imperative because the case fatality in combat casualties was five times higher in those who were coagulopathic (INR >1.5).[11]

During the course of these conflicts, the anaesthetic teams had to adapt and evolve in order to provide high-quality medical care despite the location, local threats, skill mix of staff and complexity of injuries in the received casualties. To achieve this aim, changes were made to the layout and location of operating theatres, the number of anaesthetists in theatre, anaesthetic techniques, the management of major haemorrhage- and trauma-related morbidity, drugs and equipment and by the introduction of DCR/DCS and new pain management protocols.[12] A comprehensive textbook entitled *Combat Anesthesia: The First 24 Hours* has been jointly written by UK and US military anaesthetists and offers a practical, detailed description of best practice and the clinical anaesthetic advances that have been developed during these conflicts.

This chapter will focus less on the clinical improvements, and more on the organisational structure, workload, and lessons learned by *Defence Medical Services* (DMS) anaesthetists during these conflicts.

ANAESTHETICS BEFORE *OPERATIONS TELIC* AND *HERRICK*

Before *Operations Telic* and *Herrick*, the most recent experience of similar levels of battlefield trauma had been in the Korean War (1950–1953), Falklands Conflict (1982) and, to a lesser extent, the "Troubles" in Northern Ireland (1969–2007).

Lessons from the Korean War included the trial and success of *mobile army surgical hospital* units, the establishment of a mobile blood bank and the use of body armour.[8] During the Falklands War, the nine deployed naval anaesthetists gave 652 anaesthetics: 540 at sea (on five ships) and 112 at the CSH in Ajax Bay. The deployed consultants felt that there had been a shortage of anaesthetists and mechanical ventilators but that their experience reinforced the usefulness of the *tri-service anaesthetic apparatus* (TSAA) (Figure 5.1), which functions utilising the casualty's own breath to draw volatile anaesthetic gas into their lungs.[13] For emergency anaesthesia, the anaesthetists used thiopentone or ketamine with suxamethonium as the muscle relaxant for rapid sequence inductions. On land, it was felt that the use of multiple field and advanced surgical teams expedited DCS for battle casualties, to good effect.[14]

Northern Ireland taught the DMS about blast injuries and their complexities[4] and how bombs cause multiple casualties, which can disrupt theatre lists and intensive care unit (ICU) daily workloads for weeks.[15] The Omagh bomb in 1998 also highlighted the fact that that the use of mobile anaesthetic teams was critical in keeping patient flow moving through the hospital via the emergency department (ED), radiology, operating theatres and ICU.[15]

There was undoubtedly a degree of DMS anaesthetic team skill fade in the management of combat casualties after these conflicts, which was partly off-set by sending higher anaesthetic trainees to international medical centres that experienced high levels of trauma (for example the *R Adams Cowley Shock Trauma Centre* in Baltimore, MD, USA). Other DMS theatre staff were regularly involved in annual mock hospital trauma moulage exercises (HOSPEX) on land or at sea in *RFA Argus*. *Operations Palliser* (2000) and *Silkman* (2001) in Sierra Leone helped to maintain familiarity with the team and kit in theatre. Prior to *Operation Telic*, *Exercise Saif Sareea* II in Oman (2001) and *Exercise Log Viper* (2002) helped to prepare the field medical units, but the real learning occurred during the conflicts themselves.

DEPLOYED ANAESTHETIC TEAM – *OPERATION TELIC*

Coyote district hospital

At the beginning of the invasion of Iraq in March–April 2003, *202 Field Hospital* was located near the Iraqi border in Kuwait in order to receive the large number of casualties that were anticipated.

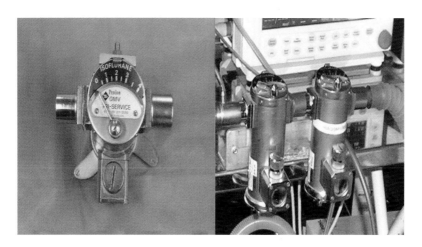

Figure 5.1 The TSAA.

There were four general operating tables in two theatres, with another two theatres reserved specifically for neurosurgery. There were 20 anaesthetists (two of whom were ICU consultants), with four ICU and four high dependency unit (HDU) beds. In all, 160 patients underwent 323 operative procedures for trauma- and non-trauma-related problems. There were 60 burns cases, including children under 18 months.[16] After a period of high intensity, the Coyote district hospital became the Role 4 facility for neurosurgical and burns cases, and the main CSH moved to Shaibah Air Base near Basrah.

Use of forward surgical groups during *Operation Telic*

During the invasion, DMS anaesthetists were an integral part of the *forward surgical group* (FSG) and worked in Role 2 facilities. Operations were usually performed in a lightweight tent with the aim of undertaking 'life-saving surgery' (Figure 5.2). The operating theatre (two bays) was small, with limited holding capacity for casualties. The FSG had laboratory facilities, X-ray facilities, ultrasound and a limited blood bank capability. The casualties were eventually transported by road or helicopter often to the CSH or primary casualty receiving facility (RFA Argus) for further treatment.[17] *3 Commando Brigade* had two FSGs: the

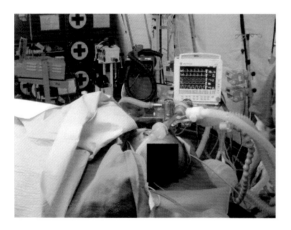

Figure 5.2 Tented field anaesthesia 2005.

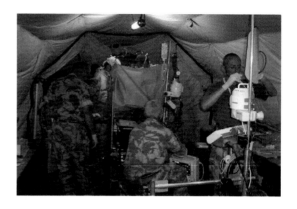

Figure 5.3 *16 Air Assault brigade* FSG undertaking an operation in the lightweight Deployable Rapid Assembly Shelter (DRASH™) tent, 2003.

first received 47 battle injured casualties and operated on 8, and the second FSG operated on 12 casualties. *16 Air Assault Brigade* also had two FSGs, each of which included an orthopaedic and a general surgeon, two anaesthetists and eight operating department practitioners. They performed 51 surgical procedures on 31 patients (Figure 5.3).

An important lesson from *Operation Telic* was that full use of the FSGs had not been made. Two FSGs reported treating several paediatric patients, highlighting the need for paediatric equipment in future military modules for Role 2 facilities: the recognition that there was a need for DMS facilities to be able to treat paediatric casualties was an issue that remained unresolved for far too long.

Combat support hospital

After the invasion of Iraq in 2003, the medical assets were amalgamated into the UK medical group at the Role 3 CSH at *Shaibah Logistics Base*. The CSH was the standard tent structure used by the Army and consisted of a long central corridor, with several tents feeding off the central spine. One of these side arm tents was a large theatre suite in which two surgical tables could be used simultaneously. The tent on the opposite side of the central corridor also had the capacity to function as an operating theatre with a further two surgical tables but was rarely used.

At the beginning of *Operation Enduring Freedom* (May 2003), the number of staff at the CSH in Shaibah reduced, although more than 100 personnel remained. Apart from the frontline medical staff, this team also included the hospital management cell; a radiology department providing X-ray, computed tomography (CT) and ultrasound imaging; a laboratory that housed blood bank, biochemistry and haematological testing facilities; a physiotherapy department; a primary healthcare facility; a dental department; a pharmacy; medical device sterilisation services facilities; a community psychiatric service; patient welfare service and mortuary facilities. The theatre team consisted of two surgical consultants (one general, one orthopaedic), a surgical trainee, with two anaesthetic consultants and a senior anaesthetic trainee.[18] Between 50 and 150 general beds were available and divided between the surgical, medical and isolation wards. This was complemented by two ICU beds and two HDU beds.

The CSH was located at the Shaibah logistics base from 2003 to 2007, when it moved 15 km to Basrah International Airport and remained until the withdrawal of UK Medical Group in 2012. During *Operation Telic 10* (2007), the logistic base was repeatedly subject to indirect fire (IDF). As a consequence, operating theatre staff often had to decide whether to abandon surgery during these alarms and place patients on the ground or to continue with the available protection.[19]

Role and work of the anaesthetist on *Operation Telic*

The role of the anaesthetist included attending the trauma calls, assisting in airway management, and participating in the daily running of emergency and elective theatre lists (Figure 5.4).

The number of cases varied but in the first few years of *Operation Telic* (2003–2006); the injures were predominantly to the thorax, head and upper and lower limbs from explosive weapons.[7]

At the beginning of *Operation Enduring Freedom*, there was a decrease in the number of emergency cases. Over a 12-month period, 524 theatre cases were undertaken at Shaibah CSH largely on personnel from the coalition military (58%; 303/524)

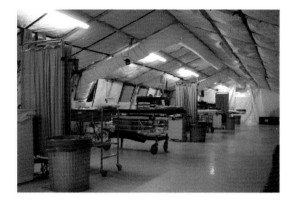

Figure 5.4 The ED in Basrah CSH, which had four resuscitation bays. The anaesthetist was a key member of the trauma team led by the ED consultant.

but also on civilian adults (35%; 186/524). The majority were elective (54%; 281/524) as opposed to emergency (45%; 239/524) cases.[18] This was thought to be due to the amount of repeat theatre trips for the civilian casualties who could not be discharged so easily back into the community and their own healthcare system, unlike coalition troops, who could be rapidly repatriated for continuing care.

During this time, the anaesthetic equipment available included the TSAA, Datex Ohmeda AS/5® patient monitor with agent monitoring, DeVilbiss 515® Oxygen concentrator and ComPac 200® ventilator. The Modular Transportable Surgical Facility had a pneuPAC 300® anaesthetic machine, piped medical oxygen, air and suction capability. Nitrous oxide gas was not available.

Most anaesthetics were general anaesthetics alone (76%; 401/524), with some having both general and regional anaesthesia (5%; 28/524). Endotracheal intubation (28%; 147/524) and laryngeal mask airways (LMA) (29%; 150/524) were the most commonly used airway techniques. Propofol was used most often as the intravenous (IV) induction agent with volatile gas (isoflurane or sevoflurane) using the TSAA for maintenance of anaesthesia. Casualties were usually spontaneously breathing (39%; 167/429) rather than ventilated (34%; 146/429). Of note, at least 5% of patients were children (29/524).[18] It must be noted that the use of sevoflurane with the TSAA for induction of anaesthesia in draw over mode may not produce a high enough concentration of volatile agent to induce anaesthesia in a timely manner.[20]

Clinical governance and significant events

The approaches used during *Operation Telic* to attain the highest standards of medical practice and clinical outcomes evolved over time, but the main efforts and improvements were made through strong leadership (for example from commanding officers [COs], DCAs and hospital clinical directors), improved patient data collection (such as the *Joint Trauma Theatre Registry*) and effective and regular communication.

During *Operation Telic*, the novel haemostatic agents, new field surgical dressings and the combat tourniquet were all introduced as a result of observing data that suggested that soldiers died of incompressible haemorrhage This data also drove the change from the ATLS® paradigm of ABC to <C> (catastrophic haemorrhage) ABC for emergency medical care.[21]

Weekly telemedicine meetings began in 2006 and included the hospital clinicians, led by the clinical director, Royal Centre for Defence Medicine surgical and ICU consultants and staff from the rehabilitation unit at Headley Court to discuss the patients recently sent back or to be repatriated that week. The progress of previous casualties and future changes that were required for patient management were considered. This was an important forum that offered a means of real-time improvement in the management of patients in theatre prior to evacuation. Indeed, the US military viewed the telemedicine conferences as being pivotal in helping to decrease mortality amongst the most seriously injured casualties.[22]

There was one published anaesthetic critical incident during *Operation Telic* that occurred during a routine elective procedure. The chemical alarm went off in camp, which meant that the breathing circuit of the spontaneously breathing anaesthetised patient had to be protected. This involved attaching the inspiratory limb of the circuit to a Pneupac compPAC 200® ventilator with a chemical and biological filter: the concern was that the respiratory resistance through the ventilator could be as high as 6 cm H_2O, which might have been problematic for the emerging,

spontaneously breathing patient. However, the patient was recovered uneventfully.[23]

OPERATION HERRICK

Camp bastion hospital

In 2006, British involvement in Afghanistan increased, and a 25-bed tented field hospital of similar structure to that used on *Operation Telic* was placed 160 km west of Kandahar city. It was staffed by 86 Tri-Service personnel and had a single surgical theatre with two tables. In 2008, a hard-standing purpose-built Role 3 hospital was created and capacity was increased to eight resuscitation bays in the ED, two theatres and a CT scanner. The fact that there were at least 200 UK casualty deaths when the operational tempo was at its peak during 2009–2010 gives an indication of the clinical workload that forced the Role 3 facility to grow and evolve to create a total of four theatres, two CT scanners and 12 ICU beds.[24]

Role and work of the anaesthetist in operation herrick

Gunshot wounds (GSWs) were the most common injury in 2006–2007. After this time, the Taliban began using ever more sophisticated and effective IEDs, which created an injury pattern typically consisting of high bilateral trans-femoral amputations with severe perineal and pelvic injuries (Table 5.1).

Between July 2008 and December 2010, severely injured casualties with an ISS mean (interquartile range) of 30 (23–37) were reaching the CSH with a mean transfer time of 58 (38–78) minutes.[10] The relatively quick arrival of severely injured casualties provided a considerable challenge to DMS anaesthetists, and it was estimated that for the initial management of the most complex trauma cases, three anaesthetists (or two anaesthetists and one ED consultant/registrar) were required: one to conduct the anaesthetic and gain an airway, one to obtain the vascular access (large bore access, arterial line and central line) and one to check, document and administer the blood products.

The Bastion complex trauma team often consisted of 17 personnel (8 of whom would normally be consultants from emergency medicine,

Table 5.1 Type and number of injured regions in UK combat casualties as defined by the abbreviated injury score by year during *Operations Telic* and *Herrick*

	Head	Face	Thorax	Abdomen	Lower extremities	Upper extremities
2003	43 (13)	25 (8)	78 (24)	41 (13)	59 (18)	25 (8)
2004	54 (21)	25 (10)	40 (15)	16 (6)	45 (17)	37 (14)
2005	13 (5)	19 (8)	27 (11)	26 (11)	50 (21)	58 (24)
2006	140 (19)	75 (10)	118 (16)	57 (8)	116 (16)	86 (12)
2007	284 (14)	224 (11)	228 (12)	179 (9)	490 (25)	321 (16)
2008	126 (8)	143 (10)	233 (16)	191 (13)	465 (31)	199 (13)
2009	282 (8)	422 (13)	414 (12)	470 (14)	842 (25)	501 (15)
2010	196 (8)	299 (12)	279 (11)	368 (14)	758 (29)	404 (16)
2011	140 (8)	194 (11)	156 (9)	177 (10)	649 (36)	326 (18)
2012	117 (9)	134 (10)	204 (15)	91 (7)	393 (29)	250 (19)
Total	1395 (10)	1560 (11)	1777 (13)	1616 (11)	3867 (27)	2207 (16)

Source: Penn-Barwell JG et al., *J Trauma Acute Care Surg* 2015;78:1014–1020.
Note: The percentages of injuries as a fraction of total injuries are presented in brackets.

anaesthesia, surgery and radiology). The success of these multidisciplinary teams was evident with at least 210 'unexpected survivors' by 2011.[25] This was thought to be largely due to the definitive clinical pre-hospital training (discussed below) and experience that had been honed in theatre, with excellent non-technical skills and clear lines of communication and leadership.

It was of note that once again, in a different operational theatre, paediatric patients represented a significant proportion of casualty numbers. Paediatric patients made up 11% of the surgical workload mainly with fragmentation and GSW injuries[26,27] and 30% of the critical care bed occupancy.[28] Twenty-five percent of paediatric admissions were ≤24 months old.[26]

Clinical governance and significant events

The weekly telemedicine conferences were as described for *Operation Telic* and provided valuable feedback to the medical teams in theatre. During 2008–2009, it was identified that there was a requirement for a *pre-deployment training* (PDT) package that was distinct from hospital exercises (HOSPEX) in order to prepare the anaesthetist and surgeons for the increased level of trauma that was occurring at Bastion at this time. This PDT included essential components such as equipment training,

human factors and clinical techniques (for example nerve catheter use), with sessions on principles, ethics and decision making. The military operational surgical training (MOST) course was pivotal in preparing surgical and anaesthetic teams for managing trauma and mitigating against human factors impacting on performance once in theatre.[29]

Also at this time, the role of the *Deployed Medical Director* (DMD) was created to work alongside the CO and *senior nursing officer* to manage the complex multidisciplinary requirements of casualties and their evacuation, whilst maintaining and developing high clinical standards within the hospital. The DMD was the interface with multinational aid agencies, allied military medical facilities and the local Afghan population. The DMD position was essential to resolving the governance issues and ethical dilemmas that arose within the hospital or during the management of individual casualties.[25]

Due to the distances and terrain involved in Afghanistan, many casualties, and almost all those who were critically injured, were brought to Bastion by helicopter. The *Medical Emergency Response Team* (MERT) began to develop from 2006 and consisted of an ED or anaesthetic consultant (or, at least initially, senior trainees), a nurse and two paramedics on board a helicopter (usually a CH-47 Chinook) to retrieve severely wounded casualties. In the 2013–2014 season, there was a significant event involving the failed intubation of a casualty retrieved by the MERT. In response, new protocols and training were introduced regarding the detection and management of failed intubations.

There was little IDF into Camp Bastion, and it was therefore safer than the tented hospital in Basrah, Iraq. However, the relentless admission of injured casualties and fatalities, many of whom were children, presented significant emotional and ethical challenges even for the experienced personnel.[25]

CLINICAL ANAESTHETIC CHALLENGES AND ADVANCES DURING *OPERATIONS TELIC* AND *HERRICK*

Airway

In 2009, 11% (56/534) casualties had advanced airway management (41 intubation, 2 LMA and 13 surgical airway) by the clinicians at Role 1 or the MERT prior to arrival at the deployed hospital.[30] Although pre-hospital cricothyroidotomy was not commonly practiced, it became more frequent as the conflicts progressed. Fourteen surgical airways were placed before arrival at Bastion over a 30-week period in 2013. The principal indication was failed intubation, and half the patients had complications or significant events related to the procedure.[31] Other indications for insertion of a surgical airway pre-operatively included trauma or burns obstructing the airway; where endotracheal intubation was not tolerated by an individual who required it; and 'can't intubate, can't oxygenate' scenarios.

A recent review of patients between 2006 and 2014 found that 86 surgical airways were inserted, primarily (>90%) by a Role 1 combat medical technician or general duties medical officer.[32] In this review, only seven devices (8%) were incorrectly placed or failed to work adequately, which is better than the civilian experience.[33]

For the receiving anaesthetist, penetrating airway injuries from IEDs or GSWs were also a hazard during this period. Clinical guidelines were written to assist in the best choice of airway and route of intubation, dependent on where the injury

was located (zones 1–3).[34] The recommended protocol for the management of penetrating airway injuries included pre-oxygenation of the casualties in a position in which they could maintain their own airway with spontaneous ventilation: this avoided the requirement for *intermittent positive pressure ventilation* and the risk of worsening the injury through tissue tearing and surgical emphysema.

Awake fibre optic intubation was considered the gold standard for securing an airway in the patient with a traumatic airway injury if it could be tolerated and was physically possible.[34] However, fibre optic intubating scopes were introduced quite late in the conflicts and, as they were non-disposable, required a lengthy journey for sterilisation. Use of the new disposable fibre optic intubating scopes may be beneficial in this context and should be evaluated in future conflicts. Practice in difficult airway drills during MOST training was critical to improving performance when in theatre.[29]

Vascular access/infusion devices

Due to protective clothing and the patterns of injuries sustained on the ground, peripheral vascular access was sometimes difficult. However, IV access was successfully augmented by the introduction of intra-osseous (IO) access for delivery of fluids and pre-hospital emergency anaesthesia (PHEA) drugs.[35] Experience demonstrated that due to the muscularity of many casualties, the longest available IO needle (yellow) was the most appropriate for routine use. Once the casualty had initial IV/IO access and had been intubated, it was important to establish large-bore IV access to allow appropriate fluid and blood product resuscitation. This was usually accessed via the internal jugular or supraclavicular vein using a trauma line or pulmonary artery catheter introducer or simply with two peripheral 14G cannulae.[36] Femoral lines were also used on occasion. Use was frequently made of ARROW™ wide bore IV access devices.

Damage control resuscitation

The Role 3 anaesthetist was involved with DCR from the moment the casualty reached the ED. The first tasks after handover from the MERT clinician were to establish that any airway device was correctly inserted and to check that large-bore IV access had been attained. Fluid resuscitation would continue with blood products and haemostatic resuscitation allowing for permissive hypotension. Blood products were used in an attempt to normalise physiology and biochemistry, and vasopressors were avoided.[37]

If the airway had not yet been secured, induction of anaesthesia in the unstable trauma patient would occur in the ED. From the ED, the casualty would either be transferred to the CT scanner or direct to the adjacent theatre depending on the severity of their injuries. DCR was partnered with DCS as a single process in a physiologically unstable patient. Additional treatment with IV calcium (to keep ionised levels above 1 mmol/L) (and recombinant activated factor VII in the earlier years) was used as appropriate to aid normalisation of the metabolic response to trauma.

The introduction in 2009 into military casualty management of near patient coagulation testing using *rotational thromboelastometry* (ROTEM)™ allowed a more detailed real-time assessment of trauma-induced coagulopathy, which occurs in more than 25% of victims of major trauma.[38] Coagulopathy was previously detected by using standard laboratory tests, taking 40–60 minutes to measure the prothrombin and activated partial thromboplastin times, which prevented timely administration of appropriate blood products, for example fresh frozen plasma (FFP) and platelets.[39] This experience has shown that in military trauma, early clotting abnormalities as assessed by ROTEM™ (within 10 minutes) can effectively predict coagulopathy and help guide blood product therapy.[39,40] The anaesthetic team responsible for their patient in the operating theatre was thus in an ideal position to request, interpret and act on ROTEM™ results. In the future, it is hoped that military trauma coagulopathy will be fully understood and that ROTEM™ testing will play a pivotal part in ensuring that casualties receive an individually tailored resuscitation package dependent on their particular injuries, coagulopathy and physiological derangements.[41]

PAIN

Pain is commonly experienced by two thirds of casualties,[42] and there were significant improvements in its management during the conflicts. During *Operation Telic*, soldiers were issued with two intramuscular (IM) 10 mg morphine auto-injectors to be used following injury in the battlefield, either by the casualty himself, by buddy-buddy aid, prior to medical assistance or by team medics after their arrival. The consensus amongst military anaesthetists and emergency medicine specialists was that this form of analgesia was far from ideal, a situation exacerbated by the entirely correct *Battlefield Advanced Trauma Life Support* (BATLS) teaching that the control of haemorrhage comes before the giving of morphine for pain.[43] This situation was addressed by trialling and then introducing the *fentanyl lozenge*[44] and the creation of new pain management guidelines. These guidelines encouraged use of an escalating 'analgesic ladder' of interventions: early simple analgesics, splinting, IV morphine and ketamine administered by a medical officer at Role 1, peripheral nerve blocks or catheters and morphine *patient controlled analgesia* (PCA) at Role 2 and the availability of epidurals delivering local anaesthetic and weak opioid at Role 3.[45]

Pain advances during the conflicts

The management of pain throughout a casualty's journey is important as, if effective, it may reduce the incidence of medical complications, chronic pain syndromes and psychological conditions.[46,47] During the conflicts, as stated earlier, battlefield analgesia for the soldier moved from the morphine IM auto-injector[48] to the use of a fentanyl citrate lozenge in 2013,[44] with seemingly good effect. Intranasal ketamine and diamorphine were also considered but were not adopted for use.[47]

Different strategies for pain management included physical methods (for example manipulation and splintage, heat/cold packs), drugs (such as IM or IV morphine, ketamine and local anaesthetics) and psychological interventions (reassurance and support), which are now part of the current management of pain from pre-hospital to aeromedical evacuation.[49,50] Pain scoring was also simplified to a 0 (no pain) to 3 (severe pain) scale to aid diagnosis by the inexperienced caregiver.[42]

The use of regional anaesthesia, including ultrasound sited continuous peripheral nerve block catheters, increased over time due to its success in reducing pain and the requirement for opiates.[51] Regional anaesthesia also proved effective, especially when repeated trips to the theatre were required (for example for debridement or burns dressings) or the patient was to be evacuated by air with complex traumatic injuries.[52] Infections did not appear to be a problem for long-term peripheral nerve catheters, and if there was a risk of compartment syndrome in a limb, pre-emptive fasciotomies were performed.[42,53] There were occurrences of plasma local anaesthetic concentrations sufficient to cause central nervous system (CNS) toxicity in humans with the use of nerve catheters in military patients, but without any apparent adverse clinical effects.[54]

Phantom limb pain affects between 50% and 80% of amputees irrespective of cause. The treatment of this neuropathic pain in military casualties was aided by the early normalisation of visual, sensory and motor input to the CNS. This was brought about by early anti-neuropathic analgesics (pregabalin and amitriptyline)[47] and early stimulation of the somatosensory cortex (for example by using mirror training and by good prosthetic use).[55] The prevention of chronic pain, neuropathic or otherwise, was taken very seriously and treated with early adjunctive pain medications and with specialist pain team input.[46] A recent study of employed military amputees found that although half had experienced phantom limb pain in the preceding month, this was a favourable incidence when compared to similar civilian pain literature.[56] More randomised controlled trials are required to answer whether the use of any particular mode of analgesia at the point of injury prevents the progression to chronic pain syndromes, the incidence of which can be as high as 77% after trauma.[57]

The UK DMS pain teams (unlike the US military) have not found opioid addiction to be a problem in trauma patients with chronic pain; this might be explained by the high levels of patient motivation, vocational rehabilitation and peer group support.[58]

Pain management challenges

Despite their perceived benefit, there was a concern that placement of nerve and epidural catheters would cause an increase in haematoma formation in coagulopathic trauma patients. Whilst no actual statistics are available, military anaesthetists put protocols in place in 2010 to avoid these complications.[59] These protocols are echoed in recent *Association of Anaesthetists of Great Britain and Ireland* (AAGBI) guidelines for the insertion of epidurals and nerve catheters (INR must be ≤1.5, APTTR ≤1.5 and platelets >80 × 10^9/L). Vascular trauma was minimised by using ultrasound guided blocks with close monitoring of casualties for new neurology post-procedure in order to identify those requiring urgent magnetic resonance imaging to exclude epidural haematoma formation.[45,60,61] An unexpected case of cervical intraspinal air (*pneumorrhachis*) following a thoracic GSW highlighted a requirement to avoid nitrous gas and to consider the possibility that this complication could cause difficulties for trauma patients requiring epidural analgesia for pain relief and aeromedical evacuation.[62]

During *Operation Herrick*, it was thought by some anaesthetists that it was difficult to estimate and titrate the required dose of opiate for Afghan trauma patients (military, International Security Assistance Force or civilian). This may have been because some locals were not 'opiate naïve'. There was also a lack of understanding of the concept of PCA in the indigenous population. In this context, the use of peripheral nerve blockade (single shot or catheter) was very useful.[52]

PAEDIATRICS

The conflict in Afghanistan showed that there was a requirement for the military anaesthetist to manage paediatric trauma. Normal paediatric anaesthetic guidelines were adapted to meet the requirements of the often undernourished children, who were almost invariably smaller than British children of the same age.[63]

In response to this lack of knowledge and experience, the *Paediatric Anaesthesia and Critical Care Specialist Interest Group* (PACCSIG) was created in 2010. They reviewed and changed the available anaesthetic equipment, protocols and guidelines and successfully instigated pre-deployment paediatric experience for deploying DMS anaesthetists at the *Birmingham Children's Hospital* prior to *Operation Herrick 13.*[26]

The new military paediatric anaesthesia guidelines (2014) provided a weight adjustment for drug calculations (age 1–5, subtract 2 kg from the estimated UK weight; if over 5 years, subtract 4 kg from the estimated UK weight). This advice included guidance that Hartmann's solution was to be used for maintenance fluids, with additional glucose if required, and that surgical airways were to be avoided in children unless all other options were exhausted, due to the demonstrably high levels of complications.

Severe bleeding in children was treated with 5 mL/kg alternative boluses of red cells and FFP until adequate resuscitation was achieved. This was complemented with 5 mL/kg platelets, 5 mL/kg cryoprecipitate and 0.2 mL/kg of 10% calcium chloride after the first 15 mL/kg of red cells and 15 mL/kg FFP.[63] The authors recommended that rapid infusion devices should be avoided in children under 20 kg, that a 50 mL syringe should be used instead and that tranexamic acid should be given as a 15 mg/kg bolus, followed by a 15 mg/kg infusion over eight hours.

EQUIPMENT AND DRUGS

Equipment changes, modernisation and re-supply of the modules were sometimes slow to materialise. Repairs and servicing of anaesthetic equipment were difficult in the beginning but became easier once Camp Bastion was more established. Examples of problems that were addressed during *Operation Herrick* included deficiencies or weaknesses in MERT physiological monitoring, deep vein thrombosis prophylaxis, cleaning and disinfection of fibre optic bronchoscopes, the availability of portable *extracorporeal membrane oxygenation* and rapid infusion warming devices. Successes included the provision of versatile ICU ventilators (Vela, Carefusion®, California), near patient coagulation testing (ROTEM™; Tem International GmbH, Switzerland), ETCO$_2$ and blood warmers on the MERT, lightweight oxygen cylinders, elastomeric pumps, nerve catheters and needles, ultrasound machines and transthoracic echo.

Anaesthesia delivery and ventilators

The TSAA (Figure 5.5) was designed by Brigadier Ivan Houghton in 1981[64] as a simple way to deliver anaesthetics in a hostile environment. It is a 'draw over' system in which the gas (oxygen and air) is pulled through the volatile Oxford Miniature Vaporiser (OMV; Penlon, Oxford, UK) by either the patient's breath or self-inflating bag. The TSAA was often used with a ventilator in the 'push over' format with the ComPac 200® ventilator (Smiths Medical, UK) and required removal of the self-inflating bag from the patient end and the ventilator to be added behind the vaporiser.[65]

A concern was raised about the prolonged recovery times after volatile isoflurane anaesthetic using the TSAA.[66] The authors hypothesised that this may have been due to a lack of nitrous oxide available at the CSH and described a case using a remifentanil infusion in an attempt to reduce the quantity of volatile agent used.[66] The authors noted that although successful, this was probably a technique to be used during enduring operations rather than during warfighting. The TSAA was also shown to be remarkably versatile in providing paediatric anaesthesia.

The comPAC 200® ventilator at its lowest settings can only provide a minimum minute ventilation of

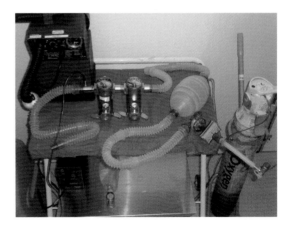

Figure 5.5 TSAA configured for spontaneous ventilation. The two small silver cylinders in the middle of the picture are the Oxford Miniature Vaporisers that produced the volatile anaesthetic vapour. The CompPAC 200 ventilator (green box) can be seen at the left of the picture.

4 L/m with a maximum respiratory rate of 30. This creates a minimum tidal breath of 130 mL, which is too large for young children under 20 kg and could cause pulmonary barotrauma. The manufacturers correctly state that it should be used in patients who are 20 kg or over. However, by placing an adjustable pressure limit (APL) valve between the ventilator and vaporiser, the ventilator can be used in a pressure controlled mode and adjusted to an appropriate level of 20 cm H_2O. This, used in conjunction with an un-cuffed endotracheal tube, provides sufficient air leak in the circuit to allow safe paediatric ventilation.[67]

The TSAA is robust, relatively light and easy to maintain but has no CE mark, carries the risk of disconnections, has a heavy valve system at the patient end, is not temperature compensated and has potential for spillage of volatile liquid during filling and general use. For these reasons, the TSAA is being phased out and may soon be replaced for 'light' capabilities with the Diamedica Portable Anaesthesia System (DPA 03™, Devon, UK).

In afloat or 'heavy' Role 2 and 3 facilities, the TSAA has been replaced in recent years by the Fabius® Tiro M (Drager, Germany) anaesthetic machine, with great success. These facilities have the necessary logistic support to provide the cylinders of oxygen and air required for modern anaesthesia.

Total intravenous anaesthetic

The recent conflicts honed the use of total intravenous anaesthesia (TIVA) for situations in which casualties were required to be intubated and ventilated outside the operating theatre. TIVA was often started for casualties in the pre-hospital environment and continued throughout their hospital journey. TIVA allows continuity of anaesthesia and sedation between the ED, CT scanner, theatre, ICU and aeromedical evacuation. TIVA may have beneficial effects on the stress response to injury and provides a favourable recovery profile with potentially less post-operative nausea and vomiting, headache and airway irritation. A range of drugs can be used, including propofol, remifentanil, ketamine and midazolam, some of which can be mixed together to simplify the anaesthetic. However, care must be taken in haemodynamically unstable patients, with

careful assessment for awareness in those who are paralysed.[68] With the requirement to replace the TSAA, TIVA may become more popular for Role 2/3 facilities in future operations.

THORACIC INJURY

Thoracic trauma was relatively common during both conflicts (9–24%; Table 5.1) and occurred in both military and civilian casualties. Anaesthetists had to remain aware of the possibility of tension pneumothorax and be prepared to perform bilateral thoracostomies if these had not been carried out before the patient's arrival in hospital. Further anaesthetic management of these injuries has been described elsewhere.[37,69]

BLOOD AND MASSIVE TRANSFUSION

Due to the nature of the trauma from IEDs, deaths on the battlefield were primarily from truncal haemorrhage.[70] US data from between 2004 and 2008 demonstrated that nearly a third of casualties required a blood transfusion, with 7% requiring a major transfusion (>10 red cell concentrate [RCC] units/24 hours).[22] The mortality rate of those receiving one to nine RCC units (16%) was lower than that of those receiving a major transfusion (21%), reflecting the severity of the injuries sustained. The authors of this study noted that after 2006, casualty mortality for the most severely injured improved because of the introduction of DCS and the use of the components of whole blood for transfusion.[22]

In a retrospective study conducted between 2008 and 2010, it was found that intra-operative resuscitation with blood products (RCC, FFP, cryoprecipitate and platelets) was vital in order to normalise the metabolic and coagulation derangements caused by severe haemorrhagic shock.[10] In order to achieve normal physiology in casualties with severe blast injury, the median quantity of blood products required per patient ($n = 59$) was 27 RCC units, 27 units FFP, two units cryoprecipitate and four pools of platelets. The casualties also received tranexamic acid ($n = 30/59$), calcium and, occasionally, recombinant factor VIIa ($n = 21/59$) or whole blood (number of patients not given).[10]

This success of the massive transfusion protocol (introduced by Surgeon General's Policy Letter in February 2009) was confirmed in a 2009 UK military retrospective review of patients; 59 received a massive transfusion (>10 RCC units) and 86% survived until hospital discharge.[71]

The AAGBI has recently (2016) published a consensus document detailing the requirement for a massive blood transfusion protocol including the early administration of FFP and platelets alongside red cells.[72] They state the importance of point of care testing (including ROTEM™) and suggest that a guide for transfusion should be FFP administration if the INR is >1.5, cryoprecipitate if fibrinogen is <1.5 g/L and platelets if the count is <75 × 10^9/L. The use of tranexamic acid and red cell salvage should be considered in cases likely to lose more than 500 mL of blood. These guidelines have been produced in part due to the recent military advances in the understanding of trauma and coagulopathy.[73]

ANAESTHETIC AND PAIN CHALLENGES FOR THE FUTURE

Manpower

Tri-service anaesthetic consultant numbers increased from 59 in 2011 to 71 in 2016, reflecting the requirement for increased consultant numbers to staff the ever-more complex needs of the DMS (including tactical *Critical Care Air Support Teams*). Yet, there still remains concern that there is a shortage of anaesthetic consultants, especially in the sub-specialties of *intensive care medicine* (ICM) and *pre-hospital emergency medicine* (PHEM). This has in part resulted from ICM becoming a specialty in its own right and from the requirement for further training, examinations and clinical experience in the fields of ICM and PHEM in order to dual accredit in either as a consultant. The inevitable losses of consultants to the National Health Service (NHS) following the end of the conflicts is likely, as it is in all specialties, to make a difficult situation even more challenging.

The number of injured or unfit medical personnel not able to deploy on operations has been highlighted as an issue, with the result that the burden of deployments inevitably falls on a smaller number of deployable anaesthetists and intensivists. It is unknown whether the high rate of attrition was in part caused by the conflicts themselves or the high operational tempo and regular deployments.

The Reserve anaesthetic force (53 in 2015–2016) is an increasingly important resource. However Reserve personnel often have difficulty in attending training courses, exercises and short-notice deployments, especially during contingency operations. Better integration of the Reserves into the Regular cadre is also required, as is greater command oversight of these valuable assets. Further development of this cadre is essential if DMS 20 targets are to be met within the context of an NHS, which is under considerable pressure.

Continuing education

Continued professional development is paramount in avoiding skill fade in the peri- and intra-operative management of the trauma victim, in maintaining knowledge of the equipment used in theatre and in the management of pain. Weaknesses in managing major trauma, ICM, thoracic surgery and neurosciences were identified early in *Operation Herrick*, and to combat these, several courses (for example MERT, Military Advanced Paediatric Life Support [MAPLS] and MOST), simulator training programmes and hospital exercises were provided for military and reserve personnel in their PDT package.[74] Membership on specialist interest groups (such as PACCSIG mentioned previously) will also help maintain cadre knowledge of the anaesthetic lessons learned on *Operations Telic* and *Herrick*.

PAIN EDUCATION

Early on in the conflicts, the DMS received negative media attention due to the poor management of patients' pain. Good pain management is brought about through a multi-disciplinary approach offering multimodal analgesia with good communication between the patients and staff.[47,75] Therefore, the concept of pain management must be recognised as a key component of clinical care. The introduction of a 'named person' to manage each patient's pain from point of injury has proved useful and should be considered in future conflicts. The use of advanced analgesics such as fentanyl and ketamine by frontline medical officers and combat medical technicians was found to be useful, but continued use must be accompanied by appropriate regular training.[76]

AIRWAY EDUCATION

Some concerns were raised about the use of advanced airways in casualties prior to their admission to a Role 3 facility. Most airway training for pre-hospital airway clinicians inevitably occurred in their NHS job, during individual continual professional development or by attendance in a BATLS course (or similar). Lessons learned during the conflicts resulted in the addition of a suitable carbon dioxide detector (colorimeter – Easycap®) to aid the recognition of failed endotracheal intubation attempts as well as the introduction of a standardised military cricothyroidotomy kit, the use of which was practiced on the BATLS course.

However, the use of $ETCO_2$ monitors to confirm correct placement of supraglottic airway devices or surgical airways is currently not mentioned in BATLS or Clinical Guidelines for Operations, an omission identified by subject matter experts.[31] It may be the case that too much reliance is put on the airway management experience that anaesthetists gain in their day job, and more could perhaps be done to regularly simulate failed intubation drills and use of a surgical airway in austere environments with the appropriate monitoring equipment.

PAEDIATRIC EDUCATION

Future PDT for consultant anaesthetists should ideally include a refresher course in paediatric trauma management as it was very evident that there was a lack of such expertise amongst DMS anaesthetists. One author has argued that all final-year anaesthetic trainees should do a mandatory six months of paediatric anaesthesia in a tertiary centre.[26]

Anaesthetic and pain research

During the conflicts, the role of the *Defence Professor for Anaesthesia and Critical Care Medicine* was created to manage the research outputs being produced by the cadre, especially in the field of trauma anaesthesia. There soon followed the development of the *Academic Department of Military*

Anaesthesia and Critical Care Medicine (2008) with the creation of several competitively appointed lecturer and senior lecturer posts ratified by the *National Institute of Academic Anaesthesia* in 2013.

To date, the UK Military *Defence Scientific and Technical Laboratories* have focussed on researching the pathophysiological and immunological impact of militarily relevant injuries, particularly blast-related injuries with haemorrhage and coagulopathy.[77] This work is part of an ongoing suite of projects within the *Combat Casualty Care Research Programme*, and a number of anaesthetists are conducting this research as part of their higher degrees. The anaesthetic and critical care academic lecturers met in May 2016 and decided on a list of key research priorities for the coming years. These included the following:

- Prolonged field care/PHEM (including determining the optimum resuscitation fluid, novel resuscitation methods and biomarkers of injury)
- Field anaesthesia (for example, is TIVA better than volatile anaesthesia, and if so, what regime is best?)
- Critical care (including the genomics of patients, resource management, diagnostics and delirium)
- Evacuation of the casualty (including in-transit pain management, feeding and pressure care)
- Pain (aspects including neuroplasticity, battlefield analgesia and the role of complementary medicine)
- Education/simulation and human factors (such as the effect of fatigue on medical performance)
- Chemical, biological, radiological and nuclear threats (including biomarkers, diagnostics, mass ventilation and the effect of chemical weapons on anaesthetic equipment)

During *Operations Telic* and *Herrick*, the US military deployed 12 dedicated research teams to further their knowledge on subjects such as traumatic brain injury, haemorrhage and coagulopathy. They learned valuable lessons about how to conduct efficient research in an austere environment, making best use of the data produced during the conflicts. The UK DMS can learn from the US experience, especially in their use of waived consent (for example plasma used for research that would otherwise be thrown away), simple research with standard operating procedures, dedicated research teams and good communication between clinicians and researchers.[78] This will ensure that data and patient information are not wasted, but captured in a timely fashion, leading to better powered studies and therefore more definitive answers on how best to manage the trauma victim.

CONCLUSION

The efforts and clinical advances in anaesthesia made by DMS anaesthetists during these conflicts have been remarkable. As such, this was recognised by the Royal College of Anaesthetists in 2010 and 2014, which awarded the *Pask Certificate of Honour* to all DMS anaesthetists who had deployed on *Operations Telic* and *Herrick*, respectively. The next conflicts are unlikely to mirror those experienced in *Operations Telic* and *Herrick*. The medical and casualty evacuation capabilities will be reduced, and this must be reflected and managed in contingency planning and training. The concept of a longer duration of casualty evacuation may become more likely, and therefore, casualty management will also change and evolve as we become accustomed to quickly mobilising a more compact medical capability to austere environments.[79]

Whatever the future challenges, a combination of intelligent tasking and efficient decision making by military medical leaders will make the best use of the current highly trained, adaptable and resourceful DMS anaesthetic cadre.

REFERENCES

1. Belmont PJ Jr., Goodman GP, Zacchilli M, Posner M, Evans C, Owens BD. Incidence and epidemiology of combat injuries sustained during "the surge" portion of Operation Iraqi Freedom by a US Army Brigade combat team. *J Trauma Inj Infect Crit Care* 2010;68:204–210.
2. BBC. UK military deaths in Afghanistan: How they died. 2016;2016.
3. DePalma RG, Burris DG, Champion HR, Hodgson MJ. Blast injuries. *N Engl J Med* 2005;352:1335–1342.
4. Harrisson SE, Kirkman E, Mahoney P. Lessons learnt from explosive attacks. *J R Army Med Corps* 2007;153:278–282.
5. Eastridge BJ, Mabry RL, Seguin P et al. Death on the battlefield (2001–2011): implications for the future of combat casualty care. *J Trauma Acute Care Surg* 2012;73:S431–S437.
6. Singleton JAG, Gibb IE, Bull AMJ, Mahoney PF, Clasper JC. Primary blast lung injury prevalence and fatal injuries from explosions: Insights from postmortem computed tomographic analysis of 121 improvised explosive device fatalities. *J Trauma Acute Care Surg* 2013;75:S269–S274.
7. Penn-Barwell JG, Roberts SAG, Midwinter MJ, Bishop JRB. Improved survival in UK combat casualties from Iraq and Afghanistan: 2003–2012. *J Trauma Acute Care Surg* 2015;78:1014–1020.
8. Baker MS. Military medical advances resulting from the conflict in Korea, part I: Systems advances that enhanced patient survival. *Mil Med* 2012;177:423–429.
9. Buckenmaier C, Mahoney PF. *Combat Anesthesia: The First 24 Hours.* Virginia, US: Borden Institute, 2015.
10. Morrison J, Ross J, Poon H, Midwinter M, Jansen J. Intra-operative correction of acidosis, coagulopathy and hypothermia in combat casualties with severe haemorrhagic shock. *Anaesthesia* 2013;68:846–850.
11. Niles SE, McLaughlin DF, Perkins JG et al. Increased mortality associated with the early coagulopathy of trauma in combat casualties. *J Trauma Inj Infect Crit Care* 2008;64:1459–1463.
12. Pruitt BA Jr., Rasmussen TE. Vietnam (1972) to Afghanistan (2014): The state of military trauma care and research, past to present. *J Trauma Acute Care Surg* 2014;77: S57–S65.
13. Bull PT. Anaesthesia ashore and afloat during the Falklands war. *J R Nav Med Serv* 1983;69:85–90.
14. Jackson D, Batty C, Ryan J and McGregor W. The Falklands war: Army field surgical experience. *Ann R Coll Surg Engl* 1983;65:281–285.

15. Lavery GG and Horan E. Clinical review: Communication and logistics in the response to the 1998 terrorist bombing in Omagh, Northern Ireland. *Crit Care* 2005;9:401–408.

16. Rew DA, Clasper J, Kerr G. Surgical workload from an integrated UK field hospital during the 2003 Gulf conflict. *J R Army Med Corps* 2004;150:99–106.

17. Rew D. *Blood, Heat and Dust: Operation Telic and the British Medical Deployment to the Gulf 2003–2009. 2nd edition.* London: Defence Medical Services Department, Ministry of Defence; 2015.

18. Bateman RM, McNicholas JJK. Overview of 12 months anaesthetic activity in a UK field hospital on enduring operations in Iraq. *J R Nav Med Serv* 2006;92:51–56.

19. Stansfield T, Hay H. Spinal anaesthetic with patient wearing enhanced combat body armour. *J R Army Med Corps* 2008;154:85.

20. Mellor A, Hicks I. Sevoflurane delivery via the Triservice apparatus. *Anaesthesia* 2005;60:1151.

21. Hodgetts T, Mahoney P, Russell M, Byers M. ABC to <C> ABC: Redefining the military trauma paradigm. *Emerg Med J* 2006;23:745–746.

22. Eastridge BJ, Wade CE, Spott MA et al. Utilizing a trauma systems approach to benchmark and improve combat casualty care. *J Trauma Inj Infect Crit Care* 2010;69: S5–S9.

23. Nordmann GR, Woolley T. Unusual critical incident: Chemical gas alert. *Anaesthesia* 2003;58:926.

24. Vassallo D. A short history of Camp Bastion Hospital: The two hospitals and unit deployments. *J R Army Med Corps* 2015;161:79–83.

25. Vassallo D. A short history of Camp Bastion Hospital: Part 2 – Bastion's catalytic role in advancing combat casualty care. *J R Army Med Corps* 2015;161:160–166.

26. Nordmann GR. Paediatric anaesthesia in Afghanistan: A review of the current experience. *J R Army Med Corps* 2010;156: S323–S326.

27. Nordmann GR, McNicholas J, Templeton P, Arul S, Woods K. Paediatric trauma management on deployment. *J R Army Med Corps* 2011;157:S334–S343.

28. Harris C, McNicholas J. Paediatric intensive care in the field hospital. *J R Army Med Corps* 2009;155:157–159.

29. Mercer S, Tarmey N, Mahoney P. Military experience of human factors in airway complications. *Anaesthesia* 2013;68:1081–1082.

30. Haldane AG. Advanced airway management – a Medical Emergency Response Team perspective. *J R Army Med Corps* 2010;156:159–161.

31. Pugh HE, LeClerc S, Mclennan J. A review of pre-admission advanced airway management in combat casualties, Helmand Province 2013. *J R Army Med Corps* 2015;161:121–126.

32. Kyle T, Le Clerc S, Thomas A, Greaves I, Whittaker V, Smith J. The success of battlefield surgical airway insertion in severely injured military patients: A UK perspective. *J R Army Med Corps* 2016;162:460–464.

33. King DR, Ogilvie MP, Velmahos G et al. Emergent cricothyroidotomies for trauma: Training considerations. *Am J Emerg Med* 2012;30:1429–1432.

34. Mercer SJ, Lewis S, Wilson S, Groom P, Mahoney P. Creating airway management guidelines for casualties with penetrating airway injuries. *J R Army Med Corps* 2010;156:S355–S360.

35. Barnard EBG, Moy RJ, Kehoe AD, Bebarta VS, Smith JE. Rapid sequence induction of anaesthesia via the intraosseous route: A prospective observational study. *Emerg Med J* 2015;32:449–452.

36. Hulse EJ, Thomas G. Vascular access on the 21st century military battlefield. *J R Army Med Corps* 2010;156:S385–S390.

37. Tarmey N, Park C, Fox M, Lowes T, Mellor A, Mahoney P. Anaesthesia for Overseas Operations: UK Military Guidelines. *Med Corps Int Forum* 2013;3:4–7.

38. Doran CM, Woolley T, Midwinter MJ. Feasibility of using rotational thromboelastometry to assess coagulation status of combat casualties in a deployed setting. *J Trauma Inj Infect Crit Care* 2010;69: S40–S48.

39. Woolley T, Midwinter M, Spencer P, Watts S, Doran C, Kirkman E. Utility of interim ROTEM (R) values of clot strength, A5 and A10, in predicting final assessment of coagulation status in severely injured battle patients. *Inj Int J Care Inj* 2013;44:593–599.

40. Keene DD, Nordmann GR, Woolley T. Rotational thromboelastometry-guided trauma resuscitation. *Curr Opin Crit Care* 2013;19:605–612.

41. Tarmey NT, Woolley T, Jansen JO et al. Evolution of coagulopathy monitoring in military damage-control resuscitation. *J Trauma Acute Care Surg* 2012;73:S417–S422.

42. Aldington DJ, McQuay HJ, Moore RA. End-to-end military pain management. *Philos Trans R Soc B Biol Sci* 2011;366:268–275.

43. Jones CP, Chauhan R, Aldington D. Use of intramuscular morphine in trauma patients. *Anaesthesia* 2014;69:796–797.

44. Aldington D, Jagdish S. The fentanyl 'lozenge' story: From books to battlefield. *J R Army Med Corps* 2014;160:102–104.

45. Tarmey N, Park C, Aldington D, Ingram M, Mahoney P. Acute pain management on overseas operations: UK military guidelines. *Med Corps Int Forum* 2014;3:40–43.

46. Mercer S, Chavan S, Tong J, Connor D, de Mello W. The early detection and management of neuropathic pain following combat injury. *J R Army Med Corps* 2009;155:94–98.

47. Keene DD, Rea WE, Aldington D. Acute pain management in trauma. *Trauma* 2011;13:167–179.

48. Gaunt C, Gill J, Aldington D. British military use of morphine: A historical review. *J R Army Med Corps* 2009; 155:46–49.

49. Flutter C, Aldington D. Pain priorities in pre-hospital care. *Anaesth Intensive Care Med* 2011;12:380–382.

50. Flutter C, Ruth M, Aldington D. Pain management during Royal Air Force strategic aeromedical evacuations. *J R Army Med Corps* 2009;155:61–63.

51. Buckenmaier CC, Rupprecht C, McKnight G et al. Pain following battlefield injury and evacuation: A survey of 110 casualties from the wars in Iraq and Afghanistan. *Pain Med* 2009;10:1487–1496.

52. Hughes S, Birt D. Continuous peripheral nerve blockade on OP HERRICK 9. *J R Army Med Corps* 2009;155:57–58.

53. Clasper JC, Aldington DJ. Regional anaesthesia, ballistic limb trauma and acute compartment syndrome. *J R Army Med Corps* 2010;156:77–78.

54. Bleckner LL, Bina S, Kwon KH, McKnight G, Dragovich A, Buckenmaier III CC. Serum ropivacaine concentrations and systemic local anesthetic toxicity in trauma patients receiving long-term continuous peripheral nerve block catheters. *Anesth Analg* 2010;110:630–634.

55. Le Feuvre P, Aldington D. Know pain know gain: Proposing a treatment approach for phantom limb pain. *J R Army Med Corps* 2014;160:16–21.

56. Aldington D, Small C, Edwards D et al. A survey of post-amputation pains in serving military personnel. *J R Army Med Corps* 2014;160:38–41.

57. Radresa O, Chauny J-M, Lavigne G, Piette E, Paquet J, Daoust R. Current views on acute to chronic pain transition in post-traumatic patients: Risk factors and potential for pre-emptive treatments. *J Trauma Acute Care Surg* 2014;76:1142–1150.

58. Jagdish S, Aldington D. The use of opioids during rehabilitation after combat-related trauma. *J R Army Med Corps* 2009;155:64–66.

59. Connor and Ingram. Regional anaesthesia in patients after trauma shock. 2011. http://wwwrespond2articlescom/ANA/forums/post/714aspx.

60. Wyldbore M, Aldington D. Trauma pain – a military perspective. *Br J Pain* 2013;7: 74–78.

61. Walker C, Ingram M, Edwards D, Wood P. Use of thromboelastometry in the assessment of coagulation before epidural insertion after massive transfusion. *Anaesthesia* 2011;66:52–55.

62. Haldane AG. Traumatic pneumorrhachis. *J R Army Med Corps* 2010;156:318–320.

63. Tarmey N, Easby D, Park C, Mahoney P, Bree S. Paediatric anaesthesia for overseas operations: UK Military guidelines. *Med Corps Int Forum* 2014;1:32–35.

64. Houghton I. The Triservice anaesthetic apparatus. *Anaesthesia* 1981;36:1094–1108.

65. Henning J. The Triservice anaesthetic apparatus – an alternative configuration. *Anaesthesia* 2006;61:1123.

66. Bateman R, Wedgwood J, Henning J. Case report: Use of a remifentanil infusion with the tri-service anaesthetic apparatus. *J R Nav Med Serv* 2005;91:48–49.

67. Ralph J, George R, Thompson J. Paediatric anaesthesia using the Triservice anaesthetic apparatus. *J R Army Med Corps* 2010;156:84–87.

68. Lewis S, Jagdish S. Total intravenous anaesthesia for war surgery. *J R Army Med Corps* 2010;156:S301–S307.

69. Round J, Mellor A. Anaesthetic and critical care management of thoracic injuries. *J R Army Med Corps* 2010;156:145–149.

70. Kelly JF, Ritenour AE, McLaughlin DF et al. Injury severity and causes of death from operation Iraqi freedom and operation enduring freedom: 2003–2004 versus 2006. *J Trauma Inj Infect Crit Care* 2008;64: S21–S26.

71. Allcock E, Woolley T, Doughty H, Midwinter M, Mahoney P, Mackenzie I. The clinical outcome of UK military personnel who received a massive transfusion in Afghanistan during 2009. *J R Army Med Corps* 2011;157:365–369.

72. Klein A, Arnold P, Bingham R et al. AAGBI Guidelines: The use of blood components and their alternatives 2016. *Anaesthesia* 2016;71:829–842.

73. Thomas D, Wee M, Clyburn P, Walker I, Brohi K, Collins P, Doughty H, Isaac J, Mahoney P, Shewry L. Blood transfusion and the anaesthetist: Management of massive haemorrhage. *Anaesthesia* 2010;65: 1153–1161.

74. Davey CMT, Mieville KE, Simpson R, Aldington D. A Proposed model for improving battlefield analgesia training: Post-Graduate Medical Officer Pain Management Day. *J R Army Med Corps* 2012;158:190–193.

75. Plunkett A, Turabi A, Wilkinson I. Battlefield analgesia: A brief review of current trends and concepts in the treatment of pain in US military casualties from the conflicts in Iraq and Afghanistan. *Pain Manage* 2012;2: 231–238.

76. Davey CMT, Mieville KE, Simpson R, Aldington D. A Survey of experience of parenteral analgesia at Role 1. *J R Army Med Corps* 2012;158:186–189.

77. Kirkman E, Watts S. Combat casualty care research programme. *J R Army Med Corps* 2014;160:109–116.

78. Hatzfeld JJ, Childs JD, Dempsey MP et al. Evolution of biomedical research during combat operations. *J Trauma Acute Care Surg* 2013;75:S115–S119.

79. Strategic Trends Programme – Future Operating Environment 2035. 2015;1:1–60.

6

Intensive care medicine

INTRODUCTION

> ICU is a product of clinical developments, technological advances, social changes and history. Military ICU reflects all of these as well as deployed operational experience.[1]

Since the late 1990s, Defence Medical Services (DMS) intensive care has undergone a radical transformation. Underlying this are two complementary narratives: the first is that this change reflects the shift that intensive care has undergone within the UK National Health Service (NHS), where there has been a growth in bed numbers, in capability and integration and in overall strategic importance[2]; indeed, the two services are contemporaneous – intensive care within the UK NHS being awarded the status of a specialty only in 1999. A second, historical, perspective puts this gain into context; Defence medical doctrine shifted radically after the end of the Cold War, with a new emphasis on ensuring that the care of ill and injured service personnel should be as least as good as that which they would receive in the NHS or in peacetime.[3] Thus, the focus needed to change from one of providing basic quality healthcare for many to providing high-quality care for a much smaller number. Deployed intensive care has been a fundamental element of this change.

This chapter explores the challenges of operational intensive care and the extraordinary clinical advances made possible in a quarter of a century. Since the first embryonic intensive care was deployed on operations to the Balkans in the late 1990s, the capability of deployed intensive care has grown. Overlapping conflicts in Iraq and Afghanistan have proved the unfortunate catalyst for much of the improvement in capability.

Successive campaigns have allowed iterative improvements across a broad spectrum of capability, including individual preparedness, clinical equipment, standards improvement, systems and process integration. Indeed, it is difficult to precisely define the individual contribution of intensive care against a background of substantial improvements in pre-hospital care and damage control resuscitation when so many specialties are so tightly integrated. This is the nature of twenty-first century military healthcare.

In spite of impressive gains within the deployed intensive care, we should be wary of placing it on a pedestal. The conflicts in Afghanistan and Iraq have raised important questions about the provision of deployed intensive care in austere environments. This chapter closes with a discussion of the political, doctrinal and clinical challenges for providing future deployed intensive care capability to Defence.

THE SPECIALTY BEFORE *OPERATIONS TELIC* AND *HERRICK*

With the end of the Cold War, there was a marked shift in perception with the return to contingency operations. Concomitant with this was a significant change to the delivery of military healthcare. Following a series of reviews throughout the 1990s, including *Options for Change, Front Line First* and the *Defence Costs*

Study 15, all military hospitals managed by the single services were closed. In their place, five *Ministry of Defence Hospital Units* were opened within existing NHS Trusts, and shortly after, the *Royal Centre for Defence Medicine* was established in Birmingham. At the same time, two regular field hospitals (*33* and *34 Field Hospitals*) were created in addition to the already established *22 Field Hospital*. Major reviews of equipment and planning within the DMS during this period put modern intensive care units (ICUs) in UK field hospitals, marking the starting point in the development of deployed intensive care over the last quarter century.[4] A summary of these changes follows.

The acknowledgement of public intolerance of poor treatment for wounded service personnel on any future operations and its consequent political unacceptability[3] led to the declaration by the then Defence chiefs that servicemen should, *wherever possible*, be offered medical care to a standard equal to that which they would receive in the United Kingdom in peacetime. Doctrinal changes in the DMS led to significant resource allocation to the critically injured with the integration of *Battlefield Advanced Trauma Life Support* (BATLS), surgical resuscitation and deployed intensive care to improve outcome. Major updates of equipment scales for medical units in the field were undertaken by the UK *Surgeon General's Department* in the late 1990s, and anaesthesia and intensive care were two areas where there were significant developments. At the same time, civilian intensive care medicine was being increasingly recognised as a specialty in its own right.[5] This led to a greater tendency to take the specialist qualifications and experience of nursing and medical staff into account when planning deployments.

Another motivator for change was an increasing sense of threat in the Middle East, in particular the potential use of chemical and biological weapons, with the expectation of critically ill casualties who would need to be managed within the theatre of operations. To counter this threat, a *biological ICU*, capable of managing the complications of severe sepsis, was scaled and equipped. Whilst untested, the concept of managing the critically ill in the field beyond the immediate post-operative period had been established.

Operation Granby – First Gulf War

The field hospitals that deployed for the 1991 Gulf War to liberate Kuwait were equipped to the scale that had been in place during the Cold War, in anticipation of a major conflict in North Western Europe. None of the field hospitals had an intensive care/high dependancy unit facility.[6] This resulted in prolonged stays in the recovery ward and in the operating theatres, delaying subsequent surgical procedures. Fortunately, the hospitals never worked to their full capacity, but this would have been a significant problem in a mass casualty situation.

Other post-Cold War deployments

22 Field Hospital had deployed a medical support team to Kuwait in 1994 (*Operation Driver*), *23 Parachute Field Ambulance* (*PFA*) deployed a field surgical team to Brazzaville in the Congo in 1997 (*Operation Determinant*) and *16 Close Support Medical Regiment* deployed to Sierra Leone in 2000 (*Operation Palliser*), yet on none of these deployments was intensive care provided at anything other than a rudimentary, improvised level.

The Balkans: Croatia and Bosnia

A number of medical units were deployed to the Balkans.[1] Critical care facilities were deployed, but the units were static in nature. During this period of multinational operations, it was possible to compare UK facilities with those of other nations. In contrast to the tented *Deployable Rapid Assembly Shelters* (DRASH™) systems in use by the United Kingdom, the latter were often of semi-permanent expandable, containerised construction. As a result, by 1997, a containerised surgical unit that included an ICU (made by GIAT industries) had been commissioned and deployed to enhance the hospital facility at Sipovo. Such changes to the physical footprint of deployed units are significant when considering the later developments at the UK Field Hospital, Camp Bastion.

The Balkans: Kosovo

Operation Agricola (former Yugoslav Republic of Macedonia and Kosovo, 1999) deployed against the background of a deteriorating political, diplomatic and humanitarian situation. The United Kingdom initially provided a medical unit based on *2 Armoured Field Ambulance*, which included a surgical resuscitation capability from *23 PFA* with an intensive care capability. The lead-in time for *Operation Agricola* allowed *23 PFA* to acquire the necessary equipment (on the shelves at the main medical supply depot and intended for the biological ICU) in order to achieve this standard of care. This supported a four-bay emergency and resuscitation department (the first time the DMS had deployed a specialist emergency physician), a two-table operating theatre and a four-bay post-operative department, including one intensive care bay (with ventilator) and one high-dependency bay (without ventilator). X-ray, diagnostic ultrasound scan and simple laboratory support were included along with a telemedicine link to the United Kingdom. Two six-bed wards were added in due course.

Accommodated in DRASH™, this unit could be set up and open to receive casualties in 90 minutes and taken down and ready to move in three hours. The equipment deployed was of a standard of sophistication that would not have been out of place in a civilian UK hospital; however, it had all been selected with simplicity of operation and versatility in terms of power supply in mind. Although not subjected to the caseload of a high-intensity battle, this unit proved itself in terms of manoeuvrability and the level of critical care it provided to seriously sick or severely injured servicemen.

In June 1999, *22 Field Hospital* was also deployed with the capacity for a 50-bed field hospital to a disused prison in Lipljan. This facility was redeployed to the British military sector in Pristina in November 1999 and remained in operation until the middle of 2001.

All of these operations informed future practice and laid the ground for developments in deployed intensive care during the subsequent conflicts in Iraq and Afghanistan.[4,7] These included the development of personnel capability (the need for intensive care trained nurses), the realisation that non-battle injury accounts for a significant proportion of the clinical burden and the acknowledgment that effective flow and rearward evacuation are crucial in maintaining operational capability. Also of note, the pattern of injuries seen in these

peace support operations (blunt trauma from road traffic accidents, mine injuries and medical admissions) was to inform planning for the conflicts in Iraq and Afghanistan.

SPECIALTY ON DEPLOYMENT

The Second Gulf War – Iraq 2003[8,9]

Operation Telic was the first major conflict in which the *Army Medical Services* deployed a significant critical care facility in order to deal with battle casualties; as discussed previously, a similar level of sophistication in terms of equipment had been deployed on *Operation Agricola*, albeit on a much smaller scale.[4] At the onset of hostilities, *202 Field Hospital (V)* had been established in Kuwait, 28 miles south of the Iraqi border. The ICU had eight beds; four Level 2 beds, and four Level 3 beds (see page xl). A further four ventilators and beds could be provided in two *Modular Transportable Surgical Facility* (MTSF) units, reserved for neurosurgical cases. Each MTSF consisted of a theatre unit with one operating table, an ICU with two beds and a support module supplying power, air conditioning, oxygen, water and medical vacuum. The unit was staffed by a team of four intensive care consultants and 21 nurses, 16 of whom had intensive care unit (ICU) qualifications and at least two years of experience in critical care. Six days after the ground conflict began, *34 Field Hospital* set up near the front line, close to the Iraqi city of Al Basrah. For the first seven days, there were two Level 2 and two Level 3 beds, expanded thereafter to four Level 2 and six Level 3 beds, respectively. Staffing was similar to that of *202 Field Hospital*.

The Royal Navy provided off-shore maritime support through *RFA Argus* and her embedded *Primary Casualty Receiving Facility* (PCRF). The PCRF was equipped with 10 Level 3 and 20 Level 2 beds. The role of RFA Argus on this campaign is discussed in more detail in Chapter 21. Of note, *RFA Argus* and other coalition naval vessels were the nearest units able to provide computed tomography (CT) scanning for *34 and 202 Field Hospitals*. As an example of capacity, the *34 Field Hospital* ICU treated 47 patients in the first month of activity. Thirty-seven were adults and 10 were children. Forty-two (89%) were trauma patients, mostly related to the conflict. Sixty-eight per cent of patients were ventilated and mortality to discharge was 6%. The average bed occupancy was five beds, and the mean duration of patient stay was 3.3 days.[9] At *202 Field Hospital*, during the war-fighting period, there were 63 admissions to intensive care. The majority were male, with an average age of 26.8 years (range, 6 months–67 years). Eleven patients were coalition military, and just over half of all patients were civilian. There were nine patients under the age of 12 (14%). Also, 44.5% were intubated and therefore categorised as Level 3 patients at some stage of their stay.[8] After the conflict (1 May to 20 July), the incidence of ballistic or burns trauma reduced to 37%, while the medical admissions including heat injury rose to 47% and road traffic collisions, resulting in blunt trauma, accounted for 16% of ICU admissions.[8]

Afghanistan – Camp Bastion

Deployed intensive care at the *British Military Field Hospital, Camp Bastion*, can be seen within the context of the overall development of the hospital, which had two phases. This has been covered extensively elsewhere[10]; an outline is given here, as it is relevant both to the development of deployed intensive care facilities and in identifying some of the clinical challenges faced by clinicians (Figure 6.1).

The first phase was the development of a tented environment. This lasted from 2006 to

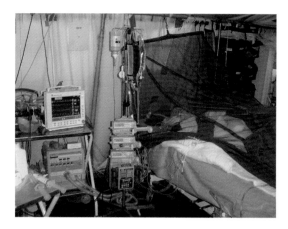

Figure 6.1 ICU in the tented field hospital, Camp Bastion.

2008 and coincided with the deployment of 3300 troops drawn mainly from *16 Air Assault Brigade* on *Operation Herrick 4*. The main base and a 25-bedded tented field hospital were constructed at Camp Bastion, some 9 km south of the main Kandahar to Jelalabad road. By 2007, it was clear that there were significant environmental issues to be contended with, and the ICU was transferred to 'tier 2 accommodation'.[11] Similar MTSFs had been deployed with *202 Field Hospital* to Iraq in 2003 for use in neurosurgical cases, where they provided a 'pleasant, albeit cramped' environment. However, those modules, which had not been fully tested in a desert environment, were extremely unreliable and usually not available for use.[8]

The second phase of the Camp Bastion development was the new build facility in use between 2008 and 2014. *243 Field Hospital (V)* was the first unit to occupy the facility. The subsequent growth of intensive care in terms of both bed numbers and physical space occurred in tandem with the growth of the hospital. Initially, the intensive care was scaled for 4 beds, although this rapidly increased to 12 and then to 16 by 2011. The intensive care also increased in absolute size and lay down, taking over the original Ward 1; this was due to the increased casualty flow through the facility, which peaked over the period 2008 to 2010 (Figure 6.2).

As an example of the ICU workload, in Camp Bastion in 2009, 636 casualties were treated on the unit. Of these, 49% were admitted following an IED explosion, 25% as a result of gunshot wounds, 15% due to disease non-battle injury, 8% following a motor vehicle collision and 4% as a result of indirect fire. The average length of stay was 2.5 days, although this ranged considerably between British military patients (1.9 days) through Afghanistan government forces (2.8 days) to enemy detainees (3.3 days). The average length of stay for children was three days. In terms of total number of ICU days, as a proportion, British military personnel (298 days) were underrepresented in comparison to Afghan civilians (688 days). In all, 40% of patients were discharged from the ICU to the ward, 34% of patients were transferred to other hospitals within the operational theatre, 18% of patients were evacuated by a critical care aeromedical evacuation team (CCAST – Chapter 7)

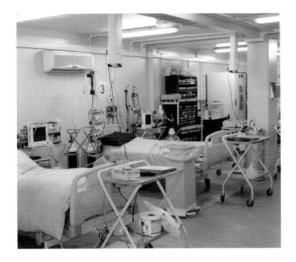

Figure 6.2 ICU in the Tier 2 field hospital, Camp Bastion.

and 3% by a non-critical-care aeromedical evacuation team. Six per cent of patients died.[12]

University Hospital Birmingham (Queen Elizabeth Hospital)

No discussion on the growth and capability of deployed ICU would be complete without mention of the Role 4 capability.[13] Following the rationalisation of the DMS, all critical care repatriations were admitted to the University Hospital Birmingham – the Queen Elizabeth Hospital. In one trauma series looking specifically at blast lung injury from a Role 4 perspective,[14] 517 blast injuries were sustained in theatre during an 18-month period. Of those, 95 (18.4%) were killed in action. Of the injured, 412 (79.7%) survived to Role 3. Thirteen Role 3 admissions (3.1%) died of their wounds, whilst 33 Role 3 admissions (8.0%) returned to duties. A total of 366 (70.8%) were evacuated to Role 4, and 259 (70.7%) of those evacuated to the Queen Elizabeth Hospital were admitted to a trauma ward, whilst 107 (29.2%) were admitted to intensive care. Four (0.8%) ICU admissions died of their wounds, whilst 103 (96.3%) ICU admissions survived to hospital discharge. This demonstrates the enormity of the workload faced by military clinicians and their NHS colleagues at Role 4 and their outstanding results.

CHALLENGES OF PROVIDING DEPLOYED INTENSIVE CARE

Unknown expectations

As has been seen, Operation Telic was the first major conflict in which a significant critical care facility was deployed. Changes in Defence doctrine and political imperative predate the deployments to Iraq and Afghanistan by only a decade, and thus, there were many unknowns, both known and unknown, before war-fighting began. Concepts of workload and utilisation were largely guided by peacetime operations. The expectation was that deployed intensive care would function as a hub for high-dependency skill and experience, enabling throughput of patients from ED and theatres whilst also supporting the wards.[15] In the event, planning for deployment to Iraq underestimated the workload; an early assessment of the case mix found that the proportion of intubated and ventilated patients (44.5%) was significantly higher than expected. As concepts of damage control resuscitation grew in tandem with injury severity, so the amount of time and resources that went into individual patient care increased beyond the expectations at that time. This was the case even after the outset of conflict in the early days of war-fighting in Iraq.[8]

Environmental

Tented field hospitals clearly have their advantages, although in both Iraq and Afghanistan, the environmental challenges associated with them became issues of operational effectiveness. This is one of the main reasons why deployed ICU was eventually containerised and later took over Ward 1 at Bastion.[11] There proved to be several issues.

TEMPERATURE CONTROL

Environmental temperature control is crucial for optimal care of the critically injured casualty, especially as sedated patients are less able to regulate their own temperature. This has a number of clinical consequences, not the least an increased tendency to haemodynamic instability with increased fluid use and the use of vasopressor support with all the risks that this entails. In 2003, 34 Field Hospital

ICU reported temperatures of over 40°C, with low humidity.[9] This led to a rapid rise in temperature in the ICU and a documented rise in patient temperatures despite cooling.

SANDSTORMS

Sand blew into the tents easily and the unit had to be damp dusted twice a day to control this. During sand storms (see colour plate 26), ventilator testing was stopped to avoid unnecessary exposure of the ventilators to sand, and a choice had to be made between the air-conditioning adding to the dust or the ICU temperature increasing.[8]

INSECTS

Insects were a concern particularly around burns and blood stained dressings. Mosquitoes were prevalent in the deployed setting in Iraq, and mosquito nets and anti-malarial chemoprophylaxis were necessary for both staff and patients. Mosquito nets were not available until later in the operation.[8]

NOISE

Noise was a major problem, from air-conditioning and generators and particularly from the tents flapping during high winds. In these conditions, clinical examination involving auscultation was impossible, leading to a greater reliance on X-ray examination. Munitions noise during the initial war-fighting in Iraq was an additional burden.[9]

WAR-FIGHTING

The close proximity of the field hospital to the conflict caused problems for *34 Field Hospital*. The use of white light outside was controlled, which made any movement of personnel or vehicles outside tents hazardous. Prisoners of war admitted to the hospital for treatment required an armed guard. Nerve agent chemoprophylaxis had to be taken by staff. Personal protective equipment needed to be carried and regular warnings of incoming indirect fire also interfered with patient care.[8,9]

A chemical attack alarm occurred during the first week of deployment for *34 Field Hospital* in Iraq. This made it necessary for staff to don protective equipment, including respirators, and then to attempt to protect their patients. Wearing full personnel protection in the heat was found to be significantly disabling for the physicians involved. Due to equipment limitations, improvised field work-arounds were employed, although it was noted that oxygen delivery to spontaneously breathing patients was compromised.[9] There was no immediate solution for the protection of casualties who were civilians or Iraqi prisoners from a vapour-borne chemical attack. The ideal would have been the provision of chemical casualty bags or the use of collective protection.[8]

LOGISTICS

Critical care is in competition with other deployed military assets for access to the logistics chain and, by its very nature, is often more reliant on logistics than other components of the deployed medical capability. Military intensive care has to be delivered with these restrictions in mind and equipment choice will reflect this.[11] In spite of this, critical incidents that affected the operating capability of the deployed intensive care did occur as a result of resource failure on both operations. For example, in the initial deployment of *34 Field Hospital*, there were 14 documented complete power failures, the longest lasting nearly two hours. All essential equipment ran on battery power except for the oxygen concentrators, requiring an urgent transfer of patients from oxygen concentrators to cylinders.[9] Of note, the field hospital intensive care ventilator at that time was the T Bird VS Ventilator™ (Bird Products Corp, Palm Springs, CA); this had internal and external batteries that lasted up to 45 minutes and around three hours, respectively.

SPECIFIC INJURY PATTERNS

A full discussion of the injury patterns in combat trauma in relation to intensive care is beyond the scope of this chapter, and excellent reviews exist elsewhere.[16–19] However, given the workload experienced by the deployed ICUs in Afghanistan and Iraq, certain specific patterns of injury and their relevance to ICU workload merit consideration. Most importantly, blast injuries became increasingly common in these conflicts as the nature of combat changed from conventional to asymmetrical warfare and counter-insurgency.

Blast lung injury

Lung injury is not infrequently a component of the polytrauma sustained by military personnel surviving battlefield blast injury,[20,21] although how common it is will depend on the nature of the explosive device and context of the detonation. In one series of *Joint Theatre Trauma Registry* (JTTR) records between 2003 and 2009, 1678 patients were injured by explosion, of whom 113 had evidence of blast lung injury. Of the 50 patients who survived to reach a medical facility, 80% required ventilatory support.[22] In another series of post-mortem CTs, 121 improvised explosive device (IED) blast fatalities in UK troops showed a 48% rate of primary blast lung injury.[23] Finally, from a Role 4 perspective at University Hospital Birmingham's critical care unit, of the 135 casualties admitted during an 18-month period, radiological chest findings were identified in 66/107 (62%), and five patients met the criteria for adult respiratory distress syndrome (ARDS).[14] The incidence of ARDS creates issues for the aeromedical evacuation of these casualties, where the hypobaric atmosphere can exacerbate (occult) injury.[24]

Burns

Burns patients also present a very significant workload for the deployed ICU, both as a result of the metabolic derangement resulting from their injury and as a consequence of the treatments that are often necessary, including debridement, escharotomy and, in some cases, amputation. A further challenge was the prevention of acute renal failure prior to transfer to a tertiary burns centre. For UK personnel – the majority of whom were resuscitated, debrided, dressed and evacuated within 36 hours of wounding – this was not a problem. For civilian or other Iraqi or Afghan casualties, it was a major issue, and domestic burns, particularly in children, offered both clinical and ethical challenges.

TREATMENT OF LOCAL NATIONALS

The doctrine underpinning deployed intensive care is for the capability to provide up to 48 hours of Level 3 treatment prior to evacuation. For local nationals, no effective onward evacuation plan existed; either the domestic healthcare system was incapable of providing the required Level 3 support or, if an evacuation was planned (as in the case of paediatric patients), each evacuation had to be negotiated on a case-by-case basis either to the United Kingdom or within the Middle East.[8]

For local nationals, this necessitated more prolonged management in the ICU until the patient was fit for transfer, with all of the resultant ethical and resources issues stemming from this. In Iraq[8] and Afghanistan,[12] this resulted in an ICU length of stay twice as long for the local national patients overall and over three times as long for local national burns patients. As the majority of both patients in both conflicts were local nationals, this had a significant effect on the bed occupancy.

PAEDIATRICS

It was not unusual for children to be brought to deployed field hospitals for medical attention, with a variable proportion of child casualties requiring treatment by deployed military personnel.[25] Papers have previously described the overall paediatric workload at the field hospital in Camp Bastion,[26] noting that around 40% of children presenting to the hospital were admitted to the ICU at some point during their stay. Paediatric issues are discussed in greater detail in Chapter 18.

During the first month of *34 Field Hospital* deploying to Iraq in 2003, 10 children were admitted to the intensive care, where no official paediatric intensive care equipment was available.[9] In one retrospective review of a case cohort at the British Military Field Hospital, Camp Bastion,[27] 112/811 (14%) admissions to the ICU were paediatric (median age, 8 years; interquartile range (IQR), 6–12 years; range, 1–16 years). Of these 112 paediatric admissions, 80 were for trauma, 13 were for burns, 4 were non-trauma admissions and 15 were readmissions. The mechanism of injury in trauma was blunt in 12 patients, blast (IED) in 45, blast (indirect fire) in 7 and gunshot wounds in 16. The median length of stay was 0.92 days (IQR, 0.45–2.65 days). Of the 112 admissions, 82 (73%) were mechanically ventilated, 16 (14%) required inotropic support and 12 (11%) died before unit discharge. Seven cases required specialist advice and were discussed with the Birmingham Children's Hospital paediatric intensive care retrieval service. Children could at times account for up to 30% of ICU bed occupancy.[28] This disproportionate ICU bed occupancy occurred because there was no rearward evacuation chain available for children.

CLINICAL CAPABILITY GAPS WHEN COMPARED TO CIVILIAN PRACTICE

At the onset of hostilities in Iraq in 2003, there was no capability or equipment within the established equipment modules for renal replacement therapy (RRT), intra-cranial pressure (ICP) monitoring or for neurosurgical, burns or paediatric care. To mitigate the latter, deploying physicians had packed some paediatric equipment. In dealing with paediatric casualties, *202 Field Hospital* also had an advantage in comparison to *34 Field Hospital* in its Territorial Army (now Reserve) composition, deploying a paediatrician (as physician), several nurses with a background in paediatrics and a midwife. None of these were capabilities were available in the regular DMS.

These three areas, RRT, total parenteral nutrition (TPN) and ICP monitoring, remained areas of much debate for the duration of the conflict in Afghanistan.

Renal replacement therapy

Historically, there are isolated case reports of RRT having been used in the deployed setting for UK Armed Forces[29]; US forces maintain the capability to provide peritoneal dialysis – mostly to local nationals in theatre.[30] However, the mainstay of treatment is still the rapid evacuation of patients requiring RRT to Role 4; indeed, this is also becoming US practice.[31] A deployed RRT service would be a significant resource burden as well as present significant ethical issues for the provision of RRT for local nationals. CCAST does maintain RRT capability,[32] and case reports of the decision to activate this facility in theatre have been published.[33] This has generally been reserved for situations in which lack of RRT prior to CCAST evacuation would be deleterious to the

patient's outcome in circumstances where CCAST has been delayed or in cases of severe metabolic derangement.

ICP monitoring

This is recognised as a capability gap. There are issues with neurosurgical availability as well as with compatibility of ICP bolts with aeromedical transfer and with existing equipment at Role 4. Allied to this are questions regarding the merits of ICP monitoring per se, which have been debated in the general ICU literature. For the present, clinical experience, monitoring and a lower threshold for repeat CT scanning are used to mitigate this risk.[34]

Total parenteral nutrition

Feeding patients enterally has been shown to improve outcomes in the general intensive care population, and early enteral feeding has been adopted for UK critical care casualties.[35,36] Debate continues concerning the commencement of feeding in theatre – particularly with regard to aeromedical evacuation. There is currently no provision for deployed TPN given the intention to rapidly repatriate UK personnel, and this capability is not supported for local nationals.[34]

Infection control

Infection control measures are as important in the deployed ICU as they are in the NHS.[37] Emphasis on infection prevention and control, including hand hygiene, isolation, cohorting and antibiotic control measures in deployed medical treatment facilities is essential to reducing healthcare-associated infections.[38,39] In one review,[40] infections occurred in 24% of those with mangled extremities, including 6% with osteomyelitis. Early recovery of *Acinetobacter* was found, with late recovery of *Staphylococcus aureus*, and there was an association between *Pseudomonas aeruginosa* and injury severity. Multi-drug-resistant infections have been found to be present in critically injured coalition soldiers being repatriated.[41] In all of these circumstances, close liaison with Role 4 microbiology advice was found to be beneficial.[42]

CLINICAL ADVANCES

Deployed intensive care mirrors changes in civilian intensive care practice. Just as the latter is no longer seen simply as a location in which to gather critically ill patients, but also as a repository for evidence and knowledge intended to aid the provision of critical care support,[2] so too is the deployed ICU. The scope of these changes is vast. Clinicians are better trained to deploy, guidelines have been standardised, volume status is targeted, there is a far better understanding of the theoretical and microvascular changes that occur in major trauma and there now exists an extensive reach back service for sub-specialty capability.

Many of the changes to the DMS as a whole can be seen in microcosm in the deployed ICU. Similarly, many of these global changes, including in the management of major trauma, in doctrine,[4] resuscitation,[18,42-44] governance[45] and in training terms,[46] have been extensively reviewed elsewhere. They are mentioned here in brief because of their pertinence to deployed intensive care.[47]

Doctrine

Since the end of the Cold War, the triad of BATLS, surgical resuscitation and the introduction of deployed intensive care has been critical to the political aspiration for improved standards in deployed healthcare.[3] Over time, Defence healthcare doctrine has evolved. Concepts such as *care under fire, tactical field care, enhanced field care, prolonged field care, progressive resuscitation, damage control*, and *enhanced diagnostics* have grown in parallel with conflict.[48,49] Indeed, post Afghanistan, the operational patient care pathway is now seen as all encompassing, seamlessly integrating pre-hospital care and deployed hospital care.[50]

Resuscitation

The concept of damage control resuscitation is characterised by the use of abbreviated interventions in tandem with ongoing resuscitative efforts.[51,52] These abbreviated interventions may be used to, for example, rapidly control haemorrhage or reduce the risk of contamination.[53-55] Following successful (operative) intervention, emphasis then shifts to the ICU, where severe physiological derangements are normalised. The patient can then be returned to theatre for further surgery: intensive care is critical to the outcome of damage control resuscitation.[18] Care is consultant led and focuses on ventilatory technique, resuscitation, rewarming, correction of acidaemia and coagulopathy,[56] whilst maintaining a high index of suspicion for the need for unplanned re-operation or for complications such as abdominal compartment syndrome.[57]

The integrated '*damage control resuscitation – damage control surgery*' sequence for the management of patients sustaining complex injuries was introduced into the UK DMS in 2007, both as a powerful tool for integrating rapid advances in pre-hospital and emergency care and as a means to assist planning.[48,58] There is now seamless integration between damage control surgical techniques and damage control resuscitation,[59] so that patients leave the operating room with their normal physiology restored.[60]

The understanding of multi-organ failure in trauma haemorrhagic shock, as well as its relationship with coagulopathy, has been extensively covered elsewhere.[61-63] A significant proportion of critically ill trauma patients develop multi-organ failure, and this leads to a significant increase in morbidity and mortality.[62,64]

In Iraq, in 2003, during the initial phase of operations, packed red blood cells were a very limited resource, platelets were not available, there was no deployed capability for coagulation testing and no adjuncts were in use.[8] Contrast this with 2009, when over 3200 units of blood products were administered as massive transfusions to severely injured UK personnel.[60,65] Improvements in the capability of the logistics cold chain and the introduction of point-of-care testing have helped to improve outcomes.[66-69]

One practical difficulty in the field ICU environment is the decision regarding when to stop the early, empirical use of predefined ratios of blood and clotting products[70-72] and revert to a conventional transfusion approach.[32] As soon as control of bleeding is achieved, current practice is to switch towards tailored transfusion, based on clinical and laboratory assessments, including point-of-care haemoglobin (i-Stat®) and coagulation testing (ROTEM™). A further difficulty is when to start chemical thromboprophylaxis, given that trauma patients have a 10-fold increase in the incidence of thrombotic events.[32]

Governance – Trauma audit and trauma scoring

There is the expectation that standards in the UK DMS are equal to those in the NHS.[73–75] Assessing the quality of deployed care requires an effective clinical governance structure. Details of all UK military deaths on operations are collected from clinical notes, post-mortem reports and incident reports. These are held on the UK JTTR.[76] There is a deliberate approach to continuous performance improvement, by a process collectively known as the *Major Trauma Audit for Clinical Effectiveness*.[77] There is also considerable interest in using this contemporary data to further improve trauma scoring.[78]

Training – HOSPEX and military operational surgical training

In order to improve trauma team preparation, military medical training has been continuously developed[79] to reflect the most recent practice.[77] At a macro-simulation level,[80] HOSPEX is one such example of this.[79] The use of high-fidelity simulation to prepare teams to deploy[81] has enabled high-calibre multidisciplinary training of medical services personnel, concentrating on non-technical skills (human factors), communication and teamworking.[82] The expectation has been that all hospital staff (including attached US, Danish, Estonian and civilian personnel) undertake two separate three-day periods at the *Army Medical Services Training Centre*. Most recently, the HOSPEX trainer been adapted to other clinical scenarios, for instance, it was rapidly transformed to prepare military civilian hospital staff deploying to Sierra Leone from October 2014 onwards to combat Ebola in West Africa.

CRITICAL CARE CLINICAL GUIDELINES

Working in an environment with clinicians from a wide variety of different critical care units in the United Kingdom, together with multinational colleagues, has driven standardisation of roles and responsibilities, equipment and most importantly the treatment of critically ill patients.

A broad range of critical care guidelines now exists. These cover the standards of critical care in the deployed environment, exploring current recommendations for goal-directed trauma resuscitation, management of severe traumatic brain injury, sedation and analgesia, venous thromboembolism prophylaxis, management and weaning of ventilation, ARDS, central venous catheter placement, brain stem death, spinal clearance, nutrition and glycaemic control in the deployed setting. Clinical governance also applies to the deployed field hospital, where there is a system of incident reporting and investigation similar to that seen in the United Kingdom,[27] including inadvertent extubations, unplanned readmissions and rates of unit acquired or associated sepsis.

Casualties with severe traumatic injury frequently suffer haemodynamic instability.[83] There is increasing evidence to suggest that targeted resuscitation solely based on the use of pressure indices correlate less well with evidence of microvascular dysfunction than algorithms based on targeted volume resuscitation.[84,85] There has therefore been considerable interest in the development of consultant-delivered, targeted resuscitation in the immediate post-injury period using targeted trans-thoracic echocardiography.[34,86]

Special interest groups

There are a variety of specialist interest groups, for example in *equipment, critical care* and *paediatric anaesthesia and critical care*. They sit within the *Department of Military Anaesthesia, Pain and Critical Care* and provide clinical guidelines, advice and recommendations on equipment and training.[87–90] Membership is drawn from UK military doctors, nurses and physiotherapists.[32]

INTEGRATION WITH UK-BASED HEALTHCARE AGENCIES

The situation in the hospital at Camp Bastion, in which children were admitted to an adult ICU, contrasts to that in the United Kingdom, where *paediatric* ICU services are centralised in a small number of regional centres. A number of strategies were developed over the course of the conflict in Afghanistan to improve paediatric care in the field hospital at Camp Bastion.[87] One of these was the provision of specialist advice by telephone from *KIDS*, the Birmingham Children's Hospital paediatric intensive care retrieval service (Birmingham, UK).

Communication and integration were also available with Role 4 in other specialties: generally in the weekly critical care case conferences and most notably for the provision of specialist microbiology liaison for intensive care. The use of telemedicine is one area of future interest.[91]

PAIN MEDICINE IN THE ICU

Together with more mainstream intravenous analgesics, neuropathic pain medications and local anaesthetic regional blocks have become increasingly popular and provide effective pain relief.[92–94] The full range of devices is to be seen within the deployed ICU and at Role 4.[95] Indeed, indwelling catheters for neuraxial and peripheral nerve blocks are now regularly placed under ultrasound guidance. The arguments surrounding the placement of block catheters in relation to possible coagulopathy and sepsis have been debated elsewhere.[32,96]

FOLLOW-UP OF INTENSIVE CARE PATIENTS

The campaign in Afghanistan also marked the introduction of a pilot follow-up clinic for military casualties who required intensive care, which was found to be helpful for the majority of clinic attendees.[97] The study highlighted rates of hallucinations (50%), occipital alopecia and pressure sores (35%) and longer-term personality change and anger issues. Among this cohort, there were also concerns around stigmatisation regarding referral to psychiatric support services. Patient diaries, which were begun on intensive care in Afghanistan and continued throughout treatment until discharge in the United Kingdom, were found to be very helpful.

CHALLENGES FOR THE FUTURE

Operations in Iraq and Afghanistan have rightly been seen as major successes for the DMS. They have become 'the envy of civilian trauma systems'.[98] The intensive care is clearly a key part of this. The British military field hospital at Camp Bastion allowed a static, stable Role 3 environment to respond to a predominant injury type over a prolonged period. It would be a major concern if this hadn't led to the types of iterative improvements laid out already.

With the closure of the UK Role 3 in Afghanistan and a return to (true) contingency operations, the focus of the UK DMS may well have to change significantly. Yet it must continue to meet the high political expectations placed upon it in terms of rates of survival among UK personnel deployed in areas of conflict and of providing similar outcomes to host nations in support of non-governmental organisations (NGOs) and environmental disasters.

Crucially, for the continuation of the success of the DMS, both in this country and in those of coalition partners,[99] the pace of operations has meant that corporate expertise has accumulated within a relatively small cadre of providers. Again, there is no guarantee, in spite of best efforts,[82] that this expertise will be transmitted to the next generation of clinicians.

Doctrinal Issues

Doctrine is guided by strategic and political imperative; there is no reason to believe that these will remain static in the next quarter century. It is fortuitous that the major conflicts in Iraq and Afghanistan were preceded by the much smaller deployed critical care presence in the Balkans and that injury patterns and severity both evolved over time. It is also fortunate that intensive care has not had cause to deploy within a chemical biological radiation and nuclear environment.[100] Deployed intensive care has been conceived as a facility intended for 48-hour holding prior to repatriation. In the future, there may well be instances of prolonged extraction times. It will be necessary to look at civilian and non-governmental organisation experience[101–104] and to the experience of other countries when developing future UK Defence doctrine.[105,106] With the potential for numerous low-level contingency operations, there are issues surrounding preparedness, local clinical governance and continuity of practice.[32]

Operational capabilities and provision of healthcare to local nationals

RRT is not feasible at present in the deployed setting, ICP monitoring is not available and TPN is not provided, nor for that matter is extracorporeal membrane oxygenation (ECMO) routinely available to UK service personnel. In future settings where prolonged holding before evacuation and long evacuation times are to be expected, how should we provide for prolonged treatment at Role 3 and what adjuncts may safely be employed to mitigate the risk of a prolonged evacuation chain? As one example, in one case series from Afghanistan, 10 combat casualties complicated by severe respiratory failure were supported on ECMO, with a one-year survival rate of 90%.[107] How can the lessons of Afghanistan be applied to contingency operations in austere environments? In providing some or all of the earlier interventions, there are also ethical considerations surrounding the justice of resource allocation to coalition and local nationals with similar injury patterns, especially in times of active war-fighting[34,108] and where different lines of evacuation and rehabilitation services exist.[32] In any future deployment of field intensive care, it will be critical to have in place clear guidelines for the treatment of local nationals and acceptable rules for onward transfer.

Unexpected survivors

With enhanced resuscitation, far greater numbers of unexpected survivors are stabilised to Role 4 and beyond. In more austere settings, where need may far outstrip resource allocation to the deployed intensive care, a better understanding of trauma scoring will be necessary.[17,73,78,109]

Provision of critical care to children and provision of palliative services

Ethical dilemmas arise when children present with very severe injuries that may radically limit quality of life or injuries known to have a poor outcome in the deployed environment. Examples include penetrating head trauma, severe burns, renal failure or multiple injuries. In the deployed operations in Afghanistan, there was evidence from survival figures in major burns for the need for early palliation.[12]

Integration with host nation healthcare

Onward movement of civilians can prove complex, particularly where host nation facilities may not be to the deployed critical care standard. Resource allocation has already been discussed, but there are also concerns of creating a 'culture of dependency' in the local population, that is to say the expectation of critical care provided by external agencies, which may undermine the development of local critical care capability.[110]

Logistics

The resource of a fully equipped hospital environment in Afghanistan has enabled significant improvements in standards of care. However, these developments have presented an increasing logistic burden. Forward operations and future entry operations will require the ICU to be able to support itself as much as possible. There will clearly be compromise with what can pragmatically be provided at short notice.[32,43,111]

Non-battle injury

It should be noted that whilst trauma care has been the overwhelming task and focus for the set of conflicts to which this book chapter relates, with differing deployed operations, different clinical conditions will manifest. These will affect deployed forces, as well as deployed nationals, and range across the full gamut of pathophysiology seen in a general critical care.[112,113]

EQUIPMENT ISSUES

The equipment used in field ICUs has to satisfy several competing needs to function in an austere environment. There have been outstanding advances in the quality of intensive care equipment in the deployed environment. This has clearly mirrored the growth of intensive care as a specialty. Changes in equipment are summarised in Table 6.1.

Improvements in the provision of ventilators, bronchoscopy, percutaneous tracheostomy, vacuum

Table 6.1 Equipment development

	Iraq, 2003	Afghanistan, 2012
Monitoring	Datex-Ohmeda S5 system (Instrumentarium Corp., Helsinki, Finland)	S/5 Compact (General Electric Healthcare, Chalfont St Giles, UK)
Ventilator	T Bird VS (Bird Products Corp, Palm Springs, CA)	Vela (Carefusion, Yorba Linda, CA)
Oxygen provision	DeVilbiss oxygen concentrators (Sunrise Medical Respiratory Products), each providing a flow rate of 5l of 93% oxygen	DeVilbiss Oxygen Concentrator (DeVilbiss, Somerset, PA)
Infusion pump	1. Braun Perfusor Compact (B. Braun, Melsungen, Germany) 2. IMED Gemini PC2 volumetric pumps (Alaris Medical, Basingstoke, UK)	Perfusor (B Braun, Melsungen, Germany)
Warming/cooling	BAIR Hugger patient warming/cooling unit (Augustine Medical Inc, Eden Prairie, MN)	
Defibrillator	Zoll M with external pacing capability	
Suction	Laederal suction units	
Fluid/warming	Hotline HL-90 (Sims Level 1 Inc., Rockland, MA)	Level 1 H-1200 Fluid Warmer (Smiths Medical, Ashford, Kent, UK) Belmont Rapid Infuser FMS 2000 (Belmont Instrument Corp, Billerica, MA)
Blood analysis	i-Stat (Abbott Laboratories Ltd, Berks, UK)	

dressings and ultrasound guidance have been extensively reviewed elsewhere.[34] Much of the increase in capability is dependent on the ability to readily sterilise equipment in the deployed environment. The new Vela ventilator offers a considerable increase in capability, including an airway pressure release ventilation mode.

RESEARCH

The umbrella for much of the integrated research in haemorrhage control, resuscitation and stabilisation, optimising casualty throughput prognostication and diagnosis over the past 12 years has been the *Combat Casualty Care Research Programme.* This has involved a close collaboration between the *Royal Centre for Defence Medicine* and the *Defence Science and Technology Laboratory* (Dstl).[114] Much of the research has concerned the pathophysiology of trauma and is therefore covered extensively elsewhere[43,114]; however, some examples are given in Table 6.2.

Table 6.2 Major clinical research strands during *Operations Telic* and *Herrick*

- Development of a hybrid resuscitation strategy
- Pre-hospital use of blood products
- Pathophysiology of trauma coagulopathy
- Pathophysiology of blast lung
- Pathophysiology of blast-induced brain injury
- Endothelial damage in blast injury
- Battlefield pain management
- Effects of opioids in simulated hypovolaemia
- Evaluation of antimicrobial wound dressings
- Developing transfusion capability without the need for frozen or short shelf-life products
- Developing trauma team training for complex decision-making
- Telemedicine and remote monitoring
- Near patient assessment

It should be noted that the conflict in Afghanistan was the first time that deployment of research teams in the intensive care environment was attempted. Towards the end of the conflict, a deployed research facility was set up and there was a significant contribution from intensive care to this.[115] As argued previously, there is also the need to develop an ethics framework to address the provision of deployed intensive care in an environment where onward care of local nationals is of poor quality.

CONCLUSION

Of all of the deployed medical specialties, intensive care is the newest in the DMS, having grown out of the changes in lay down and doctrine after the end of the Cold War. Indeed, deployed intensive care now rightly lies on the continuum of damage control resuscitation and will continue to evolve as one aspect of it.

Far removed from the tented hospitals and newly conceived equipment modules of the late 1990s and in Iraq in 2003, one of the reasons that the British military field hospital at Camp Bastion was so successful is that knowledge and understanding of damage control resuscitation (of which critical care is an integral part) have permeated throughout all the medical cadres.

This chapter has documented the expansion of deployed intensive care in the UK Armed Forces; its historical context, adaptation to the nature of conflict over the last 12 years, recent challenges and advances in operational effectiveness, research strands that have been pertinent to intensive care, and the future challenges presented by warfare and contingency operations in the first half of the twenty-first century.

REFERENCES

1. Henning J, Roberts M, Sharma D, Hoffman A, Mahoney P. Military intensive care. Part 1. A historical review. *J R Army Med Corps* 2007;153(4):283–285.
2. Borthwick M, Bourne R, Craig M, Egan A, Oxley J. *Evolution of Intensive Care in the UK*. BMA Royal Pharmaceutical Society, 2003.
3. Hawley A. Trauma management on the battlefield: A modern approach. *J R Army Med Corps* 1996;142(3):120–125.
4. Roberts M, Salmon J, Sadler P. The provision of intensive care and high dependency care in the field. *J R Army Med Corps* 2000; 146(2):99–103.
5. Vincent J-L. Need for intensivists in intensive-care units. *Lancet* 2000;356(9231): 695–696.
6. Adley R, Evans DHC, Mahoney PF, Riley B, Rodgers CR, Shanks T, et al. The Gulf war: Anaesthetic experience at 32 Field Hospital Department of Anaesthesia and Resuscitation. *Anaesthesia* 1992;47(11):996–999.
7. Hodgetts TJ, Turner L, Grieves T, Payne S. *Major Trauma Effectiveness Project: Report of Operation Agricola, Kosovo 1999*. London: Defence Logistics Organisation, 2000.
8. Roberts MJ, Fox MA, Hamilton-Davies C, Dowson S. The experience of the intensive care unit in a British Army Field Hospital during the 2003 Gulf Conflict. *J R Army Med Corps* 2003;149(4):284–290.
9. Lockey DJ, Nordmann GR, Field JM, Clough D, Henning JDR. The deployment of an intensive care facility with a military field hospital to the 2003 conflict in Iraq. *Resuscitation* 2004;62(3):261–265.
10. Vassallo D. A short history of Camp Bastion Hospital: The two hospitals and unit deployments. *J R Army Med Corps* 2015;161(1): 79–83.
11. Hoffman A, Henning J, Mellor A, Mahoney P. Military intensive care. Part 2. Current practice. *J R Army Med Corps* 2007;153(4): 286–287.
12. Johnston AM, Henning JD. Outcomes of patients treated at Bastion Hospital Intensive Care Unit in 2009. *J R Army Med Corps* 2014;160(4):323.
13. Jones C, Chinery JP, England K, Mahoney PF. Critical Care at Role 4. *J R Army Med Corps* 2010;156(Suppl 4):S342–S348.
14. Mackenzie IMJ, Tunnicliffe B. Blast injuries to the lung: Epidemiology and management. *Philos Trans R Soc Lond, B, Biol Sci* 2011;366(1562):295–299.

15. Thornhill R, Tong JL, Birch K, Chauhan R. Field intensive care – weaning and extubation. *J R Army Med Corps* 2010;156(Suppl 4): S311–S317.

16. Penn-Barwell JG, Roberts SAG, Midwinter MJ, Bishop JRB. Improved survival in UK combat casualties from Iraq and Afghanistan: 2003–2012. *J Trauma Acute Care Surg* 2015;78(5):1014–1020.

17. Keene DD, Penn-Barwell JG, Wood PR, et al. Died of wounds: A mortality review. *J R Army Med Corps* 2016;162(5):533–360.

18. Sagraves SG. Damage Control Surgery – the intensivist's role. *J Intensive Care Med* 2006;21(1):5–16.

19. Morrison JJ, Hunt N, Midwinter M, Jansen J. Associated injuries in casualties with traumatic lower extremity amputations caused by improvised explosive devices. *Br J Surg* 2011;99(3):362–366.

20. Morris MJ. Acute respiratory distress syndrome in combat casualties: Military medicine and advances in mechanical ventilation. *Mi Med* 2006;171(11):1039–1044.

21. Brogden TG, Bunin J, Kwon H, Lundy J, McD Johnston A, Bowley DM. Strategies for ventilation in acute, severe lung injury after combat trauma. *J R Army Med Corps* 2015;161(1):14–21.

22. Smith JE. The epidemiology of blast lung injury during recent military conflicts: A retrospective database review of cases presenting to deployed military hospitals, 2003–2009. *Philos Trans R Soc B Biol Sci* 2010;366(1562):291–294.

23. Singleton JAG, Gibb IE, Bull AMJ, Mahoney PF, Clasper JC. Primary blast lung injury prevalence and fatal injuries from explosions. *J Trauma Acute Care Surg* 2013;75:S269–S2674.

24. Dorlac GR, Fang R, Pruitt VM et al. Air transport of patients with severe lung injury: Development and utilization of the acute lung rescue team. *J Trauma Inj Infect Crit Care* 2009;66(Suppl):S164–S171.

25. McGuigan R, Spinella PC, Beekley A et al. Pediatric trauma: Experience of a combat support hospital in Iraq. *J Pediatr Surg* 2007;42(1):207–210.

26. Arul GS, Reynolds J, DiRusso S et al. Paediatric admissions to the British military hospital at Camp Bastion, Afghanistan. *Ann R Coll Surg Engl* 2012;94(1):52–57.

27. Inwald DP, Arul GS, Montgomery M, Henning J, McNicholas J, Bree S. Management of children in the deployed intensive care unit at Camp Bastion, Afghanistan. *J R Army Med Corps* 2014;160(3):236–240.

28. Harris CC, McNicholas J. Paediatric intensive care in the field hospital. *J R Army Med Corps* 2009;155(2):157–159.

29. Stevens PE, Bloodworth LL, Rainford DJ. High altitude haemofiltration. *BMJ* 1986;292 (6532):1354.

30. Pina JS, Moghadam S, Cushner HM, Beilman GJ, McAlister VC. In-theater peritoneal dialysis for combat-related renal failure. *J Trauma Inj Infect Crit Care* 2010;68(5):1253–1256.

31. Chung KK, Perkins RM, Oliver JD III. Renal replacement therapy in support of combat operations. *Crit Care Med* 2008;36(Suppl): S365–S369.

32. McNicholas J, Henning JD. Major military trauma: Decision making in the ICU. *J R Army Med Corps* 2011;157(Suppl 3):S284–S288.

33. Nesbitt I, Almond M, Freshwater D. Renal replacement in the deployed setting. *J R Army Med Corps* 2011;157(2):179–181.

34. Hutchings S, Risdall J, Lowes T. Intensive care in the Defence Medical Services. *J Intensive Care Soc* 2014;15(1):24–27.

35. Henning J, Scott T, Price S. Nutrition of the critically ill patient in field hospitals on operations. *J R Army Med Corps* 2008;154(4):279–281.

36. Jansen JO, Turner S, Johnston A. Nutritional management of critically ill trauma patients in the deployed military setting. *J R Army Med Corps* 2011;157(Suppl 3):S344–S349.

37. Johnston AM. Focus on sepsis and intensive care. *J R Army Med Corps* 2009;155(2): 129–132.

38. Landrum ML, Murray CK. Ventilator associated pneumonia in a military deployed setting: The impact of an aggressive infection control program. *J Trauma Inj Infect Crit Care* 2008;64(Suppl):S123–S128.

39. Hospenthal DR, Green AD, Crouch HK et al. Infection prevention and control in deployed military medical treatment facilities. *J Trauma Inj Infect Crit Care* 2011;71:S290–S298.

40. Brown KV, Murray CK, Clasper JC. Infectious complications of combat-related mangled extremity injuries in the British Military. *J Trauma Inj Infect Crit Care* 2010; 69(Suppl):S109–S115.

41. Tien HC, Battad A, Bryce EA, Fuller J, Mulvey M, Bernard K et al. Multi-drug resistant Acinetobacter infections in critically injured Canadian forces soldiers. *BMC Infect Dis* 2007;7(1):1268.

42. Shirley P. Operational critical care. Intensive care and trauma. *J R Army Med Corps* 2009; 155(2):133–140.

43. Doughty H, Woolley T, Thomas G. Massive transfusion. *J R Army Med Corps* 2011; 157(Suppl 3):S277–S283.

44. Midwinter M. Damage control surgery in the era of damage control resuscitation. *J R Army Med Corps* 2009;155(4):323–326.

45. Hodgetts TJ, Davies S, Russell R, McLeod J. Benchmarking the UK Military deployed trauma system. *J R Army Med Corps* 2007;153(4):237–238.

46. Mercer SJ, Whittle CL, Mahoney PF. Lessons from the battlefield: Human factors in defence anaesthesia. *Br J Anaesth* 2010;105(1):9–20.

47. Dawes R, Thomas GR. Battlefield resuscitation. *Curr Opin Crit Care* 2009;15(6): 527–535.

48. Hodgetts TJ. ABC to <C>ABC: Redefining the military trauma paradigm. *Emerg Med J* 2006;23(10):745–746.

49. Mahoney P, Hodgetts T, Midwinter M, Russell R. The Combat Casualty Care Special Edition. *J R Army Med Corps* 2007; 153(4):235–236.

50. Morrison JJ, Oh J, DuBose JJ et al. En-route care capability from point of injury impacts mortality after severe wartime injury. *Ann Surg* 2013;257(2):330–334.

51. Sumann GN, Kampfl A, Wenzel V, Schobersberger W. Early intensive care unit intervention for trauma care: What alters the outcome? *Curr Opin Crit Care* 2002;8(6):587–592.

52. Morrison JJ, Ross JD, Poon H, Midwinter MJ, Jansen JO. Intra-operative correction of acidosis, coagulopathy and hypothermia in combat casualties with severe haemorrhagic shock. *Anaesthesia* 2013;68(8):846–850.

53. Rotondo MF, Schwab CW, McGonigal MD, et al. Damage control. *J Trauma Inj Infect Crit Care* 1993;35(3):375–383.

54. Lamb CM, MacGoey P, Navarro AP, Brooks AJ. Damage control surgery in the era of damage control resuscitation. *Br J Anaesth* 2014;113(2):242–249.

55. Haider AH, Piper LC, Zogg CK et al. Military-to-civilian translation of battlefield innovations in operative trauma care. *Surgery* 2015;158(6):1686–1695.

56. Gentilello LM, Pierson DJ. Trauma critical care. *Am J Respir Crit Care Med* 2001;163 (3):604–607.

57. Sharrock AE, Barker T, Yuen HM, Rickard R, Tai N. Management and closure of the open abdomen after damage control laparotomy for trauma. A systematic review and meta-analysis. *Injury* 2016;47(2):296–306.

58. Hodgetts T, Mahoney P, Kirkman E. Damage control resuscitation. *J R Army Med Corps* 2007;153(4):299–300.

59. Beekley AC. Damage control resuscitation: A sensible approach to the exsanguinating surgical patient. *Crit Care Med* 2008; 36(Suppl):S267–S274.

60. Mercer SJ, Tarmey NT, Woolley T, Wood P, Mahoney PF. Haemorrhage and coagulopathy in the Defence Medical Services. *Anaesthesia* 2012;68(s1):49–60.

61. Brohi K, Singh J, Heron M, Coats T. Acute traumatic coagulopathy. *J Trauma Inj Infect Crit Care* 2003;54(6):1127–1130.

62. Hess JR, Brohi K, Dutton RP, et al. The coagulopathy of trauma: A review of mechanisms. *J Trauma Inj Infect Crit Care* 2008;65(4):748–754.

63. Tarmey NT, Woolley T, Jansen JO et al. Evolution of coagulopathy monitoring in military damage-control resuscitation. *J Trauma Acute Care Surg* 2012;73:S417–S422.

64. Gruen RL, Brohi K, Schreiber M et al. Haemorrhage control in severely injured patients. *Lancet* 2012;380(9847):1099–1108.

65. Allcock EC, Woolley T, Doughty H, Midwinter M, Mahoney PF, Mackenzie I. The clinical outcome of UK military personnel who received a massive transfusion in Afghanistan during 2009. *J R Army Med Corps* 2011;157(4):365–369.

66. Woolley T, Midwinter M, Spencer P, Watts S, Doran C, Kirkman E. Utility of interim ROTEM(®) values of clot strength, A5 and A10, in predicting final assessment of coagulation status in severely injured battle patients. *Injury* 2013;44(5):593–599.

67. Maegele M, Lefering R, Yucel N et al. Early coagulopathy in multiple injury: An analysis from the German Trauma Registry on 8724 patients. *Injury* 2007;38(3):298–304.

68. Fries D, Martini WZ. Role of fibrinogen in trauma-induced coagulopathy. *Br J Anaesth* 2010;105(2):116–121.

69. Doran CM, Woolley T, Midwinter MJ. Feasibility of using rotational thromboelastometry to assess coagulation status of combat casualties in a deployed setting. *J Trauma Acute Care Surg* 2010;69(1):S40–S48.

70. Kirkman E, Watts S, Hodgetts T, Mahoney P, Rawlinson S, Midwinter M. A proactive approach to the coagulopathy of trauma: The rationale and guidelines for treatment. *J R Army Med Corps* 2007;153(4):302–306.

71. Gunter OL Jr, Au BK, Isbell JM, Mowery NT, Young PP, Cotton BA. Optimizing outcomes in damage control resuscitation: Identifying blood product ratios associated with improved survival. *J Trauma Inj Infect Crit Care* 2008;65(3):527–534.

72. Watts S, Nordmann G, Brohi K et al. Evaluation of prehospital blood products to attenuate acute coagulopathy of trauma in a model of severe injury and shock in anesthetized pigs. *Shock* 2015;44:138–148.

73. Brooks AJ, Sperry D, Riley B, Girling KJ. Improving performance in the management of severely injured patients in critical care. *Injury* 2005;36(2):310–316.

74. Lockey D. Improving UK trauma care: The NCEPOD trauma report. *Anaesthesia* 2008;63(5):455–457.

75. Henning DCW, Smith JE, Patch D, Lambert AW. A comparison of civilian (National Confidential Enquiry into Patient Outcome and Death) trauma standards with current practice in a deployed field hospital in Afghanistan. *Emerg Med J* 2011;28(4):310–312.

76. Hodgetts T, Davies S, Midwinter M et al. Operational mortality of UK service personnel in Iraq and Afghanistan: A one year analysis 2006–7. *J R Army Med Corps* 2007;153(4):252–254.

77. Smith J, Hodgetts T, Mahoney P et al Trauma governance in the UK Defence Medical Services. *J R Army Med Corps* 2007;153(4):239–242.

78. Russell RJ, Hodgetts TJ, McLeod J et al. The role of trauma scoring in developing trauma clinical governance in the Defence Medical Services. *Philos Trans R Soc Lond B Biol Sci* 2011;366(1562):171–191.

79. Cox C, Roberts P. Hospex: A historical view and the need for change. *J R Army Med Corps* 2008;154(3):193–194.

80. Arora S, Sevdalis N. HOSPEX and concepts of simulation. *J R Army Med Corps* 2008;154(3):202–205.

81. Mercer S, Arul GS, Pugh HEJ. Performance improvement through best practice team management: Human factors in complex trauma. *J R Army Med Corps* 2014;160(2):105–108.

82. Vassallo D. A short history of Camp Bastion Hospital: Preparing for war, national recognition and Bastion's legacy. *J R Army Med Corps* 2015;161(4):355–360.

83. Butler F. Fluid resuscitation in tactical combat casualty care: Brief history and current status. *J Trauma Inj Infect Crit Care* 201;70:S11–S12.

84. Parks JK, Elliott AC, Gentilello LM, Shafi S. Systemic hypotension is a late marker of shock after trauma: A validation study of Advanced Trauma Life Support principles in a large national sample. *Am J Surg* 2006;192(6):727–731.

85. Guly HR, Bouamra O, Spiers M et al. Vital signs and estimated blood loss in patients with major trauma: Testing the validity of the ATLS classification of hypovolaemic shock. *Resuscitation* 2011;82(5):556–559.

86. Hutchings SD, Rees PS. Trauma resuscitation using echocardiography in a deployed military intensive care unit. *J Intensive Care Soc* 2013;14(2):120–125.

87. Nordmann GR. Paediatric anaesthesia in Afghanistan: A review of the current experience. *J R Army Med Corps* 2010;156(4 Suppl 1):323–326.

88. Woods KL, Russell RJ, Bree S, Mahoney PF, McNicholas J. The pattern of paediatric trauma on operations. *J R Army Med Corps* 2012;158(1):34–37.

89. Bree S, Wood K, Nordmann G, McNicholas J. The paediatric transfusion challenge on deployed operations. *J R Army Med Corps* 2010;156(Suppl 4):S361–S364.

90. Nordmann GR, McNicholas J, Templeton P, Arul S, Woods K. Paediatric trauma management on deployment. *J R Army Med Corps* 2011;157(Suppl 3):S334–S343.

91. Withnall RDJ, Smith M, Graham DJ, Morris LE. Telemedicine in the UK Defence Medical Services: Time for an upgrade? *J R Army Med Corps* 2016;162(5):318–320.

92. Stojadinovic A, Auton A, Peoples GE et al. Responding to challenges in modern combat casualty care: Innovative use of advanced regional anesthesia. *Pain Med* 2006;7(4):330–338.

93. Allcock E, Spencer E, Frazer R, Applegate G, Buckenmaier C III. Continuous Transversus abdominis plane (TAP) block catheters in a combat surgical environment. *Pain Med* 2010;11(9):1426–1429.

94. Beard DJ, Wood P. Pain in complex trauma: Lessons from Afghanistan. *BJA Educ* 2015;15(4):207–212.

95. Edwards D, Bowden M, Aldington D. Pain management at Role 4. *J R Army Med Corps* 2009;155(1):58–61.

96. Connor DJ, Ralph JK, Aldington DJ. Field hospital analgesia. *J R Army Med Corps* 2009;155(1):49–56.

97. Scott T, Davies M, Dutton C et al. Intensive care follow-up in UK military casualties: A one-year pilot. *J Intensive Care Soc* 2014;15(2):113–116.

98. *Illness Arising on Military Operations.* National Audit Office, 2010.

99. Gawande A. Casualties of war – military care for the wounded from Iraq and Afghanistan. *N Engl J Med* 2004;351(24):2471–2475.

100. Henning JDR, Lockey DJ. The protection of critically ill patients in a military chemical warfare environment. *Resuscitation* 2005;64(2):237–239.

101. Pesola G, Bayshtok V, Kvetan V. American critical care team at a foreign disaster site. *Crit Care Med* 1989;17(6):582–585.

102. Halpern P, Rosen B, Carasso S et al. Intensive care in a field hospital in an urban disaster area: Lessons from the August 1999 earthquake in Turkey. *Crit Care Med* 2003;31(5):1410–1414.

103. Owens PJ, Forgione A Jr., Briggs S. Challenges of international disaster relief: Use of a deployable rapid assembly shelter and surgical hospital. *Disaster Manag Response* 2005;3(1):11–16.

104. Parker MM. Critical care and disaster management. *Crit Care Med* 2006;34(Suppl):S52–S55.

105. Bricknell MCM, Moore GW. Health risk management matrix – a medical planning tool. *J R Army Med Corps* 2007;153(2):87–90.

106. Bricknell MC, Hanhart N. Stability operations and the implications for military health services support. *J R Army Med Corps* 2007;153(1):18–21.

107. Bein T, Zonies D, Philipp A, et al. Transportable extracorporeal lung support for rescue of severe respiratory failure in combat casualties. *J Trauma Acute Care Surg* 2012;73(6):1450–1456.

108. Henning J. The ethical dilemma of providing intensive care treatment to local civilians on operations. *J R Army Med Corps* 2009;155(2):84–86.

109. Birch K. Who benefits from intensive care in the field? *J R Army Med Corps* 2009;155(2):122–124.

110. Hodgetts TJ, Mahoney PF, Mozumder A, Mclennan J. Care of civilians during military operations. *Int J Disaster Med* 2009;3(1–4):3–24.

111. Sariego J. CCATT: A military model for civilian disaster management. *Disaster Manag Response* 2006;4(4):114–117.

112. Bar-Dayan Y, Leiba A, Beard P et al. A Multidisciplinary field hospital as a substitute for medical hospital care in the aftermath of an earthquake: The experience of the Israeli Defense Forces Field Hospital in Duzce, Turkey, 1999. *Prehosp Disaster Med* 2012;20(2):103–106.

113. Porter D, Johnston AM, Henning J. Medical conditions requiring intensive care. *J R Army Med Corps* 2009;155(2):141–146.

114. Kirkman E, Watts S. Combat Casualty Care research programme. *J R Army Med Corps* 2014;160(2):109–116.

115. Hutchings SD, Howarth G, Rees P, Midwinter M. Conducting clinical research in the deployed intensive care unit: Challenges and solutions. *J R Nav Med Serv* 2013;99(3):151–153.

7

Strategic medical evacuation – The critical care air support team

INTRODUCTION

The *Royal Air Force* (RAF) has been providing aeromedical evacuation (AE) since 1918, with ever-increasing sophistication and capability. One of the most significant developments occurred during the Balkan conflicts, with the establishment of *Critical Care Air Support Teams* (CCAST) to retrieve critically ill and injured service personnel from around the world. The mission of these teams was to provide critical care to the level expected in a UK teaching hospital, whilst operating in the austere aviation environment. Despite considerable previous experience in strategic evacuation, *Operations Telic* and *Herrick* were defining periods in CCAST's history. These campaigns produced a requirement to deliver high-quality care in non-permissive environments, during high-tempo operations. This chapter will discuss the evolution of CCAST and both the lessons identified and the advances made during this period. It will also consider the particular challenges of these campaigns.

UK AE AND CCAST

The first transfer of a British casualty by air is credited to the *Royal Flying Corps* in Sinai in 1917, when a soldier with a gunshot wound to the ankle was flown in the observer's seat of a biplane. Formal AE flights by the RAF did not begin until 1920; prior to this time, AE flights were organised on an ad hoc basis, using assets commandeered from non-medical units. It was not until the latter stages of the Second World War that the United Kingdom

began to move substantial numbers of patients by air, with 300,000 patients evacuated in 1944 from Europe and South East Asia.[1] Early evacuations were restricted by the available aircraft technology, often requiring patients to be transferred through multiple staging posts because of limits imposed by flying conditions and the range of the airframe. The introduction of jet aircraft allowed faster direct flights, the patient being accompanied by RAF nurse escorts.[2] Subsequent conflicts saw the continued evolution of this capability, with nearly 700 casualties evacuated from Montevideo to RAF Brize Norton during the Falklands Campaign.[3]

Cold War doctrine had assumed that medical care would be under mass casualty conditions, with only compassionate care available to those casualties needing intensive care.[4] However, the start of the conflicts in the former territories of Yugoslavia in 1991 saw a paradigm shift in medical planning. Responding to the changing nature of contemporary conflict and the increasing expectations of timely, high-quality care,[5] new policies aimed to deliver treatment of a quality as close to that achieved in peacetime UK hospitals as battlefield conditions would allow.[6]

At this time, critical care AE existed in a rudimentary form (consisting of what were colloquially known as 'Priority One' moves). There were no dedicated aircraft, transfer equipment was basic and few nurses were trained to deliver intensive care. Teams offered nurse-led care augmented by an anaesthetist when this was dictated by the patient's condition. Unfortunately, despite being seconded from *RAF Hospital Wroughton*, the allocated anaesthetist might never have worked with the rest of the team. As a result, and in response to evolving medical doctrine, the RAF formalised the capability during the late 1990s with the formation of the *Critical Care Air Support Team*. This team developed around a core group of RAF critical care doctors and nurses at *Tactical Medical Wing* (TMW) based at RAF Lyneham (and now at RAF Brize Norton). Following initial training in AE and transfer equipment, personnel were generally on standby at their usual place of work, unless notified of a patient retrieval by the *Aeromedical Coordination Cell* (AECC), located at RAF Brize Norton. By the time preparations were being made for *Operation Telic*, the RAF had a well-established strategic asset that could rapidly evacuate patients from field hospitals back to the United Kingdom. CCAST facilitated access to specialist care following initial surgery and stabilisation, maintaining the intensive care capacity of the deployed medical facilities by timely evacuation of their patients.

THE MISSION

The mission of the *Aeromedical Squadron* is

'to provide in-flight medical care, utilising multi-disciplinary teams, to effect the expedient and safe transfer of patients by air from any location worldwide; whilst providing training and maintaining logistic and governance processes'.

For CCAST, this means careful optimisation of physiology, close observation for signs of deterioration and appropriate timely interventions when required. To deliver this effectively requires robust training and governance pathways, ensuring that personnel and procedures are always ready and appropriate for deployment.

AE DOCTRINE AND PROCESS

AE doctrine has matured against a background of lessons learned from the conflicts in Iraq and Afghanistan and has flexibly adopted the new capabilities as they are proven and introduced. Three stages of AE and CCAST are described: *forward*, *tactical* and *strategic*. Forward and tactical AE are assets deployable to a theatre of operations as required, whilst strategic AE is a permanent commitment, manned 24 hours a day, 365 days a year (Figure 7.1).

Forward AE transports patients from the combat medics and regimental medical officers providing initial treatment under fire to Role 2 or 3

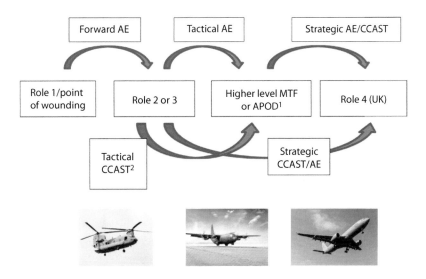

Figure 7.1 AE and CCAST (see text). [1]APOD, air point of departure. [2]Although the main Tac CCAST function was Role 2/3 to higher level MTF or APOD transfer, Tac CCAST on occasion also did Role 1 to Role 2/3 and very occasionally did Role 2/3 to Role 4 transfers for very time critical patients.

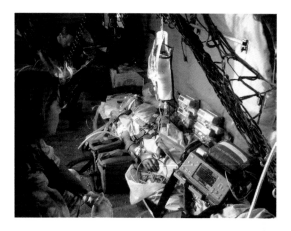

Figure 7.2 Rotary wing tactical CCAST.

facilities. Tactical AE transfers patients to higher levels of care within the joint theatre of operations area (JOA)[7] and provides access to services such as ophthalmology and neurosurgery[7] at other medical treatment facilities (MTFs). Tactical AE also conveys patients to suitable locations from where they can be transported out of the JOA by strategic AE. Destinations might include the United Kingdom, host countries for non-UK combatants or to temporary safe areas. The operational tempo will often dictate how these concepts are applied and adapted. On *Operations Telic* and *Herrick*, for example, forward AE and tactical CCAST evacuated patients from Role 1 facilities and tactical CCAST delivered the strategic role when further delay in repatriation posed significant risks to the patient or risked compromising the availability of medical capability in the AO (Figure 7.2).

Command, control and coordination

Headquarters Air Command (HQ AIR) tasks Headquarters (HQ) TMW and the *UK Strategic Aeromedical Evacuation Centre* (AECC) at RAF Brize Norton to provide and coordinate UK Strategic AE.[7] The AECC assesses risk, plans and tasks all UK strategic AE, with TMW supplying AE teams to deliver safe patient repatriation. These teams are composed of primary and secondary care personnel drawn from either the Aeromedical Squadron at TMW or from the wider RAF Medical and Nursing Services.

Command and control of forward and tactical AE are delegated to the medical commander (*Commander Medical* – the senior medical administrative officer) and the *Aeromedical Evacuation Control Officer* (AECO) deployed to the JOA. The AECO is a medical officer, supported by an *Aeromedical Evacuation Liaison Officer* (AELO) (a flight nurse or nursing officer) and, in large-scale deployments, an *Aeromedical Evacuation Operations Officer* (AEOO). These personnel assess the possesive patients' to fly[7] and provide the interface between the medical facilities and the Air Transport system.

Timelines and team composition

In a theatre of operations, medical doctrine states that critical care patients should be transferred by tactical CCAST, once it is safe to do so. The AEOO will liaise with the in-theatre *Flight Movement Coordination Cell* and *Joint Helicopter Force* to ensure that air assets are made available to meet the timeline. CCAST and AE teams do not have dedicated air assets and therefore require an airframe to be tasked. Although CCAST has a slower response time than the *Medical Emergency Response Team* (MERT), it is fully independent of the aircraft systems, making it highly flexible and able to operate on virtually any airframe and over any distance.

Strategic CCAST aims to repatriate cases within 24 hours of the request being made to the AECC[7] and to facilitate this, the first on call team (R-0) is resident at RAF Brize Norton. R-0 is on six hours *notice to move*, with the second on-call team (R-0 standby) assuming the R-0 role when the first team is tasked.

Tactical and strategic teams consist of a consultant anaesthetist (usually an intensivist), two intensive care unit (ICU) trained nurses, a medic and a medical equipment engineer with one of the ICU nurses acting as team leader. As dictated by the airframe or vehicle available, the basic team may be reduced in the *tactical* environment or at the airhead to an anaesthetist and nurse. Similarly, in the *strategic* role, the CCAST may be augmented with additional nurses and an anaesthetic trainee for multiple patient tasks (Figure 7.3).

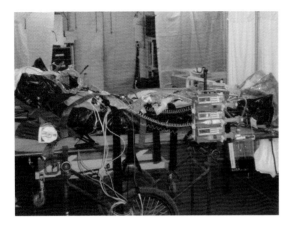

Figure 7.3 Preparing the patient for a tactical CCAST transfer – ready to go.

THE SPECIALTY ON DEPLOYMENT

Deployment of CCAST on Operation Telic

Planning for *Operation Telic* led to the deployment of aeromedical personnel to the *airport of disembarkation* (APOD) at Kuwait City International Airport (KCIA) and to RAF Akrotiri in Cyprus. Two CCASTs were deployed to KCIA alongside No 1 *Aeromedical Evacuation Squadron* (1AeVacS), which established an *aeromedical reception and staging establishment*, with an intensive care holding capability.[8] The first field hospital was located at *Camp Coyote*, approximately 70 km northwest of KCIA, before *34 Field Hospital* deployed under fire at Shiabah Logistic Base 10 days after the initial invasion.

Operation Telic was the occasion of the first deployment of forward CCAST, a flexible asset that operated in a wide variety of rotary-wing and fixed-wing aircraft, moving patients to and from the deployed MTFs, the *Primary Casualty Receiving Unit* on RFA Argus (where computed tomography [CT] and neurosurgical facilities were located) and USS Comfort (see Chapter 21). CCAST's flexibility meant that it overlapped with the *Immediate Response Team*, the forerunner of the *MERT*, providing forward MEDEVAC from the point of wounding and Role 1 facilities. The teams also provided strategic evacuation from the APOD at KCIA to RAF Akrotiri, by VC10 or C-130 Hercules.

A CCAST based at RAF Akrotiri then conducted the onward move to the United Kingdom using chartered aircraft.[8]

Enduring commitments during Operation Telic

As operations in Iraq transitioned from war-fighting to stabilisation, forward CCAST adopted the now familiar tactical role, since neurosurgery and CT scanning were not available at Shaibah until 2005. In January 2006, the field hospital relocated to the Contingent Operating Base in Basrah, where the APOD had been established after the initial fighting phase. During the interim period, strategic CCAST would land at Basrah, and retrieve casualties from Shaibah by air or road, for evacuation back to the United Kingdom. Following a brief basing at Shaibah, AE relocated to the field hospital at Basrah, simplifying both strategic and tactical transfers.

Initial operations in Afghanistan

British involvement in Afghanistan began in 2001 centred on a stability operation around Kabul and a counter terrorism task force in northern Afghanistan. During this early period, strategic CCAST evacuated a number of casualties from Kabul and Kandahar. However, it was not until the scale of the United Kingdom involvement expanded significantly in 2006 that the requirement for tactical CCAST arose.

Camp Bastion

In 2006, fresh outbreaks of violence in the South led to the creation of *Task Force Helmand* led by British Forces. Initially deploying 3000 troops[9]; this number was increased to 8000 in 2007 due to a much increased operational tempo.

The Role 2 Enhanced (Role 2 E) MTF at Camp Bastion was established by *22 Field Hospital* in April 2006. It was one of a network of field hospitals providing specialist services at different locations across the battlespace. The need to transfer critically ill patients between these MTFs for complex levels of care led to the deployment of a tactical CCAST capability to Bastion in 2006. The APOD was initially located at Kandahar, so repatriation of patients to the United Kingdom and allied nations required transfer by tactical CCAST from Camp Bastion for a ramp to ramp handover to the care of strategic CCAST. The operational tempo and casualty flows reached a peak in 2009–2010, with strategic CCAST regularly flying back-to-back missions to Camp Bastion. To alleviate some of the pressure on CCAST during this time, anaesthetic registrars were used to augment strategic AE teams and transfer ward level patients with epidurals and nerve catheters in situ.

Following the closure of the (by that time) Role 3 at Camp Bastion in September 2014, tactical CCAST moved to a US Role 2 MTF at the Bastion Airhead until the final withdrawal of UK combat troops in October 2014.

Reception arrangements and the Royal Centre for Defence Medicine

Initially casualties were flown to a variety of hospitals around the United Kingdom, as part of the *Reception Arrangements for Military Patients*

(RAMP) process, which was designed to ensure that individual hospitals were not overwhelmed and that injured service personnel were treated near to home. The *Royal Centre for Defence Medicine* (RCDM) was established in Birmingham in 2001, and from 2003, it became standard practice to repatriate all UK military casualties there. This allowed the development of expertise in managing complex military trauma and the establishment of a comprehensive welfare support system.

WORKLOAD

The number of patients evacuated by AE and CCAST is collated by AECC at RAF Brize Norton. Table 7.1 shows the numbers of patients evacuated from *Operation Telic*, *Operation Herrick* and the rest of the world since 1 January 2003, by both CCAST and general AE.

The figures in the table include UK service personnel and civilians (civilians include Royal Fleet Auxiliary as well as entitled and non-entitled civilians). They indicate only the number of personnel evacuated and do not include connecting flights

Table 7.1 AE workload data (1 January 2003 to 30 September 2016)

Year	All	Telic		Herrick		Rest of the world	
		Aeromed	CCAST	Aeromed	CCAST	Aeromed	CCAST
All	21,638	4,627	42	6470	447	10,541	59
2003	1,534	1,522		12	0		
2004	756	704		52	2		
2005	642	592		50	2		
2006	947	672	14	262	20	13	0
2007	1,149	592	26	554	31	3	0
2008 [7]	1,763	337	2	704	36	722	6
2009	2,390	175	0	1,039	104	1,176	7
2010	2,505	23	0	1,085	107	1,397	2
2011	2,263	9	0	904	69	1,350	6
2012	2,132	0	0	940	49	1,192	2
2013	1,839	1	0	578	24	1,260	8
2014	1,535	0	0	287	7	1,248	9
2015	1,167	0	0	2	0	1,165	15
2016	1,016	0	0	1	0	1,015	4

Source: Aeromedical Evacuation Control Centre (AECC).

Note: The majority of the rest of the world data begins 1 April 2008. 2016 data are up to and including 30 September 2016. CCAST data are not available between 1 January 2003 and 31 December 2005 for *Operation Telic*.

and reverse AEs. In some cases, the injury or natural cause for which a casualty was aeromedically evacuated may have occurred in a previous year. The numbers given for *Operations Telic* and *Herrick* should not be compared with the numbers published on Gov.uk, which include all AEs.

CLINICAL CHALLENGES ON *OPERATIONS TELIC* AND *HERRICK*

Airframes and interoperability

All equipment must be appropriately air-tested prior to entry into service. By using cylinder oxygen and battery-powered equipment, CCAST remains independent of the aircraft's systems,[10] which allows for greater flexibility should there be a change of vehicle, airframe or itinerary (Figure 7.4).

Tactical issues

A great variety of aircraft were used by tactical CCAST, including British *Puma HC1's*, *CH-47 Chinooks*, *Sea Kings* and *C-130 Hercules*. Furthermore, the operational tempo necessitated the employment of other coalition aircraft such as US *UH-60 Blackhawks*, US *V-22 Ospreys* and French *Super Pumas*. Flying with coalition partners often required adaptability since the Blackhawk and other airframes were too small to accommodate more than two team members and CCAST equipment was used on US aircraft under operational inter-flight agreements.

Strategic issues

The VC10 and TriStar were the predominant strategic airframes utilised during the early roulements of *Operations* Telic and *Herrick*. CCAST often worked on routine trooping flights, with limited space and patient privacy. Stretcher fit was an issue with some airframes in the RAF fleet not being compatible with the NATO stretcher; as a consequence use had to be made of wooden stretchers. The C17A Globemaster III entered service with the RAF in 2001 and quickly became the airframe of choice, with excellent all round patient access, easy stretcher loading and plenty of room for equipment and the medical team. Runway modifications

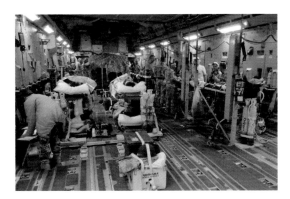

Figure 7.4 Multiple patient strategic CCAST.

allowed the C17A to land at Bastion from 2008 and the TriStar from 2011, negating the need for a tactical transfer to Kandahar for strategic CCAST.

Aviation considerations

All takeoffs and landings into and out of the JOA were performed tactically, which meant steep ascents and descents usually in darkness. Consequently, the patient, the team and all equipment had to be well secured and monitors were required to have low light displays, which would not be visible from outside the aircraft or disturb the night vision of the crews. Tactical CCAST personnel had to be very familiar with 'hot loads' (loading with the engines running) in a hot, dusty environment, again often in the dark. It was imperative that everything was well secured and that nothing could cause a hazard to the aircraft or the team. CCAST team members became well used to an 'immediate action drill' on completion of a hot load (or off load) to confirm that all equipment was functioning and that the patient was ventilating with no disconnections. Patients were provided with ear and eye protection prior to these moves.

Both tactical and strategic teams became well used to sharing the airframe with other 'cargo', which varied from munitions to food, from vehicles to post. Sadly, the teams also became familiar with the company of flag-covered coffins bearing the bodies of fallen soldiers, who were always treated with great dignity, irrespective of their nationality.

It was common for the team to request a cabin altitude restriction for certain patients because of the injuries they had sustained. The expansion of gases as an aircraft ascends can exacerbate conditions such as pneumocephalus and pneumothorax. Following bowel surgery, anastomoses may also be threatened by rapid expansion of intraluminal gas. Such a restriction requires the aircraft to fly lower to maintain the same barometric pressure as the departing airfield. This burns more fuel and prolongs transfer times, factors that need to be considered during the planning phase of the flight.

Airspace

The importance of the air-bridge to medical operations in Afghanistan was highlighted in April 2010, when it was disrupted due to the volcanic events at Eyjafjallajökull in Iceland. The resultant ash cloud caused the closure of large portions of northern Europe's airspace and briefly caused the air-bridge to close, preventing strategic AE to the United Kingdom. Deployed intensive care capacity was fortunately maintained, with rearward evacuation of patients by tactical CCAST to *Landstuhl Regional Medical Center*, a US Army hospital in Germany, until the airspace reopened.

The remote location of Afghanistan meant that for the first few hours of flight, the only possible diversion was back to the departure airfield. This made the decision to emplane critical care patients more difficult, weighing up the risks of in-flight deterioration against the risks of not moving during a window of relative stability. In retrospect, the rarity of in-flight diversions for medical reasons was testament to the skill and expertise of the damage control resuscitation and surgery performed and to the capabilities of CCAST.

Logistics

The dispersion of coalition MTFs, specialist surgical care and the APOD led to the requirement for tactical CCAST in both theatres of operation. Co-locating the team with the field hospital at Camp Bastion facilitated the rapid evacuation of patients, as transfers became almost a continuum of the resuscitation and stabilisation process and on occasion proceeded directly from the emergency department trauma bay. Teams could continue to resuscitate and prepare the patient for transfer while air assets were assigned. Lack of familiarity

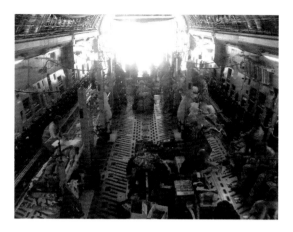

Figure 7.5 Combined multiple patient strategic CCAST and Aeromed transfer on board a C-17A Globemaster.

with coalition forward operating bases and MTFs could make retrievals more challenging, especially where there was no British medical footprint. In contrast, the commonality of equipment and consumables between the UK MTFs and CCAST led to transfers between them becoming almost seamless in comparison (Figure 7.5).

ICU capacity

The AE chain was also critical in maintaining ICU capacity in the field hospitals, which always had the potential to become overwhelmed during casualty surges. This was particularly so when beds were occupied by local nationals or enemy forces, who were difficult to transfer to a facility offering an equivalent level of care.

Environmental issues

TEMPERATURE

The desert environments of Iraq and Afghanistan are subject to extremes of temperature, with daily maximums exceeding 40°C during summer and sub-zero temperatures during winter months. Trauma patients are often pyrexial as a result of the systemic inflammatory response syndrome, and CCAST found that the wide variation in aircraft temperature made maintaining normothermia difficult. To address this and reflecting the increasing evidence that preventing pyrexia was beneficial in head injured and post-cardiac arrest patients,[11,12] a cooling system (EMCOOLS Flex.PadTM) was trialled and a heating mattress (Inditherm™) was purchased for strategic usage.

The variability in environmental and in-flight temperatures resulted in some items of equipment being operated outside the manufacturer's recommended temperature range, with the potential for malfunction. In particular, the portable blood analyser (Abbott i-STAT™) would not function when it failed to reach its minimum operating temperature, while the portable monitor (MRL Portable Intensive Care System™) frequently exceeded its maximum operating temperature, requiring a dry ice bed to keep it cool. Careful monitoring of drug temperatures was also required, as exceeding recommended thermal ranges resulted in shelf lives being considerably reduced.

NOISE

Noise levels on both fixed and rotary wing aircraft are high, and with the move to the C17A aircraft for strategic CCAST, teams were exposed to levels requiring ear protection throughout the flight. The continuous noise made verbal communication difficult, with hand signals being necessary at times, as well as having an additional fatiguing effect. Subsequently, a marked improvement was seen with the introduction of the Tru-link inter-communication system, which provided a reduction in noise levels and effective wireless communication between team members.

Clinical issues

TIMING

Despite world class management at deployed MTFs, the benefits of early rearward evacuation were clear – complex injuries were best managed at RCDM where there was access to a wide range of specialist interventions.[13] The early post-DCS period offered a window of 'relative' stability in even the most severely injured, where the balance of risk usually favoured emplaning. However, some injuries, such as multiple fasciotomies or extensive pelvic soft tissue wounds,[13] required continuing resuscitation throughout the transfer. To transfuse

and correct coagulopathies in these patients and to mitigate for unexpected bleeding, CCAST uplifted blood and blood products for the flight.

EARLY EXTUBATION

The increasing use of epidurals and peripheral nerve catheters for acute pain management led to the earlier extubation of some trauma patients, allowing expedient transfer from the ICU to the surgical ward during casualty surges.[14] These improvements in regional pain management also produced a potential cohort of level 2 (HDU) patients for CCAST evacuation. The location of tactical CCAST at the Role 3 allowed early discussions about extubation prior to a CCAST transfer. With a minimum flight time to the United Kingdom of eight hours (which was often considerably extended by altitude restrictions and routing issues), patients at high risk of re-intubation or instability in-flight generally remained intubated, as did patients with pain, which, it was anticipated, would be difficult to manage (for example from thoracoabdominal injuries).[14] This approach also facilitated second look procedures at the Role 4, as well as addressing the risk of respiratory failure in flight.

VENTILATOR-ACQUIRED PNEUMONIA

The risk of micro-aspiration is increased during CCAST transfers because of the vibration, turbulence and G forces to which the patient is exposed.[15] This may lead to an increased frequency of *ventilator associated pneumonia* (VAP). By meticulously following VAP prevention guidelines (in-line tracheal suction, chlorhexidine mouthwash, tracheal cuff pressure monitoring and maintaining a 30° head up position[11]), the risk was largely mitigated. Despite the intention to establish early enteral feeding in these highly catabolic patients, a study conducted during *Operation Herrick* showed evidence of microaspiration in-flight, and feeding was subsequently discontinued on strategic CCAST moves.

PRESSURE AREA CARE

During both conflicts, it was standard practice to transfer patients on a vacuum mattress. This helped secure the patient, any indwelling lines and monitoring equipment and allowed easier movement from bed to stretcher. It also helped splint injured limbs and immobilise the spine. An area of potential concern on long strategic transfers however, was the potential for skin breakdown and the development of pressure sores. Regular rolling and inspection were mandated to prevent this. Nonetheless, following feedback from RCDM, a gel head ring was introduced to reduce the incidence of occipital alopecia.[16] Another area of concern was the potential for endotracheal cuff pressure to vary with altitude. Given that elevated pressures reduce mucosal blood flow and increase the frequency of tracheal stenosis, intermittent cuff monitoring was routinely conducted.

RENAL REPLACEMENT THERAPY

The last two decades saw medical support planning focused on small, mobile medical units supported by rapid evacuation to Role 4 facilities by an effective evacuation chain.[17] Therefore, *renal replacement therapy* (RRT) was not provided in MTFs during *Operations Herrick* and *Telic*. A brief exception to this followed the volcanic events at Eyjafjallajökull in Iceland, referred to earlier, when CCAST deployed a Baxter Aquarius haemofilter to Camp Bastion. This was used once on a patient with fulminant hepatic failure and an acute kidney injury.[18] Providing RRT in a deployed setting is a significant logistical undertaking. Despite in-flight RRT being achieved in the 1980s,[19] modern haemofilters rely on integrated weighing scales to monitor fluid balance as well as requiring large volumes of fluid, making in-flight RRT almost impossible for CCAST. Despite these limitations, CCAST retains the ability to deploy this capability if required.

PAEDIATRICS

As well as supporting the 'hearts and minds' campaign, the Defence Medical Services had a duty of care to children injured by coalition action under the Law of Armed Conflict. Approximately 10% of admissions to Camp Bastion ICU were paediatric casualties,[20] many of whom required transfer to surgical specialties provided at other locations in the JOA. Few of the clinicians had a subspecialty interest in paediatrics, and none of the nursing staff worked in paediatric ICUs (PICUs). A package of paediatric training for the nursing staff, consisting of 75 hours in a PICU, was initiated as part of pre-deployment training, to increase familiarity with managing children. Fortunately, most of the equipment used by CCAST was appropriate for all but the smallest babies.

INFECTION CONTROL

Only the strategic airframes (C17A, TriStar and VC-10) provided hand-washing facilities with hot water, making hand hygiene a challenge since these facilities were limited and not dedicated to CCAST use. Teams had to use disposable gloves and alcohol gel, and extra care was taken to check indwelling lines and tubes before leaving the MTF, to reduce the need to insert cannulae and lines in flight.

PERSONNEL

Both tactical and strategic CCAST required personnel to work in small teams, with the tactical teams spending prolonged periods living and working together. This close proximity can forge better working relationships, improving efficiency with shared care outside of traditional doctor–nurse roles. Indeed, one of the nurses assumed the role of team leader, encouraging a flatter command structure and empowering more junior team members to challenge decisions. This could occasionally cause confusion when interacting with other personnel who might direct questions at the highest ranking team member, usually the consultant.[21] On the other hand, these enforced relationships could cause friction and exacerbate personality differences. Consequently, it was beholden on all team members to address these issues through team de-briefs and to take every opportunity for recreational activities.

Periods of high activity, with long strategic transfers in hostile environments, led to considerable fatigue amongst team members. Having two nurses per team allowed some scope for rest, and the addition of a registrar on strategic CCAST also helped reduce the workload of the consultant. Whilst there is no evidence of suboptimal care, future planning needs to consider team fatigue, allowing for direct flights without the need for refueling stops or, where possible, the completion of secondary tasks (Figure 7.6).

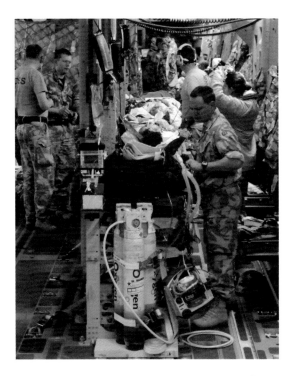

Figure 7.6 Multi-disciplinary management of the complex patient during a CCAST flight.

ROYAL CENTRE FOR DEFENCE MEDICINE

The ICU at RCDM became extremely adept at receiving CCAST patients, with senior clinicians present for handover irrespective of the time of day. Indeed, by the later stages of *Operation Herrick*, the receiving clinicians had already studied imaging and clinical information transmitted from Bastion before the patient arrived.

A particularly challenging task for CCAST was meeting the families of wounded and sick personnel, who often arrived at the hospital before the patient thanks to the excellent welfare system. CCASTs were the first contact that the families had with the clinicians and nursing staff who had directly managed their loved ones. Despite the seriousness of the injuries, this interaction was always welcomed by the families. The CCAST clinicians were always receptive to conducting these meetings, but coming at the end of a mission when fatigue was mounting, and the information conveyed was often distressing, the effects of these conversations on the doctors and nurses involved remains to be seen.

ETHICAL ISSUES

The campaign in Afghanistan presented many ethical issues for tactical CCAST. Local nationals could not generally be taken out of country for ongoing medical care, which meant that they had to be moved in country to maintain the capacity and readiness of the Role 3 for United Kingdom and allied troops. As a result, tactical CCAST had to transfer intensive care patients to the care of other agencies, which were invariably less capable than the Role 3 facility at Bastion. This was particularly difficult with burns and paediatric patients when clinicians were aware that therapeutic options were available in the United Kingdom that could not be accessed in the JOA. A limited provision for burns treatment was provided by NGO facilities.

EQUIPMENT

The heavy usage of CCAST's *Airworthy Medical Equipment* (AME) during *Operations Telic* and *Herrick* and the development of tactical CCAST contributed to the procurement of new equipment towards the end of *Operation Herrick*. The equipment used up until then had been purchased incrementally, much had reached the end of its serviceable life and upgraded equipment was required to meet CCAST's needs and modern clinical governance standards. The widespread use of peripheral nerve catheters, epidurals and patient controlled analgesia also required the procurement of specialist infusion pumps and syringe drivers. This new AME took time to undergo the necessarily rigorous air-testing required before it could be released to service on military aircraft.[22] Further careful consideration of how this equipment was to be used in flight was then required – from the safe fixing of equipment onto aircraft (using specially designed brackets, clamps and bags) to modification of screens to ensure compatibility with night vision equipment and suitability for use in the tactical environment.

ADVANCES

The Association of Anaesthetists of Great Britain and Ireland (AAGBI) released guidelines in 2006[23] and 2009,[24] setting out standards to improve the quality of civilian transfers: it was found that CCAST had been exceeding these from its inception. The nature of military operations meant that patients were moved over considerable distances and time frames, necessitating active clinical management beyond the simple transfer role. Consequently, CCAST was already delivering levels of care such as VAP prevention bundles and in-flight optimisation of patient physiology prior to the AAGBI's guidance (Figure 7.7).

Clinical care

The clinical capabilities of CCAST far exceeded those of simple civilian transfers. In-flight point-of-care blood testing enabled the management of ventilation, fluids, vasopressors, blood and blood products to be tailored to the patient. The advances in acute pain management in the MTFs using continuous peripheral nerve block catheters and epidurals allowed pain to be managed more effectively in awake patients during their flight. Equipment and compatibility issues prevented continuous intracranial pressure (ICP) monitoring

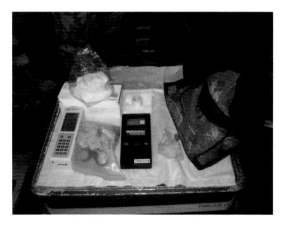

Figure 7.7 Point-of-care testing during strategic CCAST flight.

using intraparechymal monitors (or 'ICP bolts'), but patients with brain injuries were frequently flown with extraventricular drains that could be transduced in flight.[25]

Training

With each roulement of the field hospital, a course was conducted in the United Kingdom to test the readiness of the deploying unit. This exercise, HOSPEX, was identified by the RAF as a training opportunity to integrate tactical CCAST into the deployed hospital. Exercises were conducted during which CCAST retrieved and delivered patients to and from the field hospital in order to familiarise all team members with the AE process.

Governance

Clinical governance and quality improvement (Chapter 19) developed significantly during Operations Telic and Herrick, and central to this was the excellent communication that existed between theatre, the Role 4 and CCAST. An important milestone was the development of the Joint Theatre Clinical Case Conference, which was established in 2007.[26] This weekly multi-disciplinary teleconference between RCDM and the Role 2+/3 in Camp Bastion included CCAST, AECC, Headley Court and other operational theatres. The forum allowed the deployed teams the opportunity to update RCDM on patients waiting for repatriation and allowed RCDM to back brief on the patients received.[27] This forum for discussion and learning (which is still running for other areas of operation) proved an exceptional resource for improving clinical outcomes and for developing SOPs during a dynamic campaign.

A database of strategic CCAST patients was maintained at TMW to allow audit and monitoring of workload. Similarly, at the end of each operational tour, the tactical CCAST team leader provided a report to Commander Med to aid organisational learning. Cases of interest were then presented at the regular CCAST forums held at RAF Brize Norton, to share learning and to discuss challenges.

Patient follow-up

RAF critical care nurses were embedded in the ICUs in Birmingham, providing feedback during patients' critical care admissions. Additionally, RCDM developed its own ICU follow-up clinic, allowing identification and feedback of longer-term problems (Chapter 6). Morbidity such as occipital alopecia and several cases of tracheal stenosis were recognised, leading CCAST to procure gel head-rings and to develop a method of continuously monitoring tracheal tube cuff pressures in-flight.

CHALLENGES FOR THE FUTURE

Tactical environment

The RAF became accustomed to the air superiority seen over Afghanistan and Iraq,[28] allowing AE to proceed with threats limited to small arms and rocket fire. Future operations may not be conducted in such a permissive environment. This will limit access to AE and CCAST, potentially extending evacuation timelines. Any resulting extension of the 48-hour maximum hold in deployed ICUs may see strategic CCAST being unable to evacuate patients during the early window of stability. Consequently, second look procedures may need to be conducted in field hospitals, and patients may begin to develop secondary complications related to sepsis and systemic inflammatory response syndrome, such as haemodynamic instability and acute renal failure. Planners may have to consider a staged evacuation chain, with patients managed at another facility en route or with the deployment of an RRT prior to transfer.

Logistics

Tactical and strategic CCAST became accustomed to retrieving patients from UK MTFs, working to the same Clinical Guidelines for Operations (CGOs) as themselves. Patients retrieved from Camp Bastion R3 were often prepared for transfer by tactical CCAST and were well resuscitated, with compatible medical devices and consumables, making transfer to strategic aircraft relatively seamless. Future conflicts may require CCAST to provide patients managed in non-UK MTFs with periods of resuscitation and stabilisation prior to emplaning. Under these circumstances, a deployed AELO will be crucial to effective co-ordination of all the logistic elements of the transfer.

When flying out of Camp Bastion, the strategic CCAST capability was able to uplift blood products from the Role 3 that had been supplied by *UK Blood and Transplant Service*, thereby meeting UK standards of screening and preparation. Future taskings retrieving patients from foreign assets or UK MTFs during entry operations may not have access to blood products due to limited supply or differing standards. This will require CCAST to take blood from RCDM and use lyophilised plasma preparations).

Clinical

The primary clinical focus during the campaigns in Afghanistan and Iraq was trauma, with just 2.4% of patients being admitted to the ICU in 2009 as the result of *disease and non-battle injury* (DNBI).[29] However, the *Operational Patient Care Pathway*[30] considers that the 'All Hazards Environment' (chemical, biological, radiological, nuclear, explosive, environmental, endemic and trauma) and the potential burden of DNBI need to be remembered[31] with a return to contingency operations. This was emphasised by the 2014 military deployment of the Ebola virus disease treatment facility to Sierra Leone, providing assurance to UK and international healthcare workers.[32]

New airframes

The introduction to service of new airframes, such as the Voyager A330 and the Airbus A400M, brings many advantages but also requires CCAST to adapt. These aircraft are required to fulfil a multitude of roles, which means that CCASTs have to maintain their flexibility in adjusting to the new environment, such as in terms of securing and stowing kit, in order to deliver the aeromedical role.

Future capability

The recent addition of a Sonosite M Turbo™ ultra-sound machine to the CCAST module will assist in pre-flight patient assessment as well as aiding the insertion of central and arterial lines prior to transfer. This is particularly important with the increasing use of ultrasound to site lines and the use of echocardiography to assess volume status and cardiac performance. The machine can also provide the intensivist with valuable information about the patient's lung status, identifying pneumothoraces and giving information about lung water and consolidation.

Training and maintenance of skills

The retention of corporate knowledge is crucial as we return to contingency operations, with new airframes being introduced and experienced team members leaving the Service. The drastic reduction in workload seen following the UK withdrawal from Afghanistan provides the challenge of training and maintaining the skills and knowledge of new and existing personnel. This is partially addressed by high-fidelity simulation exercises conducted during the first week of the strategic on call month and during the annual CCAST (training) revalidation course. The use of real clinical cases and critical incidents to formulate scenario training helps to keep this relevant. Opportunities to exercise alongside aircrew should be embraced, as many loadmasters have worked alongside CCAST during their busiest times and understand how the teams operate. Training needs identified during *Operation Herrick* are continuing to be addressed, with nursing staff rotating through PICU placements in Oxford, in order to build confidence and maintain the skills needed to treat children.

RESEARCH

The most significant study conducted during *Operation Herrick* looked at the safety of in-flight enteral feeding. A study was conducted looking for evidence of microaspiration in CCAST patients, which was confirmed by the presence of pepsin in tracheal aspirate. As a result, enteral feeding was discontinued in-flight. Other areas of study included changes in P/F ratio, body areas at risk of pressure damage, laboratory research on the effects of pressure changes on ventilators and an audit and survey on the usage and efficacy of the EMCOOLS patient cooling system. Following several reported occurrences of tracheal injury, a study into in-flight endotracheal tube cuff pressures was conducted, resulting in the development of a method of in-flight continuous cuff pressure monitoring.

CONCLUSION

The past two decades have seen the formal establishment of CCAST in the RAF, and its role being proven in supporting medical operations. The ability to evacuate very seriously injured personnel to the Role 4 within 24 hours of injury is a considerable achievement, as is the efficiency of tactical CCAST around the JOA. The dedication and professionalism of military aircrew and medical coordinators has been remarkable. The increase in unexpected survivors will ensure that CCAST continues to play a critical role in deployed and strategic military healthcare.

REFERENCES

1. Tipping RD, Vollam J. Transfer and evacuation. In: *Ryan's Ballistic Trauma*, eds. Brookes A, Clasper J, Midwinter M, Hodgetts T, Mahoney P. London: Springer, 2011, pp. 597–611. doi:10.1007/978-1-84882-124-8_39
2. Mackie M. *Wards in the Sky – The RAF's Remarkable Nursing Service*. Stroud: The History Press, 2014.
3. Marsh AR. A short but distant war – The Falklands campaign. *J R Soc Med* 1983;76: 972–982.
4. Bricknell MCM. The evolution of casualty evacuation in the British Army in the 20th century (part 3) – 1945 to present. *J R Army Med Corps* 2003;149:85–95.

5. Hawley A. Trauma management on the battlefield: A modern approach. *J R Army Med Corps* 1996;142:120–125. doi:10.1136/jramc-142-03-09

6. Joint Doctrine and Concepts Centre. *Joint Warfare Publication 4-03*. London: Joint Doctrine and Concepts Centre, 2016.

7. Command of the Defence Council. *AP3394: The Royal Air Force Aeromedical Evacuation Service*. 4th ed. London: Ministry of Defence, 2009.

8. Rew D. *Blood, Heat & Dust: Operation TELIC and the British Medical Deployment to the Gulf 2003–2009*. 3rd ed. London: Ministry of Defence, 2015.

9. Vassallo D. A short history of Camp Bastion Hospital: The two hospitals and unit deployments. *J R Army Med Corps* 2015;161:79–83. doi:10.1136/jramc-2015-000414

10. Turner S, Ruth M, Tipping R. Critical Care Air Support Teams and deployed intensive care. *J R Army Med Corps* 2009;155:171–174. doi:10.1136/jramc-155-02-18

11. Johnston AM, Easby D, Ewington I. Sepsis management in the deployed field hospital. *J R Army Med Corps* 2013;159:175–180. doi:10.1136/jramc-2013-000089

12. Nielsen N, Wetterslev J, Cronberg T et al. Targeted temperature management at 33°C versus 36°C after cardiac arrest. *N Engl J Med* 2013;369:2197–2206. doi:10.1056/NEJMoa1310519

13. McNicholas J, Henning J. Major military trauma: Decision making in the ICU. *J R Army Med Corps* 2011;157:S284–S288. doi:10.1136/jramc-157-03s-05

14. Thornhill R, Tong JL, Birch K et al. Field intensive care – Weaning and extubation. *J R Army Med Corps* 2010;156:S311–S317. doi:10.1136/jramc-156-04s-08

15. Turner S, Ruth MJ, Bruce DL. "In flight catering": Feeding critical care patients during aeromedical evacuation. *J R Army Med Corps* 2008;154(4):282–283.

16. Scott T, Davies M, Dutton C et al. Intensive care follow-up in UK Military casualties: A one-year pilot. *J Intensive Care Soc* 2014;15:113–116. doi:10.1177/175114371401500206

17. Chung KK, Perkins RM, Oliver JD III. Renal replacement therapy in support of combat operations. *Crit Care Med* 2008;36:S365–S369. doi:10.1097/CCM.0b013e31817e302a

18. Nesbitt I, Almond M, Freshwater D. Renal replacement in the deployed setting. *J R Army Med Corps* 2011;157:179–181. doi:10.1136/jramc-157-02-11

19. Stevens PE, Bloodworth LL, Rainford DJ. High altitude haemofiltration. *BMJ* 1986;292:1354. doi:10.1136/bmj.292.6532.1354

20. Inwald DP, Arul GS, Montgomery M et al. Management of children in the deployed intensive care unit at Camp Bastion, Afghanistan. *J R Army Med Corps* 2014;160:236–240. doi:10.1136/jramc-2013-000177

21. Lamb D. Collaboration in practice – Assessment of an RAF CCAST. *Br J Nurs* 2006;15:552–556. doi:10.12968/bjon.2006.15.10.21131

22. Lamb D. The introduction of new critical care equipment into the aeromedical evacuation service of the Royal Air Force. *Intens Crit Care Nurs* 2003;19:92–102. doi:10.1016/S0964-3397(03)00010-7

23. The Association of Anaesthetists of Great Britain and Ireland. Recommendations for the Safe Transfer of Patients with Brain Injury. London: The Association of Anaestheists of Great Britain and Ireland, 2006. http://www.aagbi.org/sites/default/files/braininjury.pdf

24. The Association of Anaesthetists of Great Britain and Ireland. Interhospital transfer. London: The Association of Anaestheists of Great Britain and Ireland, 2009. https://www.aagbi.org/sites/default/files/interhospital09.pdf

25. Ralph JK, Lowes T. Neurointensive care. *J R Army Med Corps* 2009;155:147–151.

26. Vassallo D. A short history of Camp Bastion Hospital: Preparing for war, national recognition and Bastion's legacy. *J R Army Med Corps* 2015;161:355–360. doi:10.1136/jramc-2015-000465

27. Willdridge D, Hodgetts T, Mahoney P et al. The Joint Theatre Clinical Case Conference (JTCCC): Clinical governance in action. *J R Army Med Corps* 2010;156:79–83. doi:10.1136/jramc-156-02-02

28. Michell S. *Air Power 2015/16 – Securing Our Skies*. London: Royal Air Force, 2015.

29. Johnston AM, Henning JD. Outcomes of patients treated at Bastion Hospital intensive care unit in 2009. *J R Army Med Corps* 2014;160:323. doi:10.1136/jramc-2014-000263

30. Ministry of Defence. *The Operational Patient Care Pathway. Joint Service Publication (JSP) 950 Leaflet 1-4-1.* London: Ministry of Defence, 2014. https://www.gov.uk/government/publications/operational-patient-care-pathway

31. Becker G, Laundy T. A lesson not yet learned. *J R Army Med Corps* 2003;149:274–276. doi:10.1136/jramc-149-04-06

32. Rees PSC, Ardley C, Bailey M et al. Op GRITROCK: The Royal Navy supports defence efforts to tackle Ebola. *J R Nav Med Serv* 2014;100:228–230.

8

Torso trauma

INTRODUCTION

Haemorrhage is the commonest cause of potentially preventable death after combat trauma, and significant bleeding into either the chest or abdominal cavities (or both) will almost always require a surgeon to correct it. Historically, thoracic and abdominal injuries sustained during conflict have been associated with a high incidence of morbidity and mortality, despite advances in medical care.

During the *Great War (1914–1918)*, thoracic injuries accounted for 6% of all combat wounds[1] and the mortality reached 27%[2]; the mortality rate for abdominal injuries was approximately 50%. There was limited thoracic surgical intervention at the time, with very few thoracotomies being performed, as patients often arrived in haemorrhagic shock and unfit for surgery.[3] The main causes of mortality were haemorrhage (60%) and sepsis (25%). By the *Second World War (1939–1945)*, the overall mortality from thoracic injuries had decreased to 11%,[4] and that from abdominal injuries, to 36%.[5]

The post-Second World War reduction in mortality rates following thoracic trauma has largely been attributed to clinical advances such as endotracheal ventilation, the use of antimicrobial agents, tube thoracostomy and improved thoracic surgical techniques, such as removing retained clots and contamination from the pleural spaces.[6]

However, even in the more modern era, thoracic trauma in war remains a major cause of disability and death, with data from the *Vietnam War* demonstrating that 24% of those who died had a fatal chest wound. Nevertheless, by the time of the conflict in Vietnam,[6] the overall mortality rate from thoracic wounds had decreased to 2.9%,[7] and from abdominal wounds, to 10%.[5] The major factor contributing to this improvement in mortality is thought to have been the improvement in the speed of evacuation from point of wounding to surgical care, particularly associated with the use of air assets, rather than large strides in surgical technology.[4]

Over the last two decades, especially in the conflicts in Iraq and Afghanistan, the nature of warfare has changed; warfare between armies using conventional munitions has given way to asymmetric insurgency-style conflicts characterised by the widespread use of *improvised explosive devices* (IEDs).[8] The UK *Defence Medical Services* have adopted a *damage control resuscitation* (DCR) paradigm, in order to deliver an end-to-end trauma system incorporating rapid evacuation, early haemostatic resuscitation and damage control surgery (DCS) in order to improve battlefield mortality.[9]

DCR–DCS APPROACH

DCR follows a philosophy of prioritising restoration of normal physiological parameters over definitive anatomical repair. The phrase 'damage control' originates from the naval terminology of allowing the ship to continue its fight whilst simultaneously preventing it from sinking or destruction by fires. Working as a coordinated unit, the damage control team aims to prevent the lethal triad of *acidosis*, *hypothermia* and *coagulopathy* from becoming established and progressive, buying time for management of other injuries when the situation is less critical.

When *DCR* was initially described, it was seen as a process with distinct and separate stages, during which the patient was initially *resuscitated* in the emergency department (*DCR*), then underwent DCS in the operating theatre and finally was subject to physiological restoration on the intensive care unit (ICU), with repeat re-look operative interventions as required. However, with time, this paradigm changed and *DCS* was demonstrated to be an integral component of DCR, with surgery and restoration of physiology occurring concurrently.[10]

Determining which patients will benefit from DCS has been a much-debated topic. Even at the midpoint of the conflict in Afghanistan, analysis demonstrated the possible under-utilisation of DCS procedures. A review of 22 procedures demonstrated that 7 of these incorporated the DCS philosophy, whereas 15 patients underwent definitive laparotomy. Of the 15 definitive procedures, four patients underwent re-look laparotomy for anastomotic breakdown and ongoing bleeding, leading to the conclusion that DCS was still being under-utilised.[11] Current criteria for DCS include mechanism of injury and the presence of physiological derangement,[12] with recent studies also advocating the use of the *shock index* (SI) to identify high-risk patients.[13] SI is heart rate divided by the systolic blood pressure; the normal value is 0.5–0.7. A value over 0.9 is associated with an increased mortality.

When used appropriately, DCS, in particular damage control laparotomy, has demonstrated low rates of mortality when compared to definitive surgery. Rotondo et al.[14] first described this in 1993, but our recent experience in the conflicts of Iraq and Afghanistan has re-emphasised this finding. A retrospective analysis looking at a five-month deployed operative workload demonstrated that 94 out of 636 casualties underwent laparotomy. Forty-four of these patients had colonic injury and 70 had some form of hollow viscus injury, 59 of whom had repair or primary resection and anastomosis, and low levels of faecal diversion.

Unfortunately, DCS is not without its problems. Care must be taken to undertake this in the right casualties.[14] To that end, extensive studies examining imaging have been undertaken. The advent of high-resolution and rapid imaging (most frequently computed tomography [CT] scanning), along with advances in resuscitation, has enabled more casualties to undergo imaging to determine whether cavity surgery is necessary and thereby decreases negative laparotomy rates.[15,16] Imaging is important as casualties in conflict often present with polytrauma, and imaging may prevent negative explorations. As mentioned previously, DCS and negative laparotomies carry increased morbidity. The SI has been demonstrated to be a useful parameter in aiding military surgeons in triaging ballistic battlefield torso trauma, thereby assisting in the identification of patients who potentially require operative torso haemorrhage control. Unfortunately, the SI assessment requires a normal physiological response to hypovolaemia and thus should always be considered in its clinical context.[13]

One of the major drivers in DCS is arresting haemorrhage. Data from the conflict in Afghanistan demonstrated that two-thirds of dismounted fatalities had haemorrhage that may have been anatomically amenable to pre-hospital intervention implicated as a cause of death. One-fifth of the mounted fatalities had haemorrhagic trauma, which at the time and currently could only be addressed surgically. This has led to maintenance of the drive to improve all haemostatic techniques for blast casualties, from point of wounding to definitive surgical proximal vascular control, alongside the development and application of novel haemostatic interventions.[17]

SPINAL INJURY

The burden of injury to the axial skeleton as a result of the conflicts in Iraq and Afghanistan has been substantial. A coordinated treatment plan is required that begins with the first encounter on the battlefield and continues throughout the patient's management. Such systems require that issues of expediency, operational limitations and restrictions and personnel be addressed. Current staffing of advanced echelons in theatre may not include a spine-trained orthopaedic surgeon, neurosurgeon or musculoskeletal specialist. There is currently one regular neurosurgeon in the Army (the other services do not have any) as this capability otherwise lies in the Reserves. How operationally responsive this structure will be remains to be seen.

The most widely used classification systems and treatment algorithms were formed in the context of a civilian trauma setting. The ready availability of advanced medical imaging, sterile operating theatres and specialty-specific ICUs in these civilian hospitals may make modern spinal trauma classification systems less applicable to a far-forward battlefield setting. However, efforts must be made to adapt current knowledge in the pursuit of a theatre-specific, relevant pathway or philosophy of care for the spine-injured warrior, with implementation as far forward as feasible to ensure the best possible clinical outcome.[18]

Cervical spine fractures and dislocations are uncommon injuries with potentially devastating neurological consequences. These injuries require adequate stabilisation to prevent further spinal cord injury during transfer between hospitals. Evacuation from point of wounding in a combat zone often requires a combination of road ambulance, helicopter and fixed wing aircraft. All unstable cervical spine fractures should be stabilised with a halo vest prior to transfer from Role 3; as a consequence, halo rings and vests must be available at Role 3 facilities,[19] as must the capability to fit them.

THORACOABDOMINAL INJURY

The management of patients who have sustained blast injuries poses an important challenge for military healthcare professionals. The spectrum of injuries is wide and often severe. *Operations Telic* and *Herrick* generated large numbers of such casualties, and current asymmetric conflicts around the World appear to be continuing to replicate this pattern of injuries. Modern military healthcare facilities (ever more commonly followed by civilian systems) are increasingly using CT scanning to facilitate their management.[20] The military surgeon must be prepared to make a decision and open the cavity where he or she thinks the major source of haemorrhage will be but be prepared to change tack quickly if the surgical findings do not match the physiological status of the patient.[21]

Non-compressible torso haemorrhage (NCTH) remains the leading cause of potentially preventable death in military trauma,[22] even in the absence of direct abdominal injury. The majority

Table 8.1 *Department of Defence Trauma Registry* patterns of torso injury (2002–2010)

- Thoracic, including lung
- Solid organ (high-grade spleen, liver and kidney)
- Named axial vessel
- Pelvic fracture with ring disruption

of casualties with NCTH die before admission with exsanguination as the cause of death,[23] predominantly as a consequence of arterial and pulmonary injuries.[24] Four patterns of torso injury, each based on vascular disruption, were identified in US military casualties from the *Department of Defence Trauma Registry* (2002–2010) (Table 8.1).

Injuries within these categories were evaluated in the context of physiological indicators of shock and/or the need for operative haemorrhage control. Of 15,209 battle injuries sustained during the study period, 12.7% (n = 1,936) had sustained one or more categories of torso injury. Of these, 331 (17.1%) had evidence of shock or the need for urgent haemorrhage control, with a mean *Injury Severity Score* and mortality rate of 30 (standard deviation, 13) and 18.7%, respectively. Pulmonary injuries were most numerous (41.7%), followed by solid-organ (29.3%), vascular (25.7%), and pelvic (15.1%) injuries. Following multivariate analysis, the most lethal injury complexes were identified as major arterial injury (odds ratio, 3.38; 95% confidence interval, 1.17–9.74) and pulmonary injury (odds ratio, 2.23; 95% confidence interval, 1.23–4.98).[24]

The current method of obtaining definitive proximal control in major thoracoabdominal trauma, especially in cases of traumatic cardiorespiratory arrest is clamping the descending thoracic aorta via a left anterolateral thoracotomy or clamshell thoracotomy. This is, however, a maximally invasive procedure with the potential for blood-borne transmission. Analysis of data obtained from the *Joint Trauma Theatre Registry* found that one in five severely injured UK combat casualties had a focus of haemorrhage in the abdomen or pelvic junctional region, which was potentially amenable to management by *Rapid Endovascular Balloon Occlusion of Aorta*, resulting in the UK military exploring the utilisation of this adjunct.[25] It was, however, not deployed on *Operations Telic* or *Herrick* and its deployed role is not yet established.

Despite advances in haemostatic adjuncts, the mainstay remains proximal and distal control to achieve haemostasis as part of the DCR paradigm.[26] Casualties who presented to the Role 3 Bastion Hospital with traumatic lower limb amputations frequently had associated abdominal and thoracic injuries, with approximately 40% requiring laparotomy.[27]

Whilst many patients with thoracoabdominal injury will be adequately managed with tube thoracostomy and laparotomy, a significant proportion of patients will require dual cavity surgery. In a review of patients from the war in Lebanon, thoracoabdominal injuries were 1.5 times more lethal than isolated thoracic wounds.[28] In a study of 27 patients with thoracoabdominal trauma treated at the Role 3 hospital in Bastion, 9 out of the 20 (45%) patients who required immediate surgery underwent both thoracotomy and laparotomy. Thus, 74% underwent immediate operation and the remainder were initially managed without surgery. Eleven out of 27 required laparotomy and chest tube, 9/27 required thoracotomy and laparotomy. Two out of five patients presenting in cardiac arrest and undergoing resuscitative thoracotomy (RT) survived. Of the seven patients initially managed conservatively, 4/7 required a laparotomy.[29] Unsurprisingly, multi-regional injury worsens outcomes compared to patients with isolated thoracic or abdominal injury.

THORACIC TRAUMA

In war, a defining characteristic of combat injury is high and early lethality. However, prompt surgical care can save some patients who would otherwise succumb to their injuries. The *Telic* and *Herrick* conflicts demonstrated that 10% of casualties had thoracic injury, with an associated mortality of 10.5%. The mortality was highest in individuals who had a vascular injury or flail chest.[30] A description of the wounding mechanisms associated with an explosive blast event, such as an IED strike, is given in Chapter 10.

In summary, primary injuries result from the impact on the body of the 'blast wave'; which arises almost instantaneously following the detonation but declines in effect with distance. *Secondary* injury is caused by the impact of energised fragments on the body. Fragments that are components of the device are termed primary fragments and fragments of energised environmental debris are termed secondary fragments. The mass movement of air and gaseous combustion products or blast wind is responsible for *tertiary injuries*. *Quaternary blast injury* following an explosion is injury not caused by primary, secondary or tertiary blast effects such as burns and psychological effects. Despite advances in personal protective equipment and medical intervention, primary blast lung injury (PBLI) still continues to be associated with a high mortality rate, with one study reporting that 33 out of 42 vehicle mounted fatalities and 25 out of 32 dismounted fatalities had PBLI.[31] The contribution of primary blast lung injury to the cause of death was not discussed, and significantly lower rates of PBLI are seen in survivors.

Analysis of the recent *Operation Herrick* experience at the Role 3 Facility at Camp Bastion shows that 7856 patients were admitted because of trauma, 826 (10.5%) of whom had thoracic injury; 106/826 (13%) underwent thoracotomy (in a prospective study of stabbed chests at a civilian trauma centre, 14% of patients underwent sternotomy or thoracotomy, and up to 20% of patients with gunshot wounds needed operative care[32,33]; Figure 8.1). In the *Herrick* cohort, the thoracic injury-related mortality was 118/826 (14.3%); 46/106 (43%) patients who underwent thoracotomy died, and

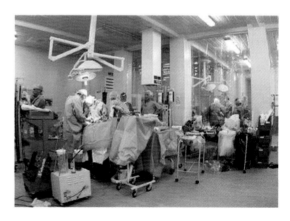

Figure 8.1 Camp Bastion operating theatre in the non-tented facility.

28/30 (93%) died after RT, meaning that the mortality for urgent thoracotomy was 18/76 (23%).[34]

When cardiac injury is proven or highly suspected, the biggest question is *which incision to use*? In cases where the patient is in a state of cardiac arrest or is peri-arrest, the safest option is a clamshell thoracotomy. However, current evidence suggests that this technique does not increase survival in the pre-hospital military setting.[35] RT following combat injury has the best outcomes if it occurs in the emergency department or on admission to hospital.[36,37]

Once the initial operative intervention has taken place, and the patient's physiology has been restored to normal parameters, evidence suggests that military casualties with complex cardiothoracic injuries have a decreased mortality if there is early engagement with specialist cardiothoracic surgeons at Role 4.[38]

A penetrating wound track through the substance of the lung with severe bleeding must be opened and any sources of bleeding and/or air leak controlled with fine monofilament absorbable sutures. Peripherally, a non-anatomic resection can be done; however, pulmonary tractotomy gives the potential for salvaging lung tissue. A proprietary gastrointestinal stapler is placed through the wound track and fired. Bleeding and air leak can be controlled under direct vision and the lung parenchyma can then be approximated with a single running locked suture. The entry and exit wounds of the missile are left open for the egress of air and/or blood and the integrity of the suture line is tested by fully inflating the lung, so that any residual air leaks can be identified and repaired.

In a review of the collective experience of 826 patients with thoracic injury treated by British surgeons in Afghanistan, 503 (61%) were managed non-operatively, 61 (7%) had thoracotomy alone, 217 (26%) had laparotomy alone and 45 (5%) underwent combined thoracotomy and laparotomy. Pneumonectomy was undertaken in only two patients and both survived, although one patient required extracorporeal membrane oxygenation for refractory respiratory failure. Lobectomy was undertaken in 16 patients, of whom 10 survived, 8 patients underwent non-anatomic resections (no survival data presented) and 4 underwent tractotomy with 100% survival.[34]

Resuscitative thoracotomy

No chapter on torso trauma would be complete without mention of RT. RT is performed on trauma patients who either have no central pulse or are peri-arrest. It is a dramatic manoeuvre, intended to facilitate the release of pericardial tamponade, control massive haemorrhage and air leaks or allow open cardiac massage and aortic control, in order to restore spontaneous circulation. RT has been thoroughly evaluated in civilian practice, with the best survival rates being observed in penetrating trauma to the thorax (8.8–33.0%) and the least favourable outcomes noted in blunt injury (0.5–1.4%).[37] In a review of 65 patients undergoing RT after combat injury, 14/65 survived (21.5%). The time from arrest to RT is obviously crucial: 10 patients (15.4%) had an arrest in the field, with no survivors; 29 (44.6%) had an arrest *en route*, with 3 survivors; and 26 (40.0%) had an arrest in the emergency department, with 11 survivors.[37]

In a prospective observational study of patients who experienced cardiorespiratory arrest after military trauma, Tarmey et al.[39] identified 52 patients: the commonest cause of the arrest was exsanguination and 8/52 (15%) survived to discharge. In a subsequent analysis of these data, it was noted that 4/12 patients who underwent RT survived and there were no survivors in the group who did not have RT. Iatrogenic complications of RT were noted, including cardiac and pulmonary lacerations.[40] The lesson from this experience is that surgery offers hope for salvage, but selection of patients must be accurate, and be made as early as possible. If the patient arrests at the scene, unless simple manoeuvres can restore circulation (such as relief of airway obstruction or tension pneumothorax), then they are highly unlikely to survive.

DIAPHRAGMATIC INJURY

Assessment of the diaphragms is a mandatory component of both trauma thoracotomy and laparotomy. Relatively easy to miss (particularly in penetrating injury), a diaphragmatic defect signals multi-compartment trauma and the potential for a significant injury on the other side of the barrier.

At best, an overlooked diaphragmatic injury can present as a later diaphragmatic hernia, sometimes many years after the index injury.

Traumatic diaphragm injuries are more commonly identified on the left side than the right. If identified from the chest, the conventional approach is to add an exploratory laparotomy in order to deal with any abdominal injuries and to repair the defect. This is best done with a heavy, non-absorbable monofilament suture, in two layers. Chest X-ray and CT scanning can be falsely negative in diaphragmatic injury and a suitable index of suspicion is required in all patients. In a cohort of 826 patients from Afghanistan with chest injury, only 6 were identified as having diaphragmatic injury.[34]

ABDOMINAL INJURY

As discussed previously, the major change in military general surgery in recent years has been the widespread adoption of the principles of DCS. In a recent review of the Joint Force Role 3 Hospital in Afghanistan, 94/636 trauma patients (15%) underwent laparotomy. Of these, 72/94 patients (77%) underwent DCS.[41] The goals of primary DCS are to undertake the minimum surgery necessary to save a life by stopping bleeding and controlling leakage from hollow organs, then to identify and document all the injuries, temporarily close the abdominal wall, document what has been done (for example maintaining a record of retained swabs), safely transfer the patient to the ICU and plan for the re-look. Planned re-look usually takes place between 24 and 48 hours after the primary laparotomy.

Combat-related injury to the major intra-abdominal vascular structures is a highly morbid injury pattern and associated with high pre-hospital mortality. There is also a high incidence of occult vascular injury in casualties exposed to blast or ballistic trauma, which can be identified on CT angiography.[42] The priority remains to obtain proximal control and secure the patient's physiology prior to anatomical repair.[43] For junctional trauma involving the pelvis, control may have to be obtained at a more proximal site.[44] In a cohort of patients with abdominal injury treated at the Bastion Hospital,

13/149 intra-abdominal injuries were to named abdominal vessels (6/13 to the mesenteric vessels and 7/13 to the iliac artery or veins).[41]

Selective non-operative management

The selective non-operative management (SNOM) of ballistic abdominal injuries is contentious, particularly in the military setting. This practice is routinely undertaken at civilian trauma centres throughout the world, and the paradigm has been slowly introduced into the military. The exigencies of military practice have traditionally favoured a more liberal approach to abdominal exploration. This paradigm is based on the perception that the risk of intra-abdominal injury is high (because wartime injuries are often caused by high-energy transfer gunshot wounds, which are more destructive) and the belief that the risk of complications from a non-therapeutic laparotomy is low.[45] Evidence from the civilian setting suggests that some of these assumptions are erroneous, and a large retrospective study of civilian abdominal gunshot injuries, both anterior and posterior, has shown that 47% had no clinically significant injuries.[46]

Most patients with pneumoperitoneum after blast injury will require laparotomy; however, as CT is increasingly used to help guide the management of patients with blast injuries, clinicians need to be aware of the phenomenon of pneumoperitoneum without visceral injury and must incorporate the possibility of this diagnosis into their treatment algorithms to enable conservative management in suitable patients.[20]

The key to successful SNOM is identifying the grade of injury in order to determine if it is amenable to this style of management, taking into account physiological parameters and clinical surveillance. Recent studies[47–49] have demonstrated that this method of management is suitable for *selected* casualties in war zones.

Imaging can be used to reduce non-therapeutic laparotomy rates in penetrating abdominal trauma, especially in patients with solid organ trauma who are not physiologically compromised.[50] This is particularly important, as non-therapeutic laparotomies are associated with increased morbidity rates.[45] However, surgeons should approach patients who have sustained ballistic or blast abdominal trauma in the expectation of having to operate, especially in the military setting. Nevertheless, SNOM of ballistic solid organ injury is safe and resource effective, in experienced hands, in a military setting, when it is supported by high-quality cross-sectional imaging and combined with diligent serial examination.[49]

Hollow viscus injury

Modern approaches to colonic injury now closely follow protocols for small bowel injury. The immediately post-World War II vogue for mandatory colostomy for colon injury has given way to an evidence-based policy of primary repair (or resection and primary anastomosis). Since the first randomised trial in 1979, multiple trials and subsequent meta-analyses have confirmed that mortality is not significantly different between diversion and repair, but primary repair is generally associated with lower morbidity.

However, colostomy formation should not be considered a failure, as the *second hit* of anastomotic failure is associated with high mortality rates. If the patient is critically wounded, with multi-visceral injury, high transfusion requirements and ongoing haemodynamic compromise, colostomy remains a good option. However, if there is indirect colonic injury, it is feasible to undertake primary repair either by direct repair or resection and anastomosis.[51]

Rectum

Penetrating rectal injury can be difficult to diagnose, as lower third rectal injuries are, by definition, not within the peritoneal cavity. Any penetrating injury of the lower abdomen, around the hip girdle or to the proximal thigh (including gluteal injury) should be considered to be associated with a rectal injury until proven otherwise. Major pelvic fractures may also be associated with rectal injury. The signature injury from the *Operation Herrick* conflict included destructive anorectal injury, and the four 'D' paradigm was shown still to be effective – *diversion, distal washout, drainage* and *direct repair.*[52]

Open abdomen

In trauma, damage control laparotomy is a well-established technique aimed at prioritising the control of haemorrhage and contamination and the preservation of physiological reserves, over restoration of anatomical congruity. A key part of the damage control laparotomy is deferment of fascial closure until after the visceral injuries have been definitively managed.[53] Over the past two decades, the use of damage control or abbreviated laparotomy has become established as a standard of care for patients with severe abdominal injury. This philosophy prevented abdominal compartment syndrome and facilitated abdominal access until further surgical episodes were no longer required and closure could be achieved. However, it resulted in a variety of temporary and early definitive abdominal closure techniques alongside the solution of planned ventral hernia and the potential for some form of reconstruction.

The management of complex abdominal problems with the *open abdomen* technique has become a routine procedure in surgery. The number of cases treated with an open abdomen has increased dramatically for a number of reasons, including the utilisation of DCS for life-threatening conditions, the recognition and treatment of intra-abdominal hypertension and abdominal compartment syndrome (which can occur in the absence of significant abdominal injury)[54] and new evidence regarding the management of severe intra-abdominal sepsis.[55]

The principal goal is to control both the abdominal contents and the opening that gives access to the abdominal cavity. This also allows the control of intra-abdominal fluid secretion and preservation of the fascia. Methods of achieving this vary from the very basic, cheap and readily available to more expensive techniques. The classical *Bogota bag*[56,57] is a sterile plastic bag used for closure of abdominal wounds. It is generally a sterile, three-litre saline bag that is opened and then sewn to the skin or fascia of the anterior abdominal wall. This is, however, a time-consuming procedure and damages the fascial edges; it has generally been superceded by vacuum closure techniques, either 'home-made' or using proprietary devices.

Topical negative pressure dressings[58] (V.A.C. Via™ and ABThera™) have been successfully utilised in the management of low exudate (V.A.C. Via™) or high exudate open abdominal wounds (ABThera™).[59] The Wittmann Patch is an artificial dressing that serves as a temporary abdominal fascial prosthesis in cases where the abdomen cannot be closed due to abdominal compartment syndrome or because multiple further operations are planned (staged abdominal repair). It consists of a sterile hook and a sterile loop sheet made from propylene.

Reported closure techniques following a damage control laparotomy for trauma have demonstrated that acute component separation and acute mesh repair are alternative techniques to delayed primary closure. Despite robust statistical analysis, Sharrock et al.[53] were unable to conclusively recommend any one particular technique due to study heterogeneity and poverty of outcome reporting. Complex operative strategies have also been employed, with success in the management of the open abdomen, including hybrid procedures, utilising negative pressure dressings, a form of tension sutures, component separation, mesh and a multi-disciplinary team approach.[53,60–63]

PELVIC/PERINEAL INJURY

Physiologically compromised patients with a mechanically unstable pelvic ring fracture continue to be a challenge to manage. These injuries are indicators of high-energy transfer into the casualty's tissues. Studies demonstrate that there should be a high index of suspicion for these injuries as they are commoner than might be initially suspected in both military and civilian trauma victims. In the management of the patient with suspected pelvic injury, it is always useful to define the common injury patterns and their likely mechanisms.

It is important to emphasise that substantial bleeding can occur with all pelvic fracture patterns; therefore, it may be the haemodynamic status of the patient that dictates the clinical strategy for advanced haemostasis rather than the pelvic radiological appearances. The three major bleeding sources that produce life-haemorrhage secondary to pelvic fractures are

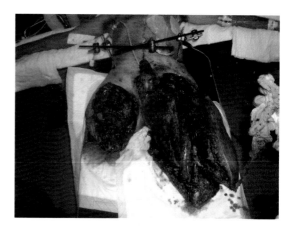

Figure 8.2 Pelvic and peritoneal injury from an IED.

fractured cancellous bone, venous laceration and arterial laceration.[64]

Appropriately sited pelvic binder placement is vital in order to maintain maximum benefit. Bonner et al.[65] suggest that up to 39% of binders are placed too high, resulting in a mean diastasis 2.8 times greater when compared to satisfactorily placed binders; there can be no doubt that high placement is common and results in suboptimal reduction of the pelvic ring.

IED-related lower limb amputation was associated with a high rate of pelvic and torso injury (Figure 8.2).[66] These casualties require early and aggressive resuscitative management, with the emphasis on early proximal control, achievement of haemostasis with a 1:1:1 blood product resuscitation regime[67] and thorough initial debridement. A scoring system has been developed to allow characterisation of the extent of pelvic injury as part of a more complex logistic regression model. The aim is that this will contribute towards a unique trauma scoring system designed to aid surgical teams in predicting fluid requirements and operative timelines.[68]

Pelvic packing has evolved from the principles of DCS. It is a means of rapidly tamponading large raw bleeding areas within the pelvic basin. To minimise the disadvantages of a trans-approach, a more controlled retroperitoneal approach has been described. However, packing can also (and may often) be performed as part of a formal laparotomy.[64]

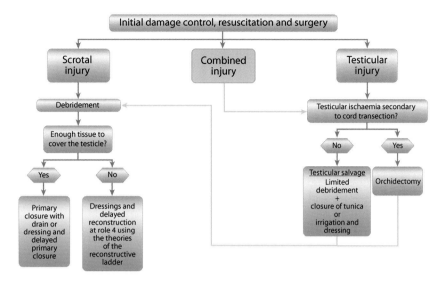

Figure 8.3 Algorithm for management of scrotal and testicular injury.

Major pelvic ring fracture due to blunt trauma resulted in lower genito-urinary injury in 10% of casualties, which subsequently led to major morbidity if unrecognised, an occurrence that is three times more common in military casualties.[69] Concurrent perineal injury with pelvic fracture had a higher rate of mortality when compared to perineal injuries in isolation. In these patients, thorough debridement, immediate faecal diversion and early enteral feeding is advocated.[70]

The signature lower extremity/pelvic blast injury from *Operation Herrick* presented with concurrent perineal injury in a small but significant number of casualties. This had significant consequences, especially if the external genitalia/testicles were affected. The Defence Medical Services, as well as helping to develop ballistic protection and providing a multidisciplinary approach and management algorithm (Figure 8.3),[71] established a pathway for casualties with devastating testicular injury to have their sperm frozen for later fertility therapy.[72–74] This initiative has now successfully resulted in pregnancy.

TRAINING FOR DEPLOYMENT

Deployed consultants for both conflicts comprised both regular clinicians and reservists. The main specialties for torso surgeons were general and vascular surgery. Initially, the *Defence Medical Services* usually deployed one consultant torso surgeon and one senior general surgery trainee, mirrored by a consultant orthopaedic surgeon and a senior orthopaedic trainee. However, as *Operation Herrick* progressed, allied forces also deployed teams to work alongside British personnel.

In the latter stages of *Operation Herrick*, the United States provided, on average, three general surgeons and three orthopaedic surgeons, but no trainees.

Relevant pre-deployment training was mandated by the single services, specialist cadres or academic departments and developed as the operations matured. The initial requirement for full-time military personnel was merely that they had to have passed the *armed services consultant appointment board* and thus were professionally and personally of a sufficient standard to be a military consultant as well as being sufficiently experienced to allow them to deal with the environment to which they were being sent. Exposure to the injury patterns seen on *Operations Telic* and *Herrick* led to a rapid evolution of medical pre-deployment training, which continued to develop for the remainder of the operations.

The pre-deployment requirement for British surgeons ideally included ongoing National Health Service (NHS) work that ensured regular exposure to emergency surgery, but given the differences in both presentation and incidence between military and civilian trauma, attendance at the *Military Operational Surgical Training* (MOST) *Course* became mandatory. Once the *MOST Course* had been completed, each deploying surgical team then attended a three-day training package provided by the Danish Military in which DCR (including surgery) was undertaken on porcine surrogates. After all the technical aspects had been addressed, the whole deploying hospital unit was required to attend HOSPEX at the Defence Medical Services Training Centre. This was undertaken in two one-week blocks. The first week was an assessment phase to determine areas of improvement, and the second was validation, which was undertaken just prior to deployment.

Such training has become even more important in the last decade as surgeons have become more specialised and less 'general' in their skill set. Most surgeons undertake less and less open surgery and the majority maintain their skill set in one cavity only. General surgeons are utilising more laparoscopic techniques and vascular surgeons are undertaking more endovascular work. This makes training packages like the *MOST Course* and the *Danish Trauma Training Course* even more valuable. To further address this need, there is an ongoing drive to divert military personnel to preferred partners in the NHS, which are generally in the main *major trauma centres*, thereby allowing military personnel to participate in the management of major trauma patients as part of their daily routine. This will allow them, at least in part, to maintain the appropriate clinical skill set for deployment.

CONCLUSION

Modern wars have seen a change in wounding mechanism towards the IED, and as a consequence, military medical care has also changed with an emphasis now on DCR and surgery. Military surgeons have always been at the forefront of advances in the care of the injured, and this has certainly been true over the last decade or so of conflicts in the Middle East and Afghanistan. Even in an era of effective body armour, the modern service person remains vulnerable, and injury within the chest or abdomen (the two largest body cavities) confers a high risk of death. Rapid assessment and decisive primary surgery can lead to excellent results, and

military surgeons must maintain the skills to open both the chest and the abdomen and to undertake a temporary or definitive vascular repair, as combat wounding mechanisms do not respect civilian professional surgical boundaries.

REFERENCES

1. Debakey ME. The management of chest wounds. *Coll Rev Int Abst Surg* 1942;74: 203–237.
2. West JP. Chest wounds in battle casualties. *Ann Surg* 1945;121(6):833–839.
3. Debakey ME, Carter BN. Current considerations of war surgery. *Ann Surg* 1945;121(5): 545–563.
4. Molnar TF, Hasse J, Jeyasingham K, Rendeki MS. Changing dogmas: History of development in treatment modalities of traumatic pneumothorax, hemothorax, and posttraumatic empyema thoracis. *Ann Thorac Surg* 2004;77(1):372–378.
5. Rignault DP. Abdominal trauma in war. *World J Surg* 1992;16(5):940–946.
6. Bellamy RF. History of surgery for penetrating chest trauma. *Chest Surg Clin N Am* 2000;10(1):55–70, viii.
7. McNamara JJ, Messersmith JK, Dunn RA, Molot MD, Stremple JF. Thoracic injuries in combat casualties in Vietnam. *Ann Thorac Surg* 1970;10(5):389–401.
8. Bird SM, Fairweather CB. Military fatality rates (by cause) in Afghanistan and Iraq: A measure of hostilities. *Int J Epidemiol* 2007; 36(4):841–846.
9. Hodgetts TJ, Mahoney PF, Kirkman E. Damage control resuscitation. *J R Army Med Corps* 2007;153(4):299–300.
10. Midwinter MJ. Damage control surgery in the era of damage control resuscitation. *J R Army Med Corps* 2009;155(4):323–326.
11. Fries CA, Penn-Barwell J, Tai NR, Hodgetts TJ, Midwinter MJ, Bowley DM. Management of intestinal injury in deployed UK hospitals. *J R Army Med Corps* 2011;157(4):370–373.
12. Lamb CM, MacGoey P, Navarro AP, Brooks AJ. Damage control surgery in the era of damage control resuscitation. *Br J Anaesth* 2014;113(2):242–249.

13. Morrison JJ, Dickson EJ, Jansen JO, Midwinter MJ. Utility of admission physiology in the surgical triage of isolated ballistic battlefield torso trauma. *J Emerg Trauma Shock* 2012;5(3):233–237.

14. Rotondo MF, Schwab CW, McGonigal MD et al. 'Damage control': An approach for improved survival in exsanguinating penetrating abdominal injury. *J Trauma* 1993;35(3):375–382; discussion 82–83.

15. Smith JE, Midwinter M, Lambert AW. Avoiding cavity surgery in penetrating torso trauma: The role of the computed tomography scan. *Ann R Coll Surg Engl* 2010;92(6): 486–488.

16. Smith IM, Naumann DN, Marsden ME, Ballard M, Bowley DM. Scanning and war: Utility of FAST and CT in the assessment of battlefield abdominal trauma. *Ann Surg* 2015;262(2):389–396.

17. Singleton JA, Gibb IE, Hunt NC, Bull AM, Clasper JC. Identifying future 'unexpected' survivors: A retrospective cohort study of fatal injury patterns in victims of improvised explosive devices. *BMJ Open* 2013;3(8).

18. Lehman RA Jr., Huddleston P, Yaszemski M. Axial spine injuries in the current conflicts in Iraq and Afghanistan. *J Am Acad Orthop Surg* 2012;20(Suppl 1):S13–S17.

19. Bird JH, Luke DP, Ward NJ, Stewart MP, Templeton PA. Management of unstable cervical spine injuries in southern Iraq during OP TELIC. *J R Army Med Corps* 2005; 151(3):179–185.

20. Bowley DM, Gillingham S, Mercer S, Schrager JJ, West A. Pneumoperitoneum without visceral trauma: An under-recognised phenomenon after blast injury? *J R Army Med Corps* 2013;159(4):312–313.

21. Bowley DM, Jansen JO, Nott D, Sapsford W, Streets CG, Tai NR. Difficult decisions in the surgical care of military casualties with major torso trauma. *J R Army Med Corps* 2011;157(3 Suppl 1):S324–S333.

22. Kisat M, Morrison JJ, Hashmi ZG, Efron DT, Rasmussen TE, Haider AH. Epidemiology and outcomes of non-compressible torso hemorrhage. *J Surg Res* 2013;184(1): 414–421.

23. Morrison JJ, Stannard A, Rasmussen TE, Jansen JO, Tai NR, Midwinter MJ. Injury pattern and mortality of noncompressible torso hemorrhage in UK combat casualties. *J Trauma Acute Care Surg* 2013;75(2 Suppl 2):S263–S268.

24. Stannard A, Morrison JJ, Scott DJ, Ivatury RA, Ross JD, Rasmussen TE. The epidemiology of noncompressible torso hemorrhage in the wars in Iraq and Afghanistan. *J Trauma Acute Care Surg* 2013;74(3): 830–834.

25. Morrison JJ, Ross JD, Rasmussen TE, Midwinter MJ, Jansen JO. Resuscitative endovascular balloon occlusion of the aorta: A gap analysis of severely injured UK combat casualties. *Shock* 2014;41(5):388–393.

26. Morrison JJ, Rasmussen TE. Noncompressible torso hemorrhage: A review with contemporary definitions and management strategies. *Surg Clin North Am* 2012;92(4):843–858, vii.

27. Morrison JJ, Hunt N, Midwinter M, Jansen J. Associated injuries in casualties with traumatic lower extremity amputations caused by improvised explosive devices. *Br J Surg* 2012;99(3):362–366.

28. Zakharia AT. Cardiovascular and thoracic battle injuries in the Lebanon War. Analysis of 3,000 personal cases. *J Thorac Cardiovasc Surg* 1985;89(5):723–733.

29. Morrison JJ, Midwinter MJ, Jansen JO. Ballistic thoracoabdominal injury: Analysis of recent military experience in Afghanistan. *World J Surg* 2011;35(6):1396–1401.

30. Keneally R, Szpisjak D. Thoracic trauma in Iraq and Afghanistan. *J Trauma Acute Care Surg* 2013;74(5):1292–1297.

31. Singleton JA, Gibb IE, Bull AM, Mahoney PF, Clasper JC. Primary blast lung injury prevalence and fatal injuries from explosions: Insights from postmortem computed tomographic analysis of 121 improvised explosive device fatalities. *J Trauma Acute Care Surg* 2013;75(2 Suppl 2):S269–S274.

32. Demetriades D, Rabinowitz B, Markides N. Indications for thoracotomy in stab injuries of the chest: A prospective study of 543 patients. *Br J Surg* 1986;73(11):888–890.

33. Demetriades D, Velmahos GC. Penetrating injuries of the chest: Indications for operation. *Scand J Surg* 2002;91(1):41–45.

34. Poon H, Morrison JJ, Apodaca AN, Khan MA, Garner JP. The UK military experience of thoracic injury in the wars in Iraq and Afghanistan. *Injury* 2013;44(9): 1165–1170.

35. Morrison JJ, Mellor A, Midwinter M, Mahoney PF, Clasper JC. Is pre-hospital thoracotomy necessary in the military environment? *Injury* 2011;42(5):469–473.

36. Morrison JJ, Poon H, Rasmussen TE, Khan MA, Garner JP. Re: Traumatic cardiorespiratory arrest on the battlefield. *J Trauma Acute Care Surg* 2013;75(2):343–345.

37. Morrison JJ, Poon H, Rasmussen TE et al. Resuscitative thoracotomy following wartime injury. *J Trauma Acute Care Surg* 2013;74(3):825–829.

38. Senanayake EL, Poon H, Graham TR, Midwinter MJ. UK specialist cardiothoracic management of thoracic injuries in military casualties sustained in the wars in Iraq and Afghanistan. *Eur J Cardiothorac Surg* 2014;45(6):e202–3207.

39. Tarmey NT, Park CL, Bartels OJ, Konig TC, Mahoney PF, Mellor AJ. Outcomes following military traumatic cardiorespiratory arrest: A prospective observational study. *Resuscitation* 2011;82(9):1194–1197.

40. Bhangu A, Nepogodiev D, Bowley DM. Outcomes following military traumatic cardiorespiratory arrest: The role of surgery in resuscitation. *Resuscitation* 2013;84(1):e23–e24.

41. Smith IM, Beech ZK, Lundy JB, Bowley DM. A prospective observational study of abdominal injury management in contemporary military operations: Damage control laparotomy is associated with high survivability and low rates of fecal diversion. *Ann Surg* 2015;261(4):765–773.

42. Watchorn J, Miles R, Moore N. The role of CT angiography in military trauma. *Clin Radiol* 2013;68(1):39–46.

43. Tai NR, Dickson EJ. Military junctional trauma. *J R Army Med Corps* 2009;155(4): 285–292.

44. Walker NM, Eardley W, Clasper JC. UK combat-related pelvic junctional vascular injuries 2008–2011: Implications for future intervention. *Injury* 2014;45(10):1585–1589.

45. Morrison JJ, Poon H, Garner J, Midwinter MJ, Jansen JO. Nontherapeutic laparotomy in combat casualties. *J Trauma Acute Care Surg* 2012;73(6 Suppl 5):S479–S482.

46. Velmahos GC, Demetriades D, Toutouzas KG et al. Selective nonoperative management in 1,856 patients with abdominal gunshot wounds: Should routine laparotomy still be the standard of care? *Ann Surg* 2001;234(3):395–402; discussion 403.

47. Jansen JO, Torso Trauma Working Group. Selective non-operative management of abdominal injury in the military setting. *J R Army Med Corps* 2011;157(3):237–242.

48. Mossadegh S, Midwinter M, Sapsford W, Tai N. Military treatment of splenic injury in the era of non-operative management. *J R Army Med Corps* 2013;159(2):110–113.

49. Wood AM, Trimble K, Louden MA, Jansen J. Selective non-operative management of ballistic abdominal solid organ injury in the deployed military setting. *J R Army Med Corps* 2010;156(1):21–24.

50. Morrison JJ, Clasper JC, Gibb I, Midwinter M. Management of penetrating abdominal trauma in the conflict environment: The role of computed tomography scanning. *World J Surg* 2011;35(1):27–33.

51. Webster C, Mercer S, Schrager J, Carrell TW, Bowley D. Indirect colonic injury after military wounding: A case series. *J Trauma* 2011; 71(5):1475–1477.

52. Brogden TG, Garner JP. Anorectal injury in pelvic blast. *J R Army Med Corps* 2013;159(Suppl 1):i26–i31.

53. Sharrock AE, Barker T, Yuen HM, Rickard R, Tai N. Management and closure of the open abdomen after damage control laparotomy for trauma. A systematic review and meta-analysis. *Injury* 2016;47(2): 296–306.

54. Lamb CM, Berry JE, DeMello WF, Cox C. Secondary abdominal compartment syndrome after military wounding. *J R Army Med Corps* 2010;156(2):102–103.

55. Demetriades D. Total management of the open abdomen. *Int Wound J* 2012;9(Suppl 1): 17–24.

56. Myers JA, Latenser BA. Nonoperative progressive "Bogota bag" closure after abdominal decompression. *Am Surg* 2002;68(11): 1029–1030.

57. Kirshtein B, Roy-Shapira A, Lantsberg L, Mizrahi S. Use of the "Bogota bag" for temporary abdominal closure in patients with secondary peritonitis. *Am Surg* 2007;73(3): 249–252.

58. Perez Dominguez L, Pardellas Rivera H, Caceres Alvarado N, Lopez Saco A, Rivo Vazquez A, Casal Nunez E. Vacuum assisted closure in open abdomen and deferred closure: Experience in 23 patients. *Cir Esp* 2012;90(8):506–512.

59. Fitzgerald JE, Gupta S, Masterson S, Sigurdsson HH. Laparostomy management using the ABThera open abdomen negative pressure therapy system in a grade IV open abdomen secondary to acute pancreatitis. *Int Wound J* 2012;10(2): 138–144.

60. Burlew CC, Moore EE, Biffl WL, Bensard DD, Johnson JL, Barnett CC. One hundred percent fascial approximation can be achieved in the postinjury open abdomen with a sequential closure protocol. *J Trauma Acute Care Surg* 2012;72(1):235–241.

61. Dietz UA, Wichelmann C, Wunder C et al. Early repair of open abdomen with a tailored two-component mesh and conditioning vacuum packing: A safe alternative to the planned giant ventral hernia. *Hernia* 2012;16(4):451–460.

62. Arul GS, Sonka BJ, Lundy JB, Rickard RF, Jeffery S. Managing combat laparostomy: Author's reply. *J R Army Med Corps* 2015;161(4):352.

63. Lamb CM, Garner JP. Managing combat laparostomy. *J R Army Med Corps* 2015;161(4): 351–352.

64. Adams SA. Pelvic ring injuries in the military environment. *J R Army Med Corps* 2009; 155(4):293–296.

65. Bonner TJ, Eardley WG, Newell N et al. Accurate placement of a pelvic binder improves reduction of unstable fractures of the pelvic ring. *J Bone Joint Surg Br* 2011;93(11):1524–1528.

66. Cross AM, Davis C, Penn-Barwell J, Taylor DM, De Mello WF, Matthews JJ. The incidence of pelvic fractures with traumatic lower limb amputation in modern warfare due to improvised explosive devices. *J R Nav Med Serv* 2014;100(2):152–156.

67. Jansen JO, Thomas GO, Adams SA et al. Early management of proximal traumatic lower extremity amputation and pelvic injury caused by improvised explosive devices (IEDs). *Injury* 2012;43(7):976–979.

68. Mossadegh S, Midwinter M, Parker P. Developing a cumulative anatomic scoring system for military perineal and pelvic blast injuries. *J R Army Med Corps* 2013; 159(Suppl 1):i40–i44.

69. Durrant JJ, Ramasamy A, Salmon MS, Watkin N, Sargeant I. Pelvic fracture-related urethral and bladder injury. *J R Army Med Corps* 2013;159(Suppl 1):i32–i39.

70. Mossadegh S, Tai N, Midwinter M, Parker P. Improvised explosive device related pelvi-perineal trauma: Anatomic injuries and surgical management. *J Trauma Acute Care Surg* 2012;73(2 Suppl 1):S24–S31.

71. Uppal L, Anderson P, Evriviades D. Complex lower genitourinary reconstruction following combat-related injury. *J R Army Med Corps* 2013;159(Suppl 1):i49–i51.

72. Davendra MS, Webster CE, Kirkman-Brown J, Mossadegh S, Whitbread T, Genitourinary Working Group. Blast injury to the perineum. *J R Army Med Corps* 2013;159(Suppl 1): i1–i3.

73. Sharma DM, Bowley DM. Immediate surgical management of combat-related injury to the external genitalia. *J R Army Med Corps* 2013;159(Suppl 1):i18–i20.

74. Sharma DM, Genitourinary Working Group. The management of genitourinary war injuries: A multidisciplinary consensus. *J R Army Med Corps* 2013;159(Suppl 1):i57–i59.

9

Limb trauma

INTRODUCTION

Limb trauma has always provided a high surgical workload in war. The Iraq and Afghanistan conflicts were no different, with surgical teams frequently at capacity, both on deployment and in the management of repatriated patients in the United Kingdom. This chapter will review advances in the management of often extremely complex upper and lower limb wounds arising from *Operations Telic* and *Herrick* at the different echelons of care, concluding with a review of current and future research areas.

LIMB TRAUMA MANAGEMENT AS A MULTI-SPECIALTY DISCIPLINE

The orthopaedic and plastic surgery cadres deployed together as part of the initial entry operation into Iraq on board Royal Fleet Auxiliary (RFA) Argus, the Primary Casualty Receiving Facility. *202 Field Hospital* was active from Day 1 in Kuwait, and a field hospital (initially *34 Field Hospital*) was quickly established at the *Shaibah Operating Base*, where it remained between 2003 and 2007, when it moved to Basrah *Air Station* and remained until withdrawal of the main element of UK forces.

The initial hospital facility in Afghanistan was at the US *Bagram Air Base*. The United Kingdom then set up a Role 2 Hospital at Camp Bastion in Helmand Province with singleton general and orthopaedic surgeons. As the tempo increased from 2007 onwards, this hospital increased in size, with plastic surgeons joining the deployed surgical cadre from 2008. The hospital was further reinforced with multinational personnel from the United States,

Denmark, the Czech Republic and Estonia, as the deploying forces in Helmand Province increased to combat the Taliban within what became known as the 'Green Zone'. At the height of operations, multiple orthopaedic and general surgeons were deployed together, at times four of each specialty. As a coalition force, provision was made for neurosurgery, ophthalmology and maxillo-facial surgical input across the area of operations.

On return to the United Kingdom, all casualties were initially seen and managed in Birmingham, first at *Selly Oak Hospital* and then from 2010 at the *Queen Elizabeth Hospital*, where highly specialised teams provided multi-disciplinary care.

CLINICAL CHALLENGES

At the outset of the conflicts in 2003, 83% of battle casualties sustained injury to an extremity.[1] An amputation rate of 16% is quoted, and these figures are supported by experience from *International Committee of the Red Cross* (ICRC) hospitals in Asia and Africa.[2] A much larger cohort of casualties was reviewed over a five-year period using the *US Joint Theater Register*, which includes UK and US casualties. This investigation[3] reviewed orthopaedic wounds sustained by service personnel deployed to Iraq and Afghanistan from 2005 to 2009. Seventy-seven percent of all casualties sustained a musculoskeletal wound, with amputations representing 6% of all combat injuries. The incidence of musculoskeletal combat casualties was 3.06 per 1000 deployed personnel per year, with fractures occurring in 3.42 per 1000 and soft tissue wounds being most common (4.04 per 1000). In this study, most musculoskeletal wounds were caused by blast mechanisms, as were nearly all the traumatic amputations.

Complex lower limb injury caused by *improvised explosive devices* (IEDs) became the signature wounding pattern of the conflict in Afghanistan. A retrospective analysis looked at a six-month period between September 2009 and April 2010. Seventy-seven consecutive patients presenting with traumatic amputations due to blast injury were reviewed.[4] In total 22% of patients who had a traumatic amputation also had an associated pelvic fracture. However, if the casualty had sustained bilateral transfemoral amputations, which was the commonest configuration in the cohort reviewed, the rate of associated pelvic fracture increased to 39%.

The initial management at point of wounding was designed to ensure haemorrhage control. The application of a pelvic binder became automatic in those casualties with a lower extremity injury following on from the Cross review.[4] The extent of initial interventions delivered by the combat medical technicians on the ground and the subsequent *Medical Emergency Response Team* is discussed in Chapter 3. Rapid transfer to a hospital facility, usually within an hour of wounding, became the norm, and thus, survival of massively injured personnel became expected, rather than exceptional.

The reception in the emergency department delivered by a consultant-led trauma team meant that the patient was soon stabilised for computed tomography (CT) scanning or the decision was made to move immediately into the operating theatre. The use of the trauma CT 'pan-scan' became invaluable in delineating the full extent of the injury patterns, and only those casualties with uncontrollable haemorrhage or arriving in traumatic cardiac arrest had their trauma CT scan delayed until they were sufficiently physiologically stable. Appropriate antibiotic therapy was given if it had not already been delivered either by those on the ground at point of injury or during the rapid transit to the hospital facility. This combination of pre-hospital and initial management, now described as the *damage control resuscitation/surgical continuum*, had the aim of rapidly restoring the patient to good physiological status, including normothermia and normal or near normal coagulation, as well as a normal (or near normal) lactate. Surgical intervention could then proceed, with the aim of achieving debridement and stabilisation of any extremity injury and re-vascularisation of any ischaemic limb, as well as primary surgery of other cavities. As the conflicts proceeded, the techniques for achieving physiological stability improved, and by the end of the conflicts, the balance required between surgical intervention and resuscitation was so frequently practiced that it became rare to have to call a halt to the primary surgery. However, on occasion, there was the requirement to maintain a balance between surgical completeness and resuscitation when the injury severity was extreme, and a surgical pause, or an interruption of several hours, occurred to allow the patient to achieve physiological stability.

For the most severely injured casualties, repatriation to the United Kingdom was undertaken rapidly, usually between 18 and 36 hours post injury. Transfer via multiple flight stages was required, with journeys taking up to 18 hours to complete. On arrival at the *Royal Centre for Defence Medicine* (RCDM), part of the Birmingham University Hospitals National Health Service Trust, casualties were immediately assessed by a multidisciplinary team and frequently returned to the operating theatre within one or two hours of arrival. This allowed reassessment of all injuries and management plans to be formulated.

ORTHOPAEDIC BLAST INJURY

Conflict in the Middle East saw a change in the warfare tactics identified in previous hostilities. The use of the IED became typical,[5] resulting in a well-documented change in the observed wounding patterns. There was a marked increase in casualties with severe lower leg injuries and associated pelvic trauma.[6] A review of UK military casualties with amputations over eight years of conflict compared those from an early time period (2003–2008) with a later one (2008–2010) and showed significant differences in the nature of the injuries, the number of multiple amputations and soft tissue perineal wounds, and a significantly higher injury severity score (ISS) in the later period.[7] This study not only clearly illustrates the sizeable burden of limb trauma in both conflicts but also demonstrates differing injury patterns with significant implications for logistical and medical support.

The term *blast injury* is given to the various effects that an explosion has on the human body.[8] This subject is covered in detail in Chapter 10; therefore, only a brief summary is given here. Following detonation of an explosive in air, a shock front (a wave travelling in excess of the speed of sound in that medium) travels away from the centre of the charge. The initial shock wave following an explosion is a special form of high-pressure stress wave, with an effectively instantaneous wave front.[9] The surrounding atmosphere is heated by the passage of this shock wave and then forced outwards and compressed by the expansion of gases formed within the explosion: the *blast wave*. Behind this blast wave are the products of the explosion; gas and fragments of debris. The blast wave travels supersonically before decaying into an acoustic wave as it loses velocity and magnitude. If the explosion is in the open and unconfined, then a simple waveform is produced. This simple wave has an almost instantaneous rise to peak overpressure, which then declines exponentially through ambient pressure to sub-atmospheric pressure, corresponding to the rarefied zone behind the blast front. Overpressure lasts for approximately 10 milliseconds, with the sub-atmospheric pressure zone lasting for considerably longer. Confinement of the explosion within a building or underwater produces a complex blast wave pattern containing multiple overpressure peaks, due to reflections of the blast wave. The biological effects of the blast wave depend on the peak overpressure and its duration.

Primary blast injury relates to the interaction of the initial shock wave with the body. Gas-containing structures such as the ear, lungs and gastrointestinal tract are at particular risk, and solid organs, including the skin, are more resistant. Secondary blast injury occurs as a result of the blast wind and is caused by bomb fragments and other projectiles energised by the explosion. Tertiary blast injury occurs as the result of gross body displacement. Traditionally, it has been thought that the combination of primary blast injury from the shock wave and tertiary injury due to body displacement leads to limb avulsion injuries. This has now been questioned and is discussed on page 199. The term *quaternary blast injury* is given to a miscellaneous collection of all other mechanisms.

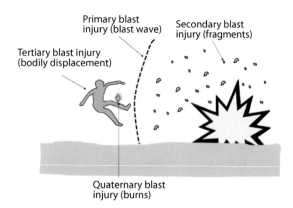

Figure 9.1 Demonstrating the modes of blast injury. (From Stapley SA, Cannon LB, *Curr Orthop* 2006;20(5):322–332.)

These include thermal injury to exposed skin caused by the radiant and convective heat of the explosion, methaemoglobinaemia, acute septicaemic melioidosis and psychological sequelae. This classification is shown in Figure 9.1.[8]

The IED encompasses a range of different explosive types.[10] In Iraq, the majority of IEDs were of the explosively formed projectile type. In Afghanistan, the IED was characterised by a high explosive content with little primary fragmentation material.[11] In the latter case, the resulting injuries were mainly the consequence of the primary blast effects and secondary fragments and typically resulted in extensively contaminated bilateral and very proximal traumatic lower extremity amputation, perineal soft tissue injuries and pelvic fractures.

The complex nature of these extremity injuries meant that a new classification system was needed to aid communication between clinicians and to assist evaluation of treatment and outcomes. As yet, this system (the *Camp Bastion system*) has not been used extensively, but in the future, it may assist in consideration of the types of injury observed. The classification was developed by a panel of surgeons with deployed experience[12] and is shown in Table 9.1.

Associated injuries are indicated by suffixes, which are applied to the main numerical injury class. For example, segmental injury is defined as the presence of potentially viable tissue distal to the proximal injury and denoted by the suffix 'S'

Table 9.1 Camp Bastion classification of lower limb injury caused by IED – the most proximal extent – and associated injuries recognised and denoted by the suffixes

Class of limb injury	Description
1	Injury confined to foot
2	Injury involving lower leg permitting effective below knee tourniquet application
3	Injury involving proximal lower leg or thigh, permitting effective above knee tourniquet application
4	Proximal thigh injury, preventing effective tourniquet application
5	Any injury with buttock involvement

Suffixes	Associated injuries
A	Intraperitoneal abdomen
B	Genitalia and perineum
C	Pelvic ring
S	Potentially viable tissue distal to the proximal injury

demonstrated in Table 9.1. The panel identified 179 IED-related lower limb injuries in 103 consecutive casualties from November 2010 to February 2011. Sixty-nine per cent of casualties had a traumatic amputation and 74% suffered significant bilateral lower limb injuries, with 49% having bilateral lower leg amputations. The spectrum of lower limb injuries recorded during the validation of this classification confirmed that the injury burden from IED-related mechanisms was extremely high, with most casualties sustaining traumatic amputations through or above the knee. Most IED-related injuries occurred in dismounted personnel whilst patrolling on foot. However, it was recognised that in-vehicle extremity injury also resulted in significant morbidity and mortality.[13]

A comparison of mounted and dismounted casualties demonstrated that a higher proportion of lower limb fractures were seen in the enclosed/mounted group (81% versus 52%), with an increased incidence of tibia, fibular and foot fractures being observed.[14]

EXTREMITY GUNSHOT WOUND

Although blast was the commonest mechanism of injury observed in both conflicts, gunshot wounds (GSWs) were the second most frequent. As yet unpublished data from Stevenson et al. has confirmed the fact that the UK burden of GSWs in the 12 years of conflict from 2003 to 2014 was significant. There were 717 casualties as a result of GSWs, of whom 540 survived. Of the survivors, 69% had GSW extremity injuries (43% lower limb and 26% upper limb). Within the UK *Joint Theatre Trauma Registry* (JTTR) database, this accounts for 2815 separate entries and, amongst the survivors, 2351 surgical episodes, either in a deployed hospital facility or at RCDM Birmingham. Overall, there was a mean length of stay per casualty of 2.3 days in the deployed facility and 14 days at RCDM.

NON-BATTLE INJURY

Non-battle extremity injury remains a significant cause of morbidity. The operational environment encourages sporting activities of all descriptions, particularly amongst those situated at the main deployed operating bases, who are not involved in direct combat-related activities. A review of primary care casualties aeromedically evacuated from Afghanistan to the United Kingdom between 1 January 2009 and 31 December 2010 found that musculoskeletal causes accounted for 183 out of 387 patients, with lower extremity, upper-extremity and spinal problems being identified.[15] Non-freezing cold injuries were also a cause of extremity injury. A review of cold-related injuries sustained between 1 October 2011 and 30 March 2012 recorded by the *UK Medical Group Environmental Health Team* found 14 patients with 13 non-freezing cold injuries and two hypothermic injuries. Of these, the feet were affected in seven cases, and the hands in six cases. Five patients were of African ethnic descent.[16]

In summary, extremity trauma, either combat related or non-combat related, remains common in war, and the recent conflicts reinforce the necessity for the orthopaedic/extremity surgeon to be available close to the conflict zone. Blast, GSW, road traffic collision, sporting and climate-induced injury patterns were observed throughout *Operations Telic* and *Herrick*.

CLINICAL ADVANCES

Haemorrhage control

Haemorrhage from extremity trauma is a well-recognised cause of battlefield mortality.[17] The focus on haemorrhage control at point of wounding has made a significant impact on reducing the number of battlefield deaths caused by exsanguination. However, at the start of the conflict, 40% of battlefield deaths were still attributable to haemorrhage.[18] Initial management protocols at point of injury within the UK Military shifted from the *ABC* to *<C>ABC* to reflect the significance of catastrophic haemorrhage on battlefield survival and the vital importance immediate haemorrhage control has on survival to an enhanced medical treatment facility.[19]

Ninety-four per cent of deaths occur within the first 30 minutes of injury, a significant proportion, as discussed earlier, from exsanguination. Jacobs et al.[12] reported that 78% of casualties with a traumatic amputation from an IED had injuries that were potentially controllable by a tourniquet.

All UK troops have carried a tourniquet since April 2006. Currently, the issued tourniquet is the *Combat Application Tourniquet, C-A-T*™ (Phil Durango LLC, USA). An extensive review of the use of the tourniquet in combat was undertaken by Brodie et al.[20] in 2007. This concentrated on the prevalence of use in combat trauma. The contribution to lives saved and complications of its use were identified. Between February 2003 and September 2007, the UK JTTR identified 70 patients who had tourniquets applied: 61/70 survived their injuries, and 64/70 had the tourniquet applied after April 2006 when the device became an individualised item of kit. Three complications were noted: two were cases of compartment syndrome secondary to a venous tourniquet, although any period of extremity ischaemia results in significant swelling and increases the potential for compartment syndrome anyway. However, it was considered that the venous tourniquet effect had occurred due to the application over a trouser pocket containing a book. This led to an immediate training refinement. The third complication was an ulnar nerve palsy in an upper extremity where there had been a significant GSW injury. The US experience in both Vietnam and Somalia suggested that 7% of combat deaths could have been prevented by the application of a pre-hospital tourniquet.[21] Thus, the use of the C-A-T™ device has been comprehensively embraced by both the US and the UK Armed Services. Despite the obvious benefits, concern has been expressed that the resulting temporary ischaemia[22] and injuries, combined with an open fracture, are associated with a significant complication rate and later risk of amputation.[23] A matched cohort study was performed reviewing members of UK Armed Forces who sustained severe limb-threatening injuries in Iraq and Afghanistan, based on the presence or absence of a pre-hospital tourniquet.[24] Nineteen patients out of a cohort of 22 with a pre-hospital tourniquet had at least one complication compared to the 15 patients out of a similar cohort of 22 with no tourniquet applied. Superficial infection was the most common complication, occurring in 50%, and there was no difference in incidence between the two groups. This is not surprising given the nature of the highly contaminated military wounds. Of more concern is the significant incidence of major complications after tourniquet use, in particular the deep infection rate of 32% in comparison to 4.5%. The study is of small numbers, and other factors may have contributed to the problems, such as implant choice for fracture fixation and also the timing and method of wound closure. A higher infection rate following vascular injury resulting in temporary ischaemia has been reported in the literature,[25] and this may be an explanation of the increased infection rate with tourniquet application.

Ultimately, the widespread use of the tourniquet within the UK military during the recent conflicts has undoubtedly saved lives. A study by Kragh et al. in 2009 demonstrated improved survival when a tourniquet was applied. Furthermore, no limb has been lost solely due to the application of a tourniquet.[26] However, it must be remembered that tourniquets may have significant complications and there remains a need to continue to prospectively review their use, to ensure that continual, accurate training is delivered to frontline personnel in their correct use, and to monitor the risk/benefit ratio.

Debridement

Adequate wound debridement and irrigation are fundamental to the initial management of complex extremity trauma. Debridement consists of wound edge excision, appropriate wound extensions, excision of unequivocally dead tissue, removal of contamination and extensive irrigation. The use of antiseptic solutions to irrigate viable but vulnerable tissue has great potential to cause further tissue destruction and thus is not recommended; normal saline is being used in preference, delivered by gravity or hand-powered devices, such as a standard giving set.[27,28] High-pressure lavage devices should not be used as there is evidence to suggest that contamination particles may be forced into the medullary canals of long bones and further into the tissue planes. If normal saline is not available, then clean water, such as bottled water, may be utilised as a substitute. Blast injuries involve significant destruction of tissue that may still be attached, but not viable, together with gross contamination by dirt, vegetation, and clothing driven deep along tissue planes. It has been found that contamination and debris driven along such planes cannot be easily washed away and excision of the epimysium is frequently required. Tissue of dubious viability should be excised unless it is part of a vital structure, the removal of which would cause significant morbidity; consideration should then be given to the probability that the structure will recover given the correct conditions and management, and a judgement call must be made. No attempt to fashion formal flaps should be made at the initial debridement, either with regard to bone or soft tissue.

A joint meeting of the *Limb Trauma* and *Wounds Working Groups* resulted in the establishment of 29 consensus recommendations for the conduct of initial extremity war wound debridement.[29] These represent the consensus opinion of orthopaedic, plastic and vascular surgeons, as well as nursing officers, from across the *Defence Medical Services* who were regularly deploying to the conflicts at the time of publication and provide useful guidance on the recommended best practices in wound debridement within the UK military. The working group agreed with the spirit of the statement from the ICRC that 'the best antibiotic is good surgery'.[30]

However, in addition to a good debridement, early administration of antibiotics is essential to reduce the risk of life-threatening infections from organisms such as Clostridia and Streptococci. The recommendations of the working group are listed in Table 9.2.

All wounds must be examined and potentially explored, but the working group agreed with the ICRC that certain low-energy soft tissue wounds can be managed with less aggressive techniques.[29] A low-energy narrow channel wound characterised by entry and exit wounds of minimal size, which has no wound cavity, no significant swelling of the intervening tissue and no other signs of injury to important structures, may be treated in a more conservative manner. It is satisfactory to excise the entrance and exit wounds and irrigate the connecting channel. Laying open the complete length of the connecting bullet track is not required.

Small superficial wounds that do not penetrate the deep fascia do not require any formal surgical intervention. These wounds can be scrubbed clean, irrigated with normal saline and left to heal by secondary intention, with consideration of the use of oral antibiotics and regular dressing changes. A review of 450 cases of GSWs in UK personnel[31] showed that high-energy firearms do not necessarily cause high-energy wounds. Simple GSWs to the limbs with no associated neurovascular or bony damage do not need to be laid open with full exploration of the tract. The wound can be treated simply with drainage and then can either heal by secondary intention or by delayed primary closure. High-energy firearms can cause simple wounds if there is low energy transfer to the tissues and the bullet passes straight through the body (*through and through* wounding). These wounds require minimal surgical intervention. In contrast, when there is high energy transfer to the wound, demonstrated by the presence of bullet fragments or fracture of a bone, then these wounds need full surgical exploration and debridement. GSWs should therefore be assessed according to the level of energy transferred, and limb wounds without the features of high energy transfer do not require extensive exploration. The assessment and identification of wounds that may be left without extensive exploration are skills that are learnt with increasing experience in military surgery. Research is currently being undertaken

Table 9.2 Consensus wound debridement recommendations

Pre-operative principles

1   Debridement of limb wounds should be undertaken as soon as practical.
2   Debridement of limb wounds should be undertaken in an operating theatre.
3   Pre-operative washing with copious volumes of warmed detergent solution is essential.
4   Pre- and post-debridement photography is an essential part of the patient record.

Surgical technique

5   Macroscopically nonviable tissue should be excised.
6   Traumatised but potentially viable tissue may be left if serial debridement is guaranteed.
7   It is not necessary to excise the skin edges in the absence of macroscopic injury.
8   Undermining skin by over generous excision of fat/fascia is to be avoided.
9   Fasciotomy should be along the full length of the muscle compartment.
10   Adequate skin bridges should be preserved between fasciotomy incisions and between traumatic
     wounds and fasciotomy incisions.
11   Wound extension dissection should be in the sub-fascial plane.
12   The use of diathermy is not recommended other than for control of bleeding.
13   Non-contractile muscle of altered consistency should be excised.
14   Formal muscle flaps should not be fashioned at the initial debridement.
15   Suture tagging of divided nerve and tendons should not be performed.
16   The status of vital structures encountered during debridement should be carefully documented.
17   It is not necessary to locate neurovascular structures solely in order to document their status.
18   Primary reconstruction of tendons and nerves should not be performed at the initial debridement.
19   Contaminated bone fragments with a very tenuous or no soft tissue attachment should be excised.

Irrigation

20   Irrigation should be performed with warmed sterile physiological saline where available.
21   Irrigation should be performed using a low-pressure delivery system such as a
     syringe, giving set or cutting the corner off a fluid bag.
22   9 L of irrigation should be used for complex blast wounds, 6 L for penetrating ballistic injury and
     3 L for superficial wounds.

Post-debridement principles

23   Dressings should be well secured to prevent displacement during evacuation.
24   Traditional sterile gauze and topical negative pressure are both acceptable wound dressings.
25   Where the surgeon is entirely happy with the debridement delayed primary closure should be
     performed at around 5 days.
26   Where traumatised but potentially viable tissue has been left the wound should be inspected in
     the operating theatre at around 48 hours.

Special circumstances

27   In the context of complex blast/explosion wounds, initial debridement should be undertaken
     whenever the opportunity permits.
28   A philosophy of serial marginal debridement is indicated for the majority of complex blast/
     explosion wounds.
29   Some low energy narrow channel and superficial soft tissue wounds do not require full surgical
     debridement.

both in the United States and United Kingdom to identify a method of quantifying when a wound does or does not require significant intervention.

Complex debridement

The close-proximity blast wound caused by a dismounted IED was the UK signature injury from the Afghanistan conflict. These devastating injuries (Figures 9.2 to 9.4), which frequently included multiple extremity amputations with pelvic and perineal injury, presented a new challenge to the *Defence Medical Services*. Injury severity on this scale had not regularly been observed before in conflict, and previously, casualties with such severe blast injury rarely reached medical facilities before succumbing to their injuries. However, immediate point of wounding care, rapid retrieval by a consultant-led team and transfer to a sophisticated medical facility allowed many such casualties to survive. The debridement of these injuries is complicated because of the fragility of the victim's physiological status and the vast degree of destruction and contamination of the injured tissues. At first, the constraints of damage control resuscitation, needed to secure improvement in physiological status, did not allow a long enough surgical window

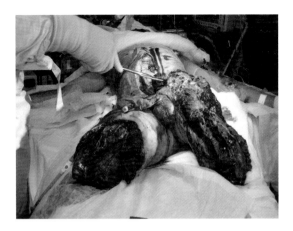

Figure 9.3 Appearance following second look of the casualty in Figure 9.2.

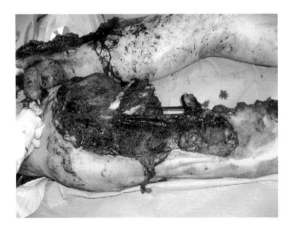

Figure 9.4 Early bilateral lower extremity injury requiring intra-abdominal proximal control.

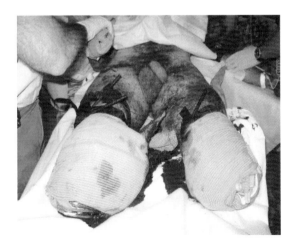

Figure 9.2 Injuries caused by the detonation of a roadside IED: on arrival at deployed hospital with tourniquets and first field dressings in place. Two tourniquets have been applied to the right leg and one to the left to achieve effective haemorrhage control.

to complete the first debridement. These patients required consistent communication between surgeons and anaesthetists in order to deliver the best possible balance between surgery and physiology. This took time to develop and perfect. From the orthopaedic view point, the principles of debridement remained but had to be undertaken with more flexibility.

At times, the initial debridement had to be limited to the removal of grossly contaminated and dead tissue. This proceeded alongside continuing resuscitation and lifesaving damage control surgery. This was made possible by having multiple teams operating on the casualty at the same time.

It was not unheard of to have two anaesthetists, two general surgeons and two orthopaedic/plastic surgeons working simultaneously. Furthermore, casualties were taken back to the operating theatre on repeated occasions following the initial interventions, in order to complete the debridement, but also because the wounds were observed to evolve over time. The nature of the contamination, especially from the wetlands of central Helmand Province, was complex and included fungal infections which did not demonstrate their presence until several days post injury, with the wounds taking on appearances not previously seen. This was first observed after the major offensive in summer 2009 and was initially considered to be associated with surgical teams in theatre not undertaking the meticulous surgery that had previously been achieved. However, further investigation and microbiological examination of samples taken from these evolving wounds demonstrated the presence of fungi that did not respond to the usual antibiotic regime.

A study looking at the change in pattern of amputations[7] showed that there was a significant difference between the limb trauma seen in Iraq and that from the later years of the conflict in Afghanistan. These injuries reflected a change in the weapons deployed against the troops and in particular the increased use of IEDs. This change in injury pattern required modifications to surgical technique as experience in blast injury management increased.

The importance of gaining proximal control cannot be underestimated. The C-A-T™ has been previously discussed. However, it became regular practice when a casualty arrived at hospital to replace the C-A-T™ with a pneumatic tourniquet as soon as resuscitation commenced. Pneumatic tourniquets were available in the emergency department. The high level of some of the injuries meant that proximal control could not be gained through the use of a pneumatic tourniquet applied to the thigh or upper arm. In these cases, haemorrhage control was obtained in the operating theatre at the level of femoral or iliac arteries or aorta for the lower extremities and axillary or subclavian arteries for the upper extremity (Figure 9.4).

It is recognised by those who delivered this level of expertise over the last 15 years that such a pattern of injuries is unlikely to be repeated in the foreseeable future, and thus, deploying personnel will have to understand and modify their expectations with regard to high-quality and prompt medical delivery. Nevertheless, some conclusions of use for future operations can be drawn.

A highly specialised team of personnel was required to deliver such success, and a combined meeting of the *Lower Limb* and *Torso Trauma Working Groups* in the Academic Department of Military Surgery and Trauma produced 25 clear, didactic statements to provide advice to the future consultant team.[32] These are given in Table 9.3.

The basic principles of the debridement of war wounds were well known prior to these latest conflicts. The very early presentation of complex wounds to the emergency department led to the development of serial marginal debridement dictated by the physiological status of the patient in line with the principles of damage control resuscitation. Topical negative pressure (TNP) dressings (see page 212) were used extensively in the management of these wounds with good effect,[33] although it is important to realise that these dressings are no substitute for a thorough debridement and meticulous surgery.

Compartment syndrome

Acute compartment syndrome is well recognised in severely injured limbs following trauma. The incidence is high in military populations and it has been reported that 16% of casualties evacuated from Iraq and Afghanistan with lower limb injury had undergone a fasciotomy.[34] Fasciotomies should be carried out if there is any clinical suspicion of, or significant potential for the development of, compartment syndrome.

There is no place for monitoring compartment pressures in a deployed hospital environment. Furthermore, the need for aeromedical evacuation from the deployed facility back to the United Kingdom, sometimes taking more than 24 hours, occurring very soon after injury, is unique to military medical practice. The patient must be optimised both physiologically and from a surgical/orthopaedic viewpoint, in the form of adequate analgesia, fracture stabilisation and extremity vascularity. Compartment syndrome initially presents with pain out of proportion to that expected from the

Table 9.3 Consensus recommendations regarding management of extremely injured patients

1	Bleeding is a surgical problem. Early proximal control is mandatory.
2	In all cases, obtain the most distally appropriate proximal control above the zone of injury.
3	Agonal (arrest/peri-arrest) junctionally injured patients mandate *in theatre* (right turn) resuscitation, immediate <C>ABCDE assessment (consider immediate bilateral subclavian trauma lines) and immediate thoracotomy for intrathoracic aortic occlusion. A urinary balloon catheter may be placed in the right atrium and connected directly to the Level 1 infuser.
4	Clear and continuous dialogue must take place, at all times, between the surgical and anaesthetic teams.
5	If multiple surgeons are operating on one patient, one surgeon must be in overall charge. If there are multiple anaesthetists working on this patient, one must also be in overall charge. These two physicians together run the team and agree end-states and end-timings.
6	Remove all CAT tourniquets in the emergency department (ED). If there is bleeding or concern over bleeding, immediately (pre-) apply a padded pneumatic tourniquet. If there is no bleeding, do not inflate the tourniquet. The implication is that ED must have its own pneumatic tourniquets ready for use.
7	For debridement of bilateral below knee injuries/traumatic amputations, retain these loosely applied uninflated bilateral pneumatic tourniquets. Ensure the tourniquet is not occluding venous outflow from the limb.
8	Our consensus is to undertake rapid but accurate surgical debridement with an inflated tourniquet when possible; main vessels are identified and either tied off or temporarily controlled prior to release of the tourniquets.
9	Tourniquets may be placed over wounded proximal areas as a temporising measure to obtain control of distal bleeding.
10	For IED/mine injuries higher than the knee, the most distal proximal control practical (above the haematoma/zone of injury) should be considered. Venous control is usually not necessary.
11	For IED/mine injuries higher than the knee; the minimal acceptable patient position is 'cruciform' on an active warming blanket, nipple to groin Betadine prep and a Bair-Hugger® Patient-Warmer replaced on top of the torso.
12	Bilateral above knee amputations (AKAs) will usually mandate double groin control. The most distal proximal control sequencing in the lower limb junctional zone is commonly femoral artery, external iliac artery, common iliac artery, aorta.
13	Uncontrollable buttock bleeding after packing may require intra-abdominal control.
14	Uncontrollable perineal bleeding after packing may require intra-abdominal control.
15	If pelvic bleeding is suspected, and a pelvic binder is in place, it must remain until proximal vascular control is obtained. Ensure the binder is placed correctly over the trochanters. If there is a pelvic fracture or ligamentous disruption, it will be seen on the initial film.
16	If the patient is stable – leave the binder on. Consider skeletal stabilisation (external fixation) for transport.
17	For pelvic injury – deal with the injuries you see. Mostly this will involve packing using a midline incision. Obtain the most appropriate proximal control you require, then 'Walk the Clamps' distally.
18	In pelvic trauma, consider urethral injury and place a suprapubic catheter.
19	In pelvic trauma, consider rectal injury and disconnect the colon – use an intestinal stapler to divide the colon and leave the ends inside the abdomen, formal colostomy is not necessary.

(Continued)

Table 9.3 (Continued) Consensus recommendations regarding management of extremely injured patients

20	All viable gonadal tissue should be preserved – wherever possible. Do not over-debride testicular tissue. Apply Vaseline gauze and moist dressings only. Gonadal placement into a thigh pocket stretches the vas deferens, compresses the epididymis and expels potentially harvestable viable sperm. It is therefore not recommended.
21	In upper limb junctional trauma, consider the intra-thoracic injury first.
22	Place patients in a crucifix position on a warming blanket and prep for a whole-chest thoracotomy. Place a Bair-Hugger over all uninjured extremities.
23	For axillary artery bleeding, obtain subclavian control.
24	For uncontrollable subclavian injury, apply direct pressure and perform a median sternotomy.
25	For uncontrollable bleeding in the root of the neck, apply direct pressure and perform a median sternotomy.

injury. It is frequently intractable, and patients are restless and agitated. Even if ventilated, their oxygen consumption rises and the need for further analgesia is identified. Nursing and medical staff in the military environment are very aware of these developing signs. If there is any concern regarding the possibility of a developing compartment syndrome, then four-compartment decompression of the extremity should be performed. It is most common in the lower leg. However, buttock, thigh, foot, forearm and hand decompressions were all undertaken during the conflicts.[24,34] Perhaps one of the most controversial areas in which compartment decompression might be performed is in association with foot injury, frequently as a result of crush or blast. Clinical experience demonstrates that the casualty's pain in such cases is uncontrollable by any conventional analgesia, including regional blockage. Although the actual procedure is unsatisfactory to the orthopaedic surgeon, if foot compartments are released correctly, the pain is rapidly relived.[35]

Although there is controversy with respect to the use of regional anaesthetic blocks in extremity trauma due to the risk of masking a developing compartment syndrome, it is our experience that the block does not mask the developing compartment syndrome if the patient is being monitored correctly. An editorial supporting this written by Clasper et al. in 2009, reviewed 100 cases of casualties with significant limb injuries. Only two casualties were identified as requiring fasciotomies after evacuation from the deployed theatre. Both were cases of late presentation, and not an acute compartment syndrome that had not been identified during initial management. The editorial recommended that

'Role 2/3 clinicians should be encouraged to use regional anaesthetic blocks. However, consideration must always be given to the risk of possible acute compartment syndrome, and thus regional techniques should only be carried out with the agreement of both the treating surgeon and anaesthetist. Patients must be closely monitored clinically and any staff responsible for the on-going care, particularly during evacuation, must receive specific training in their management'.

Patients who receive a regional block in the deployed environment are audited at the UK Role 4 facility, thus maintaining a continual overview on the outcomes, both positive and negative, following use. The recommendations regarding compartment syndrome are set out in Table 9.4.

Fracture fixation

Most fractures sustained due to a ballistic mechanism of injury are high energy and multi-fragmentary. The majority are open, associated with a severe soft tissue injury, and in addition are highly contaminated. The United Kingdom deployed hospital facilities remain austere environments and none provided or currently could provide the UK standard of an ultra-clean air theatre (defined as one in which the air contains less than 10 colony forming units per cubic metre <10 CFU/m³).[36] This was not the same for US capabilities, and the United States did have a facility that was considered satisfactory enough to perform complex fracture stabilisation procedures. However,

Table 9.4 Recommendations for compartment decompression

1   Following diagnosis, compartment decompression should be carried out as soon as practical due to the increase in complications with delay.

2   All compartments should be decompressed. In the lower leg, failure to decompress the deep posterior compartment is relatively common: Missed compartment syndrome is associated with a very high complication rate.

3   Full-length incisions must be performed. A common error is that the incision is too short; usually the decompression appears adequate, but post-operative muscle swelling leads to acute compartment syndrome recurrence due to the tourniquet effect of tight skin and fascia at the extremes of the incision.

4   Incisions should be placed with regard to later reconstructive options. If the medial incision to decompress the lower leg is placed too posteriorly, the perforating vessels may be damaged, limiting the options for local flaps.

5   All planned incisions should be pre-marked with a pen, including possible surgical extensions prior to any incision being made. It should be noted that significant swelling might obscure the normal anatomical features.

6   Any associated fracture should be reduced and stabilised. Most fasciotomies are carried out through a longitudinal skin incision. If the incision is performed in the presence of an unstable displaced fracture, particularly with rotational abnormalities, the final incision, after reduction of the fracture, may expose bone or again compromise reconstructive options. External fixation, traction and plaster of Paris are all viable options.

7   Unnecessary exposure of the bone must be avoided, as this will also compromise reconstructive options, possibly necessitating free or local flap rather than split skin graft coverage. If the medial incision to decompress the lower leg is placed too anteriorly, the subcutaneous surface of the tibia may be exposed. The upper tibia may also be over-exposed by failure to appreciate its proximal flare.

Source: Ritenour AE et al., *J Trauma* 2008;64(2 Suppl):S153–S161; discussion S161–S162.

the available results from these facilities are limited, and many of the patients they treated were returned to local host nation facilities, and thus, follow-up was not achieved. It is unlikely that the United Kingdom will have any facility that conforms to UK standards within the foreseeable future. Therefore, we must maintain the ability to treat fractures safely in the operational environment and should only utilise complex procedures in safe environments.

FRACTURE FIXATION

Basic fracture stabilisation

Experience in both conflicts supported the accepted emphasis that when addressing the bony injury in war, the adage 'less is more' remains valid. Basic splintage techniques utilising plaster of Paris remain very relevant in such environments, and simple and sometimes more complex fracture

patterns may be treated very adequately this way. Definitive fixation is not frequently achieved and should not be attempted unless the fracture pattern allows the use of basic splinting, external fixation or Kirscher wires. Internal fixation has no place in the austere environment. Bony injuries were stabilised and transferred to the Role 4 in the United Kingdom for definitive further reconstruction. Table 9.5 outlines the various stabilisation techniques available currently and considered suitable for the deployed environment.[37–40]

External fixation

The value of external fixation has been accepted by military surgeons, and it was used widely for the stabilisation of the fractures with associated soft tissue injury and/or vascular injury, where other forms of immobilisation were considered inappropriate. External fixation allows rigid

Table 9.5 Basic fracture stabilisation methods prior to definitive management

Stabilisation technique	Potential complication
1 Plaster of Paris, e.g. lower leg, foot, upper limb fracture	Difficult observing wounds; fracture may lose position
2 Thomas splint, e.g. femoral immobilisation; may be reinforced with plaster of Paris to form the 'Tobruk Splint' if evacuation likely to be particularly difficult	Pressure areas must be considered and monitored carefully, particularly at the ischial tuberosity; use contraindicated with a pelvic fracture
3 Skin traction/skeletal traction, e.g. initial management of long bone injuries, particularly of the lower extremity	Skin traction may encounter skin blistering/breakdown, particularly in children and the elderly; use difficult during evacuation to maintain position
4 Kirscher (K) wires, e.g. fixation of open foot, hand and wrist fractures	Invasive, limited reduction capability; may develop pin tract infection
5 External fixation, e.g. open extremity injuries particularly if complicated with a vascular injury; certain pelvic fractures	Invasive, limited anatomical reduction achievable; may require revision; may develop pin tract infection

fixation to be achieved and the continuation of aggressive management of the associated soft tissue injury. Direct observation of the injured limb, wound status, neurovascular status and assessment of associated muscle compartments are all possible. External fixation allows continual wound debridement and irrigation, skin grafting and dressing changes to continue without losing the alignment of the fracture configuration. It also allows for easier transportation and patient comfort during long aeromedical evacuation journeys. When combined with *TNP dressings*, external fixation reduces analgesia requirements and facilitates the management of the excess exudate, which was so apparent in these complex wounds, causing smelly, soggy wound dressings, which were potentially distressing to both patient and clinical staff.

External fixation is not without its disadvantages.[38] It can be cumbersome, may be complicated by pin tract infection and fracture can occur through pin tracts. It is also potentially expensive, difficult to apply and requires the use of an image intensifier if those applying the device are inexperienced in its use. There may be difficulties with host nation patients for whom external fixation devices may not be readily available, and thus, they may not be able to complete the entire course of treatment.

Early failure of external fixation was identified by Clasper and Phillips[38] in a small series of patients treated in 2003 during the Iraq conflict. The series was of 15 patients, of whom 86.7% required early revision or removal due to complications. Instability occurred in 67% of fixators, with particular problems being noted with bridging fixators across the knee and femoral fixators. However, it must be stated that external fixators have hugely improved since this early experience. The current UK external fixator of choice is the *Hoffman III device®*, manufactured by Stryker®, which allows for 360 degrees of freedom when applied, hugely increasing its versatility. The Schantz pins are self-drilling and self-tapping, and the system has the ability to connect the bar directly to the pin using a quick coupling device. The original Centrifix® device had significant problems with initial pin insertion, pre-drilling was required, it allowed only unilateral fixation configurations, had poor bar strength and thus delivered extremely limited fixation arrangements. It was removed from service in 2005, although some packs remained available until later in the Iraq conflict.

Internal fixation

In a series of 58 patients treated with internal fixation after war trauma,[41] 80% of fractures were open and 57% were of the femur. Forty percent of fracture sites were infected and osteomyelitis was suspected in 17%. A review of a cohort of patients treated with femoral nails in Iraq[42] concluded that in an established US Role 3 Facility, 'internal fixation may be performed with an acceptable infection risk'. However, in this publication, only 13 patients out of 22 had any follow-up, and even then, 8 of the 13 only had two months follow-up and a further 5 had six months, so these conclusions are questionable. Two thirds (68%) of these fractures were closed injuries, and 32% were combat injuries; 25% required additional later surgical procedures, with one diagnosed infection of *Staphylococcus aureus* from internal fixation, which required two further debridements. This study is atypical within the combat environment, due to the preponderance of closed injuries. Despite this, the overall complication rate was 22%, with an average follow-up of 17 months. These levels are unacceptable by UK standards. In addition to the potential for an increased infection rate, the other arguments against internal fixation in the deployed hospital care environment include the increased time required for each procedure, the increased resource commitment of internal compared to external fixation and simple splintage, the need for fracture tables and image intensifier facilities, which were shielded from other operating tables and the additional blood usage. A deployed hospital would not

necessarily have all the extra equipment needed to address the unforeseen complications of internal fixation or any unexpected perioperative complications, particularly as the fracture patterns observed will undoubtedly be complex.

In 2011, the *Limb Trauma Working Group* met to discuss the issue of internal fixation on deployment and consider the limited evidence. These discussions generated several consensus statements, which are listed as recommendations in Table 9.6.[36] These conclusions represent the unanimous views of those present and serve as clear practice guidelines for deploying UK surgeons. In summary, the consensus is that 'internal fixation should not be performed in our deployed theatres of war. The risks of internal fixation do not outweigh the benefits and the long-term consequences of these interventions must be considered even on short term operations'.

The definitive reconstruction of patients with bony limb trauma evacuated to the United Kingdom presented significant challenges to those working at the Role 4 hospital. Combined management of the injuries by orthopaedic and plastic surgeons improved the outcomes of these potentially devastating injuries.[43-45] Open fractures sustained in war differ significantly from those sustained in the civilian setting. The energy transfer tends to be greater, resulting in larger zones of injury and significantly greater contamination. However, a

Table 9.6 Recommendations regarding deployed fracture fixation

1	It is not a Role 2 or 3 function to perform internal fixation, and there should be no capability for internal fixation at these echelons of care. UK surgical teams should not perform any internal fixation on coalition troops, nor should UK troops undergo internal fixation at R2/R3 by other nation's surgical teams.
2	Civilians/local troops should be managed in a manner that is safe, ethical, effective and compatible with local infrastructure and healthcare provision. It is not acceptable to return patients to their local communities with an internal fixation device that cannot be removed. The management of children should also be governed by these principles. Captured persons should be humanely treated in accordance with the *Geneva Conventions*.
3	Open reduction and stabilisation (not fixation) of certain specific fractures may be acceptable. One example of this would be a displaced talus fracture at risk of avascular necrosis, which could be opened in order to reduce it and, if unstable, stabilised with a single K-wire prior to transport.
4	When external fixators are applied as part of fracture stabilisation, intelligent and pragmatic consideration should be given to subsequent definitive management. If an external fixator is applied as a treatment of last resort in a local civilian/local troop case, the patient must be discharged with the tool required to remove the fixator firmly strapped to the fixator frame.

combined orthopaedic/plastic surgical approach remains essential to success. A study reporting the pattern of severe open diaphyseal tibial fractures sustained by military personnel between 2006 and 2010 identified 49 patients with 57 tibial fractures.[46] The median number of orthopaedic and plastic surgical interventions was 3 (2–8). Twelve-month follow-up was complete in 91%, with 50% of the fractures uniting or progressing towards union. Poor bony healing was not associated with New Injury Severity Score (NISS) score, method of internal fixation, requirement for vascularised soft tissue coverage or the degree of bone loss. However, infection was identified in 12 of 52 tibiae (23%) and was directly associated with poor bony healing.

AMPUTATION

The accepted mechanism of blast-mediated traumatic amputation, namely that the initial primary shock wave induces a fracture followed by avulsion of the limb by the blast wind, producing a trans-osseous amputation, has been called into question during these past conflicts. Previously, blast-mediated through-joint traumatic amputations were very rare, with a published incidence of approximately 2%.[47] In addition, it was considered that through-joint traumatic amputation was generally associated with fatal primary blast lung injury. The improved survival rates, access to immediate CT scanning and the numbers of casualties identified with traumatic amputations led Singleton and co-workers in 2014[48] to examine a series of blast-mediated traumatic amputations and post-mortem CT scans in order to provide new insights into the potential biomechanics of such injury patterns. Their findings show that there is no link between primary blast lung injury and traumatic amputation and demonstrate a significantly higher rate of traumatic amputation through joints, thus challenging the role of the initial blast shock wave in causation of all blast-mediated traumatic amputations and supporting a tertiary blast injury/flail as a valid mechanism of amputation.

Between 2003 and 2014, 416 lower limb amputations were sustained by 265 UK personnel.[49] The average number of limbs lost per person was 1.6. These included a total of 32 major upper extremity amputations (Roberts et al., unpublished). The significant majority of these amputations occurred during and after 2009. A review of 77 consecutive casualties who presented to the *UK Role 3 Facility* between 2009 and 2010 with traumatic amputation was undertaken.[4] Thirty-one (40%) had a unilateral amputation, with 46 (60%) bilateral amputations. The commonest configuration was bilateral transfemoral amputations. The *Limb Trauma Working Group* made recommendations regarding the management of extremity amputation in 2007[50]; these remain extant but should be considered in association with the recommendations for debridement already listed. These recommendations are listed in Table 9.7.

The results of a review of 1694 UK military personnel injured by IEDs between 2004 and 2010 are interesting.[51] All the casualties were men with a median age of 25 years. Forty-three (2.8%) were casualties with bilateral lower limb amputations. Six of these sustained the injuries in vehicles, whilst the remaining 37 (80%) were patrolling on foot. The median NISS was 48: four patients had a maximum score of 75. The mean *Trauma Revised Injury Severity Score* probability of survival was 60% (SD, 39.4). As previously stated, bilateral transfemoral amputations were the most common amputation pattern. Nine patients (21%) had also lost an upper extremity (triple amputation). No patient survived loss of all four limbs. In upper extremity injuries, hand and forearm injuries were common, particularly loss of digits. Six patients (14%) sustained an open pelvic fracture. Perineal/genital injury was a feature in 19 (44%) patients. The median requirement for blood products was 62 units. The minimum transfusion requirement was 8 units, and the greatest was a total of 193 units of blood product. Twenty patients (47%) had an immediate laparotomy, 3 were treated with resuscitative thoracotomy while 2 required thoraco-laparotomy as part of their damage control surgery. The median stay in the intensive care unit (ICU) was 7 days (range, 0–64). The median number of orthopaedic operations per residual limb was 3 (range, 1–10), with a total median number of operations per patient of 8. These injury patterns described are at the severe end of the spectrum of survivability, and the success achieved demonstrates the role of the multi-disciplinary approach to trauma management, which has evolved over the course of the last 15 years.

Table 9.7 Recommendations regarding extremity amputation

1	The examination findings, together with the indications to amputate the limb, should be documented.
2	Existing limb salvage scores should NOT be used to determine the need for amputation.
3	Whenever possible, the decision to amputate a limb should be confirmed by a second surgeon.
4	All wounds should be photographed.
5	Radiographs should be obtained prior to amputation.
6	Neurological dysfunction (particularly numbness of the sole of the foot) should NOT be part of the criteria used to decide amputation.
7	The site of amputation should be at the lowest level possible.
8	Guillotine amputations should not be performed.
9	No fashioning of flaps at initial debridement.
10	Viable, non-contaminated bone should not be excised, even if this is distal to the soft tissue levels. This is particularly important in upper extremity reconstruction.
11	The level of any fracture should be ignored when considering amputation, particularly in the upper extremity. Only debridement of non-viable tissue should initially be undertaken. Any remaining viable tissue may assist with later reconstruction.
12	No part of the wound to be closed at initial surgery.
13	No attempt should be made to prevent skin retraction.
14	Through-knee amputation is acceptable if appropriate.

COMPLEX INJURIES

As expected, the initial management of complex injuries concentrates on obtaining haemorrhage control. As the conflicts continued and the nature of the injuries became more severe, it became routine pre-hospital practice to apply a pelvic binder to any casualty sustaining a lower limb amputation. On arrival at the hospital facility, a pelvic X-ray was performed with the binder in situ. During the course of the conflict, there was one casualty who sustained a pelvic ring injury that could not be identified on the initial antero-posterior (AP) pelvic film with the binder in situ. Thus, it remained the recommended practice to perform a CT scan before removal of the binder if the casualty was haemodynamically stable. The trauma CT scan also assisted in delineating soft tissue and visceral injuries. Without the presence of a CT scanner, a controlled binder-off AP pelvis film may be appropriate. Immediate transfer to the operating theatre was undertaken if haemorrhage was uncontrolled.

Haemorrhage from amputation below mid-thigh level can usually be controlled using a pneumatic tourniquet, as described previously.

Sometimes, the pneumatic tourniquet was initially used in combination with the C-A-T. However, the pneumatic device allows for accurate timing of application and duration, at a known pressure, and reduces the soft tissue damage sustained beneath the tourniquet, as compression is spread over a wider area. If required, surgical control may be obtained at the level of the femoral artery.

In the case of a more proximal injury, the method of haemorrhage control will depend upon whether the injury is unilateral or bilateral. With a unilateral high thigh or groin injury, haemorrhage control may be achieved via the external iliac artery using an extraperitoneal approach. However, if the amputations are bilateral and depending on the available surgical experience, more rapid control via a laparotomy to the level of the distal aorta or iliac vessels may be more appropriate. This certainly limits the blood loss from both amputation sites and any pelvic and perineal injuries. Time remains critical, and recording the distal ischaemic time should not be forgotten. Where the injury included an unstable pelvic ring injury, surgery was performed with the pelvic binder in situ. This was changed to a pelvic external fixator device, utilising iliac crest pins and allowing the binder to be removed and the extraperitoneal pelvis to be packed against the external fixator. Debridement and irrigation of the lower extremity injuries could then proceed. Ideally, this was performed by multiple personnel working on each limb simultaneously, thus reducing operating time. During this process, each muscle was inspected to assess its viability. Diathermy was utilised, on a low frequency setting, to observe muscle contraction, and muscle consistency was also considered. Contaminated particles were found frequently to have been forced proximally between the tissue planes, often far beyond expected levels. Extensive low-pressure normal saline irrigation was utilised. Relevant arteries and vessels were tied off before the proximal control at the aorta or iliac vessels was released. Other general surgical interventions were performed concurrently, for example bowel diversion if there were associated injuries to the ano-rectal margin and preservation of testicular remnants. This is discussed in Chapter 8. Urethral injuries were treated with a urethral catheter and/or a suprapubic catheter. These procedures frequently lasted many hours in order to debulk the contaminated and dead tissue.[11]

Notable figures to date from the Afghanistan conflict published by Jansen et al. in 2012[11] show that 16% of UK casualties reaching a deployed hospital facility with traumatic lower limb amputations died. Of five patients requiring a hindquarter amputation, three did not survive. The median NISS for those who did not survive was 71, in comparison to 45 for those who survived.

Another important consideration when dealing with complex extremity injury is associated head and torso injury. Morrison et al.[52] found in their review of 169 patients who reached deployed hospital care that injuries to the head and torso, which were not immediately clinically apparent, were rare. Thus, if a casualty requires proximal haemorrhage control and is haemodynamically unstable, CT scanning should be performed on completion of their surgery, en route to ICU.

The traditional teaching of the two-stage unsalvageable extremity amputation had to be modified during the Afghanistan conflict. The severity of the injuries observed required repeated debridement.

A study investigating the number of surgical procedures per stump prior to closure demonstrated a mean of 4.1. A more proximal amputation level was required in 30%. *Aeromonas hydrophila* was associated with a requirement for a more proximal amputation level and a greater number of debridements when compared to wounds without such infection.[53]

LIMB SALVAGE

Successful limb salvage is highly subjective and patient dependent.[54] Pain, function and the ability to return to work all define outcomes. Military personnel are young and active, have high degrees of pre-injury fitness and thus place increased demands upon the post injury rehabilitation process. Several scoring systems have been developed in order to guide the decision to amputate after severe lower limb trauma. The only one that has been validated in military patients is the *Mangled Extremity Severity Score* (MESS). This looks at skeletal/soft tissue injury, ischemic time, shock and age.[55] This scoring system suggests that a score of 7 or more is a positive predictor for amputation. However, Brown et al.[54] reported the largest study investigating the use of the MESS, specifically in ballistic lower extremity injuries. In this study, nine patients (10 limbs) with an MESS score of 7 were successfully salvaged. This equated to one in three limbs being unnecessarily amputated. The authors concluded that the MESS could not be utilised to determine the need for primary amputation, and thus, it is no longer taught on any of the pre-deployment training courses for medical staff. The presence of a vascular injury that required repair in a physiologically unstable patient was the main factor in the decision to perform amputation. This combination gives a MESS score of at least 8. A possible algorithm for the decision-making process was proposed and is shown in Figure 9.5.[54]

The decision to attempt limb salvage is complex and remains multifactorial, not necessarily taking into account only patient factors. During conflict, the severely injured rarely present with a solitary mangled extremity for the management of which all requirements are in place and accessible: these include optimised physiological status, a short

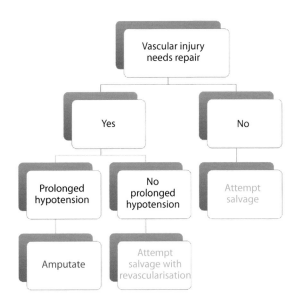

Figure 9.5 Algorithm for limb salvage.

ischaemic time, the necessary surgical expertise and the full range of necessary capabilities, as well as capacity within the clinical facility. Other patients, concomitant life-threatening injuries and the availability of resources may influence the decision making.

The huge steps forward in point of wounding care and rapid transport to a hospital facility with surgical expertise had significant effects on the status of the patient. Aggressive management to prevent coagulopathy, hypothermia and acidosis presented the team with a physiologically salvageable patient able to withstand long surgical interventions. Such patients frequently arrived more than one at a time.

Assessment of limb vascularity should be undertaken rapidly on arrival. Fox et al.[56] estimate that vascular injury represents 12% of all battlefield injury. Obviously, hard signs such as continued haemorrhage and limb ischaemia require immediate operative attention, with a relatively limited requirement for other diagnostic interventional studies, unless other injuries prevail. Other softer signs such as injury proximity to major vessels, fracture pattern, bruising or haematoma formation and the questionable presence or absence of a palpable pulse will mandate further imaging. This potentially includes CT angiography. The presence of a surgeon with vascular expertise during

these campaigns allowed rapid assessment, proximal and distal control of the vascular injury, the appropriate use of tourniquets and exploration of the injured vessel. Removal of the clot from the vessel and use of heparinised saline with the restoration of blood flow utilising a temporary shunt followed by appropriate fasciotomies were also possible. Definitive vascular repair utilising the patient's own remaining vascular tree was performed dependent upon surgical expertise and the patient's physiological status. Despite these rapid interventions, appropriate irrigation, debridement and antibiotic usage, it was observed that fractures associated with a vascular injury had a higher infection rate[23] and non-union rate (Roberts et al., unpublished) (Table 9.8).

Overall outcomes comparing limb salvage to amputation are available only to the medium term. A study published in 2015[57] comparing UK military patients who had undergone limb salvage procedures for severe open tibial injuries with individuals who had sustained a unilateral trans-tibial amputation demonstrated that in those who were contacted by telephone to perform a lifestyle SF-36 questionnaire, no difference was observed in either the physical or mental component between groups. This supports the findings of the LEAP study, performed in the United States on a civilian population over seven years asking similar questions.[58]

Overall, the surgical team was very often faced with difficult decisions in extremity trauma following ballistic injury. Despite systematic review, objective criteria were not found to aid the process of limb salvage decision making. Recommendations, already discussed in relation

Table 9.8 Factors to be considered when deciding on limb salvage

1. Devitalised and contaminated deep tissue requires surgical removal.
2. Damaged and infected tissue may respond rapidly to medical resuscitation.
3. Traumatised skin rarely requires excision.
4. Bone defects may heal from intact periosteum.
5. Joints should be spared if at all possible.
6. Through-bone amputation should be avoided if possible.

to the initial management of extremity injury earlier in this chapter, have been made, but these should be treated as guidelines rather than hard rules. Each situation will present unique challenges, which will need to be addressed in light of all the injuries sustained by the patient, the presence or absence of other casualties and the available resources (Figure 9.6).

PAEDIATRIC CONSIDERATIONS

The same basic principles apply to the child with devastating extremity injuries, although more sophisticated reconstruction techniques may be available or appropriate in a developed country with intact healthcare infrastructure.[54] A UK deployed military surgical facility is neither staffed nor trained with paediatric care in mind, and difficulties are inevitable. There is a tendency for surgical treatment of children with severe trauma to be at once overly tentative and unnecessarily aggressive. Both primary suture of a contaminated wound over necrotic tissue and an unjustifiably high tibial amputation for a foot injury from the same surgical facility have been noted. The circumstances of the injury are frequently emotive, and clinical decisions must be made in the face of an inevitable emotional response to the child from both relatives and medical carers.

It is important, therefore, to have clear surgical principles to guide decision making in these circumstances. These principles are essentially the same as for an injured adult, but with some important physiological and anatomical differences.

Growth

Limb bones grow longitudinally by interstitial growth in the specialised cartilage of the growth plates situated at either end of most long bones. The rate and extent of growth are governed by intrinsic or 'genetic' programming and by the influence of mechanical factors imparted by weight bearing and muscle action. Amputation through a long bone obviously removes one of the growth plates, but in addition, the mechanical environment changes and growth at the remaining growth plate is inhibited such that longitudinal growth of the remnant is less than would be expected.[54]

Stump overgrowth

There is another mechanism of bone growth that is significant in the juvenile amputee: appositional or intramembranous ossification from the transected bone ends. This causes problems by growing out from the bone stump in a spike, which extends into the surrounding soft tissues, causing discomfort, which may be severe. In some circumstances, the tip of the bone spike erodes the skin, exposing the bone and leading to the risk of infection. Through-bone amputation in a child may result in a short, painful stump precluding prosthetic use due to the characteristics of growing bone.[54]

Response to injury

A child's physiological response to blood loss is characterised by very effective compensation up to a critical point when circulatory collapse is rapid. Coupled with this, tissue elasticity is greater in children than in adults, and there appears to be a greater tolerance of muscle tissue to crush and hypoxia. This combination of circumstances means that following adequate resuscitation, limb damage that would be irreparable in an adult may be salvageable in a child. In addition, the healing response is more vigorous in a child so that skin and bone defects in particular have the possibility of repairing to an extent that is not seen in maturity.[54]

Fracture healing

Children's bones have a higher proportion of collagen fibre to calcified matrix than adult bone does, and the periosteum is thicker and more physiologically active. Force applied to a child's bone is dissipated more widely than in stiffer adult bone, and multi-fragmentary fractures are less common. The periosteum is strong and tends to maintain the integrity of the bone to some extent, even when fractures occur. In addition, juvenile periosteum forms new bone very readily to the extent that even in cases of extensive bone loss from open trauma, if the periosteum is preserved and the limb is stabilised, bone re-growth occurs in time. This is particularly striking in younger children.[54]

Table 9.9 Management of paediatric lower limb injuries

Injury level		Management
1.	Unsalvageable mid or hind foot injury	Amputate through ankle joint (leave epiphysis intact)
2.	Unsalvageable ankle or tibia	Amputate through tibia as distal as possible: either resect fibula at least 2 cm proximal to tibia or attempt surgical synostosis
3.	Unsalvageable proximal tibia	Through knee amputation if patella tendon cannot be preserved
4.	Unsalvageable distal femur	Amputate through femur as distal as possible

Surgical treatment of the injured extremity in children

Taking the particular anatomy and physiology into account, certain principles can be identified. The surgical sequence is similar to that of an adult. Table 9.9 details the management of the paediatric lower limb injury.[54] Decision making regarding a very high transtibial amputation is difficult and will depend to a large extent on the available local services and to some extent on the age of the child. An amputation through the proximal tibial condyle will be beneficial if the prosthetic support is sufficiently sophisticated to provide a workable below knee limb and if there are surgical facilities available to deal with any bone overgrowth that may subsequently occur. On the other hand, a young child with a high amputation living in an area with poor infrastructure will end up with a very short stump at maturity, with the risk of painful bone overgrowth and either no prosthesis or one that doesn't allow knee movement. This child would be better off with a through knee amputation.[54]

ROLE 4 EXTREMITY MANAGEMENT

The multidisciplinary team approach was considered vital for Role 4 management, and orthopaedic and plastic surgeons were present during all visits to the operating theatre. Cases were discussed at regular multidisciplinary team meetings. At the height of the conflict, these were held three times daily. A goal for the first visit to the operating theatre in the United Kingdom was to identify all the injuries and delineate the apex of the wounds in all planes, ideally removing all residual foreign material and dead tissue, as well as obtaining tissue specimens

for culture and histology. Wound progression was a common feature and did not indicate poor initial wound debridement in the operational theatre. Unless very heavily contaminated, any bone that appeared viable was maintained and not shortened at this stage. The plastic surgeons frequently utilised the Versajet™ hydrosurgery dissection device,[30] which by use of the Venturi effect, draws contamination away from the tissues; this was an extremely useful adjunct in ensuring that ingrained mud, dirt and sand were removed from the wound surface. The use of X-ray image intensification was also considered to help identify occult particulate contamination. In the early visits to theatre, drains were laid into tissue planes in order to alleviate the development of purulent collections of fluid. TNP dressings were reapplied. Antibiotic therapy was considered carefully, and was initially co-amoxiclav therapy, augmented with meropenem in those with signs of sepsis. In addition, for casualties who had been injured in the wet agricultural lands on foot patrol, ambisome and posaconazole were used.

When the tissues were seen to have stabilised, the bony element was shortened to its final length and the soft tissues were enveloped to surround it. By deferring definitive level bone resection until soft tissue closure was performed, the risk of intramedullary colonisation was reduced. Thus, the femur and tibia were often left long for some days, until necrosis and evolvement of the soft tissue envelope was observed to have ceased. Muscles were not sutured to the bone, but secured to each other using dissolvable sutures. Every effort was made to avoid strangulation of muscle by suturing remaining healthy fascia to fascia or tendon. TNP was again used in the depths of the wound, but in such a manner that it could be removed without unpicking the stump. Finally, the TNP drainage was removed, leaving a standard drain laid into a circumferential TNP dressing. This could be removed on the ward. Once debridement was complete, staged reconstruction was performed, using a variety of techniques including tissue transfer.

As the Queen Elizabeth Hospital, Birmingham, became a *major trauma centre* following the realignment of trauma services within the United Kingdom, it became possible to compare the management of the military and civilian traumatic amputation patients.[59] Of the patients reviewed over a seven-year period, statistically significant differences in age, ICU length of stay, blood product usage and number of surgical procedures were identified. Military patients had longer ICU stays and more operating theatre visits. Despite this, the time to stump closure and length of stay overall was not statistically different in comparison to the civilian patients. These observations support the combined orthoplastic approach delivered, the regular case discussions and the weekly multidisciplinary meetings, which included rehabilitation staff.

UPPER LIMB LESSONS

So far, we have tended to concentrate on the lower extremity, with little reference to the upper limb. However, it is probably the upper limb that allows the wounded soldier to maintain independence in activities of daily living if the residual extremity is managed to its optimum outcome. A total of 1949 upper limb injuries in 1067 UK soldiers occurred over the 10 years from 2004 to 2014[60] (890 in Afghanistan, 177 in Iraq; Roberts et al., unpublished). A review of all upper limb injury patterns is ongoing. The following paragraphs provide a summary of the findings to date that offer important messages for future surgeons.

Scapular injuries

Scapular injuries are relatively uncommon. UK Military personnel sustained 44 such fractures out of a total of 572 (7.7%) upper limb fractures in the 10-year period from 2004 to 2014,[60] in comparison to the civilian incidence of 0.4%.[61] By its very position, surrounded by significant musculature, high-energy injury mechanisms are required to sustain scapular damage. In our study, 40 were a result of gunshot or blast injury, 54% being open. ISSs were almost double compared to the average upper limb injury without a scapular fracture (21 versus 11). Most were accompanied by other injuries. Seventeen per cent had an associated brachial plexus injury. Brachial plexus injuries associated with GSWs had a favourable chance of recovery, but those associated with blast injury mechanisms had much poorer outcomes overall. Fixation was required in 10% for either glenoid fracture or floating shoulder; these were the result of high-velocity GSWs or mounted blast ejections. No cases of deep soft tissue infection or osteomyelitis occurred and all scapula fractures united.[60]

Vascular injuries

A total of 52 UK soldiers were evacuated from UK military facilities in the Middle East having sustained arterial injuries to the upper limb proximal to the carpus.[62] Blast injuries and GSWs were the two most frequent mechanisms of injury (33 and 16, respectively), with blast mechanisms (IEDs and rocket propelled grenades [RPGs]) producing significant fragmentation. Vascular injuries associated with IEDs occurred almost universally when dismounted (22 vs. 2). The reverse was true with RPGs when the majority of injuries were sustained whilst mounted in or on a vehicle (4 vs. 1) (Figure 9.6).

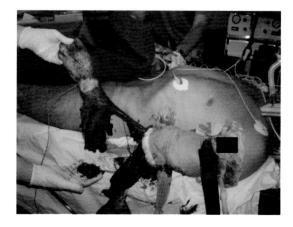

Figure 9.6 Upper limb amputation due to RPG strike. Note the field dressing and the CAT® tourniquet.

The brachial artery was most frequently injured, and alongside the ulnar artery, injuries were particularly associated with blast. Axillary artery injuries were more likely to be secondary to GSWs, but no such correlation was identified with radial artery injuries. A non-statistically significant preponderance to involvement of the ulnar side of the forearm ($p = 0.23$) and left forearm ($p = 0.13$) was noticed.[62]

Apart from three temporary shunts, all vascular injuries were treated definitively in the deployed hospital before medical evacuation to the United Kingdom. Proximal injuries were predominantly managed with long saphenous vein grafts and distal injuries with ligation, apart from combined radial and ulnar injuries, where vein grafts were utilised (Figure 9.7).

The limb salvage rate was 96%, and there were no delayed secondary amputations, following further

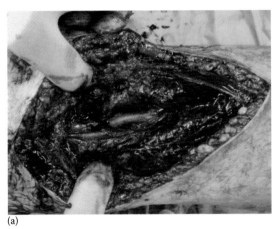

(a)

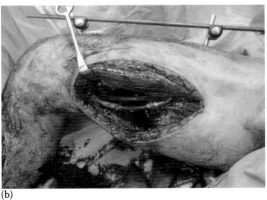

(b)

Figure 9.7 Popliteal injury. (a) Popliteal artery injury. (b) Shunt and external fixation applied.

management in the United Kingdom, as a result of vascular insufficiency, graft failure or infection.

There were five identified graft failures following repatriation (21%), including in combined radial/ulnar artery injuries. There were no subsequent perfusion issues, even in those cases treated with delayed proximal ligation. Nerve injuries were commonly associated with vascular injuries, necessitating a variety of surgical reconstruction techniques. One hundred per cent of radial fractures went onto non-union if associated with a radial artery injury. However, overall successful immediate reperfusion of a vascularly compromised upper limb correlates with excellent long-term limb survival, despite one in five grafts developing secondary failure.[62]

Amputations

Between 2004 and 2014, 28 major upper limb amputations (proximal to the carpus) occurred together with a further four peri-carpal amputations having near total loss of the hand with preservation of the thumb (3%).[63] All injuries were blast mediated, with 93% of soldiers being dismounted at the time of the blast. Of the two mounted military personnel, one was the driver of the vehicle and the other was positioned as top cover. IEDs were almost universal as the cause of injury, apart from three RPGs. Right and left arms were affected equally. The commonest level of amputation was trans-humeral (64%). One trans-humeral amputation occurred through the neck of the humerus, the remainder, at the diaphyseal level.

Excluding the peri-carpal amputations, 21 out of the 28 amputations (75%) occurred in the deployed hospital because the limb was deemed unsalvageable, and as a result, surgeons proceeded straight to completion of the primary amputation. The remaining 25% occurred at the time of injury as a direct result of the blast impact. If successful reperfusion of an ischaemic upper limb occurred in the deployed hospital, there were no delayed amputations following evacuation as a result of vascular insufficiency or infection. Despite no amputations being performed at Birmingham, there were six cases of stump-level revision from one anatomical region to a more proximal level.

The most frequent was from through-elbow to trans-humeral.[63]

Combined upper and lower limb amputations were frequent, with 22 out of the 32 amputations (69%) having at least one concomitant lower limb amputation. Eighteen of these (81%) were bilateral lower limb (triple amputee). Above knee amputations occurred in 17 soldiers (77%). There were no cases of bilateral upper limb amputation in UK personnel; however, the contralateral upper limb was frequently injured, with the injuries including fractures, peripheral nerve injuries and minor digital amputations (65%). Lower limb amputations were often associated with pelvic fractures, abdominal injuries and perineal wounds. The average ISS was 26 compared to the average upper limb ISS of 11. There was no statistical difference in ISS according to the level of upper limb amputation. Soldiers with associated bilateral lower limb amputations had significantly higher ISS (29) compared to isolated upper limb amputations (20).[63]

Every soldier's amputation stump was left open following debridement, and a *vacuum-assisted closure* dressing applied. The initial debridement frequently took place within one hour of arrival; however, this was dependent on the physiological reserve of the individual. Secondary debridement with stump fashioning was undertaken once the patient had been evacuated to the United Kingdom by specialist multi-disciplinary teams of orthopaedic, hand and plastic surgeons. Amputation stumps were not primarily closed following initial surgical debridement in Afghanistan or Iraq.

Maintaining stump length with adequate soft tissue coverage was considered a priority, and therefore, a variety of measures were employed when delayed primary closure was not technically feasible. Split skin grafts were most frequent, but local flaps were also utilised (for example the lateral arm flap). Free flaps, such as the anterolateral thigh flap, were only carried out in revision procedures following complications. In one case, vascularised radial bone lengthening of the proximal ulnar was carried out in order to maintain stump length.

COMPLICATIONS

Complications were observed in several soldiers, including superficial infections, partial graft failures, phantom limb pain, residual limb pain (neuroma formation) and heterotopic ossification (HO).

Split skin grafts interfered with prosthetic fitting in a number of ways, including through scarring, skin clefts, friable skin grafts, bony prominences and nerve tethering. Neuroma formation and residual limb pain did not correlate with the level of amputation but also had an impact on prosthetic compliance. Stump revision with neuroma excision as well as serial skin graft/scar excision with or without flap coverage improved prosthetic usage. The incidence of phantom limb pain was higher with more distal amputation levels. To improve rates of phantom limb pain, pregabalin and amitriptyline were started on the first day following repatriation even if the patient was sedated. Pain team visits occurred in the acute hospital setting and continued throughout the rehabilitation period. Targeted muscle re-innervation reduced stump pain and phantom limb pain.[63]

The formation of HO started at an early stage and was visible on one soldier's radiograph within three days of his amputation. Not all cases were symptomatic; however, the degree of HO was often extensive and reduced prosthetic tolerance. The ability to use prostheses following excision did not depend on timing of excision, and there is no indication for delaying excision, especially with the potential for inability to wear prosthetic devices. Following excision, non-steroidal anti-inflammatory drugs were given for four weeks to reduce recurrence. Functional results, symptomatic relief and patient satisfaction were all high.

Initial rehabilitation took place in one dedicated unit (*Defence Medical Rehabilitation Centre, Headley Court, Surrey, UK*) with a team of physiotherapists, psychiatrists, prosthetists and physicians. A variety of upper limb prostheses were used, including body-powered, myo-electric, hybrid and cosmetic types. Prosthetic usage varied, even at the same level of amputation, and was dependent on complications and psychological well-being. Selection was focused on the individual's needs and the extent of their injuries. Mechanical body-powered prostheses were common, incorporating a variety of adaptations for activities of daily living, including split hook, mole grip, knives and gym arm attachments. Cosmetic and myoelectric devices (for example i-limb and

Beibonic) were often used alongside body-powered mechanical prostheses, depending on the social environment.[63]

HAND INJURIES

Military deployments expose personnel to complex hand trauma, caused in part by ballistic or fragmentation injury, but also as a result of the more mundane risks associated with heavy manual work, operating machinery and heavy vehicles, training and sport.[64] Consequently, the number of observed hand injuries is significant, ranging from 9% to 18% in the published literature.[64,65] In a six-year review of UK Military personnel between 2003 and 2009, isolated hand injuries were responsible for 6.5% of aeromedical evacuations. Most of these were cases of non-battle injury.

This review will not attempt to provide an in-depth explanation of how to manage all hand injuries, as by their very nature, they are diverse. However, the aim will be to stress the importance of not ignoring hand injuries, particularly when they occur as part of multi-system trauma in the most severely injured personnel. It will often be long-term hand function that will define whether the casualty will be able to undertake some of the normal activities of daily living, thus facilitating the maximum degree of independence. A systematic sequence of management will be considered, which will include evaluation, initial treatment, reconstruction and rehabilitation, with the ultimate goal of obtaining early maximal function.[66]

The deploying surgeon should have an awareness of the biomechanical and functional properties of the hand, in order to understand its importance in the first instance.[67] The hand has four functional units: the thumb, opposable index and middle fingers, the ring and small fingers and the wrist. Prehension, the ability to grasp and manipulate objects, should be possible if there is a stable wrist joint and at least two sensate, pain-free digits that can achieve opposition.[68] The six basic components of a digit are bone, joint, skin, tendon, nerve and blood vessels. Moran and Berger[68] suggest that early amputation should be considered if any four of the six are severely damaged. However, in the early stages of management, this decision should

be left to the reconstructive surgeons as component parts might be utilisable for salvaging other digits.

Retention of the thumb has the greatest priority because of its unique ability to circumduct and oppose.[66] Loss of the thumb may reduce hand function by more than 50%. Second to the thumb in importance is the index finger, with its role in precision and directional grip as well as extension independence.[68] Loss of the index finger affects overall hand strength and leads to a 20% decrease in power grip, key pinch and supination strength.[69] The middle finger is often recruited if the index finger is damaged, and its position allows it to participate in both power and precision grips. The little finger plays an important role in the digitopalmar grip due to the mobility of its carpo-metacarpal joint. There is considerable debate regarding the little finger, and it is considered by some to have the greatest functional role after the thumb.[70]

Initial management and assessment

Hand injuries are rarely solitary when the mechanism is ballistic or fragmentation. Wounds are multiple, complex and the result of any combination of avulsion, laceration or crushing with tearing and shredding of the tissues, all frequently compounded by heavy contamination with dirt and debris, which are driven deep into the tissues. The patient is frequently physiologically unstable or in need of significant resuscitation, so the hand injury is often seen to be less of a priority.

GSW or blast fragmentation injury is often assessed according to the degree of energy transfer transmitted to the individual. Injuries to the hand are no different. The hand may sustain cavitatory defects, which are often far from apparent on initial inspection, and it contains a dense concentration of structures vital to function. These may easily be compromised by excessive initial debridement, beyond the removal of obvious contamination and non-viable tissue.

If possible, a clinical examination should be undertaken at the earliest opportunity in order to assess the extent of overall injury. As a basic minimum, the *ulnar nerve* may be tested using the first *dorsal interosseous muscle* (abduction against resistance) and sensation on the ulnar border of the little finger. *Median nerve* power is tested by *abductor pollicis brevis* function and sensation in the palmar aspect of the thumb, index and long fingers, and the radial nerve, by assessment of the *posterior interosseous nerve* with extension of the interphalangeal joint of the thumb and the metacarpal phalangeal joints of the other digits. Skin colour, skin loss, capillary refill and finger cascade should all be compared to the uninjured limb. Radiological assessment prior to surgery is paramount.

Ideally, as with any other ballistic or blast injury, assessment should be undertaken using the *ICRC System of Wound Classification*. This enables the passage of information to be consistent between clinicians. This is given in Table 9.10.

Initial surgical management

With these complex injuries, the surgeon who initially manages a wound largely determines the subsequent outcome. In the recent conflicts, the deployed capability included personnel with specialist hand experience. However, this may not be the case in the future. Staged surgical management initially described by Churchill in 1944 remains key to our practice.[71] Recent experience demonstrates the need to buy time for the injured hand, and the initial surgery should be extremely conservative as the hand contains little that may be sacrificed without significant consequence.[72] The preliminary aims should be to preserve and protect vital structures, restore viability and prevent sepsis. This may be achieved using the approach in Table 9.11.

Table 9.10 ICRC wound assessment modified for the hand

Wound characteristic	Measurement
E (Entry)	Maximum diameter in cm, including skin loss
X (Exit)	Maximum diameter in cm, including skin loss
C (Cavity)	Presence of a cavity (usually assessed with two gloved fingers in larger structures, but will be smaller within the hand muscle bulk but potentially significant)
F (Fracture)	Presence of associated fractures and bone loss, including joint injury/destruction
V (Vital Structures)	Injury to nerves, blood vessels and tendons
M (Metallic Debris)	Retention of any retained ballistic material/debris

Table 9.11 Initial approach to the injured hand

1. Thorough washout to remove contaminants and debris.
2. Release of any developing haematomas.
3. Inspection of vital structures, tagging of nerves is NOT recommended.
4. Minimal debridement; retaining tissue of marginal viability as blood supply to the hand is robust.
5. Preservation of any non-functioning but potentially viable tissue, including skin, tendon and nerve.
6. Stabilisation of unstable fractures and or joints with K wires, if re-establishing anatomical position restores viability.
7. Carpal tunnel decompression, along with the release of the muscular compartments, should be carefully considered if swelling is considerable, whilst attempting not to interfere with later flap coverage or surgical approach.
8. All wounds should be left open.
9. Dressings should include a non-adherent base layer, gauze, with the forearm and hand splinted in the position of safe immobilisation, also known as the *Edinburgh position*, with the wrist in 30–60 degrees of extension, metacarpal-phalangeal joints in 70–90 degrees of flexion and the proximal interphalangeal and distal interphalangeal joints in extension.

Delayed primary closure

Delayed primary closure is performed three to five days post initial injury. This procedure should include careful reassessment regarding tissue viability, contamination and injury demarcation, with further careful debridement if indicated. Skeletal alignment and stabilisation using K wire fixation or micro-external fixation is also performed if this was not previously achieved, or adjustment may be required. At the same time, if appropriate, nerve repair and delayed primary closure of wounds are carried out.

If at second look the wounds still appear contaminated, then delayed primary suture should be deferred for a further 48 hours. There is a balance to be met between early closure with associated infective complications and late closure that may lead to scarring and contractures. The decision making for this process remains difficult, and experience in dealing with such wounds is invaluable. Oedema often remains a significant problem at this stage, but with skeletal stabilisation, the commencement of mobilisation with measured hand therapy intervention is enabled, thus promoting reduction of swelling, assisting with pain control and inhibiting infection. Many of our recent casualties remained in intensive care at this stage post injury, and once again, the multidisciplinary approach to total casualty management cannot be stressed more forcefully. Ignoring the hand injury at this stage potentially leads to later significant deficits in function.

The use of topical negative pressure wound therapy dressings has assisted in the management of hand injury, potentially improving wound healing, optimising recipient graft sites and decreasing the overall duration of management required. TNP may also assist in the stabilisation of the hand in the initial management phase, thus reducing the need for a metal fixation device and further surgical intervention.

The overall aim of this stage of surgery is to produce a non-infected, stable environment, suitable for definitive closure or reconstruction with bone, tendon and/or nerve grafting depending upon the situation.

Definitive reconstruction

This is ideally undertaken within 7 to 14 days of the original injury, and at the earliest point possible. A combined orthopaedic and plastic surgical approach should be undertaken with careful pre-operative planning. A full explanation of all reconstructive procedures undertaken during the conflict period is outside the scope of this review.[66]

FOOT AND ANKLE

When an explosive detonates beneath a vehicle, the blast wave from the explosion causes the release of a cone of super-heated gas and soil that impacts the undersurface of the travelling vehicle. This results in rapid deflection of the vehicle floor, transmitting a very-short-duration (less than 10 milliseconds), high-amplitude load into anything that is in contact with it. Most frequently, it is the lower leg and particularly the foot and ankle complex that are injured.[73] Injuries to the foot and ankle complex are of particular interest as it has been demonstrated that patients sustaining foot and ankle injuries have significantly greater disability scores than do those without.[74,75] These effects may be even more pronounced in a young military population, who are likely to place significant functional demands on the foot and ankle complex.

Until the recent conflicts in the Middle East, clinical information relating to under-vehicle mine incidents had been limited to a single case series of injuries over a five-year period in Croatia.[76] Of the 31 survivors described in this study, only limited data were available on the pattern of lower limb injury, and there was none on clinical outcome. Due to the lack of clinical data on lower limb injuries sustained during under-vehicle explosions, mitigation engineers extrapolated data from automotive injuries in an attempt to understand the injuries they were trying to prevent. In order to address this deficit, there was thus an urgent requirement to characterise the injury profile and medium-term outcomes of casualties suffering lower limb injuries from under-vehicle explosions. The analysis of contemporary clinical data allows the development of appropriate research questions and hypotheses that drive engineers to develop a greater understanding of areas where the effectiveness of the current protection offered to vehicle occupants may be improved.

Using a prospective military trauma registry,[77] UK Service personnel who sustained lower leg injuries following an under-vehicle explosion between

January 2006 and December 2008 were identified and followed up for a mean of 33.0 months.[78] This analysis demonstrated that casualties who suffered lower limb trauma from under-vehicle explosives frequently had multi-segmental foot and ankle injuries, which resulted in an amputation rate of 30%. In addition, 75% of injured limbs were noted to have a poor clinical outcome three years following injury. A poor outcome was defined as *one* of (i) persistent chronic infection (either osteomyelitis or persistent wound infection 12 months post injury), (ii) delayed fracture healing beyond 12 months post injury (iii) symptomatic post-traumatic osteoarthritis *or* (iv) need for amputation.

Statistical modelling of the injuries demonstrated that open fractures, vascular injuries and hind-foot injuries were associated with an increased risk of amputation.[12] Further sub-group analysis of casualties with hind-foot injuries confirmed that they were associated with significantly higher amputation rates, and only 5% of patients were able to return to pre-injury levels of activity at three years post injury.[79] These data showed that attempts to protect the hind-foot from injury may reduce the risk of amputation within this cohort of casualties.

In an attempt to quantify injury and set injury criteria, military researchers have used the *Abbreviated Injury Score* (AIS) to evaluate lower limb injury. Developed for use in the automotive industry, AIS is based on the likelihood of a particular injury being fatal.[80] Hence, its use as a tool to evaluate non-lethal injuries and, in particular, to discern injuries that may result in long-term disability is less certain.[81] Using the clinical data collected, a probit analysis statistical model was created, which compared AIS with the *Foot and Ankle Severity Score* (FASS)[82] in its ability to predict either amputation or poor clinical outcome. From the results of the statistical modelling, it was demonstrated that the FASS was superior in predicting poor clinical outcome compared to AIS.[83] FASS has the advantage of showing greater resolution in differentiating between morphologies of foot and ankle injuries and so offers a better metric than AIS does for setting criteria for the evaluation of injury and mitigation from under-vehicle explosions. In addition, being an anatomical injury scoring system, it is better than the AIS in evaluating cadaveric specimens or other anatomic lower limb surrogates.

It is fundamentally important to understand the long-term outcomes of such disabling lower limb blast injuries. Although limb salvage could be considered to be advantageous over amputation, early functional outcomes in combat below knee amputees appear to be better than those undergoing limb salvage.[84] It remains unclear whether those effects will endure with longer-term follow up, and as current combat operations in the middle-east conclude, there remains a requirement to set up long-term longitudinal studies to evaluate the lasting effects of combat injury.

PLASTIC SURGERY AND RECONSTRUCTION

Plastic surgeons played a key role in the management of the complex wound. From mid-2009, a plastic surgeon was deployed to the hospital facility in Afghanistan. Whilst this was not new during larger conflicts, during *Operation Telic*, plastic surgery had not been one of the deploying specialties. This change in practice has led directly to an increase in the size of the plastic surgery cadre within the DMS.

Contemporary approaches to definitive reconstruction of military wounds

The established principles of extremity reconstruction remain and are to establish a clean and non-contaminated wound through adequate debridement of both hard and soft tissues, to stabilise and rigidly fix associated fractures and to achieve early soft tissue closure so as to deliver a useful and functional limb. The body of evidence within the civilian literature suggests that early soft tissue coverage of open fractures reduces infective complications and flap loss and shortens the time to bony union. However, the time to definitive flap coverage remains controversial. During the 1980s Byrd, Cierny and Godina published studies looking at acute phase (within days), sub-acute phase (one to six weeks) and chronic phase (after six weeks) of flap coverage of complex lower limb fractures. The most frequent complications were identified in the subacute groups in all three papers. However, the papers were considered to have bias. Initially, patients were transferred to specialised centres late, and the authors suggested that there was a definite learning curve in undertaking the flap surgery. No account was made for patient comorbidities. Other papers have replicated the findings but have failed to focus on the timing of soft tissue cover.

In the military population, many factors influence the opportunity to deliver soft tissue coverage. Almost inevitably, the patient has been injured aboard and requires transfer into the UK healthcare system. This is likely in most cases to take a minimum of 48 hours. Almost all casualties have multiple injuries, which require co-ordinated surgical interventions for their management. Casualties are often systemically compromised secondary to the massive transfusions received in resuscitation and thus must physiologically recover before complex reconstruction can proceed, usually after 72 hours. Infection and heavy contamination may also cause delay. The availability of donor sites for local or free flap soft tissue transfer following on from the extensive areas of wounding must also be considered. Reconstruction relying on local perforator flaps should be used with caution as the zone of trauma can often be underestimated. There is some suggestion that the primary blast wave may disrupt the intimal layer within the local blood vessels, although this has yet to be demonstrated in the research setting. Flap donor site selection must be carefully considered as the standard *latissimus dorsi* and *rectus abdominus* flaps have key core stability functions, and harvesting these may compromise physical rehabilitation.

In a military population, good results have been achieved when soft tissue coverage has been undertaken within the subacute stage at 7–21 days. Unpublished UK data demonstrates success with pedicle-flap and free-flap reconstruction of upper and lower extremities during this period. Pedicle-flap options for the lower limb include gastrocnemius, perforator-based fasciocutaneous flaps and sural artery perforator flaps. Free muscle flaps have been used, as well as free antero-lateral thigh flaps with success.

USE OF TNP DRESSINGS

Prior to the introduction of TNP wound treatment (TNPWT), wounds were dressed in a standard fashion involving fluffed dressing gauze followed by some form of bandage in order to fix this dressing to the patient. Non-adherent dressings were sometimes used to cover exposed neurovascular structures or partial thickness burn injury. The high volume of exudate frequently overwhelmed this construct, with leakage onto the external aspect of the dressings and bedding. Malodour, skin complications due to moisture and subjective deterioration of the wound during transfer were common.[85]

The use of TNP involves either an open cell/pore foam or gauze being placed in direct contact with the wound bed; a semi-occlusive dressing then creates a seal (iodine impregnation may reduce wound colonisation[86]). Negative pressure is applied via a pump to the wound–dressing interface and fluid from the wound is collected in a canister (Figure 9.8).

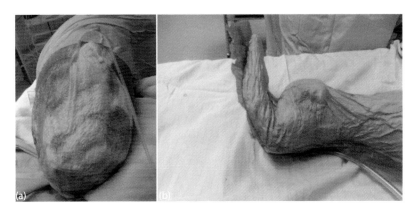

Figure 9.8 TNP therapy. (a) Lower Limb. (b) Hand.

TNP exerts beneficial effects in the damage control setting by preventing tissue from contracting (macro-deformation) and by creating a hypoxic stimulus at the centre of the wound that produces a gradient of vascular endothelial growth factor driving angiogenesis and the formation of granulation tissue. The manner in which tissue within the wound bed is altered by mechanical forces acting across it is known as micro-deformation. Exudate is removed from the wound and collected, allowing more accurate fluid balance calculations. The semi-occlusive dressing helps create a moist environment that is beneficial for wound healing and also reduces oedema. These dressings are also quick and simple to apply and require minimal training.

TNP wound therapy (TNPWT) has been shown to allow the earlier closure of fasciotomy wounds[87] and reduce the incidence of infection when used in the treatment of open fractures of the lower limb.[88] However, care should be taken in interpretation of the latter study as the numbers were low (59 patients with 63 open fractures), and inevitably, the investigators were not blinded to the dressings utilised.

In the military damage control environment and inclusive trauma systems, TNPWT facilitates movement of the patient between differing medical treatment facilities with the wound appropriately packaged. The system is deemed safe aboard fixed wing strategic aeromedical evacuation assets. In the recent campaigns, TNP applied in the operational theatre following debridement served effectively to manage the exudate and allowed the maintenance of a sealed and clean dressing during repatriation. In addition, it can further assist in minimising tissue necrosis in compromised but viable tissue by removing excessive tissue fluid and inflammatory mediators. The amount of exudate removed from these wounds was observed to be in the order of 4–5 L per day, and therefore, careful fluid management is required. This fluid also contains considerable protein, and thus, careful assessment of nutritional requirements is fundamental for these casualties.

MANAGING PERIPHERAL NERVE INJURY

The UK experience of military peripheral nerve injury in recent conflicts is excellently summarised in two papers by Professor Rolf Birch detailing their epidemiology and outcomes. These papers deal with 261 nerve injuries in 100 patients reviewed at Headley Court. They were evenly divided between the upper and lower limbs, with 82% of injuries being associated with open wounds. The most commonly injured nerves were the *ulnar*, *common peroneal* and *tibial*, and '*the nerve lesions were predominantly focal prolonged conduction block/neurapraxia in 116 (45%), axonotmesis in 92 (35%) and neurotmesis in 53 (20%)*'.[89] The theories underlying the treatment of nerve injury have not advanced since the *Second World War*, and whilst magnification and instruments have improved, tension-free repair of divided nerves by direct co-aptation or using autologous graft nurtured in a healthy infection-free soft tissue envelope remains the goal. This is more difficult to achieve in the modern military wound and patient in whom nerve graft is scarce and donor sites for fasciocutaneous cover limited.

Birch reported final outcomes graded as good in 173 cases (66%), fair in 70 (26.8%) and poor in 18 (6.9%). He confirmed previous findings that absent sensation to the sole of the foot often recovers and noted that, in some cases where results were initially poor, improvements could be made by adherence to sound principles.[89]

RESEARCH

The conflicts in Iraq and Afghanistan have refocused attention on combat casualty care and in particular on the impact of far forward resuscitation, prompt evacuation, haemorrhage control and time-limited surgery on patient outcome. Despite these improvements, a burden of significant extremity trauma remains in those who survive combat injury. This patient cohort is a result, in part, of increasing survival but is also a consequence of the nature of current combat wounding. Injury by gunshot has been eclipsed by explosive devices. The late extremity complications of skin coverage, fracture stabilisation and infection persist, and there remains a need to optimise through animal modelling the management of these disabling injuries. Simple, soft tissue wounding models based on velocity and studies of smooth projectile passage through muscle and gelatin have limited relevance to modern conflict wounding patterns.[90]

In order to care for those injured in conflict and conduct appropriate research, clinicians must be able to identify key in vivo studies, understand their weaknesses and resist the propagation of incorrectly cited and misunderstood ballistic dogma. A review by Eardley et al.[90] provides an inclusive critical overview of key studies of relevance to military extremity injury. In addition, the non-ballistic studies of limb injury, stabilisation and contamination that will form the basis from which future small animal extremity studies will be constructed are presented. The key messages of this review are demonstrated in Table 9.12.

Current military conflicts are characterised by the use of the IED. Improvements in personal protection, medical care and evacuation logistics have resulted in increasing numbers of casualties surviving with complex musculoskeletal injuries, often leading to lifelong disability. Thus, there exists an urgent requirement to investigate the mechanisms of extremity injury caused by these devices in order to develop mitigation strategies. In addition, the wounds of war are no longer restricted to the battlefield; similar injuries can be witnessed in civilian centres following a terrorist attack. Key to understanding such mechanisms of injury is the ability to deconstruct the complexities of an explosive event in a controlled, laboratory-based environment. A traumatic injury simulator, designed to recreate in the laboratory the impulse that is transferred to the lower extremity from an anti-vehicle explosion, is presented by Masouros et al.[91] and characterised experimentally and numerically. Tests with instrumented cadaveric limbs have been conducted to assess the simulator's ability to interact with the human in two mounting conditions, simulating typical seated and standing vehicle passengers. This experimental device will now allow the ability to gain comprehensive understanding of the load-transfer mechanisms through the lower limb, to characterise the dissipating capacity of mitigation technologies and to assess the bio-fidelity of surrogates.

Fundamental to designing novel mitigation strategies is a requirement to understand the injury mechanism by developing appropriate injury modelling tools that are underpinned by the analysis of contemporary battlefield casualty data. Ramasamy et al.[92] have attempted to summarise our understanding of the clinical course of lower limb blast injuries from IEDs. This is invaluable in developing unique injury modelling test-beds to evaluate and produce the next generation of protective equipment for reducing the devastating effects of blast injury. Further work on the blast injury mechanism at every level of extremity injury is required.

Identified areas for future research

Management of junctional trauma remains problematic. These very proximal injuries often involve

Table 9.12 Key messages in research modelling for military trauma

1.	Extremity ballistic injury is unique and demands individual care, based on clinical and in vivo research.
2.	Ballistic injury literature is often misinterpreted: a situation that propagates an often dogmatic approach to war surgery.
3.	Large animal models of simple projectile injury must be placed in context with and contrasted with modern combat injury patterns.
4.	Civilian small animal models of injury and infection have application to military injury modelling although they are limited in their exploitation of contaminated soft tissue injury.
5.	A need exists to further develop military specific, contaminated soft tissue small animal soft tissue models.
6.	With an awareness of both large and small animal ballistic and extremity trauma models, military surgeons are in a better position to accurately interpret pertinent literature and optimise patient care.

Source: Eardley WG et al., *J R Army Med Corps* 2013;159(2):73–83.

a perineal component and the use of standard limb tourniquets is not possible. Work continues on novel solutions including abdominal and junctional tourniquets and abdominal foams.

Long-term clinical results after combat-related orthopaedic wounds need to be evaluated. It is recognised that the debate over the choice between limb salvage and amputation is unresolved. Long-term studies in military patients comparing modern prostheses with salvaged limbs are not yet available. However, these are in progress under the combined rehabilitation and musculoskeletal teams at the Defence Medical Rehabilitation Service.

Heterotopic ossification remains a problem especially in traumatic amputation patients. Recent work by Eisenstein et al.[93] at the University of Birmingham has shown some promising results with regard to a potential chemical agent that may reduce the volume of mineralised bone that develops after a significant extremity injury, such as that following blast. However, this is in the very early stages of development, and work needs to continue to identify a delivery agent and to ensure that it does not interfere with normal bone.

There is a paucity of data regarding the use of external fixators. Papers from the early stages of the conflict in Iraq (*Operation Telic*) showed poor results and a high incidence of complications in the use of external fixation in war extremity injury, but techniques and equipment had improved considerably by the later stages of the conflicts and the results of treatment with modern external fixator systems in experienced and well trained surgeons need to be clarified.

Ballistic injury cannot be ignored. Although the results of blast injury featured much more heavily in the later stages of the conflict, GSWs were still the second commonest cause of extremity injury. A recent review by Stevenson et al.[94] has demonstrated that our overall understanding of ballistic injury is minimal and that very few published papers demonstrate ballistic GSW modelling that includes the role of clothing in the injury outcome. Obviously, foreign material injection into the wound cavity must have some effect on the overall nature of the resulting GSW, thus this is an area of study that should be continued.

CONCLUSION

Complex limb injuries due to blast from IEDs are the signature injury of recent campaigns. Many such injuries occurred in association with injuries elsewhere, especially, in the case of leg injuries, to the perineum and pelvis. Advances in resuscitation from point of wounding onwards have led to patients surviving, who, only 20 years ago, would almost certainly have died. Modern military surgery of the limbs is not only essential in the initial management of these devastatingly injured casualties but also, further down the patient's pathway, provides the basis for the rehabilitation of these predominantly young and fit patients. To achieve the best that can be achieved, limb surgery and the management of limb injuries more widely are truly parts of a multi-disciplinary process involving surgeons from various specialties and a wide range of therapists, scientists and prosthetists working together.

REFERENCES

1. Ramalingam T. Extremity injuries remain a high surgical workload in a conflict zone: Experiences of a British Field Hospital in Iraq, 2003. *J R Army Med Corps* 2004; 150(3):187–190.
2. Coupland RM. War wounds of bones and external fixation. *Injury* 1994;25(4): 211–217.
3. Belmont PJ Jr., McCriskin BJ, Hsiao MS, Burks R, Nelson KJ, Schoenfeld AJ. The nature and incidence of musculoskeletal combat wounds in Iraq and Afghanistan (2005–2009). *J Orthop Trauma* 2013;27(5): e107–e113.
4. Cross AM, Davis C, Penn-Barwell J et al. The incidence of pelvic fractures with traumatic lower limb amputation in modern warfare due to improvised explosive devices. *J R Nav Med Serv* 2014;100(2):152–156.
5. Ramasamy A, Harrisson SE, Clasper JC et al. Injuries from roadside improvised explosive devices. *J Trauma* 2008;65(4): 910–914.

6. Woodward C, Eggertson L. Homemade bombs and heavy urogenital injuries create new medical challenges. *CMAJ* 2010;182 (11):1159–1160.

7. Brown KV. Clasper JC. The changing pattern of amputations. *J R Army Med Corps* 2013;159(4):300–303.

8. Ramasamy A, Hill AM, Masouros S et al. Outcomes of IED foot and ankle blast injuries. *J Bone Joint Surg Am* 2013;95(5):e25.

9. Stapley SA, Cannon LB. An overview of the pathophysiology of gunshot and blast injury with resuscitation guidelines. *Curr Orthop* 2006;20(5):322–332.

10. Champion HR, Holcomb JB, Young LA. Injuries from explosions: Physics, biophysics, pathology, and required research focus. *J Trauma* 2009;66(5):1468–1477; discussion 1477.

11. Jansen JO, Thomas GOR, Adams SA et al. Early management of proximal traumatic lower extremity amputation and pelvic injury caused by improvised explosive devices (IEDs). *Injury* 2012;43(7):976–979.

12. Jacobs N, Rourke K, Hicks A et al. Lower limb injuries caused by improvised explosive devices: Proposed 'Bastion classification' and prospective validation. *Injury* 2014;45(9):1422–1428.

13. Ramasamy A, Masouros SD, Newell N et al. In-vehicle extremity injuries from improvised explosive devices: Current and future foci. *Philos Trans R Soc Lond B Biol Sci* 2011;366(1562):160–170.

14. Ramasamy A, Bull AM, Clasper JC et al. Blast-related fracture patterns: A forensic biomechanical approach. *J R Soc Interface* 2011;8(58):689–698.

15. Nelson TG, Wall C, Driver J, Simpson R. Op HERRICK primary care casualties: The forgotten many. *J R Army Med Corps* 2012; 158(3):252–255.

16. Mitchell J, Simpson R, Whitaker J. Cold injuries in contemporary conflict. *J R Army Med Corps* 2012;158(3):248–251.

17. Champion HR, Bellamy RF, Roberts CP, Leppaniemi A. A profile of combat injury. *J Trauma* 2003;54(5 Suppl):S13–S19.

18. Bellamy RF. The medical effects of conventional weapons. *World J Surg* 1992;16(5): 888–892.

19. Hodgetts T, Mahoney P, Russell MQ. ABC to <C>ABC: Redefining the military trauma paradigm. *Emerg Med J* 2006;23(10):745–746.

20. Brodie S, Hodgetts TJ, Lambert P et al. Tourniquet use in combat trauma: UK military experience. *J R Army Med Corps* 2007;153(4):310–313.

21. Walters TJ, Mabry RL. Issues related to the use of tourniquets on the battlefield. *Mil Med* 2005;170(9):770–775.

22. Parker PJ, Clasper J. The military tourniquet. *J R Army Med Corps* 2007;153(1):10–12.

23. Brown KV, Ramasamy, A, Tai N et al. Complications of extremity vascular injuries in conflict. *J Trauma* 2009;66(4 Suppl): S145–S149.

24. Clasper JC, Brown KV, Hill P. Limb complications following pre-hospital tourniquet use. *J R Army Med Corps* 2009;155(3):200–202.

25. Gustilo RB, Mendoza RM, Williams DN. Problems in the management of type III (severe) open fractures: A new classification of type III open fractures. *J Trauma* 1984;24(8):742–746.

26. Kragh JF Jr., Walters TJ, Baer DG et al. Survival with emergency tourniquet use to stop bleeding in major limb trauma. *Ann Surg* 2009;249(1):1–7.

27. Penn-Barwell JG, Murray CK, Wenke JC. Comparison of the antimicrobial effect of chlorhexidine and saline for irrigating a contaminated open fracture model. *J Orthop Trauma* 2012;26(12):728–732.

28. Owens BD, White DW, Wenke JC. Comparison of irrigation solutions and devices in a contaminated musculoskeletal wound survival model. *J Bone Joint Surg Am* 2009;91(1):92–98.

29. Guthrie HC, Clasper JC, Kay AR, Parker PJ. Initial extremity war wound debridement: A multidisciplinary consensus. *J R Army Med Corps* 2011;157(2):170–175.

30. Taylor CJ, Hettiaratchy S, Jeffery SL et al. Contemporary approaches to definitive extremity reconstruction of military

wounds. *J R Army Med Corps* 2009;155(4): 302–307.

31. Penn-Barwell JG, Sargeant ID. Severe lower extremity combat trauma study, gun-shot injuries in UK military casualties – features associated with wound severity. *Injury* 2016; 47(5):1067–1071.

32. Parker P. Limb Trauma Working Group. Consensus statement on decision making in junctional trauma care. *J R Army Med Corps* 2011;157(3 Suppl 1):S293–S295.

33. Penn-Barwell JG, Fries CA, Street L, Jeffery S. Use of topical negative pressure in British servicemen with combat wounds. *Eplasty* 2011;11:e35.

34. Ritenour AE, Dorlac WC, Fang R et al. Complications after fasciotomy revision and delayed compartment release in combat patients. *J Trauma* 2008;64(2 Suppl):S153–S161; discussion S161–S162.

35. Middleton S, Clasper J. Compartment syndrome of the foot – implications for military surgeons. *J R Army Med Corps* 2010; 156(4):241–244.

36. Beech Z, Parker P. Internal fixation on deployment: Never, ever, clever? *J R Army Med Corps* 2012;158(1):4–5.

37. Rowlands TK, Clasper J. The Thomas splint – a necessary tool in the management of battlefield injuries. *J R Army Med Corps* 2003;149(4):291–293.

38. Clasper JC, Phillips SL. Early failure of external fixation in the management of war injuries. *J R Army Med Corps* 2005;151(2): 81–86.

39. Dharm-Datta S, Hill G. Improvised equipment for skeletal traction on operations. *J R Army Med Corps* 2007;153(2):144.

40. Boyd MC, Mountain AJ, Clasper JC. Improvised skeletal traction in the management of ballistic femoral fractures. *J R Army Med Corps* 2009;155(3):194–196.

41. Mody RM, Zapor M, Hartzell JD et al. Infectious complications of damage control orthopedics in war trauma. *J Trauma* 2009;67(4):758–761.

42. Keeney JA, Ingari JV, Mentzer KD, Powell ET. Closed intramedullary nailing of femoral shaft fractures in an echelon III facility. *Mil Med* 2009;174(2):124–128.

43. Hertel R, Lambert SM, Müller S, Ballmer FT, Ganz R. On the timing of soft-tissue reconstruction for open fractures of the lower leg. *Arch Orthop Trauma Surg* 1999; 119(1–2):7–12.

44. Okike K, Bhattacharyya T. Trends in the management of open fractures. A critical analysis. *J Bone Joint Surg Am* 2006; 88(12):2739–2748.

45. Naique SB, Pearse M, Nanchahal J. Management of severe open tibial fractures: The need for combined orthopaedic and plastic surgical treatment in specialist centres. *J Bone Joint Surg Br* 2006;88(3): 351–357.

46. Penn-Barwell JG, Bennett PM, Fries CA et al. Severe open tibial fractures in combat trauma: Management and preliminary out-comes. *Bone Joint J* 2013;95-B(1):101–105.

47. Hull JB, Cooper GJ. Pattern and mechanism of traumatic amputation by explosive blast. *J Trauma* 1996;40(3 Suppl):S198–S205.

48. Singleton JA, Gibb IE, Bull AM, Clasper JC. Blast-mediated traumatic amputation: Evidence for a revised, multiple injury mechanism theory. *J R Army Med Corps* 2014;160(2):175–179.

49. Edwards DS, Phillip RD, Bosanquet N, Bull AM, Clasper JC. What is the magnitude and long-term economic cost of care of the British Military Afghanistan Amputee Cohort? *Clin Orthop Relat Res* 2015;473(9):2848–2855.

50. Clasper J, Lower Limb Trauma Working Group. Amputations of the lower limb: A multidisciplinary consensus. *J R Army Med Corps* 2007;153(3):172–174.

51. Penn-Barwell JG, Bennett PM, Kay A, Sargeant ID. Acute bilateral leg amputation following combat injury in UK servicemen. *Injury* 2014;45(7):1105–1110.

52. Morrison JJ, Hunt N, Midwinter M, Jansen J. Associated injuries in casualties with trau-matic lower extremity amputations caused by improvised explosive devices. *Br J Surg* 2012;99(3):362–366.

53. Penn-Barwell JG, Fries CA, Sargeant ID, et al. Aggressive soft tissue infections and amputation in military trauma patients. *J R Nav Med Serv* 2012;98(2):14–18.

54. Brown KV, Hennan P, Stapley S, Clasper JC. Limb salvage of severely injured extremities after military wounds. *J R Army Med Corps* 2011;157(3 Suppl 1):S315–S323.

55. Rush RM Jr., Kjorstad R, Starnes BW, Arrington E, Devine JD, Andersen CA. Application of the Mangled Extremity Severity Score in a combat setting. *Mil Med* 2007;172(7):777–781.

56. Fox CJ, Gillespie DL, Cox ED et al. The effectiveness of a damage control resuscitation strategy for vascular injury in a combat support hospital: Results of a case control study. *J Trauma* 2008;64(2 Suppl):S99–S106; discussion S106–S107.

57. Penn-Barwell JG, Myatt RW, Bennett PM, Sargeant ID. Medium-term outcomes following limb salvage for severe open tibia fracture are similar to trans-tibial amputation. *Injury* 2015;46(2):288–291.

58. MacKenzie EJ, Bosse MJ, Pollak AN et al. Long-term persistence of disability following severe lower-limb trauma. Results of a seven-year follow-up. *J Bone Joint Surg Am* 2005;87(8):1801–1809.

59. Staruch RM, Jackson PC, Hodson J et al. Comparing the surgical timelines of military and civilians traumatic lower limb amputations. *Ann Med Surg (Lond)* 2016;6:81–86.

60. Roberts DP, Stapley SA. A review of 10 years of scapular injuries sustained by UK military personnel on operations. In: *Upper Limb Studies*. Birmingham: RCDM, 2017.

61. Court-Brown CM, Caesar B. Epidemiology of adult fractures: A review. *Injury* 2006;37(8):691–697.

62. Roberts DP, Stapley SA. *Management and Outcomes of Major Upper Limb Arterial Injuries Sustained during Military Operations*. Birmingham: RCDM, 2017.

63. Roberts DP, Stapley, SA. *Major Upper Limb Amputation in UK Soldiers from Recent Conflicts: A Ten Year Review*. Birmingham: RCDM, 2017.

64. Penn-Barwell JG, Bennett PM, Powers D, Standley D. Isolated hand injuries on operational deployment: An examination of epidemiology and treatment strategy. *Mil Med* 2011;176(12):1404–1407.

65. Owens BD, Kragh JF Jr., Wenke JC, Macaitis J, Wade CE, Holcomb JB. Combat wounds in operation Iraqi Freedom and operation Enduring Freedom. *J Trauma* 2008;64(2):295–299.

66. Eardley WG, Stewart MP. Early management of ballistic hand trauma. *J Am Acad Orthop Surg* 2010;18(2):118–126.

67. Husum H, Ang SC, Fosse E. *War Surgery: Field Manual*. Third World Network, 1995.

68. Moran SL, Berger RA. Biomechanics and hand trauma: What you need. *Hand Clin* 2003;19(1):17–31.

69. Murray J, Carman W, MacKenzie J. Transmetacarpal amputation of the index finger: A clinical assessment of hand strength and complications. *J Hand Surg* 1977;2(6):471–481.

70. Tubiana R, Thomine J, Mackin E. *Movements of the Hand and Wrist. Examination of the Hand and Wrist*. St Louis, MO: Mosby, 1996, pp. 78–111.

71. Churchill ED. The surgical management of the wounded in the Mediterranean theater at the time of the fall of Rome – [Foreword by Brig. Gen'l Fred W. Rankin, MC]. *Ann Surg* 1944;120(3):268.

72. Brown PW. War wounds of the hand revisited. *J Hand Surg* 1995;20(3):S61–S67.

73. Ramasamy A, Bull AM, Clasper JC et al. Blast-related fracture patterns: A forensic biomechanical approach. *J R Soc Interface* 2011;8(58):689–698.

74. Tran T, Thordarson D. Functional outcome of multiply injured patients with associated foot injury. *Foot Ankle Int* 2002;23(4):340–343.

75. Turchin DC. Do foot injuries significantly affect the functional outcome of multiply injured patients? *J Orthop Trauma* 1999;13(1):1–4.

76. Radonic V, Giunio L, Biocić M, Tripković A, Lukcić B, Promorac D. Injuries from anti-tank mines in Southern Croatia. *Mil Med* 2004;169(4):320–324.

77. Smith J, Mahoney PF, Russell R. Trauma governance in the UK defence medical services. *J R Army Med Corps* 2007;153: 239–242.

78. Ramasamy A, Hill AM, Masouros S et al. Outcomes of IED foot and ankle blast injuries. *J Bone Joint Surg Am* 2013;95(5):e25.

79. Ramasamy A, Hill AM, Phillip R. The modern "deck-slap" injury – calcaneal blast fractures from vehicle explosions. *J Trauma* 2011;71(6):1694–1698.

80. Gennarelli TA, Wodzin E. AIS 2005: A contemporary injury scale. *Injury* 2006;37(12):1083–1091.

81. Poole GV, Tinsley M, Tsao AK, Thomae KR, Martin RW, Hauser CJ. Abbreviated injury scale does not reflect the added morbidity of multiple lower extremity fractures. *J Trauma* 1996;40(6):951–956.

82. Manoli A, Prasad P, Levine RS. Foot and Ankle Severity Score (FASS). *Foot Ankle Int* 1997;18(9):598–602.

83. Ramasamy MA, Hill AM, Phillip R et al. FASS is a better predictor of poor outcome in lower limb blast injury than AIS: Implications for blast research. *J Orthop Trauma* 2013;27(1):49–55.

84. Frisch HM, Hayda RA, Frisch HM et al. The Military Extremity Trauma Amputation/ Limb Salvage (METALS) Study: Outcomes of amputation versus limb salvage following major lower-extremity trauma. *J Bone Joint Surg Am* 2013;95(2):138–145.

85. Taylor CJ, Hettiaratchy S, Jeffery SL, et al. Contemporary approaches to definitive extremity reconstruction of military wounds. *J R Army Med Corps* 2009;155(4):302–307.

86. Jacobson C, Osmon DR, Hanssen A et al. Prevention of wound contamination using DuraPrep solution plus Ioban 2 drapes. *Clin Orthop Relat Res* 2005;439:32–37.

87. Yang CC, Chang DS, Webb LX. Vacuum-assisted closure for fasciotomy wounds following compartment syndrome of the leg. *J Surg Orthop Adv* 2006;15(1):19–23.

88. Stannard JP, Volgas DA, Stewart R, McGwin G Jr., Alonso JE. Negative pressure wound therapy after severe open fractures: A prospective randomized study. *J Orthop Trauma* 2009;23(8):552–557.

89. Birch R, Misra P, Stewart MP et al. Nerve injuries sustained during warfare: Part II: Outcomes. *J Bone Joint Surg Br* 2012;94(4):529–535.

90. Eardley WG, Watts SA, Clasper JC. Modelling for conflict: The legacy of ballistic research and current extremity in vivo modelling. *J R Army Med Corps* 2013;159(2):73–83.

91. Masouros SD, Newell N, Ramasamy A, et al. Design of a traumatic injury simulator for assessing lower limb response to high loading rates. *Ann Biomed Eng* 2013;41(9):1957–1967.

92. Ramasamy A, Newell N, Masouros S. From the battlefield to the laboratory: The use of clinical data analysis in developing models of lower limb blast injury. *J R Army Med Corps* 2014;160(2):117–120.

93. Eisenstein N, Richard Williams, Cox S, Stapley S, Grover L. Enzymatically regulated demineralisation of pathological bone using sodium hexametaphosphate. *J Mater Chem B* 2016;4:3815.

94. Stevenson T, Carr DJ, Stapley S. The effect of clothing on patterns of gunshot wounding in ballistic gelatin: The Naked Truth. International Symposium on Ballistics Long Beach, CA, USA, 2017.

10

Ballistic weaponry, blast and personal protective equipment development

INTRODUCTION

One of the most striking components of the medical response to the conflicts in Iraq and Afghanistan, using the term medical in its most inclusive sense, has been the dramatic improvement in personal protective equipment (PPE). Not only has PPE significantly improved, but its optimisation and development have proved exceptionally responsive to the changing threats faced by deployed personnel. This has resulted from the multidisciplinary approach adopted by Defence scientists and engineers, procurement teams, industry, academia, users of the PPE and clinicians. An essential component of this process was the dynamic and detailed system of data collection that enabled early identification of wounding patterns, of which the signature injury, of Afghanistan at least, must be considered the complex of lower limb and pelvic/perineal injuries resulting from buried *improvised explosive devices* (IEDs). This chapter discusses both the threats faced by deployed personnel and the injury prevention responses that followed.

WEAPONS USED AGAINST UK FORCES IN IRAQ AND AFGHANISTAN

The aim of this section is to provide a broad outline of those types of ballistic weaponry used against UK military forces during the Iraq and Afghanistan conflicts from November 2001 to October 2014. This will give context to the patterns of injuries treated by the Defence Medical Services

(DMS) during this period and their role in the PPE developments designed to mitigate against such weapon systems.

Improvised explosive devices

The conflicts in Iraq and Afghanistan were characterised by the use of the IED, a term that came into common usage shortly after the start of the Iraq War in 2003. IEDs are defined as 'devices placed or fabricated in an improvised manner incorporating destructive, lethal, noxious, pyrotechnic or incendiary chemicals, designed to destroy, disfigure, distract or harass and often incorporate military stores'.[1] Because they are improvised, IEDs take many forms, ranging from a small pipe bomb to a sophisticated device capable of causing massive damage and loss of life. IEDs can be vehicle borne (VBIED); carried, placed or thrown by a person; delivered in a package; or concealed at the roadside.

The effects of IEDs and the extent of damage they cause depends upon their size, construction and placement and whether or not the device incorporates a high explosive or propellant.[2] For example, VBIEDs are obviously capable of carrying significantly more explosive material and therefore do more damage, as the recent (June 2017) tragic events in Kabul have demonstrated. IEDs consist of a variety of components, including an initiator, switch, main charge, power source and a container. They may be surrounded by, or packed with, additional materials or *enhancements* such as nails, glass, or metal fragments designed to increase injury from fragments propelled by the explosion.

Enhancements may also include other elements such as hazardous materials. During the Iraq and Afghanistan campaigns, IEDs were often used in conjunction with other munitions such as the used 155 mm artillery shells rigged with blasting caps used by Iraqi insurgents. An IED can be initiated by a variety of methods depending on the intended target and may make use of many commonly available materials, such as fertiliser, gunpowder and hydrogen peroxide. Explosives must contain a fuel and an oxidiser, which provides the oxygen needed to sustain the reaction; a common example is a mixture of ammonium nitrate, which acts as the oxidiser, and fuel oil, which acts as the fuel source.

The design of the devices used in Iraq was different from those used in Afghanistan. In Iraq, the typical injury profile was related to the use of the *explosively formed projectile* (EFP – sometimes referred to as an explosive formed penetrator). These are cylindrical charges, fabricated from commonly available metal pipe, with the forward end closed by a concave metal disc-shaped liner to create a shaped charge (Figure 10.1).[3] The explosive is loaded behind the metal liner to fill the pipe.

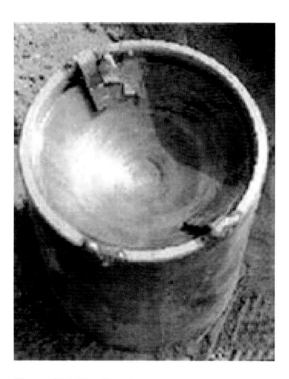

Figure 10.1 EFP from Iraq.

When the explosive is detonated, the conical metal plate (or lens) is deformed and reshaped into an aerodynamically efficient penetrator moving at high velocity (>1500 ms^{-1}). This in effect becomes a very high-energy ballistic weapon, with casualties caught in the trajectory of the EFP suffering catastrophic injuries whereas those sitting adjacent to the projectile's path were less severely injured.[4] Due to the high-energy nature of the EFP, they are able to penetrate armour protected vehicles.[5] In Iraq, there was certainly a gradual trend towards devices becoming larger as coalition forces added more armour to their vehicles.

Bullets

During both conflicts, high-velocity rifle ammunition was the second most common cause of injury to UK Service personnel during hostile action. Enemy combatants most commonly used 7.62 mm calibre ammunition (for example 7.62 × 39) and less commonly 5.45 mm calibre ammunition (5.45 × 39). UK forces primarily used individual weapons firing 5.56 mm calibre ammunition (e.g. 5.56 × 45), with the standard weapon being the SA80-A2 (Figure 10.2a).

In Iraq, the most common weapons firing 7.62 mm calibre ammunition were variants of the Kalashnikov assault rifle.[6] According to the US Army, most rifles in Iraq were Yugoslav- and Iraqi-produced weapons of Soviet design (Figure 10.2b). The most common was the AKM variant of the Kalshnikov and, to a lesser extent, the AK-47.[7] A smaller but still significant number of bolt-action rifles were also found in caches; most of them appeared to be chambered for the 303 round used by various iterations of the British Lee-Enfield rifle, which was first produced more than a century ago.[6] Most sniper rifles and machine guns circulating in Iraq shortly after the US invasion were of Soviet design and produced in Iraq or in Eastern European countries. These included the Russian Dragunov and the Romanian FPK, as well as the Iraqi Al-Kadissiya and Tabuk sniper rifles.[7]

Strong evidence existed that coalition forces were also being attacked by insurgents using US weapons, particularly the M16 assault rifle.[8] A later audit in 2014 revealed that the Pentagon had lost track of many of the 465,000 light weapons the

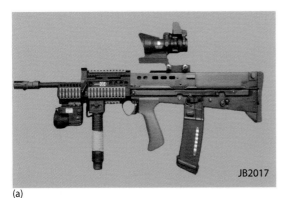
(a)

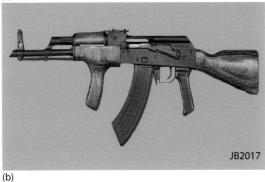
(b)

Figure 10.2 (a) SA80 rifle used by UK forces during the campaigns in Iraq and Afghanistan. Shown is the A2 L85 modification, first introduced to Afghanistan in 2001. (b) Kalashnikov AKM automatic rifle captured from insurgents in Afghanistan.

United States had supplied to the Afghan security forces, particularly of the M16.[9] The M16 has twice the effective range of the Kalashnikov variants such as the AK47 or AKM, making it particularly desired by Taliban sharpshooters.[10]

Grenades

Seized weapons caches from Iraq demonstrated that insurgent forces used both hand and rocket-propelled grenades. The majority of the items for which detailed information was available appeared to be Soviet-designed models first fielded in the 1960s and 1970s.[7] The RKG-3 anti-tank grenade became a signature weapon, being easily concealed under the robes of a dishdasha.[11] It could be thrown overhand into armoured convoys at the last moment and at very short range (Figure 10.3). The

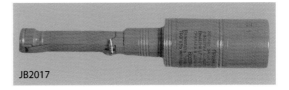

Figure 10.3 RKG-3 hand grenade captured from insurgents in Iraq.

most common grenade launcher used by the Taliban was the Soviet RPG-7 launcher.[12] The two main grenade types were anti-personnel rounds and *high-explosive, anti-tank* rounds. The types of grenade included hand, rifle and spin-stabilised. Later in the conflict, the Taliban utilised improvised ammunition, particularly making use of ball bearings, with an alleged 30 feet kill radius.[12] RPG-7 launchers and their foreign variants fire a variety of rounds.[7]

Rockets and mortars

In both Iraq and Afghanistan, mortars and mortar rounds were the most frequently encountered items found in recovered arms caches.[7] Rockets and mortars gave insurgents the ability to carry out stand-off, or 'indirect' attacks, on fixed positions such as patrol bases. Quick to set up, insurgents often fired these weapons with no direct line of sight to their targets. One weapon found repeatedly in Iraq and Afghanistan was the Type 63 Chinese 107 mm artillery rocket.[11] Unlike the longer 122 mm rockets of the 'Grad' series, the Type 63 is self-stabilising and thus can be fired from a simple ramp of dirt or rocks (Figure 10.4).

Missiles

Use of missiles against coalition forces in either Iraq or Afghanistan was infrequent during this

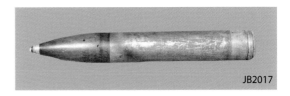

Figure 10.4 Captured type 63 Chinese 107 mm artillery rocket.

period. The most notable exception was when insurgents used a Stinger missile to bring down a US helicopter in Afghanistan; fortunately, there were no casualties.[13] Although the Iraqi military had an extensive missile development programme prior to 2003, these installations were targeted heavily by coalition air strikes, and depots of arms including missiles were systematically destroyed when they were found.[14]

Mines

Mines were laid extensively by Iraqi forces during the Iran–Iraq War (1980–1988) and therefore presented a significant risk for coalition forces.[15] The broad types found included anti-personnel and anti-armour mines, which were generally buried and sometimes linked to one another in chains.[16] Detonation was generally produced by the target or vehicle stepping on or passing over the device, but tripwires linked to the mine were also used.

Anti-personnel mines are a form of land mine and can be classified into blast mines or fragmentation mines.[17] While blast mines are designed to cause severe injury to one person, fragmentation mines are designed to project small fragments across a wider area, thereby causing a greater number of injuries.[16] Mines can be distributed by a plethora of weapon systems, including aerial delivery and *Multiple Launch Rocket Systems*, which can deliver hundreds of mines in a matter of minutes.[18]

BASIC BALLISTIC SCIENCE

Principles of explosives

An explosion is a result of a change in state from solid or liquid, to gas, and of the resulting release of energy. The explosive properties of a material are determined by its chemical composition and the speed at which energy is expelled. Low explosives react by deflagration, or burning, where the reaction is propagated by flame passing through the material at a rate significantly slower than the speed of sound. They consist of a combustible material (for example sulphur and charcoal in gunpowder), together with a source of oxygen (potassium nitrate in the case of gunpowder), and during the explosive process, there is a low rise in pressure.

Low explosives include fireworks and most commonly injure by burning; they are not a significant medical problem in modern conflicts. However, if a low explosive is contained in a hard object, such as in a pressure cooker, the internal pressure can rise to high levels before there is a sudden release of energy, and more significant injuries can occur. This is also the process used in firearms where the explosive acts as a propellant for the bullet.

In contrast, high explosives degrade via detonation, where propagation through the substance is far faster; and the resultant energy is thus expelled at very high speeds. The input of a relatively small amount of energy, via an initiator, to the explosive, results in the production of a very large volume of gas, at high temperature and pressure. This gas expands outwards at high speeds to occupy a volume far greater than that occupied by the original explosive. This outward expansion results in a pressure wave from the compressed air, which moves away from the point of detonation at supersonic speeds: the *shock wave*.

The change in surrounding pressure is described as the *blast overpressure*; there is a near-instantaneous pressure rise that then falls exponentially. In addition to the pressure wave, the expanding gases generate *blast winds*, tumbling air and hot products of combustion; these can displace large objects, including people. Thirdly, detonation of explosives may result in the expulsion of fragments. These fragments may be part of the device casing, separate material deliberately added or environmental material displaced by the blast, including body parts. It is these three mechanisms, overpressure, winds and fragments, that result in most injuries seen following explosions.

Blast injuries

Traditionally, the injurious effects from explosions have been classified after the initial descriptions by Zuckerman during the Second World War[19]; a more detailed description was subsequently produced by the US Department of Defense in 2008.[20] Whilst the classification is considered by many as definitive, it has limitations, particularly as the initial work related to free field blast (explosions in an open environment). It was acknowledged in the early literature that different environments will result in different injury patterns, and this will be considered in the next subsections. Blast injury is now generally classified into primary, secondary, tertiary and quaternary.

PRIMARY BLAST INJURY

This results from blast overpressure, which can result in direct transmission of the shock wave through the tissues of the body, as well as compression and acceleration of tissues. Differential acceleration occurs at the interface of tissues of different densities and impedance. This may result in compression, shearing forces and spallation. Blast-related lung injury (BRLI) is probably the most important effect of blast overpressure. From a pathophysiological point of view, alveolar septal rupture occurs with pulmonary haemorrhage and oedema, resulting in impaired gas exchange and hypoxia, which may be fatal. Pneumothoraces and evolving pulmonary contusions further exacerbate the effects, although the exact cause of the lung damage is not fully understood, and in addition, the microscopic and metabolic effects have not yet been described in detail. It is also believed that significant air emboli can occur, leading to cardiac and central nervous system effects; this may be the mechanism of death in fatalities with no external signs of injury. It has been proposed that emboli result from the re-expansion of compressed gasses in the lungs, which are able to access the circulation via the damaged microvasculature.

Blast bowel and tympanic membrane rupture are influenced by the environment, blast bowel being more common when the victim is in water, particularly when half-submerged such as when wearing a life vest. The impulse travels faster and further in the less compressible water than in air, presumably resulting in relative protection to the chest, which is above water. The concept that different injuries resulted from transmission of the blast wave through the different states of matter, gas, liquid and solid was recognised soon after the original classification.[21]

Although tympanic membrane damage is considered a primary blast injury, it is related to the position of the head and may also be related to any head protection that is being worn. It is associated with head injury rather than other primary blast injuries. Tympanic membrane rupture has been

shown to be unrelated to significant lung problems, which are the most serious consequence of the blast overpressure.[22]

Despite the importance of the primary blast overpressure, most survivors will have sustained secondary or tertiary injuries, and in general, only a small minority of survivors will have significant primary blast injuries, as casualties with the necessary blast loading will very often have been killed immediately from a combination of all effects. Nevertheless, due to the increasing survival of casualties with injuries that would previously have been considered unsurvivable, blast lung is becoming an issue for the intensive care clinician. Primary blast injuries are more commonly seen at postmortem, and this also appears to be related to the environment, as will be discussed below.

SECONDARY BLAST INJURY

The effects of secondary blast injury are due to fragments accelerated by the blast wind; these might be from the device itself (referred to as *primary fragments*), or other environmental objects such as stones or soil, particularly when the explosive device is buried (referred to as *secondary fragments*). In addition fragments may be deliberately placed within the device. These can include nails, bolts or ball bearings and may be embedded within the device or adherent to its exterior. Shrapnel is a specific rather than a collective term and strictly refers to pre-formed fragments contained within an artillery shell designed as an anti-personnel device. It is fragments that are generally the most lethal mechanism following explosions, with a greater radius of effect that the blast overpressure.

TERTIARY BLAST INJURY

Tertiary effects relate to the displacement of the body by the blast wind and are often similar to the effects of civilian blunt trauma, although usually with higher levels of injury. Head injuries are common (and may be fatal), as are fractures. Crush injuries and injuries from buildings collapsing are also included in this group.

As a result of the injuries seen in Iraq and Afghanistan, the concept of 'solid blast' has been re-described, having been largely ignored in the literature since the Second World War.[23] As this is related to transmission through a solid structure, such as a vehicle floor or a ship's hull from an underwater blast, it cannot be adequately classified using a free-field blast classification; however, it results in injury patterns, predominately to the musculo-skeletal system, similar to those seen from the tertiary effects of blast. Mortality from underbody blast is most commonly caused by head injury and non-compressible torso haemorrhage, including aortic disruption and liver laceration.[24]

In addition, flailing can also cause injury, often due to relative restraint or protection of one part of the body compared to another, usually a limb. Experience from Afghanistan suggests that it can also result from solid blast; at its most extreme, it seems to result in traumatic amputation of the limb, again illustrating the need to be aware of the specific situation when considering blast injury mechanism.

QUATERNARY BLAST INJURY

Quaternary effects are essentially a miscellaneous group of injuries not specifically associated with one of the other groups; this group was an addition to the original classification. Burns, inhalation injuries and other toxic effects are included in this category. The extent and distribution of burns have been reported to fall into two distinct patterns, with one group of victims sustaining burns to the exposed areas of the hands and face, which are relatively superficial flash burns from the initial detonation.[25] The second group may have more extensive, deeper burns from fires that break out after the explosion; in this group, clothing offers much less protection. The use of an incendiary component as part of the device will obviously increase the severity of associated burn injuries.

More recently, it has been proposed that *quinary* effects of blast should be included; these are specific non-explosion-related effects such as radiation and bacterial or viral infections. Such devices have been referred to as 'dirty bombs'.[26] This has been a concern with suicide bombers who may deliberately infect themselves in the hope that the infection will be transmitted from biological fragments.

Effect of environment

Most research into blast effects and injuries dates from during and after the Second World War,

particularly in relation to the effects of nuclear weapons, hence the focus on free-field blast. However, as bombs have always been a favoured weapon of terrorists, it is such incidents rather than conventional warfare that have provided the majority of the injury data. This experience has led to the understanding that the fatality rates and the patterns of injury are related to the environment in which the explosion occurs. In terms of air blast (as opposed to liquid or solid blast), these can be considered to be explosions in the open air, explosions associated with structural (building) collapse and explosions in confined spaces.

EXPLOSIONS IN THE OPEN AIR

Fragments are by far the most common cause of injury in the open environment. Blast lung and other conditions associated with primary blast injury do occur in survivors but are much less common that in *confined space explosions*. Fractures can occur from both the fragments and the casualty been thrown by the blast wind.

EXPLOSIONS ASSOCIATED WITH STRUCTURAL (BUILDING) COLLAPSE

Fragment injures are less common than with *open air explosions*, but fractures are more common, due to crushing of the casualty when the structure collapses. Head injuries are also more common for the same reason.

EXPLOSIONS IN CONFINED SPACES

When compared to the other two environments, primary blast injuries such as blast lung are far more common in *confined space explosions*. Burns are also more common, and fractures and head injuries are more common than in the other two groups. This is likely to be due to the close proximity to the blast, causing flash burns, and throwing the casualty against the sides of the structure. The energy involved in displacing the casualty can cause severe head injuries, as well as fractures. There is also a higher rate of abdominal injury to the liver and spleen, which may cause bleeding into the abdomen. However, this is still less common than penetrating injuries from fragments and much less common than blast lung. Blast wave reflection with summation is a particular problem in confined space explosions.

MEDICAL CONSEQUENCES OF EXPLOSIVE DEVICES USED IN IRAQ AND AFGHANISTAN

Protection and mitigation against EFPs was the main focus in Iraq. Buried IEDs were the predominant method used in Afghanistan and resulted in the devastating lower limb injuries with multiple amputations which characterised the survivors. Primary blast injury was less common, and secondary blast injuries were due to the close-range products of combustion and energised soil fragments, resulting in a highly contaminated shredding of tissue. In addition, there were significant tertiary effects resulting in flailing injuries in dismounted victims and a significant solid blast effect when the IED strike was against a vehicle.

The effect of the difference in the deployment of IEDs between the conflicts can be seen in an analysis of the pattern of amputations in survivors.[27] There were significant differences in the cause and site of the amputations: multiple and high amputations with soft tissue perineal wounds, as well as significantly higher *Injury Severity Scores* were present in the casualties from Afghanistan. The greater understanding of the mechanism of injury of the severely injured casualties from Afghanistan and the high survival rates are testament to the significant advances made in the management of these casualties. In addition, there was increasing understanding of the nature of these injuries and their surgical requirements, which led to changes in surgical techniques.[28] Operatively, more guillotine amputations were carried out on patients from Iraq, compared to Afghanistan, where the concept of viable tissue preservation was used.

Mechanism of traumatic amputation

At the start of the conflict in Afghanistan, the accepted mechanism of traumatic limb amputation following blast was considered to be initial bone disruption caused by *brisance*, the shattering effect of the shock wave, with the amputation completed by the blast wind tearing off the limb after the fracturing.[29] Survival following such injuries was considered unlikely due to the significant blast exposure necessary. However, this was not the experience from the conflict in Afghanistan,

with many survivors following traumatic amputation, including unprecedented survival rates in double and triple amputees.[30] These results, from a much larger group than the one on which the brisance hypothesis was based, together with a similar distribution of injuries found in fast-jet pilots, supports the theory that some traumatic blast-mediated amputations are the result solely of the tertiary effects of blast, including flailing.

DEVELOPMENT OF BLAST RESEARCH FROM IRAQ AND AFGHANISTAN

With the recognition that one of the most common causes of death on the battlefield was haemorrhage, significant changes were made to treatment protocols. These included improved training of first responders, the issuing of haemorrhage control devices such as tourniquets and haemostatic dressings and rapid evacuation to consultant delivered care at the field hospital. In addition, research initiatives were developed at *Defence Science and Technology Laboratories (Dstl) Porton Down*, specifically focusing on optimising resuscitation and limiting coagulopathy following blast (see Chapter 24). This is essentially physiologically based research, but more mechanically based research has also been developed, particularly at Imperial College London.

As a result of collaborative work on the severe foot and ankle injuries seen following blast,[23] *Imperial Blast* was formed in 2008, as a multidisciplinary group of scientists, engineers and military surgeons focussing on understanding and preventing severe blast injury. This unit expanded and *The Centre for Blast Injury Studies* (CBIS) was established in 2011 to address the disabling injuries of conflict. With funding from the *Royal British Legion* and *Imperial College London*, as well as support in kind from the Ministry of Defence, CBIS aims to 'improve the mitigation of injury through addressing specific clinical areas, and increase lifelong health and quality of life after blast injury by developing and advancing treatment, rehabilitation and recovery'.[31] Since their formation, both *Imperial Blast* and CBIS have furthered the understanding of blast-related injuries, particularly vehicle-related blast.[32,33] This has led to increased insights into severe foot and ankle injuries and traumatic amputations as noted previously and also into BRLI.

Blast lung

Blast lung is commonly thought of as a primary blast injury, with alveoli septal rupture and pulmonary haemorrhage from blast wave effects at the interface between two areas of different acoustic impedance. However, lung injury can result from all aspects of blast, and it can be difficult to differentiate primary blast effects from blunt and penetrating trauma to the torso, as well as from the effects of medical treatment such as resuscitation and ventilation.[34] In addition, it has been increasingly realised that the environment also plays a significant factor in the incidence and type of BRLI. A review of 12 separate incidents from Israel noted that explosions that occurred in buses had the highest mortality rates (21.2%), both as a result of crowding and of reflection of the blast in the confined space.[35] It is this reflection that seems to be a factor in the increased incidence of primary blast lung in these 'ultra-confined' spaces, as was seen following the 7/7 London bombings. However, as this scenario was rare in Iraq or Afghanistan, primary blast lung was also uncommon, although anatomical disruption within the chest cavity was seen in casualties from Afghanistan who were inside vehicles.[36] Further analysis has demonstrated that the blast loading inside a vehicle, when the device is outside, does not result in significant blast overpressure even if vehicle breech occurs. It can be hypothesised, therefore, that rather than the primary effects of blast, thoracic trauma in vehicles is a result of tertiary effects, including solid blast. Research of this kind is not pursued solely out of academic interest; one of the main driving forces behind work of this nature is to develop mitigation strategies, particularly in vehicle design, based on a better understanding of the mechanism of injury.

BLAST PROTECTION

Vehicle blast injury prevention

As described earlier, following detonation and propagation of the blast wave, there is a rapid

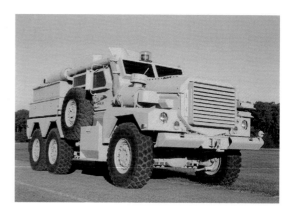

Figure 10.5 Mastiff 2 protected patrol vehicle.

reduction in the blast overpressure with distance, and so the most effective way to reduce its effect is to increase the distance of the victim from the explosion, although this is impractical in most instances. However, increasing the standoff distance is one of the most effective means of reducing the effects of buried devices deployed against vehicles. Again, as noted earlier, solid blast with the transmission of the force through the vehicle hull has been recognised as a significant mechanism of injury in vehicle blast incidents. This can be mitigated against by using V-shaped hulls, which will also redirect the energised soil, another significant injury mechanism (Figure 10.5).

Increasing the weight of the vehicle to reduce its displacement will reduce the impact of tertiary blast effects, and clearly, armour plating will reduce the effects of secondary blast. These principles were used in the vehicles deployed on the ground in the later stages of the conflict in Afghanistan. Although advances were made in vehicle design during the campaigns in both Iraq and Afghanistan, a detailed discussion is not possible for security reasons. However, *Imperial Blast* did analyse the effects of vehicle protection using historical data from Rhodesia. This demonstrated a cumulative effect and an overall reduction in mortality from 45% in unprotected vehicles to 0.8%.[37]

Personal blast injury prevention

Personnel protective equipment also uses the principles described previously, typified by the protective suits worn by *explosive ordnance disposal*

(EOD) personnel. In terms of primary blast protection, they may reflect or redirect the blast wave; this can be accomplished by a hard outer surface, although this will restrict movement. A deeper layer, often foam based, is designed to delay and reduce the transmission of the energy. Compression of the foam occurs as a result of transmission of kinetic energy, and the gross structure of the material, as well as its plastic deformation, mitigates the effect of the blast wave; honeycomb structures can absorb a considerable amount of energy. Combining materials of different densities, or acoustic impedance, will result in energy deposition in the structure, in the same way that energy is deposited in the lungs at solid and gaseous interfaces. In addition to kinetic energy, heat energy can be formed, resulting in controlled temperature rises, or even hydraulic energy, using the displacement of fluids in contained channels. EOD suits also include para-aramids to reduce fragment injuries, and their outer layers are usually made from a fire-retardant material. However, the interactions can be complex, and suits require specific testing to ensure injury is reduced rather than potentiated, which can occur if localisation of impact occurs to a particularly vulnerable area, such as the heart.

EVOLUTION OF PPE DURING THE IRAQ AND AFGHANISTAN MILITARY CAMPAIGNS

The aim of this section is to describe the evolution of some of the PPE used by UK Armed Forces during the Iraq (*Operation Telic*) and Afghanistan (*Operation Herrick*) campaigns; it will outline how evidence (including from the DMS) informed some of the key developments in the equipment and will show how some of the research and development carried out during both campaigns are shaping future PPE.

In the context of this chapter, the term *personal protective equipment* includes soft body armour (waistcoat or vest-like garments covering the torso) and its system components (collars, brassards and pelvic protection), helmets, face and eye protection (visors, glasses, goggles) and hearing protection. Body armour prevents or reduces the damage caused by ballistic projectiles to structures

within the thorax and abdomen and generally comprises 'soft' and 'hard' armours.[38] Soft armour provides resistance to perforation from fragments, and protection from high-velocity rifle bullets is provided in the form of ceramic-faced and composite backed armour plates.[39] Combat helmets protect the brain from fragments and non-ballistic impacts. Helmets are comprised of a composite shell, a foam liner, a suspension system and a retention system.[39]

The PPE issued to UK Armed Forces personnel deployed on *Operations Telic* and *Herrick* improved significantly throughout these campaigns due to the multidisciplinary approach adopted between Defence scientists and engineers, procurement teams, industry, academia, users of the PPE and clinicians. Continuous improvement and optimisation of the PPE were possible due to the ability to act positively on a change in threat and/or injury pattern through agile procurement, which was made possible through *Urgent Operational Requirements* (UORs; see Chapter 23). PPE evolved due to, for example:

- Visits by the procurement teams to operational theatres to educate and elicit direct feedback from deployed Armed Forces personnel, with subsequent action based upon direct feedback from user feedback questionnaires;
- Examination of PPE from casualties (including analysis of retained fragmentation or bullets);
- Examination of the PPE of fatalities (including analysis of retained fragmentation or bullets);
- Scientific evidence from, for example, Dstl, Defence Intelligence and academia; and
- Acting on medical evidence from deployed DMS clinicians.

PPE USED BY UK ARMED FORCES ON *OPERATIONS TELIC* AND *HERRICK*

Enhanced Combat Body Armour

When UK Armed Forces first deployed on *Operation Telic* in Iraq, they were issued with the in-service *Enhanced Combat Body Armour*

(ECBA) and the MK6 General Service combat helmet. *Combat Body Armour* (CBA) was originally introduced just prior to the Gulf conflict in 1991. CBA is a waistcoat-style fragmentation-protective soft body armour covering the torso, consisting of layers of nylon and para-aramid fabrics[38–40] encased in a waterproof cover to prevent ingress of water and ultraviolet radiation and then placed in a fabric outer carrier.[39,40] The soft armour is designed to prevent perforation of the body by fragments. CBA incorporates pockets in the front and rear of the fabric carrier, which accommodate ceramic-composite plates designed to provide protection primarily to the heart against high-velocity rifle ammunition, based on the assumption that definitive surgical care would be available within 20 minutes.[38,41,42] The exact position and shape of the plate were determined by the UK Armed Forces medical community.[40] CBA worn with plates was originally called *Combat Body Armour Internal Security*, but the ensemble (of CBA worn with ceramic-composite plates) is now referred to as ECBA.[40]

Only the outer fabric carrier of the ECBA changed during the Afghanistan campaign, from the *Desert Camouflage Pattern* (issued at the beginning of the Iraq campaign) to the *Multi-Terrain Pattern* (MTP) camouflage carrier issued in the latter stages of *Operation Herrick* (Figure 10.6). The total mass of ECBA was approximately 5 kg for a medium size, of which each ECBA plate accounted for 1.1 kg.[38,39]

Mark 6 general service combat helmet

The *Mark 6 General Service Combat Helmet* (commonly referred to as the Mk6 helmet), has been in service since 1986. It consists of a nylon composite shell with a high-density closed-cell polyethylene foam liner[39,40] and a three-point harness for securing to the head and chin.

Kestrel body armour system

In 2006, as the campaign in Iraq developed, medical evidence provided by deployed DMS personnel and information available from post-mortem examinations of repatriated UK Armed Forces personnel demonstrated that a significant proportion of injuries were to the neck, upper arm and underarm regions.[43] The ECBA vest did not provide coverage to these areas of the body, which were particularly vulnerable in 'top cover' and standing sentry roles. As a result and as part of an urgent operational requirement (see Chapter 23), the *Kestrel* body armour system was introduced to supplement ECBA for specific roles. *Kestrel* was developed on the same principles as ECBA, with a front opening tabard-style soft armour, but it also included integral neck and arm coverage (Figure 10.7).[43] The Mark 1 *Kestrel* body armour utilised front and rear ECBA plates in plate pockets on the outer cover of the vest, and the *Kestrel* system also included an *under body armour combat shirt* (UBACS),

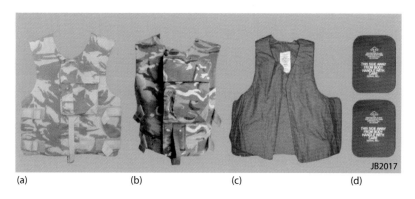

(a) (b) (c) (d)

Figure 10.6 ECBA. **(a)** ECBA in the Desert camouflage pattern as worn at the start of the Iraq campaign; **(b)** ECBA in the MTP camouflage as worn during the latter period of the Afghanistan campaign; **(c)** soft armour filler shown encased in the UVR and waterproof cover; and **(d)** front and rear hard armour ECBA plates.

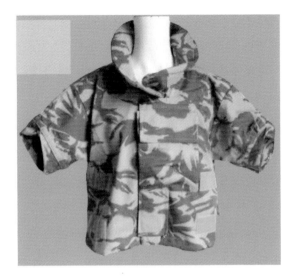

Figure 10.7 Mark 1 Kestrel Body Armour system, with pockets to insert front and rear ECBA plates.

to replace the combat shirt (to improve comfort and aid heat dissipation under the body armour), hot weather combat gloves, eye protection and an improved combat helmet (Mk6A combat helmet).

Mark 6A general service combat helmet

The Mark 6A combat helmet was introduced into operations in Iraq as part of the *Kestrel* system.[43] The Mark 6A used the same mould as the Mk6

combat helmet (and therefore is the same shape) and retained the same non-ballistic-impact protection but had a 40% increase in the level of fragmentation protection compared to the Mark 6.[43] This was due to the use of a hybrid (para-aramid and nylon) composite shell. The Mark 6A also introduced a new improved four-point chinstrap, compared to the three-point chinstrap of the Mk6.

Eye protection

On *Operation Telic*, an increase in the number of eye injuries was reported by deployed DMS clinicians. Explosive devices produced multiple small fragments capable of causing injuries, and the eyes were particularly at risk, with a number of soldiers suffering permanent blindness in one or both eyes.[44] Following a UOR for eye protection, low-impact sunglasses and medium-impact goggles were issued to Armed Forces personnel deployed on *Operation Telic* in October 2004[45] (Figure 10.8) and continued to be issued to Armed Forces personnel throughout both the Iraq and Afghanistan campaigns. Prescription lens inserts were available with both sets of eyewear.

Osprey body armour system

Concurrent with the development of the *Kestrel* body armour system, the *Osprey* system was also being developed by Defence scientists and

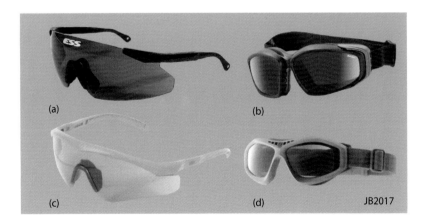

Figure 10.8 Eye protection available to UK Armed Forces personnel during the Iraq and Afghanistan campaigns. (a) Low-impact sunglasses 2006–2010; (b) medium-impact goggles 2006–2010; (c) low-impact sunglasses 2010–2014; and (d) medium-impact goggles 2010–2014.

engineers in conjunction with industry. The drive for the development of the *Osprey* body armour was to increase the ballistic performance and area of coverage provided by the ECBA plates, in response to the increase in the number of reported injuries to the thorax that were primarily outside the area of coverage of the ECBA plates. It was also recognised that *Kestrel* was unpopular with UK Armed Forces personnel in terms of its mass, bulk, mobility and lack of comfort, deployed DMS personnel also reported the difficulty they encountered in removing ECBA and *Kestrel* to treat injuries. Taking these factors into account; the modular *Osprey* body armour system was introduced in 2005 following another UOR.[38,40,43] The components of the *Osprey* system are the soft armour vest (Figure 10.9), high and low collars, brassards (Figure 10.10) and front and rear *Osprey* plates (Figure 10.11).

The *Osprey* plates provide a higher level of ballistic performance compared to ECBA plates and an enhanced multi-hit capability, as well as an increase in the area of coverage compared to the ECBA plates.[43] Medical advice from DMS clinicians stated that the *Osprey* plates should provide coverage to the heart, liver, mediastinum and spleen based on the assumption that definitive surgical care was available within one to two hours.[38]

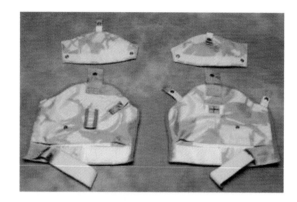

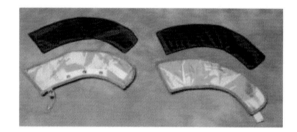

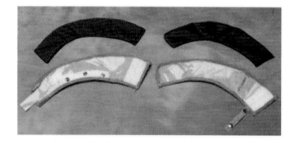

Figure 10.10 Osprey brassards (top), low collar (middle) and high collar (bottom).

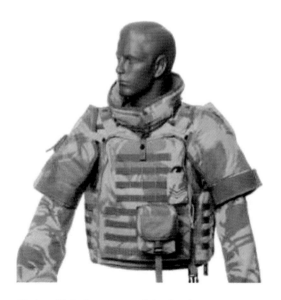

Figure 10.9 Osprey modular body armour system, worn with brassards and high collar.

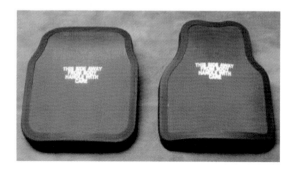

Figure 10.11 Osprey plates: Rear plate (left), front plate (right).

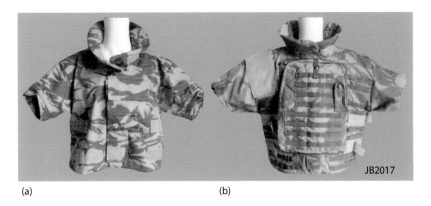

(a)   (b)

Figure 10.12 Two iterations of Kestrel for comparative purposes: **(a)** Mark 1 with fabric outer cover and used with front and rear ECBA plates and **(b)** Mark 2 with Cordura™ outer cover used with front and rear Osprey plates.

Osprey was designed as a modular body armour system, which can be adapted to increase or decrease the level of protection dependent on the user's role. For example, *Osprey* can be worn without any ballistic plates, thus providing protection against fragmentation. Wearing high or low collars and brassards will increase the area of coverage, and therefore the protection; conversely, the ECBA plates can be used instead of *Osprey* plates where there is a reduction in threat[43] (the *Osprey* vest has front and rear pockets to accommodate either the ECBA or Osprey plates), giving the user a lower level of protection (than if the *Osprey* plates were worn) but a slightly higher level of protection than if ECBA was worn. The first iteration of the complete *Osprey* system weighed approximately 15 kg,[39] and each plate weighed approximately 3 kg.

The *Osprey* soft armour provided an increase in the level of fragmentation protection compared to ECBA and contained para-aramid materials that were water repellent treated, encased in a water-resistant outer cover and placed in an outer Cordura™ carrier.[40] The carrier itself was modified from the fabric ECBA and *Kestrel* waistcoat-style to a tabard-style garment manufactured from Cordura™ to minimise the wear and tear observed in fabric outer carriers, to enable easier removal of the vest at the shoulders and to allow better access for clinicians to treat injuries since the comprehensive assessment of an injured person requires the removal of personal armour.[46] This can be challenging due to the need to immobilise the spine

until spinal injury can be excluded and because the soft body armour (comprising multiple layers of para-aramid fabrics) cannot be cut from a casualty with the standard heavy-duty scissors (Tuff-Cut™) carried by emergency clinicians. Clinicians were advised and trained to remove body armour by cutting the side webbing straps of the ECBA as this did not involve directly cutting the armour material. The modification of the *Osprey* (to a tabard-style vest) ensured easier removal of the armour at the shoulders.[39]

With the introduction of the *Osprey* body armour system, *Kestrel* Mk2 was subsequently modified to provide front and rear pockets that could accommodate either the ECBA plates, or the new *Osprey* plates, and the outer cover was modified from fabric to Cordura™ (Figure 10.12).

OPTIMISATION OF PPE THROUGHOUT THE CAMPAIGNS

The *Osprey* body armour system was continually modified throughout its use on *Operation Telic* in Iraq and *Operation Herrick* in Afghanistan: in response to the users' needs, changes in reported threats against UK Armed Forces personnel and medical data from deployed DMS personnel. In addition; personnel from the procurement teams regularly visited deployed UK Armed Forces personnel in all areas of operation in order to educate users on the correct use of the new protective equipment and to directly elicit views from the users on the ground regarding any enhancements or modifications that might be required. For repatriated UK Armed Forces personnel, all items of PPE worn at the time of a fatal injury were examined at post-mortem examination, as part of HM Coroner's investigation, and linked to the mechanism and location of injury. In-theatre policy during *Operations Telic* and *Herrick* also specified that any item of personal armour struck by projectiles or otherwise damaged in an incident where an individual was injured was recovered for assessment. Any bullets or fragments contained within the PPE as well as those removed during surgical intervention were retained as potential forensic evidence and for threat intelligence purposes. This provided assurance that the personal armour was not only meeting its protection and coverage requirement but also provided the opportunity to evaluate trends in the mechanisms and location of injuries, informing any potential PPE enhancements.

The *Osprey* body armour system was concurrently issued to Armed Forces personnel deployed in two different theatres of operation, *Operation Telic* in Iraq and *Operation Herrick* in Afghanistan. Different threats to UK Armed Forces personnel were encountered in these different theatres of operation, and the modification and optimisation of the *Osprey* body armour system ranged from relatively straightforward improvements such as those made to the *Osprey* plate pockets, to significant enhancements such as the introduction of the pelvic protection system (PPS) and the Mk 7

combat helmet. Some of these optimisations and enhancements will be discussed.

Introduction and optimisation of Osprey side plate pockets

On *Operation Telic* in 2007, due to an increase in reported injuries to the flank (side) areas, some UK Armed Forces personnel inserted their ECBA plates into the sides of the outer cover of the OSPREY body armour to increase their protection against high-velocity bullets. From this date, side plates became an integral part of the *Osprey* body armour system, and subsequent modifications of the soft armour vest allowed ECBA plates to be worn more securely and comfortably. In the *Osprey* Mk 4 iteration, the ECBA plates were inserted into a cummerbund on the outside of the *Osprey* vest, and in the Mk4A *Osprey*, separate plate pockets were provided that were attached to the *Osprey* vest (Figure 10.13).

Optimisation of Osprey front plate pockets

The external plate pocket of the original *Osprey* body armour system had a top opening zip and fastener to insert and secure the *Osprey* plate. One of the modifications to a subsequent iteration of the *Osprey* vest was changing the zip and fastener opening to the bottom of the plate pocket (Figure 10.14), as medical evidence had demonstrated that blast events from below had, on occasions,

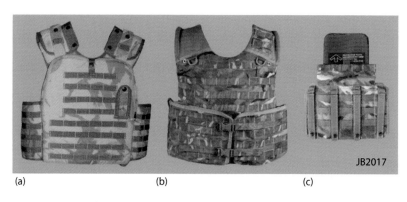

(a) (b) (c)

Figure 10.13 Side plates were slid into the vest of OSPREY Mark 1 (a), held in a cummerbund on the outside of Osprey Mark 4 (b) and inserted into separate plate pockets in Osprey Mark 4A (c).

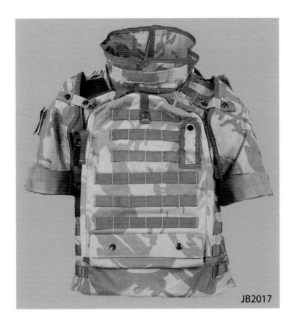

JB2017

Figure 10.14 Osprey Mk3 showing the optimised bottom zip and fastener opening of the front plate pocket.

deflected the hard armour plate upwards, causing mandibular fractures.[47]

Mark 7 general service combat helmet

In 2010, the Mark 7 combat helmet was introduced into combat operations in Afghanistan. The Mark 7 helmet is a different shape and is thinner and slightly lighter than the Mark 6 and Mark 6A.[40] The Mark 7 shell is comprised of a para-aramid composite and provides an enhanced level of fragmentation protection compared to the Mark 6 and

Mark 6A (Figure 10.15), whilst retaining the same level of non-ballistic impact protection.

Pelvic protection system

In 2009, deployed DMS clinicians reported an increase in the number and severity of genital and perineal injuries observed in UK Armed Forces casualties, from stepping on or being near a buried IED on Operation *Herrick* (Figure 10.16).

In response to this, research and development work commenced to evaluate potential options to provide protection to these vulnerable areas. As a result, additional protection to the genitals, perineum, pelvis and legs from explosively propelled debris and fragmentation was introduced in 2010 as another UOR.[48] The PPS (Figure 10.17) consists of three garments that provide

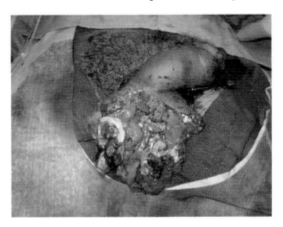

Figure 10.16 Urogenital injuries from Afghanistan caused by an IED. (From Waxman, S. et al., *International Journal of Impotence Research*, 21: 145–148, 2009.)

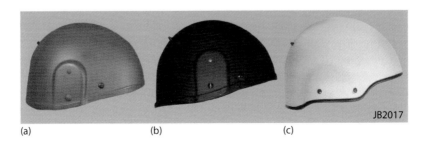

JB2017

(a)　　　　(b)　　　　(c)

Figure 10.15 General Service Combat Helmets worn during the Iraq and Afghanistan campaigns: (a) Mark 6, (b) Mark 6A and (c) Mark 7.

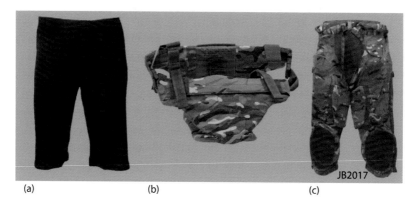

Figure 10.17 PPSs as worn by UK Armed Forces personnel in Afghanistan. **(a)** Tier 1, **(b)** Tier 2 and **(c)** Tier 3.

an incremental increase in coverage and level of protection.

Tier 1 Pelvic Protection, fielded in September 2010, was designed as a next-to-skin undergarment to be worn on a daily basis (Figure 10.17a) to provide protection against the dirt, dust, grit and debris emanating primarily from the soil/substrate in which IEDs were buried.[40,48] The knee-length garment is constructed from jersey material with two layers of high performance knitted silk stitched to the outside. The knitted silk was selected as the protective material as it provided the best balance between ballistic performance against small fragments and user acceptability.[40,48] The area of coverage of knitted silk is identical on the front and the rear of the garment. The Tier 1 Pelvic Protection can be repeatedly laundered without compromising the performance.[49] Tier 2 Pelvic Protection, fielded in February 2011, is a protective overgarment that provides coverage and protection to the groin, buttocks and some of the inner thigh and offers the same level of fragmentation protection as the *Osprey* soft body armour (Figure 10.17b). Tier 2 Pelvic Protection was intended to be worn over the combat trousers when the user was patrolling and was rolled up and secured on the back of the trousers when not in use.[40,48] Tier 3 Pelvic Protection, issued in September 2011, provides a further tier of protection and is a longer calf-length garment intended to be worn over the combat trousers and to provide enhanced protection from fragmentation to the inner thigh, femoral artery and legs (Figure 10.17c).[48] Tier 3 was designed to integrate

with tier 1 (worn underneath the combat trousers) and tier 2 pelvic protection which can be worn over or under the Tier 3. Tier 3 pelvic protection was designed for intense high-risk and short-duration tasks conducted by counter-IED (C-IED) operators and dismounted personnel conducting C-IED drills.

Patrol collar

Combat neck injury was reported as a significant cause of mortality and long-term morbidity in UK Armed Forces personnel deployed in Iraq and Afghanistan[50] despite efforts to introduce integral (*Kestrel*) and detachable (*Osprey*) collars. The detachable *Osprey* collars were routinely used in (top cover and standing) sentry roles in Iraq, and multiple instances were cited where the collars prevented potentially fatal neck wounds from ground based fragmentation whilst on mounted patrols.[43] However, the differing nature of the campaign in Afghanistan (compared to Iraq) and an increase in dismounted (foot) patrolling resulted in the collars not being routinely worn or attached to the vest but not in the correct position,[51] thereby completely negating their ballistic properties (Figure 10.18).

The collars were perceived by the users to be uncomfortable, increasing their thermal burden, reducing situational awareness and lacking integration with the helmet and rucksack.[51] Clinical and post-mortem injury analysis demonstrated that 16 UK soldiers died directly from neck wounds from energised fragments and that none

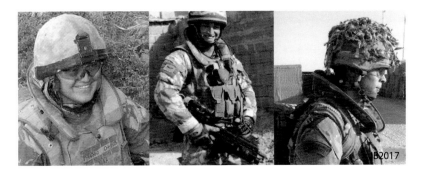

Figure 10.18 The *Osprey* neck collars were often attached but not secured correctly at the front, therefore negating their protective capability.

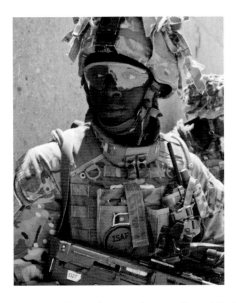

Figure 10.19 UK soldier wearing the Patrol Collar with Mark 4A Osprey whilst on foot patrol in Afghanistan in mid-2014.

were wearing their neck protection at the time.[52,53] This medical evidence provided the impetus to optimise the collar, in particular for dismounted patrolling roles, in an attempt to mitigate these injuries. After determining the anatomical structures in the neck that required protection,[54–56] prototype designs were developed (using the same level of ballistic protection as the *Osprey* soft armour, but shorter and fitting closer to the neck) and subjected to human factors evaluation. The Patrol Collar was issued to Armed Forces personnel on Operation *Herrick* in 2014 (Figure 10.19). Although shorter than the *Osprey* half collar, the Patrol Collar afforded the same coverage of vulnerable anatomical structures and attached to the *Osprey* body armour vest with the same press stud attachments as the *Osprey* collars. User acceptability, particularly in terms of equipment integration, was demonstrated to be far higher than with the *Osprey* collars (Figure 10.20).[57]

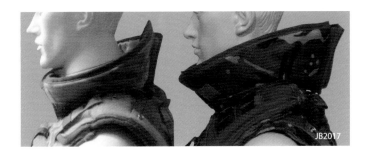

Figure 10.20 Osprey Mark 1 half (left) and Mark 4 full (right) neck collars worn on a 50th percentile anatomical mannequin demonstrating the difference in coverage of the neck and lower face.

Enhanced protection UBACS

The UBACS was introduced to replace the combat shirt as part of the *Kestrel* system and was intended to improve comfort and aid heat dissipation under the body armour. In response to the evidence of neck injury from DMS, it was recommended that ballistic protective material could be integrated into the neck collar of the UBACS (Figures 10.21 and 10.22). This concept of protection was

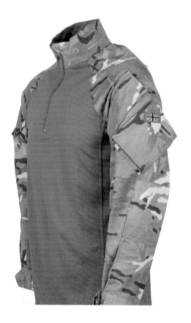

Figure 10.21 UBACS shirt in MTP pattern material.

similar to that of the tiered PPS, where a reinforced UBACS collar could provide the minimum level of protection (similar to the Tier 1 Pelvic Protection) with the option to increase the level of protection by wearing an *Osprey* neck collar (Tier 2) in situations of increased threat.[58] Enhanced Protection UBACS with a reinforced neck was introduced to Armed Forces personnel deployed in Afghanistan in February 2014.[57]

HEARING PROTECTION

Permanent *noise-induced hearing loss* (NIHL), principally through exposure to high levels of impulse noise from weapon fire, was a source of long-term morbidity to UK forces during *Operations Telic* and *Herrick*.[59,60] It was the third commonest primary care evacuation category in 2009–2010, and it accounted for significant numbers of medical discharges from all three services.[61] It was estimated that the incidence of permanent NIHL for UK service personnel returning from Afghanistan was 0.8%, resulting in approximately 15% of service personnel becoming unfit for further deployment or promotion.[59]

In 2001, hearing protection for UK Armed Forces personnel was provided in the form of foam earplugs and passive ear defenders. The *Combat Arms Ear Plug* was introduced for UK Armed Forces personnel in 2006 and provided two levels of protection determined by which colour end of the plug was inserted into the ear.[60] The

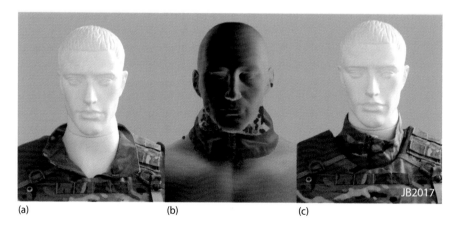

(a)   (b)   (c)

Figure 10.22 The unzipped UBACS (a) was demonstrated by *Surface Wound Mapping* (b) to provide additional coverage and potentially protect against fragmentation wounds to the neck if zipped up (c).

acceptance of these methods of hearing protection by Armed Forces personnel on deployment was generally poor, with most preferring to maintain situational awareness by not using them and running the risk of hearing loss.[60] Following a UOR, the *Personal Interfaced Hearing Protection* (PIHP) system was introduced in March 2009 for Armed Forces personnel deploying to Afghanistan. The system incorporated translucent silicone custom-moulded earplugs that attached to the in-ear headset (Figure 10.23). The headset attached to the *talk through* switch box, which in turn connected to the *Personal Role Radio* (PRR). However a study undertaken by clinicians in 2011 demonstrated that only 4% of those UK Armed Forces personnel issued with PIHP used it.[59] This was found to reflect a lack of awareness of how to use the system

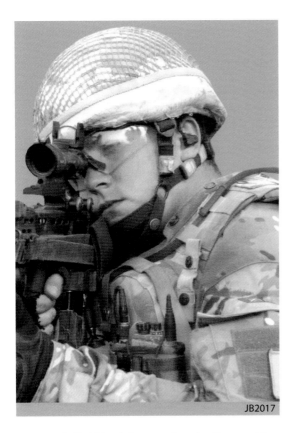

Figure 10.23 UK soldier wearing the *Personal in Ear Hearing Protection* (PIHP) system. The headset is attached to the talk through switch box, which in turn is connected to the PRR.

and a dislike of the reduction in situational awareness it caused when it was worn.

ANALYSIS OF MEDICAL EFFICACY OF PPE

Whilst discrete, individual analyses of casualties and casualty patterns throughout the Iraq and Afghanistan campaigns have demonstrated the efficacy of (some) PPE; a comprehensive analysis of the medical efficacy of all PPE issued to UK Armed Forces personnel is currently ongoing. This information, coupled with the innovations observed in combat casualty care, will assist in the optimisation and evolution of future PPE. Although undoubtedly effective at mitigating life-threatening injuries, determining the true efficacy of PPE is challenging, as PPE information in relation to casualties was not fully captured during the early stages of the Iraq campaign (this significantly improved throughout both campaigns). In addition, UK Armed Forces personnel were seldom injured whilst not wearing any PPE, particularly towards the end of the campaign in Afghanistan. However, some analyses carried out during *Operation Herrick* provided real-time evidence of the efficacy of the PPE. For example, research carried out in 2010 by the DMS demonstrated that eye protection was not only effective in mitigating eye injuries, but also that it was important in preventing potential ingress of fragments into the brain via the eye.[62] An observational review carried out to determine the effectiveness of pelvic protection on operations in Afghanistan showed that wearing pelvic protection was associated with a decreased odds ratio of genital and urinary tract injury.[63] In addition, real-time *Surface Wound Mapping* (SWM) analysis performed over a three-month period in September 2012 determined that:

- Personnel wearing a body armour vest were 4.1 times less likely to sustain a fragmentation wound to the chest or abdomen than those who were unprotected (Figure 10.24).[64]
- The odds of sustaining a head injury from energised fragments when wearing a helmet were 2.7 times lower than when not wearing a helmet (Figure 10.25).[64]
- Personnel wearing Tier 1 Pelvic Protection (only) were 9.5 times less likely, and wearing

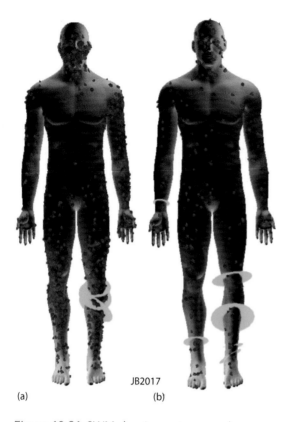

(a)   (b)

Figure 10.24 SWM showing entry wound locations from energised fragments during a prospective trial undertaken in Afghanistan in September 2012. (a) UK service personnel and (b) Afghan National Army.

both Tiers 1 and 2 Pelvic Protection were 10.1 times less likely, to sustain a fragmentation wound to the pelvis compared with those that were unprotected (Figure 10.26).[64]

LESSONS FROM *OPERATIONS TELIC* AND *HERRICK* INFORMING CURRENT AND FUTURE PPE

A significant effort of research and development (R&D) into the optimisation of PPE occurred during the Iraq and Afghanistan campaigns, yet not all the lessons were identified nor R&D efforts realised during those campaigns. However, maturation of some of the R&D efforts has been, and continues, to be realised, such as the use of computer technology, developed towards the end of the Afghanistan campaign, to visualise the actual coverage to anatomical structures provided by PPE (Figure 10.27). Developed by Dstl, with input from the DMS and Defence Equipment and Support (DE&S), PPE can now be superimposed over internal anatomical structures and visualised using the *Coverage of Armour Tool* (CoAT). Lessons learned, R&D and medical evidence from both the Iraq and Afghanistan campaigns were all used, for example to drive aspects of the design and evaluation of the new *Virtus* body armour and load carriage system, which was issued to high-readiness troops in late 2015 after the cessation of combat operations in Afghanistan. *Virtus* is a scalable system that is thinner, lighter, more streamlined and less bulky than *Osprey*. This in part is due to the procurement of

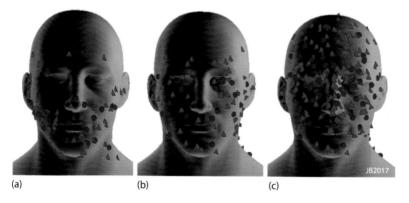

(a)   (b)   (c)

Figure 10.25 SWM clearly demonstrated the effectiveness of helmet and eye protection in mitigating the injury from energised fragments. (a) Helmet and eye protection worn; (b) helmet but no eye protection worn; (c) no helmet or eye protection worn.

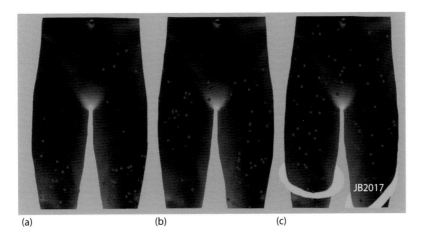

(a)   (b)   (c)

Figure 10.26 SWM demonstrating entry wound locations in casualties wounded in leg and pelvic regions: (a) UK Armed Forces personnel wounded whilst wearing pelvic protection (Tiers 1 or 2); (b) UK Armed Forces personnel not wearing pelvic protection; (c) Afghan National Army personnel not wearing pelvic protection.

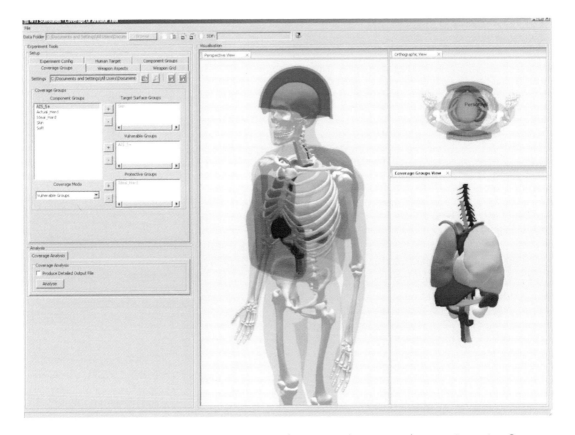

Figure 10.27 CoAT used to visualise the coverage of anatomical structures by superimposing Osprey plates and the Mk7 helmet.

Virtus as a complete system as opposed to procuring piecemeal components. Clinical analyses using the *Joint Theatre Trauma Registry* and critical analyses of the published literature carried out during both campaigns, together with SWM carried out in the Bastion Role 3 Hospital in Afghanistan, provided the medical evidence required for the *Virtus* collar and *Virtus* helmet (including face and eye protection) to be medically optimised, particularly in terms of area of coverage. The essential coverage required for a helmet was defined from a medical perspective as protection of the brain and brain stem and it was recommended that the nasion, external auditory meatus and superior nuchal line be used as anatomical landmarks to define the area of coverage.[40,65] These definitions were used when specifying the coverage requirements of the *Virtus* helmet. A quick release mechanism has been incorporated into the *Virtus* soft armour vest to aid quick and safe extraction from hazardous situations such as burning vehicles or from water.[40] The soft armour vest, after deploying the quick release, can be reassembled quickly and easily in minutes. CoAT was used to evaluate the area of coverage of the systems submitted as part of the *Virtus* competitive tender assessment in order to enssure that the systems provided the correct coverage to the internal anatomical structures.

At the time of writing, further optimisation of *Virtus* is benefitting from the lessons identified and the R&D carried out during the Afghan campaign. In fact, both campaigns have driven the medical requirements for current and future body armour systems, including, for example:

- The incorporation of visors and mandible guards on to the *Virtus* helmet to optimise eye and facial protection.[40]
- The re-definition and confirmation of the medical area of coverage for the torso in terms of essential and desirable coverage, enabling the optimisation of future high-velocity rifle ammunition protection.[38]
- The provision of further optimisation of area of coverage of other aspects of the PPE such as brassards and pelvic protection, taking into account the need to be able to apply a tourniquet

as high as possible on the arms (and legs), suggesting that the area of coverage could be reduced.[66]
- The ability to assess, visualise and compare area of coverage of PPE using CoAT in future procurement.

CONCLUSION

PPE has advanced significantly since the beginning of Operation *Telic*, through continuous optimisation of materials and components, in response to user feedback, to changes in the threats faced by Armed Forces personnel in concurrent theatres of operation, and through the multidisciplinary approach adopted by Defence scientists and engineers, procurement teams, industry, academia, users of the PPE and medical clinicians. PPE continues to evolve through further optimisation and developments in order to further increase the mobility and agility of the user. The design of any new PPE will inevitably be a compromise between the area of coverage, the level of protection and user acceptance, particularly in the assessment of any added burden versus the possible physiological and psychological impact on the user.[67]

REFERENCES

1. Department of Defense. *Joint Tactics, Techniques, and Procedures for Antiterrorism: Joint Pub 3-07.2*. 1998, pp. 1–158.
2. Ramasamy A, Hill AM, Clasper JC. Improvised explosive devices: Pathophysiology, injury profiles and current medical management. *J R Army Med Corps* 2009;155: 265–272.
3. Ramasamy A, Harrisson SE, Clasper JC et al. Injuries From Roadside Improvised Explosive Devices. *J Trauma* 2008;65:910–914. doi:10.1097/TA.0b013e3181848cf6
4. Ramasamy A, Harrisson S, Lasrado I et al. A review of casualties during the Iraqi insurgency 2006 – A British field hospital experience. *Injury* 2009;40:493–497. doi:10.1016/j.injury.2008.03.028

5. Morrison JJ, Mahoney PF, Hodgetts T. Shaped charges and explosively formed penetrators: Background for clinicians. *J R Army Med Corps* 2007;153:184–187.

6. Chivers CJ. What's inside a Taliban gun locker? *The New York Times* 2010, pp. 1–6. http://atwar.blogs.nytimes.com/2010/09/15/whats-inside-a-taliban-gun-locker/ (accessed 5 January 2017).

7. Schroder M, King B, Kelly C. Surveying the Battlefield: Illicit Arms in Afghanistan, Iraq and Somalia. Small Arms Survey. 2012, pp. 1–44. http://www.smallarmssurvey.org/fileadmin/docs/A-Yearbook/2012/eng/Small-Arms-Survey-2012-Chapter-10-EN.pdf (accessed 3 February 2017).

8. Broder J, Yousafzai S. Arming the Enemy in Afghanistan. 2017, pp. 1–5. http://europe.newsweek.com/arming-enemy-afghanistan-327451?rm=eu (accessed 5 January 2017).

9. Sopko JF. Afghan National Security Forces: Actions Needed to Improve Weapons Accountability. Special Inspector General for Afghanistan Reconstruction. 2014. https://www.sigar.mil/pdf/audits/SIGAR-14-84-AR.pdf (accessed 1 February 2017).

10. Tilstra RC. *The Battle Rifle: Development and Use since World War II*. Jefferson, NC: McFarland & Company, 2014.

11. Ismay J. Insight into how insurgents fought in Iraq. *The New York Times* 2013, pp. 1–1. http://atwar.blogs.nytimes.com/2013/10/17/insight-into-how-insurgents-fought-in-iraq/?nytmobile=0 (accessed 4 January 2017).

12. Silinsky M. *The Taliban: Afghanistan's Most Lethal Insurgents*. Santa Monica, CA: ABC-CLIO, 2014.

13. Timmerman KR. How the Taliban got their hands on modern US missiles. *New York Post* 2014. http://nypost.com/2014/06/08/how-the-taliban-got-their-hands-on-modern-us-missiles/ (accessed 13 February 2017).

14. Salo EG, Stallings FP. The US Army Engineering and Support Center, Huntsville captured enemy ammunition and coalition munitions clearance mission 2003–2008. 2013, pp. 1–181. http://www.hnc.usace.army.mil/Portals/65/docs/History/CMCHistory.pdf (accessed 2 February 2017).

15. Creamer S. (U) Iraq: Small Arms (Infantry Weapons) Used by the Anti-Coalition Insurgency. 2004, pp. 1–13. https://weaponsdocs.files.wordpress.com/2015/02/small_arms_used_by_the_anti-coalition_insurgency.pdf. US Army Ground Intelligence Centre.

16. Breeze J, Carr DJ. Energised fragments, bullets and fragment simulating projectiles. In: Bull AMJ, Clasper J, Mahoney PF (eds.). *Blast Injury Science and Engineering*. Cham: Springer International Publishing, 2016, pp. 219–226. doi:10.1007/978-3-319-21867-0_18

17. Ramasamy A, Hill AM, Hepper AE et al. Blast mines: Physics, injury mechanisms and vehicle protection. *J R Army Med Corps* 2009;155:258–264.

18. International Committee of the Red Cross. Anti-personnel Landmines – Friend or Foe? A Study of the Military Use and Effectiveness of Anti-Personnel Mines. 2006, pp. 1–100. https://www.icrc.org/eng/assets/files/other/icrc_002_0654.pdf (accessed 6 February 2017).

19. Zuckerman S. Discussion on the problem of blast injuries. *Proc R Soc Med* 1941;34:171–188.

20. Department of Defense. DOD Directive 6025.21E, July 5, 2006. 2006, pp. 1–10.

21. Draeger R, Barr JS, Sager WW. Blast injury. *JAMA* 1946;132:762–767.

22. Harrison CD, Bebarta VS, Grant GA. Tympanic membrane perforation after combat blast exposure in Iraq: A poor biomarker of primary blast injury. *J Trauma* 2009;67:210–211. doi:10.1097/TA.0b013e3181a5f1db

23. Ramasamy A, Hill AM, Phillip R et al. The modern "deck-slap" injury – Calcaneal blast fractures from vehicle explosions. *J Trauma* 2011;71:1694–1698. doi:10.1097/TA.0b013e318227a999

24. Singleton JAG, Gibb IE, Hunt NC et al. Identifying future "unexpected" survivors: A retrospective cohort study of fatal injury

patterns in victims of improvised explosive devices. *BMJ Open* 2013;3:1–8. doi:10.1136/bmjopen-2013-003130

25. Hill JF. Blast injury with particular reference to recent terrorist bombing incidents. *Ann R Coll Surg Engl* 1979;61:4–11.

26. Champion HR, Holcomb JB, Young LA. Injuries from explosions: Physics, biophysics, pathology, and required research focus. *J Trauma* 2009;66:1468–1477, discussion 1477. doi:10.1097/TA.0b013e3181a27e7f

27. Brown KV, Clasper JC. The changing pattern of amputations. *J R Army Med Corps* 2013;159:300–303. doi:10.1136/jramc-2013-000103

28. Clasper J, Lower Limb Trauma Working Group. Amputations of the lower limb: A multidisciplinary consensus. *J R Army Med Corps* 2007;153:172–174.

29. Hull JB, Cooper GJ. Pattern and mechanism of traumatic amputation by explosive blast. *J Trauma* 1996;40:S198–S205.

30. Singleton JAG, Gibb IE, Bull AMJ et al. Blast-mediated traumatic amputation: Evidence for a revised, multiple injury mechanism theory. *J R Army Med Corps* 2014;160:175–179. doi:10.1136/jramc-2013-000217

31. The Centre for Blast Injury Studies at Imperial College London. 2017, pp. 1–1. http://www.imperial.ac.uk/blast-injury/about (accessed 29 January 2017).

32. Spurrier E, Gibb I, Masouros S et al. Identifying spinal injury patterns in underbody blast to develop mechanistic hypotheses. *Spine* 2016;41:E268–E275. doi:10.1097/BRS.0000000000001213

33. Walker NM, Eardley W, Clasper JC. UK combat-related pelvic junctional vascular injuries 2008–2011: Implications for future intervention. *Injury* 2014;45:1585–1589. doi:10.1016/j.injury.2014.07.004

34. Mackenzie I, Tunnicliffe B, Clasper J. What the intensive care doctor needs to know about blast-related lung injury. *J Intensive Care Soc* 2013;14:303–312. doi:10.1177/175114371301400407

35. Kosashvili Y, Loebenberg MI, Lin G et al. Medical consequences of suicide bombing mass casualty incidents: The impact of explosion setting on injury patterns. *Injury* 2009;40:698–702. doi:10.1016/j.injury.2008.06.037

36. Singleton JAG, Gibb IE, Bull AMJ et al. Primary blast lung injury prevalence and fatal injuries from explosions: Insights from postmortem computed tomographic analysis of 121 improvised explosive device fatalities. *J Trauma* 2013;75:S269–S274. doi:10.1097/TA.0b013e318299d93e

37. Ramasamy A, Hill AM, Masouros SD et al. Accident analysis and prevention. *Accid Anal Prev* 2011;43:1878–1886. doi:10.1016/j.aap.2011.04.030

38. Breeze J, Lewis EA, Fryer R et al. Defining the essential anatomical coverage provided by military body armour against high energy projectiles. *J R Army Med Corps* 2016;162:284–290. doi:10.1136/jramc-2015-000431

39. Lewis EA, Breeze J, Malbon C et al. Personal armour used by UK Armed Forces and UK Police Forces. In: Breeze J, Keene DD, Jeyanathan J et al. (eds.). *Ballistic Trauma*. London: Springer, 2017, pp. 1–25.

40. Lewis E, Carr DJ. Chapter 8: Personal armor. In: Bhatnagar A (ed.). *Lightweight Ballistic Composites*. Cambridge, UK: Woodhead Publishing, 2016, pp. 217–229.

41. Bowditch SC, Boyd N, de Vries A et al. UOR IO4077: Improved performance body armour initial examination of rigid insert shape. *Dstl Report* 2005:1–80.

42. Breeze J, Lewis EA, Fryer R. Optimising the anatomical coverage provided by military body armour systems. In: Bull AMJ, Clasper J, Mahoney PF (eds.). *Blast Injury Science and Engineering*. Cham: Springer International Publishing, 2016, pp. 291–299. doi:10.1007/978-3-319-21867-0_28

43. Lewis E. Between Iraq and a hard plate: Recent developments in UK Military Personal Armour. Proceedings of Personal Armour Systems Symposium 2006; Leeds, UK.

44. Breeze J, Allanson-Bailey LS, Hunt NC et al. Surface wound mapping of battlefield occulo-facial injury. *Injury* 2012;43:1856–1860. doi:10.1016/j.injury.2011.07.001

45. Breeze J. Saving faces: The UK future facial protection programme. *J R Army Med Corps* 2012;158:284–287.

46. Ryan JM, Bailie R, Diack G et al. Safe removal of combat body armour lightweight following battlefield wounding – A timely reminder. *J R Army Med Corps* 1994;140:26–28. doi:10.1136/jramc-140-01-06

47. Breeze J, Gibbons AJ, Hunt NC et al. Mandibular fractures in British military personnel secondary to blast trauma sustained in Iraq and Afghanistan. *Br J Oral Maxillofac Surg* 2011;49:607–611. doi:10.1016/j .bjoms.2010.10.006

48. Lewis EA, Pigott MA, Randall A et al. The development and introduction of ballistic protection of the external genitalia and perineum. *J R Army Med Corps* 2013;159(Suppl 1):i15–i17. doi:10.1136 /jramc-2013-000026

49. Helliker M, Carr D, Lankaster C et al. Effect of domestic laundering on the fragment protective performance of fabrics used in personal protection. *Text Res J* 2014;84(12): 1298–1306.

50. Breeze J, Midwinter MJ, Pope D et al. Developmental framework to validate future designs of ballistic neck protection. *Br J Oral Maxillofac Surg* 2013;51:47–51. doi:10.1016/j.bjoms.2012.03.001

51. Breeze J. The problems of protecting the neck from combat wounds. *J R Army Med Corps* 2010;156:137–138.

52. Breeze J, Masterson L, Banfield G. Outcomes from penetrating ballistic cervical injury. *J R Army Med Corps* 2012;158:96–100. doi:10.1136/jramc-158-02-05

53. Breeze J, Allanson-Bailey LS, Hunt NC et al. Mortality and morbidity from combat neck injury. *J Trauma* 2012;72:969–974. doi:10.1097/TA.0b013e31823e20a0

54. Breeze J, Midwinter MJ. Prospective computerised surface wound mapping will optimise future body armour design. *J R Army Med Corps* 2012;158:79–81. doi:10.1136 /jramc-158-02-02

55. Breeze J, Leason J, Gibb I et al. Characterisation of explosive fragments injuring the neck. *Dstl Report* 2013;51:e263–e266. doi:10.1016/j.bjoms.2013.08.005

56. Breeze J, West A, Clasper J. Anthropometric assessment of cervical neurovascular structures using CTA to determine zone-specific vulnerability to penetrating fragmentation injuries. *Clin Radiol* 2013;68:34–38. doi:10.1016/j .crad.2012.05.011

57. Breeze J. Design Validation of Future Ballistic Neck protection Through the Development of Novel Injury Models. PhD thesis, University of Birmingham, 2015. http://etheses.bham.ac.uk/5739.

58. Breeze J, Allanson-Bailey LC, Hunt NC et al. Using computerised surface wound mapping to compare the potential medical effectiveness of Enhanced Protection Under Body Armour Combat Shirt collar designs. *J R Army Med Corps* 2015;161:22–26. doi:10.1136/jramc-2013-000220

59. Patil ML, Breeze J. Use of hearing protection on military operations. *J R Army Med Corps* 2011;157:381–384. doi:10.1136 /jramc-157-04-06

60. Breeze J, Cooper H, Pearson CR et al. Ear injuries sustained by British service personnel subjected to blast trauma. *J Laryngol Otol* 2011;125:13–17. doi:10.1017 /S0022215110002215

61. Nelson TG, Wall C, Driver J et al. Op HERRICK primary care casualties: The forgotten many. *J R Army Med Corps* 2012;158:252–255.

62. Breeze J, Allanson-Bailey LS, Hunt NC et al. Surface wound mapping of battlefield occulo-facial injury. *Injury* 2012;43:1856–1860. doi:10.1016/j.injury.2011.07.001

63. Oh JS, Do NV, Clouser M et al. Effectiveness of the combat pelvic protection system in the prevention of genital and urinary tract injuries: An observational study. *J Trauma Acute Care Surg* 2015;79(Suppl 1):4.

64. Breeze J, Allanson-Bailey LS, Hepper AE et al. Demonstrating the effectiveness of body armour: A pilot prospective computerised surface wound mapping trial performed at the Role 3 hospital in Afghanistan. *J R Army Med Corps* 2015;161:36–41. doi:10.1136/jramc-2014-000249

65. Breeze J, Baxter D, Carr D et al. Defining combat helmet coverage for protection against explosively propelled fragments. *J R Army Med Corps* 2015;161:9–13. doi:10.1136/jramc-2013-000108

66. Breeze J, Fryer R, Lewis EA et al. Defining the minimum anatomical coverage required to protect the axilla and arm against penetrating ballistic projectiles. *J R Army Med Corps* 2016;162:270–275. doi:10.1136/jramc-2015-000453

67. Carr DJ, Lewis EA. Ballistic protective clothing and body armour. In: Wang F, Gao C (eds.). *Protective Clothing: Managing Thermal Stress*. Cambridge: Woodhead Publishing/The Textile Institute, 2014, pp. 146–170.

11

Head and neck

INTRODUCTION

This chapter describes the deployed head and neck capability during *Operations Telic* and *Herrick*. The head and neck is a complex anatomical region, with no one surgical specialty having precedence in the forward operational environment. Therefore, the narrative for this chapter adopts a broad point of view in order to highlight the fundamental lessons learned and the need for closer collaboration as a 'head and neck team' rather than as individual specialties.

HEAD AND NECK TRAUMA: CONTEXT

The importance of having deployed surgeons capable of managing injuries to the head, face and neck has long been recognised. *Dominique-Jean Larrey*, often called the father of modern military medicine, observed that many soldiers died before they received medical attention and devised the concept of embedding surgical teams in forward locations to stabilise the wounded before evacuation.[1,2] An important element in the success of Napoleon's campaigns was the provision of medical care on the battlefield, which resulted in high levels of morale among the soldiers as well as returning injured troops to the fighting strength. Many of the observations that Larrey made in his *Memoirs of Military Surgery*[3] are still relevant today. Larrey, and many other surgeons of the last 200 years, provided a wealth of knowledge for the conflicts that followed, much of which involved simple but effective interventions. However, with every new conflict, these lessons have tended to be relearned rather than remembered.

Head and neck trauma, and the role of a dedicated head and neck surgical team, came to prominence during the *First World War*.[4] Soldiers with horrific jaw injuries often survived initial wounding and evacuation only to be encouraged by well-meaning attendants to lie down when they reached a place of safety, with the result that they died from an occluded airway soon after. The anatomical and functional complexity of the head and neck exceeded the skills of most general surgeons and resulted in haphazard efforts to close wounds without consideration being given to the replacement of lost tissue and the restoration of function.

After initially serving with the Red Cross in France in 1915, Harold Gillies was commissioned in the Royal Army Medical Corps and soon convinced the War Office that the only way to manage the increasing number of casualties with devastating facial and jaw injuries was to organise a dedicated unit for their treatment and rehabilitation.[4] At the end of the War, Gillies consolidated his unprecedented experience into a comprehensive study of reconstructive surgery of the face.[5,6] Many of the lessons he learned have remained as cornerstones for the management of head and neck trauma during the conflicts of the last hundred years.

In 1942, Burns and Zuckerman[7] proposed a pattern of conflict-related injuries based on body surface area. According to their system, the 'head and neck' might be expected to account for 12% of all wounds if surface area was the only factor involved. Clearly, such an assumption is too simplistic in the modern combat environment, but it does provide a notional idea of how susceptible the unprotected region should be to injury from blast and ballistic events. Dobson et al.[8] concluded that 'head and neck' injuries accounted for 16% of all wounds sustained in conflicts between 1914 and 1986. The incidence varied between, and within the phases of, individual conflicts, accounting for 4% of all injuries in World War II but more than 30% in specific campaigns of World War I. These data are now historical and are difficult to interpret in the context of modern conflict because potential confounding variables and injury-specific details are not recorded. Nevertheless, this study established that the incidence of head and neck trauma was likely to wax and wane but had the potential to account for up to a third of all injuries.

Soon after combat operations commenced in Afghanistan, it was apparent that the incidence of head and neck trauma was not only increasing compared to experience in Iraq but was also sustained. In 2006, head and neck trauma accounted for 18% of all wounds in UK Armed Forces personnel but increased to 28% in 2007 and remained at 23% in 2008.[9] The waxing and waning pattern seen in historical data was still true to some extent, but head and neck trauma was now a 'routine' pattern of injury that started to challenge deployed surgical capability.[9,10] The sustained injury levels were reflected in contemporary US data, where head and neck trauma accounted for 21–29% of all wounds.[11–16] However, Belmont et al.[17] demonstrated that during the 'surge' operation conducted by the United States in 2007, head and neck trauma accounted for 36.2% of all wounds. Hœncamp et al.[18] confirmed this sustained prevalence in a systematic review of eight cohort studies of injury prevalence for coalition forces based in Iraq and Afghanistan that included 19,750 battle-injured casualties. Despite limitations in methodological designs between the studies, the authors clearly demonstrated the high prevalence of wounds caused by explosions and explosively propelled fragments, which led to head and neck trauma in 31% of all casualties. The authors concluded that the increase in head and neck trauma was significant compared to previous conflicts.

It is generally agreed that the sustained incidence of head and neck trauma in Iraq and Afghanistan was due to improvements in the design of individual combat body armour, which afforded greater protection from penetrating injury to the abdomen and thorax, and the use of the improvised explosive device (IED) in an evolving asymmetric battlespace.[13,14,19–27] A systematic review of the literature found no evidence that the incidence of head and neck trauma increased by virtue of wearing combat body armour but rather that explosive munitions were more likely to affect those areas that were less well protected.[28] However, it is also possible that enemy forces deliberately targeted the more exposed areas of the mounted or dismounted soldier, in particular the face and neck.[29] These issues and research into future combat face and neck protection are discussed later.

One of the problems in interpreting the published literature, both past and present, is the definition of what is encompassed by the 'head and neck'. In modern clinical practice, the 'head and neck' is a broad concept that covers a range of specialties and sub-specialities. The modern head and neck multidisciplinary meeting can involve a number of surgical teams, including neurosurgeons, oral and maxillofacial or otorhinolaryngology head and neck surgeons, ophthalmologists and plastic and reconstructive surgeons, reflecting the diverse and complex anatomy of the region. The surgical teams are supported by a wealth of specialist surgical and non-surgical healthcare professionals. This collaborative aspect has driven significant advances in care but has, at times, complicated inter-specialty agreement regarding best practice. According to the *International Classification of Diseases, Ninth Revision with Clinical Modification (ICD-9-CM)*,[30] which is used in the *Joint Theatre Trauma Registry* (JTTR), the terms 'head, face and neck' should be used as a better reflection of the complex anatomy of the region.[10]

Official statistics for *Operation Telic* have not been published, and the injury data discussed in this chapter is mostly based on the published literature. However, the *Ministry of Defence* has published official statistics[31] for *Operation Herrick* covering the period from the opening of the UK Field Hospital on 1 April 2006 to its closure on 30 November 2014. A total of 7800 UK Service personnel and civilians were admitted, of whom 4220 admissions were the result of injuries. This number includes personnel who subsequently died of their wounds as well as those who survived to the point of discharge. It does not cover all injuries sustained because the level of detail recorded in the field hospital electronic data was insufficient to support coding. Of the 4220 injury admissions, roughly half were *battle injuries* and half were *non-battle injuries* (NBIs). A total of 1982 (47%) patients were admitted with injuries that required activation of the trauma team. This group sustained a total of 10,371 separate injuries. A total of 718 UK Service personnel sustained a total of 1,908 injuries involving the head, face or neck, which accounted for just under a fifth of the total wounds. An additional 9 injuries to the eyes and 15 injuries to the ears were recorded separately.

It is clear that injuries to the head, face and neck accounted for a significant part of the workload for the coalition during operations in both Iraq and Afghanistan.[12,13,19,32–35] There is every reason to expect that this pattern of injury will continue to be a significant burden for future conflicts, especially if IEDs predominate. Deployed head and neck pathology can be broadly divided into injuries of the cranium, face, neck, eyes and ears. However, a full description of the anatomy of each area and the surgical interventions, repairs or reconstructive procedures that can be used for every discrete type of wound are beyond the scope of this chapter.

CLINICAL ADVANCES AND EMERGING CONCEPTS

The lessons learned in Iraq and Afghanistan broadly encompass doctrinal changes and refinements of existing surgical concepts. The high incidence of head, face, neck and ophthalmic injuries during *Operations Telic* and *Herrick* made research into ways of reducing the burden of such injuries in future conflicts essential (Figure 11.1). Some of the changes in doctrine have been true 'paradigm shifts' that will be the cornerstone of future combat casualty care, whereas others will prove to be rather more specific to the environments of Iraq and Afghanistan. Most of the surgical lessons learned in the field of head and neck trauma have been relatively modest, but this has the benefit of making them more likely to be integrated into routine civilian practice. In other words, lessons learned will be refined and reinforced within the multispecialty head and neck surgical teams to become 'common practice' rather than a skill set that is specific to the deployed military setting.

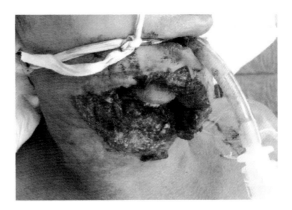

Figure 11.1 Typical combat-related penetrating neck wound.

This section describes some of the recent doctrinal models that have emerged over the last decade that have had, or will have, an impact on the management of head and neck trauma in future contingency operations.

Damage control resuscitation and surgery

One of the most important concepts to be questioned during *Operation Telic* was the conventional *ABC paradigm* for trauma care. Champion et al.[36] estimated that up to 10% of battlefield deaths were due to haemorrhage from extremity wounds and non-compressible 'junctional zones' such as the root of the neck, axillae and groins. It was recognised that combat trauma had unique features in terms of acute resuscitation, including the high energy and lethality of the wounding agents, the presence of multiple wounds and a high incidence of penetrating injury. In addition, the importance of contributing factors, such as the pervasive threat in tactical settings, the often austere or resource-constrained environments and delayed evacuation to definitive care, was also recognised.

The concept of *damage control resuscitation/ damage control surgery* (DCR–DCS) and the <C>ABC sequence were introduced in 2007 as a new paradigm for pre-hospital and hospital-based trauma care.[37,38] The purpose of DCR is to commence aggressive resuscitation as soon as the need is identified, which includes the immediate control of catastrophic haemorrhage before efforts to

Table 11.1 Damage control interventions in head and neck surgery

Haemorrhage, scalp:
- Apply direct pressure.
- Identify specific bleeding points, cauterise, clip or ligate.
- Oversew wound margin with large sutures.

Haemorrhage, soft tissues of face:
- Apply direct pressure.
- Identify specific bleeding points, cauterise, clip or ligate.
- Consider tacking sutures to approximate wound edges.

Haemorrhage, facial fractures:
- Reduce fracture(s) if possible.
- Stabilise fracture with intermaxillary fixation.
- Consider posterior nasal packs or inflated urinary catheters for ongoing posterior nasal bleeds.

Compromised airway with c-spine protection:
- Apply adjunctive airway procedures such as head lift, chin lift and jaw thrust while protecting the c-spine.
- Insert oropharyngeal or nasopharyngeal airway.
- Laryngeal mask airway.
- Endotracheal intubation.
- Emergency cricothyroidotomy.

Facial avulsion injury:
- Secure airway.
- Control haemorrhage.
- Stabilise with intermaxillary fixation.
- Pack wound if there is appreciable loss of tissue.

Facial burns:
- Secure airway with endotracheal intubation or definitive surgical airway only if evidence of impending airway compromise.
- Assess for signs of inhalation injury.

Penetrating neck wound(s):
- Secure airway.
- Control haemorrhage.
- Vascular imaging studies if available.
- Exploration of neck as soon as tactical situation and facilities are appropriate.

secure the airway. In practice, where the tactical setting and resources allow, the control of haemorrhage occurs at the same time as efforts to control the airway and protect the cervical spine. The DCS element of the combined resuscitation/surgery process occurs as soon as possible in an effort to stabilise and restore normal physiology, the DCR and DCS elements being synergistic and continuing until the casualty reaches intensive or critical care support. The *DCR–DCS* concept is now the cornerstone of modern surgical trauma care.[39]

There are no specific skills within *DCR–DCS* that are exclusive to injuries of the head, face or neck.[40] Catastrophic haemorrhage from a penetrating neck injury is difficult to control and usually fatal at the point of wounding. The primary cause of death in this region remains airway compromise, and catastrophic haemorrhage is seen much less frequently.[10] As such, the airway is usually the main concern. A set of simple damage control interventions has been proposed[40] (Table 11.1). Pre-hospital care and resuscitation are discussed further in Chapters 3 and 4.

Medical emergency response teams

The head, face and neck are rarely wounded in isolation, and although catastrophic haemorrhage can be controlled or mitigated, failure to definitively secure the airway may result in potentially salvageable casualties arriving at forward surgical locations in a non-salvageable state.[10] In recent operations, the contribution of air supremacy and rapid tactical evacuation of casualties from the point of wounding to rearward levels of advanced care cannot be underestimated. Most wounded casualties, with or without life-threatening injuries, were able to receive DCR–DCS within very short timescales.

The establishment of the *Medical Emergency Response Team* (MERT) capability was a revolution in military medical evacuation.[41] Originally conceived in Iraq as the *Incident Response Team*, the concept of advanced aeromedical evacuation was established in Afghanistan in 2006 in response to the potential for longer flight times for casualties.[42] The original MERT consisted of a critical care registered general nurse with a background in emergency medicine and a paramedic.[43]

The MERT composition was then developed to include a second paramedic and consultant, or occasionally a senior trainee, with a background in emergency medicine, critical care or anaesthesia.[44] The team structure enabled advanced trauma interventions to be performed well before arrival at Camp Bastion.[45]

Although MERT could be deployed on a number of airframes, the capabilities of the CH-47 Chinook provided a robust platform for evacuation of multiple casualties and the space to perform advanced pre-hospital care interventions. Conventional retrieval of casualties also occurred using the US *DUSTOFF* (UH-60 helicopter with combat medical technicians) and *PEDRO* (HH-60 Pave Hawk helicopter with paramedics) assets.[45] A study of casualties evacuated by all three platforms demonstrated that two thirds were well served by conventional helicopter retrieval.[45] However, casualties with severe but survivable injuries had a reduced mortality when retrieved by MERT. Understanding the injury severity at the scene may allow appropriate tasking of retrieval assets and continues to be a focus of research.

The provision of field care in the tactical combat environment is very different from that in a civilian environment. Nevertheless, the high standard of care provided to combat casualties in Iraq and Afghanistan is a testament to the assets that could be deployed in those environments, as well as to the fact that, in general, only low numbers of casualties were being taken at any one time. In the absence of air supremacy or an ability to deploy forward assets with the capabilities of MERT, it remains to be seen whether casualties with head, face or neck trauma will generate the same survival data in future conflicts.

Radiology and diagnostic imaging

Due to the limited number of personnel and low intensity of conflict, military radiologists were not deployed to *Operation Telic*.[46] Instead, multi-detector computed tomography (MDCT) images were relayed to the United Kingdom and reported back to the field hospital. The same system was employed during the early phase of *Operation Herrick*, but as the intensity of the conflict increased, remote reporting was unable to cope with the data from

multiple casualties with devastating and immediately life-threatening injuries. Therefore, from 2009, military radiologists deployed to *Operation Herrick* in order to support the emerging DCR–DCS concept.[46] The lessons learned from deployed imaging are discussed further in Chapter 13.

The use of ultrasound and MDCT imaging has become an integral part of the management of casualties during recent operations and its importance in the investigation of head and neck trauma cannot be overestimated.[46,47] Casualties were scanned as soon as they were stable enough. A consultant radiologist provided an immediate screening review for the surgical team, which identified potentially life-threatening injuries and assessment of the adequacy of pre-hospital interventions. The level of clinically relevant information provided by deployed radiologists was an invaluable decision tool during hospital-based management.

It can be argued that MDCT is the ideal asset to image the head, face and neck after injuries sustained in combat. While many fractures are usually clinically obvious, the size and position of all fragments, especially those that have been propelled into the brain or neck, can be clearly identified (Figure 11.2). Foreign bodies from secondary fragmentation injury are almost ubiquitous and

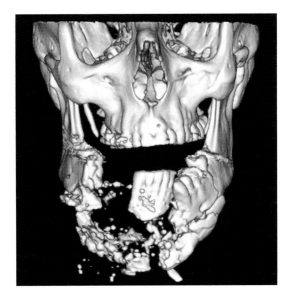

Figure 11.2 3D Computed tomographic reconstruction demonstrating a highly comminuted mandibular fracture.

can easily be missed during the primary and secondary survey in the presence of other more devastating wounds. Subdural haemorrhage can be subtle and can occur in the absence of skull fractures. Eye injuries are common and can be difficult to examine in the presence of severe facial trauma. Fragments striking the face or neck may damage any structure and may, in rare circumstances, embolise to distant locations.[48-50] MDCT allows evaluation and definition of the extent of vascular and nerve injuries and the position of fragments, which can inform the surgical team as to whether immediate surgical exploration and repair are needed before evacuation.[46,47] However, the current dilemma is whether it provides enough benefit to justify the resources needed to deploy and maintain an MDCT scanner in a potentially hostile environment. Unfortunately, this decision may have to be made with the benefit of hindsight following experience in the early stages of any future conflict.

'Left of bang' research

The traditional paradigm for medical care has been a sequence of events that proceed along a linear timeline from point of wounding, through forward surgery and evacuation to definitive care and rehabilitation. This timeline, moving from left to right, starts with the trauma, or 'bang'. In a military context, 'left of bang' describes the sequence of events preceding the incident that contributed to success or failure in its management.[51,52] However, in the context of military medicine, 'left of bang' can be described as any medical, pharmacological or surgical intervention that is delivered before the incident that serves to reduce morbidity and mortality.[53] These interventions may include wearable technologies that monitor and identify individuals at risk of injury before the injury has occurred or that can help to augment care at the point of wounding, nutritional and physiological preconditioning or, more loosely, interventions that are administered soon after wounding that mitigate the secondary physiological or psychological effects of trauma.[53]

In a broader context, 'left of bang' principles can be considered to include novel research that serves to reduce morbidity and mortality in the combat environment. This research may include personal protective equipment or equipment design. However, the 'dual-use dilemma' can arise in the sense that novel research sometimes has the potential to be harmful if it is not used for the purpose in which it was conceived.[54-56] The 'left of bang' model has now become an integral part of research and development, which means that the highest ethical standards must be followed when considering study proposals.

It remains to be seen exactly how 'left of bang' research will impact on the management of head and neck trauma in the future. However, the ability to incorporate wearable technologies into a combat helmet to monitor brain or hearing function following exposure to significant blast injury or, indeed, to mitigate the secondary effects of brain or cochlear injury near to the point of wounding is not beyond the scope of current research programmes.

CRANIOFACIAL AND NECK TRAUMA

Injuries of the head and neck are usually classified as blunt or penetrating, with the face often being described as the 'window to the brain'. Blast-related mild traumatic brain injury (mTBI) was a common injury in Iraq and Afghanistan due to the frequent use of IEDs.[57-61] Indeed, it has been referred to as one of the 'signature injuries' of these conflicts alongside the lower limb amputation/perineal injury complex.[57,58] Facial injuries can be divided into thirds when describing wound patterns.[62] Due to distinct variations in the anatomy and in protection from body armour, the three facial zones have marked differences in terms of wounding potential, morbidity and mortality. Considerable kinetic energy is required for a projectile striking the upper third of the face to penetrate the cranium. However, once the cranium is breached, only a small amount of residual energy is needed for it to pass through the brain. Middle third facial injuries generally have a low mortality, but the associated morbidity from disfigurement and ocular injury can be devastating. Lower third facial injuries also have a low mortality, but there is little published evidence for the long-term morbidity associated with military wounding patterns in this area.[63]

Traumatic brain injury

The prevalence of mTBI in UK Armed Forces personnel is lower than that of comparable US military personnel.[58,59] It is widely accepted that mTBI is a complex multifactorial disease process, not a single entity.[64] This is one of the main reasons why it is difficult to define the aetiology clearly and it explains why a constellation of physical, cognitive and emotional symptoms, collectively referred to as post-concussion syndrome, is associated with it.[65–67] The primary injury is almost certainly caused by immediate mechanical damage to brain tissue.[68] However, this process is itself complex and remains poorly understood. Mechanisms of primary injury are likely to include direct neuronal, glial and other cellular damage; macroscopic and microscopic haemorrhage from damaged blood vessels; and axonal shearing.[68] Secondary injury follows over a variable timeframe mediated by an array of neurochemical, inflammatory and neuroinflammatory mechanisms.[69,70] Modulation of these mechanisms may offer potential therapeutic options in the future.[71] Research continues to unravel the complex interactions within the brain with the hope of developing novel therapeutic interventions and improved quality of life for millions of sufferers.

Traditional military teaching is that outcome and mortality from penetrating brain injury are dependent on the *Glasgow Coma Scale* (GCS) score prior to the induction of anaesthesia.[72] However, this teaching was based on historical data that did not take into account modern advances in critical care and the marked difference in energy transmission and tissue interaction between explosively propelled fragments and gunshot wounds. As the mechanisms of injury on the battlefield have changed, so have our preconceptions evolved as historically non-salvageable wounds result in unexpected survivors.[21,73–76]

Penetrating intracranial injuries are rare in UK civilian practice.[75] In the Unites States, civilian cranio-cerebral gunshot wounds have been reported to have a mortality of 73% at the scene, with an additional 15% not surviving initial attempts at resuscitation in the emergency department.[77] The mortality from gunshot wounds is high, but the outcome for explosively propelled fragments is generally better.[75,78,79]

In a study of 813 UK Armed Forces casualties with penetrating intracranial injury sustained between 2003 and 2011, 336 (41.3%) were killed in action or died of wounds.[75] Secondary blast and explosively propelled fragments caused 625 injuries (76.9%), with the remainder attributed to gunshot wounds. No other mechanisms of injury were identified. The injury severity scores were significantly higher in the gunshot wound group, with an expected poorer survival. The earliest recorded GCS was significantly lower in the gunshot wound group. The authors attempted to mitigate the influence of extracranial injury on survival by analysing a subgroup of 157 casualties with isolated penetrating cranial injury. The blast and gunshot wound groups were almost equal in size. In the gunshot wound group, the median Abbreviated Injury Score (AIS) remained higher and was still associated with a lower survival and less favourable initial GCS. This finding remained when both groups were compared using a median AIS of 6. In other words, and as expected, higher-energy gunshot wounds that penetrate the cranium carry a higher mortality risk. And yet, the most significant aspect of these data is that even with an initial GCS of 3–5, 21% of blast-injured and 14% of gunshot wound casualties survive to hospital discharge.

While it is true that a low initial GCS is associated with poor survival, it is clear that traditional military teaching regarding penetrating intracranial injury does not necessarily hold true in the context of the high standards of medical care and evacuation that were deployed to *Operations Telic* and *Herrick*. The United Kingdom only deployed a military neurosurgeon to Camp Bastion for a few months in 2007, and from 2008, a neurosurgeon was attached to a dedicated head and neck surgical team based in Kandahar.[80] The United Kingdom provided neurosurgeons as civilian contractors and other coalition partners provided similar neurosurgical support to maintain the deployed capability. However, this arrangement would not be sustainable outside of the relative security of a facility the size of Camp Bastion. There is currently a zero liability for neurosurgery across all three Services, and the United Kingdom is therefore unable to provide any forward neurosurgical support for future contingency operations in the absence of coalition partners. This has significant implications for the care of penetrating brain injury in future conflicts. It may be possible to return to the remote telemedicine approach that was used until 2009, when military radiologists deployed to *Operation Herrick*, but that also assumes that there is the capability or willingness to deploy a head or whole-body MDCT scanner, without which diagnosis remains extremely difficult. The management of blunt or closed brain injuries is just as uncertain without diagnostic imaging and will rely on clinical signs and symptoms to guide intervention.

Until these issues are resolved, the management of both blunt and penetrating injury should be kept simple. Blunt injuries may require diagnostic burr holes, while penetrating intracranial injury should involve wound debridement and removal of loose fragments, primary closure of the wound and antibiotics. All head injuries must be considered for urgent evacuation for appropriate investigations and definitive care. For the foreseeable future, forward surgical care is likely to be achieved by non-neurosurgeons with additional pre-deployment training.

Research remains a priority and continues to be directed to improving diagnostic capabilities in forward locations on the basis that the liability for neurosurgeons is not going to increase in the future. A number of civilian research centres are supporting this work. The management of penetrating brain injury in austere environments may also benefit from the 'left of bang' research discussed previously.

Facial injury

A study of facial injuries among UK Service personnel killed or injured on *Operation Herrick* from April 2006 to March 2013 identified 633 casualties.[19] Of these 563 (88.9%) were attributed to blast injury and explosively propelled fragments, although 59 were excluded from further study as they had isolated ruptures of the tympanic membranes. Seventy (11.1%) were attributed to gunshot wounds. Therefore, of the 566 casualties with facial injuries included in the study, 405 (71.6%) survived their injuries, with 375 (92.6%) returning to the United Kingdom for further management. Isolated injury to the face was uncommon in both blast (36, 7.1%) and gunshot wound (11, 17.7%) groups. Thirty-three casualties with gunshot wounds to the

face died of their wounds or were killed in action. The presence of a facial fracture was associated with higher injury severity scores in those with blast injury, but the same pattern was not observed in the gunshot wound group. Blast-injured survivors tended to have middle third facial fractures, whereas fatalities tended to have lower third facial fractures and concurrent head injuries. This was in contrast to gunshot wound survivors who tended to have lower third facial fractures.

The data from UK and US casualties is broadly similar.[11,33] The maxilla is the most commonly fractured bone in survivors, whereas the mandible tends to be fractured in fatalities, and such fractures are likely to be attributed to the magnitude of the ground-based detonation. Lower-order explosions are likely to cause less lower limb or pelvic trauma and will cause fractures of the weaker maxilla in preference to the mandible. However, higher-order explosions are likely to cause more extensive trauma, and the more energetic blast wave will cause fractures of the mandible as well as other concurrent injuries.[81–83]

A total of six patients were transferred from the British Field Hospital at Camp Bastion to Kandahar for a specialist ophthalmic or neurosurgical procedure.[19] Facial surgery was required in 283 (70.0%) of the facial injuries. Those facial injuries that did not require surgery were either small lacerations or abrasions that could be managed in the emergency department or simple closed fractures that could be managed non-operatively, for example nasal fractures. A single procedure was needed in approximately half of those requiring surgery, with 134 (47.3%) cases requiring only simple debridement and primary closure of facial wounds. No facial infections were reported in the cohort of primary closures that were subsequently evacuated to the United Kingdom. This supports the practice of primary closure of facial wounds in austere environments.[32]

The management of facial wounds generally differs dramatically to surgery elsewhere in that primary closure can be achieved immediately.[19,32] Indeed, careful consideration should be given to preservation of tissue with minimal wound excision and retention of bone fragments with their periosteal attachments.

Temporary stabilisation of fractures can be achieved with intermaxillary fixation using drill-free bone screws.[84,85] This is a simple technique that can be performed by non-specialists with relatively limited training and equipment.[10,85] This procedure has proved to be extremely useful for the management of combat casualties and can assist with the process of minimal wound excision and retention of bone fragments. The technique is also an extremely effective form of pain relief, which can reduce the need for excessive opioid analgesia in a forward location.[10]

The study of facial injuries in UK Armed Forces highlighted the difficulty in accurately scoring the soft tissue element based on the current AIS coding used in the JTTR database.[19] In addition, scoring the severity of the facial injury using the AIS is a poor predictor of morbidity based on the eventual functional and aesthetic outcome. Isolated injuries affecting a prominent facial structure can cause substantial morbidity, for example 10 survivors scored 1 or 2 on the facial AIS component but required staged reconstructive surgery to the nose associated with longer-term physical and psychological problems. The difficulty in scoring facial injuries is not solely a military problem. Many scoring systems for craniofacial fractures in civilian trauma have been proposed in recent years.[86–90] A scoring system for facial trauma should include both skeletal and soft tissue elements and convey the severity, functional deficits and aesthetic morbidity.[91]

Despite a wealth of UK and multinational data from recent conflicts, there is still little published evidence on the outcome of facial injuries sustained in combat. Research is still needed into the longer-term outcomes of combat-related facial injuries, both in terms of physical morbidity and the associated social and psychological effects of disfigurement. A large multinational conference on future facial protection concluded that there was a need to collaborate in research to quantify the outcomes following facial injury and to highlight areas of the face that required protection in future conflicts.[92] The consensus opinion is that the combat helmet and visor should protect the brain, upper and middle thirds of the face and possibly extend to include the nose.[93]

Neck injury

Neck trauma can be divided into blunt and penetrating injuries. Blunt trauma is generally managed with close observation in the absence of hoarseness, change in voice quality, dysphagia or surgical emphysema.[10] However, casualties with significant blunt neck trauma must be considered for an early definitive airway. Penetrating neck injury is a highly lethal event on the battlefield.[94] In general, patients with penetrating neck injuries who survive to reach forward surgical care should be intubated, and if platysma has been breached, surgical exploration will be necessary to exclude more insidious injuries. This may not be necessary if an MDCT scanner is deployed.[46,47]

Fragments striking the neck can have entirely unexpected wound tracts.[24,95] Injury to the oropharynx and larynx is usually obvious due to the presence of surgical emphysema, although this may be subtle in the presence of other facial injuries. Damage to the oesophagus is often an occult injury with no surgical emphysema and can lead to significant morbidity, such as mediastinitis and sepsis.

Meticulous physical examination of the neck is mandatory.[96] The haemodynamically unstable casualty with 'hard signs' should have immediate exploration of the neck after the airway is secured, while asymptomatic casualties can be observed closely. Stable casualties with 'soft signs' can be investigated using MDCT, if available, as an initial screening tool. Selective investigation is based on the 'no zone' concept and reduces the high negative exploration rate that occurs if all penetrating neck trauma undergoes surgical exploration as a default.[96] However, as combat-related fragmentation injuries are prone to complex wound tracts, casualties with penetrating neck trauma should ideally have a panendoscopy, including an upper rigid oesophagoscopy, to exclude aerodigestive injury. All penetrating neck trauma therefore requires urgent evacuation to the United Kingdom whether or not surgical exploration has occurred. Casualties should have a nasogastric tube passed under direct vision and remain nil by mouth for at least 24 hours. Passing a nasogastric tube using an oesophagoscope is not a deployed skill set, and for injuries beyond the reach of the laryngoscope, passing a nasogastric tube blindly risks inadvertently penetrating the oesophagus with passage of the tube into the neck or chest.

OBJECTIVE ASSESSMENTS OF HEAD AND NECK BODY ARMOUR

Surface wound mapping (SWM) is a technique that records the entrance and exit wounds caused by ballistic injuries. Early attempts in World War II used two-dimensional anatomical diagrams,[97,98] but more recent studies have used three-dimensional software.[26,63,99,100] Each wound is assigned an AIS score, and so, for each casualty, SWM provides a visual representation of all wounds that can be linked to injury severity and outcome.

A retrospective SWM study for UK casualties evacuated to the United Kingdom proved cumbersome and time-consuming due to inadequate data collection methods.[101] However, retrospective analysis of detailed post-mortem records yielded much better data. Prospective SWM allows analysis of complex mechanisms of injury, such as those seen in *Operations Telic* and *Herrick*. In response, the *Defence Science and Technology Laboratory* and *Royal Centre for Defence Medicine* (RCDM) jointly developed the *Interactive Mapping Analysis Platform* (IMAP) as a prospective SWM tool to collect data as close to the point of wounding as possible.[101]

Prospective SWM can be a powerful tool for investigating the wounding potential of explosive ordnance and the protection afforded by body armour or other design enhancements, such as vehicle modifications.[101–103] The *Under Body Armour Combat Shirt* (UBACS) was issued to UK Service personnel deployed to *Operation Herrick*. It was routinely worn under the UK MkIV Osprey combat body armour. However, it had no inherent ballistic protection, as its principal function was to improve comfort by dissipating sweat and body heat. When the ballistic neck collar was worn during increased threat levels, a potential gap existed between the collar and the neckline of the body armour, which left the lower neck vulnerable to fragment injury. An *Enhanced Protection UBACS* (EP-UBACS) was designed with a standard collar reinforced with ballistic protective material, in an attempt to provide full coverage to the neck. Tests were conducted on three *EP-UBACS* prototypes using SWM based on two years of neck wound data from casualties sustained on *Operation Herrick*.[103] The IMAP tool demonstrated that all three prototypes would have prevented a large number of wounds. However, perhaps the most important feature was the ability to be able to overlay armour designs onto a standardised simulated human manikin, which allowed the neck protection to be tested from a variety of fragmentation sources. The study concluded that reinforced neck collars with the greatest stand-off from the skin provided the best protection (Figure 11.3).

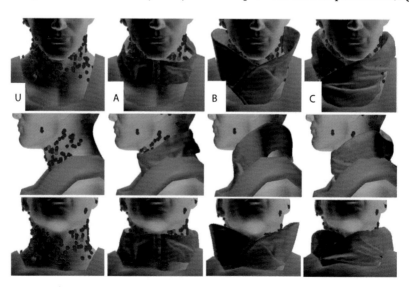

Figure 11.3 Entry wound locations visualised from anterior horizontal (upper row), lateral horizontal (middle row) and anterior ground (lower row). A standard UBACS is shown with no integral neck protection (U) along with EP-UBACS Prototypes (A–C).

A similar system to evaluate protection to specific areas of the body is the *Coverage of Armour Tool*.[104] All three models have proved to be useful tools in quantifying head, face and neck wounding patterns in UK Service personnel. Although prototypes for personal protective equipment may be validated using these models, it is important to remember that this does not necessarily equate to a design that is combat effective.[105-107] However, when integrated with a period of robust testing in simulated combat environments with the soldiers who are expected to wear them, an ideal risk–benefit balance can be established.

Combat helmet and future facial protection

The UK Mk7 combat helmet comprises a woven fabric reinforced composite shell, a non-ballistic impact protective liner, and suspension, sizing and retention systems.[108] It is designed to protect the brain from penetrating fragment injury as well as to protect the head and face from low impact 'bump' injuries. Unlike the standard-issue US combat helmet, it is not designed to withstand penetrating projectiles from handguns.

It is difficult to quantify how effective the modern combat helmet is because almost all casualties are wearing one at the time of injury.[9] Undoubtedly, the number of casualties with cranial injuries would have been higher if the combat helmet was not worn, as was observed in the different casualty rates between US and Iraqi soldiers in *Operation Desert Storm*.[109] A systematic review of military data suggests that, in the modern battlespace, approximately 20% of penetrating injuries will involve the 'head', excluding the neck.[108] These injuries account for 40–50% of combat casualties.

The neurosurgical literature indicates that helmets provide effective protection against moderate to severe head trauma likely to result in severe disability or death.[110] However, there is a lack of civilian and military data on helmet efficacy against concussion. Sone et al.[110] have suggested that patients wearing a helmet do not have better relative clinical outcomes and protection against concussion than do patients who are not wearing one. A systematic review of military head injuries found no evidence of behind helmet blunt trauma in the openly accessible literature since composite helmets were adopted as standard issue.[108] The authors discuss the difficulties that arise in attempting to compare international civilian and military data across the decades, in particular due to issues concerning the exact definition and anatomical boundaries of the 'head'. Calls to address this lack of standardisation have been made for at least 25 years.[109] From a military perspective, the 'head' is considered to be the area covered by the combat helmet, which is designed to protect the brain and brainstem.[111,112] The anatomical landmarks of the 'head' should therefore include the nasion, external auditory meatus and superior nuchal line.[111] The establishment of internationally accepted standards must be considered a priority for future research. The morbidity from mild brain injury and concussion has only recently been established and further research is ongoing to optimise the protection afforded by the combat helmet.

The face is potentially the most difficult body region to protect, resulting in a lack of international consensus and reflected in the wide range of commercial prototype designs available.[92] The UK Mk7 combat helmet provides excellent protection from fragments travelling horizontally towards the upper facial third. However, in an attempt to provide greater 'bump' protection, there is a wide gap or 'stand-off' that offers less protection from fragments travelling towards the face from ground-based IEDs. If combat eye protection is worn, a significant part of this gap is covered. Combat eye protection covers about two thirds of the anterior face. Combat visors offer better protection than goggles, both in terms of coverage to the face and greater ballistic performance. There is no doubt that an integrated visor system would reduce middle third facial injuries but the Mk7 combat helmet has no attachment options. The lower facial third is also prone to ground-based IEDs, which can be mitigated with mandible guards or ballistic neck collars if they project sufficiently far forward.

Logically, integrating a visor with modular protection for the mandible and chin would reduce the morbidity and mortality associated with fragmentation and ballistic injuries to the head, face and neck.[63,113] A number of prototype designs are available from commercial suppliers, including those with multifunctional adaptors for the attachment of visors, night vision goggles and cameras. However, despite the incontrovertible benefits of wearing eye and ear protection, which are discussed later in this chapter, the uptake of enhanced combat helmets among soldiers may be variable if there is a belief that loss of sensory perception and situational awareness occurs. A recent consensus statement proposed that the priorities for protection should be the head (brain) and eyes, possibly extending to include the nose.[93] Procurement of an alternative combat helmet may be necessary in the near future but should be part of a wider programme of equipment integration and interoperability, which can unite the combat needs of soldiers and commanders with the desire of the DMS to protect them from injury.

OCULAR TRAUMA

The potential for a wide range of traumatic and non-traumatic eye problems was recognised before deployment to the dusty environments of Iraq and Afghanistan. The eyes occupy 0.1% of the total body surface area, but their injuries cause significant morbidity and can be life-changing.[114,115] Importantly, even minor eye injuries or infections can rapidly incapacitate personnel and, if untreated, cause permanent severe visual loss. Contact lens-related problems can occur in any environment, including high altitudes.[116,117] Rare ophthalmic presentations such as external ophthalmomyiasis highlight the difficulties of deploying to austere environments.[118,119] The prompt diagnosis of ocular pathology, coupled with appropriate treatment in the field or evacuation for advanced care, can limit potential sight-threatening complications.

British military ophthalmologists were deployed to *Operation Telic* as part of the initial phase in March 2003 but were not deployed in support of operations in Iraq or Afghanistan after May 2003.[120] Thereafter, initial management of eye injuries was undertaken by the emergency medicine consultant, with patients being admitted under medicine, surgery or, occasionally, emergency medicine. Telephone advice was sought from the United Kingdom when required. Eye injuries requiring the clinical input of an ophthalmologist were treated through two routes. All such personnel

were evacuated back to the United Kingdom to be seen and treated at the RCDM in Birmingham and most were evacuated using UK assets. Some were managed in-theatre and returned via US facilities in Germany. The decision to evacuate most patients with eye injuries to the United Kingdom ensured consistent and optimal treatment.

During the conflict period of *Operation Telic*, 45 eye injuries were seen, accounting for 2% of all admissions to *34 Field Hospital*.[121] Six casualties required evacuation for definitive care. Between March 2003 and June 2007, ophthalmic presentations accounted for 1610 (5.3%) attendances at the emergency department and Role 3 Facility.[122] Only 22 (1.4%) were injuries sustained as a direct result of combat. Non-battle injuries were relatively minor, including foreign bodies and corneal abrasions. The remainder of the presentations included common causes of 'red eye', such as conjunctivitis, or conditions caused by dangers inherent to the deployed environment, such as oils, grease and chemicals being wiped or splashed into or around the eyes.[122] Unfortunately, these early data do not identify the number of casualties needing surgical intervention or their long-term outcomes in terms of loss of visual acuity or discharge from Service. However, the data do demonstrate how ophthalmic presentations varied over time and peaked during the height of hostilities in 2003. A similar peak was noted during *Operation Desert Storm* in 1991, when ophthalmic injuries accounted for 13% of all wounds.[123] Combat eye protection was therefore issued to all personnel deployed to Iraq and this is likely to have contributed to the reduction in incidence of eye injuries seen during *Operation Telic*.[13]

Another study of 630 major trauma admissions treated during *Operations Telic* and *Herrick* from 2004 to 2008 identified 63 (10%) casualties with eye injuries.[124] Nineteen casualties had bilateral injuries. Injuries were classified according to the *Birmingham Eye Trauma Terminology System*, a standardised system to describe and share eye injury information (Figure 11.4).[125-127] It is a particularly useful system for use in deployed environments, where casualties may be managed by multiple teams during assessment, treatment and evacuation.[120,124-127] As with previous US studies,[123,128] this study considered only 'significant' injuries and excluded 'minor' injuries, such as superficial foreign bodies, corneal abrasion

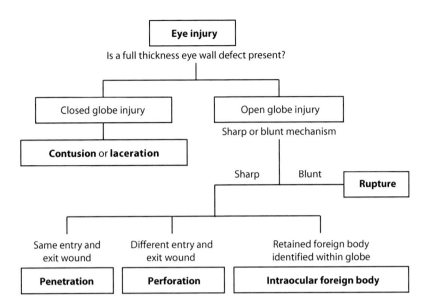

Figure 11.4 Birmingham Eye Trauma Terminology System. Terminology – *Rupture*: A full thickness defect of the sclera and cornea caused by a blunt mechanism; the impact causes a transient increase in intraocular pressure resulting in an inside–out disruption at the weakest point. *Penetration*: A single full-thickness wound caused by an in–out injury mechanism or the incomplete passage of an object through the eye wall; more than one penetrating wound implies more than one injuring agent. *Perforation*: Full-thickness defects of the eye wall caused by an injurious agent passing through the globe. *Intraocular foreign body*: A retained injurious agent within the substance of the globe (see 'Penetration'). (From Kuhn F et al., *J Fr Ophtalmol* 2004;27(2):206–210; Kuhn F et al. *Ophthalmol Clin N Am* 2002;15(2):139–143.)

and subconjunctival haemorrhage. Explosive blast injuries occurred in 54/63 patients (86%) and closed globe contusion injuries occurred in 6/63 (9.5%) cases. There were three cases of disease NBI: one following a motor vehicle collision, one from a non-combat-related aircraft incident and one associated with an electrical burn. Among the significant injuries, 40/48 (83%) were caused by explosive blast. The mean time from injury to arrival in the United Kingdom was 2.63 days for all injuries and 2.52 days for open injuries. Of the 58 severe injuries, 22 (38% of eyes) had an associated adnexal injury, for example lid lacerations, burns or orbital fractures. Facial or orbital fractures occurred in 17 of 48 patients (35%). Penetrating or closed brain injury with structural abnormality on imaging occurred in nine patients (19%); cases of mTBI/post-concussive syndrome were not included (Figure 11.5).

Isolated eye injuries occurred in nine individuals (19%), of whom one only had minor injuries. A further seven cases (two minor) were associated with soft tissue fragmentation injuries, which required no

treatment. For open-globe injuries, mean time to primary repair was 1.9 days (range 0–5), with an average of 1.57 operations per eye. The total number of ocular casualties is much lower than that reported in the US military,[123,128–131] reflecting differences in the overall number and casualty profile of UK and US military casualties. The authors conclude that British military ophthalmologists managed the challenge of providing highly technical eye care to Service personnel through good teamwork with the deployed hospitals and the aeromedical evacuation services. Despite the delay to primary surgical repair compared to civilian practice, there was no statistically significant difference in outcomes, and the efficacy of this approach seems justified in the context of *Operations Telic* and *Herrick*. Whether or not this approach can be extrapolated to contingency operations with extended timelines remains to be seen.

No statistically significant differences were found in the prevalence of mental health problems among ex-servicemen with a combat-related visual impairment compared to those with non-combat-related

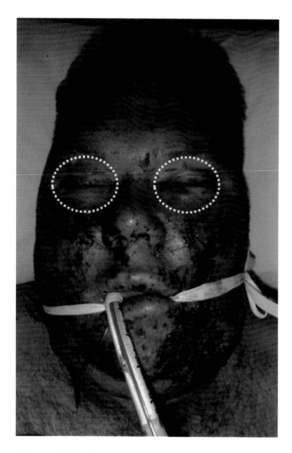

Figure 11.5 Photograph of a soldier who suffered a facial fragmentation injury. The eyes have been well protected by combat eye protection (dotted lines) but suffered a severe primary blast injury. Visual recovery was good, although near vision was reduced due to ciliary muscle atrophy.

impairment.[114] Mental health problems are prevalent among visually impaired younger ex-Service men, irrespective of the cause of their visual impairment (combat vs. non-combat). It is important that the *Defence Medical Services*, as well as the wider family of the affected soldier, are aware that visual impairment has far-reaching consequences and that optimal support must be guaranteed to ensure that such patients can adjust mentally, physically and socially. Special attention needs to be paid to the mental health of all soldiers, and research should be directed towards the best ways of providing support and care to enable the visually impaired person to cope with this traumatic,

often life-changing, event. Mental health issues are described in more detail in Chapter 15.

All facial trauma, regardless of mechanism, has the potential to result in injury to the eyes. In the deployed environment, ophthalmic injuries rarely occur in isolation, whether or not they are attributed to combat.[120] The assessment and initial management of eye injuries usually take place during the secondary survey once life-threatening conditions have been addressed.

The most important aspect is to exclude an occult or subtle globe rupture.[115,120] The clinical history must be as detailed as possible and include an examination of the condition of the eye protection (if any) worn at the time of the injury. Visual acuity must be documented at the earliest opportunity. Whilst a thorough examination of both eyes and surrounding structures is mandatory in order to exclude an open globe injury, it must be recognised that the casualty's ability to cooperate may be limited. Local anaesthetic drops may be instilled to facilitate examination after assessing the visual acuity. If there is any suspicion that an open globe injury has occurred, examination must cease and management be directed to preventing any further deterioration of the injury. Under no circumstances must any pressure be applied to the globe as this increases the risk of extrusion of the ocular contents.

The management of 'minor' closed globe injuries and disease conditions is based on simple clinical protocols, such as irrigation and the use of topical antibiotics. These are covered in Defence Medical Services doctrine and will not be discussed further in this chapter.

The majority of 'significant' open globe injuries sustained during combat are attributed to high-energy explosions and IEDs. Blanch et al.[120] identified 21 open globe injuries in their study, of which 11 had intraocular foreign bodies, 9 were rupture/perforations and 1 was a penetrating injury. Differentiating between rupture and perforation is often difficult in these cases because the eye is often severely disrupted and a mixed injury pattern is present.[120] Unlike the majority of closed globe injuries, open globe injuries need specialist assessment, investigation and surgical intervention as soon as possible.[120] This requires prioritisation for urgent evacuation. In the pre-hospital environment, tetanus prophylaxis and broad-spectrum antibiotics should be administered while the globe is protected from further injury. All foreign bodies must be left in situ and, if necessary, splinted or padded to prevent further penetration but without applying any additional pressure to the surface of the globe. It is also important to keep the casualty calm and recumbent while suppressing any nausea or vomiting. Any increase in pressure from blowing the nose, bending forwards, straining or retching increases the risk of extrusion of the intraocular contents. This is particularly important during transfers and aeromedical evacuation.

Combat eye protection

There is universal agreement that polycarbonate-based combat eye protection or 'ballistic goggles' reduces the incidence and severity of eye injuries.[115,120,131–133] An analysis of data from the Vietnam War demonstrated that if the current standard of eyewear had been issued and worn at the time, 52% of eye injuries would have been prevented.[132] In simple numbers, this equates to around 5000 eye injuries. Enforced wearing of eye protection in US military convoys in 2004 reduced the incidence of eye injuries from around 6% to 0.5%.[25] The impact of this reduction in terms of force heath protection and retained combat effectiveness cannot be overstated.

Combat eye protection was issued to all UK and US personnel in Iraq and Afghanistan, but despite the clear evidence for its effectiveness in mitigating injury, soldiers frequently chose not to wear it.[124] Many reported that the lenses became scratched or misted, which reduced their visual field awareness during dismounted operations. A study of facial trauma from 2005 to 2009 revealed that only a third of UK Service personnel were wearing eye protection at the time of wounding.[63] Most importantly, these soldiers had a 36-fold reduction in eye injuries in association with fewer facial injuries. Combat eye protection could have prevented 7 (7.8%) of the 90 deaths in this cohort of casualties, but if eye protection had comprised a ballistic visor, this may have prevented up to 19 (21.1%) deaths.[63] As discussed previously, combat facial protection is an ongoing high-priority area of research.

The need to wear combat eye protection was actively promoted on *Operation Herrick*, and the reported use gradually increased from about 30% in 2007 to 90% in 2011.[124,132] During the same period, the incidence and severity of eye injuries gradually reduced despite the intensity and pattern of combat operations remaining much the same. Additional concern was highlighted that combat eye protection was not available to Host Nation personnel.[134] A similar reduction in eye injuries was noted once 'ballistic goggles' were issued to the ANSF.

Ocular primary blast injury

Blast injury subtypes are discussed in more detail in Chapter 10. It is universally accepted that secondary blast injuries, caused by fragments of the explosive device or from exogenous debris propelled by the explosion, are the most common mechanism of ocular injury. Tertiary blast injury, caused by displacement of the casualty against solid objects, is responsible for far fewer injuries but still represents an important mechanism, particularly for blunt trauma. Ocular burns, whether chemical or thermal, are a type of quaternary blast injury and can occur in association with other subtypes of blast injury depending on the proximity to the source of the explosion. However, the evidence for primary blast injury affecting the eyes and orbits, caused solely by the blast overpressure, remains controversial (Figure 11.6).

Abbotts et al.[135] conducted a systematic review of the literature and concluded that there was limited evidence to suggest the existence of isolated *ocular primary blast injury*. The study highlighted inconsistencies in the historical literature where cases of suspected primary blast injury were reported with coexistent injuries that were probably caused by secondary blast effects.[136–140] Nevertheless, a wide range of 'peculiar' effects[140] were reported, some of which had no evidence of secondary blast-related injury.[139] For many years, it was believed that if primary blast injury was a genuine phenomenon, it occurred only at overpressures that would cause fatal injury of the lungs in humans.[135] Any pathophysiological changes due to ocular primary blast injury were masked by or, in fact, directly attributed to secondary fragmentation effects. Case

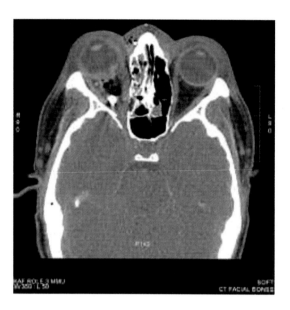

Figure 11.6 Computed tomography scan showing an occult IED fragment at the apex of the right orbit. The patient sustained an apparently trivial facial injury but was immediately and permanently blinded.

reports of convincing ocular primary blast injury continued to emerge,[141,142] and the concept gradually gained acceptance.

As body armour evolved and combat eye protection reduced the fragmentation component, a number of observations and case studies provided support for ocular primary blast injury and its acceptance gradually gathered pace throughout *Operation Herrick*.[115,142,143] Clinical features included *commotio retinae* that rapidly resolved, retinal tears leading to neurosensory detachment, corneal oedema from endothelial disruption, hypaema from damage to the iris, recession of the irido-corneal angle, post-traumatic anterior uveitis and orbital floor blowout fractures.[115,120,143] Retinal injury in any form is a potential cause of profound and intractable visual loss, and a number of animal models have been developed to enable research.[144]

A 'quinary blast injury pattern' has been described as a hyper-inflammatory state, unrelated to the complexity of injuries that manifests as hyperpyrexia, hyper-hydrosis, low central venous pressure and positive fluid balance.[145] This deranged inflammatory response may cause

or exacerbate the primary ocular event following blast overpressure injuries.[146-148]

Rossi et al.[149,150] used a finite element model of the eye to simulate the propagation of blast waves through the orbit. The model suggests that even relatively small explosive events can generate pressures in the retina, choroid and optic nerve that are likely to cause significant pathological damage. The model also demonstrated two distinct patterns of blast wave behaviour. Anterior structures outside of the bony orbit, such as the cornea and vitreous base, quickly reached a peak overpressure that decayed rapidly, as might be expected. However, posterior structures within the bony orbit reached much higher pressures and the blast wave itself appeared to oscillate within the pyramidal geometry of the orbit. This effect, first reported in 1945,[139,151] generates stress waves in the orbital soft tissues that are sufficient to cause ocular primary blast injury. It is interesting to note that blast yields significantly different pressures within the orbit depending on its incident angle. In order to achieve maximum pressure at the orbital apex, the blast wave must travel exactly along the orbital axis to converge at the apex as a result of the ideal reflection path. This was postulated in 1947[152] but never tested further despite being accepted as a theoretical possibility.[153]

Future research

There are a number of disorders of the ocular surface, including persistent epithelial defects of the cornea, acute chemical burns with long-term loss of integrity of the ocular surface epithelium and conjunctival scarring from mucous membrane disorders, that still pose a clinical challenge in ophthalmic surgery.[115,154] The cornea is the most important part of the ocular surface, providing two thirds of the focusing power and maintaining clear and useful vision due to its transparent and avascular nature.[155] Amniotic membrane, or amnion, consists of a thick basement membrane and an avascular stromal matrix. Meller et al.[154,156] demonstrated that amniotic membrane transplantation is effective in promoting corneal epithelialisation and reducing inflammation, thus preventing later scarring complications. In mild to moderate chemical or thermal burns, the authors found that amniotic membrane transplantation alone rapidly restored both the corneal and conjunctival surfaces.[156] In severe burns, amniotic membrane transplantation allowed restoration of the ocular surface without debilitating symblepharon and reduced limbal stromal inflammation but did not prevent limbal stem cell deficiency.[156] Nevertheless, these findings support the importance of intervention at the earliest possible stage for eyes with a severely damaged ocular surface.[120] The goal of ongoing research is to augment the effects of dry-preserved amniotic membrane for use as an immediate field dressing for ocular burns sustained in the deployed environment.[115]

As our understanding of ocular pathophysiology advances,[147] it is clear that combat-related eye injuries are not limited to the obvious physical manifestations of ballistic trauma to the orbits and middle third of the face. Further research is ongoing to develop models of ocular blast injury in order to measure the blunt trauma forces transmitted to the eye and optic nerve following exposure to blast overpressures.[157–165] It is hoped that neuroprotective interventions may be developed that might prevent or mitigate traumatic optic neuropathy and retinal injuries. For soldiers blinded during combat operations, current research is also looking at sensory substitution devices to allow the user to regain a representation of the World around them.

In a military context, primary blast alone can produce clinically relevant damage.[166] A review of the JTTR database identified two cases of orbital wall fractures with no damage to the globe that were highly suggestive of occult ocular primary blast injury.[167] The incidence of combat-related blast pathology is likely to be much higher than suggested by the literature. Combat eye protection, whether in its current form or integrated into a future combat helmet design as a visor, will reduce the incidence of penetrating fragment injuries but will offer little in the way of protection against ocular primary blast injury or the use of novel weapons, such as lasers, in future conflicts.[142,168] These facts must be considered in future personal armour development.

However, based on the current liability, it is unlikely that UK military ophthalmologists will be deployed on future contingency operations. The appropriate management of ocular trauma, as with many other aspects of head, face and neck trauma, will rely on non-specialist surgeons with additional pre-deployment training. The use of ultrasound to assess the eyes has been described in a deployed environment,[169] and it is an effective tool in the hands of a trained practitioner.[170] For many years, the technique found limited acceptance in the United Kingdom, despite studies showing its value in the diagnosis of globe rupture, vitreous haemorrhage, retinal detachments, retrobulbar haemorrhages[171] and raised intracranial pressure.[172,173] This reluctance is, in part, due to concern that pressure on an open globe injury may cause further damage.[169] However, no pressure is applied if an ultrasonically visible layer of gel is present between the probe and eyelid.[169] Further work is needed to establish if ultrasound can be used as an effective triage tool by deployed radiographers or other non-specialists in the absence of military radiologists and ophthalmologists. Further research is needed to establish outcomes in order to stratify the risk of injury for future conflicts once patients are evacuated for definitive care.[174]

OTOLOGIC TRAUMA

Noise-induced hearing loss

The UK Armed Forces *hearing conservation programme* was last updated in 2009.[175] UK personnel should have routine pure tone audiogram testing yearly as well as six months either side of a deployment.[176] The UK Armed Forces hearing grading system is given in Table 11.2. If an audiogram is found to be significantly impaired (H3), the functional loss may impact on role-specific responsibilities. Immediate restriction of duties may be imposed to prevent further noise exposure until full occupational and medical assessments have been carried out. A hearing grading of H4 in either ear has very significant career implications. All UK Armed Forces personnel are referred to an otolaryngologist for detailed hearing assessment when graded as H3 or H4. If H4 grading is confirmed, the soldier is unlikely to be unable to deploy abroad for the rest of his military career and will have significant restrictions to duties in the United Kingdom. In severe cases, this results in a medical discharge from the UK military.[176]

Table 11.2 Hearing standards

Grades	Sum of hearing level at low frequencies in dB	Sum of hearing level at high frequencies in dB	General description
1	Not more than 45. (RN only; No single level to be more than 20 dB)	Not more than 45. (RN only: Level not to be more than 30 dB at 6 kHz or 20 dB at any other frequency)	Good hearing.
2	Not more than 84	Not more than 123	Acceptable hearing.
3	Not more than 150	Not more than 210	Impaired hearing.
4	More than 150	More than 210	Poor hearing where continuing employment is subject to specialist assessment.
8	More than 150	More than 210	Poor hearing that has been assessed as being incompatible with continued service.

Noise-induced hearing loss (NIHL) is a well-recognised health problem in the UK Armed Forces. According to Defence statistics,[177,178] more than 300 regular Armed Forces personnel were medically discharged between 2008 and 2013 with a principal or contributing condition of hearing loss. At the same time, 3530 personnel were recorded as having impaired hearing (H3) and a further 630 personnel recorded as having poor hearing (H4), of which 470 (1.3%) and 90 (1.4%), respectively, were attributed to NIHL. This represents a significant health burden to the UK Armed Forces but also has personal, psychological, social and wider economic implications.[179-181] In the United Kingdom, hearing protection is enshrined in law as the *Control of Noise at Work Regulations 2005*.[182] The *Regulations* define an 'upper exposure action value' as a C-weighted peak sound pressure of 137 dB, a level that is exceeded by virtually all modern weapon systems and the soundscape inherent to the combat environment.[183,184] Employers are required to reduce the risk of hearing loss by limiting noise exposure where possible and taking steps that are 'reasonably practicable' to mitigate injury if the upper exposure thresholds are likely to be violated. At the same time, employees have an obligation to make use of any noise-control measures provided by their employer. The Ministry of Defence has complied with these Regulations by providing *Personal Hearing Protection* (PHP) systems and mandating their use in both training and combat operations.[176]

Combat hearing protection

During *Operation Herrick*, UK Service personnel had access to several PHP systems. All personnel were issued with basic soft polymer foam earplugs (E-A-R™ Classic, 3M™, Loughborough, Leics) and had access to a number of passive over-the-ear defenders during training exercises. In addition, personnel were issued with earplugs that could be reversed to provide protection during active and passive phases of combat operations (Dual-Ended Combat Arms™ Earplugs, 3M™, Loughborough, Leics) or hear-through earplugs with a switchable acoustic filter that did not require removal and re-insertion (Combat Arms™ Earplug, 3M™, Loughborough, Leics). The hear-through variant allowed soldiers to maintain greater situational awareness until weapons discharge occurred, at which point the rocker switch could be toggled to increase protection. Although the mechanism was simple, manually switching to greater hearing protection is cumbersome and potentially perilous when closing with enemy combatants. Many soldiers perceive the loss of situational awareness that results from wearing earplugs in the 'closed' combat state as equally perilous. As a result, the phrase 'better deaf than dead' was in common parlance among UK Service personnel.[185,186]

By the end of 2008, an urgent operational requirement had been sent to *Defence Equipment and Support* to provide a hearing system for dismounted personnel that could be worn comfortably through combat operations with minimal loss of general situational awareness while providing protection against the 'impulse noise' of blast waves or live weapons firing.[187] After rigorous testing of five systems, the Frontier1000® in-the-ear headset (Esterline Racal Acoustics, Bellevue, WA, USA) was issued to deployed personnel in 2009. This was a lightweight, rugged headset with custom-molded silicone earplugs that attached to the *personal role radio* via a talk-through switchbox. It was introduced as the *Personal Interfaced Hearing Protection* (PIHP) system.[187]

The introduction of PIHP represented an important step towards reducing the significant morbidity associated with NIHL in a combat environment with a significant threat of 'impulse noise'. However, compliance with wearing the system was initially poor.[187] PIHP was introduced to soldiers who had not undergone pre-deployment training with the system. They were unfamiliar with its use in a combat environment and, as with previously issued hearing protection systems, defaulted to an equipment state that did not reduce their combat effectiveness at the expense of increasing a perceived risk to their lives or those of their colleagues. This has been demonstrated in previous studies. Despite health promotion efforts, compliance with wearing any form of PHP remained poor in a later study.[185] The authors concluded that health promotion itself does not encourage soldiers to comply with mandatory wearing of PHP and that key to eliminating NIHL must be a greater understanding of the reasons for their choice to wear it or not.

Future research

Further research is needed to design an integrated and interoperable system for combat hearing protection that is operationally effective in the combat environment and does not reduce situational awareness. Only then can we mandate that soldiers use personal protective equipment in compliance with UK Health and Safety legislation.

The detrimental effects of noise have been well established.[188] Acoustic overexposure results in hearing loss that causes a *transient threshold shift* (TTS). The reduction in hearing sensitivity recovers after a couple of days.[189] It is generally accepted that TTS does not result from damage to the cochlear hair cells but rather a transient swelling of the nerve terminals.[190-192] The underlying assumption has been that TTS is a benign process because no residual anatomical deficit remains once the swelling resolves.[188] However, in some cases, there is no recovery of the hearing loss and a *permanent threshold shift* (PTS) occurs.[193] It has been suggested that noise damage is cumulative and that repeated exposure to 'impulse noises' sufficient to cause TTS eventually progresses to PTS. In other words, there is progressive damage to the cochlear neurons or mechanosensory hair bundles that eventually becomes irreversible.[194] For many years, this remained the prevailing opinion and it was accepted that acoustic overexposure caused progressive damage to the hair cells and that cochlear neuronal death occurred once they degenerated.[195] However, in 2009, Kujawa and Liberman[196] published a seminal paper in which they were able to demonstrate a post-exposure permanent loss of cochlear neurons in high-frequency regions despite full recovery of the hair cells and return of the TTS to pre-exposure levels. Their findings, referred to as 'cochlear synaptopathy', have been reproduced in a number of subsequent animal studies.[197-199] A detailed discussion of this emerging concept is beyond the scope of this chapter. However, recent studies have identified the fact that the ribbon synapses between spiral ganglion cells and cochlear hair cells, particularly the inner hair cells, are the likely focus for cochlear synaptopathy.[200] The exact mechanism remains elusive, but it appears that there may be deficits in the temporal coding of sound.[201-203] Some authors have referred to the process as 'noise-induced hidden hearing loss' (NIHHL).[204] The hearing loss is 'hidden' because the loss of the spiral ganglion cells takes months or years to occur, and as a result of full recovery of the hair cells, pure tone audiograms may be normal despite a significant underlying injury.[203-205]

Normal hearing is a complex process, and easy communication relies on extracting key features from audible sounds, not on sound detection.[181,206] Many people report difficulty where there are competing sound sources, but the reasons are still debated. Ruggles et al.[206] have demonstrated that people with clinically normal thresholds can have marked individual differences during a task, requiring them to focus on one speech stream when there are similar, competing speech streams coming from other directions. This may be, in part at least, due to 'cochlear synaptopathy' and represents part of a spectrum of disease including hyperacusis and tinnitus.[207–209]

Our understanding of NIHL has taken a significant leap forward over the last decade. The science is still controversial but is gradually becoming accepted as part of the pathophysiology of primary blast injury. Natural presbyacusis is likely to result in further deterioration of any combat-related hearing loss.[210] This will inevitably have a substantial impact on future health protection in both civilian and military workplaces and result in claims for compensation for many years to come. The Ministry of Defence, in conjunction with National Health Service England, has stated that it is committed to preventing hearing loss attributed to military duties but needs to clearly define the scope of the problem in order to investigate and prevent future hearing loss. While the design of operationally effective hearing protection systems is critical, these can be truly preventative only if they mitigate the entire spectrum of NIHL and NIHHL. A key research objective is the development of a remote, unobtrusive system that allows real-time monitoring of hearing during combat operations in such a way that health protection personnel can detect the earliest possible signs of hearing damage. Within the operational environment, this can be relayed to commanders so that actions can be taken to minimise further exposure to those most affected. The same system can then be used to monitor recovery and ensure that the combat effectiveness of deployed personnel is preserved.

CONCLUSION

During *Operations Telic* and *Herrick*, the head and neck have been the focus of substantial and diverse research efforts targeting everything from 'left of bang' concepts to unravelling the complex pathophysiology of blast overpressures in traumatic brain injury, optic neuropathy and 'hidden' hearing loss. It has been a stimulating period for those involved in military research despite limited funding. Our evolving knowledge base has led to enhancements in every aspect of personal protective equipment for the head and neck and numerous refinements in the management of combat-related head and neck trauma. Much of this research is ongoing and will continue to influence doctrine for contingency operations for many years to come.

Surgeons have always been integral to the care of combat casualties with head and neck trauma. Yet, increasing specialisation and loss of scope of 'general' surgery implies the need for an increasing number of deployable specialists to maintain the standards of care for wounded soldiers. Each of these specialties has skill sets specific to their civilian practice that complement those of other specialties, especially with regard to the head, face and neck. Expecting inexperienced surgeons to provide the same standard of care as a fully equipped multidisciplinary head and neck team is naïve. Indeed, such a belief risks placing unnecessary pressure on those surgeons who do deploy to forward locations if their actions are criticised with the benefit of hindsight. And yet, there exists a cadre of UK military 'head and neck' surgeons, whether they come from the domain of oral and maxillofacial surgery, otorhinolaryngology, plastic and reconstructive surgery or neurosurgery, who have the knowledge, understanding, experience and aptitude to look beyond the issues that have arisen as a result of surgical sub-specialisation and ensure that our wounded soldiers receive the care that they need on the battlefield. Resolving some of these human factors will guarantee that the DMS can continue to enhance and support combat operations in the future.

The DMS has learned a number of lessons in the last decade. However, the contingency battlespaces of the future are unlikely to be directly comparable to those of Iraq and Afghanistan, and while every lesson learned is knowledge gained, that knowledge must be applied in the context of the operational environment to ensure the highest standards of care is maintained for our wounded soldiers.

REFERENCES

1. Brewer LA. Baron Dominique Jean Larrey (1766–1842). Father of modern military surgery, innovator, humanist. *J Thorac Cardiovasc Surg* 1986;92:1096–1098.
2. Skandalakis PN, Lainas P, Zoras O et al. "To afford the wounded speedy assistance": Dominique Jean Larrey and Napoleon. *World J Surg* 2006;30(8):1392–1399.
3. Larrey DJ. *Memoirs of Military Surgery, Campaigns of the French Armies.* Hall RW (trans.). Baltimore: Joseph Cushing, 1814. Birmingham, AL, Classics of Medicine Library, 1987.
4. Martin NA. Sir Alfred Keogh and Sir Harold Gillies: Their contribution to reconstructive surgery. *J R Army Med Corps* 2006;152(3):136–138.
5. Gillies HD. *Plastic Surgery of the Face.* Oxford: Oxford Medical Publications, 1920.
6. Gillies HD, Millard DR. *The Principles and Art of Plastic Surgery.* London: Little, Brown, 1957.
7. Burns BD, Zuckerman S. *The Wounding Power of Small Bomb and Shell Fragments.* London: British Ministry of Supply, Advisory Council on Scientific Research and Technical Development; 1942.
8. Dobson JE, Newell MJ, Shepherd JP. Trends in maxillofacial injuries in wartime (1914–1986). *Br J Oral Maxillofac Surg* 1989;27(6):441–450.
9. Breeze J, Gibbons A, Shief C et al. Combat-related craniofacial and cervical injuries: Five year review from the British Military. *J Trauma* 2011;71(1):108–113.
10. Breeze J, Bryant D. Current concepts in the epidemiology and management of battlefield head, face and neck trauma. *J R Army Med Corps* 2009;155(4):274–278.
11. Chan RK, Siller-Jackson A, Verrett AJ et al. Ten years of war: A characterization of craniomaxillofacial injuries incurred during operations Enduring Freedom and Iraqi Freedom. *J Trauma Acute Care Surg* 2012;73(6):S453–S458.
12. Lew TA, Walker JA, Wenke JC et al. Characterization of craniomaxillofacial battle injuries sustained by United States service members in the current conflicts of Iraq and Afghanistan. *J Oral Maxillofac Surg* 2010;68(1):3–7.
13. Owens BD, Kragh JF Jr, Wenke JC et al. Combat wounds in operation Iraqi Freedom and operation Enduring Freedom. *J Trauma* 2008;64(2):295–299.
14. Wade AL, Dye JL, Mohrle CR, Galarneau MR. Head, face, and neck injuries during Operation Iraqi Freedom II: Results from the US Navy–Marine Corps Combat Trauma Registry. *J Trauma* 2007;63:836–840.
15. Xydakis MS, Fravell MD, Casler JD. Analysis of battlefield head and neck injuries in Iraq and Afghanistan. *Otolarynolg Head Neck Surg* 2005;133(4):497–504.
16. Bilski T, Baker B, Grove JR et al. Battlefield casualties treated at Camp Rhino, Afghanistan: Lessons learned. *J Trauma* 2003;54(5):814–821.
17. Belmont Jr PJ, Goodman GP, Zacchilli M et al. Incidence and epidemiology of combat injuries sustained during "the surge" portion of operation Iraqi Freedom by a US Army brigade combat team. *J Trauma Acute Care Surg* 2010;68(1):204–210.
18. Hœncamp R, Vermetten E, Tan EC et al. Systematic review of the prevalence and characteristics of battle casualties from NATO coalition forces in Iraq and Afghanistan. *Injury* 2014;45(7):1028–1034.
19. Wordsworth M, Thomas R, Breeze J et al. The surgical management of facial trauma in British soldiers during combat operations in Afghanistan. *Injury* 2017;48(1):70–74.
20. Breeze J, Allanson-Bailey LS, Hepper AE, Midwinter MJ. Demonstrating the effectiveness of body armour: A pilot prospective computerised surface wound mapping trial performed at the Role 3 hospital in Afghanistan. *J R Army Med Corps* 2015;161(1):36–41.
21. Penn-Barwell JG, Roberts SA, Midwinter MJ, Bishop JR. Improved survival in UK combat casualties from Iraq and Afghanistan: 2003–2012. *J Trauma Acute Care Surg* 2015;78(5):1014–1020.
22. Paquette EL. Genitourinary trauma at a combat support hospital during Operation

Iraqi Freedom: The impact of body armor. *J Urol* 2007;177(6):2196–2199.

23. Zouris JM, Walker GJ, Dye J, Galarneau M. Wounding patterns for US Marines and sailors during Operation Iraqi Freedom, major combat phase. *Mil Med* 2006;171(3):246–252.

24. Rustemeyer J, Kranz V, Bremerich A. Injuries in combat from 1982–2005 with particular reference to those to the head and neck: A review. *Br J Oral Maxillofac Surg* 2007; 45(7):556–560.

25. Gondusky JS, Reiter MP. Protecting military convoys in Iraq: An examination of battle injuries sustained by a mechanized battalion during Operation Iraqi Freedom II. *Mil Med* 2005;170(6):546–549.

26. Kosashvili Y, Hiss J, Davidovic N et al. Influence of personal armor on distribution of entry wounds: Lessons learned from urban-setting warfare fatalities. *J Trauma* 2005;58(6):1236–1240.

27. Mabry RL, Holcomb JB, Baker AM et al. United States Army Rangers in Somalia: An analysis of combat casualties on an urban battlefield. *J Trauma* 2000;49(3): 515–528.

28. Tong D, Beirne R. Combat body armor and injuries to the head, face, and neck region: A systematic review. *Mil Med* 2013;178(4):421–426.

29. Petersen K, Hayes DK, Blice JP, Hale RG. Prevention and management of infections associated with combat-related head and neck injuries. *J Trauma Acute Care Surg* 2008;64(3):S265–S276.

30. *International Classification of Diseases, Ninth Revision with Clinical Modification (ICD-9-CM)*. Geneva: World Health Organization, 2008.

31. Ministry of Defence. *Types of Injuries Sustained by UK Service Personnel on Op HERRICK in Afghanistan, 1 April 2006 to 30 November 2014*. Camberley, UK: Crown, 2016.

32. Brennan J. Head and neck trauma in Iraq and Afghanistan: Different war, different surgery, lessons learned. *Laryngoscope* 2013;123(10):2411–2417.

33. Feldt BA, Salinas NL, Rasmussen TE, Brennan J. The joint facial and invasive neck trauma (J-FAINT) project, Iraq and Afghanistan 2003–2011. *Otolaryngol Head Neck Surg* 2013;148(3):403–408.

34. Pannell D, Brisebois R, Talbot M et al. Causes of death in Canadian Forces members deployed to Afghanistan and implications on tactical combat casualty care provision. *J Trauma Acute Care Surg* 2011;71(5):S401–S407.

35. Kelly JF, Ritenour AE, McLaughlin DF et al. Injury severity and causes of death from Operation Iraqi Freedom and Operation Enduring Freedom: 2003–2004 versus 2006. *J Trauma Acute Care Surg* 2008;64(2):S21–S27.

36. Champion HR, Bellamy RF, Roberts CP, Leppaniemi A. A profile of combat injury. *J Trauma Acute Care Surg* 2003;54(5): S13–S19.

37. Hodgetts TJ, Mahoney PF, Kirkman E. Damage control resuscitation. *J R Army Med Corps* 2007;153(4):299–300.

38. Hodgetts TJ, Mahoney PF, Russell MQ, Byers M. ABC to <C>ABC: Redefining the military trauma paradigm. *Emerg Med J* 2006;23(10):745–746.

39. Lamb CM, MacGoey P, Navarro AP, Brooks AJ. Damage control surgery in the era of damage control resuscitation. *Br J Anaesth* 2014;113(2):242–249.

40. Tong DC, Breeze J. Damage control surgery and combat-related maxillofacial and cervical injuries: A systematic review. *Br J Oral Maxillofac Surg* 2016;54(1):8–12.

41. Blackbourne LH, Baer DG, Eastridge BJ et al. Military medical revolution: Prehospital combat casualty care. *J Trauma Acute Care Surg* 2012;73(6):S372–S377.

42. McLeod J, Hodgetts T, Mahoney P. Combat "Category A" calls: Evaluating the pre-hospital timelines in a military trauma system. *J R Army Med Corps* 2007;153(4):266–268.

43. Davis P, Rickards A, Ollerton J. Determining the composition and benefit of the pre-hospital medical response team in the conflict setting. *J R Army Med Corps* 2007;153(4):269–273.

44. Calderbank P, Woolley T, Mercer S et al. Doctor on board? What is the optimal skill-mix in military pre-hospital care? *Emerg Med J* 2011;28:882–883.

45. Morrison JJ, Oh J, DuBose JJ et al. En-route care capability from point of injury impacts mortality after severe wartime injury. *Ann Surg* 2013;257(2): 330–334.

46. Graham RN. Battlefield radiology. *Br J Radiol* 2012;85(1020):1556–1565.

47. Gay DA, Miles R. Use of imaging in trauma decision-making. *J R Army Med Corps* 2011;157(Suppl 3):S289–S292.

48. Nolan T, Phan H, Hardy AH et al. Bullet embolization: Multidisciplinary approach by interventional radiology and surgery. *Semin Intervent Radiol* 2012;29(3):192–196.

49. Davies EM, Boylan M, Hawker JJ, Banerjee B. Don't forget the fragment! An unusual case of occult fragment embolization following penetrating neck injury. *J R Army Med Corps* 2011;157(3):396–398.

50. Aidinian G, Fox CJ, Rasmussen TE, Gillespie DL. Varied presentations of missile emboli in military combat. *J Vasc Surg* 2010;51(1):214–217.

51. Lowden C. *Left of the Bang*. New York: HarperCollins, 2015.

52. Van Horne P, Riley JA. *Left of Bang: How the Marine Corps' Combat Hunter Program Can Save Your Life*. New York: Black Irish Books, 2014.

53. Eisenstein NM, Naumann DN, Bowley DM, Midwinter MJ. Pretrauma interventions in Force Health Protection: Introducing the "Left of Bang" Paradigm. *J Spec Oper Med* 2016;16(4):59–63.

54. Parliamentary Office of Science and Technology. *The Dual-Use Dilemma*. London: Parliamentary Office of Science and Technology, 2009.

55. Selgelid MJ. Governance of dual-use research: An ethical dilemma. *Bull World Health Organ* 2009;87(9):720–723.

56. Miller S, Selgelid MJ. Ethical and philosophical consideration of the dual-use dilemma in the biological sciences. *Sci Eng Ethics* 2007;13(4):523–580.

57. Manners JL, Forsten RD, Kotwal RS et al. Role of pre-morbid factors and exposure to blast mild traumatic brain injury on post-traumatic stress in United States military personnel. *J Neurotrauma* 2016;33(19):1796–1801.

58. Rona RJ, Jones M, Fear NT et al. Mild traumatic brain injury in UK military personnel returning from Afghanistan and Iraq: Cohort and cross-sectional analyses. *J Head Trauma Rehab* 2012;27(1):33–44.

59. Jones N, Fear NT, Rona R et al. Mild traumatic brain injury (mTBI) among UK military personnel whilst deployed in Afghanistan in 2011. *Brain Inj* 2014;28(7):896–899.

60. Terrio H, Brenner LA, Ivins BJ et al. Traumatic brain injury screening: Preliminary findings in a US Army Brigade Combat Team. *J Head Trauma Rehab* 2009;24(1):14–23.

61. Hoge CW, McGurk D, Thomas JL et al. Mild traumatic brain injury in US soldiers returning from Iraq. *New Eng J Med* 2008;358(5):453–463.

62. Breeze J. Editorial: Saving faces: The UK future facial protection programme. *J R Army Med Corps* 2012;158(4):284–287.

63. Breeze J, Allanson-Bailey LS, Hunt NC et al. Surface wound mapping of battlefield occulo-facial injury. *Injury* 2012;43(11):1856–1860.

64. Masel BE, DeWitt DS. Traumatic brain injury: A disease process, not an event. *J Neurotrauma* 2010;27(8):1529–1540.

65. Walker WC, Franke LM, McDonald SD et al. Prevalence of mental health conditions after military blast exposure, their co-occurrence, and their relation to mild traumatic brain injury. *Brain Inj* 2015;29(13–14):1581–1588.

66. Donnell AJ, Kim MS, Silva MA, Vanderploeg RD. Incidence of postconcussion symptoms in psychiatric diagnostic groups, mild traumatic brain injury, and comorbid conditions. *Clin Neuropsychol* 2012;26(7):1092–1101.

67. Fear NT, Jones E, Groom M et al. Symptoms of post-concussional syndrome are non-specifically related to mild traumatic brain injury in UK Armed Forces personnel on return from deployment in

Iraq: An analysis of self-reported data. *Psychological Med* 2009;39(8):1379–1387.

68. Gaetz M. The neurophysiology of brain injury. *Clin Neurophysiol* 2004;115(1):4–18.

69. Nizamutdinov D, Shapiro LA. Overview of traumatic brain injury: An immunological perspective. *Brain Sci* 2017;7(1):11.

70. McKee CA, Lukens JR. Emerging roles for the immune system in traumatic brain injury. *Front Immunol* 2016;7:556.

71. Gyoneva S, Ransohoff RM. Inflammatory reaction after traumatic brain injury: Therapeutic potential of targeting cell–cell communication by chemokines. *Trend Pharmacol Sci* 2015;36(7):471–480.

72. Roberts P (ed.). *The British Military Surgery Pocket Book.* Camberley, UK: Crown, 2004.

73. Bahadur S, McGilloway E, Etherington J. Injury severity at presentation is not associated with long-term vocational outcome in British Military brain injury. *J R Army Med Corps* 2016;162(2):120–124.

74. Roberts SA, Toman E, Belli A, Midwinter MJ. Decompressive craniectomy and cranioplasty: Experience and outcomes in deployed UK military personnel. *Br J Neurosurg* 2016;30(5):529–535.

75. Smith JE, Kehoe A, Harrisson SE et al. Outcome of penetrating intracranial injuries in a military setting. *Injury* 2014;45(5):874–878.

76. Russell RJ, Hodgetts TJ, McLeod J et al. The role of trauma scoring in developing trauma clinical governance in the Defence Medical Services. *Phil Trans R Soc B* 2011;366(1562):171–191.

77. Siccardi D, Cavaliere R, Pau A et al. Penetrating craniocerebral missile injuries in civilians: A retrospective analysis of 314 cases. *Surg Neurol* 1991;35(6):455–460.

78. DuBose JJ, Barmparas G, Inaba K et al. Isolated severe traumatic brain injuries sustained during combat operations: Demographics, mortality outcomes, and lessons to be learned from contrasts to civilian counterparts. *J Trauma Acute Care Surg* 2011;70(1):11–18.

79. Gönül E, Erdoğan E, Taşar M et al. Penetrating orbitocranial gunshot injuries. *Surg Neurol* 2005;63(1):24–31.

80. Eisenburg MF, Christie M, Mathew P. Battlefield neurosurgical care in the current conflict in southern Afghanistan. *Neurosurg Focus* 2010;28(5):E7.1–E7.6.

81. Morrison J, Hunt N, Midwinter M, Jansen JO. Prevalence of torso and head injuries in combat casualties with traumatic lower extremity amputations. *Br J Surg* 2012; 99(3):362–366.

82. Breeze J, Gibbons AJ, Hunt NC et al. Mandibular fractures in British military personnel secondary to blast trauma sustained in Iraq and Afghanistan. *Br J Oral Maxillofac Surg* 2011;49(8):607–611.

83. Breeze J, Gibbons A, Opie N, Monaghan A. Maxillofacial injuries in military personnel treated at the Royal Centre for Defence Medicine. *Br J Oral Maxillofac Surg* 2010;48:613–616.

84. Gibbons AJ, Hodder SC. A self-drilling intermaxillary fixation screw. *Br J Oral Maxillofac Surg* 2003;41(1):48–49.

85. Gibbons AJ, Baden JM, Monaghan AM, Dhariwal DK, Hodder SC. A drill-free bone screw for intermaxillary fixation in military casualties. *J R Army Med Corps* 2003;149(1): 30–32.

86. Sahni V. Maxillofacial trauma scoring systems. *Injury* 2016;47(7):1388–1392.

87. Ahmad Z, Nouraei R, Holmes S. Towards a classification system for complex craniofacial fractures. *Br J Oral Maxillofac Surg* 2012;50(6):490–494.

88. Catapano J, Fialkov JA, Binhammer PA et al. A new system for severity scoring of facial fractures: Development and validation. *J Craniofac Surg* 2010;21(4):1098–1103.

89. Bagheri SC, Dierks EJ, Kademani D et al. Application of a facial injury severity scale in craniomaxillofacial trauma. *J Oral Maxillofac Surg* 2006;64(3):408–414.

90. Zhang J, Zhang Y, El-Maaytah M et al. Maxillofacial Injury Severity Score: Proposal of a new scoring system. *Int J Oral Maxillofac Surg* 2006;35(2):109–114.

91. Chen C, Zhang Y, An JG et al. Comparative study of four maxillofacial trauma scoring systems and expert score. *J Oral Maxillofac Surg* 2014;72(11):2212–2220.

92. Breeze J. Obtaining multinational consensus on future combat face and neck protection – Proceedings of the Revision Military Protection Workshop. *J R Army Med Corps* 2012;158(2):141.

93. Breeze J, Tong DC, Powers D, Martin NA et al. Optimising ballistic facial coverage from military fragmenting munitions: A consensus statement. *Br J Oral Maxillofac Surg* 2017;55(2);173–178.

94. Breeze J. The problems of protecting the neck from combat wounds. *J R Army Med Corps* 2010;156(3):137–138.

95. Breeze J, Leason J, Gibb I et al. Characterisation of explosive fragments injuring the neck. *Br J Oral Maxillofac Surg* 2013;51(8):e263–e266.

96. Bagheri SC, Khan HA, Bell RB. Penetrating neck injuries. *Oral Maxillofac Surg Clin North Am* 2008;20(3):393–414.

97. Oughterson AW, Hull HC, Sutherland FA, Greiner DJ. Study on wound ballistics – Bougainville Campaign. Chapter 5 of Wound Ballistics. http://historyamed darmymil/booksdocs/wwii/woundblstcs /chapter5htm (accessed 10 February 2017).

98. Herget CM, Coe GB, Beyer JC. Wound ballistics and body armour in Korea. Chapter 12 of Wound Ballistics. http://historyamed darmymil/booksdocs/wwii/woundblstcs/ chapter12htm (accessed 10 February 2017).

99. Champion HR, Holcomb JB, Lawnick MM et al. Improved characterization of combat injury. *J Trauma* 2010;68():1139–1150.

100. Gofrit ON, Kovalski N, Leibovici D et al. Accurate anatomical location of war injuries: Analysis of the Lebanon war fatal casualties and the proposition of new principles for the design of military personal armour system. *Injury* 1996;27(8):577–581.

101. Breeze J, Allanson-Bailey LS, Hepper AE, Lewis E. Novel method for comparing coverage by future methods of ballistic facial protection. *Br J Oral Maxillofac Surg* 2015;53(1):3–7.

102. Breeze J, Midwinter MJ. Editorial: Prospective Surface Wound Mapping will optimise future body armour design. *J R Army Med Corps* 2012;158(2):79–81.

103. Breeze J, Allanson-Brown LC, Hunt NC et al. Using computerised surface wound mapping to compare the potential medical effectiveness of enhanced protection under body armour combat shirt collar designs. *J R Army Med Corps* 2015;161(1):22–26.

104. Breeze J, Fryer R, Hare J et al. Clinical and post mortem analysis of combat neck injury to inform a novel Coverage of Armour Tool. *Injury* 2015;46(4):629–633.

105. Breeze J, Midwinter MJ, Pope D et al. Developmental framework to validate future designs of ballistic neck protection. *Br J Oral Maxillofac Surg* 2013;51(1):47–51.

106. Breeze J, Clasper JC. Ergonomic assessment of future methods of ballistic neck protection. *Mil Med* 2013;178(8):899–903.

107. Breeze J, Watson CH, Horsfall I, Clasper J. Comparing the human factors of neck collars in different military body armour systems. *Mil Med* 2011;176(11):1274–1277.

108. Carr DJ, Lewis E, Horsfall I. A systematic review of military head injuries. *J R Army Med Corps* 2016;163(1):13–19.

109. Carey ME. Analysis of wounds incurred by US Army Seventh Corps personnel treated in Corps hospitals during Operation Desert Storm, February 20 to March 10, 1991. *J Trauma* 1991;40(3 Suppl):S165–S169.

110. Sone JY, Kondziolka D, Huang JH, Samadani U. Helmet efficacy against concussion and traumatic brain injury: A review. *J Neurosurg* 2017;126(3):768–781.

111. Breeze J, Baxter D, Carr D et al. Defining combat helmet coverage for protection against explosively propelled fragments. *J R Army Med Corps* 2015;161(1):9–13.

112. Carey ME, Herz M, Corner B et al. Ballistic helmets and aspects of their design. *Neurosurg* 2000;47(3):678–688.

113. Breeze J, Horsfall I, Clasper J. Face, neck, and eye protection: Adapting body armour to counter the changing patterns of battlefield injury. *Br J Oral Maxillofac Surg* 2011;49(8):602–606.

114. Stevelink SAM, Malcolm EM, Gill PC et al. The mental health of UK ex-servicemen with a combat-related or a non-combat-related visual impairment: Does the cause of visual

impairment matter? *Br J Ophthalmol* 2015; 99(8):1103–1108.

115. Scott RAH. The injured eye. *Phil Trans R Soc Lond B Biol Sci* 2011;366(1562):251–260.

116. Gibson A, McKenna M. The effect of high altitude on the visual system. *J R Army Med Corps* 2011;157(1):49–52.

117. Musa F, Tailor R, Gao A et al. Contact lens-related microbial keratitis in deployed British military personnel. *Br J Ophthalmol* 2010;94(8):988–993.

118. Dunbar J, Cooper B, Hodgetts T et al. An outbreak of human external ophthalmomyiasis due to *Oestrus ovis* in southern Afghanistan. *Clin Infect Dis* 2008;46(11):e124–e126.

119. Stacey M, Blanch RJ. A case of external ophthalmomyiasis in a deployed UK soldier. *J R Army Med Corps* 2008;154(1): 60–62.

120. Blanch RJ, Bindra MS, Jacks AS, Scott RAH. Ophthalmic injuries in British Armed Forces in Iraq and Afghanistan. *Eye* 2011;25(2):218–223.

121. Aslam S, Griffiths MF. Eye Casualties during Operation Telic. *J R Army Med Corps* 2005;151(1):34–36.

122. Ollerton JE, Hodgetts TJ. Operational morbidity analysis: Ophthalmic presentations during Operation Telic. *J R Army Med Corps* 2010;156(1):37–40.

123. Mader, TH, Aragones, JV, Chandler, AC et al. Ocular and ocular adnexal injuries treated by United States military ophthalmologists during Operations Desert Shield and Desert Storm. *Ophthalmol* 1993;100(10):1462–1467.

124. Scott RAH, Blanch RJ, Morgan-Warren PJ. Aspects of ocular war injuries. *Trauma* 2014; 17(2):83–89.

125. Kuhn F, Morris R, Witherspoon CD et al. The Birmingham Eye Trauma Terminology system (BETT). *J Fr Ophtalmol* 2004; 27(2):206–210.

126. Kuhn F, Morris R, Witherspoon CD. Birmingham Eye Trauma Terminology (BETT): Terminology and classification of mechanical eye injuries. *Ophthalmol Clin N Am* 2002;15(2):139–143.

127. Kuhn F, Morris R, Witherspoon CD et al. A standardized classification of ocular trauma. *Ophthalmol* 1996;103:240–243.

128. Thach AB, Johnson AJ, Carroll RB et al. Severe eye injuries in the war in Iraq, 2003–2005. *Ophthalmol* 2008;115(2):377–382.

129. Thach AB, Ward TP, Dick JS et al. Intraocular foreign body injuries during Operation Iraqi Freedom. *Ophthalmol* 2005;112(10):1829–1833.

130. Weichel ED, Colyer MH, Ludlow SE et al. Combat ocular trauma visual outcomes during operations Iraqi and Enduring Freedom. *Ophthalmol* 2008; 115(12):2235–2245.

131. Colyer MH, Chun DW, Bower KS et al. Perforating globe injuries during operation Iraqi Freedom. *Ophthalmol* 2008;115(11):2087–2093.

132. Thomas R, McManus JG, Johnson A et al. Ocular injury reduction from ocular protection use in current combat operations. *J Trauma* 2009;66(4 Suppl):S99–S103.

133. Cotter F, La Piana FG. Eye casualty reduction by eye armor. *Mil Med* 1991;156:126–128.

134. Parker P, Mossadegh S, McCrory CA. Comparison of the IED-related eye injury rate in ANSF and ISAF forces at the UK R3 Hospital, Camp Bastion, 2013. *J R Army Med Corps* 2014;160(1):73–74.

135. Abbotts R, Harrisson SE Cooper GJ. Primary blast injuries to the eye: A review of the evidence. *J R Army Med Corps* 2007;153(2):119–123.

136. Jamra FA, Halasa A, Salman S. Letter bomb injuries: A report of three cases. *J Trauma* 1974;14(4):275–279.

137. Mandelcorn MS, Hill JC. Orbital blast injury: A case report. *Can J Ophthalmol* 1973; 8(4):597–600.

138. Quere MA, Bouchat J, Cornand G. Ocular blast injuries. *Am J Ophthalmol* 1969; 67(1):64–69.

139. Bellows JG. Observations on 300 consecutive cases of ocular war injuries. *Am J Ophthalmol* 1947;30(3):309–323.

140. Campbell DR. Ophthalmic casualties resulting from air-raids. *BMJ* 1941;1(4199):966.

141. Beiran I, Miller B. Pure ocular blast injury. *Am J Ophthalmol* 1992;114(4):504–505.

142. Chalioulias K, Sim KT, Scott RA. Retinal sequelae of primary ocular blast injuries. *J R Army Med Corps* 2007;153(2):124–125.

143. Blanch RJ, Scott RA. Primary blast injury of the eye (letter). *J R Army Med Corps* 2008;154(1):76.

144. Blanch RJ, Ahmed Z, Berry M et al. Animal models of retinal injury. *Invest Ophthalmol Vis Sci* 2012;53(6):2913–2920.

145. Kluger Y, Nimrod A, Biderman P et al. The quinary pattern of blast injury. *Am J Disaster Med* 2006;2(1):21–25.

146. Choi JH, Greene WA, Johnson AJ et al. Pathophysiology of blast-induced ocular trauma in rats after repeated exposure to low-level blast overpressure. *Clin Exp Ophthalmol* 2015;43(3):239–246.

147. Scott RA. The science from ocular war injuries. *Acta Ophthalmol* 2014;92(s253).

148. Bricker-Anthony C, Hines-Beard J, D'Surney L, Rex TS. Exacerbation of blast-induced ocular trauma by an immune response. *J Neuroinflammation* 2014;11(1):192; erratum by same authors in *J Neuroinflammation* 2016;13(1):220.

149. Rossi T, Boccassini B, Esposito L et al. Primary blast injury to the eye and orbit: Finite element modeling primary blast injury to the orbit. *Invest Ophthalmol Vis Sci* 2012;53(13):8057–8066.

150. Rossi T, Boccassini B, Esposito L et al. The pathogenesis of retinal damage in blunt eye trauma: Finite element modeling. *Invest Ophthalmol Vis Sci* 2011;52(7): 3994–4002.

151. Wharton-Young M. Mechanics of blast injuries. *War Med* 1945;8:73–81.

152. Rones B Wilder HC. Nonperforating ocular injuries in soldiers. *Am J Ophthalmol* 1947;30(9):1143–1160.

153. Petras JM, Bauman RA, Elsayed NM. Visual system degeneration induced by blast overpressure. *Toxicology* 1997;121(1):41–49.

154. Meller D, Pauklin M, Thomasen H et al. Amniotic membrane transplantation in the human eye. *Dtsch Arztebl Int* 2011;108(14):243–248.

155. Pellegrini G, Traverso CE, Franzi AT et al. Long-term restoration of damaged corneal surfaces with autologous cultivated corneal epithelium. *Lancet* 1997;349(9057):990–993.

156. Meller D, Pires RT, Mack RJ et al. Amniotic membrane transplantation for acute chemical or thermal burns. *Ophthalmol* 2000;107(5):980–989.

157. DeMar J, Sharrow K, Hill M et al. Effects of primary blast overpressure on retina and optic tract in rats. *Front Neurol* 2016;7:59.

158. Bailoor S, Bhardwaj R, Nguyen TD. Effectiveness of eye armor during blast loading. *Biomech Model Mechanobiol* 2015;14(6):1227–1237.

159. Bricker-Anthony C, Rex TS. Neurodegeneration and vision loss after mild blunt trauma in the C57Bl/6 and DBA/2J mouse. *PloS One* 2015;10(7): e0131921.

160. Huempfner-Hierl H, Bohne A, Wollny G et al. Blunt forehead trauma and optic canal involvement: Finite element analysis of anterior skull base and orbit on causes of vision impairment. *Br J Ophthalmol* 2015;99(10):1430–1434.

161. Watson R, Gray W, Sponsel WE et al. Simulations of porcine eye exposure to primary blast insult. *Transl Vis Sci Technol* 2015;4(4):8.

162. Bhardwaj R, Ziegler K, Seo JH et al. A computational model of blast loading on the human eye. *Biomech Model Mechanobiol* 2014;13(1):123–140.

163. Bricker-Anthony C, Hines-Beard J, Rex TS. Molecular changes and vision loss in a mouse model of closed-globe blast trauma: Delayed retinal response to blast. *Invest Ophthalmol Vis Sci* 2014;55(8):4853–4862.

164. Wang HC, Choi JH, Greene WA et al. Pathophysiology of blast-induced ocular trauma with apoptosis in the retina and optic nerve. *Mil Med* 2014;179(8S):34–40.

165. Hines-Beard J, Marchetta J, Gordon S et al. A mouse model of ocular blast injury that induces closed globe anterior and posterior pole damage. *Exp Eye Res* 2012;99:63–70.

166. Sherwood D, Sponsel WE, Lund BJ et al. Anatomical manifestations of primary blast

ocular trauma observed in a postmortem porcine model. *Invest Ophthalmol Vis Sci* 2014;55(2):1124–1132.

167. Breeze J, Opie N, Monaghan A, Gibbons AJ. Isolated orbital wall blowout fractures due to primary blast injury (letter). *J R Army Med Corps* 2009;155(1):70.

168. Aslam SA, Davies WI, Singh MS et al. Cone photoreceptor neuroprotection conferred by CNTF in a novel in vivo model of battlefield retinal laser injury. *Invest Ophthalmol Vis Sci* 2013;54(8):5456–5465.

169. Ritchie JV, Horne ST, Perry J, Gay D. Ultrasound triage of ocular blast injury in the military emergency department. *Mil Med* 2012;177(2):174–178.

170. Blaivas M, Theodoro D, Sierzenski P. A study of bedside ocular ultrasonography in the emergency department. *Acad Emerg Med* 2002;9(8):791–799.

171. Blaivas M. Bedside emergency department ultrasonography in the evaluation of ocular pathology. *Acad Emerg Med* 2000;7(8):947–950.

172. Soldatos T, Chatzimichail K, Papathanasiou M, Gouliamos A. Optic nerve sonography: A new window for the non-invasive evaluation of intracranial pressure in brain injury. *Emerg Med J* 2009;26(9):630–634.

173. Sawyer N: Ultrasound imaging of penetrating ocular trauma. *J Emerg Med* 2009;36(2):181–182.

174. Chaudhary R, Upendran M, Campion N et al. The role of computerised tomography in predicting visual outcome in ocular trauma patients. *Eye* 2015;29(7):867–871.

175. Surgeon General Policy Letter SGPL number 05/2009. Assessing audiograms as part of a hearing conservation programme (HCP) and guidance on deployment of those with reduced audiogram acuity – A guide for medical staff.

176. Biggs T, Everest A. British military hearing conservation programme. *Clin Otolaryngol* 2011;36(3):299–301.

177. Defence Statistics (Health). https://www.gov.uk/government/uploads/system/uploads/attachment_data/file/253355/Public_1381235434_Redacted.pdf (accessed 20 February 2017).

178. Defence Statistics (Health). https://www.gov.uk/government/uploads/system/uploads/attachment_data/file/276357/FOI-hearing-loss-PUBLIC_1390997818.pdf (accessed 20 February 2017).

179. Alamgir H, Turner CA, Wong NJ et al. The impact of hearing impairment and noise-induced hearing injury on quality of life in the active-duty military population: Challenges to the study of this issue. *Mil Med Res* 2016;3(1):11.

180. Yong JS, Wang DY. Impact of noise on hearing in the military. *Mil Med Res* 2015;2(1):6.

181. Hill S. *Action Plan on Hearing Loss.* Joint Publication by NHS England and Department of Health, 2015.

182. The Control of Noise at Work Regulations 2005. Camberley, UK: HM Government, Crown, 2005.

183. Lwow F, Jóźków P, Mędraś M. Occupational exposure to impulse noise associated with shooting. *Int J Occ Saf Ergon* 2011;17(1):69–77.

184. Yikoski ME, Pekkarinen JO, Starck JP et al. Physical characteristics of gunfire impulse noise and its attenuation by hearing protectors. *Scand Audiol* 1995;24(1):3–11.

185. Jones GH, Pearson CR. The use of personal hearing protection in hostile territory and the effect of health promotion activity: Advice falling upon deaf ears. *J R Army Med Corps* 2016;162(4):280–283.

186. Orr L. Personal communication, 2017.

187. Patil M, Breeze J. Use of hearing protection on military operations *J R Army Med Corps* 2011;157(4):381–384.

188. Stamper GC, Johnson TA. Auditory function in normal-hearing, noise-exposed human ears. *Ear Hear* 2015;36(2):172–184.

189. Mills JH, Gengel RW, Watson CS, Miller JD. Temporary changes of the auditory system due to exposure to noise for one or two days. *J Acoust Soc Am* 1970;48(2B):524–530.

190. Wang Y, Hirose K, Liberman MC. Dynamics of noise-induced cellular injury and repair in the mouse cochlea. *J Assoc Res Otolaryngol* 2002;3(3):248–268.

191. Robertson D. Functional significance of dendritic swelling after loud sounds in the guinea pig cochlea. *Hear Res* 1983;9(3): 263–278.

192. Spoendlin H. Primary structural changes in the organ of Corti after acoustic overstimulation. *Acta Otolaryng* 1971;71(2): 166–176.

193. Clark WW. Recent studies of temporary threshold shift (tts) and permanent threshold shift (pts) in animals. *J Acoust Soc Am* 1991;90(1):155–163.

194. Wan G, Corfas G. No longer falling on deaf ears: Mechanisms of degeneration and regeneration of cochlear ribbon synapses. *Hear Res* 2015;329:1–10.

195. Liberman MC, Epstein MJ, Cleveland SS et al. Toward a differential diagnosis of hidden hearing loss in humans. *PloS One* 2016;11(9):e0162726.

196. Kujawa SG, Liberman MC. Adding insult to injury: Cochlear nerve degeneration after "temporary" noise-induced hearing loss. *J Neurosci* 2009;29(45):14077–14085.

197. Furman AC, Kujawa SG, Liberman MC. Noise-induced cochlear neuropathy is selective for fibers with low spontaneous rates. *J Neurophysiol* 2013;110(3):577–586.

198. Maison SF, Usubuchi H, Liberman MC. Efferent feedback minimizes cochlear neuropathy from moderate noise exposure. *J Neurosci* 2013;33(13):5542–5552.

199. Lin HW, Furman AC, Kujawa SG, Liberman MC. Primary neural degeneration in the guinea pig cochlea after reversible noise-induced threshold shift. *J Assoc Res Otolaryngol* 2011;12(5):605–616.

200. Song Q, Shen P, Li X et al. Coding deficits in hidden hearing loss induced by noise: The nature and impacts. *Sci Rep* 2016;6:25200.

201. Shi L, Chang Y, Li X et al. Cochlear synaptopathy and noise-induced hidden hearing loss. *Neural Plast* 2016;2016:6143164.

202. Kujawa SG, Liberman MC. Synaptopathy in the noise-exposed and aging cochlea: Primary neural degeneration in acquired sensorineural hearing loss. *Hear Res* 2015;330:191–199.

203. Moser T, Starr A. Auditory neuropathy – Neural and synaptic mechanisms. *Nat Rev Neurol* 2016;12(3):135–149.

204. Plack CJ, Barker D, Prendergast G. Perceptual consequences of 'hidden' hearing loss. *Trends Hear* 2014;18.

205. Schaette R, McAlpine D. Tinnitus with a normal audiogram: Physiological evidence for hidden hearing loss and computational model. *J Neurosci* 2011;31(38):13452–13457.

206. Ruggles D, Bharadwaj H, Shinn-Cunningham BG. Normal hearing is not enough to guarantee robust encoding of suprathreshold features important in everyday communication. *Proc Nat Acad Sci* 2011;108(37):15516–15521.

207. Hickox AE, Liberman MC. Is noise-induced cochlear neuropathy key to the generation of hyperacusis or tinnitus? *J Neurophysiol* 2014;111(3):552–564.

208. Knipper M, Van Dijk P, Nunes I et al. Advances in the neurobiology of hearing disorders: Recent developments regarding the basis of tinnitus and hyperacusis. *Prog Neurobiol* 2013;111:17–33.

209. Roberts LE, Eggermont JJ, Caspary DM et al. Ringing ears: The neuroscience of tinnitus. *J Neurosci* 2010;30(45):14972–14979.

210. Fernandez KA, Jeffers PW, Lall K et al. Aging after noise exposure: Acceleration of cochlear synaptopathy in "recovered" ears. *J Neurosci* 2015;35(19):7509–7520.

12

Internal medicine and communicable disease including diet and lifestyle

INTRODUCTION

Disease and non-battle injury (DNBI) have been the predominant causes of presentation to deployed medical services throughout military history, and disease represents the greatest challenge to overall operational effectiveness. Examples include the decimation caused by the influenza pandemic of 1918, which killed between 50 and 100 million people and the impact of trench fever on the fighting strength of allied troops during the Great War.[1] Within the medical profession, the Burma campaign of the Second World War is possibly as well known for the impact of malaria and the interventions of General Slim as for the battles that were fought.

While the military will inevitably direct their main attention towards the opposition force and their weapon systems, the challenges presented by the environment cannot be underestimated and the climate and endemic diseases of Iraq and Afghanistan made them hostile places in which to operate. This resulted in the development of a wide range of DNBI conditions that formed the majority of the field hospital workload, in terms of patient numbers, throughout the two campaigns.

At times during both operations, particular attention was paid to nutritional provision while smoking and use of supplements were ongoing health concerns that were explored by physician investigators.

THE SPECIALTY BEFORE *OPERATIONS TELIC* AND *HERRICK*

The workload of the deployed physician is dictated largely by the *population at risk* and factors including the nature of the environment, the climate, the presence of endemic disease and the availability of clean drinking water, good quality nutritional provision and adequate sanitation. The practice of medicine on deployment has largely been reliant on the clinical skills and training of the consultant physician cadre supplemented by limited diagnostic support in the form of basic radiology and simple laboratory services.

Consultant physicians were deployed throughout the Balkans conflicts but had not been an integral element of the medical support to rapid reaction forces such as the Airborne and Commando Brigades, which were largely supported by lightweight forward surgical teams. Deployment of medical assets at the enhanced Role 2 (role 2+) or Role 3 echelons would generally be required before a physician became part of the medical complement.

THE SPECIALTY ON DEPLOYMENT

Operation Telic

Physicians deployed in significant numbers to the two Role 3 medical treatment facilities that deployed into Kuwait in the spring of 2001.

Four physicians were on the strength of each of *33* and of *34 Field Hospitals*. Those who deployed with *33 Field Hospital* contributed to the establishment of the 200-bed Role 3 capability in Kuwait and saw moderate numbers of patients before handing over to *202 (Volunteer) Field Hospital* with a complement of six physicians.

34 Field Hospital moved forward into Iraq, following the initial stages of the ground invasion, and was established as a medical treatment facility (MTF) at Shaiba Logistics Base, near Basra, later moving to Basra Airbase. By July 2001, the fully established hospital at Shaiba was manned medically by a single consultant physician, supported by a junior trainee – a level of manning that was maintained throughout the operation until its end in 2009.

Operation Herrick

A single consultant physician was deployed throughout *Operation Herrick* in Afghanistan. In the latter stages of the operation, a medical registrar was deployed in addition to provide support for the consultant and a training opportunity for the registrar.

WORKLOAD DATA

On *Operation Telic*, 91% of overall admissions to field hospitals were for DNBI.[2] On *Operation Herrick*, detailed data regarding medical admissions were collected for the period April 2011–March 2013. Over this two-year period, there were 1386 admissions under the care of the consultant physician (1.9 per day; 20% of total admissions) covering a wide variety of presentations across the entire spectrum of medical specialties.[3]

This period of time coincided with a particularly kinetic phase of the operation during which battle injury was common. Overall, DNBI made up 71% of admissions to the field hospital at Camp Bastion.[4]

CLINICAL CHALLENGES ON OPERATIONS TELIC AND HERRICK

The main clinical challenges for all physicians on deployment are the breadth of possible clinical presentations (Table 12.1) and the constraints imposed by relatively limited diagnostic support in the form of imaging and laboratory services. As both operations became more established, the introduction of a computed tomography scanning capability and the increasing sophistication of the available laboratory tests improved the range of medical diagnoses that could be definitively made or, equally importantly, ruled out.

The predominant clinical challenges during *Operation Telic* were predictable, and expectations were borne out in the first 12 months during which 3044 patients were admitted under the care of physicians, representing 62.5% of the total workload. Of these, 50% were admitted with gastroenteritis and 25% with heat illness, predominantly between May and September.[5] Both of these presentations could be predicted from recent history at Bagram Airbase[6] (where there had been an outbreak of acute gastroenteritis due to Norwalk-like viruses among military personnel) and from knowledge of the climate, the environment and the nature of the living conditions – hastily erected camps with rudimentary hygiene facilities.

Prior to this structured 12-month data collection period, an outbreak of gastroenteritis had occurred at Shaibah in April 2003 involving several hundred cases, including over 100 cases on a single day. Outbreaks of a lesser scale occurred in subsequent years – usually coincident with *relief in place* time periods, when newly arrived units replaced units already in theatre before they returned to the United Kingdom.[7,8]

Throughout the remainder of *Operation Telic*, infectious gastroenteritis continued to be the main clinical challenge for physicians – remaining at 50% of the overall numbers treated, while robust acclimatisation processes limited the ongoing number of heat illness casualties,[2] which had been the focus of specific intervention early in the campaign.[9] One innovation was the establishment of a separate area within the emergency department, with its own entrance, used for the treatment of gastroenteritis patients. This prevented gastroenteritis patients mixing with other patients in the waiting room and treatment areas, as well as providing extra departmental capacity. Following assessment, patients could then be transferred to a dedicated ward without passing through the emergency department.

Table 12.1 Summary of the discharge diagnoses occurring on three or more occasions and by patient group

Ranking by frequency	British military patients Total discharge diagnoses (n = 716) Different discharge diagnoses (n = 179)		Non-UK military patients Total discharge diagnoses (n = 627) Different discharge diagnoses (n = 178)		Civilians only Total discharge diagnoses (n = 319) Different discharge diagnoses (n = 124)	
	Discharge diagnosis	n (%)	Discharge diagnosis	n (%)	Discharge diagnosis	n (%)
1	Infectious diarrhoea	138 (19.3)	Infectious diarrhoea	64 (10.2)	LRTI	41 (12.9)
2	Heat Illness	44 (6.1)	Epilepsy (inc status epilepticus)	25 (4.0)	Infectious diarrhoea	16 (5.0)
3	Volume depletion	33 (4.6)	Volume depletion	16 (2.6)	Myocardial infarction or angina	15 (4.4)
4	Acute stress reaction	23 (3.2)	Myocardial infarction or angina	16 (2.6)	Epilepsy	11 (3.4)
5	Cellulitis	20 (2.8)	Envenomation	15 (2.4)	Peptic ulcer disease and related	10 (3.1)
6	Migraine	13 (1.8)	Heat illness	14 (2.2)	Essential (primary) hypertension	8 (2.5)
7	Acute tonsillitis	9 (1.3)	LRTI	13 (2.1)	Stroke or TIA	8 (2.5)
8	LRTI	9 (1.3)	Peptic ulcer disease and related	13 (2.1)	Arrhythmia	7 (2.2)
9	Peptic ulcer disease and related	8 (1.1)	Acute stress reaction	11 (1.8)	COPD	7 (2.2)
10	Arrhythmia	7 (1.0)	Cellulitis	11 (1.8)	Calculus of kidney and ureter	6 (1.9)
11	Q fever	6 (0.8)	Migraine	10 (1.61)	Cellulitis	6 (1.9)
12	Epilepsy	6 (0.8)	Arrhythmia	10 (1.61)	Diabetes	5 (1.6)

(Continued)

Table 12.1 (Continued) Summary of the discharge diagnoses occurring on three or more occasions and by patient group

Ranking by frequency	British military patients		Non-UK military patients		Civilians only	
	Total discharge diagnoses (n = 716) Different discharge diagnoses (n = 179)		Total discharge diagnoses (n = 627) Different discharge diagnoses (n = 178)		Total discharge diagnoses (n = 319) Different discharge diagnoses (n = 124)	
	Discharge diagnosis	n (%)	Discharge diagnosis	n (%)	Discharge diagnosis	n (%)
13	Inflammatory bowel disease	6 (0.8)	Acute tonsillitis	7 (1.1)	Migraine	5 (1.6)
14	Urticarial rash	5 (0.7)	Acute pericarditis	6 (1.0)	Asthma and status asthmaticus	4 (1.3)
15	Myocardial infarction or angina	4 (0.6)	Stroke	6 (1.0)	Pulmonary embolism	4 (1.3)
16	Acute renal failure	4 (0.6)	Asthma and status asthmaticus	6 (1.0)	Acute stress reaction	3 (0.9)
17	Dental abscess	4 (0.6)	Pleural effusion	6 (1.0)	Tuberculosis	3 (0.9)
18	Infectious mononucleosis	4 (0.6)	Unspecified septicaemia	5 (0.8)	Typhoid and paratyphoid fevers	3 (0.9)
19	Stroke and TIA	4 (0.6)	Unspecified acute hepatitis	5 (0.8)	–	–
20	Pulmonary embolism	3 (0.4)	Malaria	5 (0.8)	–	–
21	Acute pericarditis	3 (0.4)	Acute renal failure	4 (0.6)	–	–
22	Asthma	3 (0.4)	Tuberculosis	3 (0.5)	–	–
23	–	–	Pulmonary embolism	3 (0.5)	–	–

Source: Cox AT et al., *J R Army Med Corps* 2016;162(1):18–22.
Note: COPD, chronic obstructive pulmonary disease; LRTI, lower respiratory tract infection; TIA, transient ischaemic attack.

During the insertion phase of the operation, individuals who had deployed into theatre with chronic disease presented a significant challenge.[11] This represented a failure of surveillance borne out of rapid deployment, which improved as *force generation* procedures matured over time.[10]

Operation Herrick presented the same predictable clinical challenges, with infectious diarrhoea and heat illness again topping the list of presentations admitted under physicians, albeit in lower proportions and balanced by a wide range of other conditions managed both at Role 3 and Role 4.[2,3,12]

An unusual cluster of cases of *undifferentiated febrile illness* cases – which became collectively known as *Helmand Fever* – was first noted in Afghanistan in 2006. Whilst not entirely unpredictable given the history of similar presentations during prior campaigns, this presented a considerable diagnostic and management challenge to the deployed physicians, and one with a wide differential diagnosis. A fever study comprising 26 cases, conducted in 2008, identified *sandfly fever, rickettsial infections* and, importantly, *Q fever* as the likely diagnoses. Q fever was responsible for six cases (26%), and given the potential long-term consequences of this infection, these findings led to new treatment protocols, including amended antibiotic regimes.[13]

Cutaneous leishmaniasis (CL), usually presenting as non-healing lesions on exposed skin following transmission by sandfly bite, has long been a threat to military personnel in a number of locations, particularly Belize (Figure 12.1). Almost half of the UK cases of CL in the last decade were in military personnel.[14] CL is endemic in Iraq, and a number of cases were seen and treated at the UK Role 4 *Military Infectious Disease and Tropical Medicine Service* at Birmingham Heartlands Hospital. There were fewer cases from Afghanistan due to the disease being more patchily endemic than in Iraq, but a single outbreak affected 20 out of 120 individuals at a camp near Mazar-e-sharif in 2004[15] and other isolated cases were reported in 2012.[16]

Respiratory illnesses formed a small part of the physician's workload within the Role 3 hospital in Helmand Province, Afghanistan, but were reported as a major problem elsewhere. So-called 'Kabul cough' was a frequent presentation to the

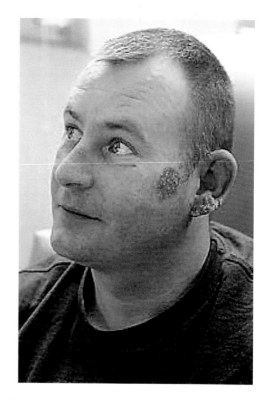

Figure 12.1 Cutaneous leishmaniasis. (Courtesy of Shutterstock.)

uniformed medical services of various nations in the capital city, and combined epidemiological and serological studies[17,18] showed that a significant number of cases were caused by infection with *Bordetella pertussis*, the bacteriological cause of whooping cough. This illustrates the dangers presented by endemic infections that are infrequently seen in the United Kingdom and the reduction in protection seen many years after vaccine administration.

Scorpion and snake bites were feared by many but in reality were an infrequent presentation with 22 cases, none of them in UK military patients, seen in two years of detailed data collection.[4] The devastating effects of snake bite were, however, seen in local civilians,[19] serving as a reminder of the enormous demand this can put on deployed healthcare services. Ensuring the availability of appropriate anti-venom for all species is challenging, and snake identification may not be possible in all circumstances. Likewise, concern about the possibility of

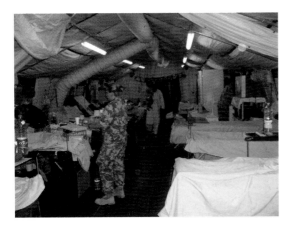

Figure 12.2 Medical ward in the tented hospital at Camp Bastion.

rabies following a bite by a local animal was an ever-present theme and forward availability of vaccine and immunoglobulin were frequently discussed. The main mitigation in these situations is, of course, prevention, and the discouragement of making pets out of local dogs was a prevailing message.

Less exotic, but equally challenging, was the management of civilian patients, including contractors who tended to be older and less fit than their military counterparts. Seventeen per cent of medical admissions on *Operation Herrick* were of civilians – spanning 23 countries of origin.[3] Ischaemic heart disease and cerebrovascular disease become more common morbidities, and the capability of the MTF needs to encompass these likelihoods (Figure 12.2).

CLINICAL ADVANCES

While the campaigns in Iraq and Afghanistan will be remembered for their enormous contribution to advances in trauma care, the incremental advances in operational medicine were comparatively small. The importance of Q fever has been discussed earlier, and the mitigation of the early burden of heat illness and enteric disease was an important achievement for commanders and public health specialists as much as physicians. The importance of antibiotic stewardship and other aspects of medicines management were apparent throughout, and a large cohort of consultant physicians gained operational experience both in the clinical role and as the *deployed medical director*.

CHALLENGES FOR THE FUTURE

The key medical challenges of the future operational space will arise from the environment including the climate, flora and fauna and endemic disease. These will vary according to the theatre of operations, as was later clearly demonstrated by *Operation Gritrock* – the deployment predominantly of medical personnel to Sierra Leone as part of a multi-agency response to the global Ebola virus disease epidemic of 2014–2015. The preparation for, and conduct of, this operation presented a series of new challenges to a force still in the final stages of drawdown from enduring operations in Afghanistan. Themes included novel training methods,[20] collaborative working across government departments,[21] risk mitigation in a threatening healthcare environment,[22] the thermal burden of personal protective equipment,[23] the dangers of mass disinfection[24] and endemic disease.[25] New technologies were embraced,[26] ethical challenges faced[27] and old experience put to new use.[28]

Equipment is a relatively minor consideration in the management of the medical patient outside the critical care environment. An important exception to this is the development of forward diagnostics. By the end of *Operation Herrick*, the hospital laboratory at Camp Bastion was highly sophisticated, although predominantly geared towards transfusion support. Microbiological diagnosis has moved rapidly from traditional techniques of culture to advanced technologies such as diagnostic polymerase chain reaction (PCR) assays, which can rapidly detect bacterial or other foreign DNA within human biological specimens. Real-time or quantitative PCR can now be performed quickly in an austere environment, and one such technology – the BioFire Film Array® – was introduced on a trial basis in Afghanistan and was subsequently highly effective in Sierra Leone.[29] This technology is a multiplex PCR system that is able to prepare the sample, amplify DNA, detect and analyse without additional operator input. Film Array panels are available for respiratory and gastrointestinal pathogens as well as blood culture identification and meningitis/encephalitis infections. Current coverage is over 100 pathogens. The prospect of portable whole genome sequencing has also since been realised,[30] and this is likely to transform outbreak tracking and control.

Other treatments used routinely in the United Kingdom were explored or discussed for introduction as the capability of the field hospital approached that of a National Health Service (NHS) unit. These included inferior vena cava filters[31] in the management of thrombo-embolic disease, renal replacement therapy[32] and bronchoscopy.[33]

TRAINING

The training of physicians is focussed on acquisition of the general and specialty specific knowledge and skills required for the award of a *certificate of completion of specialist training*. It is recognised that infectious diseases represent a significant component of the future workload of deployed consultants. Specialists in this subject will soon make up 25% of the cadre of consultant physicians and the remainder will receive regular training through the *Military Infectious Disease and Tropical Medicine* course, while others will complete the *Diploma in Tropical Medicine and Hygiene*.

The management of local national children presented a considerable challenge to all specialties throughout both operations. Humanitarian operations and other future operations in the developing world will be no different, and, in the absence of uniformed paediatricians, adult physicians must be prepared to take on a share of this workload. To this end, all physicians will undertake training and gain experience in this area. A bespoke training programme, covering these elements, and *chemical, biological radiation and nuclear (CBRN)* medicine, will be incorporated into a military medicine fellowship that aims to bridge the gap between the experience gained during specialist training in a civilian environment and to a civilian level and that required to function as a consultant physician in the deployed environment. This approach has also been adopted by other specialities and is discussed in the appropriate chapters.

A similar ethos applies to the maintenance of skills. Whatever their speciality, all consultant physicians must also complete training in *General (Internal) Medicine (G[I]M)*, a challenge in itself for some sub-specialty groups, and must maintain currency through commitment to *G(I)M*, or *Acute Medicine* as a component of their job plans. Within the NHS, however, Acute Medicine increasingly services the needs of an ageing population complicated by frailty and multiple co-morbidities: issues that are not obviously reflective of the challenges of medicine on military deployment or humanitarian missions. Refresher training in infectious diseases and CBRN medicine is mandated for physicians while the annual service physicians meeting is used as an opportunity to update the entire cadre on operational and clinical topics of importance as well as the latest research.

Military medicine manpower remained relatively stable throughout these operations, and the future operational landscape will continue to excite those who seek to use their knowledge and skills in challenging and austere environments. The establishment of a critical care cadre, drawing from both anaesthetic and medical manpower, will present both a challenge to future physician manning and an opportunity for individuals to deploy in different, or even combined, roles.

RESEARCH

Research in Medicine is overseen by the *Academic Department of Military Medicine*, established under the authority of the *Defence Medical Services* medical director (1*) and *part of the Royal Centre for Defence Medicine*.

The challenge of so-called Helmand Fever and the outcome of the study by Bailey et al. have been discussed previously.[13] Q fever was among the infections investigated in a seroconversion study[34] that showed a 1.7% seroconversion rate for deployed personnel during a six-month tour – even in the absence of symptomatic illness (figures for sandfly fever were 3.1%, and for Rickettsial infection, 2.7%.) This phenomenon, as well as the potential consequences of chronic Q infection, makes this subject an ongoing priority for research in collaboration with the *Defence Scientific and Technical Laboratories* (Dstl), *Public Health England* and other academic partners.

As discussed earlier, diarrhoea was a major cause of working days lost throughout both operations[35] and was the subject of considerable epidemiological research. The *US Navy Medical Research Centre* (USNMRC) in Maryland has an established research programme with interests aligned with the United Kingdom and collaboration has flourished, leading to a number of clinical trials exploring both the treatment and prevention of travellers' (or military) diarrhoea. This programme has included the short-term placement of a UK researcher in the USNMRC within their vaccine development research team. It is clear that enteric disease will remain a clinical challenge to deployed forces and physicians and a robust research programme remains a high priority.

As in Iraq and Afghanistan, high ambient temperature is likely to be a feature of many future operational environments. High thermal burden degrades performance and can have devastating consequences for the individual.[36] Case reports and observational studies continued to highlight this issue during the campaigns, and it is not only a problem of hot countries. Research activity has increased appropriately to make this a high-priority area for ongoing studies.

NUTRITION AND DIET

Reports in the press during the early part of *Operation Telic* questioned the adequacy of the nutritional provision for deployed personnel. This led to the establishment of the *Armed Forces Feeding Project* and the conduct of a cohort study to assess the reality of this situation. A cohort of 49 Royal Marines was assessed in detail before, during and after a six-month deployment in Afghanistan. This work was challenging in its execution[37] but delivered important data that showed minimal change in body weight and no significant change in fitness over the six-month period.[38]

The *Surgeon General's Casualty Nutrition Study* followed on from this work – assessing nutritional aspects of the recovery from critical injury. When combined with the *Steroids and Immunity from Injury through to Rehabilitation* study (Foster M, unpublished), this work has given a valuable insight into the catabolic state that follows critical injury and provides pointers towards possible mitigation

including early nutritional support and therapeutic interventions aimed at controlling the systemic inflammatory response to trauma.

Smoking has long been prevalent among serving personnel and is the focus of many strategies to reduce the health risks associated with it. Surveys during both operations assessed the incidence of established and new smoking, as well as quit rates and any relationship to operational deployment.[39] The use of dietary supplements is a more recent concern and was assessed in both operations at around the same time. These anonymous studies showed that more than one in three surveyed personnel in Iraq were using supplements to enhance the benefits of exercise, particularly body-building.[40] Similar results (40%) were found in Afghanistan in a study that also reviewed smoking rates, which remained high.[41]

Consumption of alcohol by military personnel was prohibited throughout the Afghanistan campaign and for most of the time in Iraq. Deliberate, or accidental, ingestion of methanol is an occasional presentation that can present both a diagnostic challenge and complexity in management that can rapidly challenge the limited capability of the deployed MTF.[42] In addition, although alcohol was not officially available to British military personnel, incidents related to alcohol intoxication amongst contractors were common.

CONCLUSION

Uniformed physicians were deployed throughout the operations in Iraq and Afghanistan and consistently managed a high proportion of all field hospital admissions. Much of this activity was related to infectious disease, including gastroenteritis and undifferentiated febrile illness, while the heat in both theatres of operation presented a challenge to troops, particularly during the summer months, and resulted in significant levels of heat related illness.

Research activity picked up through the campaigns and focussed on these most prevalent clinical challenges, resulting in data that have changed policy – although many of these subjects remain the subject of ongoing research.

A return to contingency operations and the forecasts for the nature of the future operational environment indicate that DNBI will continue to dominate the activity of deployed secondary healthcare, with the range of conditions managed reflecting the climate and endemic problems of the specific geographical location.

The military physician is therefore mandated to prepare for this through training that focuses on infectious diseases, environmental challenges and the relatively neglected area of CBRN medicine.

REFERENCES

1. Wilson DR. Trench fever: A relapsing fever occurring among the British troops in France and Salonica. *J R Army Med Corps* 2014;160(Suppl 1):i4–i6.
2. Bailey MS, Davies GW, Freshwater DA, Timperley AC. Medical and DNBI admissions to the UK Role 3 field hospital in Iraq during Op TELIC. *J R Army Med Corps* 2016;162(4):309.
3. Cox AT, Lentaigne J, White S et al. A 2-year review of the general internal medicine admissions to the British Role 3 Hospital in Camp Bastion, Afghanistan. *J R Army Med Corps* 2016;162(1):56–62.
4. Bailey MS. Medical and DNBI admissions to the Role 3 field hospital at Camp Bastion during Operation Herrick. *J R Army Med Corps* 2016;162(1):76–77.
5. Grainge C, Heber M. The role of the physician in modern military operations: 12 months experience in Southern Iraq. *J R Army Med Corps* 2005;151(2):101–104.
6. Brown D, Gray J, MacDonald P et al. Outbreak of acute gastro-enteritis due to Norwalk-like viruses among military personnel at Bagram airbase, Afghanistan. *MMWR Morb Mortal Wkly Rep* 2002;51(22):477–479.
7. Bailey MS, Boos CJ, Vautier G et al. Gastroenteritis in British troops, Iraq. *Emerg Infect Dis* 2005;11:1626–1628.
8. Bailey M, Gallimore CI, Lines LD et al. Viral gastroenteritis outbreaks in deployed British troops during 2002–7. *J R Army Med Corps* 2008;154:3 156–159.
9. Bolton JPG, Gilbert PH, Tamayo BCC. Heat illness on Operation Telic in summer 2003: The experience of the heat illness treatment unit in Northern Kuwait *J R Army Med Corps* 2006;152(3):148–155.
10. Cox AT, D Linton T, Bailey K et al. An evaluation of the burden placed on the General Internal Medicine team at the Role 3 Hospital in Camp Bastion by UK Armed Forces personnel presenting with symptoms resulting from previously identified disease. *J R Army Med Corps* 2016;162(1):18–22.
11. Hodgetts T, Greasley L. Impact of deployment of personnel with chronic conditions to forward areas. *J R Army Med Corps* 2003;149:277–283.
12. Glennie JS, Bailey MS. UK Role 4 Military infectious diseases at Birmingham Heartlands Hospital in 2005–9. *J R Army Med Corps* 2010;156(3):162–164.
13. Bailey MS, Trinick TR, Dunbar J et al. Undifferentiated febrile illnesses amongst British troops in Helmand, Afghanistan. *J R Army Med Corps* 2011;157:150–155.
14. Bailey MS. Tropical skin diseases in British military personnel. *J R Army Med Corps* 2013;159:224–228.
15. Bailey MS, Caddy AJ, McKinnon KA et al. Outbreak of zoonotic cutaneous leishmaniasis with local dissemination in Balkh, Afghanistan. *J R Army Med Corps* 2012;158:225–228.
16. Matheson A, Williams R, Bailey MS. Cutaneous leishmaniasis in Royal Marines from Oruzgan, Afghanistan. *J R Army Med Corps* 2012; 158:221–224.
17. Sagui E, Ollivier L, Simon F, Brisou P, Puech P, Todesco A. Outbreak of pertussis, Kabul, Afghanistan. *Emerg Infect Dis* 2008; 14(7):1173–1175.
18. Cooper NK, Bricknell MCM, Holden GR, McWilliam C. Pertussis – A case finding study amongst returnees from Op Herrick. *J R Army Med Corps* 2007;153:114–116.
19. Johnson C, Rimmer J, Mount G, Gurney I, Nicol ED. Challenges of managing snakebite envenomation in a deployed setting. *J R Army Med Corps* 2013;159(4):307–311.
20. Gibson C, Fletcher T, Clay K, Griffiths A. Foreign medical teams in support of the Ebola outbreak: A UK military model of pre-deployment training and assurance. *J R Army Med Corps* 2016;162(3):163–168.

21. Forestier C, Cox AT, Horne S. Coordination and relationships between organisations during the civil-military international response against Ebola in Sierra Leone: An observational discussion. *J R Army Med Corps* 2016;162(3):156–162.

22. Lamb LE, Cox AT, Fletcher T, McCourt AL. Formulating and improving care while mitigating risk in a military Ebola virus disease treatment unit. *J R Army Med Corps* 2017;163(1):2–6.

23. Maynard SL, Kao R, Craig DG. Impact of personal protective equipment on clinical output and perceived exertion. *J R Army Med Corps* 2016;162(3):180–183.

24. Carpenter A, Cox AT, Marion D, Phillips A, Ewington I. A case of a chlorine inhalation injury in an Ebola treatment unit. *J R Army Med Corps* 2016;162(3):229–231.

25. Quantick O, Howlett-Shipley R, Roughton S, Ross D. Malaria in British military personnel deployed to Sierra Leone: A case series. *J R Army Med Corps* 2017; 163(1):65–67.

26. Evans TO, Fominyam T, Matthews SW, Bailey MS, Hutley EJ. Use of multiplex PCR to rapidly diagnose febrile patients during a gastroenteritis outbreak among Ebola virus treatment unit workers. *J R Army Med Corps* 2017;163(1):73–75.

27. Clay KA, Henning JD, Horne S. Op GRITROCK ethics; the way of things to come? *J R Army Med Corps* 2016;162(3):150–155.

28. Ewington I, Nicol E, Adam M, Cox AT, Green AD. Transferring patients with Ebola by land and air: The British military experience. *J R Army Med Corps* 2016;162(3):217–221.

29. O'Shea MK, Clay KA, Craig DG et al. Diagnosis of febrile illnesses other than Ebola virus disease at an Ebola treatment unit in Sierra Leone. *Clin Infect Dis* 2015; 1;61(5):795–798.

30. Quick J, Loman NJ, Duraffour S et al Real-time, portable genome sequencing for Ebola surveillance. *Nature* 2016;530(7589): 228–232.

31. Parent P, Trottier VJF, Bennet DR, Charlebois PB, Schieff TD. Are IVC filters required in combat support hospitals? *J R Army Med Corps* 2009;155(3): 210–212.

32. Nesbitt I, Almond M, Freshwater D. Renal replacement in the deployed setting. *J R Army Med Corps* 2011;157(2):179–181.

33. Johnston AMcD, Batchelor NK, Wilson D. Evaluation of a disposable sheath bronchoscope system for use in the deployed field hospital. *J R Army Med Corps* 2014; 160(3):217–219.

34. Newman E, Johnstone P, Bridge H et al. Seroconversion for infectious pathogens among UK military personnel deployed to Afghanistan, 2008–2011. *Emerg Infect Dis* 2014;20(12):2015–2022.

35. Connor P, Hutley E, Mulcahy HE, Riddle MS. Enteric disease on Operation HERRICK. *J R Army Med Corps* 2013;159(3):229–236.

36. Stacey M, Woods D, Ross D, Wilson D. Heat illness in military populations: Asking the right questions for research. *J R Army Med Corps* 2014;160(2):121–124.

37. Hill N. Military nutrition: Maintaining health and rebuilding injured tissue. *Phil Trans R Soc B* 2011;366:231–240.

38. Fallowfield JL, Delves SK, Hill NE et al. Energy expenditure, nutritional status, body composition and physical fitness of Royal Marines during a 6-month operational deployment in Afghanistan. *Br J Nutr* 2014; 112(5):821–829.

39. Boos CJ, Croft AM. Smoking rates in the staff of a military field hospital before and after wartime deployment. *J R Soc Med* 2004;97(1):20–22.

40. Boos C, Wheble GAC, Campbell MJ et al. Self-administration of exercise and dietary supplements in deployed British Military personnel during Operation TELIC 13. *J R Army Med Corps* 2010;156(1):32–36.

41. Boos C, Simms P, Morris FR, Fertout M. The Use of exercise and dietary supplements among British soldiers in Afghanistan *J R Army Med Corps* 2011;157(3):229–232.

42. Barnard E, Baladurai S, Badh T, Nicol E. Challenges of managing toxic alcohol poisoning in a resource-limited setting. *J R Army Med Corps* 2014;160:245–250.

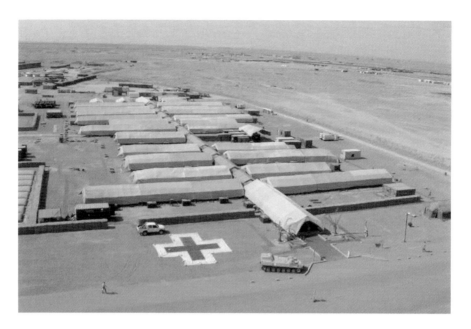

Plate 1 Tented Field Hospital *Operation Telic 4*. The main entrance is bottom right, with the two elements of the emergency department on either side of the main spine immediately beyond the ED reception tent. Other wards and departments are positioned at intervals along the corridor.

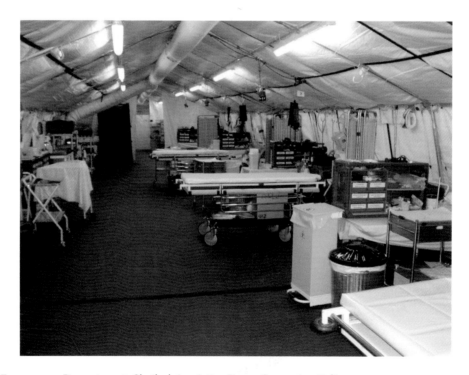

Plate 2 Emergency Department, Shaibah Logistics Base, *Operation Telic*.

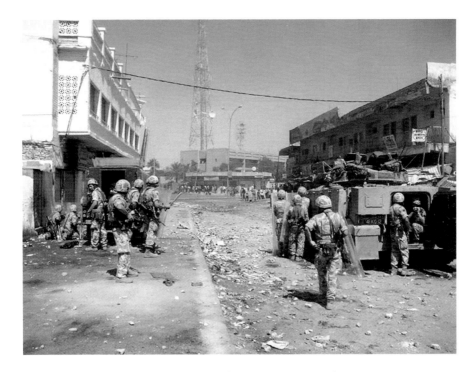

Plate 3 British troops respond to rioting in Basra during *Operation Telic 3*.

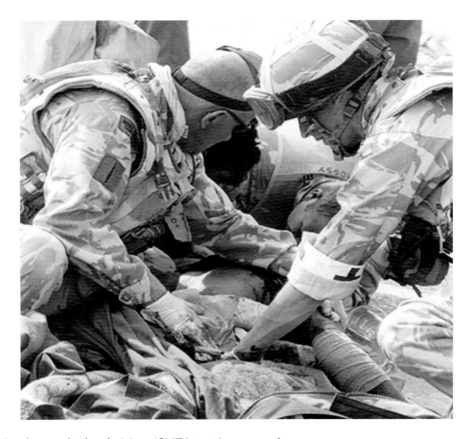

Plate 4 Combat medical technicians (CMTs) treating a casualty.

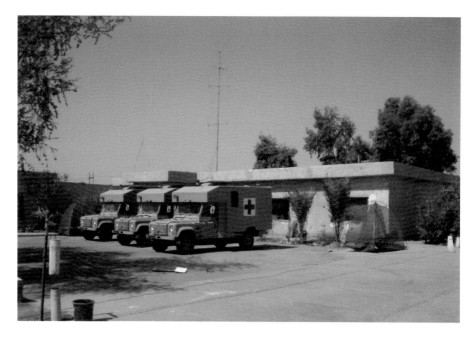

Plate 5 Regimental Aid Post, *Camp Abu Naji, Operation Telic.*

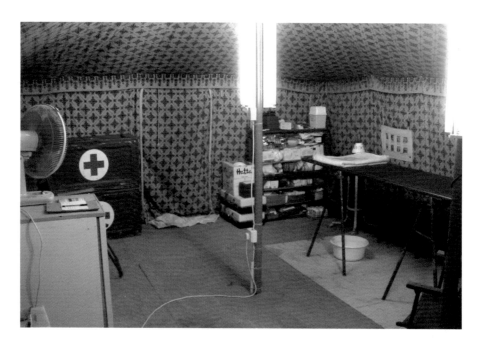

Plate 6 Company Aid Post, *Operation Telic.*

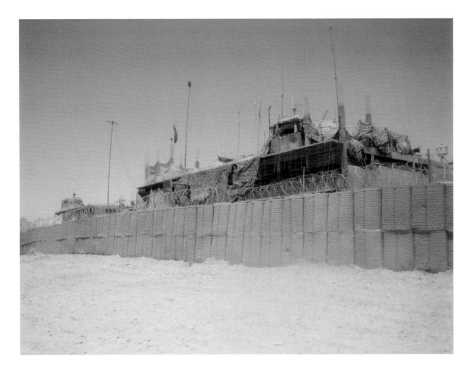

Plate 7 Forward Operating Base, *Musa Qal'eh, Operation Herrick.*

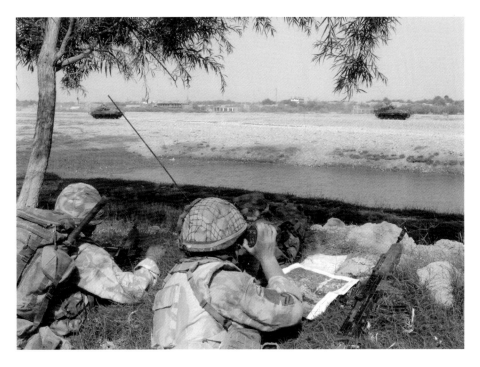

Plate 8 Operations in the 'Green Zone', *Operation Herrick.*

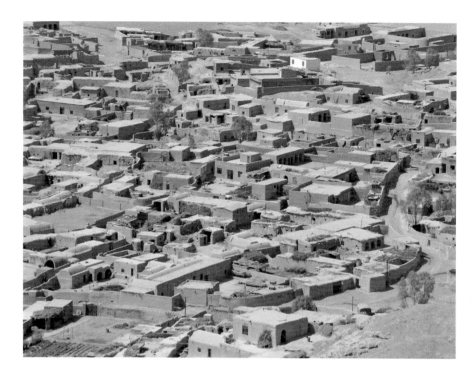

Plate 9 Typical Afghan townscape. The difficulties associated with military operations in such an environment, the potential for ambushes and booby traps and the difficulties of casualty evacuation can all be appreciated.

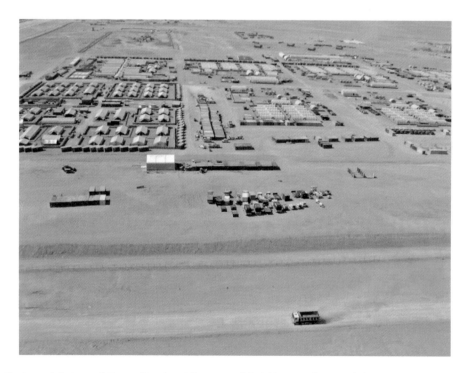

Plate 10 Early aerial view of Camp Bastion. The tented field hospital is top left. At its greatest extent, Camp Bastion covered 26 square kilometres, an area the size of Reading.

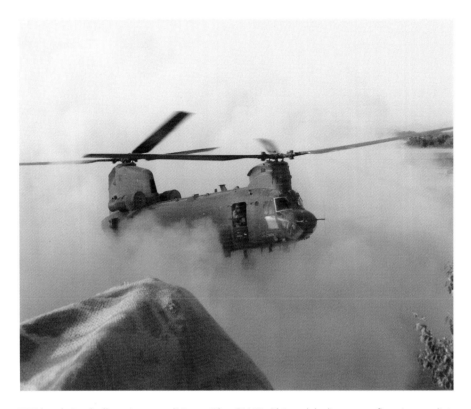

Plate 11 MERT lands in challenging conditions. The CH47 *Chinook* helicopters flew in conditions that were environmentally hostile and were frequently engaged by enemy fire.

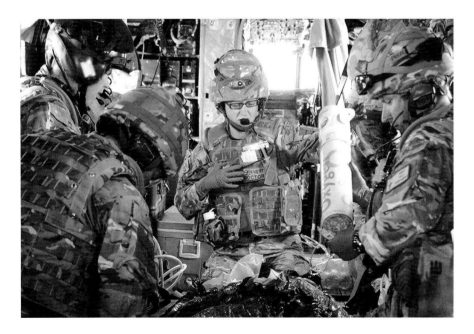

Plate 12 In-flight resuscitation on the *Medical Emergency Response Team* (MERT).

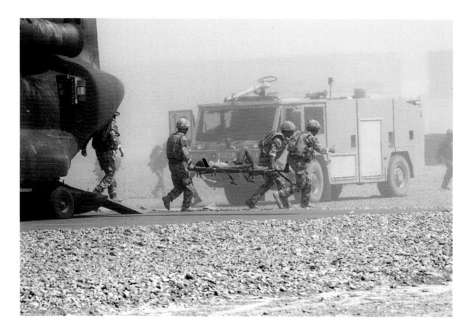

Plate 13 Evacuating an injured casualty from the MERT at Nightingale helicopter landing site, Camp Bastion.

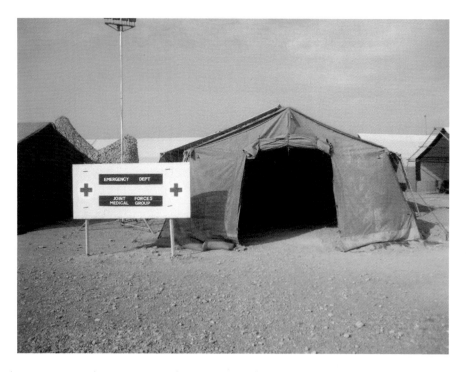

Plate 14 The entrance to the emergency department at the original tented field hospital at Camp Bastion 2006, a view instantly recognisable to anyone who has served in the military at any time since the Second World War. It is likely that this would be the appearance of any future deployed field hospital, at least in the early stages of a campaign.

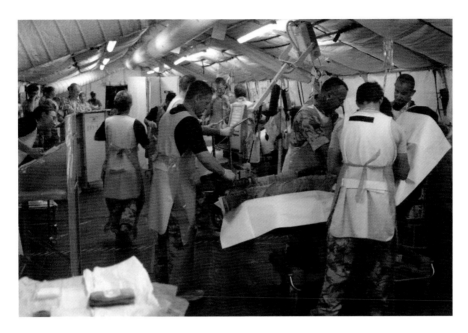

Plate 15 Resuscitation in the tented emergency department, Afghanistan 2007.

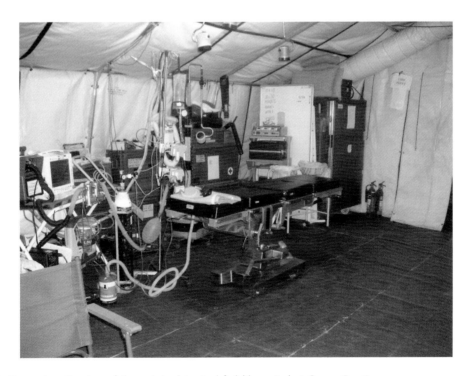

Plate 16 Operating theatre of the original tented field hospital at Camp Bastion.

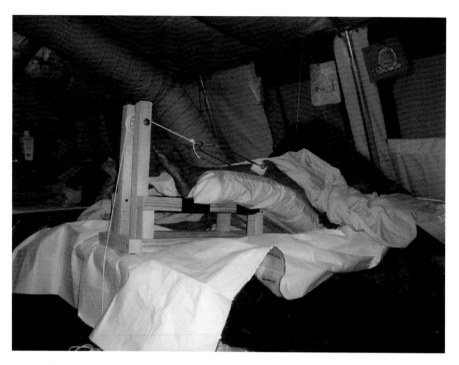

Plate 17 Improvised traction device made by military carpenters at Camp Bastion and used in the treatment of lower limb fractures. This is an early photograph from *Operation Herrick* before equipment scales matured.

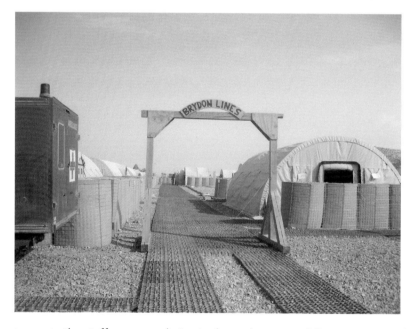

Plate 18 The entrance to the staff accommodation in the early stages of Operation Herrick. The "lines" were named after Dr Wiliam Brydon, an assistant surgeon during the First Anglo-Afghan War, who was said to be the only survivor of an army of 4,500 men and 12,000 accompanying civilians to reach safety in Jalalabad at the end of the long retreat from Kabul in 1842. Brydon was immortalized in a famous painting by Lady Butler, now in Tate Britain.

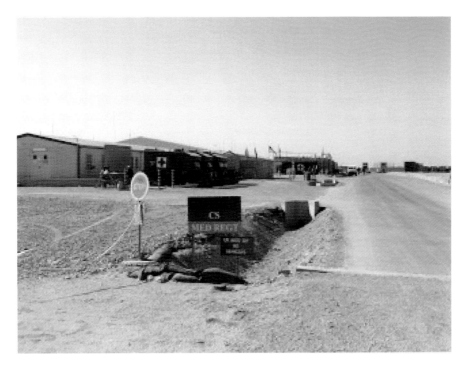

Plate 19 New Camp Bastion hospital seen from the approach road; Nightingale HLS is on the right.

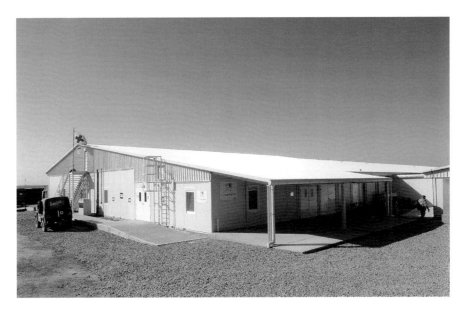

Plate 20 New Camp Bastion Hospital in its first configuration. The main entrance and entrance to the emergency department are under the canopy on the right.

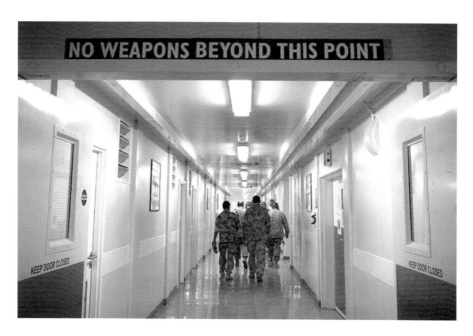

Plate 21 Main corridor of the new Camp Bastion Hospital. The military personnel are walking away from the emergency department past the entrances to the operating theatres on the left and towards the wards and primary care. The radiology department is on the right (see Figures 4.3 and 4.5 for hospital plans).

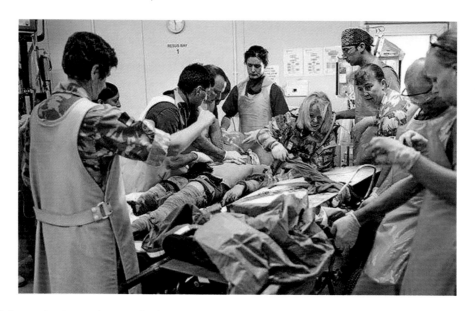

Plate 22 Resuscitation in the new facility.

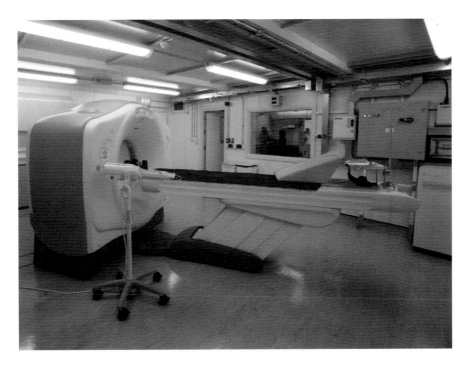

Plate 23 Bastion Hospital CT facility.

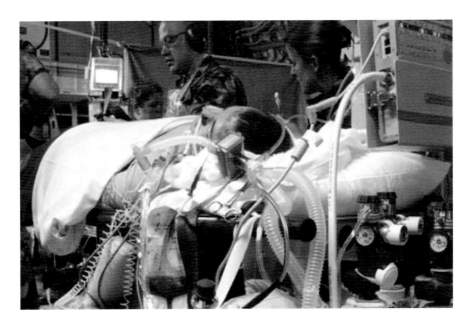

Plate 24 A patient being evacuated by the *Critical Care Air Support Team* (CCAST) to Role 4 facilities in the United Kingdom.

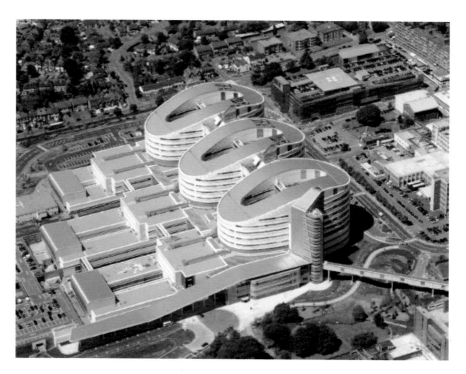

Plate 25 UK Role 4 Facility, the Queen Elizabeth Medical Centre, Birmingham.

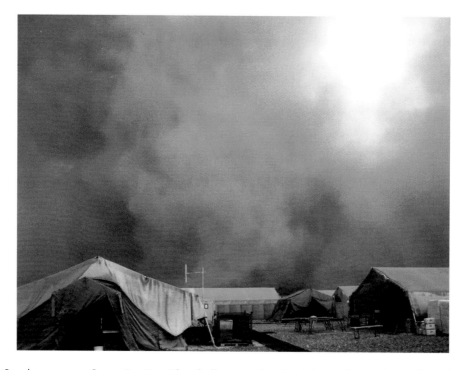

Plate 26 Sandstorm over Camp Bastion. The challenges of maintaining a dirt- and dust-free clinical environment can be readily appreciated.

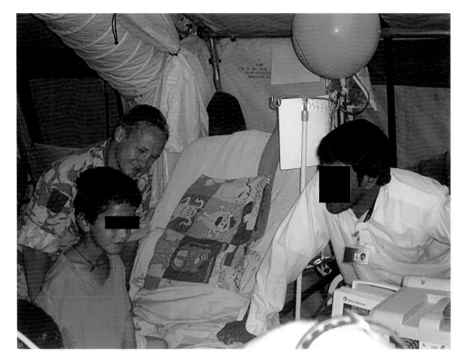

Plate 27 Managing an injured child with the help of an interpreter. The key contribution of the Afghan interpreters and the close working relationships developed with them by clinicians were vital factors in delivery of care to local nationals.

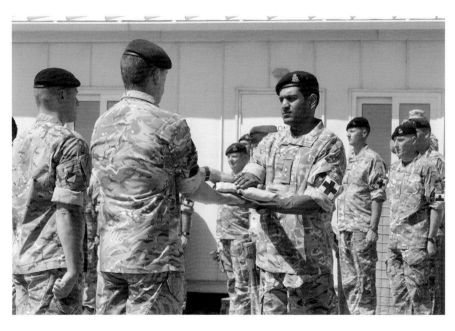

Plate 28 Lowering the flag at Camp Bastion Hospital. The Commanding Officer receives the flag as the unit is decommissioned.

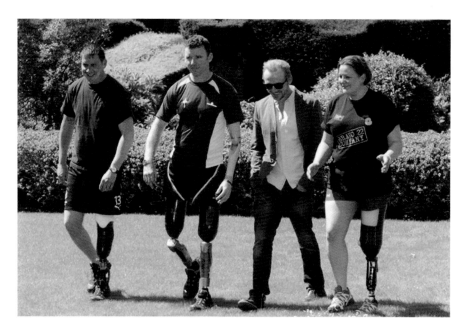

Plate 29 Actor Simon Pegg visits Headley Court. This image captures the positivity of military patients during the rehabilitation process.

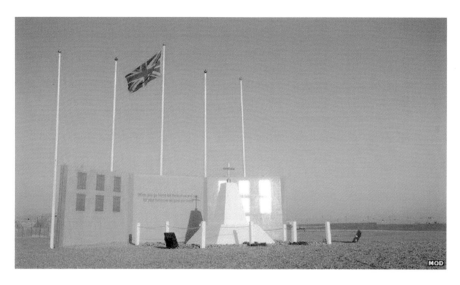

Plate 30 Third War Memorial in Camp Bastion. The first memorial cairn was established *by 16 Air Assault Brigade* in 2006. It was replaced in 2007 as casualty numbers increased, and in 2011, the memorial wall pictured was built out of blast protection wall components. The cross from the first memorial now forms part of a Garden of Remembrance in Colchester, home of *16 Air Assault Brigade*. The memorial bears the words of the Kohima Epitaph: 'when you go home, tell them of us and say, for your tomorrow, we gave our today'. The memorial has been recreated at the *National Memorial Arboretum* in Staffordshire.

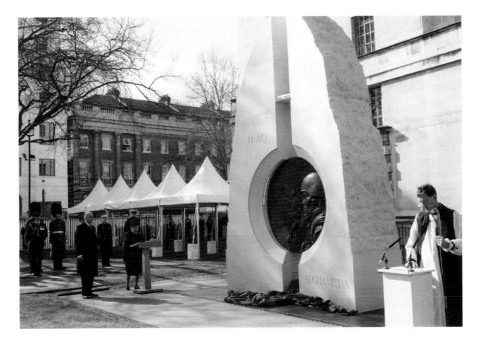

Plate 31 HM Queen Elizabeth II unveils the Iraq and Afghanistan Memorial outside the Ministry of Defence Main Building.

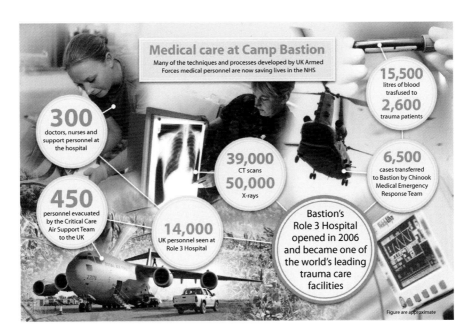

Plate 32 Summary of medical care delivered at Camp Bastion issued by the MOD at the end of Operation Herrick.

Imaging

INTRODUCTION

From the discovery of X-rays by Roentgen in 1895 and the development of plain film and fluoroscopy, there were no giant leaps in imaging until the introduction of *computed tomography* (CT) in the 1970s and nuclear magnetic resonance (now known as *magnetic resonance imaging*) in the 1980s. These modalities rapidly evolved and improved the clinical utility of imaging in civilian practice. As technology advanced, there was improved spatial and contrast resolution producing better and more accurate images.

The diagnosis of internal injury and disease became more readily available as CT became a ubiquitous radiology tool. As with the earliest use of imaging developments within the military, when X-ray was initially confined to base hospitals such as Royal Victoria Hospital Netley,[1] these newer modalities were again only approved or suitable for use within firm base hospitals and were not available in deployed hospital facilities. However, as technology advanced and became more robust, and the equipment became smaller, this new capability gradually found its way into the deployed environment.

At the outset of *Operation Telic* in 2003, land-based radiology comprised conventional plain film X-ray (Figure 13.1), mobile image intensification and rudimentary, portable ultrasound (Figure 13.2). The maritime Primary Casualty Receiving Facility, *Royal Fleet Auxiliary* (*RFA*) *Argus*, also boasted the only deployable CT scanner within the *Defence Medical Services*. By the end of operations at Camp Bastion in 2014, deployed military radiology had been transformed to include digital radiography

(DR), advanced ultrasound and 64 slice CT scanning at the Role 3 Hospital. There was also a deployed *Patient Archive and Communications System* (PACS), *Radiology Information System* (RIS) and a tele-radiology capability beyond civilian capabilities in many aspects and beyond the imaging capability of all the other coalition partners.

This chapter describes the transition from a basic deployed imaging capability to a state-of-the-art trauma imaging capability and the lessons learned along the way. The chapter follows the *Defence Lines of Development* (Table 13.1) construct with reference to both *Operation Telic* and *Operation Herrick* in each area, reflecting how improvements in one theatre could be adopted in the other.

TRAINING

Systems

The use of the military PACS and RIS in PJOBs (Cyprus and Gibraltar) and within seven UK firm base sites, including *Royal Hospital Haslar*, provided ample accessibility to the in-service applications, which ensured that all radiographers and radiologists had day-to-day familiarity with the systems in clinical use. There were also a number of advanced system administrator users within the cadre who had in-depth knowledge. These systems were in use before being deployed on *Operation Herrick*, which meant that limited additional pre-deployment training in their use was required for the regular cadre. Having numerous sites also meant that Reservist staff could more easily undergo application training and refresher

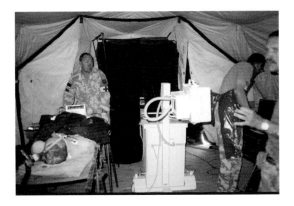

Figure 13.1 X-ray capability with 16 Med Regt during *Operation Telic 1*.

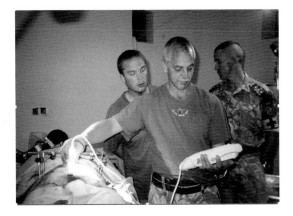

Figure 13.2 Ultrasound examination performed with Sonosite 180 during *Operation Telic 1*.

Table 13.1 Defence *Lines of Development*

Training
Equipment
Personnel
Information
Doctrine
Organisation
Infrastructure
Logistics
Clinical

Note: An important tool in capability development and management, the acronym is *TEPID OIL*. The C is sometimes added by medical planners.

training prior to deployment. With the gradual erosion and closure of these X-ray facilities, increasing numbers of staff worked in National Health Service (NHS) facilities, and more bespoke radiographer training became required to provide the skills that had been previously established and ingrained during daily clinical work. In addition, there was more limited access for Reservists to gain competency with the military systems. Heads of department and hospital information managers (HIMs) required more advanced training to be able to manage the deployed PACS/RIS, particularly when there were issues with connectivity. A robust business continuity plan was clearly required. This administrator access had the potential to corrupt the data irreparably, highlighting the vulnerability of the system without dedicated trained radiographers and information technology (IT) staff. AGFA delivered and validated this training rather than using a conventional military train-the-trainer approach due to its complexity and importance. The PACS/RIS system application requires bespoke training as part of pre-deployment training (PDT), which in the future will be achievable only in the Centre for Defence Radiology (CDR) or Defence Medical Rehabilitation Centre. The role of head of department for imaging will require more advanced administrator-level access to troubleshoot difficulties whilst remote but full administrator rights will remain with CDR.

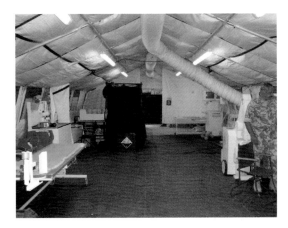

Figure 13.3 Radiology department, *Operation Herrick 5*.

Equipment training

At the outset of operations, radiography was conventional with wet film processing (Figures 13.3 and 13.4). Everyone in the cadre had been trained in wet film processing, but computed radiography (CR) was becoming the mainstay of imaging within the NHS, where radiographers were now trained following the loss of the degree course at Shrivenham. Although radiographers were being well trained in radiography techniques, they no longer had the skills to wet process films on operations. The *Rad Op Training Course* was developed to bridge this knowledge gap but could never provide the experience that comes with using chemical processing in daily practice.

The validation and collective training exercises at the Army Medical Services Training Centre (AMSTC) were useful in allowing the cadre to understand and develop their role within resuscitation scenarios and, in particular, during major incidents. Having the specific equipment to replicate the deployed capability was important. It was also important for the clinical team leaders to recognise that at times there were only two or three radiographers within the facility and to realise that this meant that effective prioritisation of requests was essential. What became evident early in the roulement cycles was the importance of recent operational experience and the necessity for the most recently returned staff to deliver the training, regardless of rank. What exercises in AMSTC did not provide was live training with exposures and clinical experience using the deployed equipment.

Later roulements used the DRagon™ portable X ray capability. which incorporated a digital viewing screen allowing 'real-time' review of X-ray images by clinicians (Figure 13.5). The DRagon™ was essentially bespoke and not used within the

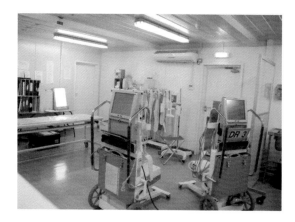

Figure 13.5 Original Xograph DRagon machines in the X-ray department of the Role 3 hospital, Camp Bastion.

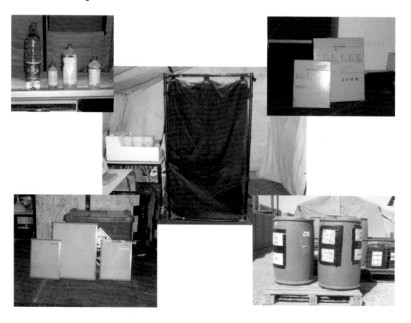

Figure 13.4 Wet film processing paraphernalia used until 2007.

NHS, although later versions of the heavier DaRt™ are used in some NHS Trusts. As a result, there was a confidence gap in the training and knowledge of this capability.

Live training on CT was possible but required careful management. All the deploying regular radiographers had basic familiarity with CT scanning as part of their job plans and, as part of PDT, had dedicated time on an identical scanner in use within the NHS. This was contractually agreed and carried a training budget. At the outset of early operational deployments, it was clear that not all reservist radiographers had civilian roles, which encompassed the spectrum of expertise that would be required. Additional training and earlier mobilisation alleviated some of these skill gaps. The radiographer job specifications were therefore rewritten to reflect the requirements for future deployments. Future planning will need to ensure clinical experience with the specific equipment being deployed, including live exercising with military radiography equipment (if no equivalent is used within NHS).

Despite the effort put into developing courses for training the cadre to be as well prepared as possible in safely and effectively using all the operational imaging modalities before deployment, these efforts were, at times, undermined by the requirement to train coalition radiographers in theatre. The US Rad Tech is not necessarily drawn from a hospital facility and may not be clinically current, and the qualification, which is not degree level, is considered by some as an 'ad qual', an additional qualification for someone whose main role lies elsewhere. Only a handful of the deploying US radiographers were CT trained and only one had previous experience on the scanner used in theatre. At times of high clinical tempo, this training requirement, with effectively reduced team numbers, placed additional strain on the trained personnel. That said, many of the coalition team were extremely competent, often with more advanced qualifications: most quickly picked up the basics of CT scanning, which was very much protocol driven and were fully integrated into the team. Patient safety, particularly with radiation exposure in CT, has to be of the highest standard, and radiographers deploying from coalition partners to UK medical treatment facilities (MTFs) had to

be competent in the use of the modalities within the facility prior to arrival in theatre, in the same way UK military staff operate. In essence, radiographers operate to UK guidelines within UK facilities and the expectations of coalition deploying clinicians must be tempered to work within this framework.

Medical device sterilisation services (MDSS) were a crucial cog in maintaining the effective running of the radiology equipment. Warranties on some high-cost items meant that the MDSS were often restricted to diagnostics or elementary repairs, but good contracts were in place for replacement equipment, and with regular flights, it was possible to obtain smaller items of equipment easily and quickly. The CT scanners, however, were installed and managed by contractors, and therefore, there was no requirement for an expensive training package for the MDSS personnel. Throughout Operation Telic and during the first few years in Afghanistan, the contracted engineer was not based in theatre but in the United Kingdom. Remote, dial-in diagnostics were not available for security reasons, and as a result, in the event of breakdown, the nature of the fault or failure could not be assessed until the engineer arrived in theatre, nor could the parts be shipped. This meant that the CT scanner could be unserviceable for many days at a time. Fortunately, this was not common, but when it occurred, it had a significant impact on the capability of the MTF, with only one CT scanner in each theatre at that time.

From 2010, with the rebuild of the CT facility and the installation of a second scanner in the Camp Bastion hospital, there were in-theatre qualified engineers who could maintain and repair the scanners. This provided a much more reliable service, and the scanners were more reliable in part due to regular maintenance and minor fault fixing. Having trained and qualified MDSS technicians or contracted engineers in theatre to maintain and repair high-value radiology equipment will be essential in future deployments in order to maintain a reliable capability, particularly in remote locations.

These were the first major conflicts where CT had been deployed, and with the improving point-of-wounding care, enhanced assets for patient retrieval and novel resuscitation techniques, patients were being imaged with degrees of injury never before seen. As such, there was little or no reference material to use in understanding and interpreting the images that were being produced. However, radiology clinical training was possible as all the images and reports were archived in the military PACS and became an accessible resource for deploying radiologists who were able to use them to familiarise themselves with the appearances of the prevalent injury patterns.

EQUIPMENT

At the outset of operations, the X-ray equipment was basic with a Siemens Mobilett™, a dark room and automated film processor. Other than the use of automated rather than manual wet-film processing, there had not been a huge change in capability in the preceding 100 years, although the newer equipment was more reliable and robust. There were issues with chemicals going off in the extreme temperatures, but the capability was relatively simple, easily maintained and reliable. However, the process was labour intensive and slow. An audit of times from acquisition to review in the emergency department (ED) in Iraq in 2005 confirmed that it could take five to six minutes to return a diagnostic image. This time could be doubled if there was an error or fault. This simple assessment of the patient care pathway was the evidence required to upgrade the radiography equipment.

This analogue technique produces a single original film. It was necessary therefore for patients to be evacuated with their images and there was no retained copy. Images could be lost, misplaced or damaged anywhere along the evacuation chain and were not necessarily archived by the final receiving NHS Trust. To expedite reporting of studies from *Operation Telic*, rather than return whole packets of films to the United Kingdom regularly, images were digitised with an urgent operational requirement (UOR) procured digitiser and transmitted back via the dedicated satellite link installed at the time of the CT scanner installation. Images could now be seen more readily in the United Kingdom, albeit with a degradation in image quality.

CR, a technique in which a digital cassette is processed and read electronically, was in general use within the NHS and in the US military. This had the advantage of producing a digital image,

and although the image could be printed using a laser printer, it was now possible to archive electronically. This was considered in the proposal for a radiography upgrade; however, the processing step remained a delay. This review coincided with the development of the earliest mobile digital radiograph (DR) machines. In essence, these were the digital cameras of the radiography world, producing a reviewable image within a few seconds after exposure and at the bedside; however, they were more expensive than CR. The clinical requirement case was won and DR was procured (Figure 13.5). This put British military radiography at the forefront of technological capability across the North Atlantic Treaty Organization (NATO) allies and in advance of most NHS hospitals. Our allies have now adopted DR over CR for the same reasons and with technological advances as available.

The introduction of DR resolved the issue of wet film processing as well as the Control of Substances Hazardous to Health issues relating to chemical replenishment, storage and disposal. However, additional training was required with upgrades of equipment relating to different operating systems on new models. DR also removed the processing requirement of the cassette, which thereby reduced the size and weight of the department, an important consideration when deploying a military medical facility. It is worth observing that all electro-medical items, including X-ray, have published environmental operating parameters, which need to be met in the deployed environment as at home in the United Kingdom.

Radiographers now had to manage data and rather than printing films, they were burning discs. Resupply of discs was an issue at times as they were considered non-essential items and as stationery items were not part of a medical module or medical resupply. Disc burning became time consuming and utilised one of the workstations almost constantly, which impacted on other clinical activity. Ultimately, a UOR for a disc burner was accepted and the device installed in Camp Bastion; however, although this is an ongoing requirement, it has not yet been brought into core for funding (see Chapter 23).

Although DRagon™ was a major advance in capability, bespoke changes were required to improve the hydraulic arm, to alter the wheel sizes to make the machine maneuverable over uneven terrain in the departments and corridors of the tented facility and ultimately to supply it in green(!). This has remained the workhorse X-ray capability for Role 2 and Vanguard Field Hospital and has gone through numerous iterations to reach the current model. The building of the tier 2 hospital in Camp Bastion with an even and strong floor allowed the deployment of a hospital standard heavier DR capability, the DaRt™. This allowed improved imaging capability but is not suitable for deployment on uneven or less robust flooring.

Ultrasound has similarly been through numerous models over the last 14 years. All have been Sonosite™ machines, which are ruggedised and drop tested, making them suited to the rough and tumble of the deployed environment. Initially, *Sonosite 180*™ and 180+™ machines were deployed, then *Micromaxx*™ and *Nanomax*™ machines. The Defence Medical Services (DMS) now has a fleet of *M-Turbos*™. The 180 series machines were relatively old technology with a small screen, and the *Micromaxx*™ provided a larger screen with an enhanced imaging capability, but at the cost of increased weight. Although the *Nanomaxx*™ was trialled and several procured, the screen was too reflective for use in the bright conditions of the resuscitation room. As a consequence, despite being heavier and not as ergonomically friendly, the *M-Turbo*™ was brought into service. Varying software capabilities were introduced within the fleet – the basic *Focused Abdominal Sonography in Trauma* (FAST) machine, a machine with Doppler capability and a highly sophisticated model for radiologist use, although none were capable of echocardiography (ECHO). Each therefore required a different procurement number, and the management of the machines became exceptionally complicated. Eventually, a capability review was conducted that standardised the base units and all had their software unlocked, ultimately providing an ECHO capability for the later years of *Operation Herrick*. By standardising the software capability of the entire fleet of *M-Turbo*™ ultrasound machines, rationalising the distribution of probes and bringing all machines into the radiology modules, it was therefore possible to achieve improved interoperability, to reduce the fleet size and to improve capability without cost.

Careful deployment or replacement of equipment as part of fleet management is required. As new versions or upgrades of existing DR equipment have come into service, there has not been whole fleet refresh for reasons of cost, although there can be widely varying differences between different versions. For example, some machines have wireless detached plates or can operate wirelessly; more significant is a difference in the operating systems and control panels. This has the potential to lead to mistakes and has training issues if different versions of the machine are deployed concurrently.

It is worth commenting that procurement of equipment without proper consideration for other users has led to problems with integration in the recent past. Various ED trolleys have been employed over the last 14 years. Although some may be more comfortable for patients, particularly with long waits in NHS departments in mind, these may not be suitable for X-ray imaging. Some designs had mid-table supports preventing placement of the cassette under the patient table. Placing the plate directly under the patient risks damage to the very expensive plate and rendering the equipment unusable. Others could take conventional sized cassettes but could not accommodate the larger DR plates. Others still sat too low to the ground, preventing the front wheels and support for the DRagon™ passing beneath and making it impossible to take any meaningful images. Each of these problems would have been manifest had there been an integration trial. In this same vein, lightweight theatre tables have been procured that are neither radiolucent nor allow the image intensifier underneath to allow on-table imaging. Likewise, a small change in wheel size can cause tremendous difficulty, and such minor alterations were not necessarily declared by the commercial provider or apparent at first glance. Integration testing by, or on behalf of, subject matter experts (SMEs) such as the Defence Consultant Advisors (DCAs) or Defense Specialty Advisors (DSAs) of all relevant groups should therefore be mandatory before the procurement of any complex equipment. The evolution of the Clinical Materiel Advisory Group has helped to minimise these interoperability issues (see Chapter 23).

The single greatest leap in imaging capability came with the deployment of the CT scanner, initially into Shaibah Log Base in 2005 in support of *Operation Telic*. This was the first time the United Kingdom had deployed CT on operations in a land environment (Figure 13.6). During *Operation Telic 1*,

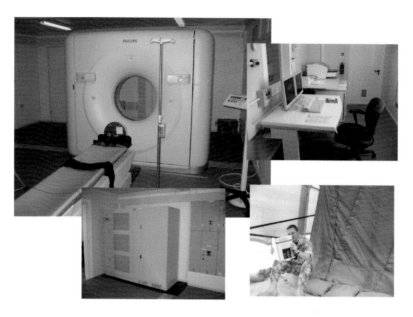

Figure 13.6 Original Philips CT scanner on *Operation Telic* also showing a small control room, uninter-ruptable power supply and a radiologist.

the CT scanner on RFA Argus provided the only deployed cross-sectional imaging capability, but during the offensive and the subsequent couple of years, patients requiring CT were transferred by tactical CCAST to Kuwait. The deployment of the scanner to the hospital provided clinicians with an appropriate investigation tool to improve decision making. The scanner was a Phillips 16-slice scanner but operated as an 8-slice scanner to provide some redundancy. A similar scanner was installed in the Tier 2 build in Camp Bastion before being replaced by two 64-slice GE scanners.

The scanners were built into the infrastructure by contractors, but with the closure of Shaibah Log base, there was a requirement to move the scanner to the new hospital facility within the *Contingency Operating Base* at Basra Airport. This was a consid-erable engineering project, which meant that there was a loss of capability for a number of weeks to allow the dismantling, move and re-assembly and testing to take place. The original location of the CT scanner on *Operation Telic* was less than ideal, and in the future, it should always be placed as near as possible to the ED and the operating theatres. Access to the hospital's main corridors allowing easy transfer from the wards and intensive care unit (ICU) is also essential.

Deploying a containerised CT scanner (CCTS) in the entry operation or early phase of an endur-ing operation provides the clinical capability from the outset, and its installation does not rely on a large engineering project. This capability, unlike the built versions, can be moved or removed easily. Once operations become enduring, consideration can then be given to building a Tier 2 CT scanner room and withdrawing the CCTS.

PERSONNEL

The numbers of radiographers and radiologists deployed varied throughout *Operation Herrick*, although numbers had remained relatively unchanged for the duration of *Operation Telic*.

During *Operation Telic 1*, all the regular con-sultant radiologists and some Reservists deployed. Each field hospital deployed with two radiologists and further radiologists were deployed on *RFA Argus* and at the military hospital at Akrotiri, Cyprus. After the offensive period passed, the radi-ologists returned to United Kingdom. By the end of 2003, there were only four consultants across the three Services. The deployment of the CT scanner required tele-radiology support. *RH Haslar* was still a functioning hospital, and with the ongoing level of clinical activity, remote reporting worked well. Even with the communications link in 2005, it was possible to get a CT head study back to the *Centre for Defence Imaging* (CDI) in RHH (now CDR in the Royal Centre for Defence Medicine) within 10 minutes and a verified report back in theatre within a further 10 minutes. The bulk of the reporting and imaging was plain film work. This workload was manageable by the two deployed radiographers with remote reporting by the serving radiologists.

Uptake in the use of the scanner was gradual. Many of the deploying radiographers were competent but not experts in CT. For this reason, there were defined protocols to constrain the requests with limited scan protocols to prevent radiographers being placed in a difficult position by senior clinicians. As the deployment progressed, the skills of the radiographers improved and there was more scope for complex scanning. It took some time to reach 100 scans,[2] which was a very

different story on *Operation Herrick* (Figure 13.7 and Table 13.2).

Operation Herrick saw the deployment of its first scanner in 2007. This was installed in the Tier 2 build before the rest of the complex was built. Having learned from the Iraq experience that the scanner was effectively immovable, it was built recognising that patients would have to be moved by ambulance from the tented facility, which was sited alongside the location of the new build to the new CT suite and then back again following the scan. The same on-call military radiologist in the United Kingdom covered reporting for both theatres. Until later in 2007, only the two radiologists in RH Haslar provided reporting capability 24 hours a day. Between 2007 and 2009, networking improved, reporting from home became possible, and the other radiologists contributed to the on-call commitment.

It is clear from Figure 13.8 and Table 13.3 that there was a significant increase in clinical activity in Camp Bastion compared to Iraq, and despite a

Table 13.2 Figures demonstrating annual recorded activity by modality

Modality	Op Telic – Number of examinations each year						
	2003	2004	2005	2006	2007	2008	2009
CT	0	1	121	108	218	124	32
X-ray	64	768	2131	1988	2033	1315	499
II	0	0	8	13	13	7	0
US	0	16	32	74	49	28	1
FAST	0	0	0	0	0	20	0

Source: Figures retrieved from RIS.

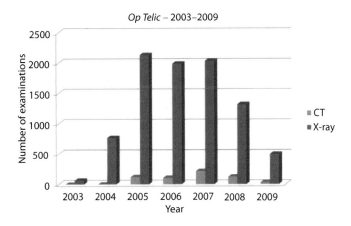

Figure 13.7 Representation of radiological activity on *Operation Telic* by year.

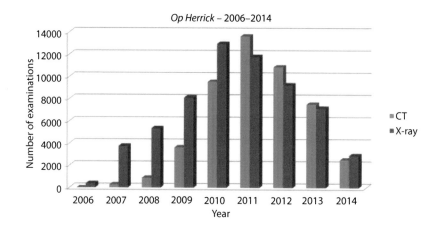

Figure 13.8 Representation of radiological activity on *Operation Herrick* by year. (Note the change of scale from Figure 13.7.)

Table 13.3 Figures demonstrating annual recorded activity by modality

	Op HERRICK – Number of examinations each year								
Modality	**2006**	**2007**	**2008**	**2009**	**2010**	**2011**	**2012**	**2013**	**2014**
CT	0	280	889	3645	9551	13643	10887	7530	2515
X-ray	398	3772	5359	8129	12970	11794	9248	7173	2906
II	2	13	4	147	205	312	272	138	27
US	2	5	2	357	595	661	514	461	190
FAST	0	0	0	74	569	1773	1268	968	328

Source: Figures retrieved from RIS.

dedicated satellite being in place by 2008, it was not possible to effectively keep up with reporting in a timely fashion. The cadre was now of sufficient size to deploy and from late spring 2009 radiologists deployed on *Operation Herrick*. Radiologists have a clear deployed role when CT or CCTS is deployed, providing contemporaneous reporting for complex trauma CT scans (Figure 13.9), which would otherwise be significantly delayed on high-latency communication links, particularly if multiple 1.5 GB studies are performed.

The initial deployments in 2009 were as singleton radiologists. Unlike some other clinical roles that were either trauma, surgically or medically focused and where there was often more than one deployed clinician, the sole radiologist took requests from all these clinical areas, and during periods of high or moderate tempo, there were extended periods with only limited rest. Anecdotally, this did not necessarily correlate to

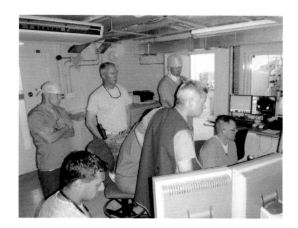

Figure 13.9 A deployed radiologist providing a contemporaneous initial report to surgeons and EM clinicians before the patient has left the scanner.

the frequency of trauma calls. Tour lengths were initially for six to eight weeks, which was considered the ceiling at that time for a busy singleton role. There was tele-radiology support providing some plain film reporting and second opinions where necessary. As the tempo increased in 2009 and into 2010, a US radiologist was deployed and UK tour lengths increased to three months. This worked well for the radiology cadre. Although some skill fade was experienced in niche areas of subspecialty practice during deployment, general and emergency care knowledge rose. This knowledge and expertise then fed back into NHS practice on the clinician's return.[3,4]

Radiographers faced slightly different manning challenges. Manning related also to the throughput of clinical activity, not bed capacity as originally determined, and whether or not CT was present. A simple but effective formula evolved, recognising that the two radiographers initially deployed could manage up to 500 examinations per month using DR but that for every additional 250 examinations per month, an uplift of one radiographer was required. Effort went into ensuring that there was an appropriate skill mix amongst the deploying radiographers. The junior non-commisioned officers (NCOs) developed in clinical roles earlier than their civilian counterparts, particularly in CT expertise, but the radiographers were also working more independently from radiologists than would be expected in the NHS. Clear guidelines and policies were developed to support the radiographers and to smooth the investigation pathway. As the radiographers were also all *Radiation Protection Supervisors*, they were further empowered beyond *Ionising Radiation (Medical Exposures) Regulations* to control the use of ionising radiation. Having small independent military X-ray departments in the firm base military hospitals allowed the junior NCOs and senior NCOs to develop their management skills and to have the confidence to run a department without a superintendent or radiologist present. With the draw down and closure of military departments, this opportunity for experience before deployment has been lost.

During reliefs in place, it was essential that there was a staggered transition of the radiography team. The head of department roulement was deliberately four weeks out of sync with the other members of the tour to ensure that there was a continuity of practice and minimal loss of corporate knowledge, recognising that collective training cannot cover all aspects of the role.

When there were so few radiographers deployed, they were busy most of the time either with clinical work, departmental administration or cleaning and maintenance. In addition, there was no opportunity to run a shift system when only two were deployed, as both would be required for any significant cases. It was an important step when the hospital management recognised their work pattern and they were only employed in their deploying role and not for other military takings. Shifts became necessary with the larger deployed numbers and higher tempo of activity.

INFORMATION

Radiology has evolved from an analogue capability to a very-high-specification digital capability during this period of operations. Not only did the imaging modalities become digital, but the archiving and reporting capabilities also transformed from paper to electronic records. There is a legal requirement to safely retain the images and reports,[5] but despite having satellite links to the United Kingdom and the CDR PACS/RIS, it became necessary to have a deployed PACS archive. This provided an in-theatre backup archive for the operational images during the later *Operation Herrick* deployments. With this expansion of technology, there was increasing reliance on radiographers becoming IT specialists, a role many were not trained for, despite personal interests, until HIMs were deployed. The HIM, *communications and IT team* and radiographers worked together, pooling their individual areas of knowledge, to overcome many of the technical issues that were experienced; however, there was still a requirement for commercial IT support from AGFA™, the PACS supplier.

Unlike civilian practice where commercial companies such as AGFA™ can remotely dial into servers to perform diagnostics, upload patches or upgrades and perform repairs, this is not possible on military servers sitting on Defence Infrastructure.

The *Ministry of Defence* (MOD) must therefore pay a premium for specific vetted engineers to access the network, with permissions, via CDR. This can cause significant delays in resolving IT issues on operations.

Even with the development of digital images, there was still an initial requirement for hard-copy films to be produced or for clinicians to come to the radiology department to view the images. Not until an appropriate network was built with viewing monitors in theatres, ED, ICU and the wards, was the requirement for hard-copy film finally abolished. This networked solution, however, provided the clinicians with easy access to all the previous imaging.

DR was deployed to *Operation Herrick* initially as part of a UOR, but there was no appropriate communication link to transmit the images. Ironically, the communications from Iraq were such that the hard-copy analogue images, once digitised, could be easily transmitted to CDI. As the Role 3 matured in Camp Bastion, the communications improved. Although the link was described as dedicated, it became apparent when the link slowed that other information system (IS) users were accessing the link without permission. The transmission of images ahead of the patient to staging Role 3 or Role 4 hospitals was extremely valuable; it ensured that the receiving clinicians had as much information as possible to use in planning management and surgery and it reduced the requirement for repeat imaging on repatriation, to the benefit of the patient. As well as optimising the transfer of patient imaging and, thus, patient management, a dedicated communications link to the United Kingdom ensured archiving of all images and provided scope for second opinions. A minimum 4 MB link is required and the operational *Information Exchange Requirement* should clearly articulate the hospital IT requirements, including reach-back, at the outset.

As well as the requirement to transfer images from a theatre of operations to CDR, there was also a need to transfer images to coalition MTFs in theatre. The US patients' images and reports were transferred to their military network for archiving in slow time. There was also a requirement to be able to transfer clinically urgent scans to Kandahar, the nearest neurosurgical unit. This was fraught

with difficulty due to security requirements. In an ideal world, there would be a switch between networks, but UK IT security could not sanction any hardwiring. The only possible way was employing an air-gap by burning the images to a disc and uploading them onto the US network, Medweb, using a node installed in the radiology department. This was time-consuming and labour-intensive, but no other approved mechanism could be found. CDR procured a Medweb unit in an attempt to find a solution and explored the possibility of moving to the US system; however, the clinical capabilities of the system were considered suboptimal by the DCA Radiology at the time. The US military also recognises the deficiencies of the system and does not use Medweb within their firm base hospitals, only for operations. Interoperability with coalition IT infrastructure should be declared when operational requirements are being defined so appropriate security resources can provide the solution.

Information governance is extremely important,[6–8] and the MOD is required to comply with the statutory policies. All archives are therefore password protected to minimise access to patient identifiable information. There is an exception, however, with burning of discs for patient transfer. No encryption is applied to these discs, which travel with the patient. This allows images to be easily accessed in any MTF should the patient be unexpectedly diverted.

Modalities and archives, by definition, hold patient identifiable information. However, to comply with JSP440,[9] the equipment must be encrypted or the system erased to a standard to ensure that the hard disks with the data are allowed to transfer across borders. This became a major issue during the draw down from *Operation Herrick*. To be able to decommission the CT scanners, the hard disks, including the operating system, had to be replaced to ensure that the data could never be accessed. This carried a significant cost. Likewise, the laptops for the imaging modalities had to be encrypted and carried by hand by the radiographers, but the hardware needed Defence courier transfer, again at significant cost. Removing patient identifiable information from current equipment on each occasion would require the removal of the operating system and render the machine unserviceable and effectively worthless.

One solution may be a second hard drive, but it is not possible to access and remove hard drives without invalidating warranties. Future high-capital-cost imaging equipment needs to be procured with a mechanism for patient identifiable information to be safely removed in accordance with JSP440 without interfering with the operating system.

Having all the imaging and reports on dedicated PACS and RIS provides the MOD with a secure single data source of all operational images for future reference and research. Research exploitation of the data from this unique archive is already being undertaken.

In order to be able to image numerous patients quickly in mass casualty events, pseudonyms were pre-loaded onto the RIS and available almost instantly on the X-ray devices. The pseudonyms were attached to the blank hospital numbers prepositioned in the trauma bays. This had the advantage of creating an additional patient identifier and reduced the risk of mistaken identity during the 'confusion' of overwhelming patient numbers. Only once patient identification was confirmed and any transfusion completed could the electronic radiology record be amended to reflect the correct details. At times, images were transmitted back to Role 4 with the pseudonym in use (because of ongoing blood requirements), although the patient had been correctly identified. This had the potential to cause confusion of identity for the clinical team in Role 4 and result in an inability to reconcile any demographic changes on images and reports.

CONCEPTS AND DOCTRINE

The deployment of CT required for the management of trauma patients complies with the standards expected by the *Royal College of Radiologists*.[4] The success of the scanners on *Operations Telic* and *Herrick* cannot be measured directly, but their positive influence on decision making for patient management is beyond doubt. The use of whole-body traumograms was adopted, and evidence from Europe suggests that this technique changed outcomes.[10,11] More recent work is less convincing on early mortality outcomes[12]; however, this work relates to typical civilian patterns of injury and not to blast or populations with significant proportions of penetrating injury. What is well recognised within military radiology is the benefit of whole-body CT for the identification of occult injury, and the REACT2 study confirms the benefit of this technique[13] in detecting significant incidental findings. With deployed radiologists, there was discretion to amend the scan protocol. Certainly, from the UK point of view, having a consistent policy and technique simplified the situation for the radiographers, some of whom were very junior and some trained in theatre, thereby improving the overall standard of examination. Currently, the land-based deployable CCTS is a Role 3 capability, consistent with NATO doctrine. There is, however, no practical reason beyond logistics why this capability cannot deploy in support of smaller MTFs. The connecting tentage is compatible. There would, however, have to be a suitable power supply and an additional radiographer, MDSS technician and radiologist.

Although not strictly a matter of doctrine, it is appropriate to mention the importance of standard operating procedure (SOPs) and imaging protocols at this juncture. Because of the independent practice of radiographers that evolved, by necessity, in the early years of the operations clear, unambiguous guidelines were developed for the radiographers and clinicians to follow. The DCA's radiographic guidelines provided the radiographers with the appropriate images to take and when it was appropriate to image. These were (and are) similar to the Royal College of Radiology CR guidelines[14] but reflect practice where there may not be access to a CT scanner. The guidelines also provided permissions to undertake CT scans for specific reasons, predominantly for trauma, to avoid delays whilst a remote, UK-based radiologist was contacted. Pragmatic approaches to practice supported the deployed radiographers and meant that appropriate imaging was carried out promptly.

Development of protocols evolved for postmortem imaging and for veterinary imaging (Figure 13.10) during these operations. These documents were constantly evolving to reflect changes in equipment and improving techniques. Department-specific SOPs should be retained from previous operations in order to provide a basis for future operations.

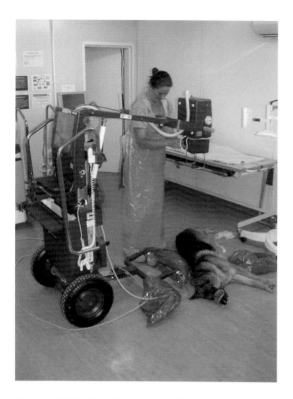

Figure 13.10 Veterinary plain films on a military working dog using Dragon™ X-ray equipment.

ORGANISATION

The *Centre for Defence Radiology* was, and still is, the de facto single point of contact for clinical radiological queries, but it also provides support for deployed radiographers and clinicians with access to SMEs concerning issues of governance, assurance, radiation protection and technical equipment queries. Having a cadre single point of contact for subject matter experts available 24/7 for all operations was invaluable for the deployed radiographers and radiologists. In any future operational planning, these positions must be considered in addition to the deploying operational manpower requirements. Although the deployed radiographers are responsible to the deployed command structure, it is important that open communication with CDR and the SMEs is encouraged and not prevented. Minor issues can be easily overcome and quickly rectified, but the head of department must inform the deployed headquarters of any such communication. The deployed radiographers

are not necessarily SMEs and as such may not be able to provide the best strategic advice to the command team on radiography or radiology. DCA Radiology and DSA Radiography, as well as the Single Service Clinical Advisors, should be considered as sources of advice regarding such queries.

INFRASTRUCTURE

The high-tech equipment of twenty-first century imaging has specific infrastructure requirements in order to comply with the manufacturers' warranties. The most sensitive modalities were the CT scanners, with a requirement for the temperature to remain between 19°C and 24°C and the need to minimise dust ingress. The latter was relatively easily managed with regular cleaning; however, a power draw was required to run the air-conditioning virtually 24 hours a day to ensure a stable temperature was maintained. Nevertheless, appropriate environmental control must be achievable for effective use of equipment and is likely to require additional power.

Experience suggests that power requirements will forever be a constraint on capability and a headache for the quartermaster. These recent operations benefitted from the generous power supply provided by the hospital CAT generator farm. Despite this, there were still fluctuations in power, particularly during *Operation Telic*, and there was a need for a large *uninterruptable power supply* (UPS) to be installed. This provided a smooth power supply and sufficient power to safely shut down the scanner if there was a power outage mid scan. It was not sufficient to complete the scan, however. Neither was the UPS installed in an air-conditioned room, which led to early degradation and damage to the UPS.

Newer versions of DR equipment have been procured, which have the advantage of being man-portable and of operating from a battery rather than a mains supply. This may be the basis of a solution to the intermittent issues of power supply compatibility with DRagon™.

The provision of power sources compatible with all imaging equipment must be considered and ideally should utilise CAT generators. Depending on the physical construct of the MTF, a different imaging capability may be deployed. If the flooring is uneven, temporary or not well supported and unsuitable for heavy weights, then the heavy DR kit (DaRt™) will not be appropriate in that environment.

LOGISTICS

Moving the equipment to and from the theatre of operations always carries a risk of equipment damage in transit. Everything possible is done to ensure that the equipment is packaged securely in the bespoke original packing. Foam cutouts provide additional protection, as do pallets inside containers for the heavy X-ray apparatus. The cases are all well marked and fork points and securing points are clearly labelled. Despite all these precautions, accidents still happen and equipment can be damaged.

CLINICAL

The experience of imaging in the recent campaigns has been challenging and educational for all involved. Like many other specialties, the collective experience, development of techniques and understanding of injuries has had benefits beyond military practice, with techniques being incorporated into civilian practice in the United Kingdom and Unied States. The injury patterns, mechanisms of injury and severity of injury were very different from the traumatic injuries normally experienced in the NHS and have led to extensive work in trying to further understand blast and ballistic injury.[15]

In UK civilian trauma practice, blunt trauma is the norm, with only 11.8% of patients sustaining penetrating injuries; the rates of penetrating injury in US forces on operations reached up to 68.3%.[16] Traumatic amputation is unusual in civilian practice, but on one day in 2009, the most common presenting complaint to Role 3 ED was bilateral lower extremity amputation, with five cases recorded. Neither was there a reference book or illustrated guide to understanding the CT appearances of high-velocity gunshot wounds and blast injury. Much of the early learning was correlating the images with surgical or pathological findings.

One of the early imaging changes was the introduction of a modified Baltimore dual-phase contrast bolus for trauma CT scans (Table 13.4). Conventionally, scans were performed during different arterial and portal venous phases following intravenous contrast administration. These scans required more planning by the radiographer, took longer to prepare and ultimately led to a higher radiation dose to the patient.[17] The dual-phase continuous contrast injection allowed for a single acquisition of the torso (from base of skull down) starting at 70 seconds, which could continue through the lower extremities, providing angiography down to the feet if necessary.[18] The torso enhancement of the arterial and portovenous system was good, whilst angiography was excellent. Such scope of scanning was not possible using the traditional contrast technique. This was further refined to provide a similar adapted protocol for paediatric patients. Defence radiology remains

Table 13.4 Dual-phase bolus dose and timings for trauma CT

Estimated weight	Contrast dose (mL)	Dual-phase contrast doses and rates
6 kg	12 mL	8 mL @0.2 mL/sec then 4 mL @0.4 mL/sec
10 kg	20 mL	14 mL @0.3 mL/sec then 6 mL @0.5 mL/sec
15 kg	30 mL	20 mL @0.4 mL/sec then 10 mL @0.8 mL/sec
20 kg	40 mL	26 mL @0.5 mL/sec then 14 mL @1.0 mL/sec
30 kg	60 mL	40 mL @0.7 mL/sec then 20 mL @1.6 mL/sec
40 kg	80 mL	54 mL @0.9 mL/sec then 26 mL @2.1 mL/sec
50 kg	100 mL	66 mL @1 2 mL/sec then 34 mL @2.4 mL/sec
60 kg	120 mL	8 mL @0.2 mL/sec then 4 mL @0.4 mL/sec
70 kg	140 mL	8 mL @0.2 mL/sec then 4 mL @0.4 mL/sec
75 kg +	150 mL	8 mL @0.2 mL/sec then 4 mL @0.4 mL/sec

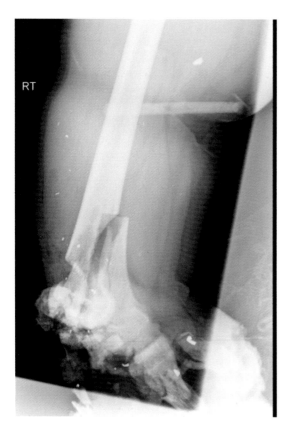

Figure 13.11 Plain film of dismounted lower extremity blast injury with CAT™ tourniquet applied mid-thigh.

cognisant of paediatric radiation dose and the paediatric trauma protocols[19]; however, the same arguments apply with children often exposed to the same battlefield injuries and having a requirement for the whole body traumogram.[20] Providing the clinicians, most of whom were not paediatric surgeons, with as much information as possible was the priority, and as such, whole-body CT was performed when justified.[19] The dual-phase contrast bolus was adjusted for weight. This chart was originally colour coded to correspond with Broselow tape colours.

An added advantage of speed using this protocol was minimising the time the patient spent in the CT scanning suite. An audit of patients in 2012 demonstrated a 1° temperature drop, on average, whilst in the scanner. The scanner had to be kept cool for operating purposes, so the air-conditioning was always on; speed was therefore of the essence. Trauma teams became very efficient at safely and rapidly transferring seriously injured patients into and out of the scanners.

The development of novel medical devices also evolved, with the use of intra-osseous needles, pelvic binders, needle thoracostomy and tourniquets, both CAT™ and pneumatic, and comments on their location and use were pertinent.[21] Both tourniquets produce characteristic soft tissue changes when applied (Figures 13.11 and 13.12a and b).

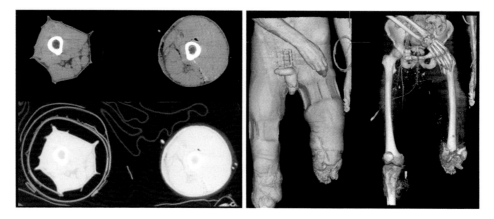

Figure 13.12 CT scan of bilateral lower limb amputation with pelvic binder in situ and bilateral inflated pneumatic tourniquets. (a) Axial images at the level of the right tourniquet. (b) Surface shaded rendering and CT angiogram with 3D reconstruction.

Collaboration between the radiologist, surgeon and anaesthetist was normal at the time of scanning to determine if the tourniquet should be released to provide angiography. This was done only with the anaesthetist's knowledge and consent in order to reduce the risks of an adverse physiological response whilst in the scanner. Pelvic

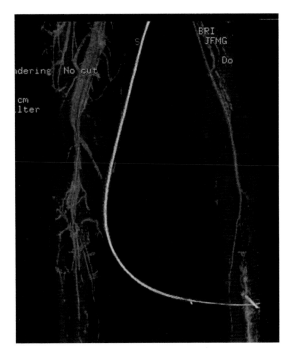

Figure 13.13 CT angiogram (posterior aspect) demonstrating hyperaemia in the left leg relative to the normal right in a patient following release of left thigh tourniquet for a complex open calcaneal injury following improvised explosive device explosion.

binders similarly altered the clinician's perception of injury, and instability could be missed on imaging if no clinical examination or imaging with the binder released was performed.[22] CT angiography with tourniquets released at the time of scanning facilitated assessment of vascularity and localised vascular injury but required consent from the anaesthetist because of the increased threat of haemorrhage and a hypotensive response. There can be a profound hyperaemia following release of tourniquets, which should not be confused with traumatic arteriovenous fistula (Figure 13.13).[23]

Patients with pelvic binders require clinical assessment of pelvic stability as well as imaging without the binder *if the binder-on CT appearances are normal* (Figure 13.14a and b).

FAST was adopted as a useful tool, particularly in the rapid triage of multiple casualties but also to provide an early indication of the presence of free intraperitoneal or pericardial fluid in any trauma patient.

It is well recognised that a positive FAST has a high specificity for intraperitoneal blood in the presence of trauma,[24,25] although a negative FAST does not exclude significant injury. It certainly helped prioritise patients for theatre and for CT scanning (Figure 13.15).

Following resuscitation, there were times when FAST was repeated in mass casualty events to re-triage patients awaiting theatre or CT scanning. In experienced hands, it can also be used to assess for large a haemothorax or pneumothorax. During *Operation Herrick*, FAST was performed by the radiologists, allowing the trauma team leaders to concentrate on their task in hand.

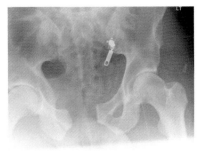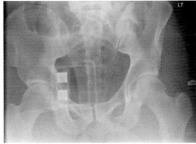

Figure 13.14 Unstable pelvic fracture with (a) binder off and (b) binder on demonstrating anatomical reduction.

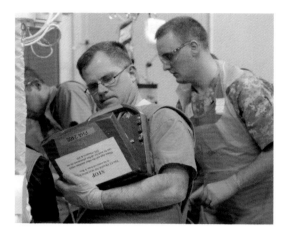

Figure 13.15 Consultant radiologist performing FAST with M-Turbo ultrasound machine.

When the CT scanner was unserviceable, clinicians had to resort to more old-school conventional imaging. Although plain films of the skull are no longer indicated in trauma, if there is no access to CT, then they are advocated. Similarly, the use of intravenous urethrography has virtually ceased in civilian practice, yet without the CT scanner, it remains an effective assessment for ureteric calculi. Radiologists and radiographers trained in the last five years are unlikely to have performed intravenous urograms or trauma skull series. These are skills that are being incorporated into the *Rad Op Training Course* for the radiographers lest they are completely consigned to history.

Post-mortem CT imaging developed as a change of practice from plain film to CT in support of imaging for the Home Office registered forensic pathologists investigating operational deaths. It also provided imaging evidence for more severe injury patterns in blast- and ballistic-related deaths as well as imaging the boots, helmet and body armour in many cases, allowing assessment of the effectiveness of such equipment. This imaging, along with the post-mortem examination and in the context of the events surrounding each of the deaths, has been instrumental in better understanding blast injuries and battlefield deaths.[26–28] These unique cases and this experience have transferrable utility in the investigation of terrorist-related events, and the military radiology cadre provides support to the Home Office

and numerous constabularies through the *Military Assistance to Civil Authorities* process.

The comprehensive catalogue of operational imaging stored in the military PACS is a unique collection. It has provided, and continues to provide, a wealth of information as one of the DMS's valuable research resources. The cadre has collaborated extensively with other specialties, including general surgery,[29] T&O,[30] maxillofacial,[31] neurosurgery (Figure 13.16), anaesthetics,[32] emergency medicine,[33] intensive care[34] and ophthalmology,[35,36] developing a better understanding of battlefield injuries and their management and outcomes. Collaboration is also ongoing with Royal British Legion Centre for Blast Injury Studies,[37–41] Cranfield University[42] and Defence Science and Technology Laboratories,[43–45] with various aspects of battlefield injury and imaging.

Veterinary imaging was performed only in the presence of the requesting vet, with the military working dogs (MWDs) often requiring sedation. MWDs were highly prized animals and much loved by the troops, and not only for their ability to detect improvised explosive devices. Most of the imaging on MWDs related to orthopaedic conditions and tail trauma; however, several animals were CT scanned as part of their investigation after more significant trauma or exposure to blast. As a

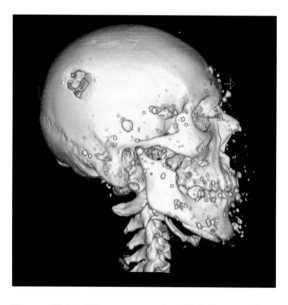

Figure 13.16 3D reconstruction CT following blast injury with depressed skull fracture, penetrating brain and penetrating ocular injuries.

result, comprehensive SOPs have been developed to assist with imaging MWDs in the future.

Not only has there been collaboration across specialties, but also there has been effective international co-operation, particularly with our American colleagues. There also has been well-described work on blast injuries, including the identification and description of acute peri-traumatic pulmonary thrombus.[46]

CONCLUSION

Military radiology has undergone a transformation in technological capability during recent conflicts as well as a transformation in standing amongst other specialties. It is now recognised as an integral component in the early investigation[47] and management planning of patients following severe trauma. It is acknowledged to be a vital asset in deployed healthcare. Advances in military imaging, particularly CT, have informed and transformed civilian trauma practice. Nevertheless, effective imaging requires complex and expensive equipment and an effective and integrated procurement process, which much be in place, funded and supported *before* it is needed on deployment.

REFERENCES

1. Thomas AM. The first 50 years of military radiology 1895–1945. *Eur J Radiol* 2007; 63(2):214–219.
2. O'Reilly DJ, Kilbey J. Analysis of the initial 100 scans from the first CT scanner deployed by the British armed forces in a land environment. *J R Army Med Corps* 2007;153(3):165–167.
3. Royal College of Radiologists. *Standards of Practice and Guidelines for Trauma Radiology in the Severely Injured Patient.* London: Royal College of Radiologists, 2011.
4. Royal College of Radiologists. *Standards of Practice and Guidelines for Trauma Radiology in the Severely Injured Patient.* 2nd ed. London: Royal College of Radiologists, 2015.
5. Royal College of Radiologists. *Retention and Storage of Images and Radiological Patient Data.* London: Royal College of Radiologists, 2008.
6. Data Protection Act 1998. London: The Stationery Office.
7. Freedom of Information Act 2000. London: The Stationary Office.
8. Department of Health. *Records management: NHS Code of Practice.* London MOD: 2006.
9. *Defence Manual of Security (JSP440).* 2001.
10. Huber-Wagner S, Lefering R, Qvick LM et al. Working Group on Polytrauma of the German Trauma Society. Effect of whole-body CT during trauma resuscitation on survival: A retrospective, multicentre study. *Lancet* 2009;373(9673):1455–1461.
11. Smith CM, Woolrich-Burt L, Wellings R, Costa ML. Major trauma CT scanning: The experience of a regional trauma centre in the UK. *Emerg Med J* 2011; 28(5):378–382.
12. Sierink JC, Treskes K, Edwards MJ et al. REACT-2 Study Group. Immediate total-body CT scanning versus conventional imaging and selective CT scanning in patients with severe trauma (REACT-2): A randomised controlled trial. *Lancet* 2016;388(10045):673–683.
13. Treskes K, Bos SA, Beenen LFM et al. REACT-2 Study Group. High rates of clinically relevant incidental findings by total-body CT scanning in trauma patients; results of the REACT-2 trial. *Eur Radiol* 2017;27(6):2451–2462.
14. Royal College of Radiologists. *iRefer: Making the Best Use of Clinical Radiology.* 8th ed. London: Royal College of Radiologists, 2017.
15. Singleton JA, Gibb IE, Bull AM, Clasper JC. Blast-mediated traumatic amputation: Evidence for a revised, multiple injury mechanism theory. *J R Army Med Corps* 2014;160(2):175–179.
16. Eastridge BJ, Costanzo G, Jenkins D et al. Impact of joint theater trauma system initiatives on battlefield injury outcomes. *Am J Surg* 2009;198(6):852–857.
17. Ptak T, Rhea JT, Novelline RA. Radiation dose is reduced with a single-pass whole-body multi-detector row CT trauma protocol compared with a conventional

segmented method: Initial experience. *Radiology* 2003;229(3):902–905.

18. Watchorn J, Miles R, Moore N. The role of CT angiography in military trauma. *Clin Radiol* 2013;68(1):39–46.

19. Royal College of Radiologists. *Paediatric Trauma Protocols*. London: The Royal College of Radiologists, 2014.

20. Borgman M, Matos RI, Blackbourne LH, Spinella PC. Ten years of military pediatric care in Afghanistan and Iraq. *J Trauma Acute Care Surg* 2012;73(6 Suppl 5):S509–S5513.

21. Blenkinsop G, Mossadegh S, Ballard M, Parker P. What is the optimal device length and insertion site for needle thoracostomy in UK Military casualties? A computed tomography study. *J Spec Oper Med* 2015;15(3):60–65.

22. Bonner TJ, Eardley WG, Newell N et al. Accurate placement of a pelvic binder improves reduction of unstable fractures of the pelvic ring. *J Bone Joint Surg Br* 2011;93(11):1524–1528.

23. Fishman EK, Horton KM, Johnson PT. Multidetector CT and three-dimensional CT angiography for suspected vascular trauma of the extremities. *Radiographics* 2008;28(3):653–665; discussion 665–666.

24. Gaarder C, Kroepelien CF, Loekke R, Hestnes M, Dormage JB, Naess PA. Ultrasound performed by radiologists-confirming the truth about FAST in trauma. *J Trauma* 2009;67(2):323–327; discussion 38–329.

25. Smith IM, Naumann DN, Marsden ME, Ballard M, Bowley DM. Scanning and war: Utility of FAST and CT in the assessment of battlefield abdominal trauma. *Ann Surg* 2015;262(2):389–396.

26. Singleton JA, Gibb IE, Hunt NC, Bull AM, Clasper JC. Identifying future 'unexpected' survivors: A retrospective cohort study of fatal injury patterns in victims of improvised explosive devices. *BMJ Open* 2013;3(8). pii: e003130. doi: 10.1136/bmjopen-2013-003130.

27. Singleton JA, Gibb IE, Bull AM, Mahoney PF, Clasper JC. Primary blast lung injury prevalence and fatal injuries

from explosions: Insights from postmortem computed tomographic analysis of 121 improvised explosive device fatalities. *J Trauma Acute Care Surg* 2013;75(2 Suppl 2):S269–S274.

28. Breeze J, Gibbons AJ, Hunt NC et al. Mandibular fractures in British Military personnel secondary to blast trauma sustained in Iraq and Afghanistan. *Br J Oral Maxillofac Surg* 2011;49(8):607–611.

29. Morrison JJ, Clasper JC, Gibb I, Midwinter M. Management of penetrating abdominal trauma in the conflict environment: The role of computed tomography scanning. *World J Surg* 2011;35(1):27–33.

30. Spurrier E, Gibb I, Masouros S, Clasper J. Identifying spinal injury patterns in underbody blast to develop mechanistic hypotheses. *Spine (Phila Pa 1976)* 2016; 41(5):E268–E275.

31. Breeze J, Leason J, Gibb I et al. Characterisation of explosive fragments injuring the neck. *Br J Oral Maxillofac Surg* 2013;51(8):e263–e266.

32. Scott TE, Kirkman E, Haque M et al. Primary blast lung injury – A review. *Br J Anaesth* 2017;118(3):311–316.

33. Ritchie JV, Horne ST, Perry J, Gay D. Ultrasound triage of ocular blast injury in the military emergency department. *Mil Med* 2012;177(2):174–178.

34. McDonald Johnston A, Ballard M. Primary blast lung injury. *Am J Respir Crit Care Med* 2015;191(12):1462–1463.

35. Gay DA, Ritchie JV, Perry JN, Horne S. Ultrasound of penetrating ocular injury in a combat environment. *Clin Radiol* 2013;68(1): 82–84.

36. Chaudhary R, Upendran M, Campion N et al. The role of computerised tomography in predicting visual outcome in ocular trauma patients. *Eye (Lond)* 2015;29(7): 867–871.

37. Singleton JA, Walker NM, Gibb IE, Bull AM, Clasper JC. Case suitability for definitive through knee amputation following lower extremity blast trauma: Analysis of 146 combat casualties, 2008–2010. *J R Army Med Corps* 2014;160(2):187–190.

38. Ramasamy A, Hill AM, Masouros S et al. Outcomes of IED foot and ankle blast injuries. *J Bone Joint Surg Am* 2013;95(5):e25.

39. Eardley WG, Bonner TJ, Gibb IE, Clasper JC. Spinal fractures in current military deployments. *J R Army Med Corps* 2012;158(2):101–105.

40. Ramasamy MA, Hill AM, Phillip R, Gibb I, Bull AM, Clasper JC. FASS is a better predictor of poor outcome in lower limb blast injury than AIS: Implications for blast research. *J Orthop Trauma* 2013;27(1):49–55.

41. Ramasamy A, Hill AM, Phillip R, Gibb I, Bull AM, Clasper JC. The modern "deck-slap" injury – Calcaneal blast fractures from vehicle explosions. *J Trauma* 2011;71(6):1694–1698.

42. Ramasamy A, Hill AM, Masouros S, Gibb I, Bull AM, Clasper JC. Blast-related fracture patterns: A forensic biomechanical approach. *J R Soc Interface* 2011;8(58):689–698.

43. Mahoney PF, Carr DJ, Delaney RJ et al. Does preliminary optimisation of an anatomically correct skull-brain model using simple stimulants produce clinically realistic ballistic injury fracture patterns? *Int J Legal Med* 2017;131:1043–1053.

44. Breeze J, Leason J, Gibb I, Hunt NC, Hepper A, Clasper J. Computed tomography can improve the selection of fragment simulating projectiles from which to test future body armor materials. *Mil Med* 2013;178(6):690–695.

45. Breeze J, Hunt N, Gibb I, James G, Hepper A, Clasper J. Experimental penetration of fragment simulating projectiles into porcine tissues compared with stimulants. *J Forensic Leg Med* 2013;20(4): 296–299.

46. Lundy JB, Oh JS, Chung KK et al. Frequency and relevance of acute peritraumatic pulmonary thrombus diagnosed by computed tomographic imaging in combat casualties. *J Trauma Acute Care Surg* 2013;75(2 Suppl 2):S215–S220.

46. Gay DA, Miles RM. Use of imaging in trauma decision-making. *J R Army Med Corps* 2011;157(3 Suppl 1):S289–S292.

14

Transfusion medicine

INTRODUCTION

Massive haemorrhage is the most immediate threat to the injured service person. The mortality rate after massive haemorrhage in trauma is high unless it is actively managed from the time of wounding. Recent military campaigns in Iraq and Afghanistan have seen increasing rates of survival from massive and complex injuries, which would previously have been considered lethal. These increasing survival rates have been the products of a military healthcare system to which transfusion medicine has been a key contributor.

This chapter narrates the development of transfusion support during recent operations. The developments have occurred during a period of dramatic changes in the regulatory environment. The account is written in sections. The order is chronological, starting first with an account of *Operation Telic 1*. The sequence continues through the developments of Defence transfusion policy, practice, logistics, safety and pre-hospital care. The final sections review the research programmes and legacy to wider healthcare.

OPERATION TELIC

Preparation for war-fighting

Preparation for desert war-fighting started in early autumn 2001 with *Exercise Saif Sarreea II* in Oman. The exercise enabled many senior clinicians to rehearse field surgery in desert conditions. However, the exercise also highlighted the fact that many lessons identified on *Operation Granby* (the First Gulf War) had not been actioned. Lessons

had been lost or forgotten: a recurring theme in military medicine. The lead-in to *Operation Telic* was short and the operation would involve the deployment of large numbers of reservists, including three haematologists. The UK Defence Medical Services (DMS) did not, and do not, include serving regular haematologists, a capability contained within the Reserves (then termed the Territorial Army [TA]). A few months after *Saif Sarreea*, *202 Field Hospital* practiced relief in place (RIP) with *34 Field Hospital* during *Exercise Log Viper* at the Army Medical Services training centre near York. The two field hospitals were then mobilised; *34 Field Hospital* as a 50-bed and *202 Field Hospital* as a 200-bed hospital. RIPs with *34 Field Hospital* occurred twice, firstly in *Camp Coyote* and then in Shaibah. *202 Field Hospital* received casualties in the theatre of operations 17 days after mobilisation. The formal war records were lost, but this section describes the experience of the *202 Field Hospital* from field diaries.

People and places

The *202 Field Hospital* laboratory was deployed with a full complement of eight staff consisting of two technical officers and a biomedical scientist (BMS) drawn from seven TA units. In addition, there was an infection control nursing officer, and there were two consultant haematologists. Local arrangements also provided a combat medical technician to act as a medical laboratory assistant. The transfusion capability formed part of a multidisciplinary laboratory. The unit took out a full-scale of Role 3 equipment using the established equipment modules. However, the reagent stock at the time of handover was only 60%. One of the biggest challenges during *Operation Telic 1* was resupply, especially the resupply of consumables. Diagnostic triage was required from the outset, particularly for microbiology. Diagnostic developments for the blood sciences included *point-of-care testing* (POCT) and semi-automation. A Column Agglutination System (DiaMed®) had been introduced before deployment as a semi-automated transfusion system to replace test tube testing for ABO and RhD testing. The Sysmex® platform provided coagulation testing (PT, APTT and fibrinogen). The work horse for clinical chemistry remained the dry chemistry system D60 (Ortho Diagnostics). The handheld iSTAT® system provided POCT for haemoglobin, clinical chemistry and blood gas testing. Later, a HemaCue® module was available for more accurate POCT for haemoglobin. The standard canvas general service tentage and the hot and dusty environment were challenges to the provision of a laboratory service. Most automated systems will not perform in temperatures over 35°C. The conditions were improved with the introduction of sun shields, which helped reduce the load on an overburdened air-conditioning system. The newly introduced Diamed® worked well in the difficult environment; however, considerable efforts were required to provide sufficient environmental control for the Sysmex® and iSTAT®. Despite these restrictions, the laboratory provided an 18-hour service for haematology, chemistry and microbiology and a 24-hour transfusion service.

Workload and blood use

The fighting phase lasted seven weeks, from 20 March to 31 April 2003. During this phase, the hospital processed 2930 patients through the emergency department. The surgical team handled 139 patients and undertook 333 surgical procedures. The laboratory received 2214 groups of pathology requests on 1137 patients, and 354 red cell units were cross-matched. Forty-seven patients were transfused. The blood components issued were: 249 units of SAGM blood, 45 units of fresh frozen plasma (FFP), 6 units of platelets and 10 units of cryoprecipitate. Most red cell units were cross-matched, with only 7 of the 47 transfused patients receiving group-specific blood. Blood

supply was from the English *National Blood Service*, supplied through the *Blood Supply Depot, Medical Supplies Agency* (MSA), and distributed in theatre by *84 Medical Support Squadron*, part of the Royal Logistic Corps. Resupply was extremely reliable for red cells and frozen products; however, there was no transport of platelets. Platelets were subsequently provided by the use of fresh blood and *Host Nation Support* (HNS). Blood component storage facilities in the field hospital were subsequently augmented during the tour to include two field blood fridges, two freezers and one platelet incubator.

The pattern of transfusion workload during the fighting phase is shown in Figure 14.1. Transfusion activity approximate mirrors the surgical workload, which is shown in Figure 14.2.

Multi-disciplinary care

The lessons learnt from *Exercise Saif Sarreea II* in Oman were being applied during *Operation Telic*, with proper debridement and cutting back to 'healthy bleeding tissue'. However, the fall in haemoglobin was being underestimated during surgery. Five bleeding patients were found to have post-operative haemoglobins of less than 5.0 g/L. On investigation, amongst the causative factors identified were the fact that the theatre table was a stretcher, which was both concave and absorbent, allowing unseen blood to pool under the body and seep through, that swabs were not weighed and that irrigation increased the volume of material

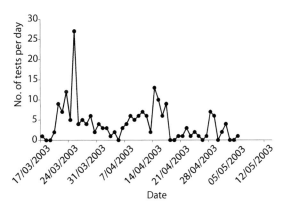

Figure 14.1 Transfusion requests during the fighting component of *Operation Telic 1.*

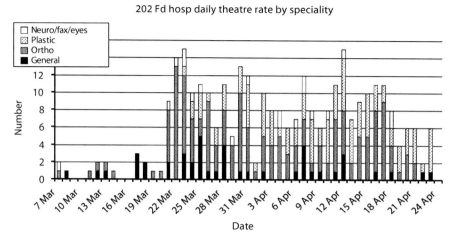

Figure 14.2 Surgical workload during *Operation Telic 1*.

collected during suction, confounding accurate measurement of the volume of blood collected.

Following this early experience, a multi-disciplinary approach to the bleeding patient was adopted. At this time, UK guidelines advised the use of laboratory testing before the use of plasma and platelets. However, it became clear that a more proactive approach was required. Some of the strategies introduced were as follows:

- Proactive correction of coagulopathies and transfusion of red cells
- Staging of surgery with re-assessment and physiological catch-up
- Careful control of haemorrhage, including the use of diathermy
- Maintenance of normothermia
- Active management of metabolic problems
- Prevention and early treatment of infection
- Notifying the laboratory if a surgical case was likely to require plasma or platelets.

Problems with platelets

There was an excellent supply of frozen materiel from the United Kingdom; the problem was platelets. Platelet support was traditionally indicated when there was micro-vascular bleeding due to thrombo-cytopenia. However, a higher count would be a useful buffer where there was ongoing consumption and dilution of platelets following major trauma, especially in association with inflammation or sepsis.

The limited shelf-life of platelets and the transport requirements prevented supply from the United Kingdom. The available alternatives to UK platelets were HN supply and the use of fresh whole blood using an *emergency donor panel* (EDP). HN supply was known to be a useful medical force multiplier in operations other than war. A supply of platelets was established from the Kuwait Central Blood Bank, a facility accredited by the American Association of Blood Banks. As the lines of communication were extended beyond the Kuwait border, a relay point was set up at in Northern Kuwait Hospital, with laboratory staff collecting platelets as required.

Caring for civilians

Following the fighting phase, many of the patients cared for in the field hospital were Iraqi, both prisoners of war and civilians. The civilians included women and children, both groups who presented transfusion challenges. Patients were often unable to provide consistent name spelling and dates of birth, so a unique alpha-numeric identifier was required. The case mix included primary and revision surgery for limb injuries and burns. However, care was complicated by pre-existing conditions and malnutrition. Many of the female patients appeared to have pre-existing microcytic anaemia. Haematologically, this was consistent with a combination of iron deficiency and beta thalassaemia trait. Both sickling haemoglobin (HbS) and thalassaemias are common in the Middle East.

It is worth noting that two patients tested positive for HbS. Another genetic variant common in this area is G6DP deficiency, which is characterised by a precipitous fall in haemoglobin following oxidative stress due to trauma, sepsis and drugs such as ciprofloxacin. The transfusion of children required small volumes of blood and plasma. The use of whole adult units was predicted to cause wastage. A more appropriate stock mix was required, including a group mix change and paediatric units.

Blood stock management

During *Operation Telic 1*, blood components were prepared for 84 patients; 47 patients received red cells. The mean dose was 5.3 units, with a range of 100 mL for a one-month child to 42 units required for a patient with deep seated infection of a gunshot wound (GSW). Most of these patients were cared for on intensive care unit (ICU). The diagnoses of ICU patients requiring blood were battle trauma (58.5%), burns due to domestic incidents (34.5%) and medical causes (6.9%). Caring for the local population had a considerable impact on blood stock management. Central planning assumptions had resulted in an initial blood stocks mix of blood groups O and A rather than the standard North Atlantic Treaty Organisation (NATO) mix. Table 14.1 shows the distribution of blood groups in the Iraqi patients contrasted with those of both a 'NATO' mix and the initial 250 units issued. Blood group B is more common in this region, and the lack of group B blood places pressure on the demand for group O.

UK red cells were issued with the usual 35-day shelf life, extended to 42 days on concession. The red cell stock was reduced from 250 to 150 units as it became clear that surgical activity was reducing. Traditionally, military units had offered blood to the host nation when the shelf life has reduced to approximately seven days. This was no longer permissible. During this period, 354 units were incinerated, including time-expired units from 84 Medical Supply Squadron. The impact of out of date blood must be considered when planning liquid clinical waste disposal.

Emergency donor panels

The EDP was used only once during the first seven weeks. Thirty-five donors had been screened during mobilisation before leaving the United Kingdom; others were screened in theatre. The first emergency bleed took place on day 1 of hostilities. Fresh whole blood was used to supply platelets following surgery for massive limb injury with evidence of microvascular bleeding and a platelet count of 30 × 10^9/L. Traditionally, the EDP contained only Group O donors, both Rhesus D positive and negative. However, with access to a full laboratory, a decision was made to bleed donors of the same blood group as the recipient where possible. The panel was actively managed, with new hospital staff being screened and tested following changeover of personnel. This required a postal service that could deal with biological material for definitive testing and an ability to communicate the results. The ability to collect whole blood in an emergency was also used by forward surgical teams with no access to haemostatic blood components.

2004: The tipping point

STOP THE BLEEDING

The lessons identified in Iraq by both the United States and United Kingdom appeared to have led to a 'tipping point' in modern military medical care. The experience from *Operation Iraqi Freedom*

Table 14.1 Distribution of ABO blood group in blood stocks and patients

	Initial stocks (%)	NATO mix (%)	Patient blood group (%)	Blood group of issued units (%)
O	60	50	27	36
A	40	42	37	38
B		8	29	26
AB			7	

had identified that haemorrhage was the cause of death of many 'survivable casualties'.[1,2] A Director General Army Medical Services (DGAMS) report following the Advanced Technology Applications to Combat Casualty Care (ATACCC) conference in August 2004 was subtitled 'Increasing survival on the battlefield as a result in advances in medically related technology'. The report summarised content from two conferences in Summer 2004 in the United States together with insights from other sources such as the Israeli Defence Forces. These programmes focused on advances in personal protection and pre-hospital care that could successfully deliver a range of tools to the front-line soldier. Such tools included new bandages and tourniquets and the need to gain better circulatory access with the 'Bone Injection Gun'. At the same time, the optimal use of fluids was being explored with the investigation of hypotensive resuscitation and the use of hypertonic solutions. In addition, novel haemostatics offered the promise of pre-hospital haemostasis. 'Stop the bleeding' would be both physical and physiological.

TRAUMA-INDUCED COAGULOPATHY

During this period, the historic view of the lethal triad was being replaced by epidemiological and molecular evidence for a distinct syndrome of *trauma-associated coagulopathy*. One of the earliest papers was the seminal work by Brohi et al. 2003,[3] which described the phenomenon that one third of civilian trauma patients had abnormal clotting on admission to hospital. The coagulopathy appeared to be an independent marker of morbidity and mortality and needed to be addressed during the clinical management of patients. The cause of the early coagulopathy was no longer thought to be only due to consumption, dilution of clotting factors and platelet dysfunction.[4] Evolving work introduced the concept that hypoperfusion, hyperfibrinolysis, activation of protein C and up-regulation of thrombomodulin pathways all contributed significantly to this early coagulopathy. These processes, as well as endothelial activation and subsequent coagulation changes, were thought to be mediated by hypoperfusion and tissue hypoxia.[4,5] The integrity of the hypoxic vascular endothelium controls fluid shifts and coagulation, but the exact details have yet to be determined. The consensus opinion

was that this was a tri-modal phenomenon with an immediate hypercoagulable state,[5] followed by a hypocoagulable period, and ending in a hyper-coagulable state. The haematological challenge was to support haemostasis in order to stop bleeding, without exacerbating hypercoagulability. A range of protocols were being adopted in 2005.[6,7] The policy maker's challenge was to agree on a simple, safe and standardised protocol.[8]

TRANSFUSION PROTOCOLS

UK policy for the management of massive haemorrhage on operations was developed during 2006 and issued as a Surgeon General's Operational Policy Letter in July 2007 and 2009.[9] The policy letter provided a brief rationale for the proactive use of blood and a new massive transfusion protocol (MTP). The policy recognised current definitions of massive transfusion, such as 10 units of red cell concentrate (RCC) in 24 hours. However, it introduced more relevant criteria such as rates of blood loss, mechanism of wounding and physiology in order to identify the casualty at risk. The primary clinical assessment would trigger the call for a 'shock pack'. Shock packs were pre-prepared packs of *red blood cells* (RBCs) and *thawed FFP*. Blood components were to be released initially as universal groups, and red cells were to be less than 14 days old where possible to minimise the effects of the red cell storage lesion.[10] This fixed formula approach contrasted with traditional civilian laboratory-based guidelines.[11] The perceived limitations were the delay in return of laboratory results and the limitations of conventional coagulation testing. The new approach was cautiously adopted by the European community,[12] but guidelines noted that the supporting evidence was limited to retrospective studies. The largest of these was the collation of US experience in Iraq by Borgman et al. 2007.[13] Civilian trauma centres reviewed their own data and increasingly supported the early use of plasma.[14-16] All agreed on rapid assessment and delivery, but controversy continued about component ratios and the use of novel haemostatics.

NOVEL HAEMOSTATICS

The new massive haemorrhage policy introduced the use of activated recombinant factor seven (rFVIIa). rFVIIa is a manufactured version of factor VIIa and is licensed to control bleeding in patients with haemophilia and clotting factor inhibitors. The drug was also available off-licence for use in the treatment of acquired coagulopathy. A multicentre randomised controlled trial had examined the efficacy of rFVIIa[17] and found that treatment with rFVIIa in blunt trauma produced a significant reduction in massive transfusion requirement in patients surviving for more than 48 hours. The first recorded UK military use of the drug had been described in 2005.[18] Although there were proponents, European guidelines recommended a cautious approach. UK military guidance for use was provided in 2007[19] and incorporated into policy. rFVIIa was to be considered only after first-line therapy had failed. When used, it was given alongside haemostatic substrate and normalisation of physiology, including core temperature. Later, a Cochrane review concluded that the use of rFVIIa as a haemostatic drug remained unproven. The Ministry of Defence (MOD) use of rFVIIa declined considerably following further developments in damage control resuscitation (DCR).[20]

BLOOD AND BOMBS

Experience derived from field hospital resuscitation of severely injured patients led to the development of DCR in both military and civilian practice. The new concepts were tested in a mass casualty event when, on 7 July 2005, the London transport network was subjected to a series of terrorist attacks. The bombings led to 56 deaths and 700 people being injured. Many hospitals activated their major incident plans. Approximately 360 casualties were received in emergency departments and 110 were admitted to five hospitals. By midnight, 23 patients, 3% of the total injured, had required transfusion with 338 units of red cells, 103 units of FFP, 235 pools of cryoprecipitate and 31 adult doses of platelets. Blood requirements continued over several weeks, with small peaks at day 5 and day 7. The subsequent review paper[21] points out that the use of blood components had not been emphasised previously in disaster planning. This was possibly due to many countries not having ready access to components, especially platelets. The review noted that the fixed formula approach was beginning to be used in the larger civilian trauma centres. The ratio of RCC and FFP used was nearer to 3:2, with

additional platelet and cryoprecipitate support as required.[22] An internal report to the blood service observed: 'The move towards haemostatic resuscitation and fixed formula shock packs in the UK since 2005 may lead to higher demand and use of components. The challenge will be not only the supply of group O D negative red cells, but also the provision of AB FFP and A D negative platelets'. External advice given to hospitals[23] highlighted the need for early communication with the blood bank and Blood Service. Systems must also maintain blood traceability and the cold chain in mass casualty events.

RULES AND REGULATIONS

Blood traceability and cold chain management were just two of the requirements of the new transfusion regulations. European Directive 2002/98/EC[24] had set standards of quality and safety for the collection, testing, processing, storage and distribution of blood. Directive 2004/33/EC[25] provided further technical guidance and required member states to bring into force the necessary laws, regulations and administrative provisions by 8 February 2005. The *Blood Safety and Quality Regulations 2005* (BSQR)[26] were laid before Parliament on 18 January. The regulations designated a competent authority, which was to be the *Medicines & Healthcare Products Regulatory Agency*, and authorized Blood Establishments to carry out the activities referred to in the regulations. A meeting was held in Birmingham on 23 February 2006 to discuss the details of the implementation of BSQR 2005 in the Armed Forces. The meeting proposed that *Blood Establishment Authorisation* would be required for distribution and that Officer Commanding *Blood Supply Team* (BST) would be the quality lead overseeing the new document control system. The most significant change was the requirement for a *Responsible Person (Blood)* as the licence holder on behalf of the Surgeon General. Full traceability of all blood leaving the United Kingdom would be required. Initially, this would be paper based, with an aspiration for an electronic system. The new transfusion stationery, including the three-part form FMed 692(01/06), was launched in 2006. An adverse events policy was already in place and all relevant reports would be filtered through the BST. The new regulatory framework and the increasing demand for blood would place an enormous burden on the newly formed BST.

FROM BIRMINGHAM TO BASTION

BST had previously been a part of the MSA based at Ludgershall. In the summer of 2004, ministerial approval had led to a fundamental restructuring resulting in MSA's transformation into the *Medical Supplies Integrated Project Team* (Med S IPT) on 1 April 2005. This change built on the transfer of the MSA from *Surgeon General's Department* (SGD) to the *Defence Logistics Organisation*. A small BST was created in Birmingham with blood provision, and testing contracted to the English *National Blood Service* with a civilian consultant adviser. NBS became part of *NHS Blood and Transplant* (NHSBT) on 1 October 2005 alongside UK Transplant. A close partnership developed between the three-man BST and Birmingham NHSBT. New developments in 2006 included the availability of BST and NHSBT staff 24/7, 365 days a year, to package military shipments, planning arrangements supporting supply surges and enhanced support for EDPs. Throughout the next decade, the blood supply partnership provided a global, safe and secure supply of blood to military personnel whilst fully complying with EU and UK standards. The partnership was awarded the Military Civilian Health Partnership Deployed Healthcare Award in 2011 for the successful delivery of 'Blood to the Battlefield'.

OPERATION HERRICK

Capability and capacity

In 2006, the entry into Helmand Province heralded an era of military medical response to increasingly complex and severe injuries.[27] During *Operation Herrick*, the laboratory at the newly established Camp Bastion started in a tent but finished in a modern spacious laboratory in a Tier 2 build. The introduction of the new transfusion policy required the handling of multiple components together with frequent monitoring. The casualty load was increasing, and there appeared to be no limit to the amount of blood that an individual could receive and survive.[28] As the workload increased, an increase in both capacity and

capability was required. Laboratory staffing was steadily increased from four to eight and laboratory services were increasingly automated as part of the massive transfusion capability (MTC).

Blood demand and stock management

The most significant impact of the changes in clinical policy and workload was the demand for blood components. An important early development was the introduction of a *Laboratory Information Management System* (LIMS) in 2009. LIMS, together with bar code readers, transformed the speed and accuracy with which staff could issue large amounts of blood components. The blood issued to theatre and BST activity from 2006 to 2014 is shown in Figures 14.3 and 14.4.

By 2014, the red cell use in Camp Bastion equated to that of a large district general hospital. However, there were significant differences. A large proportion of the components used were 'universal', for example group O negative RBC and group AB thawed FFP. In addition, red cells were issued with a shelf life of less than 14 days wherever possible. These demands stressed the supplying blood services and risked increasing wastage. One area of improvement that both reduced wastage and improved speed of delivery was the introduction in 2007 of a five-day post-thaw storage period for plasma. This increase, from 24 hours, was quite radical at the time and was not introduced into UK civilian practice until 2016.

Finally, there was the complexity of running a dual inventory with segregated US and UK components within the same laboratory. Most NATO countries traditionally provide their own transfusion support especially if large volumes are required. However, agreements exist to permit the use of blood from other nations during combat operations. An interesting consideration during this period was the potential impact of Variant Creutzfeldt–Jakob disease (vCJD) in Europe, first reported in 1996. Many countries presumed that infection might be transmissible via transfusion, and steps were taken to reduce the risks. From late 1999 onwards, all UK donations had undergone removal of white cells (leucodepletion) in order to reduce the risk of vCJD. The use of pre-thawed plasma was enabled through

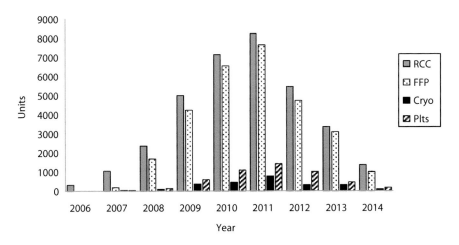

Figure 14.3 Total number of components transfused. Cryo: cryoprecipitate; FFP: fresh frozen plasma; Plts: platelets; RCC: Red cell concentrate.

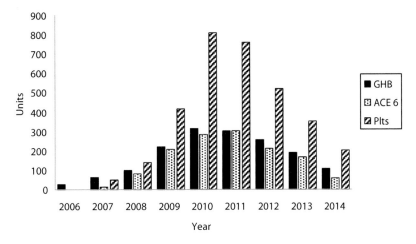

Figure 14.4 Number of boxes shipped by BST. The three temperature controlled transport systems are GHB for red cell, ACE 6 for frozen, Plts for platelet boxes.

the continuing use of the Sahara® convection heater, which had served well in Iraq.

More problems with platelets

The increasing severity of injury highlighted the need for a platelet supply. Work between BST and NHSBT had enabled a supply of fresh platelets from Birmingham three times a week from 30 May 2007. In addition, there was access to supplies from the United States at Kandahar. However, both relied on the air bridge from Kandahar Air Field to Bastion. Resilience necessitated the scoping of a local supply. The main options considered

were a frozen programme or a platelet apheresis programme based on the US model. The latter was selected as the best option. The first planning meeting was convened on 24 September 2007. Apheresis was introduced by the three-man team in the two theatres, Iraq and Afghanistan, with a full operating capacity declared in April 2008.

Apheresis is an automated system of component collection using a cell separator. It permits the collection of plasma and platelets whilst returning the red cells to the donor (Figure 14.5). The selected platform was the Haemonetics MCS®, which was being successfully used by the US programme. The capability was complex, requiring multiple lines of

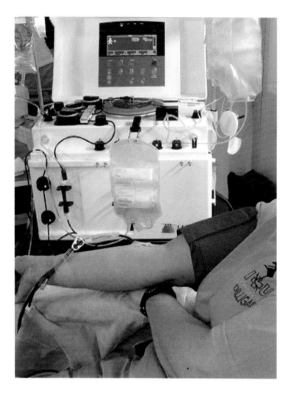

Figure 14.5 Platelet apheresis from a volunteer donor.

development. The EDP was expanded to recruit suitable group A donors to give repeat single donations at monthly intervals. However, in May 2009, there was the threat of a pandemic influenza in the United Kingdom, which threatened the potential blood supply to Bastion. Further resilience was required. It was met by the expansion of the EDP and introduction of double platelet doses.

Massive transfusion capability

The MTC was developed as an *Urgent Operational Requirement* (UOR) programme. The original papers were written in January 2010. However, many of the transfusion developments had started before that date as separate UORs. The programme continued through to October 2013. The purpose was to deliver transfusion support as an integrated part of resuscitation delivered as far forward as possible. It was an extraordinarily ambitious programme that covered both laboratory and clinical capability. Examples of the clinical elements included fluid delivery systems

and items for hypothermia mitigation. The concept of employment (definition of operational role) described four sub-capabilities that together delivered the MTC. These were the following:

- Blood product generation, including platelet apheresis and microbiology testing
- Blood product transport and storage
- Blood product delivery, including blood warmers and rapid infusers
- Blood testing: laboratory and near patient testing

The novel element was apheresis, and the *Automated Blood Culture Analyser* provided greater safety for these locally collected platelets.

GOLDEN HOUR BOXES

Cold chain management was one of the main elements of the MTC. Blood components require carefully monitored transport and storage, within specified temperature ranges. New introductions included the Acutemp RCB42P® fridge/freezer. One of the most significant advances in cold chain capability was the introduction of a new generation of passive transport containers that could maintain temperature without power.[27] These were sealed containers consisting of a fabric outer case and a vacuum insulated chamber with an inner, removable thermal isolation compartment. The type used was the Golden Hour Box® (GHB) (Minnesota Sciences and Credo). The main model was capable of maintaining storage temperatures of 2–8°C for up to 72 hours in external temperatures of 45°C. The storage temperature was continuously monitored using the TempIT® tag, a temperature indicator together with single-use time-temperature indicators WarmMark® and ColdMark®. The platelet version of the box was introduced to maintain temperatures at 22°C (±2). These boxes and the cold chain monitoring revolutionised the transport and storage of blood components and enabled blood to be projected forward.

Operation Vampire – Blood on board

The UK *Medical Emergency Response Team* (MERT) was an advanced medical retrieval platform based on a Chinook helicopter. In addition to standard en-route care, the physician-led team could administer resuscitation fluids using the intraosseous and central or peripheral intravenous routes, perform chest decompression and employ drug-assisted airway management. Blood had become the resuscitation fluid of choice in the hospital but would require temperature control to take it forward. The new generation of passive transport containers offered the promise of providing temperature control within the climatic challenge of the Helmand helicopters. The initial validation of the GHBs was completed jointly by NHSBT and BST during May and June 2008, and they were introduced shortly afterwards.

The introduction of the GHB® enabled the MERT teams to carry up to four units of packed RBCs and thawed FFP, for pre-hospital transfusion.[29] The call for MERT blood was affectionately termed *Operation Vampire*. O'Reilly's review of the initial experience of military pre-hospital transfusion showed that the mortality of matched patients who received pre-hospital blood transfusion was halved (8.2% vs. 19.6%).[30] The pre-hospital transfusion package became a part of the continuum of transfusion care through to goal directed therapy.

Goal-directed therapy

As transfusion developed, there was an increasing effort from 2008 onwards to individualise transfusion support after the initial pre-designated sequence. The challenge was whether to use standard laboratory diagnostic testing or to re-explore visco-elastic methodology. These old whole blood techniques promised to give a more dynamic interpretation of whole blood clotting and diagnose specific issues such as hyperfibrinolysis.[31] One of the drivers for introduction was that the bespoke treatment would minimise unnecessary use of blood components, thereby reducing donor exposure and preserving blood stocks. *Rotational thromboelastometry* (ROTEM™) was deployed to Afghanistan as a field trial in 2009 to determine its usefulness and reliability.[32] The investigators concluded that the machine was robust enough to be used in a field environment and was useful in detecting coagulopathy and improving outcomes.[33] The field trials demonstrated that the early A5 and A10 values were able to predict hypocoagulation, with sensitivities and specificities of 0.98/0.69 (A5) and 0.97/0.78.[34]

Ironically, the introduction of ROTEM™ increased rather than reduced the demand for platelets and cryoprecipitate.

Paediatric practice

Considerable attention and energy had been directed towards improving the treatment of injured troops. However, an unfortunate and inevitable outcome of war fighting as noted in previous sections was the presence of civilian casualties, including children. The causes included legacy munitions, enemy and coalition warlike activity. The paediatric workload in the military environment during recent conflicts was estimated to be 4% during *Operation Telic* (Iraq) and 8% for *Operation Herrick* (Afghanistan).[35] The figure for admissions to US *Combat Support Hospitals* was 10%. Previous military massive transfusion policies were adult-based guidelines, and there were few civilian examples. A Paediatric Anaesthesia and Critical Care Special Interest Group was therefore established. In 2010, the group published a paediatric massive haemorrhage protocol.[35] This was incorporated into *Clinical Guidelines for Operations* (CGOs) and training modules. The guidelines for children were similar to those of adults but based on body weight. In addition, there was emphasis on the practicalities of safe delivery of massive transfusion and on accurate monitoring.

Belmont buckets and cell salvage

Technology continued to play a part in the delivery of transfusion. One challenge in adults had been the need to deliver high-volume infusion of blood and plasma at physiological temperatures.[20] The Belmont FMS 2000® Rapid Infuser System was selected with use of the 3.0 L reservoir or 'bucket'. The use of this reservoir enabled red cells and plasma to be pre-mixed 1:1, sometimes referred to as 'Bastion Pink'. This equipment could deliver controlled flow rates of up to 750 mL/min of fluid at 37°C. The first save with the Belmont was described in an email to the author:

> …when the surgeons did their proximal control, he didn't bleed and his bowel looked white. We managed to get

800 ml of blood into him within the first 2 min via a single trauma line. He then proceeded to get a further 4 L of product (1:1) in the bucket in the next 8 min and 14 L overall in theatre in his 2 hr DCS procedure. His initial BE was −22, pH 6.8 and ROTEM was flat. He left theatre with a BE (base excess) of 1 and normal ROTEM. The Belmont® behaved impeccably with no stoppages or changes in giving sets.

Patients in military settings often require high volumes of blood products.[27] The logistic implications of use of blood from the United Kingdom are considerable and the need for resilience well demonstrated. *Intra-operative blood salvage* (IBS) offers the potential to reduce dependency on donated blood supply and may reduce allogeneic infectious risks. In November 2011, a small study showed that IBS was feasible in a military hospital in the combat environment.[36] It appeared to be more successful in cavity injuries and injuries associated with GSWs but required further microbiological and economic evaluation.

Tranexamic acid

An additional approach to reducing blood demand was the use of anti-fibrinolytic agents. These had long been shown to reduce blood loss in surgery without the risk of thrombotic complications.[37] Renewed interest and experience in civilian practice led to early adoption of tranexamic acid (TXA) as part of battlefield resuscitation.[20] However, it was the CRASH-2 trial (see list of trials, Table 14.2),[38] a global randomised controlled trial, that led to the wider adoption of TXA. The findings of the trial showed that TXA safely reduced the risk of death in bleeding trauma patients, that the all-cause mortality was reduced and that the risk of death from bleeding was reduced by 0.8%. CRASH sub-analysis suggests that it is the early use of TXA, within three hours, that delivers benefit. Despite some reservations about this study, there was emerging evidence for its use in combat-related haemorrhage. In August 2011, TXA was added to the US Joint Theatre Trauma System Clinical practice guidelines. The MATTERs study was published the following year. It confirmed not only the contribution from TXA but also the probable

Table 14.2 Summary of Transfusion Trials

CRASH 2 (Clinical Randomisation of an Antifibrinolytic in Significant Hemorrhage 2) A randomised controlled trial and economic evaluation of the effects of tranexamic acid on death, vascular occlusive events and transfusion requirement in bleeding trauma patients.

CRYOSTAT A multi-centre randomised controlled trial evaluating the effects of early high-dose cryoprecipitate in adult patients with major trauma haemorrhage requiring major haemorrhage protocol activation.

E-FIT (Early-Fibrinogen in Trauma) A multi-centre, randomised, double-blind, placebo-controlled trial evaluating the effects of early administration of fibrinogen concentrate in adults with major traumatic haemorrhage.

MATTERS (Military Application of Tranexamic Acid in Trauma Emergency Resuscitation) A study designed to characterise contemporary use of tranexamic acid in combat injury and to assess the effect of its administration on total blood product use, thromboembolic complications and mortality.

MICROSHOCK An observational study of the effects of traumatic injury, haemorrhagic shock and resuscitation on the microcirculation.

PROMMTT (Prospective, Observational, Multicenter, Major Trauma Transfusion) A study designed to relate in-hospital mortality to early transfusion of plasma and/or platelets and time-varying plasma:RBC and platelet:RBC ratios.

PROPPR (Pragmatic, Randomised Optimal Platelet and Plasma Ratios) A study designed to evaluate the difference in 24-hour and 30-day mortality among subjects predicted to receive massive transfusion (defined as receiving 10 units or more red blood cells within the first 24 hours).

synergy with higher fibrinogen levels. TXA was added to the CGOs[39] and its use was supported by NATO.[40]

Changes in practice

A retrospective UK audit documented the changes in component use during the first six years of this period[41] (Figure 14.6). Blood use per individual increased over time, as did survival. Overall, 28% of patients admitted for trauma required a transfusion. However, the percentage of patients transfused increased from 13% in 2006 to 32% in 2011. Massive transfusion increased fivefold over the period of study, from 4% in 2006 to 20% in 2011. The use of platelets and cryoprecipitate increased in the period of 2008–2009 and appears to correlate with the increased availability of those components and the introduction of ROTEM™. By the end of 2011, the mean component use for patients at the UK Role 3 with an Injury Severity Score of >16 was as follows: RCC 16, FFP 15, platelets 2 adult therapeutic doses and one pool (five doses) of cryoprecipitate. This initial transfusion was the start of a long transfusion journey, often continuing over several years during repeated revision surgery.

Massive transfusion was credited with contributing to the improved survival of the severely injured. It was, however, only one part of a carefully

considered and co-ordinated approach to the battlefield casualty. The increasing ability to provide transfusion support at all stages of the patient pathway emphasised the continuity of transfusion care.

BLOOD AND TRANSFUSION SAFETY

Blood safety

Blood transfusion is an essential part of modern healthcare. Although transfusion is associated with clinical risks, these are obviously low compared with those associated with combat injury. UK blood services have invested considerable efforts in blood safety with the introduction of universal leucodepletion for vCJD and nucleic acid testing for blood-borne viruses (BBVs). The introduction of male-only plasma was intended to reduce the risk of *transfusion-related acute lung injury*. The minimal residual risks were related to immune and other complications such as circulatory overload.[42] The focus of the UK haemovigilance system was on a safety culture designed to minimise human error. However, the past ghosts of hepatitis and human immunodeficiency virus (HIV) still loomed large in the minds of the press and the public.

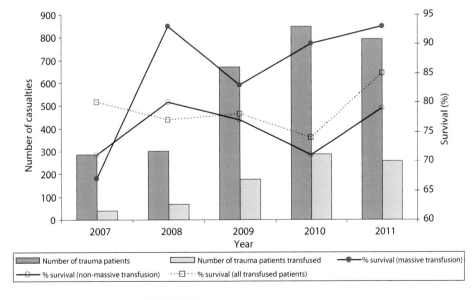

Figure 14.6 Changes in blood use 2007–2011.

'A bloody disgrace'

UK military donors are normally fully screened before emergency donation. However, it is recognised that transfusion may be life-saving and pretested donors may not be available. In January 2008, the British Press reported that 24 British soldiers and military contractors were undergoing HIV and hepatitis tests following revelations that the United States failed to screen donors who gave them emergency transfusions. Eighteen soldiers and six civilian contractors had been seriously wounded in Iraq or Afghanistan and received emergency blood sourced from the US military. The donors were not immediately tested after they gave blood, leaving the British unsure whether it was safe. A national look-back and counselling exercise was triggered, which met with considerable adverse press coverage. This was despite the fact that all donors had by then been tested and shown to be acceptable and that all transfusions were lifesaving. Representatives of the 'Tainted Blood' campaign, which represents thousands of haemophiliacs infected with HIV and hepatitis C after receiving contaminated blood in the late 1970s and 1980s, condemned the blunder as an 'absolute disgrace'. It was a valuable lesson in communication and expectation management.

Point-of-care testing

Emergency blood donors should be well at the time of donation, have an acceptable medical and lifestyle history and should be vaccinated against hepatitis B.[43] Some nations have additional safety measures, such as routine testing regimes for HIV. Options for operational blood testing include POCT of donors and post-donation testing of donors and recipients. The 'tainted blood' incident and the increasing need for platelets stimulated the scoping of POCT for locally collected blood and platelets. Funding was secured to commission a study from the *Health Protection Agency* in 2009 designed to evaluate commercially available methods for *donor testing* in the military environment. The challenge was to find CE marked tests with suitable sensitivity to detect infectious disease with a very low prevalence. High sensitivity may be associated with low specificity and

give rise to false-positives. Any positives, true- or false-positive, require very careful counselling and management when the donor is deployed. The DMS successfully introduced POCT tests for syphilis, hepatitis B and HIV1/2.

Pathogen inactivation and Parliamentary questions

An alternative approach to blood safety is pathogen inactivation, treatments designed to inactivate a range of pathogens rather than testing for individual ones. Techniques had been developed for the plasma fractionation industry, but new approaches were required for cellular components. Pooled, solvent detergent plasma was already available, and clinical trials had been completed for treatment of platelets. Most of the methods developed were effective against lipid-enveloped viruses and bacteria, but less so for non-enveloped viruses. In addition, most techniques had some impact on function. The UK blood services and, therefore, the DMS have not yet adopted pathogen inactivation. However, this did not stop a series of enquiries on this topic under the Freedom of Information Act and Parliamentary questions during November 2010 and January 2011. Pathogen inactivation technology continues to develop for plasma-rich components. More recently, the techniques have been applied to red cells. Whereas blood safety technology may become suitable for larger more permanent facilities, the current focus in DMS remains transfusion safety.

Transfusion safety

The biggest risk in transfusion is the transfusion of ABO incompatible blood. This is most likely to happen where blood of different groups is available, for example within the field hospital setting. Transfusion of the wrong blood to the wrong patient can result from errors made anywhere in the transfusion process, from blood sampling to the administration of blood. There were remarkably few events in theatre and no patient deaths due to transfusion; a considerable achievement, especially given the large number of components used in these recent conflicts. However, a sentinel event in 2011 in Bastion led to a Permanent Joint Headquarters transfusion review on 14 July 2011. The review confirmed that events were uncommon and most were reported soon after RIPs. As a consequence, a series of additional patient safety measures were initiated in 2011. The new measures included the establishment of a Defence transfusion committee: formalisation of training requirements including access to a national e-learning package,[44] a transfusion aide-memoire[39] and local clinical standard operating procedures. Transfusion reporting was further integrated into the new Defence electronic event reporting system. Most reported events were minor, related to process rather than transfusion reactions. However, it was recognised that there was a risk of under-reporting because the symptoms of *acute transfusion reactions* (ATRs) may be masked by the underlying condition. A new CGO was introduced in 2012[45] to reflect recent national guidance for the recognition and management of ATRs.[46] 2012 was the first complete year of electronic event reporting. The number of transfusion events fell from an estimated 1 per 1900 components transfused in 2012 to 1 per 3625 in 2013.[45] The key to success was training.[47]

Training

The requirement for the multi-disciplinary delivery of an operational transfusion capability was recognised. The UK solution was to use the civilian national framework supplemented by operational tools such as the Transfusion Aide Memoire. The Aide Memoire covered the 'vein-to-vein' process from blood sampling to care of the transfused patient. Transfusion was also formalised as a core operational competency for nursing staff, with transfusion *Operational Performance Statements* for both patient care and apheresis. Nursing was the key to the delivery of the apheresis capability. The training for apheresis nurses was enhanced in 2012 with training placements within NHSBT. The operational training package for *biomedical scientists* (BMS) was also enhanced. However, collective training was an essential element of mission rehearsal. Laboratory and clinical staff exercised together to deliver massive transfusion in a simulated, stressed but safe environment.

Transfusion committees

The increased complexity of transfusion services and the renewed emphasis on transfusion safety highlighted the organisational requirements for good governance. Under the chairmanship of the Defence Consultant Advisor (DCA), the DMS introduced a national DMS Transfusion Committee. The format was based on civilian structures,[48] with a multi-disciplinary committee answerable to the DMS Medical Director through the DMS Clinical Committee. The committee is unusual in that its remit covers all aspects of clinical transfusion practice, including donor care. It includes a number of civilian subject matter experts. The most important of these is the Civilian Adviser for Regulatory Affairs. The first holder of this appointment was from the Welsh Blood Service. The DMS transfusion community has a policy of open and transparent reporting and actively participates in national haemo-vigilance. The DMS experience of transfusion support for both trauma and pre-hospital care has actively informed civilian transfusion safety policy and practice.

Laboratory matters

The BMS community had implemented the new transfusion regulations within operational constraints, and many had deployed. They were supported by constantly improving operational laboratory training. In addition, the cadre were increasingly involved with the training of other staff. The contribution of the pathology community was all the more remarkable when some of the structural changes that were taking place at the same time place are recognised. In September 2007, the arrangements for the retained services at the Royal Hospital Haslar (RHH) were promulgated. Pathology posts that were on the RHH establishment were to be moved to MDHU Plymouth. However, this was an interim position pending the incremental build-up of the *Centre of Defence Pathology* (CDPath) in Birmingham. DCA Pathology, in conjunction with Commandant Royal Centre for Defence Medicine, produced a plan for the creation of the Centre for Defence Pathology in Birmingham.

In April 2016, the *Centre for Defence Pathology* was 'realised' and the Blood Supply Team returned to the DMS.

2009 – TAKING TRANSFUSION FORWARD

Role 2 review 2009

Transfusion support was now being delivered throughout the patient pathway from the MERT to Role 4. However, the use of fresh and frozen blood components ties the user to a base hospital. Thawed plasma constrains the configuration of retrieval assets and medical facilities and is not suitable for ground-based users working remote from the base. A Role 2 Transfusion Capability decision conference was convened on 16 July 2009. Representation included the three single-service commands and Director Special Forces. The rationale was that the improvements in resuscitation had led to significantly improved casualty survival rates for major trauma. Major determinants within the continuum of resuscitation were blood component replacement and the MTP. Advances in technology and the desire to deliver the optimum level of patient care quickly and as near to the point of wounding as possible led to experimentation designed to assess the feasibility of delivering an advanced transfusion capability at the Role 2 (Light manoeuvre) R2 (LM) MTF.[49] There was an expectation that this could include access to platelet support.[50] The record of decisions of the conference stated that the transfusion capability was to be RCC and FFP; that in exceptional cases, platelets might be available from an R2E/R3 hub; and that work should continue to determine the suitability of lyophilised plasma.

Freedom from frozen

The provision and re-supply of standard blood components have considerable logistic demands. Greater freedom can be provided by freeze-dried products. An important question is whether to use whole plasma or combinations of plasma fractions. During the decade of conflict, a number of lyophilised whole plasma products had been developed and successfully fielded.[51,52] These plasmas provided a balanced mix of clotting factors and fibrinogen in a volume of 200 mL when reconstituted.[53] The main disadvantage was that they were presented in glass bottles. LyoPlas-N, made by the German Red Cross (Deutsches Rotes Kreuz [DRK]), was available for procurement as an unlicenced drug in the UK (Figure 14.7). The scoping exercise and preparation of procurement process had taken place during 2010 including presentation to the Advisory Group on Military Medicine .

LyoPlas-N was introduced into service in January 2011, and the first documented use was in 2012.[54] The next step in the *Freedom from Frozen strategy* would be the introduction in 2016 of fibrinogen concentrate for forward resuscitation.

Moving forward

DMS experience in Afghanistan and Iraq helped to refine transfusion support to enduring medium scale operations. However, there was an increasing awareness that medical forces must be continually prepared for entry operations and for small-scale operations where patients may be held far longer than the doctrinal timeline of two hours. In addition, medical personnel would continue to be required to support discrete elements as well as deployed conventional forces. These requirements drove a clear requirement for medical treatment facilities to be able to deploy at all scales of effort

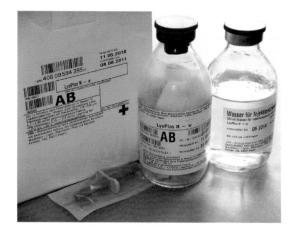

Figure 14.7 LyoPlas-N. A lyophilised single donor whole plasma.

and concurrency. The delivery of transfusion outside the hospital presents challenges, chiefly relating to the constraints of logistics. However, the demand for blood components can be reduced by optimising physical and physiological haemorrhage control. Drugs as well as blood are essential in haemostatic resuscitation; they also reduce the demand for blood. Examples of drugs incorporated into the 2010 Naval and Land policies include TXA, calcium and rVIIa.

EXPERIENCE AT SEA

Role 2 afloat

Previously, policy for Role 2 only provided for a basic transfusion and diagnostic capability. However, recent anti-piracy operations led to a request to revisit transfusion support at Role 2 afloat. The main considerations for forward deployment both on land and at sea are environmental control, weight, size, power and re-supply. Some degree of environmental control is required for laboratory equipment and consumables both during storage and transit. Equipment should be protected against a wide range of ambient temperatures, humidity and high levels of dust. Consideration must be given to a reliable power supply for automation. A ship-borne capability will also require robust connections to the on-board power source that can withstand potential repeated movement when subjected to the pitch and roll of the vessel. Role 2 afloat (Role 2A) platforms provided a stable environment but were constrained for space. In addition, if the resupply of red cells necessitated regular trips ashore this would inevitably remove the ship from its mission.

Maritime re-supply

Haemostatic resuscitation had led to the expectation that blood components would be provided for the duration of the mission. On land, this can be met by redistribution within theatre. Alternative sourcing can also be considered, such as coalition forces, HNS or contractors. However, these options do not fully address the challenge of providing haemostatic resuscitation in the maritime or isolated environment. The shelf life of components is likely to be shorter than the time at sea. In this environment, therefore, the priority was the re-supply of red cells as there are no available red cell substitutes. The feasibility of air-dropping blood was examined in 2012 and 2013; the challenge was not so much the mechanics of air-drop and sea recovery, but demonstrating the integrity of the red cell membrane during storage for up to 35 days. Tasking for the investigation was by the *Maritime Warfare Centre* (MWC) and successfully conducted in partnership between *JADTEU* (Air Warfare Centre), Blood Supply Team and NHSBT. The resulting TACNOTE was released by MWC in 2014 (MWC TACNOTE 11-2014).

LATER STAGES OF *OPERATION HERRICK*

Hook of Helmand

During the later stages of the Afghanistan campaign, ground-based Role 1 medical teams worked at *point of injury* (POI) and also on forward medevac platforms providing en-route care from POI to hospital. For most units, evacuation times were short; however, the pre-hospital emergency care capability evolved once more in order to meet a need for prolonged evacuation times as the geographical focus of military activity changed, extending south of previous areas of operations. Previously, Wild et al.[55] had described the equipment that enabled a Role 1 team to carry a vehicle-based blood capability on long-range mobility patrols. Gokhale et al.[54] then described the use of LyoPlas® carried and delivered on patrol by medics on the ground away from a firm base. Subsequently, a UK Role 1 medical team supporting a *helicopter assault force* based in southern Afghanistan delivered TXA, red cells and LyoPlas-N as a man-portable capability while awaiting CASEVAC. In a two-year audit, Aye Maung et al.[56] demonstrated that a Role 1 team, dislocated from a hospital laboratory, could maintain the cold chain required for forward blood products for prolonged periods.

The GHB system worked well within the austere environment; however, it was not designed as a man-portable system and required modification. In addition, a transfusion capability at this point in the medical chain imposes an additional logistic, training and governance burden, which has to be considered during medical planning.

Blood brothers

In 2015, a Blood Products Working Group was established to advise the MOD and military units on matters relating to the provision, use and storage of blood-related products. The working group offers an operationally focussed panel for development of clinical practice, equipment and training requirements. The group reports to the DMS Clinical Faculty Meetings and helps shape product development and research. Their recommendations for forward transfusion support concerned early use of TXA, RCC holdings based on the casualty estimate and resupply, plasma, a source of fibrinogen, calcium and rFVIIa, together with appropriate POCT. However, Role 1 capability will require further developments of the EDP if the capability is to have real utility in small isolated teams.[57] UK doctrinal notes were updated to reflect the use of a 'Blood Buddy' matrix for whole blood within a small team.[58] Changes in this programme based on international developments have also provided the initiative for subsequent military and civilian blood component research. Developments to allow the delivery of remote[59] or tactical[60] DCR have relevance to many remote or widely dispersed communities, as well as in disaster medicine. DMS investment in medical innovation is needed not only in the basic sciences but also in further translational research, operationalisation of new components, equipment and education.

GOING FORWARD

The evolution of military transfusion practice remains closely linked to the emergence of new evidence and developments in capability. Questions still remain and, with them, the requirement for well conducted research. The outcome of research and lessons identified must be tightly coupled with, and translated into, operational capability. The current military hospital model demonstrates that considerable integration is required to successfully deliver transfusion for combat care. Continuing partnership will be key to projecting the transfusion capability and meeting the requirements of future contingency operations.

Research

BACK TO THE BEGINNING

It is useful to return to the DGAMS report following ATACCC in August 2004 mentioned earlier in this chapter. DGAMS had highlighted the need to maintain an overview of current research in order to identify the areas that the United Kingdom could complement. The themes of the programme included organisational issues, command and control and managing bleeding. Subsequent advances in pre-hospital care have successfully delivered a range of tools to the frontline soldier. The need to gain better access has been met by the introduction of a variety of inter-osseous devices. Delivery has been further enhanced by warming devices and rapid fluid delivery systems. The debate regarding fluids is the province of others. However, artificial 'blood' has not progressed. Whole blood and blood components have increasingly been adopted as the best way to meet the needs of volume, oxygenation and haemostasis. Conversely, team training is mature and access to clinical decision support was delivered in 2016.

FROM PIGS TO PEOPLE

The themes of ATACCC were reflected in the early *Combat Casualty Care* research programme co-ordinated by the Defence Science and Technology Laboratories (Dstl). This research programme was focussed on the medical management of battlefield casualties from all non-CBRN weapons, characterisation of injury mechanisms and contributions to vulnerability and survival studies. The work started in 1 April 2006 and was scheduled to run in the first place to 31 March 2011, and then to 31 March 2013. Research activities were targeted through four *principal project areas*: resuscitation and stabilisation, haemorrhage control, diagnostic/prognostic tools and reduction in treatment times in order to maximise casualty throughput. The principal project area pertinent to transfusion medicine was haemorrhage control. It included not just haemostatic dressings but also resuscitation after blast injury and haemorrhage. The annual review 2008–2009 released in March 2010 showed that the findings from novel resuscitation studies had already informed doctrine, and coagulopathy studies provided the recommendations for field trials in direct support to operations. The activity had secured *Science and Technology Rapid Assistance to Operations* (STRATOS) support and, together with the revised Battlefield Advanced Trauma Life Support, was saving lives on operations. Although the programme had been planned in advance, it was clear that it was sufficiently agile to respond to direct drivers from the four principal project areas. It delivered rapid, innovative work where 'big wins' were possible. There was always a balance between completing pre-agreed programmes and maintaining horizon scanning of recent developments in medicine and basic science. The next challenge was to establish an infrastructure for deployed research (Table 14.2).

Deployed research

By 2012, the Role 3 Medical Treatment Facility (Field Hospital) in Camp Bastion was acknowledged to be one of the busiest dedicated trauma facilities in the world. Casualties typically presented with severe injuries and in physiological extremis. The casualties formed a unique cohort representing the most relevant population for evaluating the effectiveness of treating battlefield injuries. A deployed research article by Nordmann et al.[61] described four separate but related research projects that had been undertaken in Camp Bastion. Most of them were related to the haemostatic resuscitation element of the *Combat Casualty Care Research Programme*. Areas investigated included the aetiology and evolution of acute trauma coagulopathy; the alteration in platelet function in acute trauma coagulopathy; CRYOSTAT-MIL, the military arm of CRYOSTAT[62] (a randomised control trial looking at the feasibility of using cryoprecipitate early in the treatment of traumatic haemorrhage); and MICROSHOCK. The purpose of the paper was to describe and discuss some of the problems encountered and share the solutions that made research possible in an operational theatre.

The paper concluded that conducting research on deployed operations is challenging but possible with the right organisation and trained staff. Research becomes more feasible the longer a campaign continues.

Pre-hospital research

The deployed research paper focused on the Role 3 facility. The pre-hospital environment was more challenging. Important work was undertaken in partnership with US colleagues to look at the impact of pre-hospital interventions, including transfusion.[30,63] These retrospective studies had limitations, and the rationale for pre-hospital transfusion on short transfer remains unclear.[64] David O'Reilly stated 'Retrospective comparisons of outcome will be difficult because of confounding differences in other aspects of prehospital care and deficiencies in recording prehospital observations. In military practice, national differences and the operational environment exacerbate these concerns'.

One research group that focuses on the pre-hospital environment is the *Trauma Hemostasis and Oxygenation Research Network* (THOR). There has been a close affiliation between this group based in Bergen in Norway and individuals with an interest in resuscitation and transfusion. THOR is an international multidisciplinary group of investigators with a common interest in improving outcomes and safety in patients with severe traumatic injury. The network's mission is to reduce the risk of morbidity and mortality from traumatic haemorrhagic shock, in the pre-hospital phase of resuscitation through research, education and training. Following its third annual symposium in June 2013, the group produced a position statement that identified the major knowledge gaps in the field and provided a road map for future basic and applied research.[65]

People and partnership

One of the themes that run through the formal and informal research programmes is the benefit of collaborative effect. Dstl reports recognised the military academic partnerships of the *Academic Department of Military Emergency Medicine*,

Academic Department of Military Surgery, Academic Department of Military Anaesthesia and Critical Care and the DCA Transfusion Medicine. The collaborative association resulted in the integration of basic and applied science to provide the SGD with a source of relevant and timely advice. Other collaborations were made with institutes within the United Kingdom, especially where Defence personnel were already working with other organisations. Themed working groups also provided a valuable coordinating function. Examples include the Massive Transfusion and Thromboprophylaxis Working Group and the Pre-Hospital Blood Products Meeting in November 2013.

Innovation and implementation

Most of the applied Transfusion Medicine requirements have been organised with the *English National Blood Service* and its successor *NHSBT*. A contract was established with the Microbiology Reference Laboratory through STRATOS managed at Dstl. The work delivered a prioritised assessment of commercially available methods for POCT for BBVs. The results were reported to the stakeholders in September 2009 and immediately fielded. Subsequent work included validation of transport containers completed between BST and NHSBT Birmingham, which was immediately applied to the carriage of blood by MERT(E), and platelet transport. More recently, funding was secured by MWC to contract the NHSBT Components Development Laboratory to analyse the integrity of red cells dropped by parachute in the maritime environment. This work, in collaboration with a range of stakeholders, has been immediately translated into operational capability (Figure 14.8).

INDUSTRIAL AND INTERNATIONAL COLLABORATION

Partnerships for basic and applied research have also been international. Links with industrial partners have provided additional opportunities and resources. International research collaboration has been primarily exploited through *The Technical Cooperation Panel*, which avoids unnecessary duplication of effort. At DCA level, there has been collaborative effort through the NATO Blood Working Group. The spring 2014 meeting

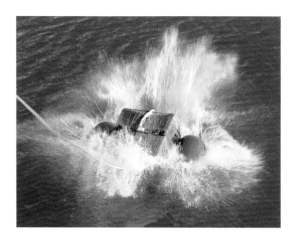

Figure 14.8 Airdrop trials for blood delivery in the maritime environment.

of this NATO group took place in Birmingham, together with a parallel research session chaired by the Defence Professor of Military Surgery. This was the first time that research had been integrated into what was primarily a policy and operationally focused group. The US representative was selected to collate the national priorities for research. The list of UK collated research priorities, dated 13 August 2014, included organisational developments and operational improvements. The main operational priorities were studies to underpin a transfusion capability within the austere environment. The first of the three formal research priorities was the evaluation of the early use of fibrinogen concentrates and cryoprecipitate in traumatic haemorrhage. This evaluation is currently being addressed through the E-FIT 1 and CRYOSTAT-2 studies co-ordinated by the NHSBT *Clinical Trials Unit*. The second priority was the ongoing evaluation of both blood products and drugs such as erythropoietin or statins during early resuscitation in order to determine the impact on coagulopathy, endotheliopathy and inflammation. The investigation of novel components and platelet enhancers continues within Dstl, and scoping studies are planned within NHSBT for the introduction of whole blood.

NEXT CHAPTER

Transfusion medicine continues to work closely with all of the defence professors, and the closest affiliation remains with the Department of

Military Anaesthesia and Critical Care. Transfusion research continues to be focused on determining why, how and when to use blood products; what alternatives may be available; and how the use of those products may impact on the delivery of DCR. The programme will continue to work closely with international collaborators, the DCA in Transfusion Medicine, the NATO Blood Working Group and the newly established *Centre of Defence Pathology* to design and deliver future capabilities. An example of the collaborative effort is a planned prospective UK–US observational study of haemostatic and immune-inflammatory changes during DCR in military trauma. The participant list reads like a Who's Who of modern trauma research.

LASTING LEGACY

Overview

Transfusion has become an essential element of combat care. In 2011, the survival of casualties who received massive transfusion was 93%. This success must be placed in the context of injury severity and the whole healthcare system, especially pre-hospital care. Combat stimulates innovation. Military developments are often based on emerging evidence and pragmatism. Many of the lessons identified from military medical and transfusion care were informally adopted in response to the 2005 London bombings[21] and the 2012 Olympics.[66] However, as the evidence base has developed, there has been a wider adoption of military transfusion practice.[67] The changes in transfusion practice started in 2003 were formally adopted in the 2016 National Institute for Health and Care Excellence guidelines for trauma.[68] This section reflects on some of the recent developments in civilian practice and the reasons for success.

Blood on board

During operations in Iraq and Afghanistan, transfusion support in the form of RCC and pre-thawed FFP together with TXA was successfully projected into the pre-hospital arena. The capability was developed in the context of severely injured patients recovered by helicopter-borne medical teams with transfer times of one to two hours. Retrospective studies of blood transfusion en route suggested a survival advantage from the advanced care in transit.[30] The London-based *Helicopter Emergency Medical Service* team introduced RCC as 'blood on board' in 2012, just before the London Olympic Games. There has been increasing interest in the use of pre-hospital blood.[69] The air ambulance service in Wales extended their capability to include a wide range of haemostatic products. The value of pre-hospital transfusion for short transfers is debated. Midwinter et al. have argued that prospective studies are required before routine introduction into civilian practice.[64]

Trauma: who cares?

The UK Major Trauma Network was created in 2012 and adopted many military practices. Major trauma already had excellent, long-term audit data from the *Trauma Audit and Research Network*, which has informed peer review of the new services. The 2015 round of peer review, undertaken between January 2015 and March 2015, noted that the probability of survival from trauma had significantly improved over the previous three years. All UK major trauma centres and networks are now required to have a massive haemorrhage protocol. Evolving UK transfusion guidelines from 2010[70–72] onwards have emphasised early haemorrhage control, use of TXA and a foundation of RCC and FFP in a 2:1–3:2 ratio followed by goal-directed therapy. The early involvement of senior experienced clinicians, well-rehearsed teams and trauma registries was acknowledged as essential. However, the evolution of knowledge and continuing uncertainties reinforce the need for quality research to be embedded into routine practice.[73]

Transfusion guidelines

Recently completed trials in traumatic haemorrhage include PROMMTT,[74] published in 2013, and PROPPR.[75] Despite perceived limitations, these trials appear to be the tipping point for the change in UK civilian transfusion guidelines. In 2015, the *British Committee for Standards in Haematology*[72] supported the early use of plasma-rich protocols in haemorrhage in RCC:FFP ratios of 3:2 to 1:1.

The implications for practice were important, as the immediate demand for plasma has highlighted some of the delays associated with using frozen plasma. The introduction of five-day pre-thawed plasma[76] has provided 'plasma now' and should reduce one of the practical barriers to the timely delivery of plasma in civilian practice. The complexities of component therapy for haemorrhage have led to the demand to revisit the use of whole blood. Whole blood would provide physiological resuscitation and reduced donor exposure and can be supplemented with fibrinogen if appropriate. It is an interesting direction for future development for both civilian and military practice.

Demand planning

The wider use of 'Massive Transfusion' protocols has led to an increased initial demand for 'universal' components such as group O negative RCC and AB FFP as well as an increased demand for platelets and cryoprecipitate. Such trends need to be factored into local and national demand planning. The technical annex of the 2015 transfusion guidelines endorsed the use of group A HT (high titre) negative plasma as an alternative universal product.[72] Likewise, it is anticipated that the 2017 guidance for the use of red cells will support the use of O D positive blood for males and older women. Both of these national guidelines will in turn impact on military practice. Recent trial results have changed the military guidance for the age of blood in shock packs. The age of RCCs in military transfusion 'shock packs' had been less than 14 days. There was a theoretical basis for this practice, but the clinical evidence was equivocal. The reduced shelf life risked shortfall in availability and increased outdating. The outcomes of studies such as the *Age of Blood Evaluation* trial showed no advantage in the use of 'young blood'.[77]

Mass casualty events

The recent terrorist incidents in Paris and Brussels remind us that the UK civilian population is not immune from the challenges seen in military medicine. The care of the critically ill patient is demanding; however, this is particularly complicated in the mass casualty situation. The recent bombings have led to a review of UK major trauma services and blood services and their ability to respond to such a threat. Preparation has included study days, modelling and table top exercises. Mass casualty events may result in a demand for blood that cannot be immediately met. Therefore, blood supply should be part of civilian emergency planning. Whereas sporting events, such as the Olympics, and other mass gatherings can be planned for, mass casualty events such as bombings require resilience within the wider health service system, including pre-hospital haemorrhage control.[78]

CONCLUSION

Transfusion support has contributed enormously to the Defence capability framework. Defence can now better protect military personnel by providing timely test results to guide clinical interventions and by ensuring a resilient supply of vital blood products. The provision of a digital results and blood component records archive has enhanced access, not only delivering best practice but also supporting research and audit opportunities. This has in turn supported evidence-based medicine, leading to peer-reviewed publications and improvements in medical care. The speed of improvement has been due to a tri-service, multi-disciplinary approach to operational capability. Financial investment has been important. However, more important has been the work with strategic partners. Tactical combat casualty care (TCCC), begun in 2001, led the way in pre-hospital care. Much of its success has been due to strong partnerships with other organisations. Likewise, within the transfusion communities, partnerships have not only permitted rapid development but have also benefitted the wider healthcare community. The legacy of recent conflict is better trauma care for all.

REFERENCES

1. Kelly JF, Ritenour AE, McLaughlin DF et al. Injury severity and causes of death from Operation Iraqi Freedom and Operation Enduring Freedom: 2003–2004 versus 2006. *J Trauma* 2008;64(2):S21–S27.

2. Butler FK Jr, Blackbourne LH. Battlefield trauma care then and now: A decade of tactical combat casualty care. *J Trauma Acute Care Surg* 2012;73(6 Suppl 5):S395–S402.

3. Brohi K, Singh J, Heron M, Coats T. Acute traumatic coagulopathy. *J Trauma* 2003;54(6):1127–1130.

4. Allen SR, Kashuk JL. Unanswered questions in the use of blood component therapy in trauma. *Scand J Trauma Resusc Emerg Med* 2011;19:5. doi:10.1186/1757-7241-19-5.

5. Ganter MT, Cohen MJ, Brohi K et al. Angiopoietin-2, marker and mediator of endothelial activation with prognostic significance early after trauma? *Ann Surg* 2008;247(2):320–326.

6. Johansson PI, Hansen MB, Sørensen H. Transfusion practice in massively bleeding patients: Time for a change? *Vox Sang* 2005;89(2):92–96.

7. Holcomb JB, Jenkins D, Rhee P et al. Damage control resuscitation: Directly addressing the early coagulopathy of trauma. *J Trauma Inj Infect Crit Care* 2007; 62(2):307–310.

8. Malone DL, Hess JR, Fingerhut A. Massive transfusion practices around the globe and a suggestion for a common massive transfusion protocol. *J Trauma* 2006;60 (6 Suppl):S91–S96.

9. Surgeon General. Surgeon General's Operational Policy Letter: Management of massive haemorrhage on operations. SGPL Number: 10/07 2009.

10. Lelubre C, Piagnerelli M, Vincent JL. Association between duration of storage of transfused red blood cells and morbidity and mortality in adult patients: Myth or reality? *Transfusion* 2009;49(7):1384–1394.

11. British Committee for Standards in Haematology, Stainsby D, MacLennan S, Thomas D, Isaac J, Hamilton PJ. Guidelines on the management of massive blood loss. *Br J Haematol* 2006;135(5):634–641.

12. Spahn DR, Cerny V, Coats TJ et al. Management of bleeding following major trauma: A European guideline. *Crit Care* 2007;11(1):R17.

13. Borgman MA, Spinella PC, Perkins JG et al. The ratio of blood products transfused affects mortality in patients receiving massive transfusions at a combat support hospital. *J Trauma* 2007;63(4):805–813.

14. Gunter OLJ, Au BK, Isbell JM, Mowery NT, Young PP, Cotton BA. Optimizing outcomes in damage control resuscitation: Identifying blood product ratios associated with improved survival. *J Trauma* 2008; 65(3):527–534.

15. Sperry JL, Ochoa JB, Gunn SR et al. An FFP:PRBC transfusion ratio >1:1.5 is associated with a lower risk of mortality after massive transfusion. *J Trauma* 2008; 65(5):986–993.

16. Duchesne JC, Hunt JP, Wahl G et al. Review of current blood transfusions strategies in a mature level 1 trauma center: Were we wrong for the last 60 years? *J Trauma* 2008;65(2):272–276; discussion 276–278.

17. Boffard KD, Riou B, Warren B et al. NovoSeven Trauma Study Group. Recombinant factor VIIa as adjunctive therapy for bleeding control in severely injured trauma patients: Two parallel randomized, placebo-controlled, double-blind clinical trials. *J Trauma Inj Infect Crit Care* 2005;59(1):8–15; discussion 15–18.

18. Williams DJ, Thomas GOR, Pambakian S, Parker PJ. First military use of activated Factor VII in an APC-III pelvic fracture. *Injury* 2005;36(3):395–399.

19. Hodgetts TJ, Mahoney PF, Kirkman E. Damage control resuscitation. *J R Army Med Corps* 2007;153(4):299–300.

20. Dawes R, Thomas GOR. Battlefield resuscitation. *Curr Opin Crit Care* 2009; 15(6):527–535.

21. Glasgow SM, Allard S, Doughty H, Spreadborough P, Watkins E. Blood and bombs: The demand and use of blood following the London Bombings of 7 July 2005 – a retrospective review. *Transfus Med* 2012;22(4):244–250.

22. Davenport R, Khan S. Management of major trauma haemorrhage: Treatment priorities and controversies. *Br J Haematol* 2011;155(5):537–548.

23. Doughty H, Allard S. Responding to major incidents – lessons learnt from July 2005 London bombings. *Blood Matters* 2006; 2006(20):14–15.

24. Directive 2002/98/EC of the European Parliament and of the Council 27 January 2003 Standards of quality and safety for the collection, testing, processing, storage and distribution of human blood and blood components.

25. Directive 2004/33/EC of the European Parliament and of the Council 22 March 2004 Certain technical requirements for blood and blood components.

26. BSQR. Blood Safety and Quality Regulations 2005 UK Statutory Instrument No. 50. www.opsi.gov.uk.

27. Doughty HA, Woolley T, Thomas GOR. Massive transfusion. *J R Army Med Corps* 2011;157(3 Suppl 1):S277–S283.

28. Allcock EC, Woolley T, Doughty H, Midwinter M, Mahoney PF, Mackenzie I. The clinical outcome of UK military personnel who received a massive transfusion in Afghanistan during 2009. *J R Army Med Corps* 2011;157(4):365–369.

29. O'Reilly DJ, Morrison JJ, Jansen JO, et al. Special report: Initial UK experience of prehospital blood transfusion in combat casualties. *J Trauma Acute Care Surg* 2014;77(3 Suppl 2):S66–S70.

30. O'Reilly DJ, Morrison JJ, Jansen JO, Apodaca AN, Rasmussen TE, Midwinter MJ. Prehospital blood transfusion in the en route management of severe combat trauma: A matched cohort study. *J Trauma Acute Care Surg* 2014;77(3 Suppl 2): S114–S120.

31. Martini WZ, Cortez DS, Dubick MA, Park MS, Holcomb JB. Thrombelastography is better than PT, aPTT, and activated clotting time in detecting clinically relevant clotting abnormalities after hypothermia, hemorrhagic shock and resuscitation in pigs. *J Trauma* 2008;65(3): 535–543.

32. Doran CM, Woolley T, Midwinter MJ. Feasibility of using rotational thromboelastometry to assess coagulation status of combat casualties in a deployed setting. *J Trauma Inj Infect Crit Care* 2010;69(Suppl 1): S40–S48.

33. Doran CM, Doran CA, Woolley T et al. Targeted resuscitation improves coagulation and outcome. *J Trauma Acute Care Surg* 2012;72(4):835–843.

34. Woolley T, Midwinter M, Spencer P, Watts S, Doran C, Kirkman E. Utility of interim ROTEM® values of clot strength, A5 and A10, in predicting final assessment of coagulation status in severely injured battle patients. *Injury* 2013;44(5):593–599.

35. Bree S, Wood K, Nordmann GR, McNicholas J. The paediatric transfusion challenge on deployed operations. *J R Army Med Corps* 2010;156(Suppl 4): S361–S364.

36. Bhangu A, Nepogodiev D, Doughty H, Bowley DM. Intraoperative cell salvage in a Role 3 combat support hospital: A prospective proof of concept study. *Transfusion* 2013;53(4):805–810.

37. Henry DA, Moxey AJ, Carless PA et al. Anti-fibrinolytic use for minimising perioperative allogeneic blood transfusion. *Cochrane Database Syst Rev (Online)* 2001;(1):CD001886.

38. CRASH-2 Trial Collaborators. Effects of tranexamic acid on death, vascular occlusive events, and blood transfusion in trauma patients with significant haemorrhage (CRASH-2): A randomised, placebo-controlled trial. *Lancet* 2010;376(9734): 23–32.

39. Royal Centre for Defence Medicine (Academia & Research) MDJMCobotSG. Joint Service Publication 999 (Clinical Guidelines for Operations). 2013. https://www.gov.uk/government/publications/jsp-999-clinical-guidelines-for-operations.

40. Heier HE, Badloe J, Bohonek M et al. Use of tranexamic acid in bleeding combat casualties. *Mil Med* 2015;180(8):844–846.

41. Jansen JO, Morrison JJ, Midwinter MJ, Doughty H. Changes in blood transfusion practices in the UK role 3 medical treatment facility in Afghanistan, 2008–2011. *Transfus Med* 2014;24(3):154–161.

42. Bolton-Maggs PHB, Poles D et al., on behalf of the Serious Hazards of Transfusion (SHOT) Steering Group. The 2014 Annual SHOT Report. 2015. www.shotuk.org.

43. Doughty H, Thompson P Cap A. A proposed field emergency donor panel questionnaire and triage tool. *Transfusion* 2016;56(S2):S119–S127.

44. Graham JE. Transfusion e-learning for junior doctors: The educational role of 'LearnBloodTransfusion.' *Transfus Med* 2015;25(3):144–150.

45. Scorer T, Doughty H. Acute transfusion reactions: An update. *J R Naval Med Serv* 2014;100(3):316–320.

46. Tinegate H, Birchall J, Gray A et al. Guideline on the investigation and management of acute transfusion reactions Prepared by the BCSH Blood Transfusion Task Force. *Br J Haematol* 2012;159(2): 143–153.

47. National Blood Transfusion Committee. Requirements for Training and Assessment in Blood Transfusion. Version 1 March 2016. Accessed 19 April 2016. www.NBTC%20 Requirements%20for%20Training%20 and%20Assesment%20FINAL%20(1).pdf.

48. Department of Health. Better Blood Transfusion. Appropriate Use of Blood. Health Service Circular HSC 2002/09 2002.

49. HQLF. 16 Med/G5/5065. Dated 5 Feb 2009.

50. Path/Admin 1.26. Platelet transfusion support to Role 2 medical treatment facility. Dated 5 May 2006.

51. Martinaud C, Ausset S, Deshayes AV, Cauet A, Demazeau N, Sailliol A. Use of freeze-dried plasma in French intensive care unit in Afghanistan. *J Trauma Inj Infect Crit Care* 2011;71(6):1761–1765.

52. Noorman F, Strelitski R, Badloe J. Lyophilized plasma, an alternative to 4°C stored thawed plasma for the early treatment of trauma patients with (massive) blood loss in military theatre. *Transfusion* 2012;52(Suppl s3):55A.

53. Shuja F, Shults C, Duggan M et al. Development and testing of freeze-dried plasma for the treatment of trauma-associated coagulopathy. *J Trauma Inj Infect Crit Care* 2008;65(5):975–985.

54. Gokhale SG, Scorer T, Doughty H. Freedom from frozen – the first British military use of lyophilised plasma in forward resuscitation. *J R Army Med Corps* 2016;162(1):63–65.

55. Wild G, Anderson D, Lund P. Round Afghanistan with a fridge. *J R Army Med Corps* 2013;159(1):24–29.

56. Aye Maung N, Doughty H, MacDonald S, Parker P. Transfusion support by a UK Role 1 medical team – a two year experience from Afghanistan. *J R Army Med Corps* 2016;162:440–444.

57. Parker P, Nordmann G, Doughty H. Taking transfusion forward. *J R Army Med Corps* 2015;161(1):2–4.

58. Establishment and management of emergency blood donor panels [pamphlet]. JSP 950 Leaflet 2-24-3. Defence Medical Services. 2014.

59. Jenkins D, Stubbs J, Williams S et al. Implementation and execution of civilian remote damage control resuscitation programs. *Shock* 2014;41(Suppl 1):84–89.

60. Fisher AD, Miles EA, Cap AP, Strandenes G, Kane SF. Tactical Damage Control Resuscitation. *Mil Med* 2015;180(8): 869–875.

61. Nordmann G, Woolley T, Doughty H, Dalle Lucca J, Hutchings S, Kirkman E. Deployed research. *J R Army Med Corps* 2014; 160(2):92–98.

62. Curry N, Rourke C, Davenport R et al. Early cryoprecipitate for major haemorrhage in trauma: A randomised controlled feasibility trial. *Br J Anaesth* 2015;115(1):76–83.

63. Morrison JJ, Oh J, Dubose JJ et al. En-route care capability from point of injury impacts mortality after severe wartime injury. *Ann Surg* 2013;257(2):330–334.

64. Smith IM, James RH, Dretzke J, Midwinter MJ. Prehospital blood product resuscitation for trauma: A systematic review. *Shock* 2016;46(1):3–16.

65. Jenkins DH, Rappold JF, Badloe JF et al. Trauma hemostasis and oxygenation research position paper on remote damage control resuscitation: Definitions, current practice, and knowledge gaps. *Shock* 2014;41(Suppl 1):3–12.

66. Glasgow SM, Allard S, Rackham R, Doughty H. Going for gold: Blood planning for the London 2012 Olympic Games. *Transfus Med* 2014;24(3):145–153.

67. Doughty H. Recent developments in military transfusion and the impact on civilian practice. *Blood Transplant Matt* 2014;42:4–5.

68. National Institute for Health and Care Excellence (NICE). Major trauma: Assessment and initial management (NG39). NICE Guideline 2016. nice.org.uk/guidance/ng39.

69. Weaver AE, Thompson J, Lockey DJ. The effectiveness of a simple 'Code Red' transfusion request policy initiated by pre-hospital physicians. *Scand J Trauma Resusc Emerg Med* 2012;20(Suppl 1):O1.

70. Thomas D, Wee M, Clyburn P, et al. Blood transfusion and the anaesthetist: Management of massive haemorrhage. *Anaesthesia* 2010;65(11):1153–1161.

71. Klein AA, Arnold P, Bingham RM et al. AAGBI guidelines: The use of blood components and their alternatives 2016. *Anaesthesia* 2016;721:829–842. doi:10.1111/anae.13489.

72. Hunt BJ, Allard S, Keeling D, Norfolk D, Stanworth SJ, Pendry K, on behalf of the British Committee for Standards in Haematology. A practical guideline for the haematological management of major haemorrhage. *Br J Haematol* 2015;170(6):788–803.

73. Doughty H. Transfusion guidelines: Mind the gap (Editorial). *Anaesthesia* 2016;71(7):743–747.

74. Holcomb JB, del Junco DJ, Fox EE et al. The Prospective, Observational, Multicenter, Major Trauma Transfusion (PROMMTT) Study: Comparative effectiveness of a time-varying treatment with competing risks. *J Am Med Assoc Surg* 2013;148(2):127–136.

75. Holcomb JB, Tilley BC, Baraniuk S et al. Transfusion of plasma, platelets, and red blood cells in a 1:1:1 vs a 1:1:2 ratio and mortality in patients with severe trauma: The PROPPR Randomized Clinical Trial. *JAMA* 2015;313(5):471–482.

76. Green L, Cardigan R, Beattie C et al. Addendum to the British Committee for Standards in Haematology (BCSH): Guidelines for the use of fresh-frozen plasma, cryoprecipitate and cryosupernatant, 2004 (*Br. J Haematol* 2004,126,11–28). *Br J Haematol* 2017;178(4):646–647.

77. Lacroix J, Hébert PC, Fergusson DA, et al. Age of transfused blood in critically ill adults. *N Engl J Med* 2015;372(15):1410–1418.

78. Doughty H, Glasgow S, Kristoffersen E. Mass casualty events: Blood transfusion emergency preparedness across the continuum of care. *Transfusion* 2016;56(S2): S208–S216.

15

Mental health

INTRODUCTION

This chapter describes the mental health impact of UK military operations in Iraq and Afghanistan based on original, mostly United Kingdom or international, collaborative research published during the period of the deployments in Iraq and Afghanistan. The account is structured according to the phases of deployment, namely pre-deployment preparation, participation in operations and post-deployment recovery. Military mental health is a broad concept that extends far beyond the boundaries of clinical care; therefore, within each of the three domains, mental health research conducted among UK Armed Forces personnel is used to explore the prevalence of psychological disorders, the detection of mental health problems, mental health and well-being support measures and remedial interventions.

Although they are but a component of deployed mental health support, and the bulk of mental healthcare is undertaken by deployed primary healthcare services; deployed specialist clinical services are the sole source of dedicated frontline mental healthcare on operations. This chapter therefore offers a brief overview of the *Field Mental Health Teams* (FMHTs) deployed in support of operations in Iraq and Afghanistan before providing an in-depth account of deployment mental health and well-being.

MENTAL HEALTH SUPPORT TO UK FORCES DEPLOYED IN IRAQ AND AFGHANISTAN

Background

When undertaking operational deployment, UK Armed Forces units are supported by mental health professionals who deploy as *FMHTs*. The FMHT typically consists of *community mental health nurses* (CMHNs) and psychiatrists. FMHT staff include regular and reserve personnel drawn from the three Service branches: Royal Navy, Army and Royal Air Force (RAF). Regular forces CMHNs offer a clinical service to serving regular and reserve personnel in the non-deployed setting, which allows them to acquire and rehearse a number of clinical competencies, including the use of evidence-based therapies such as *trauma-focused cognitive and behaviour therapy* and *eye movement desensitisation and reprocessing* therapy,[1] which they can utilise during deployment. Prior to deployment, military psychiatrists spend time acquiring skills in diagnosis, prescribing and clinical and occupational risk assessment for a clinical population that is markedly different from that found in civilian practice.

Reserve forces CMHNs and psychiatrists work in civilian mental healthcare settings where they are able to develop their clinical skills with supplementary annual military training and intensive, mission-specific, pre-deployment preparatory training. Many undertake attachments to regular forces mental healthcare facilities during peacetime. In the deployed setting, military CMHNs work autonomously, carrying out face-to-face assessments, discussing management decisions with the senior medical officer responsible for units in their area of operations and with intermittent support from visiting military psychiatrists deploying from the firm base. CMHNs are the backbone of the FMHT, and their autonomy allows them to deploy flexibly across a range of locations with remote access to advice from non-deployed psychiatrists in the United Kingdom when telecommunications and electronic communications allow. Deployed mental healthcare is necessarily brief or time limited and is organised around the doctrine of 'forward psychiatry'[2] using the principles of PIES,[3] which, although not an intervention per se, continues the occupational health framework used in the non-deployed setting. Within the PIES concept, *proximity* demands that intervention takes place close to the battle area, *immediacy* encourages early active management, *expectancy* refers to the notion of recovery and return to duty and *simplicity* relates to the use of brief, uncomplicated intervention(s). Interestingly, 2016 was the 100th anniversary of the UK Armed Forces adopting PIES and forward psychiatry during the Somme campaign of the First World War. World War I was the original setting for the development of a number of modern National Health Service (NHS) mental health interventions, including crisis care and home treatment services, even if it is rarely acknowledged as such.

In addition to clinical intervention, FMHT personnel conduct psychoeducation for newly deployed personnel during their orientation training immediately after arrival in theatre, which seeks to promote good self-management, encourage peer support and raise awareness of mental health matters for at-risk groups such as combat personnel and those undertaking unpleasant duties or frequently dangerous roles. A similar briefing is repeated at the end of deployment, often during a period of decompression conducted away from the operational area. The FMHT provides a mental health advisory service for padres, medical

officers, their staffs, commanders at all levels, civilian contractors and other deployed civilians.

FMHT in Iraq

During the initial ground and air campaign, each Brigade formation deployed integral psychiatric assets. *16 Close Support Medical Regiment (CSMR)* deployed an FMHT comprising four mental health nurses and one psychiatrist who supported *16 Air Assault Brigade* during the *relief in place* (RIP – replacement of one military unit by another) operation in the Rumaila oil field and then during follow-up operations in and around Al Amarah in Maysan province. *5 General Support Medical Regiment* deployed one psychiatrist and two mental health nurses supporting the 1st Division rear area. Following the ground assault, a *Battle Group Recuperation Centre* was opened by the 5 general support team, which was supported by one CMHN. *1 CSMR* deployed one psychiatrist and four mental health nurses supporting *7 Armoured Brigade* units. The Role 3 hospital capability consisted of psychiatric departments located in *34 and 33 (Regular) Field Hospitals* and *202 (Volunteer) Field Hospital*; each hospital department was staffed by one consultant psychiatrist and at least two community psychiatric nurses. *202 (V) Field Hospital* relieved 33 *Field Hospital* in North Kuwait prior to the invasion and performed an RIP for *34 Field Hospital* at Shaibah airfield in Iraq before handing over to *33 Field Hospital* and returning to the United Kingdom. Following cessation of the ground war phase of *Operation Telic* and the transition to *Operation Telic* 2, all in-theatre support from military psychiatrists was withdrawn and a team of five mental health nurses deployed within Shaibah Logistic Base to provide the bulk of the clinical effort, at the theatre airhead to deliver arrival and departure briefs, within Basra Palace and deployed to Al Amarah to support the forward Battle Group.

The Royal Navy deployed a mental health team as part of the *Primary Casualty Receiving Facility* (PCRF) aboard *Royal Fleet Auxiliary Argus* to support the commando amphibious/ground assault on the Al Faw peninsula and to provide broader mental health support to maritime forces. The team consisted of one psychiatrist and three mental health nurses. On cessation of the initial ground campaign, the deployed Royal Navy capability was withdrawn; however, Royal Navy mental health nurses continued to contribute personnel intermittently to the FMHT. *3 Commando Brigade* was supported on land by a naval mental health team consisting of two nurses. *3 Commando Brigade* was the only formation to provide a sizeable and integral *Trauma Risk Management* (TRiM) capability. TRiM is a peer support programme that aims to connect personnel experiencing persistent psychological trauma to the right support at the right time.

Throughout the deployment to Iraq, the RAF provided a call-forward aeromedical evacuation capability of two aeromedically trained mental health nurses, based in the forward operating base established in RAF Akrotiri; their mission was to transport mental health casualties home. Throughout the deployment to Iraq, the FMHT was predominantly regular Army led, with strong support from the reserves; as the *Telic* deployment progressed, the RAF contributed a small number of mental health nurses to the FMHT, as did the Royal Navy when *3 Commando Brigade* led the phase of deployment.

As operations during *Telic* progressed, mental health operations were focused on the contingency operating base in Basrah with peripatetic 'clinics' held in Baghdad and more isolated locations. Until the end of operations in Iraq, the mental health effort in theatre was delivered by two to four mental health nurses, the number fluctuating with the operational tempo. Supervision and clinical and command support were provided by visiting psychiatrists throughout the deployment.

FMHT in Afghanistan

In contrast to operations in Iraq, Afghanistan deployments were never characterised by the deployment of divisional strength assets. Beginning with the deployment of a single mental health nurse from *16 CSMR* in the Afghanistan capital Kabul with additional mental health assets deployed at Bagram Air Base, the FMHT remained a singleton post until the operation expanded beyond Kabul and into the Helmand region. From that point, the FMHT fluctuated, consisting of three or four mental health nurses, supported by psychiatrists

and senior mental health nurses at home in the United Kingdom when communications allowed. During the deployment into Helmand Province, the FMHT was located in Camp Bastion, whilst individuals delivered peripatetic clinics in forward locations including patrol bases and check points. Visiting clinics were also conducted in Kabul and Kandahar.

In addition to the continued presence of nurses in Camp Bastion, uniformed psychiatrists undertook frequent short visits to theatre to provide clinical supervision, general mental health support and advice to command regarding theatre policies and procedures associated with the promotion of mental health and well-being. During the deployment in the Helmand region, a singleton mental health post was established at Kandahar Airfield, which was largely staffed by RAF personnel who provided a link for incoming aeromedical evacuation flights. Although the mix of service backgrounds varied with the phase of deployment, in a similar manner to Iraq, mental health support during *Operation Herrick* was broadly a tri-Service effort.

Research into the effectiveness and activity of the FMHT is scarce, but some studies and service evaluations have been published. These are detailed in the section of this chapter dealing with deployment mental health support. As with any field of study in mental health, focusing upon the activity of clinical teams and drawing conclusions about the whole of the UK Armed Forces are likely to result in a skewed picture. It is therefore important to try to understand the overall pattern and determinants of mental health in a range of locations and settings and across the UK Armed Forces so that deployment mental health can be understood in the context of general military mental health.

UNDERSTANDING THE SCOPE OF MILITARY MENTAL HEALTH

Up to the mid-1990s, the scale of mental health problems among UK Armed Forces personnel was largely unknown, and the broader field of military mental health was under-researched. In the non-deployed setting, estimates of numbers requiring mental health support were based upon the proportions of the population at risk in a defined geographical area presenting for treatment to the military community mental health department providing a clinical service in that area. This did not take account personnel who were symptomatic but who chose not seek help, those with somatic rather than overt mental disorder presentations and those with lower levels of symptoms who were dealt with in primary care; of course, some personnel choose to seek help from non-specialist or alternative care services; in other words, existing data would have seriously underestimated the true extent of the problem. Clearly, there was a need for a better estimate of the scale of the problem in order to provide comprehensive mental health support. Although it is accepted that the UK Armed Forces have a mental health support requirement just like any other large organisation, the emergence of so called 'Gulf War Syndrome' in the 1990s triggered executive interest in the health consequences of contemporary operational deployment. It became painfully apparent that robust data to support studies of military problems such as Gulf War Syndrome were unavailable. The establishment of the *Gulf War Study Group* at King's College London was a direct consequence of the belated recognition of this shortcoming. Researchers set about comparing health outcomes among three groups of UK military personnel: those deployed to the Persian Gulf, those deployed to the early stages of the deployment in the Former Yugoslavia and a further sample of personnel who had not deployed to either area. Although personnel deployed to the Persian Gulf had a higher symptom burden, there was no evidence to support the notion of a 'Gulf War Syndrome'[4]; in other words, no unique syndrome was associated with Gulf War service. Given the ongoing military activity

in and around the Persian Gulf, the Ministry of Defence recognised that there was a need to further develop population-level mental health surveillance in order to facilitate research following potential future deployments in the region and elsewhere. The *King's Centre for Military Health Research (KCMHR)* was established to begin the task of establishing a military cohort so that the impact of deployment and broader military service could be properly studied. In preparation for full roll-out, a 'screening study'[5] tested whether large-scale military mental health surveillance was feasible, with the aim of developing the surveillance strategy to be used in the main phase of the study. In total, a sample of approximately 4500 personnel participated, representing a 67% response rate. The screening study successfully showed that large-scale military health surveillance was possible and that with much effort, including robust contact tracing, a respectable response rate was achievable. Researchers from King's College London therefore made the necessary preparations for establishing the military cohort, the main phase of which was formally started in 2004. The numbers of people participating and the study timelines are shown in Figure 15.1. Phase 1 of the cohort study compared aspects of mental health between two randomly selected groups. Group 1 comprised around 10% of the personnel, both regular and reserve, who deployed to Iraq between January and April 2003.

A second group included serving personnel who had not deployed to Iraq, termed the 'Era' group by the researchers. Given the successful implementation of the initial phase of the cohort study, a second follow-up phase was planned. During phase 2, the study group (termed the 'follow-up

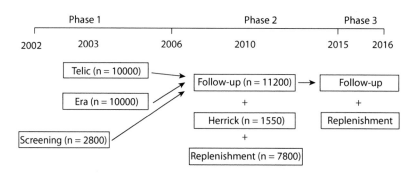

Figure 15.1 KCMHR cohort.

sample') included personnel who had become military veterans since participating in the earlier study and reserves (the latter were oversampled); the response rate for phase 2 was 59%. A randomly selected sample of personnel who deployed to Afghanistan was included to reflect ongoing operations in the region, and a 'replenishment sample' was added to maintain the survey's representative nature; the latter sought to encompass newly recruited trained-strength personnel who would have had an opportunity to deploy. Some of the original screening study participants were recontacted in later phases of the cohort survey and continue to provide longitudinal data. A further phase of follow-up study was planned for 2015 to 2016 with the aim of surveying those included in previous cohort phases and to incorporate a new replenishment sample.

The earlier screening study was serendipitous in that it took place immediately prior to the combat deployment in Iraq, and the subsequent cohort survey, carried out when the deployment was over, included a substantial number of screening study respondents. It was therefore possible to assess whether screening prior to deployment would have been effective in predicting whether Service personnel would develop post-deployment mental health problems. Of 2820 personnel from the three services who completed the pre-deployment screening survey, 69% also returned post-deployment surveys during the cohort study. Comparing mental health measures at the two survey points led the researchers to conclude that although psychological symptoms and alcohol misuse were both highly prevalent,[6] screening for common mental disorders (CMDs) symptoms before deployment would neither have reduced subsequent mental health-related morbidity nor have predicted who would develop post-traumatic stress disorder (PTSD) following deployment, at least with anything like the degree of accuracy and precision necessary.[7] The lack of effect for screening was attributed to the complex and multiple factors associated with mental health outcomes following deployment, with pre-deployment psychological health being only one amongst many candidate determinants.[8] As a result, it could be concluded that the screening process itself was feasible but too inaccurate to be useful. It would have wrongly identified

four people for every person correctly identified, clearly an unsustainable, impractical and indeed unethical process.

The power of maintaining a military cohort was further demonstrated by a study where data collected during the Iraq deployment (*Operation Telic*) was compared with health measures collected during the 'Gulf War Syndrome' study. The outcomes suggested that although those deployed on *Operation Telic* were somewhat more symptomatic,[9] increases in physical symptoms in this group were overall minimal. Furthermore, not only was there no 'Iraq War Syndrome', there was not even the significant increase in non-specific symptomatic ill-health that was so clearly demonstrated after *Operation Granby* (the first Gulf War of 1981).[10] While this is of considerable interest, it is beyond the scope of this chapter and has been reviewed in depth in a Royal Society supplement entirely devoted to Gulf War illnesses.[11]

IRAQ AND AFGHANISTAN DEPLOYMENT, MENTAL HEALTH SYMPTOM PREVALENCE AND ALCOHOL USE

Historically, contemporary, robust estimates of mental disorder symptoms and alcohol misuse prevalences within the UK Armed Forces have not been available to inform policies and procedures, which were influenced more by prevailing popular press narratives. PTSD was seen by many as the most significant mental health challenge to deployed personnel. In addition, charitable mental healthcare providers voiced their fears of a 'tidal wave' of PTSD,[12] a narrative that was adopted by British politicians who, even from the start of the conflicts, began to talk of a potential mental disorder 'bow wave'.[13] Such an effect was indeed soon found in US military research, a conundrum that remains controversial to the present day. In parallel to the developing narrative, public support for the two concurrent deployments was reportedly waning. This was potentially important as historically, military psychological well-being has been linked to prevailing levels of public support for the Armed Forces. British Social Attitude Survey data confirmed that public opinion of the Iraq and Afghanistan missions turned largely negative following the initial deployment.[14] This was not confined to the United Kingdom; Sweden, which also supplied personnel for the mission in Afghanistan, experienced similar low levels of public backing. Furthermore, and in contrast to the United Kingdom, where public support for the Armed Forces was and remained high,[15] Swedish support for the military was lacking, with little appetite for undertaking military missions overseas.[16] The missions in Iraq and Afghanistan therefore took place in the context of an internationally toxic atmosphere, which could easily have impacted on the military will to fight. Fortunately, in both the United States and United Kingdom, the public seemed very capable of distinguishing between support for the war (which was soon lacking) and support for those who were serving in the wars (which was not). It is perhaps also helpful at this stage to note that research conducted among UK military personnel suggested that many aspects of deployment to the Iraq mission were quite rewarding and most negative perceptions of deployment were largely explained by the presence of mental disorder symptoms.[17]

The King's cohort study was therefore being developed at a time when a military mental health crisis was widely anticipated. The findings from the initial phase of the cohort survey were therefore somewhat counterintuitive yet not unexpected, given a PTSD prevalence of 2.5% found in the screening study described earlier, low levels of psychological distress reported in a pre-/post-deployment study conducted during the very first deployment in Afghanistan[18] and other early UK military observational studies.[19,20]

Despite low public support for two potentially psychologically threatening deployments, the military cohort outcomes suggested that UK Armed Forces personnel were generally psychologically robust. The prevalence of PTSD was 4.4% among personnel deployed to Iraq and 3.5% in non-deployers; the difference in prevalence was not significant and the rates were only marginally above the 3% rate reported in a UK civilian population survey.[21] The prevalence of PTSD was higher (5.7%) among combat personnel and around 6% among deployed reservists. Thus, there was a deployment effect for those engaged in combat duties, a finding common to the armed forces of other nations,[22] and deployed reservists appeared to fare less well

than their non-deployed counterparts, a finding replicated in a detailed clinical interview study conducted among cohort participants.[23]

Nevertheless, expressing the problem of PTSD as a simple percentage does not adequately capture the complex pattern of morbidity or the problems encountered by those with symptoms. There is evidence that functional impairment is substantial among sufferers; furthermore, such impairment is not confined to those with the highest symptom levels.[24] There is also some evidence that the sexes are unequally affected by military service. Although the deployment effect among women was similar to that found among men, a UK study of psychological symptoms among female service members suggested that posttraumatic stress, physical symptoms and alcohol misuse were all commoner among non-deployed women than men working in the non-deployed setting.[25,26]

Contrary to widely held popular views about military mental health, the prevalence of *common mental disorder* (CMD) symptoms, including anxiety and depression, was substantially higher than that of PTSD at approximately 20%; furthermore, the level of CMD symptoms was higher than that found among an age- and gender-matched general population sample. These results should be interpreted with caution as there is compelling evidence that surveys conducted in an occupational context appear to yield substantially higher prevalence rates than surveys where non-employed people are included.[27] Symptoms of mental disorder are only a component of military mental health: arguably, a more pressing concern given its potential adverse impact on military functioning and longer-term health is alcohol misuse. In the cohort study, potentially harmful alcohol use had a prevalence of around 13%, with evidence that recently deployed personnel misused alcohol more commonly (16%) than non-deployed personnel (11%), with the effect being particularly marked among combat-deployed personnel.[28] Readers should note that alcohol use was defined as consumption potentially harmful to health; if the lower threshold 'hazardous drinking' definition were to be used, around two thirds of UK Armed Forces personnel would be defined as having a drink problem.

As described earlier, the substantial negative mental health impact of deployment emerging from US research played its part in giving impetus to the development of military health surveillance in the United Kingdom. Having a properly established, representative UK military research cohort has had the additional benefit of allowing comparison of military health experiences and research outcomes between the United Kingdom and other nations, particularly the United States, Canada, Holland, Denmark and Australia. Although much research has taken place since the initial deployment to Iraq, early US studies reported a post-deployment PTSD rate of 12.6% using the same instrument and case definition as that used among UK Armed Forces personnel[29]; subsequent studies continue to demonstrate a higher PTSD prevalence among US forces. A comparison of similar samples of United States and United Kingdom deployed combat personnel suggests that some of the difference in PTSD is related to differing levels of self-reported combat exposure[30]; however, it is likely that a complete explanation for differing prevalences is more complex than this. Some commentators have cited as an explanation the UK Armed Forces' occupational health system, which is used to continuously assess whether an individual's health allows him or her deploy and if so, in what capacity. Furthermore, personnel with poorer mental health are debarred from deployment. So, lower prevalences may in part reflect the 'healthy warrior effect'.[31]

Initial research conducted among deployed Australian forces generated a PTSD prevalence rate of 8.3%, while Canadian forces were found to have a prevalence of 2.3%[32]; however, more recent research suggests that PTSD prevalence has risen to 5.3% among Canadian military personnel.[33] Both the Canadian and Australian research used a structured clinical interview rather than a survey instrument, so direct comparison is less robust than comparisons with US research outcomes.

The second round of surveillance using King's cohort methodology started in 2006.[34] This suggested that, despite continued deployment to Iraq and Afghanistan, the mental health of the UK Armed Forces was broadly stable. PTSD prevalence was 4.0% and CMD was 19.7%, and 13.0% of personnel were drinking potentially harmful amounts of alcohol. Alcohol misuse was significantly associated with deployment for regulars, while PTSD was still significantly associated with deployment among reserves. Overall, mental health appeared very similar to the profile observed in 2003/2004.

As before, the risk of developing PTSD was highest among regular forces deployed in a combat role and there was evidence of a small but significant rise in PTSD rates among regulars with increasing time since returning from deployment. The picture was again more complex than headline figures might suggest; for instance, within the overall findings, some subgroups such as commando and airborne units had a significantly lower incidence of mental health problems than line infantry units.[35]

Although overall rates of PTSD were low in the context of substantial combat deployments, the CMD rates were more difficult to contextualise. So CMD rates obtained during phase 1 were compared with CMD rates reported by civilian respondents to the *Health Survey for England*.[36] This study suggested that when socio-demographic factors were accounted for, serving military personnel were significantly more likely to report greater levels of CMD than randomly chosen civilians. Whatever one makes of this rather surprising finding, there is still no room for complacency despite the low levels of PTSD reported by military personnel.

The second phase of the King's cohort study provided longitudinal data that gave the first opportunity to study change over time. *Delayed-onset PTSD* (DOPTSD) is defined as starting at least six months after experiencing a traumatic event. Using data provided by cohort participants at both phase 1 and 2, participants were identified who were not defined as PTSD cases at phase 1 but became cases at phase 2. Using these criteria, 3.5% exhibited DOPTSD. However, at phase 1, subthreshold PTSD, CMD, poorer perceived health, multiple physical symptoms and the onset of alcohol misuse or CMD between phases 1 and 2 were associated with the development of DOPTSD.[37] It seems likely that a substantial proportion of DOPTSD is accounted for by delayed presentation rather than delayed onset. Although limited by a low response rate, a further UK longitudinal study suggested that probable mental health disorder and functional impairment were significantly associated and that both mildly increased over time following return from deployment. Higher mental disorder symptom levels at follow-up were associated with more difficulties with transition from deployment, family and relationship problems.[38] It seems, therefore, that a small but important group experience problems sometime after deployment; given the complexity of aetiology and some reluctance to self-identify among sufferers (addressed later in this chapter), engaging them with appropriate support or clinical care may prove to be a challenge.

The King's cohort has been useful for studying not only military mental health but also deployment-related physical health outcomes. Using cohort data, UK researchers demonstrated that deployment was associated with a reduced risk of experiencing mild headache, although deployment had no impact upon moderate to severe headache; the more severe forms of headache were significantly associated with mental disorder symptoms and functional impairment.[39] Diarrhoea is a common health problem during deployment, particularly in austere conditions, and was a substantial problem during the expeditionary phases of deployment in both Afghanistan and Iraq. Although the acute phase of such illness is well understood, the longer-term outcomes are less well known. In a study of previously deployed cohort respondents, 59% reported diarrhoea and vomiting during deployment and 6.6% were classified as having probable irritable bowel syndrome at follow-up. Experiencing diarrhoea and vomiting during deployment, along with additional mental health factors, was significantly associated with the presence of irritable bowel syndrome at follow-up.[40]

From knowing little about the mental health burden of deployment and the impact of military service on health and well-being at the start of the deployments to Iraq and Afghanistan, UK researchers are now in a position to provide accurate information about the psychological health of UK Armed Forces personnel, due in large part to the establishment of the King's military cohort. Having provided a general picture of UK military mental health, this discussion now turns to mental health and supportive interventions at various stages of the deployment cycle, beginning with the build-up to operational tours in Iraq and Afghanistan.

PRE-OPERATIONAL PREPARATION

Regulating deployment mental health

The UK *Defence Mental Health Services* assist in ensuring that personnel are psychologically fit for deployment and maintain good mental health during their operational tour. This happens within an occupational health framework where a system of medical classification allocates individuals to medical employment categories that govern the way in which they deploy. As an inevitable result, some individuals will be debarred from deployment on health grounds. When personnel are mentally unwell, they are protected from deployment while their illness or mental disorder is managed effectively. For some personnel, discharge from the UK Armed Forces is arranged on medical grounds when the restrictions are enduring and mean that the person cannot be employed in any military capacity. Studies of occupational mental healthcare are rare, and at the time of the current major deployments, published data were largely unavailable. A single published study conducted in one UK military mental healthcare department during the period of deployment in Iraq and Afghanistan suggested that 68% of personnel returned to their unit following mental healthcare in a fully employable capacity and were therefore fit for deployment.[41] When this figure is multiplied across all departments providing such services, within a small volunteer military, there is clearly a substantial mental health challenge in maximising the numbers of personnel who are mentally fit for deployment.

Mental health therapies and help-seeking in the non-deployed setting

Attendance rates at military mental healthcare facilities are published as open source material[42] and include some information about deployment to Iraq and Afghanistan. These reports are often used to plan services and are sometimes quoted as an index of the mental health of the UK Armed Forces. Of course, military personnel seek help from a wide variety of sources, including primary care facilities, while others, especially officers, contravene service healthcare guidelines by sometimes seeking help outside the Armed Forces. Many more suffer mental health problems but do not seek care. The level of help-seeking for mental health reasons in these circumstances is not captured in the aforementioned reports (although many journalists seem unaware of this), and even less is known about symptomatic personnel who do not seek help. In an attempt to inform this area, during phase 1 of the military cohort, an additional in-depth telephone interview was carried out among selected respondents who reported substantial mental health symptoms on a general health questionnaire[43]; the latter were compared with personnel who scored below the chosen cut-off score. Of 1083 eligible participants, 821 then took part in structured diagnostic interviews. The samples were composed of regulars and reserves in equal measure, half of whom had deployed to Iraq. Participants completed depression and PTSD measures and answered a series of questions about help-seeking and subsequent treatment. Only 23% of symptomatic serving personnel were receiving professional medical help; help-seekers were more likely to access informal sources of support. Three quarters of serving regulars who sought formal help were seen in primary care, most commonly receiving medication or some form of psychological support. Few regular personnel were receiving *cognitive and behavioural therapy*; receipt of therapy and help-seeking mirrored levels found in the general population. Subsequent cohort-based studies replicated these early findings; seeking mental healthcare from medical sources was uncommon (around 29%) and was usually related to having more complex needs. Alcohol-related help-seeking mostly occurred when personnel were experiencing symptoms of mental ill-health.[44]

Pre-operational mental health briefing

Mental healthcare can help only those who choose to seek help; the results of previously mentioned cohort studies confirmed that there is a pool of unmet mental health need among the wider UK military population. UK Armed Forces commanders have sought to mitigate any potentially detrimental psychological effects of military service using pre-deployment mental health briefing.[45,46] Mass pre-deployment mental health briefing has the advantage of reaching large numbers of personnel in groups with a minimal time commitment from trainers; in this regard, it is probably cost-effective given that it appears to have some short-term psychological benefits, which are described

later in this chapter. But what does it consist of? In a review of coalition partners' mental health provision during deployment to Afghanistan, common areas of practice included attempts to foster mental resilience, self-regulation and psychological empowerment at various stages of the deployment cycle. Effective leadership and peer support were cited as being crucial to the delivery of such interventions, to military mental health generally and to reducing barriers to care.[47] In general, the briefing content related to minimising personal stress; however, during the campaigns in Iraq and Afghanistan, pre-operational training developed to accommodate the concept of cultural stress,[48] that is stressors arising from cultural and linguistic differences between service personnel and the local populations.[49]

Does pre-deployment briefing do any good? A UK study conducted in Iraq demonstrated that personnel who deployed without receiving a pre-deployment mental health brief reported worse mental health during their deployment than those who did,[50] and UK cohort-based studies have suggested a similar outcome.[51] Furthermore, surveys conducted in Afghanistan in 2010 and again in 2011 both suggested that non-receipt of a pre-operational brief was associated with poorer deployment mental health.[52] It is important to bear in mind that none of these studies were randomised, so it always possible that those who attended such briefings had better mental health than did those who did not attend. Likewise, not all research has demonstrated a positive effect of pre-deployment mental health briefing; a comparison of UK Armed Forces personnel who did and did not receive a mental health briefing immediately prior to the ground offensive in Iraq suggested that there was no significant benefit to the briefing.[53] It is likely that the impact of a briefing is small; however, it might still be a worthwhile activity given that the intervention is very low cost.

Content and format are not the only important mental health briefing components; the quality of delivery also appears to have a direct effect upon outcome. In a survey of 1559 Royal Navy personnel, 47% of respondents reported having received a stress brief during their military service. Briefing recipients had significantly better general mental health than non-recipients did; however, when the quality of the brief was taken into account, only those who received a subjectively useful brief had significantly better mental health while subjectively poor-quality briefs had a similar mental health effect to receiving no briefing at all.[54]

Mental health and medical countermeasures

In addition to mental health preparations for deployment, a number of medical countermeasures seek to protect personnel from known or anticipated health threats. Poorer health among some service personnel who deployed to the first Gulf War was often blamed on medical countermeasures by either the personnel themselves or the media. Among the numerous candidate agents were the various vaccinations administered prior to deployment. Based on the results of the Gulf War studies already mentioned, prior to the Iraq deployment in 2003, the UK Ministry of Defence modified its approach to the use of the anthrax vaccine in particular, administering it without the accelerant pertussis, introducing much better information and insisting on informed consent. Using data linkage (possible because of improvements in electronic data recording), the King's research team were able to carry out better studies on the short- and medium-term side effects of the anthrax vaccine administered prior to the Iraq deployment. Uptake of the anthrax vaccination was high at the start of the war (72%). Nearly all personnel thought that they were somewhat or very likely to be exposed to chemical or biological agents during the forthcoming conflict. In a series of studies, no association was found between receiving either anthrax or multiple vaccination and poorer longer-term health[55,56]; however, the protocol for delivering the vaccination may have induced concern about potential health threats among some recipients,[57] in particular the elaborate method of gaining informed consent.[58] The exception was where health outcomes were compared between personnel who self-reported multiple vaccinations and personnel with confirmed multiple vaccinations in their medical record. In this case, recall bias and other subtle cognitive distortion may have accounted for greater symptoms rather than actual multiple vaccination; this was a particularly significant observation because it probably accounted for the previously observed link between multiple vaccinations and symptoms after the First Gulf War. The level of side effects appeared to be related to how people thought about the vaccine and whether they perceived that that they had been pressurised to receive it.

Changes in the way in which anthrax immunisation was administered may have had unintended consequences. Personnel were required to give informed consent, in the form of a detailed explanation of the need for, and potential effects of, receiving the vaccination or were even required to view a video presentation. This caused some people to question why such measures were taken with anthrax when they were not required for other forms of vaccination, leading them to conclude that anthrax was particularly likely to have harmful effects. Finally, uptake of the anthrax vaccine declined with time, largely because personnel started to question the likelihood of encountering biological weapons.

This programme of research helped restore confidence in the anthrax vaccination after considerable uncertainty following the so-called 'Gulf War Syndrome' saga. Should the threat level from anthrax increase, and uptake of the vaccine become essential, the results of these studies will allow much better risk assessment and compliance, as well as reducing subjective side effects.

DEPLOYMENT MENTAL HEALTH

Operational mental health needs evaluation study

Most studies of deployment mental health use retrospective accounts collected during surveys and interviews conducted after returning home from deployment. Although initial recall of deployment experiences and associated emotions appear to be largely accurate, the passage of time inevitably results in memory distortion and other forms of cognitive bias. Following the example of the US Mental Health Advisory Team surveillance of deployment mental health,[59] UK military researchers undertook the *Operational Mental Health Needs Evaluation* (OMHNE) series of studies between 2009 and 2014, where data were obtained from around 4200 personnel working in the operational area.

The OMHNE survey is an innovative research procedure undertaken in circumstances where completing a programme of health surveillance will always be secondary to operational considerations. The key element in successful delivery was effective and extensive liaison with key deployed commanders and logisticians prior to the visit, in order to ensure that support for the survey team was in place from the outset. A detailed visit plan was constructed in advance and was modified in response to factors such as personnel moving around the operational area or changing base location, restricted access to air and ground transport and so forth; flexibility and using work-arounds were key features of each OMHNE. Unlike other research, the OMHNE teams included senior non-commissioned officers from the regular UK Armed Forces. These team members proved to be invaluable as they were able to exert military influence where researchers may not have been able to. OMHNE survey team members were required to be self-reliant and completed visit schedules alone in order to maximise movement around the operational area and minimise the impact of any potential difficulties arising from transport problems, logistical difficulties and the impact of combat operations.

Each OMHNE survey involved a representative sample of the deployed force. A power calculation was carried out before deployment to decide the minimum number of personnel required; this usually amounted to around 15% of the deployed force. Each OMHNE also over-sampled potential high-risk groups. The core of the survey was retained between OMHNEs to enable comparisons between the studies. Completed surveys were electronically scanned so that the survey team could directly export and analyse data immediately following collection. The software effectively 'read' the completed boxes on the questionnaire and converted them to numerical information, which was transferred to a statistical software package after having been cleaned by the team. This allowed the survey team to provide operational commanders with 'immediate' anonymised, pooled mental health and support information. A key objective of the OMHNE survey was to complete the process in

the shortest possible time to minimise the impact upon those in operational areas who provided support for the mission and to deliver a full report to the force commander at the end of the visit. The OMHNE is therefore highly pressurised, and efficiency is the key to delivery.

The first OMHNE (OMHNE I) surveyed deployed military personnel in Iraq. It found that the mental health of UK Armed Forces personnel on deployment was similar to that reported during surveys of home-based personnel; 20.5% of deployed personnel reported symptoms of probable CMD and 3.4% reported probable PTSD symptoms.

OMHNE I took place during the last phase of the UK's military operations in Iraq, during which the operational threat level, although still heightened, was decreased compared to previous years. This contrasted with the combat intensity experienced by UK military personnel deployed in Afghanistan at that time. So, to understand the mental health impact of prolonged operations in a high-threat area, a survey was carried out in the winter of 2010 amongst 1431 personnel deployed in Afghanistan (the survey was termed OMHNE A1). In this study, 2.8% of personnel were experiencing symptoms of probable PTSD and 17.0% reported symptoms of probable CMD.

To understand how changes in operational support and how the deployed environment may have impacted upon mental health, a further survey of deployed personnel was carried out in Afghanistan during July and August 2011 (termed OMHNE A2). Unlike the OMHNE A1, the A2 survey was undertaken during the Afghan summer to take account of different climactic conditions and seasonal variations in combat intensity. During OMHNE A1, the study team was unable to carry out as much forward sampling as had been planned prior to deployment. A major coalition offensive operation was underway, and access to transport assets, particularly helicopters, was limited; no such restrictions were present during A2. Given that being in a forward area limits access to potential sources of prevention, including medical and welfare support, the study team assessed whether location and combat environment had impacted upon mental health by concentrating on more austere, forward locations away from the main base areas. On this occasion, the PTSD rate was 1.8% and the CMD rate was 16%.

The last Afghanistan-based OMHNE (A3) took place in 2014 when the final preparations for leaving Helmand province were underway. This study was needed because the final phase of a drawdown period of operations, where rapidly reducing manpower levels and changes in the mission format from combat to a manpower and logistical extraction phase might impact upon the mental health of deployed personnel in a different way to the more kinetic deployment phases. OMHNE A3 examined the mental health of deployed personnel and mental health support efforts during the final drawdown phase of current operations in Afghanistan and made comparisons with earlier land-based OMHNE findings. Overall, rates of PTSD reduced from 3.5% to 1.4% over time and CMD rates reduced from 20.1% to 14.4% over the course of the OMHNE studies (Figure 15.2).

The OMHNE series was designed to produce data that could be used to explore a range of outcomes. Several studies have exploited OMHNE data; in all studies, leadership appeared to be crucial to maintaining mental health during deployment,[60] while family and home front problems had a similar and additive psychological impact to combat exposures.[61] This important finding bolstered the case for robust and visible support for the families of deployed personnel, especially for more isolated families living 'off base', and among deployed reserves, a group known to have unmet family welfare needs.[62] A component of the welfare package that improved over the course of the deployments in Iraq and Afghanistan was communication with home; however, researchers cautioned that such well-intentioned improvements can have paradoxical effects.[63]

Given that US commentators described *mild traumatic brain injury* (mTBI), otherwise known as concussion, as the 'signature injury' of the Iraq deployment, mTBI was assessed and found to be relatively rare during deployment, while symptomatic mTBI was rarer still.[64] PTSD symptoms were significantly associated with mTBI, indeed it is entirely possible that some cases of PTSD were probably being mislabelled as mTBI. Other King's cohort studies have similarly demonstrated low levels of mTBI in UK personnel and a strong association with pre-morbid PTSD symptoms and alcohol use when it was present.[65] Further UK studies appear to confirm that mTBI symptoms are relatively non-specific as symptoms and severity were both associated not only with self-reported exposure to blast, which was expected, but also with a wide range of other deployment exposures, which was not. In all UK studies, PTSD and CMD symptoms were strongly associated with mTBI symptoms.[66] The major strength of the OMHNE study was that the mTBI data were collected very close to the point of injury and were not subject to increases in symptoms with time or increased recall of traumatic exposures as time passed; both potential confounders have been a feature of mTBI research.

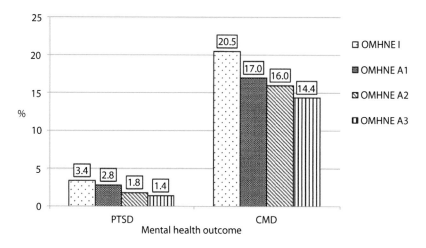

Figure 15.2 Land OMHNE studies – mental health outcomes.

Over-sampling high-risk groups allowed the OMHNE team to reassure commanders that occupational groups such as the counter-IED task force, were at no greater psychological risk than groups such as infantry personnel and medical personnel.[67] Medical personnel are consistently cited as being at heightened risk of psychological injury as a result of their experiences during deployment; however, the OMHNE and other studies suggest that this occupational group are not at substantially higher risk compared to other deployed personnel; the burden of psychological symptoms is concentrated among those deployed in a forward combat-orientated medical role.[68,69]

Maritime OMHNE

To extend the scope of OMHNE, a further survey was undertaken among approximately 1250 Royal Navy personnel participating in patrols in both the Persian Gulf (the largest sample) and South Atlantic. In contrast to the land OMNHEs, and somewhat surprisingly, there was a considerable burden of mental health symptoms: 41.2% of respondents reported probable CMD, 7.8% reported probable PTSD and 17.4% reported potentially harmful alcohol use.[70]

The OMHNE studies emerged as a valuable tool for assessing military mental health among deployed personnel where contemporaneous mental health data were largely absent and difficult to obtain. Over the course of the OMHNE study series, military academics have developed OMHNE expertise among members of the wider defence mental health community and can deliver a rapidly deployable survey capability that yields prompt results. This is particularly useful to deployed commanders at all levels, who can use OMHNE data to better understand the mental health of their command.

Effects of cumulative deployment

Historically, longer duration of time spent engaged in combat is well known to be associated with psychological break down[71]; however, overall length of deployment has been less well studied. In an attempt to reduce breakdown, the UK Armed Forces introduced 'Harmony Guidelines', which effectively placed a cap on the cumulative duration of time deployed within a given period. Examining cumulative deployment in 2005, UK researchers demonstrated that personnel deployed for periods of 13 months or more within a three-year period were more likely to fulfil the criteria for PTSD and CMD, multiple physical symptoms and severe alcohol problems, particularly when deployed in a combat role and when the length of deployment was longer than forecast.[72] In a separate study, length of deployment was also associated with mTBI.[73] In a follow-up study conducted in 2008 encompassing personnel who had deployed to Iraq and Afghanistan, breaches of Harmony Guidelines had reduced by half; however, among personnel who experienced such breaches, there continued to be a significant association with poorer physical health and greater problems at home while deployed.[74] These data were subsequently used by both US and UK senior military leaders when determining optimum deployment length.

Deployment clinical support

Little is known about mental health clinical support for deployed personnel, probably because of the difficulty of conducting robust studies while carrying out combat operations; however, some contemporary studies have been completed. A study of aeromedical evacuation for mental health conditions to a UK secondary care facility during the first year of the campaign in Iraq suggested that 69% of cases of mental disorder were found among non-combatants, while 21% of evacuations occurred among reserve forces; 37% of those evacuated had a history of contact with mental health services. In over 85% of cases, evacuation was for low mood attributed to separation from friends or family or difficulties adjusting to the operational environment.[75] Assessing the relative contribution to longer-term mental health of being evacuated home with illness and with injury, UK researchers reported that illness had at least as great a mental health impact as injury, although support for those with illness following evacuation was less well organised than for injury.[76]

Turning to deployed healthcare, during the initial ground campaign and early follow-up operations in Iraq, one UK Role 3 hospital-based FMHT assessed 170 new mental health cases.[77] The commonest presenting problem was adjustment disorder (68%, $n = 116$), 77 of which were related to theatre factors while 39 were associated with events occurring at home. Overall, 72% of cases returned to their operational unit. Cases of depressive disorder or intentional self-harm were usually aeromedically evacuated. Similar low levels of psychiatric casualties were experienced in the divisional rear area.[78] Most UK deployment mental health studies use a marker of occupational fitness or an occupational outcome as an index of success, such as returning to duty or the ability to work without medically imposed restrictions. A deployment mental healthcare study conducted among 825 UK military personnel deployed in Iraq over several years of the long-running campaign reported a return to duty rate of 72%, although a quarter of those treated during deployment subsequently underwent unplanned or premature discharge from military service.[79]

Reserve forces mental health

The King's military cohort studies suggested that deployed UK Reserve Forces personnel consistently reported higher rates of psychological health problems than deployed regular forces did.[80] Differences in mental health outcomes were related in part to socio-demographic variations between regular forces and reserves. A large proportion of the deployed reserves participating in mental health and well-being studies were undertaking a deployed medical or welfare role. The greatest mental health effect related to substantial numbers of reserves experiencing problems at home both during and following deployment. If psychological problems occur for members of the regular forces following deployment, personnel have access to dedicated military mental health assessment and treatment services. Historically, this was not the case for reserves who were required to seek help from the NHS. As a consequence of perceived heightened need and fewer dedicated services for recently demobilised reserve personnel, the *Reserves Mental Health Programme* (RMHP) was established in 2006. The RMHP provided assessment and treatment for reserve personnel with mental health problems that were deemed to be

attributable to deployment in Iraq or Afghanistan after 1 January 2003; these were termed *operationally related mental health problems* (ORMHP). RMHP attendees underwent a structured mental health assessment in a dedicated facility. All referred reservists completed a number of mental health measures and participated in a comprehensive clinical assessment. If they were found to have an operationally attributable mental health problem, treatment was then arranged in a regular forces military healthcare facility as close to their home as possible. Those found not to have an ORMHP were offered simple reassurance and referred on to an appropriate NHS provider, usually through their general practitioner (GP). All attendees were offered a personal management plan when assessment was complete. The plan detailed key assessment findings and suggestions about how any mental health condition might be managed. A copy of the mental health and welfare needs assessment was also sent to the family doctor. Occupational outcomes among reserve forces personnel who used the RMHP after deploying to Afghanistan and Iraq suggested that 76.5% of those who received treatment returned to full fitness for deployment and experienced substantial improvements in their mental health.[81]

Operational rest and recuperation

Providing a dedicated period of rest and recuperation (R&R) leave at home during an operational deployment is an important component of health and well-being support allowing personnel to rest out of line and access social support from family and friends. However, little is known about the mental health impact of R&R. UK researchers carried out such a study.[82] Baseline measures of mental health and alcohol use were obtained from 304 personnel as they embarked upon R&R and a further 232 personnel completed the same measures and an R&R experience scale at the end of their time at home. A total of 42 subjects completed measures at both points. Levels of probable CMD, PTSD and hazardous alcohol use were not significantly different between the pre- and post-R&R groups and between the pre- and post-R&R measures in those completing both surveys. Approximately 90.0% of those returning to deployment expressed strong satisfaction with the overall experience of R&R. Principal components analysis of the R&R experiences scale[83] generated five key factors: the ability to mentally disengage from events in Afghanistan, the ability to rest and access social support, travel experiences, physical recovery and relaxation. The ability to engage with the restful and recuperative elements of the time at home and to derive satisfaction from R&R were both associated with better mental health when returning to the operational area and lower levels of alcohol use while at home.

Despite relatively low levels of both CMD and PTSD among R&R study participants given recent high levels of combat exposure, around half of personnel drank hazardously while they were at home. Greater combat exposure and longer pre-R&R deployment length was associated with reduced satisfaction with R&R, more alcohol misuse and functional impairment arising from mental health symptoms. Combat fatigue may well have impaired engagement with R&R and might also explain why some personnel reinstated their alcohol use so rapidly during the brief period spent at home as they misguidedly sought to improve their state of mind. R&R therefore appears to be less restorative for those with greater combat exposure, unfortunately the very group that R&R seeks to help the most.

Although PTSD rates appeared to be unaffected by R&R, individuals who had experienced a greater frequency of thoughts of impending death and injury reported significantly greater satisfaction with R&R as they returned to the operational area. R&R may therefore have constituted an opportunity to discuss or process concerns about death and injury in a physically and psychologically safe environment.

Overall, R&R was reported to be highly satisfying for at least 90% of respondents, and the majority of respondents would value R&R during future deployments. The majority of personnel reported that they were able to relax and interact with their friends and loved ones, which is an important outcome irrespective of any mental health effects. Given its popularity, R&R may have had a positive effect upon morale, in which case it could represent an important component of deployment mental health support, given that there is a strong correlation between high morale and good mental health.

Greater satisfaction with travel, in particular, was associated with lower rates of hazardous alcohol use during R&R. It has been previously reported that travelling to and from Afghanistan is complex, often disrupted, and the air link can sometimes be fragile; as a consequence, frustration with travel is substantial.[84] It might be useful to see if allowing personnel to take a brief period of rest before boarding the aircraft, without shortening the duration of R&R, could improve engagement and reduce the use of alcohol during R&R.

Although there was no overall positive mental health effect from taking R&R, it remains a popular deployment activity that requires careful management. There was some evidence that engaging with and deriving satisfaction from R&R was associated with better mental health; if more personnel could achieve this rather than consuming large amounts of alcohol whilst at home, then R&R might well have a more positive overall impact upon mental health.

Trauma risk management

The period immediately following exposure to a distressing operational or combat event could theoretically represent an opportunity to offer support and in particular to provide assistance to those suffering from acute combat stress reaction or other persistent psychological symptoms. Preventing symptom chronicity is arguably the most important component of any early intervention. In recent decades, a number of early interventions have been proposed and tested; *critical incident stress debriefing* (CISD), sometimes known as *psychological debriefing* (PD), is an example of structured postincident support; however, this intervention has not fared well when subjected to empirical testing. A Cochrane database review published in 2002[85] and subsequent studies suggested that early intervention of this kind not only fails to prevent psychological injury[86] but actually makes things worse.[87] Given CISD's apparent lack of effectiveness and the potential to cause harm for some, the PD approach was proscribed in the UK military in 2006.

Anticipating the gap that would result from moving away from CISD and PD, military mental health practitioners developed TRiM, a voluntary, peer-support based early intervention that seeks to facilitate access to support for personnel suffering persistent psychological symptoms related to trauma exposure.[88] This is important because it is difficult to predict who will develop persistent PTSD following trauma exposure and only a proportion of those with persistent PTSD symptoms will seek help.[89] TRiM was developed in collaboration with the Royal Marine Commandos but has now been adopted across the UK Armed Forces with certain Service-specific adaptations, and its use has spread to international militaries, including those of the United States.[90] TRiM was designed to overcome a number of factors in addition to the limitations of CISD and PD. UK military personnel often deploy in remote locations where access to professional mental health support is restricted, the number of mental health specialists may be limited in the operational setting and affected personnel may be unwilling to approach mental healthcare providers because of fear about the possible negative consequences of help-seeking.[91]

The *National Institute for Health and Care Excellence* advocates a process of 'watchful waiting' as the central feature of a psychological trauma response based on the finding that most people will recover spontaneously from psychological trauma without external assistance.[92] In practice, this translates to a process where initial symptoms are monitored and specialist mental health intervention happens only in the context of persistent, worsening or delayed symptoms. The process of TRiM follows just such a path. Initially, commanders, local welfare and care providers and senior TRiM practitioners consider the index event or events and decide whether to offer intervention or not.[93] Those involved in the combat or traumatic event may be offered a structured individual or group-based, peer-led evaluation of the level of risk of developing future psychological symptoms. While participation in the TRiM process is voluntary, all personnel involved in the index event, including those on the periphery, are offered the opportunity to attend an informative briefing event that details what happened, potential psychological consequences (including recovery) and how to manage any potential mental health effects.[94] The individual or group risk assessment

is repeated one month later and the outcomes of the two assessments are compared. Personnel who are believed to be at increased risk of developing psychological symptoms or who report deteriorating mental health are encouraged to seek help from healthcare professionals who may offer further mental health intervention; this constitutes the main aim of TRiM.

TRiM has been subjected to study and has been found to be an acceptable intervention across military ranks,[95] although for this to happen, the provision of TRiM must be supported by the chain of command and not merely represent an item on a management checklist.[96,97] Research conducted during deployment suggests that TRiM has high visibility among operational commanders and medical practitioners[98] and is considered to be a viable early intervention option among this group.

Research studies have suggested that TRiM receipt may be associated with greater social support when units deploy with an integral TRiM capability[99]; when a police force used TRiM to respond to an intense and long-lasting traumatic crime scene, TRiM recipients may have experienced lower levels of sickness absence.[100] A positive mental health and anti-stigma effect has also been reported among TRiM practitioner trainees.[101] A *randomised controlled trial* (RCT) is considered to be a gold standard test of any intervention. A cluster RCT examined the use of TRiM on Royal Navy ships and found no significant difference in mental health status or reported mental health stigmatisation between trained and non-trained ship's companies over an 18-month period. However, comparison samples became fragmented and contaminated during follow-up, making it difficult to formally assess outcomes, and furthermore, participants experienced overall low levels of traumatic exposure, thus providing few opportunities to test TRiM 'in anger'. Despite the lack of a clear mental health advantage following receipt of TRiM, the results of the RCT suggested that having access to the TRiM capability might be occupationally helpful[102]; TRiM-trained ship's companies experienced better levels of discipline than non-TRiM-trained companies did, which was interpreted as an indirect marker of a better overall mental health environment in the TRiM-trained ships. Despite some limitations, TRiM remains an important item in the mental health support toolkit for commanders deploying personnel in a high-threat or combat environment.

FINISHING DEPLOYMENT – THE PSYCHOLOGICAL IMPACT OF THIRD LOCATION DECOMPRESSION

During the deployments in Afghanistan and Iraq, concern was raised about personnel finishing their period of deployment and directly embarking on leave without any intervening gap and without the support of their peers. *Third location decompression* (TLD) represents an attempt to introduce a pause between deployment and the return home. TLD takes place during the immediate period after leaving the operational area. TLD is thought to function as a primary preventative intervention in that it is intended to promote better post-deployment readjustment to homecoming and, by implication, better mental health. TLD aims to allow military personnel to begin to psychologically 'unwind' after operational deployment through the provision of a brief period of structured rest and is a discrete component of the comprehensive *post-operational stress management* (POSM) process.[103,104] TLD formally marks the transition from being deployed on operations to peacetime duties. During recent UK deployments to Afghanistan and Iraq, TLD took place in Cyprus; this constitutes the 'third location' in that it is geographically removed from the area of deployment but is not home. For the majority of personnel who are members of formed units (FUs) that deploy together, TLD has been mandatory since 2007.[105] When initially established as a routine component of the POSM process, TLD aimed to ensure that FU personnel who had deployed together were able to unwind together, the rationale being that it would enable individuals to make use of support from their peers in a neutral and stress-free setting. However, the popularity of TLD among commanders as a brief, structured stress-reduction intervention resulted in a change in policy. Since early in 2011, it has been Ministry of Defence policy that all personnel who deploy for periods in excess of 30 days will undertake TLD. The standard TLD package lasts for approximately 24–36 hours, during which time attendees undertake a pre-planned

and standardised schedule of activities including social events. In addition, two short, distinct and mandatory psycho-educational briefings are delivered. The briefings take two forms; the first is a 'coming home' brief usually delivered by a padre or faith leader, who discusses common readjustment problems and potential ways to overcome them. The second briefing includes formal psycho-education that seeks to help personnel to identify mental health disorder symptoms both in themselves and in others. This briefing effectively 'signposts' to appropriate sources of help those whose initial symptoms fail to remit. The two briefings are intended to assist post-deployment re-adjustment, including reintegration with family and friends and to facilitate the homecoming transition. In addition, the post-deployment briefing is used to cascade various stress-reduction strategies through military units by way of peer-to-peer communication and is often standardised with remarkably similar approaches being used by various nations contributing personnel to contemporary military campaigns.[106] Recognising the high prevalence of alcohol misuse in the UK military, during TLD, an opportunity is provided for the limited consumption of alcohol so that its effects can be experienced in a controlled environment following a prolonged period of abstinence.

Other nations contributing military forces to contemporary campaigns, such as the Netherlands, France and Canada, all made use of decompression in a variety of forms, but only Canada has published a review of their decompression arrangements.[107,108] Canada delivered a three- to five-day package in Cyprus where personnel were accommodated in hotels and were given spending money; French arrangements were for three days in Cyprus; the Dutch provided three days in Crete; Australia provided rest within the operational area with a psychologist interview when deployment was over; and the United States provided a period of 'normalisation' in the home garrison prior to taking post-deployment leave. Some early attempts were made to evaluate TLD. UK military researchers distributed surveys to approximately 13,000 TLD attendees returning from Iraq or Afghanistan, which were completed by 11,304 personnel. The outcome measure was how useful returnees found the TLD process.

The survey results indicated overwhelming support for TLD, with around 91% of respondents finding it moderately or very useful. This figure contrasts sharply with pre-attendance at TLD, where around 80% of respondents reported being ambivalent or not wanting to go through TLD prior to arrival at the decompression facility. The desire to participate in forthcoming TLD was the strongest predictor of perceived helpfulness when the process was complete. Personnel who found TLD less helpful included those who had been through the process before, combat arm personnel and non-commissioned officers. Twelve per cent reported substantial concerns about re-establishing relationships or settling down to 'normal life' after returning home; those reporting more adjustment concerns were more likely to perceive TLD as helpful. Although TLD was well received by personnel following arduous combat deployment, the process was not equally acceptable to all, and alterations to the TLD programme for certain sub-groups such as junior commanders and repeat attenders might well be required.[109]

The TLD survey included a box in which attendees could write comments about their experience of the process. A total of 6734 free text comments were available for further analysis. Responses were largely positive regarding the overall experience of TLD; however, significant numbers of personnel indicated that decompression could be improved by allowing personnel more choice in the activities that they participated in rather than following a fixed agenda. A major source of dissatisfaction was the quality and reliability of the air transport link. A substantial number of participants recommended greater flexibility in the TLD programme so that activities could be better harmonised with the operational role and military characteristics of decompressing units; for instance, combat units might wish to attend a social event as a group, whereas small specialist role units might wish to spend some quiet time together away from the larger gathering.[110]

Given that the majority of personnel completing the early TLD surveys were serving in FUs where personnel deployed with their peers, in a follow-on study, the subjective impressions of *individual augmentees* (IAs) were sought.[111] Usually because of their specialist role (for example many medical

and nursing personnel deployed as IAs), IAs typically deploy alone or join an FU for the duration of an operational tour before returning to their parent home unit; generally, the results of the survey suggested that there were no significant differences in mental health impact between those who deployed as IAs and FU personnel.[112] In keeping with the earlier FU survey, the strongest predictor of perceived utility was the desire to participate prior to arrival at the TLD facility. FU personnel were more likely to want to participate in TLD than IAs before arrival (60% vs. 30%); however, on completion, IAs reported high utility ratings, with 78% of IAs and 84% of FU personnel finding it useful or a little useful.

Despite being a standardised and closely managed procedure, TLD does not have an underlying theoretical basis and is largely about structured, supervised rest with some mental health input. Despite this, among military commanders, it is widely promoted as a positive mental health strategy and its distinctive features are broadly representative of a primary preventative mental health intervention. Given that TLD has been widely used within the UK Armed Forces following combat operations for a number of years without any evaluation of its effect upon mental health, military researchers used King's cohort study data to assess whether TLD had any significant positive psychological impact and whether it assisted in promoting better post-deployment readjustment.

Cohort study data were used to identify personnel who either engaged in TLD following deployment before they returned home or went directly back to their home base with no additional transition activity.[113] As these data were observational, *propensity scores* were generated so that the study data could be used to mimic some of the characteristics of an RCT in subsequent analyses. A range of mental health outcomes and post-deployment re-adjustment problems were compared between those who did and those who did not transition through TLD at the end of their operational tour. The results suggested that TLD had a positive impact upon two out of five assessed mental health outcomes; these were PTSD and reporting substantial levels of physical symptoms. In addition, TLD attendance was associated with overall reduced levels of harmful alcohol use. A small number of indicators of post-deployment readjustment were examined that were characterised by experiencing homecoming problems, difficulty readjusting to being at home and difficulty resuming normal social activities. There was no evidence to suggest that TLD promoted better transition from operations to the peacetime environment. However, when the samples were stratified by levels of combat exposure experienced during deployment, although post-deployment re-adjustment was similar for all exposure levels, personnel experiencing low and moderate levels of combat exposure experienced the greatest positive mental health benefits following participation in TLD. Through the study of TLD, it has been possible to show that it appears beneficial to mental health and has a limiting effect upon alcohol use; however, through conducting studies of subjective utility, it is also clear that while popular and useful, TLD is not a 'one-size-fits-all' procedure. The most heavily combat-exposed personnel benefit less from TLD, the approach needs to be refreshed for repeat attenders and it is unclear whether the mental health briefings are best delivered during TLD or would be better scheduled for the post-deployment normalisation period when personnel have started to process their deployment experiences.

Depleted uranium exposure

Depleted uranium (DU) was cited as a potential factor in the emergence of poor health after deployment during *Operation Granby* and became part of the Gulf War Syndrome saga. US forces carried out surveillance of soldiers with embedded DU fragments resulting from so-called friendly fire incidents that occurred during *Operation Desert Storm*. They found that contaminated personnel continued to excrete DU in their urine some 15 years following initial exposure; however, they did not experience any significant health problems that might be explained by DU contamination.[114] Following the end of the 2003 deployment in Iraq, KCMHR conducted a study among personnel deemed to be at substantial risk of DU exposure, for instance those involved in clean-up operations where DU weapons had been deployed and those manoeuvring among destroyed enemy vehicles. Among 341 personnel, no evidence was found for increased levels of urinary DU[115] and no adverse health effects were detected. A further study suggested that those who most wanted DU screening were the most anxious people, not those who were most likely to have been exposed to DU during deployment.[116]

POST-DEPLOYMENT MENTAL HEALTH

Battlemind training

Battlemind is a comprehensive training package developed for use in the US Army.[117,118] The intervention can be delivered at various stages of the deployment cycle, including the post-deployment period. The content of post-deployment *Battlemind* is similar to the standard mental health briefing delivered to UK personnel when they finish deployment; however, they differ in some important respects. Both interventions make use of a group delivery format; however, in contrast to UK stress briefing, *Battlemind* is designed to be interactive rather than didactic, and participants are encouraged to share their experiences with other training group members. The training uses an acronym where each letter of 'Battlemind' represents a unique set of skills, which are abilities, behaviours or states of mind that personnel relied upon during deployment. *Battlemind* training demonstrates the way in which personnel can successfully transition each of the deployment skills to the home environment. For example, the second T in *Battlemind* stands for 'tactical awareness', which is very useful in the deployment setting, however, it can come to represent hypervigilance when at home, a cardinal feature of PTSD. Through interaction with *Battlemind* participants, trainers use the varied experiences in the audience and their own suggestions to illustrate ways in which each of the 10 deployment skills can be transitioned to the home setting.

Battlemind training has some research support. In a US cluster RCT, Adler et al. compared post-deployment *Battlemind* training with stress education and PD in small groups versus large groups of US Army personnel. Although no overall significant effect of *Battlemind* training was found, among personnel who had experienced high levels of combat, *Battlemind* recipients experienced significantly lower levels of PTSD symptoms, depression and sleep problems compared to high combat stress brief recipients; group size did not have a significant effect upon outcome.[117]

Given that a small but significant advantage was gained from receiving US post-deployment *Battlemind* training, UK military researchers designed a study to assess the effect of training on UK Armed Forces personnel.[119] The acronym was re-designed and associated training adjusted to account for language, culture and differences in mental disorder prevalence between US and UK military personnel, producing an anglicised version of the training package.

Anglicised group-based, post-deployment *Battlemind* training was compared with the standard stress and homecoming briefing package in a cluster RCT. Both interventions were delivered to groups up to company size who were transitioning the TLD facility upon return from Afghanistan. Incidences of PTSD, CMD, depression, alcohol use and stigmatising beliefs about mental health and healthcare represented outcome measures in the study.

A total of 2443 military personnel participated in the study, 66.1% of whom completed the follow-up study measures approximately six months after receiving either *Battlemind* or standard end-of-tour stress briefing. Both forms of briefing were equally well received. No statistically significant differences were detected between the two interventions for PTSD, CMD, depression, sleep or levels of mental health stigmatisation. The effect on alcohol use was of borderline significance, and binge drinking was significantly lower among *Battlemind* recipients who also had better sleep quality at follow-up. To assess whether the US findings regarding combat exposure were relevant to the UK study, mental health outcomes and stigma were compared between study arms stratified by combat exposure; there was no effect. *Battlemind* training is a prime example of an intervention that is coherent and attractive in terms of its simplicity and appears instinctively useful; however, when subjected to rigorous testing, it was only marginally more effective than a standard briefing approach. One important finding arising from this research is that when introducing a novel approach, no matter how useful it appears, programme developers should always try to incorporate a robust evaluation process. As the *Battlemind* study demonstrated some positive effect upon alcohol use, this aspect of *Battlemind* training has now been incorporated into routine post-deployment stress briefing for UK personnel.

Reserves

The available evidence suggests that reserve forces personnel experience disproportionate deployment-related negative mental health effects compared to their regular forces counterparts. Reserves deployed to Iraq and/or Afghanistan were significantly more likely to feel unsupported by the military and were more likely to report impaired social functioning after returning home. Perceived lack of support from the military was significantly associated with the development of PTSD symptoms and alcohol misuse. Poor social support and lack of engagement with available support were additionally associated with CMD symptoms.[120] Reserve personnel who had deployed to Iraq were compared with non-deployed reserves; five years after baseline assessment, deployed reserves were twice as likely to experience PTSD symptoms and were significantly more likely to report actual or serious consideration of separation from their partners.[121]

MILITARY FAMILIES

Relationships

Until recently, UK military families have received little research attention despite being crucial to the military effectiveness of personnel serving in Iraq and Afghanistan and pivotal to successful reintegration post-deployment. Recent UK studies suggest that among King's military cohort participants, the majority had few relationship difficulties despite the rigours of military service[122] and that most problems were unrelated to deployment.[123] Among those participants who did report relationship problems, personal vulnerability, limited support from their partner, being in an unmarried relationship, financial problems and Harmony Guideline breaches were key determinants of perceived relationship quality. A further qualitative study exploring military relationships generated five themes, each representing practical, emotional and cultural dilemmas that UK soldiers (this was a single service study, not involving the Royal Navy or RAF) must balance in order to maintain successful marriages and Army careers. The authors suggested that practical and emotional solutions suggested by soldiers could be used to inform relationship resilience-building interventions.[124]

Children

UK research data exploring the effects of military life upon children's mental health is not well developed. Using cohort data, UK researchers explored military life with and without deployment to assess the impact upon children. Over half of all surveyed personnel reported a negative impact of military service upon their children, with regular forces describing a greater impact than reserves. Cumulative deployment length, the presence of mental disorder symptoms and promotion above junior rank were all associated with reporting a greater impact upon children.[125] Using funds provided by the US Department of Defense, during the period of deployment in Iraq and Afghanistan, UK researchers conducted a series of mixed-method studies examining the mental health effects of having a mentally ill father among children of service families. Although yet to be published, the study outcomes suggest that there were no adverse psychological consequences arising from paternal deployment. However, when the father came back with PTSD symptoms, there was a substantial impact on the child's emotional and social functioning. The latter was especially evident among boys and those aged less than 11 years old.

Families of wounded, injured and sick personnel

The military family has a critical role to play in the psychological recovery from physical ill-health and injury, including combat and operational trauma. *Wounded, injured and sick* (WIS) personnel are at increased risk of discharge from the UK Armed Forces on medical grounds, and additionally, a study monitoring the mental health of UK battle-injured personnel highlighted a substantial risk of developing mental health symptoms post-injury[126]; those sustaining genital injury are thought to be at substantial risk of poor mental health.[127] A series of mixed-method studies examining the support needs of WIS personnel and their families suggested that while many services were provided to support such families, a single access point for information and sign-posting guidance was notably absent. Additionally, there were few restorative mental health support services for family members with mental health needs and little robust evaluation of current support mechanisms. A further study investigated the impact of caring for WIS personnel upon the employment experiences of family members. The following themes were identified: (1) disruption of employment and career pathway; (2) excessive demands upon the caregiver; and (3) supportive and unsupportive factors in the work environment. Family studies are potentially the weakest area of UK military mental health research, and more studies of the role of military families in sustaining mental health are warranted.[128]

MENTAL HEALTH STIGMATISATION AND PERCEIVED BARRIERS TO CARE

A key feature of mental health support following the deployments in Iraq and Afghanistan is to promote appropriate help-seeking among those with persistent mental disorder symptoms. Studies of mental health and help-seeking suggest that a substantial proportion of military personnel do not seek support or treatment despite experiencing psychological distress and mental disorder symptoms. Among the potential factors influencing the decision to engage with and fully participate in mental health treatment programmes[129] are the effects of stigmatising beliefs (stigma) and perceived *barriers to care*.[130] Mental health stigmatisation is complex; however, some research suggests that it is both socially determined and an individual cognitive construct that helps to avoid receiving both a mental illness label and the social damage perceived to accompany such a label; the result being avoidance of help and non-adherence to therapy.[131] Research suggests that stigma is commonplace among military personnel,[132] that it is ubiquitous, comparable in character within various international armed forces,[133] and that it may also affect civilians in equal measure.[134,135]

Some researchers cite potential stigmatisation as a major influence on the willingness to disclose symptoms among military personnel.[136] Work from King's College London has shown that rates of reporting stigma fluctuate over time; exploration of the patterns of reporting suggests that self-stigmatisation generally correlates with current levels of subjective stress, work overload and mental health symptoms.[137] Substantial PTSD symptoms are strongly related to greater levels of stigma and reduced help-seeking.[138] Stigma may not be the only determinant of reduced help-seeking; research conducted among Canadian military personnel found that many simply fail to recognise that they are ill and that this is the major reason for not seeking help rather than the inhibiting effects of stigma.[139] Some military personnel assume that seeking support will lead to them being ostracised by peers and leaders with an accompanying loss of social position, or that within the military, occupational restrictions might ensue from declaring a mental health problem.[140] Military culture has been cited as a factor that may unintentionally foster mental health stigmatisation,[141] and military personnel frequently report negative views about mental health treatment.[142] Even though factors other than stigma may exert an influence, the weight of research evidence is that stigma and perceived barriers to care are important factors in mental health-related help-seeking.[143,144] So the relationship between current mental health status, prevailing levels of stigma/barriers to care and help-seeking is complex. Furthermore, stigmatisation might differ in character to perceived barriers to care, and each factor may exert both overlapping and unique influences upon help-seeking and mental health.

The military of many nations, including the United Kingdom, have sought to reduce stigma/barriers to care, mostly through group-based, public health activities such as psycho-education.[145] Educational interventions often incorporate mixed media campaigns and peer support programmes.[146] The effectiveness of adopting such approaches is at best mixed, with some outcome studies reporting substantial and durable positive effects upon stigma-related knowledge,[147] while others suggest that background levels of stigmatising beliefs remain largely unaffected.[148,149] Intervention-based approaches appear to have limitations, and military studies suggest that a more fruitful approach may be to attempt to modify the behaviour of leaders as there is some evidence suggesting that stigma can be positively influenced by the attitudes and behaviour of middle-tier military commanders.[150]

UK MILITARY STIGMA RESEARCH

The UK military provides high-quality mental healthcare services that are readily accessible; but as research demonstrates, military personnel often fail to do just that – access them. Using data obtained from the OMHNE study series, a principal component analysis study suggested that reduced help-seeking may be related to two main concerns: firstly, potential loss of trust and credibility among military peers and commanders, and secondly, fear of negative occupational consequences.[151] A systematic review suggested that the two most commonly reported stigmatising beliefs were 'My unit leadership might treat me differently if I had a mental health problem' and 'I would be seen as weak if I declared a mental health problem'.[152]

Comparing data obtained during decompression following deployment to Afghanistan and then approximately six months later, positive perceptions of leadership and better unit cohesion were both significantly associated with lower mental health stigmatisation levels, while greater unit cohesion was significantly associated with awareness of and willingness to discuss mental health matters.[153] Other studies have similarly shown that unit cohesion is an important determinant of mental health.[154] A study based on the same dataset examined the association of stigma and barriers to care with mental health and help-seeking. Both mental health symptoms and harmful alcohol use were significantly associated with higher levels of stigma over time. Stigma levels were correlated with changes in mental health symptom levels, suggesting that mental health symptoms, stigma and barriers to care have a reciprocal relationship. Of particular note was the finding that personnel who recovered from probable mental disorder reported significantly lower levels of stigma/barriers to care than did those with no symptoms or stable symptoms, whereas those with new-onset probable mental disorder symptoms reported significantly higher rates of stigma and barriers to care. So perhaps personnel with remitted symptoms might be in a good position to deliver a meaningful stigma reduction message.[155]

UK military researchers undertook a study examining the relationship between stigmatising beliefs, perceived barriers to care and probable PTSD among 23,101 military personnel deployed to Afghanistan and Iraq both before and after deployment and in a smaller group some six months later.[156] Overall, stigma levels were significantly higher during deployment than upon immediate exit from theatre. In a smaller group assessed six months post-deployment, stigma had increased significantly but was still lower than the levels found during deployment. Overall, men, more heavily combat exposed personnel and those with higher levels of PTSD symptoms reported the most stigma. Although the exact cause for the high levels of stigma found during deployment remained unclear, perhaps stigma may have helped to motivate personnel to complete their operational deployment without recourse to help-seeking, whilst they may be more moderate in their views of mental ill-health when the pressure is off, for instance during decompression.

In the latter study, the main stigmatising belief related to fear of being treated differently by commanders and to loss of trust among peers. The reporting of stigma/barriers to care reduced significantly over multiple sampling points and across several years. The study findings could have been related to the UK Armed Forces' anti-stigma campaigns conducted during the period of data collection, although this has not been formally demonstrated. The authors suggested that during deployment, a careful balance must be struck between encouraging help-seeking and maintaining the operational effectiveness of deployed personnel.[157]

In a UK study of 484 Army personnel awaiting deployment to Afghanistan, 40% of probable mental health cases and 70% of alcohol misusers had not sought any form of help. Significantly raised levels of stigma and barriers to care were found among personnel with probable mental disorder symptoms but not among alcohol misusers. When personnel sought help, non-medical help sources were accessed more frequently than military medical services. Friends or family were the most commonly preferred and actual source of support, while unit commanders were among the least preferred but the second most commonly accessed. Reinforcing the importance of stigma and barriers to care in help-seeking, interest in receiving help while not actually seeking it was significantly associated with heightened stigma and barriers to care. The authors recommended that military stigma reduction strategies should focus upon reassuring personnel and their families that adverse consequences are not inevitable and that seeking help from any source may be a useful step in addressing mental health problems, while alcohol misusers may benefit from a strategy that helps them to view their alcohol use as potentially socially and occupationally problematic.[158]

Given that anti-stigma interventions appear to have a small effect, UK military researchers used a novel approach comparing a comedy show containing an embedded positive mental health and stigma-reduction message with a comedy show with no such content. Both shows were viewed by military personnel in a garrison setting while they awaited deployment to Afghanistan. After the show, the mental health message group reported significantly less stigmatisation and answered mental health-related questions more accurately than the standard comedy show group. At follow-up, neither difference was maintained; however, mental health message recipients were statistically significantly more likely to have discussed mental health matters and to have advised others about mental health; however, adjusted analyses suggested that this was related to factors other than comedy show type.[159]

In summary, stigma and barriers to care are substantial among military personnel, although no different in character and magnitude to those found among civilians. Military stigma and barriers to care have reduced over time for reasons that are not clear, but remain a significant problem and appear somewhat resistant to stigma-reduction strategies. The weight of evidence suggests that they may well have a role to play in inhibiting help-seeking.

Alcohol

It may be unsurprising that there is a tradition of heavy alcohol use in the military stretching back generations; however, in modern times, attitudes to the use of alcohol have been mixed, with some viewing drinking as harmful to health, occupational and social functioning, whilst some research suggests that alcohol has a potentially positive influence on morale and cohesion, both key features of a successful military.[160] This is not necessarily a positive finding as further studies suggest that, although heavy drinkers were significantly more likely to report high levels of comradeship within their unit, they experienced significantly more negative views of their unit leadership and a greater number of major problems at home during deployment.[161]

Until recently, the scale and pattern of contemporary UK military drinking behaviour remained largely unknown; however, the current research effort driven by the Iraq and Afghanistan deployments has provided some answers. The King's cohort has been instrumental in studying alcohol use among military personnel. The cohort survey instrument included the *Alcohol Use Disorders Identification Test*, an alcohol measure widely used in research. It has been possible to compare regular and reserve forces and the three Services with the UK general population and to study changes over time. The results suggested that both men and women under the age of 35 have at least double the rate of alcohol misuse compared to an age- and sex-matched sample of the UK general population, the effect being particularly marked in younger military women. Among the younger age groups, military personnel were more than twice as likely to binge drink as their civilian counterparts; this may be important in a military context as alcohol misuse is frequently co-morbid with PTSD.[162,163] Alcohol misuse was particularly associated with youth, male sex and junior rank and with service in the Army. Those with a parent with an alcohol or drug problem were at heightened risk, and members of the Royal Navy appeared to be at particular risk of drinking heavily.[164] The use of alcohol appeared to decrease with increasing age, reaching parity with levels similar to the UK general population by the age of 35.

At the start of the campaigns in Iraq and Afghanistan, alcohol consumption and the prevalence of binge-drinking continued to increase over time, especially among personnel who had deployed and particularly among those who perceived that their life was in danger during their period of deployment.[165] More recent studies have suggested that, although hazardous alcohol consumption levels remain high, there has been a small but significant decrease in overall levels of use; this was mostly predicted by remission from mental health disorder symptoms, stopping smoking and beginning a new relationship. Increases in alcohol consumption were associated with new-onset or persistent PTSD symptoms and ending a loving relationship.[166] Cohort data suggest that overall, there may be a significant relationship between deployment and alcohol use with around a 20% increase in alcohol misuse following return from operations. It appears that personnel re-institute and accelerate their drinking after a period of operational abstinence before returning to a more consistent pattern of use.

As heavy drinking is mostly concentrated in younger members of the military, chronic alcohol dependence is not commonly seen. Furthermore, regular 'dry' deployments are also likely to mitigate the development of classic dependence. That does not mean that there is immunity from the age-related effects arising from sustained heavy drinking, a topic of current study. There is some evidence that perceived functional impairment may only affect military personnel with possible alcohol dependence or levels of use that might cause alcohol related-harm; therefore, interventions targeting those with lower level, but potentially concerning, alcohol use may not resonate with this large sub-group.[167]

Risky driving

The KCMHR cohort study used a number of survey questions to ask about various risk-taking behaviours such as driving too fast, driving without wearing a seat belt and driving under the influence of alcohol. The survey results suggested that there was an impact upon risk-taking post-deployment, which affected Army personnel in particular, occurring most frequently among young, single junior ranks undertaking a combat role who experienced combat during their period of deployment. Irrespective of whether they had deployed or not, 19% of UK Armed Forces personnel were categorised as risky drivers.[168] Among reserves, the overall prevalence of risky driving was 11%, and again, deployment was significantly associated with risky driving.[169] It is possible that risky driving is related to a failure to decouple from the operational driving mindset or a tendency to engage in sensation-seeking in the period of relative calm following intense operational experiences. Concern for safety following return from deployment prompted action to reduce the rate of accidents after deployment using an educational, video-based campaign. Although it is not possible to attribute changes to the campaign alone, based upon data from phase 2 of the King's cohort study, the prevalence of risky driving reduced from 18% to 14% over approximately three years. The incidence of new-onset risky driving was 7% and was associated with younger age, being single and harmful alcohol use; personnel who deployed after the road safety campaign was introduced were significantly less likely to engage in risky driving following deployment compared with those deployed before its introduction.[170]

Offending

In preparation for a large-scale study, a systematic review of military criminal offending was undertaken, which indicated that post-deployment violence was a potentially significant problem in military personnel and appeared to be related to combat exposure, PTSD symptoms and alcohol misuse.[171] In the first study of its kind, KCMHR researchers managed, not without effort, to link together data from the Kings cohort with criminal justice records (*Police National Computer* records).[172] The first finding might surprise some; overall rates of convictions were lower amongst military personnel than in an age-matched civilian cohort[173] even before adjusting for the fact that the Armed forces recruit people from disadvantaged backgrounds who are already at higher risk of offending. So overall, a military career positively improved the life trajectory of a disadvantaged group, but unfortunately, there is no such thing as a free lunch, because there was a significant exception. Violent offending

rates were higher, especially amongst men younger than 30 years of age. Serving in a combat role and experiencing traumatic events during deployment, post-deployment alcohol misuse, PTSD and self-reported aggressive behaviour were associated with violent offending although deployment alone was not.[174] Although a substantial proportion of violent offending appeared to be related to past conduct disorder,[175] increased violent offending was one of the clearest adverse outcomes of combat exposure.

International military interest in domestic violence (DV) is increasing, and there is some evidence that poorer mental health among military personnel may be associated with DV.[176] This does not appear to be a unique association as poorer mental health was also associated with other forms of in-service offending and subsequent poorer adjustment following discharge from service once a military prison term was completed.[177,178]

Although it does not always have a direct link with violence, anger can be an important component of mental ill-health. Among 9885 King's cohort participants, there was a moderate to strong association between anger and sub-clinical PTSD, CMD symptoms, multiple physical symptoms, alcohol misuse, combat role, childhood adversity and childhood antisocial behaviour.[179] Such study findings have important implications for clinicians, and further studies assessing the outcome of anger management interventions in particular are clearly warranted, but as yet, none have been completed within the UK military.

Given that the UK Armed Forces and, in particular, the Army recruit from areas of deprivation where exposure to crime and violence whilst growing up may be substantial, coupled with the requirement among the 'teeth arms' to use controlled violence while deployed, violent offending is an important area of study.

LONGER-TERM CONSEQUENCES OF DEPLOYMENT

Service leavers, veterans and wounded or injured personnel

Robust research among those who have left service is relatively sparse; however, many military cohort study participants, large numbers of whom have undertaken deployment to Iraq or Afghanistan, are followed up into civilian life and continue to provide data to inform this area. Although veterans are often characterised in press and popular narrative as 'damaged' by their military service, particularly from a mental health perspective, the reality may not reflect this, with the majority remaining mentally well and gaining full employment.[180] Using data extracted from the *Adult Psychiatric Morbidity Survey*, military veterans were no more likely than the general public to be mentally unwell or less engaged with mental health treatments and therapies,[181] although King's cohort data suggest that military veterans may well have higher rates of PTSD than serving regulars. Furthermore, a large sample comparison of veterans and non-veterans suggested that veterans had significantly higher rates of first-episode mental disorder and the risk for such an outcome was higher among those with shorter service careers and highest amongst those who failed to complete basic training.[182] Further studies suggest that only about half of ex-Service personnel with a mental health problem seek help, mostly from their GP, with few consulting mental health specialists.[183] There are, however, sub-groups of service leaver who may fare less well than others. Using King's cohort data, a comparison of service leavers and serving personnel was made, the outcome of which suggested that, compared to those remaining in service, leavers reported less social participation outside work, general disengagement with military social contacts and an increased likelihood of being mentally unwell. Levels of mental health were partly related to reduced levels of social integration among service leavers. Service leavers who maintained social networks in which most members were still serving were more likely to experience alcohol misuse and to be mentally unwell.[184]

King's researchers produced the 'Counting the Costs' study,[185] which provided a crude estimate of current and future veteran care needs, calculating that there are substantial unmet physical and psychological needs for physical and mental healthcare among ex-service personnel; one possible reason for the under-utilisation of veteran-specific care arrangements is that around 50% of ex-Service personnel do not consider themselves to be 'veterans'.[186]

To better understand the care requirement of minority disability groups, research was undertaken for *Blind Veterans UK* to evaluate the health needs of personnel rendered sightless during their military service. Not surprisingly, their mental health needs were substantial,[187] although there were no differences between those blinded by combat and those blinded by non-combat events.[188] In sub-group analyses, the psychosocial well-being of female ex-Service personnel was adversely affected by visual loss, although over time, women developed strategies to cope with the various visual impairment challenges and limitations.[189]

The veteran's charity *Combat Stress* is a major provider of care for UK ex-Service personnel; the charity previously reported considerable latency between leaving service and seeking care; however, there is now mounting evidence that veterans of the conflicts in Afghanistan and Iraq are seeking help at an accelerating rate post-service,[190] with a four-fold increase in the number of referrals to Combat Stress during the period of deployment to Iraq and Afghanistan. The available evidence therefore suggests that veterans from Iraq and Afghanistan are seeking help more quickly after finishing service than are veterans from previous conflicts.[191]

One category of veteran, namely the *early service leaver*, appears to be particularly difficult to help as they often have complex support needs[192] and higher levels of childhood adversity, a risk factor for PTSD in military personnel.[193] Indeed, there is some suggestion that a substantial proportion of mental illness among UK military personnel may be related to pre-enlistment vulnerability rather than in-service experiences.[194] Early service leavers leave service before they have completed their elective service term. Given that they have short periods of service, they may not have deployed; however, due to pressure to fully populate the order of battle during the periods of deployment in Iraq and Afghanistan, they may well have deployed early after completing their initial military training further compounding existing vulnerability.

CONCLUSION

At the outset of the campaign in Iraq and the subsequent deployment to Afghanistan, little was known about the mental health of the modern UK Armed

Forces. Some research had been undertaken with veterans of the earlier deployment to the Persian Gulf, the research programme being driven by concern that military personnel's health may have suffered as a result of the deployment. This early research effort has been further developed into a comprehensive programme that owes much of its success to the close working relationship forged between the UK Ministry of Defence and university academics; the 2016 Chilcot report examined in detail decision-making in the UK Government in relation to operations in Iraq immediately prior to and during operation Telic, and although many of the findings were critical, the mental health research effort and medico-welfare support were singled out for praise.

The research continues, and it is possible that a different picture of UK military mental health might emerge in the future; indeed, at the time of writing, KCMHR researchers are busy contacting personnel who responded to earlier phases of the military cohort study along with a group of new cohort recruits. So far, despite the protracted wars in Iraq and Afghanistan, the majority of UK Armed Forces personnel remain mentally healthy; however, important sub-groups are at increased risk of developing symptoms of mental disorder as a result of deployment, namely personnel deployed in a combat role and reserve forces personnel. There is therefore no room for complacency, and those who deliberately place themselves in harm's way deserve to have their mental health and well-being properly evaluated, understood and fully supported. Combat personnel are not the only group at risk of adverse mental health outcomes. Although many may not have deployed, early service leavers represent a challenging group who appear to suffer substantially more problems after discharge from the UK military than those who complete their elective term of service and are likely to be difficult to locate and less likely to engage with helping services after returning to the civilian world.

The programme of research described in this chapter identifies a number of areas that require attention. Alcohol misuse remains a substantial problem, and it appears that attempts to limit alcohol intake have been largely unsuccessful. Great effort has been expended in trying to ameliorate the adverse effects of deployment; however, the great majority of mental health support interventions have a small effect, although their cumulative impact may well be more profound. The majority of service personnel and veterans do not seek help when symptomatic despite the widespread delivery of educational and stigma-reduction campaigns; the challenge of connecting the right personnel to the right sources of help at the right time remains. At the time of writing, UK Armed Forces deployments to trouble spots around the world continue, albeit in reduced numbers, so the threat to military personnel's mental well-being remains. There is no available comprehensive solution that can eradicate all risks associated with military service, and psychiatric injury will continue to pose a management challenge to military commanders and health providers. The current programme of research will continue to assist in clarifying the extent of such injury, identifying important predisposing, precipitating and maintaining factors and will help to test the efficacy of mental health support initiatives.

REFERENCES

1. UK National Institute for Health and Clinical Excellence (NICE) Guidelines National Institute for Health and Clinical Excellence, 2005 http://www.nice.org.uk/Guidance/CG26.
2. Jones E, Wessely S. "Forward psychiatry" in the military: Its origins and effectiveness. *J Traumatic Stress* 2003;16(4):411–419.
3. Jones E, Thomas A, Ironside S. Shell shock: An outcome study of a First World War 'PIE' unit. *Psychol Med* 2007;37(2):215–224.
4. Unwin C, Blatchley N, Coker W et al. Health of UK servicemen who served in Persian Gulf War. *Lancet* 1999;353(9148):169–178.
5. Rona RJ, Jones M, French C, Hooper R, Wessely S. Screening for physical and psychological illness in the British Armed Forces: I: The acceptability of the programme. *J Med Screen* 2004;11(3):148–152.
6. Jones M, Rona RJ, Hooper R, Wessely S. The burden of psychological symptoms in UK Armed Forces. *Occup Med* 2006; 56(5):322–328.

7. Rona RJ, Hooper R, Jones M et al. Mental health screening in armed forces before the Iraq war and prevention of subsequent psychological morbidity: Follow-up study. *BMJ* 2006;333(7576):991.

8. Rona RJ, Hooper R, Jones M et al. The contribution of prior psychological symptoms and combat exposure to post Iraq deployment mental health in the UK military. *J Traumatic Stress* 2009;22(1):11–19.

9. Horn O, Sloggett A, Ploubidis GB et al. Upward trends in symptom reporting in the UK Armed Forces. *Eur J Epidemiol* 2010; 25(2):87–94.

10. Horn O, Hull L, Jones M et al. Is there an Iraq war syndrome? Comparison of the health of UK service personnel after the Gulf and Iraq wars. *Lancet* 2006;367(9524): 1742–1746.

11. *Philos Trans R Soc Lond B Biol Sci* 2006: 361(1648).

12. Harding T. Medical journal warns of 'tidal wave' of mental trauma among servicemen. *The Telegraph*, 2012. http://www.telegraph.co.uk/news/uknews/defence/7716014/Medical-journal-warns-of-tidal-wave-of-mental-trauma-among-servicemen.html

13. Hopkins N. Number of UK war veterans seeking help for mental health issues on the rise. *The Guardian*, 2014. https://www.theguardian.com/uk-news/2014/may/12/uk-war-veterans-mental-health-issues-rise

14. Gribble R, Wessley S, Klein S, Alexander DA, Dandeker C, Fear NT. British public opinion after a decade of war: Attitudes to Iraq and Afghanistan. *Politics* 2015;35(2): 128–150.

15. Hines LA, Gribble R, Wessely S, Dandeker C, Fear NT. Armed forces understood and supported by the public? A view from the United Kingdom. *Armed Forces Soc* 2016;41:688–713 (original doi: 10.1177/0095327X14559975. *Armed Forces Soc* 42(2):478).

16. Berndtsson J, Dandeker C, Yden K. Swedish and British public opinion of the Armed Forces after a decade of war. *Armed Forces Soc* 2015;41(2):307–328.

17. Sundin J, Fear NT, Hull L et al. Rewarding and unrewarding aspects of deployment to Iraq and its association with psychological health in UK military personnel. *Int Arch Occup Environ Health* 2010;83(6): 653–663.

18. Campion BH, Hughes JH, Devon M, Fear NT. Psychological morbidity during the 2002 deployment to Afghanistan. *J R Army Med Corps* 2006;152(2):91–93.

19. Hughes JH, Cameron F, Eldridge R, Devon M, Wessely S, Greenberg N. Going to war does not have to hurt: Preliminary findings from the British deployment to Iraq. *Br J Psychiatry* 2005;186(6):536–537.

20. Jones N, Greenberg N, Fear NT et al. The operational mental health consequences of deployment to Iraq for UK Forces. *J R Army Med Corps* 2008:154(2):102–106.

21. McManus S, Meltzer H, Brugha T, Bebbington P, Jenkins R. Adult psychiatric morbidity in England, 2007. NHS Information Centre for health and social care. 2009. www.ic.nhs.uk/pubs.

22. Hines LA, Sundin J, Rona RJ, Wessely S, Fear NT. Posttraumatic stress disorder post Iraq and Afghanistan: Prevalence among military subgroups. *Can J Psychiatry* 2014;59(9):468–479.

23. Iversen AC, van Staden L, Hughes JH et al. The prevalence of common mental disorders and PTSD in the UK military: Using data from a clinical interview-based study. *BMC Psychiatry* 2009;9(1):1.

24. Rona RJ, Jones M, Iversen A et al. The impact of posttraumatic stress disorder on impairment in the UK military at the time of the Iraq war. *J Psychiatr Res* 2009;43(6):649–655.

25. Rona RJ, Fear NT, Hull L, Wessely S. Women in novel occupational roles: Mental health trends in the UK Armed Forces. *Int J Epidemiol* 2007;36(2):319–326.

26. Woodhead C, Wessely S, Jones N, Fear NT, Hatch SL. Impact of exposure to combat during deployment to Iraq and Afghanistan on mental health by gender. *Psychol Med* 2012;42(9):1985–1996.

27. Goodwin L, Ben-Zion I, Fear NT, Hotopf M, Stansfeld SA, Wessely S. Are reports of

psychological stress higher in occupational studies? A systematic review across occupational and population based studies. *PLoS One* 20138(11):e78693.

28. Hotopf M, Hull L, Fear N et al. The health of UK military personnel who deployed to the 2003 Iraq war: A cohort study. *Lancet* 2006;367:1731–1741.

29. Hoge CW, Castro CA, Messer SC et al. Combat duty in Iraq and Afghanistan, mental health problems, and barriers to care. *N Engl J Med* 2004;351:13–22.

30. Sundin J, Herrell RK, Hoge CW et al. Mental health outcomes in US and UK military personnel returning from Iraq. *Br J Psychiatry* 2014:204(3):200–207. doi:10.1192/bjp.bp.113.129569

31. Wilson J, Jones M, Fear NT et al. Is previous psychological health associated with the likelihood of Iraq War deployment? An investigation of the "healthy warrior effect". *Am J Epidemiol* 2009;169(11):1362–1369.

32. Sareen J, Cox BJ, Afifi TO et al. Combat and peacekeeping operations in relation to prevalence of mental disorders and perceived need for mental health care: Findings from a large representative sample of military personnel. *Arch Gen Psychiatry* 2007;64(7):843–852.

33. Zamorski MA, Bennett RE, Rusu C, Weeks M, Boulos D, Garber BG. Prevalence of past-year mental disorders in the Canadian Armed Forces, 2002–2013. *Can J Psychiatry* 2016;61(1 Suppl):26S–35S.

34. Fear NT, Jones M, Murphy D et al. What are the consequences of deployment to Iraq and Afghanistan on the mental health of the UK armed forces? A cohort study. *Lancet* 2010;375:1783–1797.

35. Sundin J, Jones N, Greenberg NRRJ et al. Mental health among commando, airborne and other UK infantry personnel. *Occup Med* 2010;60(7):552–559. doi: 10.1093/occmed/kqq129.

36. Goodwin L, Wessely S, Hotopf M et al. Are common mental disorders more prevalent in the UK serving military compared to the general working population? *Psychol Med* 2015;45(09):1881–1891.

37. Goodwin L, Jones M, Rona RJ, Sundin J, Wessely S, Fear NT. Prevalence of delayed-onset posttraumatic stress disorder in military personnel: Is there evidence for this disorder?: Results of a prospective UK cohort study. *J Nerv Ment Dis* 2012;200(5):429–437.

38. Banwell E, Greenberg N, Smith P, Jones N, Fertout M. What happens to the mental health of UK service personnel after they return home from Afghanistan? *J R Army Med Corps.* 2016;162:115–119. doi:10.1136/jramc-2015-000425.

39. Rona RJ, Jones M, Goodwin L, Hull L, Wessely S. Risk Factors for headache in the UK military: Cross-sectional and longitudinal analyses. *Headache J Head Face Pain* 2013;53(5):787–798.

40. Goodwin L, Bourke JH, Forbes H et al. Irritable bowel syndrome in the UK military after deployment to Iraq: What are the risk factors? *Soc Psychiatry Psychiatr Epidemiol* 2013;48(11):1755–1765.

41. Gould M, Sharpley J, Greenberg N. Patient characteristics and clinical activities at a British military department of community mental health. *Psychiatr Bull* 2008;32(3):99–102.

42. Gov.uk. UK armed forces mental health annual statistics: Index. https://www.gov.uk/government/collections/defence-mental-health-statistics-index

43. Iversen AC, van Staden L, Hughes JH et al. Help-seeking and receipt of treatment among UK service personnel. *Br J Psychiatry* 2010;197(2):149–155.

44. Hines LA, Goodwin L, Jones M et al. Factors affecting help seeking for mental health problems after deployment to Iraq and Afghanistan. *Psychiatr Serv* 2014;65(1): 98–105.

45. SPEG 19/04 OROSM – 29 September 2004.

46. JSP 770, Pt2, Ch 3 – Tri Service Operational and non-operational welfare policy.

47. Vermetten E, Greenberg N, Boeschoten MA et al. Deployment-related mental health support: Comparative analysis of NATO and allied ISAF partners. *Eur J Psychotraumatol* 2014;5. doi.org/10.3402/ejpt.v5.23732.

48. Azari J, Dandeker C, Greenberg N. Cultural stress: How interactions with and among foreign populations affect military personnel. *Armed Forces Soc* 2010;36(4):585–603.

49. Greene T, Buckman J, Dandeker C, Greenberg N. The influence of culture clash on deployed troops. *Mil Med* 2010;175(12):958–963.

50. Mulligan K, Jones N, Woodhead C, Davies M, Wessely S, Greenberg N. Mental health of UK military personnel while on deployment in Iraq. *Br J Psychiatry* 2010;197:405–410.

51. Iversen AC, Fear NT, Ehlers A et al. Risk factors for post-traumatic stress disorder among UK Armed Forces personnel. *Psychol Med* 2008;38(04):511–522.

52. Jones N, Mitchell P, Clack J et al. Mental health and psychological support in UK armed forces personnel deployed to Afghanistan in 2010 and 2011. *Br J Psychiatry* 2014;204(2):157–162.

53. Sharpley JG, Fear NT, Greenberg N, Jones M, Wessely S. Pre-deployment stress briefing: Does it have an effect? *Occup Med* 2008; 58(1):30–34.

54. Greenberg N, Langston V, Fear NT, Jones M, Wessely S. An evaluation of stress education in the Royal Navy. *Occup Med* 2009;59(1): 20–24.

55. Murphy D, Hull L, Horn O et al. Anthrax vaccination in a military population before the war in Iraq: Side effects and informed choice. *Vaccine* 2007;25(44):7641–7648.

56. Murphy D, Hotopf M, Marteau T, Wessely S. Multiple vaccinations, health and recall bias in UK Armed Forces deployed to Iraq. *Br Med J* 2008;337:a220.

57. Murphy D, Marteau T, Wessely S. Longitudinal study of UK personnel offered anthrax vaccination: Informed choice, symptom reporting, uptake and pre vaccination health. *Vaccine* 2012;30:1088–1094.

58. Murphy D, Dandeker C, Horn O et al. UK Armed Forces response to an informed consent policy for anthrax vaccination: A paradoxical effect? *Vaccine* 2006;24:3109–3114.

59. Department of the Army. Operation Iraqi Freedom (OIF) Mental Health Advisory Team (MHAT) Report. December 2003.

http://www.pbs.org/wgbh/pages/frontline /shows/heart/readings/mhat.pdf (accessed 7 November 2012).

60. Jones N, Seddon R, Fear NT, McAllister P, Wessely S, Greenberg N. Leadership, cohesion, morale, and the mental health of UK Armed Forces in Afghanistan. *Psychiatry* 201275(1):49–59.

61. Mulligan K, Jones N, Davies M et al. Effects of home on the mental health of British forces serving in Iraq and Afghanistan. *Br J Psychiatry* 2012;201(3):193–198.

62. Dandeker C, Eversden-French C, Greenberg N et al. Laying down Their rifles: The changing influences on the retention of volunteer British Army reservists returning from Iraq, 2003–2006. *Armed Forces Soc* 2010;36(2). doi: 10.1177/0095327X09344068.

63. Greene T, Greenberg N, Buckman J, Dandeker C. How communication with families can both help and hinder service members' mental health and occupational effectiveness on deployment. *Mil Med* 2010;175:745–749.

64. Jones N, Fear NT, Rona R et al. Mild traumatic brain injury (mTBI) among UK military personnel whilst deployed in Afghanistan in 2011. *Brain Inj* 2014;28(7):896–899.

65. Rona RJ, Jones M, Fear NT et al. Mild traumatic brain injury in UK military personnel returning from Afghanistan and Iraq: Cohort and cross-sectional analyses. *J Head Trauma Rehabil* 2012;27(1):33–44.

66. Fear NT, Jones E, Groom M et al. Symptoms of post-concussional syndrome are non-specifically related to mild traumatic brain injury in UK Armed Forces personnel on return from deployment in Iraq: An analysis of self-reported data. *Psychol Med* 2009;39(8):1379–1387.

67. Jones N, Thandi G, Fear NT, Wessely S, Greenberg N. The psychological effects of improvised explosive devices (IEDs) on UK military personnel in Afghanistan. *Occup Environ Med* 2014;71(7):466–471.

68. Jones M, Fear NT Greenberg N et al. Do medical services personnel who deployed to the Iraq war have worse mental health than other deployed personnel? *Eur J Public Health* 2008;18(4):422–427.

69. Cawkill P, Jones M, Fear NT et al. Mental health of UK Armed Forces medical personnel post-deployment. *Occup Med* 2015;65(2):157–164.

70. Whybrow D, Jones N, Evans C, Minshall D, Smith S, Greenberg N. The mental health of deployed UK maritime forces. *Occup Environ Med* 2016;73:75–82 doi:10.1136 /oemed-2015-102961

71. Anderson RJ. Shell shock: An old injury with new weapons. *Mol Interv* 2008;8(5):204–218.

72. Rona RJ, Fear NT, Hull L et al. Mental health consequences of overstretch in the UK armed forces: First phase of a cohort study. *BMJ* 2007;335(7620):603.

73. Rona RJ, Jones M, Fear NT, Sundin J, Hull L, Wessely S. Frequency of mild traumatic brain injury in Iraq and Afghanistan: Are we measuring incidence or prevalence? *J Head Trauma Rehabil* 2012;27(1):75–82.

74. Rona RJ, Jones M, Keeling M, Hull L, Wessely S, Fear NT. Mental health consequences of overstretch in the UK Armed Forces, 2007–09: A population-based cohort study. *Lancet Psychiatry* 2014;1(7):531–538.

75. Turner MA, Kiernan MD, McKechanie AG et al. Acute military psychiatric casualties from the war in Iraq. *Br J Psychiatry* 2005;186:476–479.

76. Forbes HJ, Jones N, Woodhead C. What are the effects of having an illness or injury whilst deployed on post deployment mental health? A population based record linkage study of UK Army personnel who have served in Iraq or Afghanistan. *BMC Psychiatry* 2012;12(1):1.

77. Scott JN. Diagnosis and outcome of psychiatric referrals to the Field Mental Health Team, 202 Field Hospital, Op Telic 1. *J R Army Med Corps* 2005;151:95–100.

78. McAllister PD, Blair SPR, Philpott S. Op Telic – a field mental health team in the general support medical setting. *J R Army Med Corps* 2004;150:107–112.

79. Jones N, Fear NT, Jones M, Wessely S, Greenberg N. Long-term military work outcomes in soldiers who become mental health casualties when deployed on operations. *Psychiatry* 2010;73(4):352–364.

80. Browne T, Hull L, Horn O et al. Explanations for the increase in mental health problems in UK reserve forces who have served in Iraq. *Br J Psychiatry* 2007;190:484–489.

81. Jones N, Wink P, Brown RA et al. A clinical follow-up study of reserve forces personnel treated for mental health problems following demobilisation. *J Ment Health* 2011;20(2):136–145.

82. Jones N, Fertout M, Parsloe L, Greenberg N. An evaluation of the psychological impact of operational rest and recuperation in United Kingdom Armed Forces personnel: A post-intervention survey. *J R Soc Med* 2013;106(11):447–455. 0141076813491085.

83. Parsloe L, Jones N, Fertout M, Luzon O, Greenberg N. Rest and recuperation in the UK Armed Forces. *Occup Med* 2014;64(8):616–621.

84. Burdett H, Jones N, Fear NT, Wessely S, Greenberg N. Early psychosocial intervention following operational deployment: Analysis of a free text questionnaire response. *Mil Med* 2011;176(6):620–625.

85. Rose SC, Bisson J, Churchill R, Wessely S. Psychological debriefing for preventing post traumatic stress disorder (PTSD). *Cochrane Database Syst Rev* 2002;(2): CD000560.

86. Sijbrandij M, Olff M, Reitsma JB, Carlier IV, Gersons BP. Emotional or educational debriefing after psychological trauma randomised controlled trial. *Br J Psychiatry* 2006;189(2):150–155.

87. Mayou RA, Ehlers A, Hobbs M. Psychological debriefing for road traffic accident victims. Three-year follow-up of a randomised controlled trial. *Br J Psychiatry* 2000; 176(6):589–593.

88. Jones N, Roberts P, Greenberg N. Peer-group risk assessment: A post-traumatic management strategy for hierarchical organizations. *Occup Med* 2003;53(7):469–475.

89. Rona RJ, Jones M, Sundin J et al. Predicting persistent posttraumatic stress disorder (PTSD) in UK military personnel who served in Iraq: A longitudinal study. *J Psychiatr Res* 2012;46(9):1191–1198.

90. Keller RT, Greenberg N, Bobo WV, Roberts P, Jones N, Orman DT. Soldier peer mentoring care and support: Bringing psychological awareness to the front. *Mil Med* 2005;170(5):355–361.

91. Sharp ML, Fear NT, Rona RJ et al. Stigma as a barrier to seeking health care among military personnel with mental health problems. *Epidemiol Rev* 2015;37:144–162. mxu012.

92. National Institute for Clinical Excellence. *The Management of Post Traumatic Stress Disorder in Primary and Secondary Care.* London: NICE, 2005.

93. Whybrow D, Jones N, Greenberg N. Corporate knowledge of psychiatric services available in a combat zone. *Mil Med* 2013;178(2):e241–e247.

94. Greenberg N, Cawkhill P, March C, Sharpley J. How to TRiM away at post traumatic stress reactions: Traumatic risk management – now and the future. *J R Navy Med Serv* 2005;91:26–31.

95. Greenberg N, Langston V, Iversen AC, Wessely S. The acceptability of 'Trauma Risk Management' within the UK Armed Forces. *Occup Med* 2011;61(3):184–189.

96. Greenberg N, Henderson A, Langston V, Iversen A, Wessely S. Peer responses to perceived stress in the Royal Navy. *Occup Med* 2007;57(6):424–429.

97. Langston V, Greenberg N, Fear N, Iversen A, French C, Wessely S. Stigma and mental health in the Royal Navy: A mixed methods paper. *J Ment Health* 2010;19(1):8–16.

98. Whybrow D, Jones N, Greenberg N. Corporate knowledge of psychiatric services available in a combat zone. *Mil Med* 2013;178(2):e241–e247.

99. Frappell-Cooke W, Gulina M et al. Does trauma risk management reduce psychological distress in deployed troops? *Occup Med* 2010;60(8):645–650.

100. Hunt E, Jones N, Hastings V, Greenberg N. TRiM: An organizational response to traumatic events in Cumbria Constabulary. *Occup Med* 2013;63(8):549–555.

101. Gould M, Greenberg N, Hetherton J. Stigma and the military: Evaluation of a PTSD psychoeducational program. *J Traumatic Stress* 2007;20(4):505–515.

102. Greenberg N, Langston V, Everitt B et al. A cluster randomized controlled trial to determine the efficacy of TRiM (Trauma Risk Management) in a military population. *J Traumatic Stress* 2010;23(4):430–436.

103. Joint Services Publication Number 770, Part 2, Chapter 3 – Tri Service operational and non-operational welfare policy. HM Stationary Office.

104. Hacker Hughes JGH, Earnshaw M, Greenberg N et al. The use of psychological decompression in military operational environments. *Mil Med* 2008;173(6):534–538.

105. Fertout M, Jones N, Greenberg N, Mulligan K, Knight T, Wessely S. A review of United Kingdom Armed Forces' approaches to prevent post-deployment mental health problems. *Int Rev Psychiatry* 2011;23(2):135–143.

106. Foran HM, Garber BG, Zamorski MA et al. Postdeployment military mental health training: Cross-national evaluations. *Psychol Serv* 2013;10(2):152–160.

107. Zamorski MA, Guest K, Bailey S, Garber BG. Beyond Battlemind: Evaluation of a new mental health training program for Canadian Forces personnel participating in third-location decompression. *Mil Med* 2012;177(11):1245–1253.

108. Garber BG, Zamorski MA. Evaluation of a Third-location decompression program for Canadian Forces members returning from Afghanistan. *Mil Med* 2012;177(4):397–403.

109. Jones N, Burdett H, Wessely S, Greenberg N. The subjective utility of early psychosocial interventions following combat deployment *Occup Med* 2011;61(2):102–107.

110. Burdett H, Jones N, Fear N, Wessely S. Early psychosocial intervention following operational deployment: Analysis of a free text questionnaire response. *Mil Med* 2011;176:620–625.

111. Fertout M, Jones N, Greenberg N. Third location decompression for individual augmentees after a military deployment. *Occup Med* (Lond) 2011;62:188–195.

112. Sundin J, Mulligan K, Henry S et al. Impact on mental health of deploying as an individual augmentee in the UK Armed Forces. *Mil Med* 2012;177(5):511–516.

113. Jones N, Jones M, Fear NT, Fertout M, Wessely S, Greenberg N. Can mental health and readjustment be improved in UK military personnel by a brief period of structured postdeployment rest (third location decompression)? *Occup Environ Med* 2013;70(7):439–445.

114. Squibb KS, McDiarmid MA. Depleted uranium exposure and health effects in Gulf War veterans. *Philos Trans R Soc Lond B Biol Sci* 2006;361(1468):639–648.

115. Bland D, Rona R, Coggon D et al. Urinary isotopic analysis in the UK Armed Forces: No evidence of depleted uranium absorption in combat and other personnel in Iraq. *Occup Environ Med* 2007;64(12):834–838.

116. Greenberg N, Iversen AC, Unwin C, Hull L, Wessely S. Screening for depleted uranium in the United Kingdom armed forces: Who wants it and why? *J Epidemiol Commun Health* 2004;58(7):558–561.

117. Adler AB, Bliese PD, McGurk D, Hoge CW, Castro CA. Battlemind debriefing and battlemind training as early interventions with soldiers returning from Iraq: Randomization by platoon. *J Consult Clin Psychol* 2009;77(5):928–940.

118. Adler AB, Castro CA, McGurk D. Time-driven battlemind psychological debriefing: A group-level early intervention in combat. *Mil Med* 2009;174(1):021–028.

119. Mulligan K, Fear NT, Jones N et al. Postdeployment battlemind training for the UK. Armed Forces: A cluster randomized controlled trial. *J Consult Clin Psychol* 2012;80(3):331–341.

120. Harvey SB, Hatch SL, Jones M et al. Coming home: Social functioning and the mental health of UK Reservists on return from deployment to Iraq or Afghanistan. *Ann Epidemiol* 2011;21(9):666–672.

121. Harvey SB, Hatch SL, Jones M et al. The long-term consequences of military deployment: A 5-year cohort study of United Kingdom reservists deployed to Iraq in 2003. *Am J Epidemiol* 2012;176(12):1177–1184.

122. Keeling M, Wessely S, Dandeker C, Jones N, Fear NT. Relationship difficulties among UK military personnel: Impact of sociodemographic, military, and deployment-related factors. *Marriage Fam Rev* 2015;51(3):275–303.

123. Rowe M, Murphy D, Wessely S, Fear NT. Exploring the impact of deployment to Iraq on relationships. *Mil Behav Health* 2013;1(1):13–21.

124. Keeling M, Woodhead C, Fear N. Interpretative phenomenological analysis of soldier's experience of being married and serving in the British Army. *Marriage Fam Rev* 2016;52:511–534.

125. Rowe SL, Keeling M, Wessely S, Fear NT. Perceptions of the impact a military career has on children. *Occup Med* 2014;64(7):490–496. doi: 10.1093/occmed/kqu096.

126. Internal MoD report prepared by ADMMH. The Battle-Injured Mental Health Monitoring Pathway (BIMHMP) evaluation, dated 27 March 2015.

127. Frappell-Cooke W, Wink Pand Wood A. The psychological challenge of genital injury. *J R Army Med Corps* 2013;(Suppl 1):i–52–i56.

128. Verey A, Keeling M, Thandi G, Stevelink S, Fear NT. *TIN 2.025(B) Support to Families of Wounded, Injured, or Sick (WIS) Service Personnel – An Investigation of Current Service Provision and Potential Gaps.* London: Ministry of Defence, 2015.

129. Keeling M, Knight T, Sharp D et al. Contrasting beliefs about screening for mental disorders among UK military personnel returning from deployment to Afghanistan. *J Med Screen* 2012;1–6. doi: 10.1258/jms.2012.012054.

130. Paykel ES, Hart D, Priest RG. Changes in public attitudes to depression during the Defeat Depression Campaign. *Br J Psychiatry* 1998;173:519–522.

131. Kessler RC, Berglund PA, Bruce ML et al. The Prevalence and Correlates of Untreated Mental Illness. *Health Serv Res* 2001;36:987–1007.

132. Britt TW, Greene-Shortridge TM, Castro CA. The stigma of mental health problems in the military. *Mil Med* 2007;172(2): 157–161.

133. Gould M, Adler A, Zamorski M et al. Do stigma and other perceived barriers to mental health care differ across Armed Forces? *J R Soc Med* 2010;103:148–156. doi: 10.1258/jrsm.2010.090426.

134. Forbes HJ, Boyd CF, Jones N et al. Attitudes to mental illness in the UK Military: A comparison with the general population. *Mil Med* 2013;178(9):957–965.

135. Woodhead C, Rona RJ, Iversen A et al. Mental health and health service use among post-national service veterans: Results from the 2007 Adult Psychiatric Morbidity Survey of England. *Psychol Med* 2011;41:363–372.

136. Seal KH, Bertenthal D, Maguen S, Gima K, Chu A, Marmar CR. Getting beyond "Don't ask; don't tell": An evaluation of US Veterans Administration postdeployment mental health screening of veterans returning from Iraq and Afghanistan. *Am J Public Health* 2008;98(4):714–720.

137. Britt TW, Greene-Shortridge TM, Brink S et al. Perceived stigma and barriers to care for psychological treatment: Implications for reactions to stressors in different contexts. *J Soc Clin Psychol* 2008;27(4):317–335.

138. Iversen AC, van Staden L, Hughes JH, The stigma of mental health problems and other barriers to care in the UK Armed Forces. *BMC Health Serv Res* 2011;11(1):1.

139. Zamorski M. *Towards a Broader Conceptualization of Need, Stigma, and Barriers to Mental Health Care in Military Organisation: Recent Research Findings from the Canadian Forces.* Ottawa: NATO, 2011.

140. Langston V, Gould M, Greenberg N. Culture: What is its effect on stress in the military. *Mil Med* 2007;172:931–935.

141. Britt TW, McFadden AC. Understanding mental health treatment-seeking in high stress occupations. *Contemp Occup Health Psychol Global Perspect Res Pract* 2012;2:57–73.

142. Elnitsky CA, Chapman PL, Thurman RM, Pitts BL, Figureley C, Unwin B. Gender differences in combat medic mental health services utilization, barriers, and stigma. *Mil Med* 2013;178(7):775–784.

143. Kim PY, Britt TW, Klocko RP, Riviere LA, Adler AB. Stigma, negative attitudes about treatment, and utilization of mental health care among soldiers. *Mil Psychol* 2011;23(1):65–81.

144. Pietrzak R, Johnson D, Goldstein M, Malley J, Southwick S. Perceived stigma and barriers to mental health care utilization among OEF-OIF veterans. *Psychiatric Serv* 2009;60(8):1118–1122.

145. Zinzow HM, Britt TW, McFadden AC, Burnette CM, Gillispie S. Connecting active duty and returning veterans to mental health treatment: Interventions and treatment adaptations that may reduce barriers to care. *Clin Psychol Rev* 2012;32(8):741–775.

146. Ben-Zeev D, Corrigan PW, Britt TW, Langford L. Stigma of mental illness and service use in the military. *J Ment Health* 2012;21(3):264–273.

147. Dalky HF. Mental illness stigma reduction interventions: Review of intervention trials. *Wes J Nurs Res* 2012;34(4):520–547.

148. Abraham A, Easow JM, Ravichandren P, Mushtaq S, Butterworth L, Luty J. Effectiveness and confusion of the Time to Change anti-stigma campaign. *Psychiatrist* 2010;34(6):230–233.

149. Luty J, Umoh O, Sessay M, Sarkhel A. Effectiveness of Changing Minds campaign factsheets in reducing stigmatised attitudes towards mental illness. *Psychiatr Bull* 2007;31(10):377–381.

150. Britt TW McFadden AC. Understanding mental health treatment-seeking in high stress occupations. *Contemp Occup Health Psychol Global Perspect Res Pract* 2012;2:57–73.

151. Fertout M, Jones N, Keeling M, Greenberg N. Mental health stigmatisation in deployed UK Armed Forces: A principal components analysis. *J R Army Med Corps* 2015;161 (Suppl 1):i69–i76.

152. Sharp M-L, Fear NT, Rona R et al. Stigma as a barrier to seeking health-care among military personnel with mental health problems. *Epidemiol Rev* 2015;15,37:144–162.

153. Jones N, Campion B, Keeling M, Greenberg N. Cohesion, leadership, mental health stigmatisation and perceived barriers to care in UK military personnel. *J Ment Health.* 2018;27(1):10–18 doi: 10.3109/09638237.2016.1139063.

154. Du Preez J, Sundin J, Wessely S, Fear NT. Unit cohesion and mental health in the UK Armed Forces. *Occup Med* 2012;62:47–53.

155. Jones N, Keeling M, Thandi G, Greenberg N. Stigmatisation, perceived barriers to care, help seeking and the mental health of British Military personnel. *Soc Psychiatry Psychiatr Epidemiol* 2015;50(12):1873–1883.

156. Osório C, Jones N, Fertout M, Greenberg N. Perceptions of stigma and barriers to care among UK military personnel deployed to Afghanistan and Iraq. *Anxiety Stress Coping* 2013;26(5):539–557.

157. Osorio C, Jones N, Fertout M, Greenberg N. Changes in stigma and barriers to care over time in UK armed forces deployed to Afghanistan and Iraq between 2008 and 2011. *Mil Med* 2013;178(8):846–853.

158. Jones N, Twardzicki M, Fertout M, Jackson T, Greenberg N. Mental health, stigmatising beliefs, barriers to care and help-seeking in a non-deployed sample of UK Army personnel. *J Psychol Psychother* 2013:3:129. doi: 10.4172/2161-0487.1000129.

159. Jones N, Twardzicki M, Ryan J et al. Modifying attitudes to mental health using comedy as a delivery medium. *Soc Psychiatry Psychiatr Epidemiol* 2014;49(10): 1667–1676.

160. Jones E, Fear NT. Alcohol use and misuse within the military: A review. *Int Rev Psychiatry* 2011;23(2):166–172.

161. Browne T, Iversen A, Hull L et al. How do experiences in Iraq affect alcohol use among male UK armed forces personnel? *Occup Environ Med* 2008;65(9):628–633.

162. Debell F, Fear NT, Head M et al. A systematic review of the comorbidity between PTSD and alcohol misuse. *Soc Psychiatry Psychiatr Epidemiol* 2014;49(9):1401–1425.

163. Head M, Goodwin L, Debell F, Greenberg N, Wessely S, Fear NT. Post-traumatic stress disorder and alcohol misuse: Comorbidity in UK military personnel. *Soc Psychiatry Psychiatr Epidemiol* 2016;51(8):1171–1180.

164. Henderson A, Langston V, Greenberg N. Alcohol misuse in the Royal Navy. *Occup Med* 2009;59(1):25–31.

165. Hooper R, Rona RJ, Jones M, Fear NT, Hull L, Wessely S. Cigarette and alcohol use in the UK Armed Forces, and their association with combat exposures: A prospective study. *Addict Behav* 2008;33(8):1067–1071.

166. Thandi G, Sundin J, Ng-Knight T et al. Alcohol misuse in the United Kingdom Armed Forces: A longitudinal study. *Drug Alcohol Depend* 2015;156:78–83.

167. Rona RJ, Jones M, Fear NT, Hull L, Hotopf M, Wessely S. Alcohol misuse and functional impairment in the UK Armed Forces: A population-based study. *Drug Alcohol Depend* 2010;108(1):37–42.

168. Fear NT, Iversen AC, Chatterjee A et al. Risky driving among regular armed forces personnel from the United Kingdom. *Am J Prev Med* 2008;35(3):230–236.

169. Thandi G, Sundin J, Dandeker C et al. Risk-taking behaviours among UK military reservists. *Occup Med* 2015;65(5):413–416.

170. Sheriff RJ, Forbes HJ, Wessely SC. Risky driving among UK regular armed forces personnel: Changes over time. *BMJ Open* 2015;5(9):e008434.

171. MacManus D, Rona R, Dickson H, Somaini G, Fear N, Wessely S. Aggressive and violent behaviour among military personnel deployed to Iraq and Afghanistan: Prevalence and link with deployment and combat exposure. *Epidemol Rev* 2015;37:196–212.

172. MacManus D, Dean K, Jones M et al. Violent offending by UK military personnel

deployed to Iraq and Afghanistan: A data linkage cohort study. *Lancet* 2013;381(9870): 907–917.

173. MacManus D, Fossey M, Watson S, Wessely S. Former Armed Forces personnel in the Criminal Justice System. *Lancet Psychiatry* 2015;1:121–122.

174. MacManus D, Dean K, Al Bakir M et al. Violent behaviour in UK military personnel returning home after deployment. *Psychol Med* 2012;42(08):1663–1673.

175. MacManus D, Dean K, Iversen A, Hull L, Fahy T, Wessely S, Fear N. Influence of pre-military conduct problems on behavioural outcomes among male UK military personnel. *Soc Psychiatry Psychiatr Epidemiol* 2012;47:1353–1358.

176. Trevillion K, Williamson E, Thandi G, Borschmann R, Oram S, Howard LM. A systematic review of mental disorders and perpetration of domestic violence among military populations. *Soc Psychiatry Psychiatr Epidemiol* 2015;50(9):1329–1346.

177. Van Staden L, Fear NT, Iversen AC, French CE, Dandeker C, Wessely S. Transition back into civilian life: A study of personnel leaving the UK armed forces via "military prison". *Mil Med* 2007;172(9):925–930.

178. van Staden LN, Fear N, Iversen A, French C, Dandeker C, Wessely S. Young military veterans show similar help seeking behaviour. *BMJ* 2007;334(7590):382.

179. Rona R, Jones M, Hull L, Fear N, MacManus D, Wessely S. Anger in the UK Armed Forces: Strong association with mental health, childhood antisocial behavior and combat role. *J Nerv Ment Dis* 2015;20: 15–22.

180. Iversen A, Nikolaou V, Greenberg N et al. What happens to British veterans when they leave the armed forces? *Eur J Public Health* 2005;15(2):175–184.

181. Woodhead C, Rona RJ, Iversen AC et al. Health of national service veterans: An analysis of a community-based sample using data from the 2007 Adult Psychiatric Morbidity Survey of England. *Soc Psychiatry Psychiatr Epidemiol* 2011;46(7): 559–566.

182. Bergman BP, Mackay DF, Smith DJ, Pell JP. Long-term mental health outcomes of military service: National linkage study of 57,000 veterans and 173,000 matched nonveterans. *J Clin Psychiatry* 2016;77(6): 793–798.

183. Iversen A, Dyson C, Smith N et al. 'Goodbye and good luck': The mental health needs and treatment experiences of British ex-service personnel. *Br J Psychiatry* 2005;186(6):480–486.

184. Hatch SL, Harvey SB, Dandeker C et al. Life in and after the Armed Forces: Social networks and mental health in the UK military. *Sociol Health Illn* 2013;35(7):1045–1064.

185. Diehle J, Greenberg N. Counting the Costs. A report commissioned by Help for Heroes. 2015. http://www.helpforheroes.org.uk /together-rebuilding-lives/research-counting-the-costs/ Accessed 23 Feb 2016.

186. Burdett H, Woodhead C, Iversen AC, Wessely S, Dandeker C, Fear, NT. "Are you a Veteran?" Understanding of the term "Veteran" among UK ex-service personnel: A research note. *Armed Forces Soc* 2013;39(4):751–759. doi:0095327X12452033.

187. Stevelink SA, Malcolm EM, Fear NT. Visual impairment, coping strategies and impact on daily life: A qualitative study among working-age UK ex-service personnel. *BMC Public Health* 2015;15(1):1118.

188. Stevelink SA, Malcolm EM, Gill PC, Fear NT. The mental health of UK ex-servicemen with a combat-related or a non-combat-related visual impairment: Does the cause of visual impairment matter? *Br J Ophthalmol* 2015;99:1103–1108. doi:10.1136 /bjophthalmol-2014-305986

189. Stevelink SA, Fear NT. Psychosocial impact of visual impairment and coping strategies in female ex-Service personnel. *J R Army Med Corps* 2016;162(2):129–133. doi:10.1136/jramc-2015-000518.

190. van Hoorn LA, Jones N, Busuttil W, Iraq and Afghanistan veteran presentations to Combat Stress, since 2003. *Occup Med* 2013;63(3):238–241.

191. Murphy D, Weijers B, Palmer E, Busuttil W. Exploring patterns in referrals to combat stress for UK Veterans with mental health difficulties between 1994 and 2014. *Int J Emerg Ment Health Human Resil* 2015;17(3): 652–658.

192. Buckman JE, Forbes HJ, Clayton T et al. Early Service leavers: A study of the factors associated with premature separation from the UK Armed Forces and the mental health of those that leave early. *Eur J Public Health* 2013;23(3):410–415.

193. Jones M, Sundin J, Goodwin L et al. What explains post-traumatic stress disorder (PTSD) in UK service personnel: Deployment or something else? *Psychol Med* 2013;43(08):1703–1712.

194. Iversen A, Fear NT, Simonoff E et al. Pre-enlistment vulnerability factors and their influence on health outcomes in UK Military personnel. *Br J Psychiatry* 2007;191:506–511.

16

Primary care

INTRODUCTION

Primary care is a broad church. It is the cornerstone of *National Health Service* (NHS) and *Defence Medical Services* (DMS) healthcare, encompassing all clinical contacts in the community before a patient reaches hospital or acute mental health services. As such, primary care is usually the first point of contact for most people, resulting in some 300 million consultations and 800 million prescriptions per year in NHS England alone and accounting for some 85% of all DMS patient contacts.

NHS and DMS primary care is delivered through multidisciplinary teams that include general practitioners (GPs), dentists, nurses and allied health professionals such as pharmacists and physiotherapists.

DMS primary care is based upon the Ministry of Defence's (MOD's) 'Whole Force' approach, where regular service personnel, Reservists and civilians work together in partnership to deliver the required effect: *'One team, one vision, one goal'*. The DMS GP cadre includes military GPs (who are all commissioned medical officers), civilian medical practitioners employed by the MOD to provide essential clinical and educational continuity (who do not deploy) and, increasingly, reservists. All DMS GPs are vocationally trained and undertake the same licensing processes as NHS GPs. In a specific difference from the NHS, DMS GPs deliver general practice and occupational medicine within the same consultation. Like the NHS, the DMS primary care nursing cadre includes advanced nurse practitioners and nurse prescribers. DMS allied health professionals include pharmacists and physiotherapists, all of whom are also subject to the same national licensing processes as their civilian peers.

DMS primary care also benefits from the contributions of other military-specific groups not found in the NHS. These include *general duties medical officers* (GDMOs) (qualified doctors who work in primary care whilst gaining military experience between completing their Foundation Years and starting higher specialist training), pharmacy technicians, exercise rehabilitation instructors (non-medical staff trained to support patients' rehabilitation pathways) and 'medics'. Medics are the backbone of Defence's operational primary care capability. The Royal Navy (RN) and Royal Marines (RM) have *medical assistants,* the Army has *combat medical technicians* (CMTs), the Royal Air Force (RAF) has *RAF Medics*. All these cadres provide hands-on clinical care, complete medical administrative tasks and manage primary care facilities much as an NHS practice manager would. The UK Armed Forces also have *Health & Care Professions Council* registered paramedics.

Whilst remaining under full command of their single Services, to increase efficiency and reduce duplication, RN, RM, Army and RAF primary care resources came together to form *Defence Primary Healthcare* (DPHC), a Joint military primary care delivery organisation, as part of the 2010 *Strategic Defence and Security Review*. DPHC includes medical centres, primary care rehabilitation facilities, regional rehabilitation units, regional occupational medicine departments and departments of community mental health.

The strategic intent of the Surgeon General (SG) is for every serviceman and woman to enjoy a level of health that is appropriate for the tasks they are required to perform by the chain of command. Whilst generalists require a breadth of knowledge, and specialists require a depth of knowledge, DMS primary care clinical staff require a good deal of both in order to deliver SG's intent, prepare those elements of the Armed Forces on standby for deployment (*force elements at readiness*), maximise the number of UK Armed Forces personnel fit for task and provide health and well-being advice to commanders.

The World Health Organisation model of primary care describes the need for all service delivery organisations to consider the whole person in the context of their family, community, wider society and culture and to try to optimise equity, access and quality of care in order to realise improved patient outcomes. Whilst the hospital consultation model is necessarily disease orientated in order to achieve an objective diagnosis and appropriate management, the primary care model is more holistic. It looks to treat the person as well as the disease and incorporates health education, promotion and prevention in addition to managing the presenting complaint. Educationalists Stott, Davis, Pendleton and Neighbour have devised primary care consultation models to help facilitate long-lasting doctor–patient relationships, but NHS and DMS primary care continue to be underpinned by patient centredness, patient advocacy and an ability to address a broad range of potentially compounding physical, psychological and social problems.

Each primary care consultation is unique, but the *Royal College of General Practitioners* motto 'Cum scientia caritas' (science with compassion) provides an overarching philosophy. In his 1971 Royal College of General Practitioners (RCGP) James Mackenzie lecture, Dr. D.L. Crombie, a GP in Birmingham and then director of the Birmingham Research Unit, highlighted how compassion is complex and extends beyond the pure scientific methods that logically link identifiable causes with effects. Today, Birmingham is the home of the MOD's *Royal Centre for Defence Medicine* and its *Academic Department of Military General Practice.*

SPECIALTY BEFORE *OPERATIONS TELIC* AND *HERRICK*

This chapter describes how, in recent years, DMS primary care's efforts have been focused upon supporting the *International Security Assistance Forces* (ISAF) in Iraq and Afghanistan. Concurrently, however, DMS primary care has also continued to provide healthcare to entitled Service personnel in the Firm Base and within overseas *Permanent Joint Operating Bases* such as Cyprus, Germany, Gibraltar and Naples. On behalf of the NHS, the DMS also delivers primary care to Service dependants and civilians eligible to register. Additionally, DMS primary care has contributed to standing strategic responsibilities, such as defending the Falkland Islands since the 1982 conflict, North Atlantic Treaty Organisation (NATO) operations such as in Bosnia Herzegovina (1992–2004) and Kosovo (1999–2012), UK Special Forces missions, anti-piracy initiatives around the Horn of Africa, counter-narcotic operations in the Caribbean and humanitarian assistance whenever and wherever the need arises. Examples include the aftermath of the 2004 tsunami, the 2005 Kashmir earthquake, the 2007 flooding in Central Africa and as part of the UK response to the Ebola outbreak in West Africa (2013–2016 *Operation Gritrock*).

Due to the diverse healthcare needs of patients in these settings, DMS primary care has evolved beyond the normal NHS scope to include formal leadership and management skills, environmental medicine, tropical medicine, sports and exercise medicine, pre-hospital emergency care and community mental health.

Pre-hospital emergency care by non-specialists on the battlefield is not new.[1] Battle injuries during the First World War (1914–1918) were treated at regimental aid posts (RAPs), where regimental medical officers (RMOs) successfully stopped bleeding, splinted broken limbs, prevented disease and evacuated casualties.[1] During the Second World War (1939–1945), the time and distance between the point of wounding and definitive care increased, but RMOs' surgical capability remained relatively unchanged.[2]

The form of battle, challenging topography, inclement weather and limited availability of aeromedical evacuation during the Falklands Conflict (1982) led to an increased requirement for trauma care closer to the point of wounding. This approach to care became known as 'Role 1', a phrase that endures. Primary care teams performed triage and provided fluid resuscitation. Torso injuries were still associated with high mortality, but more casualties with injuries to the extremities survived to be evacuated.[3] During peace-keeping operations in the Balkans in the 1990s, Role 1 capability improved significantly as junior medical officers started to routinely deliver advanced life support, as evidenced following the Nis Express bus bombing.[4]

Sadly, throughout history, mental health issues on the battlefield have not been so well addressed.[5] In the First World War, thousands of soldiers were labelled as having 'shell shock'. Battlefield doctors categorised soldiers as 'wounded' if a shell-blast was thought to have caused their symptoms. If not, individuals were classified as 'sick' or 'unfit for military service'. Some were regarded as cowards. A small number were executed for desertion.[6] During the Second World War, doctors on the battlefield still attributed psychiatric symptoms to physical infirmity such as 'effort syndrome' or 'combat exhaustion'.[7] Sufferers once again faced accusations of cowardice and malingering. Famously, General Patton once slapped a soldier suffering from a post-conflict syndrome, calling him a 'gutless bastard'.[8] It is sometimes forgotten that this incident cost General Patton his command until he was reinstated in time for D-Day. In 2002, the *South Atlantic Medal Association* claimed that more UK Servicemen who served in the Falklands Conflict had committed suicide than were killed in action there. Although a 2013 study confirmed 95 Falklands veterans had taken their own lives since 1982 compared with 255 killed in battle, small studies *have* demonstrated poorer mental health outcomes among those who served in the Falklands.[9]

As the fighting lasted only 100 hours and there were minimal UK casualties, acute combat stress reactions were not prevalent during the 1990–1991 Gulf War. However, by the end of the twentieth century, UK Armed Forces personnel involved in the 1990–1991 Gulf War were presenting to DMS primary care more often. The commonest complaints were headache, depression, anxiety, fatigue, pain, low mood, concentration difficulties, memory problems and general malaise. Such symptoms became known as 'Gulf War syndrome', although it remains unclear where this phrase originated and no evidence of any unique Gulf War syndrome has been found.[10–12] UK personnel exposed to combat in the Gulf are twice as likely to report symptoms suggestive of post-traumatic stress disorder (PTSD) and alcohol misuse[13] and slightly more likely to report multiple physical symptoms, but the actual numbers remain low.[14] Most Gulf War veterans, even those with more physical symptoms, do not have mental health disorders.[15]

Since the '9/11' attack on the *World Trade Center* in New York on 11 September 2001, *counterinsurgency* (COIN) operations have become the cornerstone of the international military effort against global terrorism. COIN activities are complex and expose military personnel to unfamiliar stressors.[16] Although modern reconfigurations have reduced the size of the UK Armed Forces and the risk of large-scale casualties, the number of patients with long-term ill health presenting to primary care has not fallen. Military GPs now recognise that just like war fighting, COIN operations and even peacekeeping activities can also lead to psychological trauma and potential adverse mental health outcomes.

Mental health lessons learned during *Operation Telic* and *Operation Herrick* are covered in a separate chapter of this book (Chapter 15). Nevertheless, 100 years on, 'shell shock' still stands as a powerful emblem of the suffering of war[5] and reinforces the importance of high-quality primary care at the point of physical and/or psychological wounding.

PRIMARY CARE ON DEPLOYMENT

The role of the MOD is 'to deliver security for the people of the UK and Overseas territories by defending them, including against terrorism, and to act as a force for good by strengthening international peace and security'. For as long as the UK Armed Forces are sent into harm's way, DMS primary care will be a key component of Defence medical assets. The versatility of DMS primary care enables it to support Her Majesty's Government's policies at home and overseas across the full spectrum of military tasks.

Deployed capability

Assuming they are fit to do so, all Regular service personnel working in primary care and some categories of RN reservists, Army Reservists and Royal Auxiliary Air Force Squadron personnel are deployable. DMS primary care prepared the 46,000 personnel who deployed at the onset of *Operation Telic* (Figure 16.1) and remained in Iraq throughout the campaign, including during the *Iraqi Training and Advisory Mission* (19 March 2003–22 May 2011).

DMS primary care was embedded throughout the Joint Area of Operations (JOA), including in the

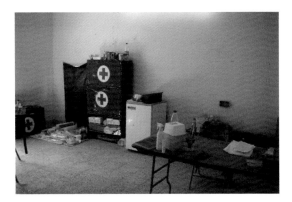

Figure 16.1 Company aid post on *Operation Telic*.

three-star tri-Service headquarters within *US Central Command* in Qatar, aboard the flagship aircraft carrier *HMS Ark Royal* and as organic medical support within the major deployed units listed in Appendix A. Primary care to other units was provided at Shaibah Logistics base and later at the COB Basra. There were also DMS primary care elements in Kuwait, Bahrain and Saudi Arabia. In the very early stages of the conflict, primary care was provided afloat pending the establishment of effective facilities on land (Figure 16.2).

Following *Operation Fingal*, after which Britain handed command of the ISAF force to Turkey, *Operation Herrick* began in 2002. At this point, the UK contribution was scaled back from 2100 to approximately 300 personnel, but DMS primary care elements remained to support the ongoing security effort around Kabul and the UK Afghan National Army Training Team. Organic primary care was enhanced in 2003, when two *Provincial Reconstruction Teams* and a rapid reaction force were established. In January 2006, the worsening situation in the south of Afghanistan led the UK Government to announce the deployment of a task force of approximately 3300 personnel to Helmand Province.

DMS primary care was embedded throughout the JOA within the resultant formations and sub-formations headed listed in Appendix B. Primary care was also delivered to the personnel at Camp Bastion, including the staff of the Role 3 hospital facility.

Figure 16.3 simplifies the laydown of the medical network on *Operation Herrick*. Factors affecting the decision of a medical officer (MO) to deploy forward from a patrol base (PB) included the location of personnel, the permissiveness of the environment

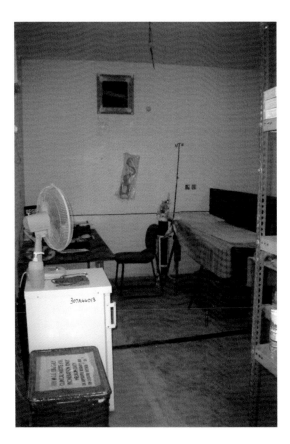

Figure 16.2 Interior of an RAP, *Operation Telic*.

including the local threat level and type, the casualty evacuation route and method, whether an advisory role was required and the clinical timelines (Figure 16.4).[17]

Medical officers were usually located somewhere easily accessible to the majority of their population at risk. In a company-level operation, this was likely to be forward of the PB, although the likelihood of sustaining casualties varied markedly depending upon the patrol route, type and local threat level. In care-under-fire situations, MOs were unable to enhance the pre-hospital emergency care capability afforded by CMTs. In more permissive environments, MOs could deliver more effective prolonged field care and so were usually 'forward-mounted' to a checkpoint closer to the area of clinical risk. Forward deployment of an MO was considered to provide additional clinical value if casualty care on the ground was likely to extend beyond 20 minutes from the point of wounding. As medical advisors, many DMS primary care staff also

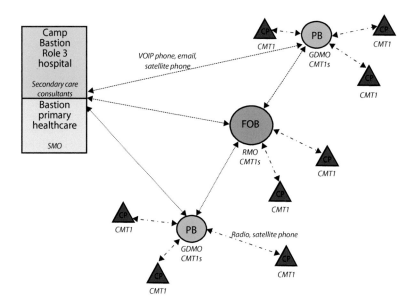

Figure 16.3 Schematic diagram (simplified) of the medical network on Op HERRICK showing the communication pathways between the personnel at different types of medical facility. CMT1, CMT Class 1; CP, checkpoint; FOB, forward operating base; SMO, senior medical officer; VOIP, voiceover internet protocol. (From Gumbley AE et al., *J R Army Med Corps* 2013;159:68–72.)

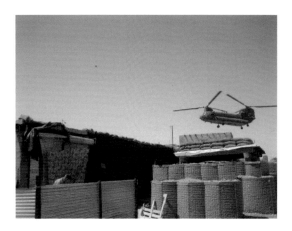

Figure 16.4 Resupply operations to *FOB Musa Qal'eh*.

found it beneficial to move with the company commander in order to gain situational awareness, which might inform their clinical opinions.[17]

In both *Operations Telic* and *Herrick*, DMS primary care tour lengths varied from two to twelve months. Rest and recuperation leave was afforded to DMS primary care personnel serving more than four months in theatre. DMS primary care personnel either deployed as formed units, non-formed units or individual augmentees to United Kingdom and coalition, mainly the United States, formations (Figures 16.5 and 16.6).

Evacuation processes

Prior to the successful development of *Medical Emergency Response Teams* (MERTs) as a consultant-led service, DMS primary care personnel conducted tactical casualty evacuation (CASEVAC). Where the medical plan involved evacuating casualties straight from the point of wounding via an emergency helicopter landing site (HLS), the MO moved forwards from the PB to supervise the evacuation. If CASEVAC was to occur from the PB's own HLS, the MO usually remained at the PB and casualties were brought to them (Figure 16.5).[17]

DMS primary care staff also held patients in bedded facilities at the aeromedical points of departure and supported the strategic aeromedical repatriation of patients not described as *seriously ill* (SIL) or *very seriously ill* (VSIL) (terms used to classify the degree of injury of illness of evacuated personnel). SIL and VSIL patients were repatriated to the United Kingdom by *critical*

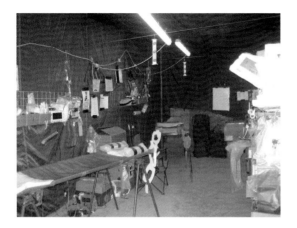

Figure 16.5 Company Aid Post, *Operation Herrick FOB Musa Qal'eh*. (Courtesy of *US News*.)

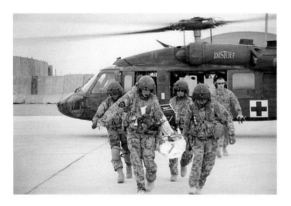

Figure 16.6 Evacuation of a casualty by US Dust-off Helicopter.

care aeromedical specialist teams. Primary care *Aeromedical Evacuation Liaison Officers* were embedded at key points along the strategic repatriation pathway, such as in Cyprus and Germany.

Workload data

A total of 179 UK Armed Forces personnel died serving on *Operation Telic* between March 2003 and the end of combat operations in July 2009: 136 in hostile incidents and 43 under non-hostile circumstances.[18] Non-fatal casualty records indicate that from 1 January 2006, 3598 UK Armed Forces personnel were wounded, injured or fell ill.[19] Of these, 1971 required aeromedical evacuation facilitated by DMS primary care.[20]

From 7 October 2001 until 28 February 2015, a total of 616 UK Armed Forces personnel were seriously or very seriously injured during *Operation Herrick*, 2209 more were wounded in action and 5598 sustained disease or non-battle injury. A total of 7477 personnel required aeromedical evacuation.[20]

Despite robust aeromedical evacuation pathways, throughout *Operations Telic* and *Herrick*, the DMS aimed to provide the best possible healthcare to wounded service personnel as soon as possible and as close to the point of wounding as possible through the delivery of *Battlefield Advanced Trauma Life Support* (BATLS). RAPs were very busy, as illustrated by a GDMO and two CMTs managing 29 significant trauma casualties (4 of whom had life- or limb-threatening injuries) and two UK fatalities over an 11-day period.[5] One study indicated that 97% of all GDMO clinical contacts on *Operation Herrick* were primary care, rather than trauma or acute medical emergencies.[21]

Patient morbidity data from a prospective case series of all 1903 patients presenting to an RAP during a six-month summer tour in Afghanistan (April 2009–October 2009) illustrated the breadth of presenting complaints and highlighted that patients came from a variety of backgrounds including UK military personnel (66.4%); Afghans (32.8%); UK civilians, for example personnel from the *Foreign and Commonwealth Office* (0.7%); and others (0.2%).[21] Of the Afghan patients, 18.2% were Afghan National Army, 4.6% interpreters, 3.5% Afghan National Police, 2.8% locally employed civilians, 2.0% local nationals, 1.1% local national children, 0.2% Afghan Government personnel and 0.2% individuals who did not fall into one of the other groups.[21]

Disease surveillance was undertaken through the recording of EpiNATO data (although this does not capture preventative health measures). EpiNATO is the NATO health surveillance system. The 15 most common presentations are given in Table 16.1.[21] Overall, 53% of cases required the input of a medical officer and could not be dealt with by a medic alone.[21] One of the strengths of DMS primary care is its ability to preserve and maintain the fighting strength. Almost 85% of patients seen at Role 1 could be returned to duty immediately.[21]

'Routine' GDMO referral rates from Role 1 occurred at a rate of 0.9 referrals per GDMO each

Table 16.1 Common presentations to primary care

- Dermatological conditions (23.5%)
- Injuries not due to hostile action (10.2%)
- Disorders of the digestive tract (9.3%)
- Intestinal infectious diseases (7.1%)
- Ear, nose and throat complaints (6.9%)
- Diseases of the teeth and oral cavity (5.4%)
- Musculoskeletal disorders excluding the knee and back (5.4%)
- Disorders of the back (3.7%)
- Injuries due to hostile action (3.5%)
- Eye disorders (3.0%)
- Respiratory tract infections (2.7%)
- Sexually transmitted diseases including HIV (1.7%)
- Knee disorders (1.2%)
- Climatic injuries (0.6%)
- Injuries due to sport (0.6%)

week.[22] The main reasons for referral were dental problems, musculoskeletal injuries, abdominal pain of unknown cause and ano-genital problems. Factors that influenced referrals were the junior doctors' inexperience in the treatment of a particular condition, lack of access to investigations, the potential for clinical deterioration and the fact that there was limited, if any, availability of forward projected services such as dentistry and physiotherapy.[22] The referral decision process was also affected by the patient's importance to the mission, manpower availability at the deployed location, the availability of flights and aircraft (influenced by the weather, enemy action and the schedule of the routine air bridge) and the timing of the complaint in relation to the patient's tour dates. DMS primary care staff often found themselves pressured by their patients who 'wished to remain at the front so they did not let down their Regiment'.[22]

CLINICAL CHALLENGES ON *OPERATIONS TELIC* AND *HERRICK*

Analysis of qualitative data from DMS primary care clinicians deployed in Role 1 medical facilities on *Operation Herrick* suggested a number of significant issues affecting the quality of clinical performance; these were standards of care, record keeping, the operating environment and situational pressures.

Standards of care and record keeping

CASE MIX

It is recognised that newly deployed GDMOs have steep medical and military learning curves and that good clinical outcomes are dependent on primary care teams' early understanding of the medical re-supply process, the management of environmental health threats, medical planning and the casualty evacuation process. In general, GDMOs on *Operation Telic* or *Operation Herrick*, did not have the pre-requisite knowledge, skills, experience or equipment to deliver the care required to the unexpectedly large numbers of medical and traumatic paediatric cases. They were also unprepared for the ethical and moral decision-making required when trying to equate local nationals' needs with the deployed eligibility matrix. Both these issues are addressed in detail elsewhere in this volume.

PAIN MANAGEMENT

Effective pain management was not always achieved. MOs and CMTs reported skill fade in acute pain management during peacetime primary care delivery. This was compounded by a paucity of pre-deployment analgesia management training available to MOs and CMTs. As a consequence, clinicians arriving at Role 1 did not feel confident to consistently provide parenteral analgesia, particularly in the context of the environment in which they were working. Available analgesia included midazolam, ketamine, fentanyl, Entonox™, local anaesthetics and morphine. CMTs were anxious about the risk of causing harm if they administered IM morphine (despite naloxone also being available). MOs had a clearer understanding of the analgesia ladder than CMTs did.[23-25]

FLUID REPLACEMENT

Intravenous access was established in 6.5% of all Role 1 attendees, for reasons including trauma, heat illness, dehydration, abdominal pain and septic shock,[21] but not all CMTs were trained in obtaining intravenous (IV) access. Fluid replacement was hampered by difficulty obtaining parenteral access and lack of familiarity with IV equipment outside the training environment. Fluids were sometimes given inappropriately or in volumes in excess of protocols. Some clinicians chose not to obtain IV or intraosseous access because the casualty was stable at the time of assessment despite them having significant injuries.

ROLE 1 RECORD KEEPING

Accurate and comprehensive medical records are a recognised requirement for the provision of safe, effective primary care. The General Medical Council's 'Generic Medical Standards for speciality training including GP Training',[26] the Academy of Medical Royal Colleges'[27] and RCGP[28] national standards for record keeping require an up-to-date clinical summary to be kept (considered essential) as well as an acceptable record keeping system that provides the right information, in the right place at the right time (considered desirable). An audit of the quality of medical records available to deployed DMS primary care clinicians and benchmarking of DMS record keeping against the GMC standards found that documentation of the quality of care at Role 1 facilities between the point of wounding and evacuation by MERT helicopter was often lacking.[29] Unlike the US military, the Unuted Kingdom did not have a continuous electronic medical record in which to record primary care interventions from the battlefield to definitive care.[30]

A lack of connectivity between the *Defence Medical Information Capability Programme (Deployed)* (DMICP[D]) electronic medical records system and its Firm Base equivalent resulted in DMS primary care staff usually having no direct access to their patients' medical history. Only 22% of patients' medical records had been imported onto DMICP(D) and only 1% of those patient records available in-theatre had an up-to-date summary.[29] Written documentation was often reported as being successfully completed but was then seemingly misplaced. The quality of in-theatre record keeping also fell below the RCGP's national standards, with key components of the medical history being recorded only in a minority of cases, including medical history (recorded in only 26% consultations), drug history (in 20%), allergies (in 16%) and summary (in 2%).

The format 'ATMIST' (as shown in Table 16.2) was universally popular and described as being a

Table 16.2 ATMIST tool

Age
Time of incident and expected arrival at ED
Mechanism of injury in detail where known
Injuries suspected
Signs: vital signs including improvement and deterioration
Treatment given

practical and efficient form of clinical documentation for the operating environment. The form was often completed by a non-medical assistant.

MEDICAL MATERIEL

Medical re-supply was managed by the normal logistic supply chain, but individuals within it often were unfamiliar with the management of medicines and medical materiel. This led to delays and errors in re-supply, which, on occasion, constrained clinical delivery.

Operational environment

Operational stress causes significant morbidity and may reduce individuals' military effectiveness. As an example, UK military helicopter aircrew (UK MHA) in Iraq and Afghanistan may have been at increased risk of operational stress as they were amongst the UK's most frequently deployed military personnel[31]; UK MHA support a wide variety of military tasks.[32] During *Operations Telic* and *Herrick*, their responsibilities included collecting wounded personnel, often whilst under fire; supporting infantry troops in contact with hostile forces; moving personnel around the combat zone; and delivering food, water and ammunition

In the first DMS, primary care quantitative and qualitative assessment of adverse mental health outcomes amongst UK Armed Forces aircrew following exposure to operational stress, 736 male UK MHA were compared with a matched comparison group of 4313 male non-helicopter UK military personnel (administrators, cooks, drivers, engineers, police and physical education staff). UK military helicopter *front crew* (pilots) were also compared to UK military helicopter *rear crew* (other helicopter personnel such as load masters and door gunners who do not have hands on control of the aircraft). The adverse mental health outcomes measured were common mental disorders (using the *Multiple Physical Symptoms* checklist), depressive symptoms (using the *General Health Questionnaire*), PTSD and alcohol misuse (using the *Alcohol Use Disorders Identification Test*).

Although the UK MHA had deployed to Iraq and Afghanistan more often and for longer, no statistical difference was measured in operational stress between the UK helicopter aircrew and those service personnel in the comparison group or between pilots and non-pilots, despite their obligatory reactivity to strategic stressors. These stressors included *leadership decisions* and frequent exposure to possible *operational, administrative* and *domestic* stressors (described by the acronym LOAD). It is possible that group-sharing of risk, effective *communications*, good military *leadership*, a mutually *supportive working environment*, effective training delivering *professional aptitude* and *psychological reward* through a feeling of making a difference and working within small, highly skilled teams (summarised by the acronym CLEAR) may have reduced the likelihood of adverse health outcomes.[33] These factors are summarised in the LOAD–CLEAR model (shown in Figure 16.7), which illustrates that leadership may have a positive (good leadership) or negative (poor leadership) influence upon the mental well-being of patients presenting to Role 1.[34] Within the prospective case series of patients presenting to an

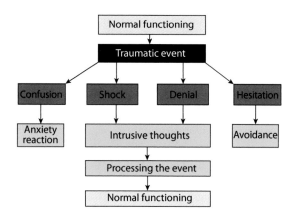

Figure 16.8 Normal psychological response to traumatic events.

RAP, stress accounted for only 0.4% of presentations, and a formal EpiNATO recording of a 'mental health disorder' was made in only 0.2% of cases.

Realistic pre-deployment training, which addressed educational needs as well as the physical stressors commensurate with an austere environment, has a positive effect on clinical performance and mental well-being of patients presenting to Role 1. Such training may help individuals to normalise their psychological responses to their environment and the proximity of traumatic events (Figure 16.8).[35]

Situational pressures

TIME TO EVACUATION

Fewer than one-quarter of cases seen at Role 1 required immediate medical evacuation (MEDEVAC). MEDEVAC was usually provided by helicopter, activation of which required an accurate '9-liner' and MIST report[36] (see Chapter 3). Factors including time management, battle space situational awareness and exposure to significant risk influenced clinical delivery. The MERT was inappropriately tasked on several occasions because primary care staff on the ground had incorrectly categorised casualties when using the 9-liner. Clinicians also felt time-pressured by the early arrival of the MERT, opting in some cases to omit interventions or procedures to ensure that the casualty was prepared for evacuation.

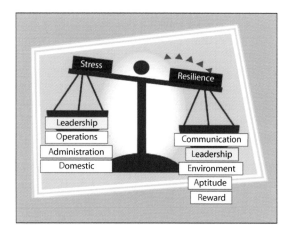

Figure 16.7 LOAD–CLEAR stress–resilience model.

MASS CASUALTY SITUATIONS

DMS primary care clinicians were occasionally overwhelmed by the number and severity of the casualties. Triage was sometimes poor, with individuals treating patients as they found them rather than by clinical priority.[37] In Musa Qal'eh, as part of the 5 Scots (formerly the Argyll and Sutherland Highlanders) RAP, one GDMO supported only by one med sergeant and three CMTs was responsible for approximately 1000 soldiers distributed across 10 PBs. The GDMO had missed much of the regimental pre-deployment training and had not had an opportunity to train or develop the RAP team. The RAP had deployed with limited medical equipment, and re-supply was tenuous. Nevertheless, the RAP soon found itself dealing with three mass casualty events and a gastroenteritis outbreak that incapacitated 43 personnel.[37]

Primary care lessons identified for the future

TRAINING

The report 'Putting Role 1 First: The Role 1 Capability Review',[38] collated as a cross *Defence-Lines of Development* analysis, combined the specific experience of *1 Medical Regiment's* hybrid foundation training, mission-specific training and deployment cycle with the analysis of questionnaire studies, subject matter expert consultation and documentary evidence. The review generated 77 recommendations and 38 sub-recommendations. The recommendations of this and other reviews offer some important messages for deployed primary care. The major messages of the *Role 1 First* review included observations that inadequate experience for CMTs in *Firm Base* primary care undermines their operational preparedness, that DMS GP manning requires re-evaluation as an operational pinch point and that the best practice template created for Role 1 healthcare governance must endure.[38] It is also clear from recent experience that pre-deployment training should emphasise the importance of using triage tools when managing multiple casualties, including the correct use of '9-liners' and MIST protocols, and include human factors training to assist delivering BATLS in a high-threat, high-stress environment.[37]

In the future there will also need to be greater emphasis on analgesia training and the use of pain scales to assess patients' analgesic needs, including a four-phase educational model providing a factual basis for military MOs to manage casualties' analgesic requirements.[24] Although the prevalence of kinetic injuries is likely to fall, the DMS must work to secure a corporate memory that ensures that primary care experience gained in pain management in Iraq and Afghanistan is not lost.

On future operations, a reduction in 'routine' referrals from Role 1 may be achieved by the introduction of clinical guidelines for common conditions and the provision of quick-reference information sheets for GDMOs.[21] As dermatological conditions were the most common presentation, colour photographs could be usefully added to the reference information to assist clinical diagnoses and decision-taking.[21] Although GDMOs receive basic dental training, additional skills (such as how to place a temporary filling) may be useful. Increased training in musculoskeletal injuries would also be beneficial, especially in preparation for deployment to locations where there is no ready access to allied health professionals. Improving primary care referral guidelines for operations could also help preserve manpower, reduce costs and minimise the risk to evacuation aircraft. There should, in addition, be increased familiarity with paediatric algorithms, including WETFAG and fluid requirements (Table 16.3).[39]

In the future, medical officers should complete the same pre-deployment training at the same time as the medical team and unit, preferably including the combined force, company and medical liaison officers.[38] This training should encompass the communication protocols required to initiate casualty evacuation, familiarisation with the infectious and tropical diseases prevalent in the area of operations, environmental health assessment and management and operational medical planning. Prior experience in the Field Army, including participation in a major battlegroup exercise, was considered invaluable by GDMOs.[38] An MO should ideally work with the same group of CMTs both prior to, and on deployment in order to better understand their individual and group capabilities and invest in their development.[38] CMTs benefited greatly from pre-deployment hospital attachments, and also and especially from high fidelity training with 'Amputees in Action'.

Table 16.3 (a) WETFAG paediatric aide-memoire and (b) paediatric fluid requirement aide-memoire

(a)

	Parameter	Calculation
W	Weight (kg)	2 × (age + 4)
E	Energy (J)	4 J/kg
T	Tube (ETT-internal diameter)	4 + age/4
F	Fluid bolus	20 mL/kg/crystalloid
A	Adrenaline	0.1 mL/kg/1 in 10,000
G	Glucose	5 mL/kg 5% dextrose

(b)

Body weight	Fluid requirement/day	Fluid requirement/hour
First 10 kg	100 mL/kg	4 mL/kg
Second 10 kg	50 mL/kg	2 mL/kg
Third 10 kg	20 mL/kg	1 mL/kg

Source: Fear NT et al., Lancet 2010;375(9728):1783–1797.

Equipment

Most MOs felt happy with the equipment provided to them, but the medical daysacks were incompatible with the body armour, making access to medicines and equipment more difficult. During *Operation Herrick*, a radical review of the Role 1 modules was undertaken by a multidisciplinary committee under the chairmanship of Defence Consultant Advisor in emergency medicine in order to bring them into line with expected clinical competencies. It is essential that medical officers are also familiar with equipment and medicine management protocols and re-supply processes. At the beginning of the deployment, most RAPs were not scaled to assess or treat sick children, but MOs were uncertain how to demand the equipment they required.[18]

Personnel

The UK Armed Forces are now amongst the most operationally experienced in the world. However, from the perspective of potential adverse mental health outcomes, this is not necessarily a good thing. Although some individuals, especially male officers, report more desirable effects of military service (for example mastery, self-esteem and coping skills) than undesirable ones, both the positive and negative effects of military service increase linearly with combat exposure.[39,40] Serving in the Armed Forces is inherently stressful, and all military personnel are at risk of developing adverse psychological outcomes.[7] Psychological distress is associated with duration of deployment, but newer forms of psychological injury may be less predictable, less well understood and harder to manage.

Portrayals of the UK's involvement in Iraq and Afghanistan have made 'operational stress' almost synonymous with PTSD. In reality, UK Armed Forces personnel most commonly present to their military GPs with symptoms suggestive of common mental disorders (such as anxiety, panic attacks and depression, 19.7%) and alcohol misuse (13.0%). The prevalence of probable PTSD remains low (4.0%). Many UK Armed Forces personnel have served in Afghanistan several times. There is no association between the number of deployments and mental health issues, but reporting of probable PTSD does increase with time after return to the United Kingdom.[39] With the correct degree of support from their DMS GPs, peers and military leaders, individuals affected by operational stress may recover swiftly. Nevertheless, the pace and frequency of military operations may lower morale, place strain on relationships and adversely impact upon the health of service personnel and their families.[40] DMS primary care is often the first port of call in such storms, and key to mitigating such risks by delivering high-quality care to military personnel on and off the battlefield, and support to registered families at home. If morbidity patterns since the Boer War persist in the future wars that 'should be expected', even if the prevalence of kinetic injuries reduces, adverse mental health outcomes after exposure to operational stress are likely to continue. Mental illness is the leading cause of disability worldwide. In the United Kingdom, 20% of the total burden of disease is attributed to mental illness, compared with 17.2% for cardiovascular disease and 15.5% for cancers.[41] Approximately 11 million people of working age in the United Kingdom experience mental health problems and about 5.5 million have a common mental disorder. Nearly one-third of NHS GP consultations include a mental health component, and mental health problems occupy one-third of an NHS GP's time. DMS primary care staffs must also be able to assess and address the mental health risks of all UK Armed Forces personnel (including medical staff) in order to provide or signpost appropriate mental healthcare in a suitably timely manner.

Information technology/health informatics

As discussed earlier, good medical record keeping is a foundation to the delivery of high-quality clinical care. During *Operation Telic* and *Operation Herrick*, DMICP(D) did not have the necessary connectivity to ensure continuity of the medical record. Furthermore, medical record entries made in-theatre did not meet national standards. Improved communication (electronic, written and verbal) regarding a casualty's progress should promote continual improvement of patient care. To enable this, operational record keeping should form part of a medical pre-deployment training package. Such training should emphasise the importance of ensuring that patient-specific records follow the evacuation of the casualty to maintain coverage of the whole patent care pathway.

Programme Cortisone[42] *is the* MOD project to develop a commercial off-the-shelf information management system to support the Defence Medical Service including electronic radiology management functions. It is intended to function as an integrated system delivering what are described as evidence-based medical, dental and healthcare functions across Defence. Interoperability is a key element of the programme. *Programme Cortisone* should allow healthcare information from multiple

treatment facilities in an austere, operational environment to be made available in real-time to support healthcare delivery. The *Role 1 Capability Review* advocated the use of a dynamically updated dashboard as an effective means of conveying risk across the Role 1 network by capability of care for each medical treatment facility (MTF).[38] This ability to review key data in real-time is a critical foundation for clinical governance and assurance.[43] It is especially pertinent in the military, as it enables assurance to be delivered remotely, reduces the reliance on assurance visits to uncertain operational environments and fosters developmental and supportive approaches that engage DMS primary care clinicians.[44] The review did not define the future dashboard but suggested that it could comprise anything from a series of simple tables to more complex comparative, interactive tools.[44] DMS primary care users' preference was for a dashboard to be a single screen information display providing management oversight of all important clinical data.[44]

Since its inception in April 2013, the DMS *Continuous Assurance Framework* (CAF) has become a useful tool for the real-time communication, assurance and management of pre-hospital healthcare activity in both the Firm Base and on operations.[44] It documents quality markers within domains and sub-domains, including audit, training, staff qualifications, significant event reporting, patient satisfaction and risk management. DMS primary care formations grade themselves over four levels of risk and self-rate their level of assurance against each sub-domain. These grades are assessed periodically through external assurance visits. Digitising the CAF on portable, hand-held devices (Figure 16.9) could enhance its operational utility and provide medical officers with an overarching 'traffic light' dashboard of their area of responsibility as illustrated by Grant and Wheatley's model.[44]

Doctrine/policy

Increased pre-deployment consideration of the future character of military medicine (as shown schematically in Figure 16.10),[45] which may differ from the primarily kinetic campaigns seen in Iraq and Afghanistan, is recommended in order that DMS primary care staff may 'train hard and fight easy'.

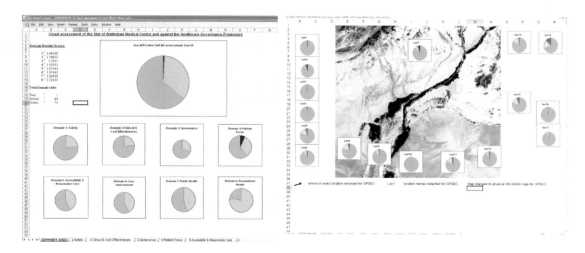

Figure 16.9 Electronic CAF. (From Grant S, Wheatley RJ, *J R Army Med Corps* 2014;160:298–303.)

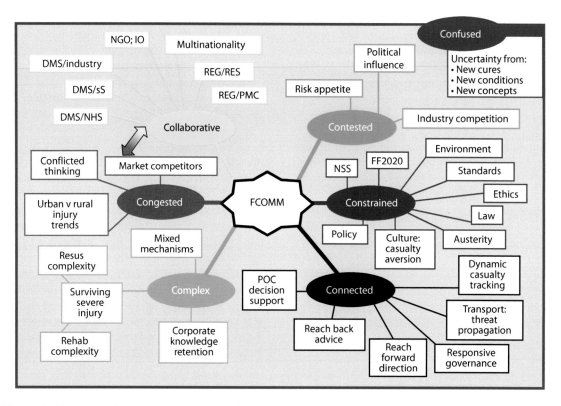

Figure 16.10 Future character of military medicine. (From Hodgetts TJ, *J R Army Med Corps* 2012;158(3): 271–278.)

Organisation

During recent campaigns, clinicians felt that feedback on the care delivered was important in terms of professional development and psychological closure of the episode. Organisational change is required to ensure that those on the frontline are updated on the progress of their casualties.

CONCLUSION

DMS primary care's contribution to *Operations Telic* and *Herrick* was significant and sustained. Role 1 interventions across a broad range of clinical domains, including what would conventionally be classed as pre-hospital emergency care, saved lives between the point of wounding and hospital care. Nevertheless, through the experiences gained and lessons identified before and during *Operations Telic* and *Herrick*, and within the concurrent activities that DMS primary care continued to support during these two campaigns, conditions were set for systematic change to enhance future DMS primary care capability. Such development began in earnest with the 2012 'Putting Role 1 First: The Role 1 Capability Review'[38] informed by multimodal data about DMS primary care's deployed capabilities, evacuation processes and workload. *Operations Telic* and *Herrick* identified clinical challenges resulting from the case mix and learning needs regarding pain management, fluid replacement, Role 1 record keeping and medical materiel. The austere and often psychologically challenging kinetic environment focused attention on adverse mental health outcomes as well as physical injury. Resilience models, including LOAD-CLEAR, were developed to better enable normal functioning despite exposure to frequent and sometimes severe psychological stressors and situational pressures, including mass casualty events and tight evacuation timelines. Pan-*Defence Lines of Development* opportunities for improvement were recognised, especially concerning training, equipment, personnel, information technology/health informatics, doctrine and policy.

Significant capability enhancements such as *Programme Cortisone*,[42] which will deliver the next-generation DMS global health informatics platform, are progressing well. The *DMS Change Programme* and single Service employability, deployability and sustainability work strands are optimising the preparation and availability of DMS primary care force elements at readiness. The DMS GP Specialty Trainee residential course has been refocused upon teaching enhanced clinical skills required in the deployed Role 1 space that are beyond the scope of the NHS national GP curriculum. The development of novel biosensors, wearable technologies, smart textiles and telemetry will assist both reach back and reach forward.

It is vital that such innovations continue. For as long as the UK Armed Forces are sent into harm's way, DMS primary care is likely to be found on the frontline. History shows that both capability and corporate memory tend to dip following a period of intense deployed activity. Any such dip in Role 1 capability or corporate memory with the end of *Operations Telic* and *Herrick* will have a detrimental impact upon DMS primary care delivery at the start of the next campaign, a price that could be repaid in service personnel's lives. Even in the fog of future war, science, compassion and patient centeredness will remain as applicable on the battlefield as they are in the peacetime consulting room.

REFERENCES

1. Blackham R, Blake T. The regimental medical officer: His powers and duties. *BMJ* 1920;02:971–973.
2. Poszner H. Regimental medical practice. *BMJ* 1941;1:412–413.
3. Marsh A. A short but distant war – the Falklands campaign. *J R Soc Med* 1983;76: 972–982.
4. O'Reilly D, Konig T, Tai N. Field trauma care in the 21st century. *J R Army Med Corps* 2008;154:260–264.
5. Wessely S. Risk, psychiatry and the military. *Br J Psychiatry* 2005;186:459–466.
6. Linden SC, Hess V, Jones E. The neurological manifestations of trauma: Lessons from World War I. *Eur Arch Psychiatry Clin Neurosci* 2012;262(3):253–264.
7. Wooley CF. Where are the diseases of yesteryear? DaCosta's syndrome, soldiers heart, the effort syndrome, neurocirculatory asthenia – and the mitral valve prolapse syndrome. *Circulation* 1976;53(5):749–751.
8. Iversen A, Dyson C, Smith N et al. 'Goodbye and good luck': The mental health needs and treatment experiences of British ex-service personnel. *Br J Psychiatry* 2005;186:480–486.

9. Orner R, Lynch T, Seed P. Long-term traumatic stress reactions in British Falklands War veterans. *Br J Clin Psychol* 1993;32: 457–459.

10. Cherry N, Creed F, Silman A et al. Health and exposures of United Kingdom Gulf War veterans. Part 2: The relationship of health to exposure. *Occup Environ Med* 2001;58(5):299–306.

11. Everitt B, Ismail K, David AS, Wessely S. Searching for a Gulf War syndrome using cluster analysis. *Psychol Med* 2002;32(8): 1371–1378.

12. Simmons R, Maconochie N, Doyle P et al. Self-reported ill health in male UK Gulf War veterans: A retrospective cohort study. *BMC Public Health* 2004;4:27.

13. Stimpson NJ, Thomas HV, Weightman AL et al. Psychiatric disorder in veterans of the Persian Gulf War of 1991. Systematic review. *Br J Psychiatry* 2003;182:391–403.

14. Hotopf M, Hull L, Fear NT et al. The health of UK military personnel who deployed to the 2003 Iraq war: A cohort study. *Lancet* 2006;367(9524):1731–1741.

15. Ismail K, Kent K, Brugha T et al. The mental health of UK Gulf war veterans: Phase 2 of a two phase cohort study. *BMJ* 2002; 325(7364):576.

16. Applewhite L, Keller N et al. Mental health care use by soldiers conducting counterinsurgency operations. *Mil Med* 2012;177(5):501–506.

17. Gumbley AE, Claydon MA, Blankenstein TN, Fell TH. Medical provision in forward locations in Afghanistan: The experiences of General Duties Medical Officers on Op HERRICK 15. *J R Army Med Corps* 2013;159: 68–72.

18. Ministry of Defence. Operations in Iraq: British Fatalities. 21 November 2007.

19. http://www.mod.uk/NR/rdonlyres/CE1302FF -C47C-4F83-B616-2FF9645A2FB2/0 /OpTelicCausaltyTables.pdf

20. https://www.mod.uk/government/uploads /system/uploads/attachment_data /file/503022/20160222_op_Herrick _Casualty_tables_Feb_16_REVISION.pdf

21. Hawksley O, Jeyanathan J, Mears K, Simpson R. A survey of primary health care provision at a Forward Operating Base in Afghanistan during Operation HERRICK 10. *J R Army Med Corps* 2011;157(2):145–149.

22. Driver JM, Nelson TG, Simpson RG, Wall C. To refer or not to refer: A qualitative study of reasons for referral from Role 1. *J R Army Med Corps* 2012;158(3): 208–212.

23. Hodgetts TJ, Aldington D, Henning J et al. *Battlefield Analgesia Review.* Birmingham: Royal Centre for Defence Medicine, 2006.

24. Davey CMT, Mieville KE, Simpson R, Aldington D. A proposed model for improving battlefield analgesia training: Post-graduate medical officer pain management day. *J R Army Med Corps* 2012;158(3):190–193.

25. Davey C, Mieville K, Simpson RG, Aldington D. A survey of the experience of parenteral analgesia at Role 1. *J R Army Med Corps* 2012;158(3):186–189.

26. General Medical Council. Generic Standards for specialty training including GP training. 2010: 10–11.

27. Royal College of Physicians, London. The Academy of Medical Royal Colleges. A clinician's guide to record standards Part 1. 2008:8. http://www.rcplondon.ac.uk /clinical-standards/hiu/medical-records.

28. Department of Health, Royal College of General Practitioners and British Medical Association. The Good Practice Guidelines for GP electronic patient records (Version 4). 2011:137–139. http://www.gov.uk/publications.

29. Batham DR, Wall CM. An audit of the quality of deployed DMICP records on Operation HERRICK 14. *J R Army Med Corps* 2012; 158(3):213–216.

30. Gaynor M, Myung D, Gupts A, Moulton S. A standardised pre-hospital electronic patient care system. *Int J Electron Health* 2009;5:102–136.

31. Air Power Under Pressure http://www.raf .mod.uk/purpose/airpowerunderpressure .cfm

32. 'Delivering Security in a Changing World.' Defence White Paper 03, Para 2.1. http://www.mod.uk/NR/rdonlyres/147C7A19-8554-4DAE-9F88-6FBAD2D973F9/0/cm6269_future_capabilities.pdf

33. Withnall RDJ, Fear NT, Wessely S. Do UK military helicopter aircrew exhibit resilience factors that protect against the development of operational stress? *Commander Joint Helicopter Command Review Paper.* July 2011.

34. Brien LS, Hughes SJ. Symptoms of post-traumatic stress disorder in Falklands veterans five years after the conflict. *Br J Psychiatry* 1991;159:135–141.

35. Finnegan A. A Mental Health Service after major trauma. *Prof Nurse* 1999;15: 179–182.

36. JDP 4-03.1. *Clinical Guidelines for Operations.* Ministry of Defence. 2008.

37. Cooper DJ. A personal view – six months in a FOB. *J R Army Med Corps* 2010;156(1): 57–63.

38. Hodgetts TJ, Findlay S. Putting Role 1 first: The Role 1 capability review. *J R Army Med Corps* 2012;158:162–170.

39. Fear NT, Jones M, Murphy D et al. What are the consequences of deployment to Iraq and Afghanistan on the mental health of the UK Armed Forces? A cohort study. *Lancet* 2010;375(9728):1783–1797.

40. Adams G, Durand D, Doris B et al. Direct and indirect effects of operational tempo on outcomes for soldiers and spouses. *Mil Psychol* 2005;17(3):229–246.

41. World Health Organization. *The World Health Report 2004: Changing History.* Geneva: WHO, 2004. www.who.int/whr/2004/en/

42. http://cui2-uk.diif.r.mil.uk/r/473/FutPlns/CORTISONE%20IGBC/20141131-CORTISONE_Prg_Def_v3_0-OS-Cmrcl.docAreCliniciansEngagedInQualityImprovement.pdf 2011.

43. Wilkinson J, Powell A, Davies H. Evidence: Are clinicians engaged in quality improvement? The Health Foundation http://www.health.org.uk/sites/health/files/AreCliniciansEngagedInQualityImprovement.pdf 2011

44. Grant S, Wheatley RJ. A system for the management, display and integration of pre-hospital healthcare activity in the deployed environment. *J R Army Med Corps* 2014;160:298–303.

45. Hodgetts TJ. The future character of military medicine. *J R Army Med Corps* 2012;158(3):271–278.

17

Defence rehabilitation

INTRODUCTION

During the conflicts in Iraq and Afghanistan, *Defence Rehabilitation* was able to respond to the casualty reception demands because it had a robust model of care, supported by an infrastructure that, although designed in peace, could be adapted for war. Although it required significant adaptation – most importantly the realignment of services to provide a rapid and effective response to complex trauma cases – the presence of a consistent and coherent clinical approach to rehabilitation through the *Defence Medical Rehabilitation Programme* (DMRP) undoubtedly enhanced outcomes and reduced clinical and presentational risk.

Defence Rehabilitation had to provide Role 4 and deployed operational support during the course of both operations whilst continuing to support an increased musculoskeletal (MSK) injury burden at home and in locations across the globe.

The main lesson learned from these conflicts is that Defence must maintain a highly adaptable medical rehabilitation service capable of managing high volumes of poly-trauma cases at short notice, as the National Health Service (NHS) does not have this capability and will not have it in the foreseeable future.

DEFENCE MEDICAL REHABILITATION PROGRAMME

The DMRP provides the rehabilitation services for all injured or ill Service personnel. It depends on a network of rehabilitation facilities and the referral of patients to the appropriate level of care within the network. During the conflicts, DMRP had the following components:

- *Primary Care Rehabilitation Facilities* (PCRF), staffed by physiotherapists and exercise rehabilitation instructors (ERI) to provide primary care rehabilitation.
- *Regional Rehabilitation Units* (RRU), designed to deliver intermediate-level, intensive, inpatient exercise-based rehabilitation.
- The *Rehabilitation Team* at the *Royal Centre for Defence Medicine* (RCDM) including a rehabilitation coordination officer, military physiotherapists and an ERI.
- The *Defence Medical Rehabilitation Centre* (DMRC – during this period Headley Court, Epsom) was the secondary/tertiary care referral centre for inpatient rehabilitation and outpatient assessment delivered by consultant based multi-disciplinary teams (MDTs).
- *Deployed Medical Rehabilitation Teams* (DMRTs) providing operational support from Roles 1 to 3 based in Iraq and Afghanistan.

This system provides a tiered approach to the Services' rehabilitation needs. The PCRFs see patients referred by the unit medical officer with physiotherapy and rehabilitation needs. The PCRFs are now managed by *Defence Primary Healthcare* on a regional basis with a tri-service role but at the time of the conflicts were under single Service lead.

RRUs

There were 15 RRUs at the time of the war fighting, distributed across the United Kingdom and with two in Germany (where there is now one). These units are designed to provide intermediate rehabilitation for patients who require group-based exercise therapy or a higher level of clinical input and access to investigations and surgery. They deliver the following: multidisciplinary injury assessment clinics – with rapid access to diagnostic imaging, 'fast-track' surgical interventions for easily remediable conditions and in-patient residential exercise-based rehabilitation.

Headley court

Defence has a unique requirement for a centralised secondary care facility; throughout the conflicts the *DMRC* at Headley Court (Figure 17.1) provided consultant-level opinions with the additional facilities and therapy staff required to manage patients with more complex rehabilitation needs. This included complex trauma cases and severe brain injuries, which rose in number as a result of the two conflicts. However, the bulk of patients seen at DMRC, even during the conflict, were those with more complicated MSK injuries unrelated to conflict, who could not be managed in the lower tiers of the rehabilitation chain.

A specialist centre is required because of the geographically widespread nature of the relatively small population at risk (PAR), the complexity of conditions requiring specialist services that can best be provided by concentration in one unit and because a single site generates the 'critical mass' of

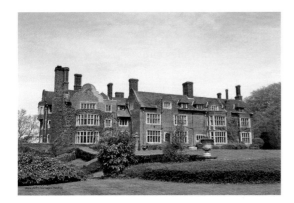

Figure 17.1 DMRC Headley Court.

expertise needed to generate new developments through research and best clinical practice. In addition, welfare and support services can be more easily co-located at the site, and such a unit can host a research capability.

The establishment required for these units was calculated from standards based on the PAR set by *the Directorate of Defence Rehabilitation* and published in the Surgeon General's policy letter for the DMRP. The Director of Defence Rehabilitation acts as the Defence Consultant Advisor for Rheumatology and Rehabilitation as well as Sport and Exercise Medicine and is therefore responsible for the training, standards and career management of the consultants in these specialities, military physiotherapists, civilian allied health professionals (AHPs) and exercise rehabilitation instructors. The Directorate is now responsible for policy and clinical leadership across all of Defence Rehabilitation, but at the time of the conflicts, this was less clear and the Directorate has never had command of any of the assets.

Rehabilitation across Defence was coordinated by the *Rehabilitation Executive Committee*, chaired by the 2 star Commander Joint Medical Command. The Director of Defence Rehabilitation chaired the Sub-*Rehabilitation Executive Committee*, which coordinated, through a number of other committees, the day-to-day policy and plans of Defence Rehabilitation.

The DMRP has two principal roles:

a. To support *force generation* for operations by returning the injured and ill to operational fitness – supporting the *physical component* of fighting power.
b. To rehabilitate seriously injured service personnel in support of the *moral component* of fighting power.

Delivering these roles satisfactorily requires a combination of adequate resources, excellent training, collective military ethos and complete engagement with the Chain of Command. The outputs of Defence Rehabilitation had to be responsive to the requirements of the Chain of Command in generating a force fit to fight and also in discharging the Armed Forces' duty of care to their wounded. If the Chain of Command loses confidence in the process, then the effectiveness of the pathway is jeopardised.

During these conflicts, it was critical to effectively link all elements of the DMRP – deployed operational teams with Role 4 and the permanent establishments. Even during the height of the conflict, there was no single chain of command, which led to inefficiencies and difficulty in providing a strategic solution for the number and complexity of returning battle casualties. The challenge was that staff and infrastructure resources required for Role 4 were simultaneously required to support the routine rehabilitation effort and provide personnel for deployed operations. An increased throughput of operational casualties at Headley Court required the reallocation of patients with MSK injury to the rest of the DMRP – but the absence of an overarching control mechanism for achieving this generated considerable administrative and command difficulties.

The DMRP provides a tiered service attempting to meet the individual clinical needs of the patient at any given time. It also acts as a 'reservoir' of rehabilitation services, which can be relied upon at different phases of a patient's treatment. For example, a patient with complex injuries early in the course of their treatment may require admission to the secondary care centre. After initial treatment, they may be released home for continued rehabilitation locally at the PCRF before returning to secondary care. This allows the patient to have respite at home whilst continuing treatment. It also releases resources for the treatment of other patients in secondary care. At later stages of rehabilitation, they may require support from the intermediate care services – the RRU.

Rehabilitation capability

Defence has been, and must remain, at the forefront of clinical developments in rehabilitation. This is achieved through horizon scanning, having the freedom to trial new equipment and techniques (within appropriate governance frameworks), liaison with stakeholder nations, particularly the United States, and conducting clinical evaluations and research.

The success of battle casualty rehabilitation was built on the breadth of capabilities developed by Defence Rehabilitation during peace time, which include the need to provide the capabilities listed in Table 17.1. In the future, there will also be a requirement to provide (or be able to provide) chemical, biological, radiation and nuclear injury rehabilitation.

Table 17.1 Rehabilitation capabilities

- Musculo-skeletal rehabilitation
- Complex trauma rehabilitation
- Neuro-rehabilitation
- Rehabilitation for complex medical disorders
  - Pain management
  - Spinal cord injury
  - Peripheral nerve injury
  - Chronic fatigue
  - Cardio-respiratory rehabilitation
  - Burns
  - Environmental injury – heat/cold
  - Non-freezing cold injury
  - Arthropathy – including osteoarthritis
- Occupational therapy – including vocational OT
- Podiatry and gait assessment
- Prosthetic/orthotic/wheelchair services
- High functional outputs/late stage rehabilitation – e.g. Special Forces.

Physiotherapy

Military physiotherapists are now trained in two cadres:

- MSK physiotherapy in support of Roles 1 and 4 and ongoing demands
- Critical care – for deployment in support of Role 2/3

each with a military senior clinical lead. All MSK physiotherapists prior to deployment are now updated in basic critical care management, but specialists are still required. At the start of these conflicts, experience in critical care physiotherapy was limited and there was insufficient expertise amongst military physiotherapists to support critical care clinicians in the field.

Support from other defence medical services cadres and civilian AHPs

Defence Rehabilitation is reliant on expertise from other military cadres, including nursing (there is no specialist cadre, which had implications for resources and quality of care at peak casualty numbers), mental health, pain services (military-led acute and chronic pain services developed during the conflict), trauma and orthopaedic, general and burns and plastic surgery. Support from civilian staff was also critical to rehabilitation services, in particular from physiotherapists, occupational therapists, social workers, prosthetic services (including contracted prosthetists and prosthetic technicians), psychology services (neuro-psychology, pain management and mental health), rehabilitation workshop services (combined military and civilian personnel) and podiatrists.

Exercise rehabilitation instructors

The ERI is critical to the delivery of exercise-based group therapy; this is a deployable capability, which cannot be adequately sourced from civilian practice. By treating large groups of patients simultaneously, the ERI acts as an important rehabilitation service force multiplier. An ERI was very effectively introduced to the acute Role 4 facility in Birmingham and was used at both Role 1 and Role 3 on operations in Afghanistan. The ERI increases the 'dose' of rehabilitation delivered to the patient, contributes to the early mobilisation of the patient from bed, improves morale and re-introduces a military ethos early in the course of recovery.

Scrutiny

The level of ministerial, parliamentary, senior military and press scrutiny should not be underestimated. It places significant logistic, professional and emotional burdens on the clinical providers at Role 4. The high level of press, public and charity scrutiny put the government of the time, and hence the Defence Medical Services (DMS), under significant pressure to deliver a high-quality outcome. Senior leaders often perceived the management of political expectations as the priority, hence placing increased pressure on clinical staff.

OPERATIONAL SUCCESS OF DEFENCE REHABILITATION DURING *OPERATIONS TELIC* AND *HERRICK*

Defence Rehabilitation successfully achieved its aims during the conflicts in Iraq and Afghanistan. It developed a national and international reputation

for the management of around 1000 seriously injured complex trauma or neurological casualties, providing the most sophisticated rehabilitation techniques available and expediting transfer from the casualty receiving hospital, the *Queen Elizabeth Hospital Birmingham* (QEHB).

Defence Rehabilitation developed an entirely new approach to rehabilitation, whilst maintaining the throughput of routine non-battle injuries. The Role 4 rehabilitation response to operations has been influential at a national level, with senior military clinicians informing NHS developments and designing the rehabilitation components of the *Major Trauma Networks*. However, there remains a lack of NHS commitment to the development of rehabilitation services, which has implications for future military capability and capacity.

It was clear that the NHS had neither the clinical capability nor the capacity to manage the volume or complexity of the casualties received by RCDM. Had there not been a successful response, there would have been major clinical, presentational and political repercussions. This success was a consequence of having the DMRP in place before the commencement of hostilities. Loss of this capability within the military system cannot be regrown within the short timescales expected for future expeditionary conflicts. Any further conflict could quickly produce a similar number of casualties and the advances in surgical and resuscitative techniques are likely to generate increased survival and further clinical complexity.

The DMRP has never been short of work – over time, it has merely refocused its efforts on the varying rehabilitation requirements of the Armed Forces. As complex trauma became a priority, other services were exported to the RRUs or not delivered – for example recruit training injury prevention and management and late stage rehabilitation.

Operational commitment

Defence Rehabilitation is required to provide support to operations in all medical Roles:

- Deployed – operational Roles 1–3
- Role 4 operations in the United Kingdom
- Support to force generation and 'business as usual'

Manning levels during these operations meant that staff employed on deployed operations, as a contingent component of a deployed unit, were taken from their normal role. Although the most effective way to provide rehabilitation services would be to have an establishment sufficient for all phases of the care pathway, the resources were not present for this, nor will they be in future. There are consequently risks to clinical continuity, waiting times to support force generation increase and there are costs in backfilling posts. There was no Role 4 doctrine until late in the conflict.

NHS capability

At the start of the Iraq conflict, there was a presumption that the NHS, as part of the reception arrangements for military patients process, would fulfil much of the Role 4 rehabilitation capability. It became clear early on that the NHS had neither the capability nor the capacity to manage the rehabilitation of these patients, particularly given the complexity and number of battle casualties and the rate at which they returned from theatre. The NHS remains unable to fulfil this role, and therefore, any future planning for operations must be based on the premise that the DMS must retain a secondary care rehabilitation capability.

Table 17.2 is taken from the National Audit of Rehabilitation Services across NHS England performed in 2016.[1] It shows the total bed capacity and approximate proportion of trauma admissions within each level of service. The service levels described are all commissioned by NHS England

and are specialist services, with Level 1 being the most sophisticated.

During the conflict period, Headley Court was operating at a level equivalent to 1a/b. Therefore, in 2014–2015, there were approximately 994 occupied beds for specialist rehabilitation in England. Across all services, 19.4% of admissions were for trauma cases, giving a total of about 195 beds used for trauma patients in the whole of England. However, it is not known what proportion of these were actually admitted from the major trauma centres (MTCs) or trauma units. About 5% of cases treated in MTCs subsequently receive specialist rehabilitation. With an average length of stay of approximately 75 days, each bed accommodates about five admissions per year; this total provision allows for 950 admissions to specialist rehabilitation per year for trauma for NHS patients in England. Therefore, across the whole of England, there is currently the same capacity for trauma admissions annually, which Headley Court was managing in the conflict in 2011–12. These casualty levels subsequently increased. These figures do not, however, tell the whole story. This NHS bed capacity is mainly targeted at managing patients with post-acute traumatic brain injury (TBI). These facilities do not have the capability or expertise to manage early trauma rehabilitation, including multiple limb loss, complex MSK injury, spinal cord injury or burns and in particular the multiple combinations of these injuries. The capacity of the NHS to expand and take on more trauma rehabilitation cases is negligible, and it would be unable to

Table 17.2 Total capacity and proportion of trauma patients in 2014–2015

Service level	No. of units	Total OBDs[a] 2014–2015	No. of beds[b]	Admissions for trauma, %	No. of trauma beds
Hyper-acute	3	8,281	23	7%	2
1a	7	56,740	155	19%	30
1b	6	38,062	104	33%	34
1c	3	8,681	24	29%	7
2a	13	95,820	263	17%	45
2b	33	155,161	425	18%	77
Total	65	362,745	994	Overall 19.5%	195

Source: National Clinical Audit of Specialist Rehabilitation for Patients with Complex Needs Following Major Injury. HQIP Report. 2017 https://www.hqip.org.uk.
[a] OBDs = occupied bed days.
[b] The number of beds was calculated as OBD/365, rounded to whole numbers.

deliver the rehabilitation services needed after one episode of multiple casualties arising from a terrorist attack such as that which occurred in Paris on November 15. It still does not have the capacity and capability to deliver battle casualty rehabilitation on the scale required during the conflicts in Iraq and Afghanistan.

Casualty numbers

Figure 17.2 shows the steady increase in casualty numbers treated at Headley Court from 2006 at the start of the increasing demand for complex

trauma rehabilitation. Operations in Afghanistan such as *Panther's Claw* (the International Security Assistance Force operation launched in June 2009 to establish a firm presence in Helmand Province) generated an increased burden on the organisation with a rapid increase in bed numbers generated without warning to the Role 4 rehabilitation services. Figure 17.3 indicates the sudden increase in demand for services that arose as a result of this one operation.

In 2006, when the concept of complex trauma was developed, there were four ward-based beds and no staff specifically allocated to this role. Staff were shared with other therapy teams. Within six months, there was one consultant-led team and approximately 20 beds. Panther's Claw caused a rapid demand in rehabilitation capacity, including bed spaces. In July 2009, there were 30 complex trauma beds and two teams, by September 2009, this had grown to 45 beds, and by January 2010, there were 60 beds.

At the peak of the conflict, there were 75 complex trauma beds, four teams and approximately 100 staff. Bed occupancy ran at between 85% and 95%. This was in addition to the neuro-rehabilitation team which had 20 beds and the general MSK teams that were managing approximately (depending on demand, resource management and case mix) 110 hostel-type beds. This was the largest rehabilitation centre in the United Kingdom.

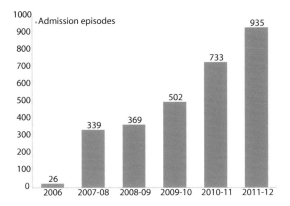

Figure 17.2 Admission episodes to complex trauma teams at Headley Court.

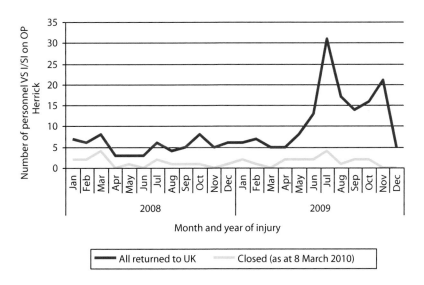

Figure 17.3 Aeromedical evacuations related to Panther's Claw.

Figure 17.4 shows the increase in clinical activity through Headley Court, with the increase in operational casualties being the biggest driver of clinical activity; however, the number of cases arising from non-operational reasons (usually MSK training injuries) also increased, probably as a result of an increased pre-deployment training

(PDT) tempo. It needs to be recognised, therefore, that in preparation for war, there is a need to manage the increased demands arising from training for battle as well as the battle casualties themselves.

Figure 17.5 demonstrates that the new patient numbers reached a peak at RCDM in July 2010. The RRUs were predominantly seeing cases 'discharged

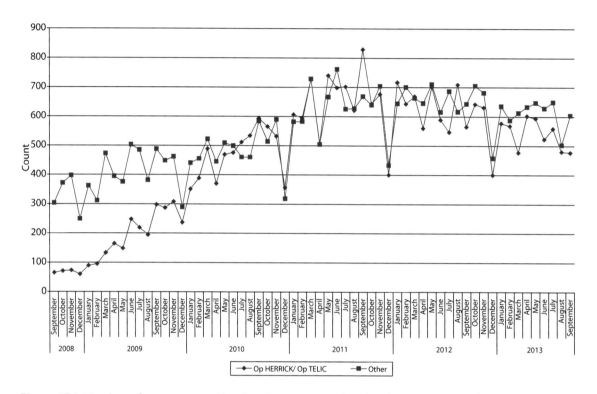

Figure 17.4 Number of cases seen at Headley Court – operational and non-operational.

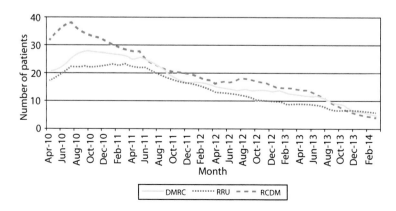

Figure 17.5 New patients with battle injuries seen at Headley Court, RRUs and RCDM.

at air-head' to ensure that a rehabilitation pathway was in place. It needs to be recognised, however, that although there was a decline in the number of new patients arriving at Headley Court (Figure 17.5), because of the length of the care pathway (a triple amputee on average took 44 months from wounding until leaving the Service) and the need to repeatedly admit patients to the unit, in-patient clinical activity did not reach a peak until mid 2011 (Figure 17.6).

Figure 17.6 also demonstrates that the intense operational commitment continued at Headley Court long after the casualty numbers fell elsewhere at Role 4.

The prosthetic service at Headley Court was not set up with specific reference to the war fighting in Iraq but because NHS shortcomings in provision were identified when a senior officer suffered a traumatic amputation. The contract to provide prosthetic services at Headley Court was awarded to Blatchfords in 2006. At that time, there was an estimated need for one half-time prosthetist. At the peak of clinical activity, there were 11 full-time prosthetists, comprising the largest centre in the United Kingdom. The relationship between this company and Defence Rehabilitation has been a model of contractor/ Defence working relationships – with a genuine sense of team-working and commitment to the mission rather than a focus on the contract. Figure 17.7 illustrates the increased demand placed on the prosthetic and rehabilitation services as a result of the different wounding patterns experienced in Afghanistan with pressure-plate improvised explosive devices (IEDs).

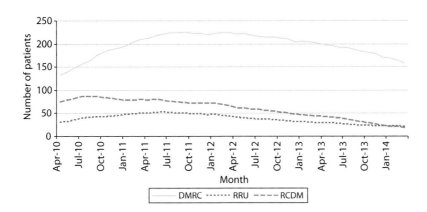

Figure 17.6 Patients with battle injuries seen at Headley Court, RRUs and RCDM, 13-month moving average.

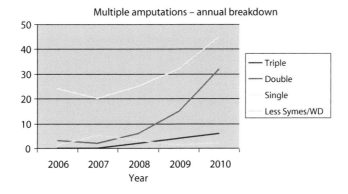

Figure 17.7 Prosthetic demand at Headley Court – incidence and type of prosthetic case.

REHABILITATION AT HEADLEY COURT

Introduction

The aim of military rehabilitation is to take a casualty from point of wounding through surgical and medical management and return him to the highest possible levels of function and integration back into military or civilian society. The recent conflicts have challenged combat casualty care providers, military rehabilitation services and society as a whole.

Rehabilitation in this group of patients is complicated by a number of factors. There are frequently multiple injuries, which cross organ and other traditional classification boundaries and include the MSK and neurological systems as well as the skin, sensory organs and urogenital system. It is therefore not possible to compartmentalise patients within one treatment group. The NHS is organised according to a system that delivers rehabilitation based on single-organ damage, such as brain injury, spinal cord injury or limb loss. Military patients frequently require therapeutic interventions from all these services simultaneously and cannot be managed in the stove-piped services in the NHS (Figure 17.8).

Psychological factors are a major influence on the long-term success of rehabilitation. Exposure to psychological trauma prior to injury, the death of colleagues, the near-death experience itself, disfigurement and perceived disability will complicate rehabilitation outcomes. Patients with similar injuries from similar circumstances may have widely different outcomes because of the individual's emotional response to the traumatic event. Similarly, even mild TBI (mTBI) can have devastating consequences as it can impact on cognition and adaptability to life-changing events.

PRINCIPLES OF MILITARY REHABILITATION

The key principles of the rapid and successful rehabilitation of patients injured in conflict are given in Table 17.3.

Early assessment

Assessment of a patient needs to occur as soon after wounding as possible in order to identify rehabilitation needs and to initiate the earliest stages of physical rehabilitation. This will mean assessment on the intensive care unit where necessary.

At the start of the conflict, Service critical care physiotherapy had suffered from a focus on MSK injuries within Defence Rehabilitation. Physiotherapists deployed on operations were meant to be skilled in critical care as well as MSK injuries. This was clearly untenable and the development of a specialist cadre of critical care physiotherapists was initiated. This aided the management of cases on intensive care units (ICUs) but also ensured good communication between deployed trauma rehabilitation services and home-based

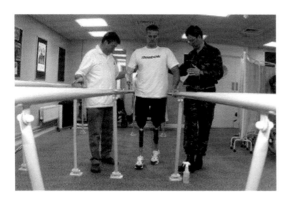

Figure 17.8 Rehabilitation at Headley Court.

Table 17.3 Principles and context of military rehabilitation

Principles
- Early assessment
- Multi-disciplinary team (MDT) approach
- Active case management
- Exercise-based rehabilitation
- Rapid access to further specialist opinion and investigation

Which need to be delivered in a military environment that will encourage:
- Military discipline
- Competitiveness
- Compliance
- Peer support

Role 4 services. There is a difference between the services provided by UK physiotherapists and US respiratory technicians. The UK physiotherapist provides management of the chest (although not usually ventilator settings), together with positioning and mobilisation of limbs to reduce contractures and other factors that might otherwise limit recovery, whereas respiratory technicians manage the ventilation of the patients alone. Both sets of skills are needed.

The doctrine of forward rehabilitation, using DMRTs in medical regiments, field hospitals or further forward to manage minor to moderate MSK injuries and to initiate rehabilitation, was particularly helpful not only in initiating early rehabilitation but also in ensuring that the chain of command was engaged in the rehabilitation pathway.

Use of the MDT

The medical consultant-led MDT is vital in complex cases. The complexity and multi-system nature of these injuries means that they cannot be allocated to single therapy teams. The MDT includes medical staff, physiotherapists, occupational therapists, social work/welfare workers, exercise therapists, prosthetists, podiatrist/orthotists and mental health and psychology support. There were regular MDT meetings with goal setting and treatment planning for each patient.

Active case management

Active case management means that patients' care pathways are planned from the point of arrival at medical care throughout their acute management until they are discharged from rehabilitation. Relying on multiple external agencies, particularly the NHS, to coordinate a patient's activities is unrealistic and frequently leads to failure of the pathway. The rehabilitation MDT is key to facilitating the ongoing medical and social management of the patient. There is a need to coordinate medical care (including ongoing surgical review), investigations, equipment (for example wheelchairs) and social and welfare support. This may include planning for resettlement into supported living environments.

Exercise-based rehabilitation

Exercise-based rehabilitation is based on the physical training of the injured body to enhance function, improve well-being and generate confidence. This relies on an understanding of tissue healing processes and exercise physiology and the ability to modify exercise programs to suit patients with multiple concomitant injuries. In the UK military, uniquely, physical training instructors undergo additional training in the delivery of exercise-based rehabilitation to groups of patients with similar levels and types of condition: these exercise rehabilitation instructors are critical to the delivery of the intense rehabilitation required to produce the enhanced outcomes expected of military patients.

Rapid access to further specialist opinion

After the initial trauma surgery, there is a need for follow-up surgical procedures including orthopaedic, plastic, urological and other reconstructive surgery. This draws upon the skills not only of the original surgical teams at Birmingham but also on other specialist units around the country. During the conflicts, alternative specialist units with experience in neuro-urology and peripheral nerve injury and plastic surgery were called upon as required to support the rehabilitation process.

The key elements required of secondary care were expertise and speed of access. NHS waiting times for an opinion and surgery were inadequate for managing the needs of these casualties. Delay in having further surgery would in turn impact on the ability to progress their rehabilitation so that they could return to Service or be discharged into civilian life.

Mental health services and psychological support were essential and commenced in Birmingham but were also available at Headley Court. Although mental health professionals were important in this environment, the key psychological support appears to have arisen from the patients' peers, their relatives and the therapeutic environment in which they were placed. An important element, both for patients and relatives, seems to have been having a clear understanding of the direction of travel of their care, the rehabilitation pathway and expected outcomes, early in the course of their injuries. Conversations with relatives whilst their family members were on the ICU seemed to have a positive effect in reassuring them that everything possible would be done. There was a policy whereby all complex trauma patients had a mental health assessment on admission to Headley Court, although the benefits of this were hard to quantify as real issues tended to arise out with this assessment.

REHABILITATION EFFECT

The rehabilitation effect relied on all elements of the DMRP. Although the main specialist rehabilitation unit at Headley Court was at the core of battle casualty rehabilitation, considerable support was provided by the RRUs and the PCRFs. Not all trauma rehabilitation required secondary care services, and as patients spent more time at home and work, they relied increasingly on primary care support. In retrospect, it is clear that the majority of this burden fell on the PCRFs, with relatively few battle casualties undergoing rehabilitation at the RRUs, although many were assessed there.

Rehabilitation was an interactive process, with patients attending for three- to four-week periods of treatment, then a period of recovery or consolidation at home or work, followed by readmission to provide further rehabilitation and a more intense level of therapeutic exercise or intervention. The rehabilitation process consisted of the structural elements listed in Table 17.4

Table 17.4 Key structural elements of the military rehabilitation process

- Patient tracking
- Patient assessment
- Goal-setting
- Treatment planning
- Exercise-based rehabilitation
- Case management
- Discharge–readmission cycle
- Discharge planning
- Vocational rehabilitation
- Reintegration into society
- Follow-up

Patient tracking

Effective rehabilitation depends on the ability to deliver the appropriate care package to the right patient at the right time. At the start of the conflict, there was no effective way of tracking patients who returned to the United Kingdom and were discharged at the airhead – with relatively minor injuries – or those patients who were discharged by NHS staff from the casualty receiving hospital in Birmingham. Patients who were discharged from the unit without being properly identified by Defence Rehabilitation and the patients' chain of command risked being sent home with no proper follow-up as a consequence. Some relatively severe cases were not entered into the rehabilitation pathway until much later in the course of their injury, with a negative effect on their physical, psychological and social outcomes. This was also a significant presentational risk.

The most seriously injured passed through RCDM to undergo definitive trauma surgery and required intensive care. The patient was therefore identified from the outset, and a rehabilitation programme was set in motion. Less seriously injured patients may have had only transient periods in the secondary care facility before being discharged to local physiotherapy services. The risk in this process is that apparently minor injuries with significant functional sequelae are passed to inexperienced services. These cases may have been at greater risk of severe psychological disturbance than the more severely injured. There is a tendency to underestimate the severity of some injuries, and the psychological consequences of even minor trauma may be significant.

To avoid the loss of patients from rehabilitation services, the Headley Court team developed a patient tracking system. This required a cell at Headley Court to receive a signal detailing all aeromedical evacuation cases. A consultant would triage them and any case likely to be discharged at the air head was allocated to an RRU – which was required to identify and see the patient within five working days of landing to ensure an appropriate level of care was delivered. This was labour intensive but ensured that the patients were getting to the right place in the care pathway. It took a few years before headquarters Surgeon General felt that this should be a centrally led DMS capability, with instigation of the *Defence Patient Tracing Agency.*

The experience of civilian trauma centres – particularly in moments of extreme demand – suggests that similar tracking systems need to be in place to ensure that patients are correctly referred for rehabilitation.

Patient assessment

The medical team played a critical part in the initial stages of the rehabilitation process when the patients were not medically stable. Rehabilitation commenced on ICU, but for the patients to be able to make significant progress, they had to be medically stable, free from life-threatening infection and not undergoing frequent medical procedures, which would interfere with the continuity of rehabilitation. It took some time to realise that wound or skin contamination with organisms such as methicillin resistant *Staphylococcus aureus* (MRSA) *did not* exclude rehabilitation but that mitigation could be taken to minimise the risk of cross-contamination. Conversely, it rapidly became apparent that pain needed to be controlled early and an understanding of pain management including neuropathic pain is vital. The introduction of a military-led acute pain management service in QEHB made a dramatic difference in the pain presenting during rehabilitation

KEY ELEMENTS IN THE HISTORY

There were a number of key elements that needed to be established in determining the history of patients requiring rehabilitation: the nature of the wounding (including the presence of single or multiple entry wounds and the level of energy transfer), the history of impairment or loss of consciousness, the nature and degree of pain, the time spent on intensive care, the nature of surgical and medical interventions and the patient's perception of their injuries. A social history detailing their home support, medical history and current medication also needed to be established. Other essential elements included any history of psychological disturbance (in particular nightmares, flashbacks, intrusive thoughts and changes in mood), the presence of cognitive deficits (word finding difficulties, memory, concentration and

executive skills) and any sensory (tactile, visual and auditory) deficits.

EXAMINATION SKILLS

It was essential that the medical teams had the skills and knowledge in both MSK and neurological examination to diagnose deficits, record impairments and monitor change.

MULTI-DISCIPLINARY ASSESSMENT

A multi-disciplinary assessment was vital. Assessments by doctors, physiotherapists, occupational therapists, social workers, exercise therapists and nursing staff informed the rehabilitation plan. After an assessment, good communication in an MDT meeting produced a problem list from which goals were set and the treatment plan was derived.

Goal setting

Goal setting is an important element of the rehabilitation programme. Goals need to be set over the long (six months), medium (two to three months) and short (three to four weeks) term (Table 17.5). The SMART (*Specific, Measurable, Achievable, Realistic* and *Time bound*) model is generally used. Critically, goals need to be set in discussion with the patient, although frequently, patients, particularly service personnel, need to be given guidance so as to avoid setting unattainable goals in unrealistic time frames. Alternatively, their goals may be very general making extrapolation of a treatment plan difficult – 'I want to return to running'.

Once long-term goals were set, the shorter-term goals were developed. Goals were set in accordance with the patient's wishes and personal aims.

Table 17.5 Example of rehabilitation goal setting

Long-term goal	In six months, I will return to part-time sedentary work.
Medium-term goal	In three months, I will be walking on my prosthetic for 1 km using one stick.
Short-term goal	At the end of this one-month admission, I will be wearing my new prosthesis for 3 hours/day.

Soldiers may not immediately grasp the importance of taking control of their treatment goals and rehabilitation, as the service spends much of their careers attempting to disempower them from decision-making. However, those with the greatest levels of self-efficacy usually made the greatest progress.

It was sometimes necessary to determine goals over even shorter periods, such as a week, in order to demonstrate to the patient measurable improvement in their function when they were sceptical of their progress. Alternatively, patients, on occasion, needed short-term goals in order to rein in over-enthusiastic activity that could have been detrimental to their outcome. Patients needed encouragement and support to improve their performance, but many cases required limitations to be placed on their activity, particularly in high-achieving military or sporting personnel.

Goal setting should focus on occupational outcomes when dealing with people capable of returning to functional employment. A lack of focus on this aspect of rehabilitation will limit overall vocational outcome. Returning patients to work de-medicalises them and reaffirms their usefulness to society and family.

Treatment planning

Treatment goals were set after discussion between the therapy staff, doctors and the patient. Patient involvement was critical to success and sometimes required involvement of the family and their employer. Ideas, concerns and wishes were explored, and an explanation of the treatment and the prognosis improved patient concordance and compliance. A joint treatment plan was produced that included the timelines for treatment and indicated the external agencies to be involved, including employers and social services. Decisions were recorded on a shared MDT document (initially paper records – later on Defence Medical Information Capability Programme [DMICP]) and actions identified for individual therapists and doctors to perform.

Once rehabilitation commenced, weekly MDT planning meetings were essential and progress was recorded and discussed with the patient. Regular review of the patient was essential, particularly in the early acute phase, and planning for discharge took place as soon as the patient was admitted. At discharge, there was readmission planning and selection of goals to be achieved whilst the patient was at home or at work. This allowed for continued progression and improved progression on return.

Exercise-based rehabilitation

The UK military is unique in that rehabilitation is undertaken over short periods, up to four weeks at a time, and much of the structure of rehabilitation focuses on exercise, which is frequently delivered in a group setting.

GROUP THERAPY

Exercise therapy was usually delivered in groups, with each group being composed of patients having similar injuries and level of function. All groups completed a varied daily program of five hours of exercised-based activity that included: class therapy, hydrotherapy, postural re-education, walking/running and gait re-education and recreational therapy with individually tailored treatment programmes. Many of the outcomes rely on the training benefits of exercise and are therefore dependent on the intensity, frequency and duration of exercise.

Peer support is important in overcoming the psychological consequences of trauma, and group therapy is a major contributor to this. Being surrounded by injured patients from similar backgrounds and experiences aided concordance with treatment and improved recovery. External social interactions were vital at an early stage in the rehabilitation to improve long-term social integration.

PHYSIOTHERAPY

Physiotherapy is a key component of the rehabilitation service provided for patients with severe physical injury. Treatments typically take place on a one-to-one basis. Core skills include manual therapies such as mobilisation, manipulation, soft and deep tissue massage and scar tissue mobilisation. Physiotherapists will provide orthotics, correct gait abnormalities and muscle imbalance and provide stretches, exercise therapy and advice on progression. They supervise the exercise therapy and may use acupuncture and a number of electrotherapy modalities, particularly for pain relief.

SOCIAL WORK

Specialist medical social workers played a key role in the rehabilitation process and benefitted from the hospital social work model of care now no longer seen in the NHS. Experience in the health-related issues that individuals or families may experience following trauma or illness was important, and an understanding of the Defence Welfare environment were vital. At the start of the conflict, the welfare support to the injured was not well organised and there was a 'turf war' between various agencies (charitable and within Defence). Having an in-house social work team was critical to the outputs of Defence Rehabilitation. They offered the following services:

Assessment and counselling: Social workers guided the patient and their family through the process of adjustment, providing support and assisting the individual and their relatives to plan for change.

Care and discharge planning: Social workers provided information about resources such as resettlement and retraining opportunities, housing, welfare benefits and access to legal advice.

Advocacy: One of the roles of the social workers was to represent the patient's view at clinical meetings and meetings with outside agencies such as housing departments or welfare agencies. Considerable time was spent negotiating with the *Armed Forces Compensation Scheme* authorities on the appropriate tariff for compensation. This eventually contributed to a major review of the compensation levels for these patients.

Resettlement: Social workers, in conjunction with occupational therapists, advised patients on opportunities for vocational assessment and retraining.

OCCUPATIONAL THERAPY

Occupational therapists enabled patients to be as independent as possible in the activities of daily living, their chosen occupations or leisure. They provided a remarkably wide range of services and assistance to the injured as follows:

Education and advice: Occupational therapists were a key source of education and practical advice about the nature of the patient's injuries

and how they could deal with the effects on their lives. They also offered advice on work, personal care and leisure activities.

Activities of daily living: Occupational therapists undertook the assessment and treatment of limitations of personal care. This often involved home visits to advise on equipment or adaptations that were required to improve safety and aid independence or, alternatively, liaising with local services to do the same. It became obvious early in the course of the battle casualty reception process that – well-meaning – agencies were authorising and adapting houses in an expensive and inappropriate way before the extent of the impairment or final home destination had been agreed. Our teams subsequently resisted this.

Provision of equipment: Provision of specialised equipment to solve the problems of temporary or permanent disability such as wheelchairs, bathing aids, pressure garments and cushions is an essential element of rehabilitation.

Community living skills: Occupational therapists undertook assessment and training in community living skills such as travelling on public transport, shopping and accessing local community facilities, as well as performing driving assessments and offering advice on equipment and adaptations to enable individuals to return to driving.

Emotional support: Occupational therapists were an important source of practical support and coping strategies to help patients adjust to their limitations and explore their concerns.

Cognitive rehabilitation: Cognitive rehabilitation included the assessment and treatment of the functional impact of cognitive problems such as memory, concentration and processing in brain injury.

Work skills: Unsurprisingly, a major component of the role of the occupational therapists was assessment of skills and advice on strategies and adaptations that could be implemented to improve return to work. Through a graded programme of work hardening, individuals were gradually introduced back to their trade. If they were unable to work, recommendations were made regarding future employment, training or rehabilitation. A specialist team of vocational rehabilitation occupational therapists was developed whose role was to help re-integrate soldiers returning to duty in the military by developing links and gradual return-to-work programmes and liaising with units and line managers.

NURSING TEAM

A named nurse was responsible for a nursing care plan for each patient and for supporting the patient through his rehabilitation. The nursing team required nurses knowledgeable in orthopaedics, neurological rehabilitation, amputee care, spinal injury, sexual dysfunction, mental health and continence care. Of particular importance was tissue viability expertise for multiple wounds, split skin grafts, reconstructive flaps and burns. Nursing staff assisted patients with the activities of daily living in order to promote and encourage independence.

The unit struggled to man the rehabilitation wards with nurses experienced in rehabilitation or tissue viability. There was a reluctance within the nursing services to allow the development of a specialist rehabilitation nursing cadre, as it wasn't considered an operational role. However, consideration should be given to having a burns and plastics nurse attached to the nursing team in any further conflicts.

NUTRITIONAL SUPPORT

Nutritional support is critical in enhancing the recovery of patients who have been in a highly catabolic state for many weeks and who need nutritional supplementation during periods of intense physical activity. Percutaneous endoscopic gastrostomy feeding may be required in more dependent patients. This is an area, on the whole, where we were weak. Access to good dietetic management was difficult, and those clinicians who were obtained were often insufficiently skilled to manage these cases. The effect of *systemic inflammatory response syndrome* was not well understood at that time, but the catabolic effect on patients was dramatic and a better understanding of the metabolic consequences of wounding and subsequent rehabilitation will be imperative in future conflicts. Weight tends to fluctuate with catabolism, recovery, immobility, intense physical activity followed by recuperation at home and sometimes calorie and alcohol overindulgence. Consequently, there were effects on prosthetic limb fitting and there may be long-term metabolic syndrome effects.

Case management

At all times, the rehabilitation programme focussed on vocational outcome and reintegration of the patient into society, work or home. Coordination of external agencies was required, including social services, local authorities, the health services, the employer and housing agencies. Ongoing specialist medical investigations and treatments were required (for example urodynamics to inform bladder management in the spinal cord injured patients or bone infection management). The consultant, who led the MDT, was responsible for the case management in this situation and had to ensure that the rehabilitation process was a smooth as possible.

Discharge: Readmission process

The scheme in Figure 17.9 demonstrates the programme for serial admissions to a complex trauma rehabilitation team. Patients were admitted for approximately four weeks at a time, longer for a first admission. Within 10 days, the goals for that period were stated, agreed and written in the MDT summary. At discharge, *readmission goals* were set for the patient to achieve while they were away and for the first 10 days of their next admission. At the end of the first admission, long-term outcome goals were set to determine what was expected to be the clinical outcome after six months. In this way, a series of admissions could be conducted with increasingly

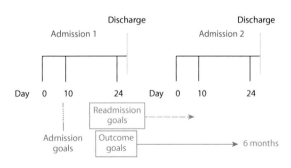

Figure 17.9 Discharge–readmission process.

long periods of time away on sick leave or, later, back at work. This system allowed for a greater through-put of cases. Patients supported it because it allowed them extended periods of time at home or work. It also reinforced the impression of being on a course. This was useful in order to consolidate and practice rehabilitation lessons learnt at Headley Court and most importantly to stop the patients becoming stale, fatigued or developing secondary injuries.

This approach has been one of the significant differences between UK and US rehabilitation processes. The US military posted wounded personnel adjacent to their centres for rehabilitation and ongoing care. This had the benefit of having all the patient facilities located next to the medical facilities, but it did remove the patients and their families from their established home and social support. It also meant that whilst US casualties could attend rehabilitation as outpatients on a sessional basis, UK service personnel attended for time-bonded in-patient courses. This allowed them to focus on their rehabilitation for a short, intense period before returning home to a normal life. This was, in many ways, similar to their pre-morbid lifestyle and improved compliance with treatment.

The admission–readmission cycle was also important in enhancing the availability of beds for new casualties. It relied on the 'reservoir' of rehabilitation services other than Headley Court (mainly the PCRFs, occasionally the NHS) to take on some of the responsibilities for maintenance of physical therapy whilst at home.

Discharge planning

The MDT worked closely with the patients, their family and outside agencies to co-ordinate a package of care that met the needs of the patient. This often involved liaising with health authorities, social services and other external organisations to negotiate the appropriate level of support for the individual. A key focus of the rehabilitation process was on returning to work, and to facilitate this, *Vocational Occupational Therapists* liaised between the MDT, the patient and their employer to ensure that the maximum number of patients returned to meaningful employment. Where appropriate, the patient was sent to their workplace for a period of work assessment; if this was not possible, each patient was supported with further vocational rehabilitation options, later in the course of the conflicts in liaison with the single Service *Personnel Recovery Units* (PRUs). Prior to the instigation of PRUs, there was a focus on returning the individual to their unit in some form of employment. This was generally successful (Figure 17.10).

Reintegration into society could be difficult and depended on a number of factors, including the physical, mental and cognitive status of the patient; the family support received by the individual; and the support from society itself.

The most significant benefit arising from the development of the new Forces charities – particularly 'Help for Heroes' – was the generation of a groundswell of public support and recognition

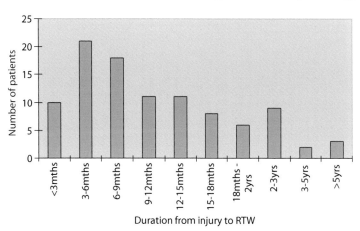

Figure 17.10 Duration from injury to return to work following final discharge from the complex trauma team.

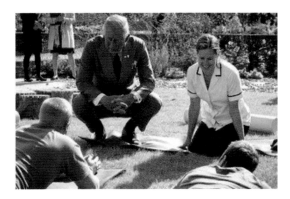

Figure 17.11 HRH The Prince of Wales visits patients at Headley Court.

for the severely wounded. Social outings arranged by charities, meetings with the Royal Family, VIPs and celebrities helped reassure the patients of their worth to society (Figure 17.11).

Measuring outcome

Outcomes were measured in a number ways, including the success of the team in accurately predicting goals, using goal attainment scaling, repeated measurements of standardised physical tests (for example the six-minute walk test, multi-stage fitness tests and Y-balance test), patient-reported outcome measures (such as 36-Item Short Form Survey [SF-36] Reintegration to Normal Living Index), measures of independence, validated questionnaire-based therapist-completed outcome measures (Special Interest Group in Amputee Medicine mobility grading (SIGAM), Amputee Mobility Predictor (questionnaire) (AMP Q), Mayo-Portland Adaptability Inventory 4 (superior to Functional Independence and Functional Assessment Measure [FIM-FAM] in this patient population[2]) and return to work data. It was clear that no one single outcome measure could encapsulate the progress or otherwise of all the domains of the patient experience or capture the variety of injuries and severity of presentation. Therefore, multiple outcome measures were reported, having undergone a standard assessment and validation approach applicable across the whole of the DMRP.

The main problem was the lack of resources available in terms of staff to code diagnoses, record outcomes and analyse the data. DMICP was not a sufficiently agile tool to analyse these data. In the

future, resources should be allocated for data collection and analysis as a means of capturing important early lessons to inform clinical planning

ROLE 4 REHABILITATION AT RCDM

Due to the improvement in battlefield first aid and acute medical care, a substantial number of service personnel survived injuries that would otherwise have been fatal, with consequently increasingly complex patterns of devastating injuries.[3] All UK service personnel who sustained major trauma on operations were aeromedically evacuated to QEHB, for definitive treatment once stabilised and the immediate threat to life had been abated. QEHB encompassed the RCDM, where military rehabilitation enhanced the NHS therapy services provision. Rehabilitation was delivered at QEHB until the patient was medically and surgically suitable for transfer for ongoing rehabilitation at Headley Court. Close liaison between the rehabilitation teams at RCDM and DMRC ensured joined-up care throughout the rehabilitation pathway.

Rehabilitation was identified as one of the top priorities for improvement when *MTCs* were established in the United Kingdom, with military coordination used as an example of good practice.[4] It is fair to say that civilian rehabilitation services lag behind the military capability and that this gap has increased following the innovations arising from these conflicts.

Early rehabilitation

Previous conflicts have identified the importance of following rehabilitation principles as early as possible, creating centres of excellence, limiting convalescent leave and introducing recreational and motivational activities.[5]

At RCDM, survivors of severe trauma were assessed on arrival at QEHB by the rehabilitation team in the critical care unit. In addition to standard therapeutic interventions to reduce cardio-respiratory and neuro-muscular complications, an 'early rehabilitation team' was introduced at QEHB in 2012. Led by NHS physiotherapists, the team delivered early physiotherapy-led mobilisation, which consisted of sitting on the edge of the bed, sitting out and walking (even if the patient was still ventilated). Evidence supports this use of early rehabilitation in critical care as soon as patients are physiologically stable,[6,7] with early interventions shown to reduce hospital length of stay,[8] reduce mortality[9–11] and improve longer-term functional outcomes.[12] These findings were replicated at QEHB with the introduction of the early rehabilitation team.[13]

The rehabilitation team supported the military pain ward rounds, issued compression garments and provided specialist equipment and bespoke splints. Exercise therapy was delivered in critical care by physiotherapists and the military ERI, a key additional member of the team. This enhanced exercise therapy included the use of the MOTOmed®, an over bed bike, provision of exercise bands, mobile weights stands holding adjustable Bowflex® Selectech® dumbbells or taking patients to the rehabilitation gym from the intensive care setting. Gym attendance was found to be particularly beneficial in the critical care setting for the long-stay, severely wounded patients in reducing the well-documented deleterious effects of prolonged bed-rest[14,15] and social isolation.

Early function

Intensive rehabilitation aimed at restoring function has been shown to demonstrate a positive effect on both pain and functional level.[16] However, patients often presented with a number of obstacles to early intervention such as language barriers, visual and auditory loss and mTBI. Communication, nutritional status, sleep pattern and pain control issues had to be addressed concurrently when commencing intensive rehabilitation. Therapists and patients used a number of innovative problem-solving strategies to achieve their goals, constantly balancing the benefits of independence with risk.

Injured Service personnel had high expectations of care and outcomes. They placed ever-increasing demands on themselves, their rehabilitation team and the healthcare system, with their outcome expectations outweighing any traditional civilian equivalent standard. Public opinion has also required facilities and services to adapt and cater for the outcomes demanded, constantly pushing the boundaries of clinical services.

The core therapy working practices that evolved at QEHB during the recent conflicts in Iraq and Afghanistan are summarised in Table 17.6. Although not all interventions were novel, the combination exceeds that found in other rehabilitation services.

Patients were taught and practised problem-solving in preparation for leaving the controlled hospital environment, for example teaching the patient and family members what to do if a fall from a wheelchair occurred. This allowed increased confidence and greater control and facilitated earlier excursions from hospital. It also protected carers and family from unsafe lifting techniques.

Upper limb prosthetics

Upper limb injury and amputation were commonly seen in association with lower limb amputation in casualties from IEDs on dismounted foot' patrols, in particular of the left arm, elevated and flexed at the elbow to support a weapon. The use of early prosthetic limb-fitting for upper limb amputees has been shown to improve final outcome.[17] The prosthetics team at Headley Court established that military patients who received their prosthetic upper limb later in their rehabilitation pathway were less likely to fully utilise their prosthesis; consequently, regular visits by a prosthetist from the Headley Court team were implemented. Patients' stumps were casted on the trauma ward as soon as wound healing allowed, with the aim of producing and fitting an upper-limb prosthesis within two weeks of amputation and prior to discharge from acute management at QEHB. It was felt that this policy improved prosthetic use; however, prospective research with an adequate sample size is needed to support these observations.

Pain management

Medical management of acute pain evolved considerably during the war-fighting period and resulted in the early use of anti-neuropathic pain medications, epidurals and nerve blocks.[18–21] The rehabilitation team at RCDM established close links with the military pain team, attending military pain rounds with the aim of achieving maximal

Table 17.6 Core therapy practices

Area	Issue	Solution/impact
Transfers	Type of mattress	Early adoption of optimal mattress firmness as Waterlow scores dictated improve early mobility and lead to a reduction in pressure-relieving mattress requirements
	Bed mobility	Appropriate provision of high–low hospital bed/cot sides/grab handles to facilitate independent bed mobility
	Dependent transfer required	Bed to plinth day 1 post-surgery if no contra-indications, such as wounds, skin grafting or pressure concerns, on wide Bobath plinths with appropriate slide sheet use. Improved motivation from leaving ward and attending gym.
		Encouragement of health and well-being, even if unable to independently transfer
		Development of use of forwards–backwards transfer method to allow early seating and encourage patient independence. Use of one-way glide sheets to remain in chair and early issue of 'banana' transfer boards.
		Nursing staff taught transfers to encourage out-of-hours use
	Hoisting amputee patients	Procurement, training and use of appropriate amputee slings with manual handling risk assessments. Stock kept to ensure no delay in waiting for amputee sling
	Complex soft-tissue injuries	Use of Vicair ® AllRounder for patients with significant blast injuries to the buttock/pelvis to allow early mobility while protecting weight-bearing skin and reducing friction during transfers. It also facilitated sitting balance for hemi-pelvectomy patients
		Liaison with burns and plastics team, including substantial use of topical negative pressure (TNP) dressings to reduce shearing forces, and increase early mobilisation, e.g. five days for skin graft, not always necessary
Gym	Attendance	Early daily attendance at gym with combined physiotherapy, occupational therapy and military ERI starting day 1.
		Plinth exercises when patient would normally be undertaking bed exercises on the ward
	Clothing	Normalisation of behaviour rehab by wearing PT kit or attending gym.
		Kept in stock with versatile Velcro seams
		Use of a rucksack over wheelchair to independently carry attachments, e.g. TNP (clothing provided by TroopAid charity)
	Tolerance	Split rehabilitation, i.e. exercise therapy session/CV fitness a.m. and therapy intervention or functional rehabilitation p.m. Adapted depending on exercise tolerance
		Focussed on strength and ROM to improve function
	Motivation/group therapy	Recreational and group therapy led by ERI, including competitive games and distraction, e.g. bi-lateral amputees playing Nintendo Wii whilst sitting on a BOSU® trainer/Swiss gym ball

(Continued)

Table 17.6 (Continued) Core therapy practices

Area	Issue	Solution/impact
Seating	Limited by external-fixators (ex-fix)	Regular liaison with surgeons to re-/position pelvic ex-fix bars to facilitate seating positions and transfers that may otherwise be restricted.
		Adaptations to chairs – tilt and space recline/removal of arm supports
		Two plinth gapped bridge to allow prone lying for amputees with pelvic ex-fix and stretch psoas/avoid hip flexor contractures (or Thomas test stretch).
		Side lying at side of plinth to allow ex-fix to hang over edge
	Standard seating unsuitable	Facilitated bespoke specialist seating procurement and pressure mapping as early as possible, e.g. for hemi-pelvectomy patients
Function	Prone nursing	Prone wheeled trolley made by military medical engineers (similar to spinal injuries design) to allow independent mobility for patients who required prone nursing due to significant buttock wounds
	Wheelchair independence	Early assessment and provision of wheelchair (designated stock), including short-term provision of electric wheelchair to facilitate early independence, even if the patient will progress to self-propelled chair quickly
		Unconventional transfer methods taught, e.g. wheelchair to shower chair, in/out bath, on/off floor into a wheelchair balancing independence vs. risk
	Amputee mobility	Plinth under parallel bars to practise sitting for bilateral amputees. Bridging work using wedge/BOSU® trainer to balance residual limb/s
		Early use of floor to plinth/chair/bed transfer and step/blocks transfers
		Negotiation of weight-bearing status with surgeons, balancing multiple injuries and function, e.g. early kneeling on through-knee amputations or upper limb stump lever use to facilitate independence with transfers
		Tilt table with Femurett/pneumatic post-amputation mobility aid weight bearing, progressed to parallel bars to allow early standing
		Innovative ways to enable stairs use (patients often declined stair lift in house) such as seated stairs manoeuvres balancing risk vs. Independence
	Outdoor mobility	Exposure to outdoor/multi-terrain obstacles in preparation for discharge, incorporating trips away from the hospital to allow integration into society

analgesia during rehabilitation periods, ensuring that patients were able to participate in early therapy and thus preventing secondary complications, such as loss of range of motion.[6]

Phantom limb pain (PLP) and *residual limb pain* were shown to occur in 70% and 75%, respectively, of military amputees at QEHB.[22] PLP is multifactorial and can be difficult to treat,[23,24] with fewer than 50% of patients describing a lasting benefit from conventional medical management.[25] There is also limited success reported in the literature to date supporting rehabilitation interventions for PLP. Consequently, with no single treatment proven to be clinically effective, RCDM rehabilitation focussed on returning physical function, with therapeutic modalities attempting to alleviate PLP often based on patient choice or therapist preference. Treatments included *transcutaneous electrical nerve stimulation* (TENS), mirror therapy, exercise therapy, graded motor imagery (GMI), compression socks, massage, desensitisation, distraction and acupuncture.

A military pain management hierarchy was developed using the available evidence and detailing potential techniques to aid in the management of PLP.[26] Experiential evidence built upon this work and enabled the early rehabilitation team to identify which techniques might be beneficial to patients. It is accepted that these observations are based on individual case studies. Selecting the appropriate therapeutic modality for PLP centred on the patient's ability to engage in active therapy. Figure 17.12 illustrates what factors were considered in the clinical reasoning process at RCDM. The aims were to provide an appropriate active treatment regimen and to give the patient tools and coping strategies to self-manage. If a patient was initially unable or unwilling to actively engage, then more passive interventions were employed.

Long-term pain outcomes were encouraging. Most battlefield trauma amputees at the end of their Headley Court rehabilitation either had no pain or pain that was controlled by analgesia or other forms of self-management (Figure 17.13).

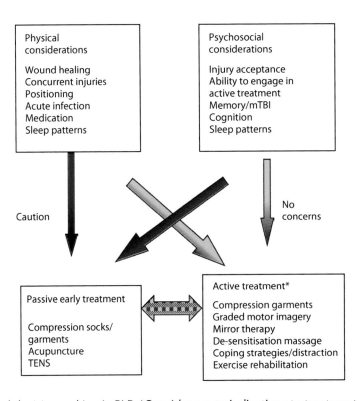

Figure 17.12 Clinical decision making in PLP. *Consider contraindications to treatment, for example acupuncture with infection.

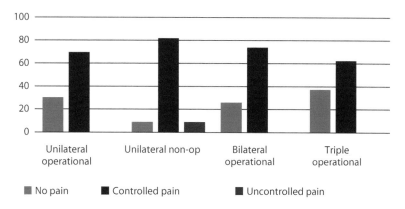

Figure 17.13 Pain at the end of the Headley Court Rehabilitation programme.

Most analgesia was rapidly discontinued in this patient group. Those who had their amputations for non-operational reasons, usually for chronic pain such as chronic regional pain syndrome, were the only ones with cases of uncontrolled pain.

Passive treatment modalities

At RCDM, the early use of amputee stump compression socks (JUZO® or Ottobock) or compression garments aided stump re-modelling and was the first stage in non-pharmacological management of pain. Due to the level and irregularity of some amputations, 'off-the-shelf' compression garments did not always fit and RCDM trialled compression shorts (suitable for use with hemipelvectomies). 'Medipro® Relax Night Care socks', made from a metallurgically knitted textile, were also used for those who complained of pain mainly at night,[27] with some anecdotal success. A systematic review found no general consensus on the use of stump compression garments[28]; however, management at RCDM was to apply compression.

Western acupuncture, in its infancy in the management of PLP,[29] was also used, with some positive results. This intervention tended to be an early option when dressings were still 'bulky', when there was no available contralateral limb to use for mirror therapy or when the patient could not participate in active intervention. Challenges remain regarding the availability of acupoints, the risk of infection and the optimum use and timing of the intervention. Of note, the 'battlefield acupuncture' technique[30] was trialled by one therapist at

RCDM with positive anecdotal evidence reported. It involved early use of up to five specific auricular points, therefore being used away from the zone of injury. Further work to examine the use of acupuncture, battlefield acupuncture and potentially electro-acupuncture in the complex trauma patient is required to fully evaluate this modality.

TENS was used in an attempt to modulate PLP. High frequency (90–130 Hz), pulse width (20–50 µs) TENS spinal pad placement to target sensory distribution, was found to be most effective. High-frequency peripheral nerve local stump application was also used, and contralateral limb placement, when available, was tried using low frequency (2–5 Hz) mirroring the pain distribution. The efficacy was mixed, with anecdotal evidence of some initial relief of acute pain. RCDM kept a stock of charity-purchased TENS units that could be issued immediately to patients. Long-term self-directed use of TENS appeared limited, suggesting accommodation to the treatment over time. There is a lack of robust evidence and there are no randomised controlled trials supporting the efficacy of TENS for treating PLP.[31]

Active treatment modalities

The vast majority of amputee patients were highly motivated and able to take ownership of their own rehabilitation pathway. This allowed the therapist to select an appropriate active treatment, taking all physical limitations into account. One such modality, GMI, uses a specific motor imagery programme working through an intensive process of limb laterality recognition exercises, followed by imagined movements and, finally, mirror therapy. Used within chronic pain management and, more recently, for PLP,[32,33] it is proposed that this graded process provides neural retraining in a manner that one intervention or a single concept does not. However, the current studies are underpowered for PLP and combine results with other pain pathologies, such as chronic regional pain syndrome, with the result that no firm conclusions can be drawn regarding its effectiveness.

Small studies have also provided evidence supporting significant reductions in PLP with mirror therapy alone,[34,35] especially in the upper limb.[36] Mirror therapy aims to alleviate pain by correcting cortical reorganisation, a suggested potential mechanism of PLP.[37] A pertinent study including 22 US military single lower limb amputees with PLP reported that phantom pain decreased in 100% of participants assigned to the mirror therapy group.[34] However, four participants were unaccounted for and potential biases were not fully addressed. At RCDM, although mirror therapy was provided for specific patients – balanced against challenges during the acute phase of rehabilitation, such as the potential for a grief reaction and having a contralateral limb without injury to use – we were unable to reproduce this success rate. Mirror boxes were procured through the charity TroopAid and were readily available for single patient issue. Virtual reality options for bilateral amputees were explored by anaesthetic colleagues at QEHB and research is ongoing in this area.

Interestingly, several patients reported that mirror therapy provided relief or restored movement for previously 'fixed' limbs, often 'stuck' in the position immediately after injury. However, there is a lack of research supporting this proprioceptive memory theory.[38] A further limitation of mirror therapy research for PLP is that training involves concurrent exercise. It may be that exercise itself provided the positive effects on PLP. Similarly, concurrent desensitisation massage taught as standard at RCDM, with the rationale of helping acceptance of the residual limb as well as normalising sensation and pain responses, may have affected responses to treatment. There is conflicting evidence regarding the efficacy of exercise or desensitisation as a treatment for PLP.[39–41]

Patients often reported that symptoms were worse at night, with minimal PLP during rehabilitation sessions, highlighting that any intervention may act as a short-term 'distraction therapy'. In reality, pain management is likely to involve a combination of interventions all affecting the complex bio-psychosocial model of pain. For example, peer support and input from the mental health team (MHT), including various coping strategies or post-traumatic stress disorder responses, may all have influenced pain outcomes.

Multi-disciplinary working

The documented benefits of a well-trained MDT[42] are particularly necessary when working with critical care[43] and complex trauma patients.[44] Although not a new concept, the RCDM and QEHB MDT evolved to find new and improved ways of working together.

The early intervention of rehabilitation specialists in the care of amputee patients and the need to educate members of the surgical team regarding prosthetic considerations has been recognised[45]: as a result, subject-matter experts fed back on a weekly basis. This included a Headley Court consultant attending the trauma ward rounds and, latterly, a weekly tele-conference led by the *Rehabilitation Co-ordination Officer* (RCO) between RCDM and Headley Court medical and rehabilitation teams. A move towards having only a small team of rehabilitation consultants directly involved in managing the complex trauma and neurological rehabilitation cohort of patients also made a positive difference to patient continuity and MDT relationships.

A valuable member of the rehabilitation team at RCDM was the ERI, who facilitated exercise-based rehabilitation. The advantages of undertaking group therapy include the opportunity to provide group peer support, as well as the accepted benefits of exercise. The ERI conducted regular group and recreational therapy to complement and augment the more formal therapy time. This encouraged patients to develop routine and independence and allowed graded exposure in order to build exercise tolerance in preparation for inpatient rehabilitation at DMRC.

Other rehabilitation centres found that running support groups and organised training could be successful in mitigating the chronic stressors experienced by staff exposed to complex trauma.[43] Stress management sessions were instigated by the RCDM therapy team to recognise and formalise peer support.

Functional outcome measures

In order to fully assess the influence of rehabilitation in the early stages, it was important to be able to effectively measure change. A lack of early outcome measures has been highlighted in a review of MTCs[4] and also by the military rehabilitation centre.[45] The *British Association of Chartered Physiotherapists in Amputee Rehabilitation* has collated recent work to effectively measure outcomes post amputation.[46] A limitation of the research is that most validated outcome measures focus on ambulation, and therefore, research studying both civilian and military amputee populations has also concentrated on this outcome.[47]

In the RCDM military amputee population, ambulation cannot be measured in the acute rehabilitation phase as lower limb prosthetic management occurs later at DMRC. Furthermore, the level of injury for some battle casualties means that ambulation may never be an appropriate outcome measure and early rehabilitation focuses instead on regaining a functional level for basic tasks, for example bed mobility, transfers from bed to wheelchair, eating, drinking and washing. The rehabilitation team at RCDM highlighted this gap in both current literature and clinical practice regarding acute rehabilitation of the amputee. It has also been observed that, despite the number and variety of available outcome measures, most were insensitive and inappropriate for use with this patient population.[41,46] Later in the course of rehabilitation, standard civilian outcome measures were inappropriate because of the 'ceiling effect', with service personnel reaching levels of function that could not be recorded successfully using civilian scales.

It was therefore decided to produce a local tool at RCDM to allow the measurement of acute outcomes. Named the *Pre-Prosthetic Functional Outcome Measure* (PPFOM), it was developed and piloted. The PPFOM was audited with the *Clinical Outcome Variability Scale* (COVS), which has been validated to be used with amputees in the acute setting.[47] The results showed that, overall, the PPFOM demonstrated a 50% increase in functional outcome from admission to discharge within this patient group when compared with the COVS ($n = 21$). The PPFOM is undergoing validation; however, the early signs are that PPFOM helps guide interventions for specific areas in a patient's function and outcomes for discharge.

REHABILITATION CO-ORDINATION

Trauma network models have been found to increase effectiveness and improve outcomes.[48] The RCO was a position established in 2008 to contend with the increasing number of casualties from the Afghanistan and Iraq conflicts. The RCO introduced a structured approach to managing complex rehabilitation, ensuring holistic delivery of care and improved formal communication regarding the patient's current rehabilitation and future care requirements. The RCO led the planning and co-ordination of the early rehabilitation pathway for operational casualties, with the role being used as an example of best practice and recommended as a standard position in setting up UK MTCs. Additionally, the RCO led the implementation of a standardised protocol increasing the number of direct transfers to DMRC, instigated to ensure a safe and effective discharge and avoid delays in the rehabilitation process. The organisation and co-ordination of rehabilitation by a senior, experienced leader ensured the delivery of an effective rehabilitation service with a strong focus on outcomes.

Overview

The influx of military casualties during the recent conflicts in Afghanistan and Iraq has led to substantial advances in rehabilitation practises at RCDM/QEHB. Dealing with complex injuries presentations that are not routinely seen in civilian practice has required the development of innovative therapies, combinations of treatments and management strategies. With an emphasis on optimal outcome rather than merely survival, early rehabilitation contributed to the high levels of outcome achieved by our patient population. It is important to note that no one intervention is responsible for these results and that they derive from a combination of factors, not only from rehabilitation but also from the entire process, including the exceptional resilience and motivation of the patient group. The rehabilitation team at RCDM did, however, change attitudes towards early rehabilitation as part of the MDT by enhancing provision, driving improvement, enabling function and independence and, therefore, making a difference to the patient.

SPECIALIST REHABILITATION ISSUES

Amputee rehabilitation

Rehabilitation of the patient who has sustained an amputation as a result of a blast or ballistic injury requires special consideration. The majority of cases of amputation in the developed world are in older populations, over the age of 50, and due to diabetic or vascular causes. The population affected by battlefield trauma is younger and has higher levels of physical function and expectation of recovery. Most of the experience of this type of patient has been in the developing world, where warfare and mine strikes have contributed to a high level of traumatic amputation. Because access to medical care, patient expectations and availability of equipment are different from our military population, there are very few transferable lessons. The increase in disabled sport, particularly in response to the Paralympic Movement, has demonstrated the high level of functional outcome attainable from these patients and has set the bar higher for clinical success.

The improvements in the technical provision of prosthetic components have revolutionised the prognosis for patients with amputations. In particular, socket–suspension system developments have significantly improved comfort and practical function.

Principles of prosthetic fitting

There are seven elements to a prosthetic prescription depending on the level of amputation.[49]

STRUCTURE

In developed societies, the usual structure is the endoskeletal form of prosthesis, which consists of a metal or composite material (for example carbon fibre) strut attached to the end fittings, which may

be covered by a cosmesis. The structure holds the socket in the correct linear and angular orientation.

SOCKET

The socket transmits the forces between the residual limb and the prosthesis, vertically for weight-bearing in the stance phase, with some suspension in the swing phase and horizontally and rotational about the long axis. The socket shape is usually a modification of the residual limb shape as it has to take into account the contained skeleton, the consistency of the soft tissues, the limb volume and pressure sensitive areas.

SUSPENSION

This may come from the socket shape and from material or additional belts. More commonly in the military patient population, the use of silicon suspensory sleeves with ratchet or vacuum suspension systems represented the gold standard. These systems give the patient more freedom of movement and greater comfort, are well tolerated and are robust. Their selection is usually based on personal preference and tolerance.[50] They allow good suspension, particularly for high-performance amputees in whom residual limb shape or scarring is less than optimal. They may increase sweating, but this frequently adapts and can be corrected by better fitting or treated with aluminium-based deodorants or botulinum injection.

ANKLE AND FOOT

These are usually considered as one unit and have to transfer forces between the prosthesis and the ground as well as modifying this transfer in the gait cycle. This may be provided by a mechanical uni-axial joint providing movement in one plane only or a flexible bush allowing multi-axial movement, an assembly of spring components producing multi-axial movements or compression wedges at the heel. High-performance limbs for running may use a spring system like the carbon fibre Flex-run® or Cheetah® systems.

MICROPROCESSOR-CONTROLLED KNEE JOINTS

These joints may be uni-axial or polycentric, and although there are many available knees, including the simplest locked systems only released for sitting, our patient population in this situation usually require high-performance prosthetics. The most significant innovations of recent years for the trans-femoral amputee have been the introduction of microprocessor controlled knees such as the C Leg®, the Genium® or the X3®. These systems have revolutionised knee control and, hence, clinical outcomes, particularly where stability is critical, for example in the bilateral trans-femoral amputee.

These systems use a knee-angle sensor to measure the angular position and angular velocity of the flexing joint. There are also moment sensors, using multiple strain gauges, to determine exactly where the force is being applied to the knee from the foot and the magnitude of that force. Measurements are taken 50–100 times a second. A microprocessor receives signals from each sensor and determines the type of motion and phase of gait of the amputee. The microprocessor directs a hydraulic cylinder to control the knee motion accordingly.

These systems can provide a close approximation to an amputee's natural gait and increase their walking speeds. Variations in walking speed are detectable by the sensors and communicated to the microprocessor, which can alter the swing through stance phases of the prosthesis. The knee system allows the amputee to walk downstairs with a step-over-step approach, rather than the one-step-at-a-time approach used with mechanical knees, and can deliver additional stability in other contexts, including recovery from stumbles.

The microprocessors, however, are expensive (a Genium® knee system at the time cost in the region of £27,000), are limited by battery time, are susceptible to water damage and require a lot of patient training. Nevertheless, they can dramatically help the bilateral trans-femoral amputee, significantly increasing their physical activity during daily life and offering an improved quality of life.[51]

There was considerable resistance from NHS providers to the introduction of microprocessor knee (MPK) systems initially as it was felt that they were expensive, unsustainable in the NHS and produced very few gains in clinical outcomes. Fortunately, the resistance to this progress was overcome, and the benefits of these systems have been demonstrated. In 2017, the NHS in England agreed to commission these systems for selected patients, but still not the most up-to-date systems such as the Genium®. Defence has found the Genium® particularly beneficial in improving function, including gait, standing posture and back pain secondary to postural issues.

HIP JOINT

In the event of hip disarticulation or trans-pelvic amputation, a hip joint is required. Fortunately, this is a relatively rare phenomenon as the functional limitation on such patients may be severe. The hip joint will need to be mounted onto the anterior inferior surface of the socket, in order to allow the patient to sit. It may be uni-axial or polycentric or incorporate one of the microprocessor joints described for use in the knee. Given the severity of the injury, initial mobilisation is relatively straightforward as the shallow nature of the hip disarticulation socket means that the patient, for all practical purposes, 'sits' on the socket when walking.

MISCELLANEOUS UNITS

Axial units will allow rotation about the long axis of the prosthesis against resistance, provide greater freedom of action and reduce the torque applied between the socket and residual limb. This is of particular use in highly functional patients, for example in those who wish to play golf where a rotational motion would aid the swing.

The successful provision of a prosthetic limb for an amputee relies on close interdisciplinary working with all members of the team. The prosthetists, prosthetic technicians and physiotherapists must work closely to provide equipment that fits and that the patient knows how to use. The particular prosthetic skill is in the provision of a comfortable, well-aligned socket.

Residual limb volume changes rapidly in the earliest stages of rehabilitation, and volume may continue to decrease for up to two years after amputation. Early use of compression socks such as Juzo® will aid this and reduce healing time. The rapid loss of volume will lead to a need to use additional socks to ensure a comfortable fit with the prosthesis. When the volume has changed significantly, a socket change should be carried out as rapidly as possible so that time is not lost from rehabilitation and the patient does not become frustrated or disillusioned. This can be expensive and time-consuming, as sockets may need to be changed every six weeks.

POWERED JOINTS

In the latter stages of the war fighting, powered joint systems were trialled. These differ from the MPKs in that the joint comes with a battery-powered motor, which provides a propulsive force as opposed to a joint stabilisation system. These systems are bulky and heavy and can be noisy and expensive but for the right case provide the propulsion in gait that considerably aids walking. The most successful system that the DMS used was the BiOM Advantage® ankle, which was useful in complex multiple lower limb amputations, particularly in very high amputations, such as a unilateral hind-quarter amputation.

Upper limbs

There were fewer amputees requiring upper limb prosthetics. Those who did often went for the most functional and least intrusive solutions for their needs, including not wearing any prosthesis; if the prosthesis was cumbersome and did not provide any additional functional benefit, then it was entirely reasonable to support this approach. If clinically appropriate, an attempt was made to offer an upper limb prosthesis to the patient within two weeks of injury, as it is known that delays in first using a prosthesis can lead to a rejection of long-term prosthetic use.

Upper limb options included purely cosmetic solutions, body-powered hook and myoelectric systems. The latter included multi-grip upper limb prosthetics such as the *Touch Bionic iLimb®*. This device generates a hand function more in keeping with normal hand movement but had a weight penalty and limited battery life, and its function does not approach that of a normal hand. Although some military patients used them, they were less popular than might be imagined because of functional limitations. The NHS will currently not commission them.

NEUROLOGICAL REHABILITATION

Blast and ballistic injury can affect any aspect of the peripheral and central nervous systems. The most devastating are the consequences of TBI. The neurological rehabilitation team at Headley Court managed the majority of the TBI cases arising from operations. They provided the comprehensive assessment, rehabilitation and management of neurologically injured cases. The same principles apply to treatment whether there has been a closed or open injury to the brain. Interestingly, apart from a relatively short period, the incidence of TBI did not increase dramatically during *Operations Telic* and *Herrick*. This may be a reflection of better head protection or possibly a high mortality rate. Figure 17.14 shows that through most of the conflict, the majority of cases managed in the unit were from non-battle injuries, usually due to road traffic collision or assault. The increased rate of battle injury TBI appears to have occurred as a result of an increase in trauma due to gunshot wounds from snipers.

The aim of the neurological rehabilitation team is to provide an intensive programme of rehabilitation, including vocational assessment, which is delivered by a specialised and experienced MDT. The structured programme of therapy addressed the physical, cognitive, communication, psychosocial, vocational and daily life issues. Involving families and carers in the patient's recovery has been essential.

The principles of management are identical to other areas of rehabilitation, but the length of treatment required was longer and the pace of treatment slower. A key worker was assigned to each patient to co-ordinate their treatment and to

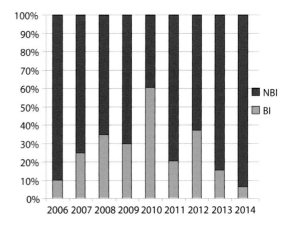

Figure 17.14 Proportion of TBI cases as a result of battle injury (BI) and non-battle injury (NBI).

liaise with the patient and their family regarding any areas of concern.

Cognitive deficits frequently overshadow physical deficits as the cause of difficulties in social adaptation, independent living, family life and vocational activity. Without appropriate intervention, cognitive deficits can lead to frustration, anxiety, depression and social withdrawal. Cognitive rehabilitation is provided by specialist occupational therapists. It focuses on regaining those cognitive skills which are lost or altered as a result of neurological trauma or illness. The process includes gaining skills through direct retraining, learning to use compensatory strategies and education about cognitive skills.

Mild traumatic brain injury

An increased awareness of mTBI developed over the course of the conflicts. This had fallen out of the US observation of an increased incidence of neuro-cognitive symptoms, after exposure to blast in the absence of evidence of other ballistic trauma. The symptoms were compatible with a concussive effect, and a causative relationship was inferred. This has generated a significant degree of medical controversy,[52,53] not the least because of confusion over terminology. A severe brain injury may leave a patient with major cognitive and other impairments, but the outcome is highly unpredictable. It is possible for a severe acute injury to leave a patient with only mild functional impairment; conversely, a minor injury can produce socially devastating consequences.

CLINICAL LESSONS LEARNT IN REHABILITATION FROM RECENT CONFLICTS

Attempted limb salvage

There are frequent debates following ballistic trauma concerning whether a limb can be salvaged. It has been accepted practice to attempt to preserve an injured limb, if possible, so as to allow further surgical interventions and rehabilitation, with the aim of maximising function and minimising pain over a period of time before a judgement is made by the patient some months later. Painful

limbs of limited function can be removed at a later date, if necessary. Most patients are glad to have the opportunity to make an informed decision for themselves at a later date. Prior to these conflicts, the literature is inconclusive about whether limb salvage or amputation is more effective in terms of hospital stay, pain and functional outcome.[54]

However, recent data from Headley Court has shown that patients with an initial unilateral amputation demonstrated a significant functional advantage over limb salvage patients. Patients electing for amputation after failed limb salvage achieved superior functional gains in mobility compared to prolonged limb-salvage patients and experienced no functional disadvantage compared to those patients who received an immediate amputation. The mental health outcomes are comparable to the general population. It therefore seems reasonable to continue with the practice of limb salvage in the knowledge that – in this population – a later amputation will not leave them disadvantaged.[55] This presupposes that the patients are fit; motivated; exposed to high-quality, intense rehabilitation; and have access to good, well-fitting prosthetics. Another innovation was the development of the energy return lower limb orthotic – developed by Blatchfords from an idea used in the US military. This is a carbon fibre structure known as the Momentum® Brace (Figure 17.15).

This has been shown to improve quality of life, pain and function. It increases walking speed by 22% and stride length by 12%. Power generation increases at the hip, knee and ankle. This orthotic is indicated in the complex hind-foot injuries seen in incomplete detonation of pressure plate IEDs or blasts coming up through a vehicle floor.

Ideal stump

The technology now available for fitting limbs in this patient population allows a wide degree of flexibility in response to stump length, quality and scarring. Healed split skin grafts will usually tolerate the silicon sleeves and suspension systems well. In the trans-tibial amputation, an optimal range is 12–16 cm when measured from the medial joint line, and in trans-femoral, 14–21 cm measured from the crotch or 23–30 cm measured from the tip of the greater trochanter. Ideally, the optimal

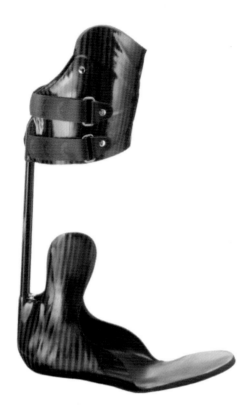

Figure 17.15 Momentum brace.

stump length should be proportional to the overall stature of the patient. An 'ideal' length of 16 cm in someone with short legs may not leave enough ground clearance to fit in the total length of the modular components in the prosthesis. This may be particularly critical in the high-performance amputee, where the prosthetic componentry may need to be longer. In a trans-tibial amputee, an approximate guide is for 8 cm of stump length per metre height. Anything shorter than 7 cm in a trans-tibial amputee is very difficult to fit. In the trans-femoral patient, a gap of 15 cm above the medial tibial plateau is described as ideal for fitting a knee joint system in place whilst retaining a sufficient lever arm. Often of greater difficulty is the management of a bulbous residual limb. A residual limb with a distal circumference greater than that measured at the level of the patella tendon can be difficult to fit. In the case of complex trauma, the choice of the residual limb length may not be open to the clinician and prosthetists have to deal with what they are given. It is important in planning

any amputation to consider the relative leg length of the patient, their height and co-existing injuries.

Post-operative oedema can be reduced with stump shrinkers and early mobilisation with PAM-aids (pneumatic aid to mobilisation). However, excess muscle bulk is the main source of the problem. This more commonly occurs in a posterior flap rather than a skew flap, a technique that produces a more conical shape and that allows better prosthetic fitting. However, these are decisions for the cold light of day rather than the battlefield and over-long or badly scarred stumps can be revised at a later date.

Through-knee disarticulation can be a very effective amputation

There was considerable bias against the use of knee disarticulation as a surgical option in trauma. This was based on poor experience of the procedure in civilian practice and reflects real concerns, albeit ones that are not always applicable to military practice.[56] The Gritti-Stokes procedure, involving reattachment of the patella to the articular surface of the femoral condyles, has fallen out of fashion and a simple disarticulation has many benefits. The main advantage of the through-knee amputation is an end weight-bearing stump. Once the prosthesis has been fitted, the patient can make rapid progress to high-level weight-bearing activity and a level of function, including running, in excess of that expected from a trans-femoral amputation. The disadvantages are mainly cosmetic, as the knee system will sit at a level below that of the contralateral knee. On sitting, the knee joint on the prosthetic limb will protrude further forward than the non-affected side. Lowering the centre of rotation of the joint may produce a minor biomechanical disadvantage, but this is more than compensated by the stability and control gained from the long lever arm, deep socket and polycentric knee joint combined with hydraulic swing phase controls.

Silicon suspension systems allow prosthetic fitting of most stumps

The new systems of suspension give improved comfort and function and are sufficiently robust for servicemen to use on operational deployments. A small number of patients have returned to operational roles, mainly in support roles but also in forward infantry roles. The limbs are tolerated well and survive the extreme environments to which they are exposed.

Concomitant injuries may be the factor limiting recovery rather than the amputation

The functional performance of the lower limb prostheses in many military amputees is so good and the socket–stump interface so effective in many that the main limitation to mobilisation is frequently the concomitant injury. Fractures have a rate of healing considerably slower than prosthetic fitting, and multiple fractures in a contralateral limb, particularly in the foot, can have a considerable slowing effect on the rehabilitation process. This frequently leads non-amputees with protracted rehabilitation due to delayed fracture union to request an early amputation. This requires careful counselling informed by the considerations discussed earlier.

Aggressive treatment of neuropathic and phantom pain is critical: Non-pharmacological methods of pain control are important

Clinical experience at RCDM and Headley Court would indicate the importance of early, aggressive treatment with analgesics to prevent the development of neuropathic pain. This includes the use of opiates and drugs such as gabapentin, amitriptylline and pregabalin as well as specialist techniques such as nerve blocks. There should be no hesitation in using maximum doses of all these medications to obtain complete control of pain. Audit of military practice shows that, once in the rehabilitation setting, the requirement for analgesia rapidly diminishes and very few patients require long-standing medication for phantom pain control. Education, reassurance, peer support and physical distraction all play a part in this. Wearing the socket and physical activity often dramatically improve the pain. Other modalities such as mirror therapy and acupuncture can be very effective in certain cases, although carry over can be limited (Figures 17.16 and 17.17).

Early assessment of peripheral nerve injury with surgical repair will reduce pain and limit disability

It is important to avoid a nihilistic approach to peripheral nerve injury. Early expert assessment is important following primary repair and follow-up is vital. Persisting pain following brachial plexus or peripheral nerve injury warrants consideration of surgical exploration and repair or grafting if needed. Monitoring the progress of nerve re-growth allows interventions to be carried out rapidly if the graft or repair is failing. There may be a later requirement for tendon transfer to return function, which further mandates expert follow-up.[57]

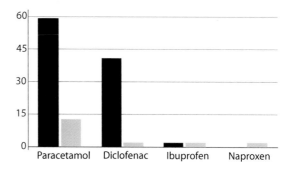

Figure 17.16 Percentage of amputees taking simple analgesics when they initially presented to Headley Court and the last entry in their notes (black bars initial reading; grey bars, final). (From Aldington DJ et al., *Philos Trans R Soc B Biol Sci* 2011;366(1562):268–275.)

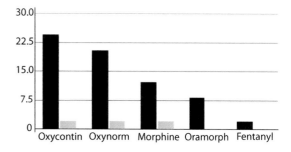

Figure 17.17 Percentage of amputees taking strong opioids when they initially presented at Headley Court and the last entry in their notes (black bars initial reading; grey bars, final). (From Aldington DJ et al., *Philos Trans R Soc B Biol Sci* 2011;366(1562):268–275.)

The psychological component to rehabilitation has an influence on outcome

It is evident that the psychological status of the patient has a major influence on physical outcome. Self-efficacy is associated with good outcomes in spinal rehabilitation and probably these very complex injuries also. Depression, persistent adjustment reactions and post-traumatic stress disorder are all detrimental to recovery. What is remarkable is the low level of psychological morbidity detectable in these patients.[58] Peer support is an important factor in this, as is the patient having a clear sense of the long-term pathway for recovery. Many patients have mild to moderate psychological morbidity in the early stages of their rehabilitation, but the long-term outcomes are unknown.

Concomitant TBI is a major prognostic determinant of polytrauma outcome

In assessing outcomes from polytrauma and amputation, there is a tendency to dwell on the surgical and physiological factors. Additional injury, particularly brain injury, may not be apparent at review but can have a major effect on physical outcome, including donning and doffing the prosthesis, ability to understand rehabilitation instruction, balance and return to work. Likewise, psychological distress is a major determinant of outcome in TBI.

Urogenital injury

Urogenital injury had a very significant impact on patients, their families and the clinical staff attempting to mitigate the consequences of the injury. Although there were a relatively small number of patients with catastrophic urogenital injuries, there were many more with partial injuries or fertility problems as a result of battle trauma: there also appeared to be a concussive effect in some patients with intact genitalia. Identification and description of the injuries at both the rehabilitation and acute management phase allowed personal protective equipment to be designed to prevent further injuries – particularly for future high-risk operators – such as search teams.

The injuries included partial or complete testicular loss, with consequent effects on fertility and also testosterone deficiency. Patients were initially under-treated with transcutaneous testosterone. This highlighted the importance of checking serum testosterone to achieve therapeutic levels. Under-treated patients tended to be apathetic, slow to reverse their catabolic state during rehabilitation and prone to delayed healing and infection.

Penile loss had implications for micturition, continence and sexual function – the latter a very important component of the psychological state of the soldier. Considerable skill was required to offer counselling and provide a urological solution as well as a plastic surgical reconstruction of the penis for cosmetic and functional reasons. The skills to reconstruct penises usually lay with those surgeons involved in transgender surgery. This was complicated by the lack of normal tissue to provide flaps for reconstruction.

Significant gains were made in the fertility treatment of these cases where there was even a small residual part of testicular tissue available. Semen was extracted from the testes as early as possible – whilst on ICU at QEHB – with several successful pregnancies arising from this intervention.

DEPLOYED REHABILITATION

The DMRT – now known as the *Force Medical Rehabilitation Team* (FMRT) – provided an MDT approach to rehabilitation for all injuries on operations. The DMRT was part of the Medical Regiment but often also had physiotherapy assets embedded with it, to support a co-located Role 2 or 3 facility.

The principal aim of the DMRT was to provide rehabilitation support to Role 1 assets through services closely attached to a medical centre. It also provided peripatetic services to remotely located medical treatment facilities, using the *Role One Rehabilitation Team* (RORT), now the *Forward Rehabilitation Team*. DMRTs were deployed on *Operations Telic and Herrick* in order to provide integral multi-disciplinary rehabilitation support at Role 1.

The DMRT, through early assessment and treatment of MSK injuries, sustained the deployed force's fitness for operations. It informed local commanders of the activities that were at risk of compromising their force's fitness to fight and hence protected the force from further degradation by MSK injury.

Organisation

The DMRT comprised a consultant in rheumatology/sport and exercise/rehabilitation medicine (OF4/OF5), physiotherapists (OF2–3) and exercise rehabilitation instructors (OR 6–8 sergeant to warrant Officer Class 2 or other service equivalent). These personnel were within the general support and forward support squadrons of the armoured medical regiment and the close support squadron of the medical regiment. This was in addition to the physiotherapist and ERI held on strength within each of the forward support squadrons of the Med Regt.

During deployments, the team provided consultant level advice on rehabilitation and injury prevention to the chain of command, rehabilitation services for the *Primary Care Medical Centre,* an in-theatre rehabilitation service for those patients with more complex needs and RORT (peripatetic Role 1 rehabilitation teams visiting forward locations). The DMRT also ensured that the patient care pathway was followed in accordance with the DMRP and assisted in the management of rehabilitation of patients returned from theatre.

The consultant deployed only when the operational tempo and other commitments allowed, usually for a 6- to 12-week tour towards the beginning of a roulement. This was a challenge when the same consultants were required to support Role 4 activities at home, where the more complex clinical cases lay. The principal benefits of having the consultant in the deployed role were to ensure that the DMRP was being adhered to, in particular ensuring that those destined to be aeromedically evacuated for discharge at the airhead were assessed within five working days at the RRUs; liaison with the medical chain of command and local commanders over the best deployment of rehabilitation assets in theatre and with the deployed hospital team (regarding complex rehabilitation patients, particularly those of local forces or civilians not being aeromedically

evacuated); providing clinical guidance and ultrasound diagnostic services for more complex MSK patients and offering guidance on local and NGO resources required for the rehabilitation of local troops and civilians. The DMRT was also capable of providing support to the three layers of primary healthcare (PHC) provision across the deployed Brigade as shown in Table 17.7.

The DMRT and RORT operated closely with the other PHC deliverers. They provided advice and support to the senior medical officer (SMO), local commanders, commander medical and the Role 2–3 unit when co-located. Advice was also provided to the *medical liaison officer* for battle groups within their area of responsibility. There was a close working relationship with partner nations that often did not have the rehabilitation resources of the UK Forces. Even US Forces often had relatively limited rehabilitation resources in theatre.

The DMRT aided commanders in deploying a fit, responsive force where the impact of common MSK injuries on the force's ability to operate was minimised. Through the provision of a peripatetic service forward, the RORT operated by supporting PHC clinicians in both remote and basic medical teams. The service was highly regarded by force commanders, not least because it reinforced the moral component of fighting power by demonstrating that the medical services were invested in the MSK health of the force. The DMRT and its RORTs were under the command of the CO of the deployed medical regiment. The DMRT remained under the command and control of the forward support medical squadron, but its component RORTs were under the command of the close support squadron when deploying forward. The brigade medical liaison officer and the SMO had sight of injury numbers and trends in forward locations through liaison with PHC clinicians in remote locations and basic medical teams throughout the brigade AOR. This allowed the DMRT and RORT to identify the priority locations to visit. The DMRT and RORTs collected data on injury trends, which informed decisions regarding the health needs of the organisation and helped direct future force development. The use of DMICP in the deployed environment was effective in places like Camp Bastion, but in forward locations, contemporaneous medical records were made as paper

Table 17.7 Rehabilitation support to primary healthcare

Ser	R1 healthcare layer	PHC/pre-hospital emergency care (PHEC) provision	Rehab support
(a)	(b)	(c)	(d)
1	Remote Medical Teams	Small teams of remotely located clinicians providing PHEC and PHC, e.g. combat medical technician in the patrol base/forward operating base	Combat medical technicians (CMTs) at these locations were taught to assess and treat acute and some chronic MSK injuries in line with clinical guidelines for operations. The RORT deployed forward to provide a service to assess, treat, advise PHC on the management of their cases and refer patients to DMRT for further assessment, diagnostic investigation (ultrasound) and residential management. The Theatre Intensive Rehabilitation Service (TIRS) was developed to support patients with more resistant MSK problems who needed more intense fulltime rehabilitation back at base – such as Bastion.
2	Basic Medical Teams	General practitioner/general medical duties officer/nurse practitioner and small team providing PHEC and PHC	The RORT deployed forward to these locations to provide support by assessing and treating patients and identifying cases that would benefit from TIRS.
3	Comprehensive Medical Teams	R1 SMO and PHC team (nurse and CMTs) providing a PHC Hub within deployed operating base) – set up as a Medical Reception Station	Base location for the DMRT and RORT. The DMRT had enhanced diagnostic capability using X-ray and MSK ultrasound available locally. Close liaison with SMO and MHT on determining which cases were remediable and which required aeromedical evacuation The TIRS delivered an intensive short-term rehabilitation programme in an attempt to retain service personnel in their operational role in theatre – taking into consideration theatre holding policy at the time.

copies before being summarised on DMICP when back at base.

The aspiration was to have the DMRT attached to brigade throughout the *preparation–deployment cycle*, in which case the DMRT would have the capability to support the brigade during pre-deployment training – informing training programmes, reducing training errors, generating injury-specific prevention strategies and treating MSK cases early in the care pathway. The DMRT would also be charged with training PHC clinicians during the PDT and deployment phases, through compliance with the MSK 'first aid' component of clinical guidelines for operations (CGOs) (JSP 999) in order to ensure compliance with accepted best practice. The DMRT deployed as an integral component of the medical capability and projected its RORTs forward to support and advise PHC clinicians in remote and basic medical teams. The number of peripatetic clinics was sometimes constrained by geography, security and the tactical situation, but the primary aim was to treat patients as far forward as possible, maintaining the force in remote and isolated locations.

The delivery of a DMRT requires the provision of professionally qualified, operationally ready consultants, physiotherapists and ERI staff. The restrictions on manning mean that all these staff also have full operational roles in garrisons or medical units or Role 4 facilities. Consequently, if drawn for deployment, such commitments may not be met without appropriate backfill.

Reservist support to these teams was limited. Exercise rehabilitation instructors are not trained in civilian practice nor are there consultants available in civilian practice with the necessary unique competencies and skill mix. Physiotherapy reservists may not have the skill set to deploy in this role and could not be reliably force generated, although there were a few exceptions. The aim to provide support to a brigade throughout the deployment–recovery cycle cannot be met with current resources.

In Camp Bastion, clinical activity was usually high, with 140 to 150 new and 350 to 400 review outpatient appointments each month. There were between 85 and 100 new in-patient episodes and 90 to 100 in-patient reviews per month. A review of the clinical effectiveness of the DMRT in November 2011 showed that 211 personnel presented to the DMRT during a four-month period in Camp Bastion who were unfit for all duties in theatre (and therefore liable to aero-medical evacuation). Following treatment, 165 injured personnel (78%) returned to duty in theatre. Of these, 108 (51%) were returned fully fit and 57 (27%) remained in theatre, fit for role.

A reduction in the number of aeromedical evacuations by 165 in one four-month period is a significant contribution to operational effectiveness. It reduced the *battle casualty replacement*

requirement and consequently reduced the demand on the operational air bridge. A consultant was reinforcing the DMRT during this period.

These data strongly support the role of the DMRT in force preservation in operational theatres. These data are similar to those reported on *Operation Telic*, in Kosovo and in Bosnia. DMRT input prevented 168 personnel, who were unfit for role on presentation, requiring aeromedical evacuation out of theatre. This is the equivalent of saving *one and a half companies* of manpower in a four-month period.

OUTCOMES

The recent conflicts in Iraq and Afghanistan have helped develop and test the systems described earlier. Enhanced survivability on operations, as a result of improved combat casualty care, has, by increasing the number of 'unexpected survivors', resulted in considerable rehabilitation challenges. The multidisciplinary clinical teams at RCDM and Headley Court have worked to enhance the outcomes of these severely injured UK battle casualties. A summary of the current data on outcomes was captured in a recent letter to *BMJ*.[59]

Table 17.8 illustrates the injury severity of a sample of amputees whose outcomes have been retrospectively analysed. The *New Injury Severity Score* (NISS) has been used in this group as a measure of injury complexity and rehabilitation challenge. The mean NISS for amputees was 40 and for triple amputees was 57. It is worth recognising that an Injury Severity Score (ISS) of 15 or greater is considered major trauma. These are some of the most severely injured cases described in the world rehabilitation literature.

This table also illustrates the mean number of admissions to Headley Court during the course of their treatment and the average duration of treatment for these patients. Amputees therefore were usually admitted between 11 and 13 times, for roughly a month at a time, with a total time in rehabilitation of 33 to 44 months. These data are important for future conflicts in understanding the time it takes to rehabilitate complex patients. There was, at times, pressure from senior officers to decrease the time spent in rehabilitation for these patients before discharge from their Service. There

Table 17.8 NISS scores for military patients

Injury characterisrics	Amputee groups				
	Unilateral	Unilateral non-op	Bilateral	Triple	Total amputees
Injury severity					
NISS (mean ± SD)	28 ± 11.3	N/A	44 ± 11.7	57 ± 5.6	40 ± 15
NISS (95% CI)	23 – 33	N/A	39 – 50	52 – 61	35 – 44
Number of admissions (mean ± SD)	11 ± 5.2	8 ± 4	13 ± 4.3	12 ± 3.7	11 ± 4.7
Length of rehab months (mean ± SD)	39 ± 15.2	20 ± 10.6	33 ± 10.2	44 ± 8.5	34 ± 14

was failure to recognise the time spent on other interventions – such as plastic and reconstructive surgery, mental health treatments, management of chronic infection and resettlement activities.

On discharge from Headley Court, 95% (n = 62) of these complex trauma patients were independent in all activities of daily living, sometimes with an aid or adaptation. Over 90% (n = 59) of amputees, around half those with multiple limb loss, walked independently over all terrains, and 75% (6) of triple amputees did not require a wheelchair for daily activities. This dispels the popular view that these seriously injured patients are likely to become dependent on the state for long-term social care and civilian rehabilitation services.

Amputees showed an average walking speed and energy expenditure comparable to a normal, age-matched, healthy population (Figure 17.18).[60] Only for bilateral transfemoral amputees was the walking speed significantly slower (1.12 m/s vs. 1.29 m/s; p = 0.025) and cadence reduced. The oxygen costs of walking for unilateral trans-tibial amputees were the same as controls and only 35% greater for bilateral transfemoral amputees compared to controls. This is in contrast to the view before these data were available that energy expenditure for bilateral trans-femoral amputees was approaching 250% greater than a healthy population (Figure 17.19).

Amputees were also assessed for their walking endurance by measuring the distance they were capable of travelling in six minutes. For

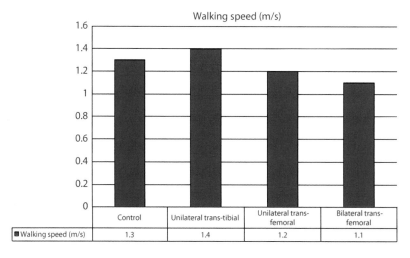

Figure 17.18 Amputee walking speeds.

comparison, subjects capable of community ambulation would be expected to walk 132 to 342 m and healthy age-matched groups 459 to 738 m in six minutes. It can be seen from Table 17.9 that bilateral amputees were, on average, very close to the lower end of normal – with a wide spread of results.

From a mental health perspective, combat amputees had PHQ-9 (Patient Health Questionnaire) scores compatible with moderate to severe depression in only 3.1% of cases, compared with 1.6% of the general population (Table 17.10). GAD-7 (Generalised Anxiety Disorder Questionnaire) (anxiety and depression test) scores indicating severe anxiety and depression were present in 1.5%, compared with 1.3% of the general population (Table 17.11).

In TBI, an important lesson learnt was that the severity at presentation was not an indication of the long-term prognosis.[61] Of 34 TBI patients admitted to Headley Court between 2008 and 2012, 42% of casualties had a GCS of 3 and 47% of casualties had an ISS score of 75 (considered at the time as incompatible with survival).

Table 17.10 PHQ-9 scores

PHQ-9	General population	DMRC amputees
Number	5018	65
Mean ± SD	2.9 ± 3.5	3.1 ± 4.5
Major depression		
Moderate (≥10) (%)	6.7	10.8
Moderate to severe (≥15) (%)	1.6	3.1

Forty-seven per cent (16) of these patients were fully independent at the conclusion of their rehabilitation and 41% (14) were fully independent in their own homes but needed help with some activities. Seventy-nine per cent (27) returned to either full-time or part-time work – 11 of these to military duties. Of these 11, 2 had ISS = 75.

Most of those with the worst possible ISS and GCS injury scores at presentation were able to return to work. Of the 11 with a GCS of 3, 91% returned to work. Of the 16 with an ISS of 75, 93% returned to work. Very severe brain injuries

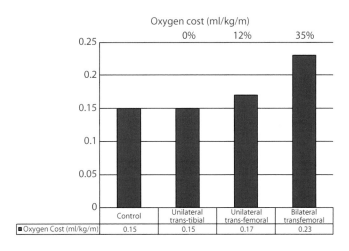

Figure 17.19 Activity oxygen costs for amputees.

Table 17.9 Six-minute walk test

	Amputee groups				
	Unilateral	Unilateral non-op	Bilateral	Triple	Total amputees
6 MWD (meters) (mean ± SD)*	544 ± 98.5*	544 ± 114.4	445 ± 103.6	387 ± 99.1	489 ± 116.6

Table 17.11 GAD-7

GAD-7	General population	DMRC amputees
Number	5030	65
Mean ± SD	2.95 ± 3.4	3 ± 4
Major GAD		
Moderate to severe (≥10) (%)	6	7.7
Severe (≥15) (%)	1.3	1.5

characterised by low levels of consciousness and multiple injuries at presentation can still be compatible with high-quality lives. Similar findings were described in a population of battle- and non-battle-related TBI. Of 91 patients with moderate to severe brain injury, 87% (79) were living independently and 92% (84) were in some form of employment four months after discharge.[62]

The determination of relevant outcome measures for a military population with TBI has bedeviled the assessment of these patients for many years. The traditional FIM + FAM measure has not been useful because of a ceiling effect. The total motor score showed a marked ceiling effect, with 42% of patients scoring the maximum on admission rising to 80% at discharge. The Mayo-Portland Inventory Score (MPAI-4) did not show significant ceiling effects. The other sub-scales of FIM + FAM and MPAI-4 were generally comparable; as a result, the MPAI-4 has been adopted as the global outcome measure for military brain injury.[63]

These outcomes are encouraging and indicate high-quality trauma care, including specialist rehabilitation. This has significant implications for the lifelong physical, mental and vocational outcomes of these patients and will have major economic benefits for the individual and the nation as a whole.

To determine the long-term outcomes of these cases and, in particular the long-term cardiovascular risk of trauma, UK Defence Rehabilitation will determine the 20-year outcomes of this cohort. The *Armed Services Trauma Rehabilitation Outcome* (ADVANCE) Study will investigate the 20-year outcomes of battlefield casualties from the Iraq and Afghanistan campaigns. The medical, physical, and psychosocial outcomes of this cohort will be compared with service personnel who did not sustain injuries

during operations. The study is led by a team from the *Academic Department of Military Rehabilitation*, Headley Court, supported by collaborating partners from Imperial College, the King's Centre for Military Health Research and Bournemouth University.

CONCLUSION

The campaigns in Iraq and Afghanistan have presented huge challenges for the rehabilitation specialists of the DMS. The systems that have been developed are complex and designed to allow the reception of complex poly-trauma cases early in the course of their *post-damage control surgery* phase. Nevertheless, sustainable flexibility remains essential, and future services must be able to respond to new patterns of wounding and the complex needs of patients.

Future systems require better coordination of rehabilitation services across the whole of the DMRP preferably through one chain of command. Inevitably, rehabilitation is a sensitive subject and the patients it serves generate close scrutiny from senior officers, politicians, the press, charities and the public, not always to the patients' advantage. Neurological rehabilitation played a critical role in supporting operations. Although the numbers were relatively small, these patients were often the most severe cases with the highest media profile and considerable emotional investment.

Patient tracking will be an essential component of any future system, and the post of *rehabilitation coordination officer* at the RCDM and electronic patient records across the DMRP have already proved their worth. As in all other specialities, the need for constant horizon scanning for new equipment and techniques cannot be over-emphasised.

Rehabilitation is an immensely collaborative specialty. Close and proactive liaison with allies, including the US and the NATO, and with welfare agencies, local authorities, charities and the NHS is a vital component of present and future service provision. Effective systems must also understand and provide for the needs of relatives.

Unfortunately, current Ministry of Defence (MOD) business models fail to react swiftly enough to provide staff, buildings, equipment and materiel for operations in the United Kingdom and not all NHS providers view the Service patients' priorities as their own. Peacetime business processes do not support war-time operations.

During the recent campaigns, research was not resourced in concert with the clinical load; as a consequence, scientific lessons have been lost. Research was tasked to busy clinicians without the resources required. DMRP staff were expected to simultaneously provide support to force generation at home, deploy to Role 1–3 and provide Role 4 support. This generated the requirement for locums, at considerable financial expense and clinical risk.

The Role 4 teams have been working in support of operations continuously for 10 years. For some staff (particularly civilians), there has been no respite from operational casualties during this time. Many have received no recognition for this. Fatigue, burnout and disillusionment are a risk to the continued support of these sorts of operations. Good local clinical leadership helps, but senior recognition of the personnel issues was sometimes absent. On completion of this phase of operations, many face losing their jobs.

There is a need for flexibility in response to newly developed training requirements that the cumbersome MOD training endorsement process fails to deliver in anything like a reasonable timeframe. There needed to be training for exercise rehabilitation instructors in complex trauma and neurological rehabilitation. Paediatric training is important for deployment, and as in other specialties, the need was not acknowledged and the provision was inadequate. There was a failure to involve Defence Rehabilitation in the casualty estimation – which could have had serious consequences for the Role 4 pathway. Those casualties undertaking rehabilitation in the United Kingdom continued to require military medical input – to maintain discipline, focus and ethos.

Operations Herrick and *Telic* demonstrated the continued effectiveness of the DMRT and of the deployed consultant in retaining operationally fit personnel in theatre. As on these campaigns, so in the future, physiotherapists, appropriately trained in critical care therapy, must be deployed embedded with the field hospital at the appropriate readiness. In the recent campaigns, an incorrect assumption was made that allied nations would provide a similar level of care with differently trained therapists.

The effectiveness of simple treatment guidelines for MSK injuries available to combat medical technicians and general medical duties officers through CGOs was also confirmed.

There remains a need for a proper structure for the force generation, training and governance of the *DMRT* (now FMRT). Whilst conflicts overseas are ongoing, 'peacetime' rehabilitation requirements persist. The DMRP must concurrently support the force generation effort – as during operations, there is an increased training tempo with a consequent rise in injury levels. There is thus benefit in having rehabilitation embedded into units during their PDT.

Defence Rehabilitation was placed under unprecedented operational pressure during the 10 years of conflict that are the subject of this book. It had to rapidly expand its capacity and develop new capabilities as a result of the types and complexity of injuries seen. A constant stream of the most severely injured casualties being admitted for rehabilitation had, at times, significant effects on the morale of the team working on the unit. By a combination of factors, including good-quality small group leadership, an examination of measures of 'burnout' at the end of the operations showed no areas for concern.

The quality of care improved as operations progressed, and at the end of the war-fighting, the outcomes were outstanding and have been described as a model for trauma rehabilitation. The data on outcomes are as good, or better, than any other published international data. The lessons learnt have slowly been adopted by the NHS, but there remains a considerable gap between the rehabilitation capability available in the NHS and a Defence capability will be required as long as injuries in the military continue to occur.

REFERENCES

1. National Clinical Audit of Specialist Rehabilitation for Patients with Complex Needs Following Major Injury. HQIP Report. 2017 https://www.hqip.org.uk.
2. McGilloway E, Mitchell J, Dharm-Datta S, Roberts A, Tilley H, Etherington J. The Mayo Portland Adaptability Inventory-4 outcome measure is superior to UK FIM + FAM in a British military population. *Brain Inj* 2016;30(10):1208–1212

3. Shirley P. Operational critical care. Intensive care and trauma. *J R Army Med Corps* 2009;155(2):133–140.

4. *Regional Networks for Major Trauma.* NHS Clinical Advisory Groups Report. 2010.

5. Besemann M. Physical rehabilitation following polytrauma. The Canadian Forces Physical Rehabilitation Program 2008–2011. *Can J Surg* 2011;54:S135.

6. Burtin C, Clerckx B, Robbeets C et al. Early exercise in critically ill patients enhances short-term functional recovery. *Crit Care Med* 2009;37(9):2499–2505.

7. Needham DM, Truong AD, Fan E. Technology to enhance physical rehabilitation of critically ill patients. *Crit Care Med* 2009;37(10):S436–S441.

8. National Audit Office. *Major Trauma care in England.* London: The Stationery Office, 2010.

9. McWilliams DJ, Atkinson D, Carter A, Foex BA, Benington S, Conway DH. Feasibility and impact of a structured, exercise-based rehabilitation programme for intensive care survivors. *Physiother Theory Pract* 2009;25(8):566–571.

10. McWilliams D, Pantelides K. Does physiotherapy led early mobilisation affect length of stay on ICU. *Respir Care J* 2008; 40:5–11.

11. Morris PE, Goad A, Thompson C et al. Early intensive care unit mobility therapy in the treatment of acute respiratory failure. *Crit Care Med* 2008;36(8):2238–2243.

12. Kress JP. Clinical trials of early mobilization of critically ill patients. *Crit Care Med* 2009;37(10):S442–S4S7.

13. McWilliams D, Weblin J, Atkins G et al. Enhancing rehabilitation of mechanically ventilated patients in the intensive care unit: A quality improvement project. *J Crit Care* 2015;30(1):13–18.

14. Brower RG. Consequences of bed rest. *Crit Care Med* 2009;37(10):S422–S428.

15. Hodgin KE, Nordon-Craft A, McFann KK, Mealer ML, Moss M. Physical therapy utilization in intensive care units: Results from a national survey. *Crit Care Med* 2009; 37(2):561–566.

16. D'Alleyrand J, Fleming M, Gordon WT, Andersen RC, Potter BK. Combat-related hemipelvectomy. *J Surg Orthop Adv* 2011;21(1):38–43.

17. Roeschlein R, Domholdt E. Factors related to successful upper extremity prosthetic use. *Prosthet Orthot Int* 1989; 13(1):14–18.

18. Aldington DJ, McQuay HJ, Moore RA. End-to-end military pain management. *Philos Trans R Soc B Biol Sci* 2011;366(1562):268–275.

19. Devonport L, Edwards D, Edwards C, Aldington DJ, Mahoney PF, Wood PR. Evolution of the role 4 U.K. military pain service. *J R Army Med Corps* 2010;156(4 Suppl 1):398–401.

20. Ilfeld BM. Continuous peripheral nerve blocks: A review of the published evidence. *Anesth Analg* 2011;113(4):904–905.

21. Edwards D, Bowden M, Aldington DJ. Pain management at role 4. *J R Army Med Corps* 2009;155(1):58–61.

22. Small C, Hankin E, Edwards D, Frazer S, Aldington D. Phantom limb phenomena: Acute findings in British armed forces amputees. *Br J Anaesth* 2013;111(4):686.

23. Flor H. Phantom-limb pain: Characteristics, causes, and treatment. *Lancet Neurol* 2002;1(3):182–189.

24. Lotze M, Flor H, Grodd W, Larbig W, Birbaumer N. Phantom movements and pain – an MRI study in upper limb amputees. *Brain* 2001;124:2268–2277.

25. Moriwaki K, Shiroyama K, Sanuki M. Combination of evidence-based medications for neuropathic pain: Proposal of a simple three-step therapeutic ladder. *J Pain Manag* 2009;2:129–134.

26. Le Feuvre P, Aldington D. Know Pain Know Gain: Proposing a treatment approach for phantom limb pain. *J R Army Med Corps* 2014;160(1):16–21.

27. Kern U, Altkemper B, Kohl M. Management of phantom pain with a textile, electromagnetically-acting stump liner: A randomized, double-blind, crossover study. *J Pain Symptom Manage* 2006;32(4): 352–360.

28. Nawijn S, Van Der Linde H, Emmelot C, Hofstad C. Stump management after transtibial amputation: A systematic review. *Prosthet Orthot Int* 2005;29(1):13–26.

29. Bradbrook D. Acupuncture treatment of phantom limb pain and phantom limb sensation in amputees. *Acupunct Med* 2004;22(2):93–97.

30. Niemtzow RC. Battlefield acupuncture. *Med Acupunct* 2007;19(4):225–228.

31. Johnson MI, Mulvey MR, Bagnall A-M. Transcutaneous electrical nerve stimulation (TENS) for phantom pain and stump pain following amputation in adults. *Cochrane Database Syst Rev* 2015; (8). http://onlinelibrary .wiley.com/doi/10.1002/14651858.CD007264 .pub3/abstract.

32. MacIver K, Lloyd DM, Kelly S, Roberts N, Nurmikko T. Phantom limb pain, cortical reorganization and the therapeutic effect of mental imagery. *Brain J Neurol* 2008;131 (Pt 8):2181–2191.

33. Moseley GL. Graded motor imagery for pathologic pain – a randomized controlled trial. *Neurology* 2006;67(12):2129–2134.

34. Chan BL, Witt R, Charrow AP et al. Mirror therapy for phantom limb pain. *N Engl J Med* 2007;357(21):2206–2207.

35. Sumitani M, Miyauchi S, McCabe CS et al. Mirror visual feedback alleviates deafferentation pain, depending on qualitative aspects of the pain: A preliminary report. *Rheumatology* 2008;47(7):1038–1043.

36. Grünert-Plüss N, Hufschmid U, Santschi L, Grünert J. Mirror therapy in hand rehabilitation: A review of the literature, the St Gallen protocol for mirror therapy and evaluation of a case series of 52 patients. *Br J Hand Ther* 2008;13(1):4–11.

37. Diers M, Christmann C, Koeppe C, Ruf M, Flor H. Mirrored, imagined and executed movements differentially activate sensorimotor cortex in amputees with and without phantom limb pain. *Pain* 2010;149(2):296–304.

38. Anderson-Barnes VC, McAuliffe C, Swanberg KM, Tsao JW. Phantom limb pain – a phenomenon of proprioceptive memory? *Med Hypotheses* 2009;73(4):555–558.

39. Ulger O, Topuz S, Bayramlar K, Sener G, Erbahceci F. Effectiveness of phantom exercises for phantom limb pain: A pilot study. *J Rehabil Med* 2009;41(7):582–584.

40. Brodie EE, Whyte A, Niven CA. Analgesia through the looking-glass? A randomized controlled trial investigating the effect of viewing a 'virtual' limb upon phantom limb pain, sensation and movement. *Eur J Pain* 2007;11(4):428–436.

41. Pasquina PF, Bryant PR, Huang ME, Roberts TL, Nelson VS, Flood KM. Advances in amputee care. *Arch Phys Med Rehabil* 2006;87(3):34–43.

42. Black CJ, Kuper M, Bellingan GJ, Batson S, Matejowsky C, Howell DC. A multidisciplinary team approach to weaning from prolonged mechanical ventilation. *Br J Hosp Med* 2012;73(8):462–466.

43. Goldberg CKF, Green B, Moore J et al. Integrated musculoskeletal rehabilitation care at a comprehensive combat and complex casualty care program. *J Manipul Physiol Ther* 2009;32(9):781–791.

44. Knowlton LM, Gosney JE, Chackungal S et al. Consensus statements regarding the multidisciplinary care of limb amputation patients in disasters or humanitarian emergencies: Report of the 2011 Humanitarian Action Summit Surgical Working Group on amputations following disasters or conflict. *Prehosp Disaster Med* 2011;26(6):438–448.

45. Deathe B, Miller WC, Speechley M. The status of outcome measurement in amputee rehabilitation in Canada. *Arch Phys Med Rehabil* 2002;83(7):912–918.

46. Atkin K, Cole M, Cumming J, Donovan-Hall M, I. BACPAR Outcome Measure Tool Box. http://www.csp.org.uk/documents/bacpar -toolbox-outcome-measures-version-12010.

47. Campbell J, Kendall M. Investigating the suitability of the clinical outcome variables scale (COVS) as a mobility outcome measure in spinal cord injury rehabilitation. *Physiother Can* 2003;55(3):135–144.

48. Celso B, Tepas J, Langland-Orban B et al. A systematic review and meta-analysis comparing outcome of severely injured patients

treated in trauma centers following the establishment of trauma systems. *J Trauma Acute Care Surg* 2006;60(2):371–378.

49. Marks LJ, Michael JW. Clinical review – science, medicine, and the future: Artificial limbs. *BMJ* 2001;323(7315):732.

50. Coleman KL, Boone DA, Laing LS, Mathews DE, Smith DG. Quantification of prosthetic outcomes: Elastomeric gel liner with locking pin suspension versus polyethylene foam liner with neoprene sleeve suspension. *J Rehabil Res Dev* 2004;41(4):591–602.

51. Kaufman KR, Levine JA, Brey RH, McCrady SK, Padgett DJ, Joyner MJ. Energy expenditure and activity of transfemoral amputees using mechanical and microprocessor-controlled prosthetic knees. *Arch Phys Med Rehabil* 2008;89(7):1380–1385.

52. Hoge CW, McGurk D, Thomas JL, Cox AL, Engel CC, Castro CA. Mild traumatic brain injury in U.S. Soldiers returning from Iraq. *N Engl J Med.* 2008;358(5):453–463.

53. Fear NT, Jones E, Groom M et al. Symptoms of post-concussional syndrome are non-specifically related to mild traumatic brain injury in UK Armed Forces personnel on return from deployment in Iraq: An analysis of self-reported data. *Psychol Med* 2008;23:1–9.

54. Saddawi-Konefka D, Kim HM, Chung KC. A systematic review of outcomes and complications of reconstruction and amputation for type IIIB and IIIC fractures of the tibia. *Plast Reconstr Surg* 2008;122(6):1796–1805.

55. Ladlow P, Phillip R, Coppack R et al. Influence of immediate and delayed lower-limb amputation compared with lower-limb salvage on functional and mental health outcomes post-rehabilitation UK military *J Bone Joint Surgery Am* 2016;98:1996–2005. http://dx.doi.org/10.2106/JBJS.1501210.

56. Met R, Janssen LI, Wille J et al. Functional results after through-knee and above-knee amputations: Does more length mean better outcome? *Vasc Endovasc Surg* 2008; 42(5):456–461.

57. Birch R, Misra P, Stewart MP et al. Nerve injuries sustained during warfare: Part II: Outcomes. *J Bone Joint Surg Br* 2012;94: 529–535.

58. Ladlow P, Phillip R, Etherington J et al. Functional and mental health status of United Kingdom military amputees postrehabilitation. *Arch Phys Med Rehabil* 2015;96:2048–2054. doi:10.1016/j.apmr.2015.07.016.

59. Etherington J, Bennett AN, Phillip R, Mistlin A. *BMJ* 2016;354:i4741 doi: 10.1136/bmj.i4741-6.

60. Jarvis H, Baker R, Bennett A, Twiste M, Phillip R. Kinematics, kinetics and gait profile score in highly functional amputees. *Prosthet Orthot Int* 2015. http://poi.sagepub.com/content/39/1_suppl/2.full#sec-406.

61. Bahadur S, McGilloway E, Etherington J. Injury severity at presentation is not associated with long-term vocational outcome in British Military brain injury. *J R Army Med Corps* 2016; 162:120–124. doi:10.1136/jramc-2014-000393.

62. Dharm-Datta S, Gough MRC, Porter PJ et al. Successful outcomes following neurorehabilitation in military traumatic brain injury patients in the United Kingdom. *J Trauma Acute Care Surg* 2015;79 (Suppl 2):S197–S203. doi:10.1097/TA.0000000000000721.

63. McGilloway E, Mitchell J, Dharm-Datta S, Roberts A, Tilley H, Etherington J. The Mayo Portland Adaptability Inventory-4 outcome measure is superior to UK FIM + FAM in a British military population. *Brain Inj* 2016;30(10):1208–1212.

18

Paediatrics

INTRODUCTION

Historically, the British Military has frequently been required to provide emergency care to children presenting to deployed military treatment facilities. Whatever the nature of the deployment, children will find a way into the military healthcare system regardless of eligibility rules. During operations in Iraq and Afghanistan, between 3% and 18% of patients presenting to Roles 2 and 3 were children.[1-8] This resulted in challenging situations for care providers and difficult decisions for the chain of command. The combination of inexperience and the emotive nature of dealing with sick and injured children results in disproportionate anxiety for the military provider and can have both positive and negative effects on unit effectiveness. Treating children is hugely rewarding but can be emotionally destructive, particularly if there is a perception of inadequate capability and readiness, both at a unit and individual level. It is important that the military commander recognises the impact that children can have on a military treatment facility and that appropriate preparation is undertaken to exploit success and to mitigate risk to patients, personnel and organisational reputation alike.

The requirement to establish and maintain a paediatric capability is described in the Geneva Conventions and North Atlantic Treaty Organization (NATO) doctrine.[9,10] Following the *Strategic Defence Review*,[11] the presence of Regular paediatric medical and nursing personnel was extremely limited. By the time the British Military deployed to *Operation Telic*, there was one only Regular general paediatrician, there were no specific paediatric

training posts and there was no significant supporting British Military policy or doctrine. By the onset of *Operation Herrick*, there was no regular paediatric skill base other than a handful of nurses and medical officers with chance paediatric training or sub-speciality training and ad hoc paediatric exposure within primary and secondary care roles. In the whole secondary care cadre, there was one consultant with formal sub-specialty training in emergency paediatrics. The lack of acceptance or recognition at the highest level of the inevitability of paediatric casualties during all forms of deployed operations was a handicap from which the Defence Medical Services (DMS) never fully recovered and which adversely effected delivery through both campaigns. Its effects continue even now. Due to the lack of policy, there was no driver to address equipment, manning and training deficiencies. In 2008, the Surgeon General's Policy Letter 04/08 *Treatment of Non-Entitled Children on Operations* was published and provided a brief framework for the provision of care to children. This was followed in 2010 by a competency framework produced by Permanent Joint Headquarters (PJHQ). However, the requirements specified were not described as essential to force generation and the infrastructure for the provision of training was inadequate.

Children presented to military treatment facilities regardless of the eligibility matrix, which was often less than clear in any case. Whilst the majority of these were trauma cases directly related to combat, we cannot console ourselves that this is all we will have to deal with. Presentations during *Operations Herrick* and *Telic* included burns, electrical injury, drowning, congenital disease

441

including cardiac abnormalities, infectious diseases and the complications of treatment at other facilities.

Regardless of the challenges presented, there were many examples of outstanding care delivered to children on operations, and outcomes were comparable to civilian paediatric major trauma centres.[6] Great improvements in capability were made over the duration of operations in Iraq and Afghanistan. Preserving that paediatric capability will be the next challenge to Defence.

CARE OF CHILDREN ON OPERATIONS

Throughout *Operations Telic* and *Herrick*, a highly variable but significant number of paediatric patients presented to the UK Role 2+ and Role 3 facilities. During the initial war-fighting phase of *Operation Telic* (March to May 2003), around 3% of all patients presenting to *33 Field Hospital* emergency department were under 16 years old, of whom more than half were burns cases. Only one in five were fit for discharge, the rest required admission; 17% were medical patients.[8] The youngest child seen during *Operation Telic* was six days old, and trauma aside, presentations included the complications of spina bifida and congenital heart disease.

During a 10-year period in Afghanistan, children represented 5.8% of admissions to US facilities; importantly, the average Injury Severity Score (ISS) in children was higher than that in injured coalition force personnel. The commonest mechanism of injury was blast, and more than 500 children on the trauma database met the criteria for tranexamic acid administration. Between January 2011 and January 2013, 281 children were seen in the UK Role 3 emergency department at Camp Bastion.[12] The admission rate to the intensive therapy unit (ITU) was up to 79%,[12] accounting for 14% of all intensive care unit (ICU) admissions but 30% of bed days[13,14]; 30% of children had an ISS greater than 25.[6] Children tended to be resource heavy; there were 112 theatre episodes for 61 patients with a median stay of 2 days, although stays of up to 26 days were recorded.[6] The mean length of stay during a three-month study of *Operation Herrick* 8b/9a was 10.5 days, with over 10% of theatre cases

being paediatric.[15] In addition, the resources used by children are disproportionately higher than the absolute numbers alone might suggest.

As a deployed specialty, paediatric capability was ad hoc and limited to the incidental presence of relevant experience and training, accredited or otherwise. Units were not required to deploy with paediatric expertise for either *Operation Herrick* or *Operation Telic*, and as such, there was no formal lay down of capability. It became clear in later *Operation Herrick* tours that coordination of all inpatient paediatric care was required and it became practice for one clinician to be a single point of contact for all clinical issues regarding children in the hospital. It is strongly recommended that this is continued on future operations. The most appropriate consultant clinician should have nominal clinical responsibility for inpatient paediatric care to ensure that the distinct needs of this group are met. During *Herrick*, duties included attending general ward rounds, a separate daily paediatric ward round, providing advice to general duties medical officers and the supervision of paediatric prescribing. Paediatric decision-making was supported by access to the *Kids Intensive Care Decision Support* line, which facilitated conference calling with relevant paediatric specialties at the *Birmingham Children's Hospital*.

Emergency care

Our most robust area of paediatric capability during this period was emergency medicine. All military emergency medicine consultants have regular exposure to sick and injured children, and some have formal subspecialty training in paediatric emergency medicine. Currently (2017), approximately 10% of the cadre holds a certificate of completion of training in paediatric emergency medicine or is in subspecialty training, and during and after the conflicts, the Defence Consultant Advisor (DCA) was clear regarding the importance to deployed activity of this reservoir of experience and expertise. This meant that the deployed emergency consultant was often the only deployed clinician with current and frequent paediatric experience. During *Operations Herrick* and *Telic*, this resource was not only key in the resuscitation phase but also important as an additional resource for the rest of the military treatment facility. Whereas there was combined experience between specialities of paediatric trauma care, emergency physicians were the only clinician group who routinely had experience of 'medical' paediatrics. During 2011, 179 children presented to the emergency department, of whom over 90% were admitted to the hospital.[12]

Anaesthesia

Many deployed anaesthetists had experience in the provision of paediatric anaesthesia, at least in older children. A smaller number of deployed consultants were subspecialists in paediatric anaesthesia, providing a higher level of expertise. However, there were significant numbers of clinicians who were not routinely anaesthetising children in their civilian practice. This was particularly the case with younger children, and nearly 50% of paediatric trauma admissions on *Operation Herrick* were under six years old.[15] This skill gap was mitigated to an extent by individual and collective pre-deployment training and the introduction of paediatric anaesthesia guidelines. Since the end of *Operation Herrick*, DCA Anaesthesia has recommended that 10% of the consultant anaesthesia cadre is subspecialty trained in paediatric anaesthesia and that all deploying consultants maintain an appropriate level of paediatric capability to meet their deployed scope of practice.

Surgery

A considerable amount of paediatric surgery was performed during both operations, practically all of which was performed by surgeons in adult National Health Service (NHS) practice (the DMS had and has only one paediatric surgeon). Between July 2008 and November 2012, 766 paediatric patients were recorded on the *Joint Theatre Trauma Registry* as having been admitted to the Role 3 facility at Camp Bastion. These accounted for 3390 surgical and resuscitative procedures, including 120 exploratory laparotomies, 329 thoracic procedures and 177 vascular procedures.[16] These data illustrate well the requirement for the deployed military surgeon to be competent and comfortable operating on children. The paper illustrates the paediatric skill sets required but

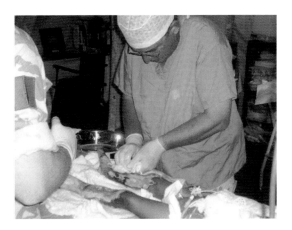

Figure 18.1 Consultant general surgeon changing a burn dressing on an Afghan child.

also concludes that none of the procedures performed were specific to the paediatric population. This serves to reassure us that adult surgeons can transfer skills to this group of patients. Nordmann et al.[14] discuss the overall management of paediatric trauma, and whilst individual procedures are common to both adults and children, decision-making has subtle differences, for example in the case of non-operative management of solid organ injury in children. As is the trend, children account for a disproportionately high resource use. Between 1 January and 29 April 2011, 61 children accounted for 112 theatre episodes. Over 50% of children required more than one trip to theatre.[6] Again, evidence from *Operation Herrick* highlights the need for the military surgeon to maintain individual capability in paediatric surgery. DCA Surgery's direction is now that military scope of practice should be reflected in the appraisal and revalidation process (Figure 18.1).

Medicine

Although not defined in policy, the medical care of children on the ward fell to the internal medical cadre. Children frequently had longer ward stays compared with coalition troops because of difficulties in transferring them to host nation or non-governmental organisation (NGO) facilities. Aside from post-operative complications, common conditions requiring treatment included sepsis, parasitic infestations and developing world illnesses including typhoid. It is clear that the deployed medical consultant requires some basic training and competencies in the recognition and treatment of the sick child, in particular in tropical and infectious diseases.

Nursing

Defence does not currently, and has not for some considerable time, supported paediatric nurse training amongst the Regular Cadre. Aside from emergency department and primary care nurses who are likely to see children in their UK practice, theatre, ICU and ward nurses do not routinely treat children. Whilst there may be a number, largely not quantified, of paediatric nurses in the Reserves, there are very few specific deployed roles that require this experience. As a result, almost all paediatric nursing care was delivered by adult trained nurses with the ad hoc, intermittent and serendipitous presence of military nurses who had previous paediatric nursing experience. In the case of nurses, as of doctors, many clinicians' main experience of managing children came from their experience as parents. During *Operation Herrick*, a number of civilian nurses were contracted to provide paediatric nursing support in the ward environment and were able to step forward to the emergency department if required. This allowed support in key areas such as drug and fluid administration, nutrition and observation of the child and helped meet the distinct physical and emotional needs of the sick or injured child.

In the emergency setting, nursing personnel required an understanding of how to provide trauma care to the paediatric patient, as described by Pearce.[12] As an example of this, the application of massive transfusion protocols and use of transfusion equipment in children are specialist skills that require familiarity with both equipment and the paediatric population. This is discussed in the clinical advances section (Figure 18.2).

Pre-hospital emergency care

Although it was not unusual for local national parents to arrive at the Bastion camp gates carrying a sick or injured child and requesting more

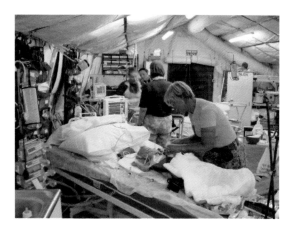

Figure 18.2 Nursing a baby on the ICU during *Operation Herrick 5*.

advanced care than could be obtained in local facilities, the first point of contact for an injured child would often be Role 1 dismounted assets or, less frequently, the Medical Emergency Response Team (MERT). Since the MERT consisted of an emergency nurse, two paramedics and either an emergency physician or anaesthetist, with the exception of the anaesthetist, the team could be expected to have a reasonable level of paediatric experience based on their UK clinical exposure. This experience would prove to be vital given the significant paediatric workload that presented to the MERT. Walker et al.[17] reviewed a 20-month period of MERT activity in 2006/7 during which 78, over 7%, of all MERT patients were children. Of these children, 88% were T1 or T2 casualties. The interventions performed included intraosseous access, haemorrhage control, PHEA and fluid resuscitation. The paper concluded that all military pre-hospital providers require appropriate paediatric training and experience.

External agency support

External agency support was available at various times. During *Operation Telic*, charitable funding was available to treat burns patients evacuated to the United Kingdom. An infant with *Tetralogy of Fallot* who presented to the hospital at Shaibah Log Base was evacuated to the United Kingdom and received cardiac surgery from the *Chain of Hope* children's charity. During *Operation Herrick*, evacuation of local nationals to Role 4 was not permitted, although one child with a gunshot wound to the head was evacuated out of country but not to the United Kingdom. *NGO* and host nation facilities were present throughout *Operations Telic* and *Herrick*, and there was access to ongoing care for paediatric patients. This access was, however, variable and depended on a number of factors, including security and capacity. Difficult ethical and clinical decisions had to be made when considering whether it was appropriate to transfer a child to a facility offering a lower level of care. In addition to treatment facilities, in the latter part of *Operation Herrick*, there was 24-hour access to specialist paediatric advice via Birmingham Children's Hospital paediatric intensive care unit, a resource that remains available at the time of writing.

Defence paediatric special interest group

In the absence of a formal deployed specialty and no paediatric cadre or specialty board, paediatric capability development was extremely difficult. As the burden of paediatric care became clear, reactive solutions to equipment, clinical guidance and policy deficits were produced. There was a clear need for coordinated subject matter expert (SME) advice. During the later years of *Operation Herrick*, the anaesthetic cadre set up the *Paediatric Anaesthetic and Critical Care Special Interest Group*. This was an informal group whose primary role was to provide SME input on equipment as well as clinical guidance. A number of items of paediatric equipment were introduced as urgent operational requirements (UORs) rather than brought into core as part of the hospital modules (see Chapter 23). Clinical guidance, for example regarding paediatric anaesthesia and massive transfusion, was produced in order to improve the care delivered by non-paediatric trained or experienced clinicians. Specific paediatric training was introduced into the *Military Operational Surgical Trauma* (MOST) course and supported by the group members. The group also reviewed any paediatric *serious event reports* and produced recommendations for the medical director and inspector general.

The group was subsequently opened to emergency medicine membership and over a period of time became the *Defence Paediatric Special Interest Group* (DEPSIG). This group is now formally recognised and multidisciplinary and has representation from all areas of the DMS. It has representation at several other Defence committees such as equipment, nursing and resuscitation and it reports to the medical director via the DMS Clinical Committee. It has become the central point of access and coordination for all paediatric issues, bringing together the paediatric expertise that exists within Defence. It advises on manning, policy, equipment and training and has produced training packages and clinical guidance to the DMS supporting training for pre-hospital emergency care (PHEC), Defence Primary Healthcare and Defence secondary care.

CLINICAL CHALLENGES ON *OPERATIONS TELIC* AND *HERRICK*

DMS personnel deployed on *Operations Telic* and *Herrick* were required to overcome the gap between the available capability and the clinical needs of severely injured or unwell children. As described earlier, the absence of experienced personnel, coupled with heightened anxiety regarding treating children, often resulted in very challenging situations, not just clinically but emotionally too. There is significant risk in not manning, equipping and preparing adequately for paediatric patients when in a remote and unsupported setting. The risk affects not only the patient but also the deployed individual, the unit, the DMS and the reputation of the British Military.

Training

Paediatric training requirements were not defined until 2008, when the SGPL 04/08 *Treatment of Non-Entitled Children on Operations* was released; this document is now found in formal military guidance in a *Joint Service Publication* (JSP 950). In addition, PJHQ produced a draft paediatric competency framework. These documents detailed the implications for commanders of their failure to deploy paediatric capability but also specifically highlighted the fact that failure to achieve the direction laid out would not be a bar to deployment: gaps would be taken at risk. Some cadres were not represented in the document. Despite the difficulties, a number of training opportunities were enabled, including the MOST Course, the *Advanced Life Support Group Online Virtual Learning Environment Paediatric Life Support (PLS) level 1* (developed by DEPSIG) and military PLS, Prehospital Paediatric life Support and Advanced Paediatric life Support packages. Much of this work was led by the single consultant in paediatric emergency medicine. How much of it will endure remains to be seen.

Equipment

Without specific paediatric equipment modules, the availability of paediatric materiel relied on Broselow™ bags and a small amount of 'dual-role' equipment such as some smaller airways, cannula and intraosseous needles. There was a good range of equipment for children in the emergency medicine modules, introduced by the emergency medicine cadre despite the lack of recognition of paediatric casualties; however, although this was probably sufficient for initial resuscitation, it was not adequate for subsequent theatre, intensive care and ward stays. Much of the deficit was made up with UORs and as a result has not been sustained, requiring a programme of uptake into the care modules under the statement of requirement (SOR) process. In fact, following the decision not to continue to procure the Broselow™ system and spending restrictions leading to slowing of the SOR process with prioritisation of individual requests for equipment, current paediatric equipment availability is worse than it was prior to *Operations Telic* and *Herrick*. Subsequent work on the paediatric content of Roles 1, 2, 3 and aeromedical evacuation equipment modules has been undertaken by DEPSIG and endorsed by command, but funding remains unconfirmed.

Work load

The numbers of paediatric patients and their use of resources were discussed earlier in this chapter. Case mix, as could be predicted, was predominantly trauma. However, around 5% of admissions

during *Operation Herrick* and 20% of admissions during *Operation Telic* were non-trauma admissions. The mean ISS of paediatric patients on *Operation Telic* was 14.7 and *Herrick* was 13.47.[18] However, up to 45% of patients had an ISS greater than 15, and up to 30%, greater than 25.[6,18]

Outcomes

Because paediatric patients were never British Nationals, follow-up after discharge was to all intents and purposes impossible. As a result, 28-day survival and long-term neurological or functional outcome is not known. Crude mortality rates were around 10%, including emergency department deaths.[6,12] This is comparable to other coalition data.[5,19] By comparison with UK TARN data, our crude mortality rates were higher; the mortality rate for children with an ISS of greater than 15 in the United Kingdom facility in 2012 was 7.6%. Our higher mortality rate probably represents the higher ISS seen, resource constraints and ethical issues in commencing treatment.

Ethics

Although ethical decision-making in patient care and the framework that is applied in doing so are not unique to deployed patient care, there were inevitably special considerations in the deployed environment. In the United Kingdom, it would rarely, if ever, be decided not to commence treatment on an injured or unwell child unless he or she was on an end-of-life pathway; likewise, there is a very high threshold for discontinuing care. In the deployed setting, considering the appropriateness of commencing treatment and deciding when it is humane to stop it or withdraw it is vital. In the remote setting, resource management includes considering futility. The limited facilities to which children can be transferred and the feasibility of ongoing long-term care will, and must, influence decision-making. The child with severe burns offers an example. For children in the United Kingdom, there is no upper limit of body surface area burned which would cause treatment not to be started. In Afghanistan, where there is little or no prospect of effective ongoing paediatric burns care and there is no option to remain in a UK medical treatment facility (MTF), the limit is much lower, probably in the region of 40%. Severe head injury decisions were similarly influenced by the complete lack of neurological critical care in country. In the same way, the absence of effective community services such as primary care, physiotherapy, equipment provision, pharmacy and social support meant that patients requiring long-term intensive support would sooner or later succumb to the complications of their condition. Examples of challenging scenarios included patients who would be wheelchair bound, would require repeated specialist surgery for burns and contractures or would need long-term management of infection or continence problems.

Given the emotive nature of acute paediatric care, it was vital that all deployed personnel understood the process and rational behind ethical decisions. Such decisions were made by discussion amongst the clinicians involved. Bernthal et al.[20] performed a qualitative study of ethical issues faced by commanders and stated in their paper that 'caring for children was categorised as one of the most challenging decisions faced by clinicians. Ethical decisions came up more often than was expected and were not dealt with in PDT'. As in all areas of training, ethical training should include the issues arising from the management of children to best prepare commanders for deployment.

CLINICAL ADVANCES

The advances in paediatric trauma care progressed in conjunction with the improvements made in the care of the military population at risk more generally. It is difficult to pick out a single area of change that influenced outcome. Mortality rates were similar throughout the deployments. There are, however, three examples of specific areas of development that have influenced civilian practice. The *Camp Bastion Contrast Calculator* was developed to calculate the intravenous contrast requirements to perform a biphasic computed tomography traumagram and is now widely used in UK civilian practice.[21] Secondly, the development of a paediatric massive transfusion protocol[22] in order to apply the military principles of haemostatic transfusion has influenced the development of paediatric massive transfusion policy in UK paediatric major trauma centres. Lastly, although no specific

guidelines were developed during the Afghanistan or Iraq deployments, a review of cases of paediatric traumatic cardiac arrest showed a 14.8% survival rate (and a return of spontaneous circulation in 39% of patients),[23] and this has gone on to influence recent work towards producing UK consensus guidelines.

RESEARCH

A number of academic papers on the care of children were published during and following *Operations Herrick* and *Telic*, the majority of which were descriptive or epidemiological in nature, recording the volume, nature and impact of paediatrics on operations.

Significant challenges to research

The challenges to paediatric research on deployment are considerable. The absolute numbers of children in our data sets are low, especially when looking at a particular intervention such as the use of tranexamic acid. Accurate weight or age was rarely known and rarely recorded, resulting in incomplete data sets and an inability to accurately define the study population. Obtaining informed consent from children and their parents is also a challenge, tends to be a verbal process and is generally not practicable in the deployed situation amongst populations with little, or more usually no, English.

The assumption prior to military deployment (other than new entry operations or humanitarian and disaster relief operations) is usually that the eligibility matrix will prevent significant numbers of children attending an MTF. Whilst retrospectively we know this is not correct, it is also not conducive to planning paediatric research, securing funding and obtaining ethical approval. Unless there is a more than tacit acceptance that children will be treated, it will continue to be very challenging to capitalise on the research potential of this population.

Ongoing research

Away from the deployed environment, research is ongoing into the use of tranexamic acid in the paediatric trauma patient in collaboration with

Alberta Children Hospital, Calgary, Canada. Other areas that have been identified as potential avenues for research include data comparison work with the Trauma Audit and Research Network, detailed analysis of MERT paediatric activity and thorough analysis of the whole paediatric data set held by the Joint Theatre Trauma Registry, in particular of demographic detail and outcomes.

FUTURE CAPABILITY

The key message from the paediatric literature arising from *Operations Telic* and *Herrick* is that regardless of eligibility, the DMS will always be faced with injured and unwell children. Whilst absolute paediatric numbers are likely to be small, the impact will almost certainly be high. Therefore the requirement to generate and maintain a paediatric capability remains. However, despite excellent experiential learning on *Operations Herrick* and *Telic* there has been very little significant secured and funded change in paediatric policy, manning, training or equipment. With the loss of corporate memory of deployed experience and the lack of paediatric exposure in the firm base, Defence paediatric capability will continue to decline. Although reserve paediatricians without deployed experience and experts taken up from the NHS are undoubtedly capable of operating an effective deployed paediatric capability given time and exposure, they cannot offer the expertise based on experience that is needed to predict or identify problems before deployment and ensure that mitigation is in place. Only a regular paediatric consultant presence can do this. The inevitable consequence will be the need to relearn the same lessons next time.

In October 2016, the DMOCG endorsed the following Single Statement of User Need for the DMS. 'The ability to triage, treat, stabilise and package for evacuation, children (0 to 18 years old) in all environments on operations including within the PHEC, primary healthcare, deployed hospital care and medical evacuation components'.

The Geneva Convention and NATO doctrine details the requirement for a deployed force to treat, when necessary, non-combatants, including children. With the increased likelihood of British military involvement in humanitarian, disaster relief and evacuation operations, children will continue to be part of our workload for the foreseeable future in nearly all military operations. Bricknell and Nadin describe the need to '*train to treat the entire patient suite*'.[24] Following *Operations Herrick* and *Telic*, the British Military have deployed in support of the UN and NATO in non-combat roles and have seen and treated significant numbers of children. UK military policy needs to enable the commander to deliver the care required by all patients, including children. At the time of writing, a paediatric concept of operations is in development, and from this, new and updated policy should follow. Only with sufficient policy and doctrine to support the capability requirement will the DMS be able to develop and maintain deployed paediatric capability.

The key to future paediatric capability is ensuring that our policy, manning, equipment, training and professional development reflect our deployed scope of practice which *will* in future deployments include children. We *must* strive to develop and sustain capability in this area.

REFERENCES

1. Heller D. Child patients in a field hospital during the 2003 Gulf conflict. *J R Army Med Corps* 2005;151:41–43.
2. Beitler AL, Wortmann GW, Hofmann LJ et al. Operation Enduring Freedom: The 48th Combat Support Hospital in Afghanistan. *Mil Med* 2006;171:189–193.
3. McGuigan R, Spinella PC, Beekley A et al. Pediatric trauma: Experience of a combat support hospital in Iraq. *J Pediatr Surg* 2007;42:207–210.
4. Creamer KM, Edwards MJ, Shields CH et al. Pediatric wartime admissions to US military combat support hospitals in Afghanistan and Iraq: Learning from the first 2,000 admissions. *J Trauma* 2009;67:762–768.
5. Borgman M, Matos RI, Blackbourne LH et al. Ten years of military pediatric care in Afghanistan and Iraq. *J Trauma Acute Care Surg* 2012;73(6 Suppl 5):S509–S513.
6. Arul GS, Reynolds J, DiRusso S et al. Paediatric admissions to the British military hospital at Camp Bastion, Afghanistan. *Ann R Coll Surg Engl* 2012;94:52–57.

7. Reavley PD, Black JJ. Attendances at a field hospital emergency department during operations in Iraq November 2003 to March 2004 (Operation Telic 3). *J R Army Med Corps* 2006;152:231–235.

8. Gurney I. Paediatric casualties during OP TELIC. *J R Army Med Corps* 2004;150: 270–272.

9. Geneva Convention (1), Chapter II, Article 12 (accessed 9 November 2016). https:// ihl-databases.icrc.org/applic/ihl/ihl.nsf /7c4d08d9b287a42141256739003e636b /fe20c3d903ce27e3c125641e004a92f3.

10. Allied Joint Publication 4.10(B): Allied Joint Doctrine for Medical Support 1-3.1.1 dated May 15 (accessed 9 November 2016). https://www.gov.uk/government /uploads/.../20150824-AJP_4_10_med_spt _uk.pdf

11. The Strategic Review White Paper RP 98-91. October 1998. Available at: researchbreifings .files.parliament.uk/documents/RP98-91 /RP98-91.pdf

12. Pearce P. Preparing to care for paediatric trauma patients. *J R Army Med Corps* 2015;161(Supp 1):i52–i55.

13. Inwald DP, Arul GS, Montgomery M et al. Management of children in the deployed intensive care unit at Camp Bastion, Afghanistan. *J R Army Med Corps* 2014;160:236–240.

14. Nordmann GR, McNicholas JJ, Templeton PA. Paediatric trauma management on deployment. *J R Army Med Corps* 2011; 157(3 Suppl 1):S334–S343.

15. Nordmann GR. Paediatric anaesthesia in Afghanistan: A review of the current experience. *J R Army Med Corps* 2010; 156(4 Suppl 1):S323–S326.

16. Mckechnie PS, Wertin T, Parker P et al. Pediatric surgery skill sets in Role 3: The Afghanistan experience. *Mil Med* 2014;179(7):762–765.

17. Walker N, Russell RJ, Hodgetts TJ. British military experience of pre-hospital paediatric trauma in Afghanistan. *J R Army Med Corps* 2010;156(3):150–153.

18. Woods KL, Russell RJ, Bree S et al. The pattern of paediatric trauma on operations. *J R Army Med Corps* 2012;158(1):34–37.

19. Creamer KM, Edwards MJ, Shileds CH et al. Pediatric wartime admissions to US military combat support hospitals in Afghanistan and Iraq: Learning from the first 2,000 admissions. *J Trauma* 2009;67(4):762–768.

20. Bernthal EM, Draper HJ, Henning J et al. 'A band of brothers' and exploration of medical ethical issues faced by British senior military clinicians on deployment to Afghanistan: A qualitative study. *J R Army Med Corps* 2017;163(3):199–205.

21. *Paediatric Trauma Protocols*. London: Royal College of Radiologists, 2014.

22. Bree S, Wood K, Nordmann GR et al. The paediatric transfusion challenge on deployed operations. *J R Army Med Corps* 2010;156(4 Suppl 1):361–364.

23. Hillman CM, Rickard A, Rawlains M et al. Paediatric traumatic cardiac arrest: Data from the Joint Theatre Trauma Registry. *J R Army Med Corps* 2016;162:276–279.

24. Bricknell MC, Nadin M. Lessons from the organisation of the UK medical services deployed in support of Operation TELIC (Iraq) and Operation HERRICK (Afghanistan). *J R Army Med Corps* 2017;163(4):273–279.

19

Trauma governance: Scoring and data analysis

INTRODUCTION

The unexpectedly large numbers of severely injured casualties that occurred in Iraq and later, and to a greater degree, in Afghanistan inevitably led to the recognition of new treatment challenges and to the need to develop solutions. A means of identifying patterns of injury in order to develop protective countermeasures and of assessing the validity and effectiveness of therapeutic interventions was therefore essential from the very early stages of the campaigns. Thus, the concept of *clinical governance* (CG) was rapidly adopted as a core function of the *Defence Medical Services* (DMS).[1-3] During *Operations Telic* and *Herrick*, a trauma governance system developed that not only provided assurance to the *chain of command* of the quality of the assessment, treatment and evacuation of Service personnel but also proved (or on occasion disproved) the effectiveness of the rapid developments in clinical trauma practice and continues to be the bedrock of research within the DMS. The early stages of this sophisticated system and culture of organisational governance were outlined by Hodgetts et al.[4] and Smith et al.[5] Russell et al.[6] described further developments. At the same time, the services offered by the DMS were scrutinised by the *Care Quality Commission (CQC)*, providing a degree of external validity to quality assessment. This chapter will provide a further update and demonstrate how weaknesses in performance could be rapidly identified and resolved by instigating guidelines, training, or equipment changes.

TRAUMA NURSE COORDINATORS

The *Joint Theatre Trauma Registry* (JTTR) at the *Royal Centre for Defence Medicine* (RCDM) holds data on all casualties treated by a trauma team at one of the deployed hospitals and, since 2007, all injured patients repatriated for in-patient treatment in Birmingham. The JTTR has been at the centre of governance and research activity at the *RCDM* since 2003. The scope of the military trauma CG system is shown in Figure 19.1.

A critical success factor for any system that uses information, whether for monitoring or research, is data quality. The DMS has used *trauma nurse coordinators* (TNCs) at both Role 3 field hospitals and the Role 4 receiving hospital in Birmingham since 2001 and before that at Ministry of Defence Hospital Unit (MDHU) Frimley Park from 1997. The deployed TNCs facilitated quality data collection, identified governance concerns and managed the weekly *Joint Theatre Clinical Case Conference* (JTCCC). In the United States, TNCs are an essential requirement for the grant of Level 1 status to a Major Trauma Centre (MTC), but they were rare in the National Health Service (NHS) before 2012 and the advent of UK MTCs.

The TNCs initially worked as part of the *Academic Department of Military Emergency Medicine* (ADMEM) at RCDM before becoming the basis for the *Clinical Information Exploitation* (CLIX) team there. In the United Kingdom, they collected Role 4 clinical information from the point of entry of casualties into the hospital on the intensive care unit or military ward. This was combined

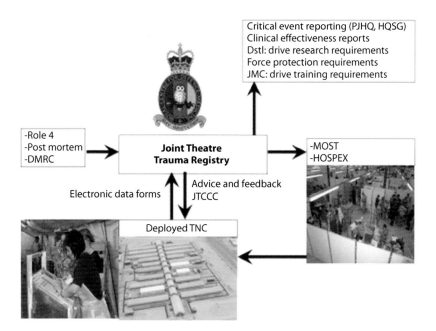

Figure 19.1 Military trauma CG.

with data sent from the deployed TNCs and sifted for governance concerns (clinical and force protection issues). The Role 4 TNCs developed and provided pre-deployment training for the Role 3 TNC posts and provided day-to-day support to them once deployed, via secure telephone and e-mail.

JOINT THEATRE TRAUMA REGISTRY

The JTTR was initiated at the then MDHU Frimley Park in 1997 as a local trauma governance tool and collected its first military casualties on *Operation Agricola* (peace keeping operations in Kosovo)[7] in 2000 before moving to RCDM. JTTR consists of three separate independent databases:

- Major trauma Audit for Clinical Effectiveness (*MACE*);
- Medical Emergency Response Team (*MERT*) data; and
- Operational Emergency Department Attendance Register (*OpEDAR*).

JTTR provides data both for quality assurance and for research. In this latter role, it has underpinned and enabled the flourishing output of the academic departments at RCDM since 2003,

providing data, to select a small number of examples, regarding features associated with wound severity in UK soldiers suffering gunshot wounds,[8] outcomes following limb salvage for severe open tibia fracture,[9] mortality and morbidity analysis from combat neck injury[10] and soft tissue injuries.[11]

OpEDAR captured all patients (with injury *or* illness) attending the emergency department of a deployed UK field hospital from 2003 onwards.[12] The collection *of OpEDAR* data was stopped in 2010 with the introduction of the *Whole Hospital Information System* (WHIS) at Bastion. It is unlikely, however, that WHIS will be used on future operations and OpEDAR may be required again depending on the development of other information systems.

The combination of the three streams enabled the formation of a complete picture of all seriously injured casualties treated at UK medical field facilities from the point of wounding, through pre-hospital treatment and evacuation, to the care given at the field hospital. For UK military casualties, the continuing pathway of evacuation by air to Role 4 and definitive treatment was also captured. The MERT database was the record of patients treated by the UK's *Medical Emergency Response Team* (physician-led helicopter-borne pre-hospital team). A separate database was required as MERT delivered patients to treatment facilities other than the UK Field Hospital, and as a result, their data would not have appeared in *MACE* unless they re-entered the UK system later on. In addition, patients with illness rather than injury were also transported by MERT but would not appear on *MACE*. Patients may have appeared in *MACE* without appearing on OpEDAR or the MERT database if they had received their initial treatment in a non-UK field hospital, prior to evacuation to Birmingham. This is the case currently for all serious non-operational casualties being repatriated to RCDM from operations around the world.

The provision of feedback is an essential part of the CG process. Feedback systems were developed at several levels to identify, recognise and reinforce good performance and to improve sub-optimal practice: in both cases, as a result, important lessons were learnt. Immediate feedback could be relayed via Permanent Joint Headquarters (PJHQ) following the arrival of a patient at Role 4 or a post-mortem; short-term feedback was relayed at the weekly JTCCCs[13] and longer-term feedback by the *Mortality Peer Review* panel[14] with formal academic review of performance during specified periods of an operation.[7,15–17]

A further application of JTTR was the academic evaluation of complex organisational changes and challenges, including the effectiveness of tourniquets,[18] the effectiveness of battlefield analgesia,[19] the required competencies of the MERT[20] and the relationship of timelines to outcomes.[21] Data were used to improve and shape clinical doctrine, research priorities and changes to the acute care training curricula.

POST-MORTEM DATA

Vital medical intelligence will be lost if data from only the surviving casualties are analysed for lessons.[22] A member of the ADMEM team (now CLIX) attended all military operational post-mortem examinations from 2007 onwards. All but a few of these were carried out at Oxford, enabling a good working relationship to develop with the forensic pathologists and their teams. The necessary clinical and military contexts were therefore available to the pathologist, and the performance of personal and vehicle protective systems and

clinical personnel could be assessed. Scientific advisers from Defence Science and Technology Laboratories also attended, allowing new patterns of wounding and the impact of changes in weaponry and bomb-making to be rapidly identified. The effectiveness of individual techniques could be determined together with their effects on patient outcome. When a technique had failed or was performed inadequately, the training message was fed back through the *Medical Directorate* and PJHQ and was immediately reinforced.

MORTALITY REVIEW

Collective data are as important as those from individual cases, and a group of casualties who are commonly excluded from clinical review in other trauma systems are those who die immediately or before receiving any medical help and certainly before reaching a medical treatment facility. This gap was closed using the post-mortem results to carry out regular mortality reviews. These were undertaken by a panel of senior clinicians from emergency medicine, anaesthetics and intensive care, general surgery and orthopaedic surgery, together with the Home Office forensic pathologist who undertook the majority of the post-mortem examinations.[14] Defence scientists and tactical experts were also included in order that they could offer advice on protection systems and the operation and tactical situation on the ground. All operational deaths were reviewed at these meetings regardless of the time and location of wounding and death.

A judgement was also made regarding whether each casualty was salvageable: that is, were the injuries treatable within the accepted capabilities of contemporary best practice had the injury taken place within easy reach of a trauma centre? Each patient was graded as *definitely* (S1, <5% chance of death), *probably* (S2) or *possibly* salvageable (S3, <5% chance of survival), or *unsalvageable* (S4). In cases other than S4, a second decision was then made regarding whether the death was preventable, this time informed by weapons intelligence and other reports. A death was classified as preventable or not for tactical, equipment or clinical reasons.

This analysis of deaths in batches at regular quarterly meetings offered another opportunity to identify emerging injury patterns and weapon trends and assess clinical effectiveness. Hodgetts et al.[23] first reported on operational deaths between April 2006 and March 2007 and concluded that the majority of lethal injuries were to the head and chest, that mathematical trauma scoring would miss classifying some survivors as 'unexpected' who would have been identified by clinical review and that 'clinical salvageability could not be reviewed in isolation from tactical constraints and overall preventability'. This analysis helped to inform the approach of the Mortality Peer Review Panel that ran on a three to four monthly basis until the end of Operation Herrick. Russell et al.[6] expanded on the need for clinical review of mathematical trauma scoring systems in order to avoid missing 'unexpected outcomes', which are important as they act as flags of either good or sub-optimal performance. Seventy-five clinically validated unexpected survivors were identified over two years between 2006 and 2008.

In 2014, an analysis of the proceedings of the Mortality Peer Review Panel that looked at all UK service personnel operational deaths between January 2002 and November 2013 was published.[14] Of the 621 deaths recorded on JTTR, 517 (83.3%) were due to hostile action, with a killed in action (no signs of life at any point after arrival at a medical treatment facility) to died of wounds ratio at 6.28:1. Explosive mechanisms were responsible for 55.65% of deaths, and penetrating mechanisms, 28.71%, with an average of 10.56 injuries per casualty affecting multiple body regions; 91.1% of deaths were judged unsalvageable. This figure is high compared to figures rating 75.7% of US combat deaths as un-survivable,[24] but direct comparisons are not possible due to different methodologies.

Keene et al.[25] conducted an in-depth review of all the operational deaths classified as died of wounds as a result of having vital signs at some point after arrival at a medical treatment facility. None were felt to have had salvageable injuries and the majority died in the first 24 hours after wounding. Forty-seven per cent had suffered isolated head injuries, with a further 18% un-survivable head injuries combined with other wounds suggesting a need for improved head protection. A further 21% died following severe lower limb trauma in conjunction with abdominal and pelvic injuries secondary to an improvised explosive device (IED).

The need for increased head protection had been emphasised by Singleton et al.[26] following a review of 121 deaths of UK servicemen killed by IEDs between 2007 and 2010. Three hundred and fifty four separate fatal injuries were identified in this group; 50% of those mounted in vehicles at the time of wounding died as a result of traumatic brain injury, with a further 20.2% suffering a fatal intracavity injury. Of those on foot, 42.6% suffered fatal extremity injuries; 22.2%, junctional haemorrhage; and 18.7%, traumatic brain injury.

HOSPITAL EXERCISE (HOSPEX)

A further application of JTTR data was the use of cases taken from the JTTR at HOSPEX, the exercises undertaken at the Army Medical Services Training Centre (AMSTC) by field hospital units in preparation for deployment. Anonymised casualty data were used to construct case scenarios, which, being genuine, contemporary and played out in real time with simulated live casualties in a realistic duplicate environment, helped achieve exercise face and content validity. Essential confidence was also inspired in those deploying for the first time. These scenarios also decreased the initial shock of encountering critical combat wounded in the field hospital. Morris et al.[27] showed the effectiveness of this training by demonstrating that there was no change in mortality at the UK Field Hospital in Camp Bastion between the month before a hospital handover when teams could be expected to be at their most effective and the month following, when responsibility had passed to the new team.

JOINT THEATRE CLINICAL CASE CONFERENCE

Another important pillar to the CG structure enhancing and accelerating the feedback process was the JTCCC. This structured weekly teleconference coordinated from RCDM was begun in 2007 and continues even when operations are not in progress in order to capture information on UK military casualties from around the world on exercise and other activities. Participants include

RCDM (military and civilian clinicians), deployed field hospitals, the *Defence Military Rehabilitation Centre*, RAF Brize Norton, AMSTC, the Inspector General's department and PJHQ. The DMS *Inspector General* is a senior officer with overall responsibility for standards and governance within the DMS.

During *Operations Telic* and *Herrick*, near real-time feedback was provided on the progress of casualties admitted to RCDM during the previous two weeks. Feedback was not given over a longer period, unless specifically requested by the clinicians in Afghanistan, due to the large number of casualties. Case summaries were forwarded the day before via a secure e-mail system. Any issues with the initial management were clarified, which enabled immediate modification of practice where appropriate and the RCDM clinicians to understand the initial context and decision-making process better. Casualties awaiting evacuation were also presented by the deployed clinicians, which allowed receiving medical teams advance warning and planning time.

As well as discussing patients, JTCCC allowed deployed clinicians to highlight clinical practice, equipment and training issues and proved the catalyst for rapid policy change.[13] Confidentiality was assured by referral to patients only by their admission numbers and distribution of two separate types of minutes across the DMS. Clinical addressees received a full set of minutes, but non-clinical addresses had copies with the clinical details removed. Commanding officers and deployed medical directors (DMDs) of medical units about to deploy also received copies of the minutes so that they developed and maintained institutional memory.

Willridge et al.[13] reported on the issues raised in the first year of the JTCCC. A total of 207 issues were raised, which encompassed every step in the casualty care pathway and every North Atlantic Treaty Organization 'J' category (Table 19.1), with J3 *Operational* (31.9%) and J6 *Communications* (21.7%) being the most frequent; 23% were raised for 'information only', but of the others, action was taken to close 68.1% within three weeks.

As *Operation Telic* ended and *Operation Herrick* matured, the number of issues raised outwith casualty feedback declined, but the *JTCCC* has

Table 19.1 NATO 'J' classification of staff duties

J1 Personnel
J2 Intelligence and security
J3 Operations
J4 Logistics
J5 Plans
J6 Communications
J7 Education and training
J8 Finance and contracts
J9 Civil-Military Co-operation (CIMIC)

remained a valuable governance tool, proving its worth during *Operation Gritrock* (the UK anti-Ebola intervention), when many similar issues required and received rapid resolution.

BENCHMARKING AGAINST NHS TRAUMA CARE

The quantity, type and complexity of trauma seen on operations are of a higher level than those seen in the NHS. The development of major trauma systems in the United Kingdom since 2012 has focused the reception and further management of trauma onto the MTCs. Prior to this, in 2007, reports from both National Confidential Enquiry into Peri-Operative Deaths[28] and the Royal College of Surgeons of England[29] criticised NHS trauma care and found that many NHS emergency departments were receiving fewer than one major trauma case a week, with some treating only one to two cases in a 12-week sampling period. Only 12/183 (6.6%) hospitals treated more than one major trauma case per week. Performance was directly related to experience in dealing with major trauma, as those hospitals with a higher caseload (more than 20 major trauma cases in 12 weeks) delivered a higher standard of care.

By comparison, over a comparable period in 2007, the DMS treated 314 major trauma cases in Iraq and Afghanistan, an average of 4.25 per week (51.0 over 12 weeks).[4] Thereafter, the frequency of major trauma in Afghanistan substantially increased, reaching a peak in 2010 and 2011. According to the same report, 56.3% of NHS major trauma patients were the result of motor vehicle collisions (MVCs). Blast or gunshot were not separately coded and were included in 10.3% of 'other' mechanisms; in the matched DMS cohort, only 5.1% of major trauma was the result of MVCs, with 53.8% being from blast/fragmentation and 29.9% from gunshot injuries. Banding the Injury Severity Score (ISS) results demonstrated that the DMS cohort was significantly (χ^2; $p < 0.0001$) more severely injured than the NHS cohort (ISS 16–24, NHS = 56.5%, DMS = 26.4%; ISS 25–35, NHS = 35.1%, DMS = 22.3%; ISS 36–75, NHS = 8.4%, DMS = 51.3%).

During the peak period in Afghanistan, a similar study was carried out on *Operation Herrrick 9*. Henning et al.[30] found that over a 12-week period, there were 226 casualties requiring trauma team activation; 93.7% were accompanied to the field hospital by a doctor with advanced airway skills (although only 6.2% required this particular intervention), 100% were received by consultants in emergency medicine and anaesthesia, 93.6% of cases had a computed tomography scan within 60 minutes, and of those requiring operative care, 98.1% had this carried out by a consultant surgeon. These are figures that MTCs are struggling to match even today.

One advantage enjoyed by the DMS is the multi-disciplinary 'ownership' of the trauma system, with all care providers feeling a personal responsibility towards the military casualties and the performance of the trauma system treating them. In the deployed field hospital, there is a full consultant-based team (consultants from each of the specialties of emergency medicine [team leader]), anaesthesia, general surgery and orthopaedic surgery resident 24 hours a day and immediately available for the reception of any seriously injured patient. At that time in the NHS, the trauma patient was rarely received by a senior doctor: 118/183 (64.5%) hospitals did not have a consultant trauma team leader during a specific sample period (the early hours of Sunday morning) and in only 6/183 (3.3%) hospitals was the consultant team leader resident.[28,29] This contributed to incorrect clinical decision-making and lack of appreciation of the severity of injury. This situation has now been partially mitigated at MTCs, but it would still be very unusual even at the time of writing (2017) to have a full team of consultants ready to receive a trauma patient at an MTC.

CQC AND NATIONAL AUDIT OFFICE

Although there is no statutory requirement for DMS services to be registered under the *Health and Social Care Act* and subject to review by the *CQC*, the CQC has, on a number of occasions, been invited by successive Surgeons General to undertake reviews of deployed and home base medical and dental care. These inspections foster a culture of openness and drive service improvements by identifying areas of concern. The press release from the 2012 CQC report into care for those injured in Afghanistan, is given in Appendix E. This relationship continues, and further reviews will be carried out in the future. The DMS were also subject to assessment by the National Audit Office, albeit using different criteria for satisfactory performance. Extracts from their 2010 report *Treating Injury and Illness Arising on Military Operations* given in Appendix F.

FUTURE DEVELOPMENTS AND MODELS

In order to monitor and help drive constant improvements in casualty care, CG mechanisms must also continue to evolve and improve. One way of achieving this is to develop improved trauma modelling and scoring systems so that *gold standards* of performance can be identified and used as comparators for clinical practice. This will allow more accurate determination of unexpected outcomes, both positive and negative. The former point to excellent practice, which holds lessons to be disseminated, the latter to sub-optimal outcomes, which need to be further investigated.

One current limitation of trauma scoring and modelling is that it uses a binary outcome: the casualty either lives or dies. There have been many survivors of serious or life-threatening injuries from *Operations Telic* and *Herrick*, and yet there is currently no way of measuring whether the care they received produced the best possible outcome for them. It has been noted that traditional trauma scoring methods (*Trauma Score-Injury Severity Score* and *A Severity Characterisation of Trauma*) were developed prior to chaos theory and use linear statistical methods which are not effective at analysing complex systems with many variables such as trauma.[6] Studies using Bayesian theory and networks are being conducted by RCDM in conjunction with other institutions and are showing promise.[31]

Whilst novel scoring systems and models are developed, old ones can be analysed and improved. An example of this is the adaptation of the triage sieve used in civilian major incident practice for use by the military to include conscious level as a variable which makes it more sensitive.[32] Further studies of the physiological parameters used within such systems are being carried out and will bring further refinements.

No CG system or trauma registry can produce useful output if the data are not collected or are not accurate. A lot of the focus on improving casualty outcome has been on advanced care, whether taken to the patient at the point of wounding (MERT) or at the hospital. Data from these interventions are comprehensive. However, there are gaps in the data for casualty care before the arrival of advanced care, and it is this time where there is most potential for improvement in the future, along with the greatest potential for preventative and protective measures. For the effect of any improvements in lower levels of care (for example first aid, buddy aid or team medic intervention) to be measured, it will be necessary to develop a system of reliable data collection from the frontline troops administering the care. This is a challenge for the Chain of Command and not purely a medical issue.

CONCLUSION

Effective governance is an essential component of any complex clinical system. At its simplest, it is often seen as a way of identifying problems and errors; in practice and when used appropriately, it is much more than this. This chapter has discussed the role of CG in identifying good practice, as well as poor, in guiding changes in the management of groups of patients as well as individuals and in identifying priorities for research and development. The development of effective and rigorous CG during the campaigns in Iraq and Afghanistan was responsible for significant improvements in the mortality and morbidity of those servicemen and women injured during the campaigns and continues to influence clinical management to this day.

REFERENCES

1. SGPL 09/00. *Clinical Governance in the Defence Medical Services.* London: Ministry of Defence, 2000.
2. SGPL 01/03. Clinical Governance in the Defence Medical Services. London: Ministry of Defence, 2003.
3. SGPL 18/04. Quality Assurance of Clinical Governance on Deployed Operations. London: Ministry of Defence, 2004.
4. Hodgetts TJ, Davies S, Russell RJ, McLeod J. Benchmarking the UK military deployed trauma system. *J R Army Med Corps* 2007;153:237–238.
5. Smith J, Hodgetts TJ, Mahoney PF, Russell RJ, Davies S, McLeod J. Trauma governance in the UK Defence Medical Services. *J R Army Med Corps* 2007;153:239–242.
6. Russell RJ, Hodgetts TJ, McLeod J, Starkey K, Mahoney PF, Harrison K, Bell E. The role of trauma scoring in developing trauma clinical governance in the Defence Medical Services. *Phil Trans R Soc B* 2011;336:171–191.
7. Hodgetts TJ, Turner L, Grieves T, Payne S. Major Trauma Clinical Effectiveness Project: Report of Operation AGRICOLA, Kosovo. London:MOD, 1999.
8. Penn-Barwell JG, Sargeant ID. Gun-shot wounds in UK military casualties – features associated with wound severity. *Injury* 2016;47:1067–1071.
9. Penn-Barwell JG, Myatt RW, Bennett PM, Sargeant ID. Medium-term outcomes following limb salvage for severe open tibia fracture are similar to trans-tibial amputation. *Injury* 2015;46:288–291.
10. Breeze J, Allanson-Bailey LS, Hunt NC, Delaney RS, Hepper AE, Clasper J. Mortality and Morbidity from combat neck injury. *J Trauma* 2012;72(4):969–974.
11. Ollerton J, Hodgetts TJ, Russell RJ. Operational Morbidity analysis of Soft tissue injuries during Operation TELIC. *J R Army Med Corps* 2007;153:263–265.
12. Russell RJ, Hodgetts TJ, Ollerton J et al. The Operational Emergency Department Attendance Register (OpEDAR) – a new

epidemiological tool. *J R Army Med Corps* 2007;153:244–251.

13. Willridge DJ, Hodgetts TJ, Mahoney PF, Jarvis L; JTCCC. The Joint Clinical Case Conference (JTCCC): Clinical Governance in Action. *J R Army Med Corps* 2010;156: 79–83.

14. Russell RJ, Hunt N, Delaney R. The Mortality Peer Review Panel: A report on the deaths on operations of UK Service personnel 2002-2013. J R Army Med Corps 2014;160:150–154.

15. Academic Departments of Military Emergency Medicine and Military Surgery & Trauma. *Operational Mortality Analysis Op HERRICK & Op TELIC 01 April 2006–31 March 2007 (Confidential internal report)*. Birmingham: Royal Centre for Defence Medicine, 2007.

16. Hodgetts TJ, Hill DA, Russell RJ, Russell MQ. *Major Trauma Audit Clinical Effectiveness Report of Clinical Effectiveness on Operation TELIC 1: War Phase 2003*. Birmingham: Royal Centre for Defence Medicine, 2005.

17. Hodgetts TJ, Russell RJ, Stannard A, Massetti P. *Major Trauma Audit for Clinical Effectiveness Report on Clinical Effectiveness on Operation HERRICK 4*. Birmingham: Royal Centre for Defence Medicine, 2006.

18. Brodie S, Hodgetts TJ, Ollerton J, McLeod J, Lambert P, Mahoney P. Tourniquet use in combat trauma: UK military experience. *J R Army Med Corps* 2007;153:310–313.

19. Hodgetts TJ, Aldington D, Henning J, Mahoney PF, DeMello W. *Battlefield Analgesia Review*. Birmingham: Royal Centre for Defence Medicine, 2006.

20. Hodgetts TJ. *Forward Deployed Medical Emergency Response Team: Interim Report*. Birmingham: Academic Department of Military Emergency Medicine, 2007.

21. Hodgetts TJ. *Medical Emergency Response Team Database Analysis: OP HERRICK 01 May 06 to 18 Jun 07*. Birmingham: Academic Department of Military Emergency Medicine, 2007.

22. Sharma BR, Gupta M, Harish D, Singh VP. Missed diagnoses in trauma patient vis-à-vis significance of autopsy. *Injury* 2005;36:976–983.

23. Hodgetts TJ, Davies S, Midwinter M et al. Operational Mortality of UK Service Personnel in Iraq and Afghanistan: A one year analysis 2006–7. *J R Army Med Corps* 2007;153:252–254.

24. Eastridge BJ, Mabry RL, Seguin P. Death on the Battlefield (2001–2011): Implications for the future of combat casualty care. *J Trauma Acute Care Surg* 2012;73:S431–S437.

25. Keene D, Penn-Barwell JG, Wood PR et al. Died of wounds: A mortality review. *J R Army Med Corps* 2015;2015(0):1–6.

26. Singleton JAG, Gibb IE, Hunt NCA, Bull AMJ, Clasper JC. Identifying future "unexpected survivors": A retrospective cohort study of fatal injury patterns in victims of improvised explosive devices. *BMJ Open* 2013;3:e003130.

27. Morris TJ, Lovell A, Groves P, Russell RJ. Impact of personnel turnover on survival at a major combat hospital in Afghanistan. Proceedings of the 99th American College of Surgeons Clinical Congress, Washington, DC, 06–10 October 2013.

28. National Confidential Enquiry into Patient Outcome and Death. *Emergency Admissions: A Journey in the Right Direction?* London, England: HMSO, 2007.

29. Royal College of Surgeons of England. *Report of the Working Party on the Management of Patients with Major Injury*. London: Royal College of Surgeons of England, 1998.

30. Henning DCW, Smith JE, Patch D, Lambert AW. A comparison of civilian (National Enquiry into Patient Outcome and Death) trauma standards with current practice in a deployed field hospital in Afghanistan. *Emerg Med J* 2011;28:310–312.

31. Mossadegh S, He S, Parker P. Bayesian scoring systems for military pelvic and perineal blast injuries: Is it time to take a new approach? *Mil Med* 2016;181:S127–S137.

32. Horne S, Vassallo J, Read J, Ball S. (2011) UK Triage – an improved tool for an evolving threat. *Injury* 44:23–28.

20

Ethics, legal and humanitarian issues

INTRODUCTION

Iraq and Afghanistan saw operations enduring over years, carried out *among the people*. In both campaigns, the need to engage with and operate amongst the local population to defeat the insurgency led to conditions of long-term engagement with a multitude of civilian populations, agencies (both governmental and non-governmental) and local and international military partners. Combined with better information systems and 24-hour media coverage, these interactions cast into sharp focus the non-clinical aspects of medical operations that appeared more prominent, and under greater scrutiny, than in previous campaigns.

Context of operations

The main themes affecting military operations in these challenging environments are listed in Table 20.1 and explained in the next subsections.

INEQUALITY

The ethical context of providing medical care in a challenging and hostile situation, where levels of healthcare provision were radically different from those of the United Kingdom, was inevitably complex. An absolutely fundamental issue was the fact that patients were suffering patterns of injury rarely seen in peacetime civilian practice and that the severity of such injuries was demonstrably worse than the vast majority of civilian trauma. In addition, civilians suffered the same injuries as combat personnel, but their own healthcare system was unable even to approach western standards of care, or achieve the same outcomes of treatment.

UNCERTAINTY

The improvements in trauma care that have arisen wholly or in part from military experience have been extensively discussed and form a significant part of the narrative of this book. These developments, in pushing the boundaries of successful treatment, and consequently the level of injuries that might be considered survivable, have resulted in their own ethical challenges. Similarly, developments in rehabilitation have redefined what injuries may be compatible with a good quality of life afterwards.

CONSTRAINT

The resources needed to achieve these outcomes are vast – so that while capability is high, capacity is limited and operational effect depends not only on implementation of *Medical Rules of Eligibility* at the point of entry to the health care system but also on return of civilians to their own healthcare system as soon as possible.

DUTY OF CARE

The treatment of captured personnel has been a subject of considerable legal, ethical and media interest, especially with regard to the conflict in Iraq (*Operation Telic*): ethical issues, particularly concerning the medical oversight of captured persons detained by the military, have become a lodestar for the moral acceptability of military intervention, and one against which the UK Military have, on occasion, been found wanting. There were also duty of care issues regarding local nationals (LNs) and enemy combatants who entered the treatment process.

Other issues that will be discussed in this chapter include the challenges of maintaining standards and effective relationships in a multinational,

Table 20.1 Ethical themes

- Inequality
- Uncertainty
- Constraint
- Duty of care

multiagency environment, the problems of managing medical major incidents, where multiple casualties arrive at isolated low-capacity facilities, and the issues associated with engagement with humanitarian agencies, naturally cautious regarding the development of links with uniformed and armed forces. The question of how the military impacts on the 'humanitarian space' is far from decided, even after more than a decade of engagement.

This chapter aims to address the developments in the ethical and managerial aspects of deployed medical operations that arose as a result of the Iraq and Afghanistan campaigns.

HARD CALLS AND RUFFLED FEATHERS: THE DEPLOYED MEDICAL DIRECTOR

Clinical governance was a key area of concern, and issues became apparent very quickly. The systems put in place to deal with governance issues have been discussed in Chapter 19, but a particular issue was how to maintain standards during periods of transition when staff were rotating through on a constant three- to six-month cycle over many years.

The *deployed medical director* (DMD) has become an established role within field hospitals. It developed, at least in part, through a need to support and guide clinicians less familiar with the deployed clinical environment once roulements of staff became established in what was clearly a long-term campaign. Initially, this was the job of the *clinical director*, an experienced clinician in an active medical position, such as the lead surgeon or consultant anaesthetist, but who was also identified as the individual to go to for guidance with complex decision-making. However, it soon became clear that the non-clinical workload precluded a significant clinical role at the same time and the role of DMD was introduced in 2009.[1]

The main function of the DMD was to maintain standards by ensuring that there was always a senior clinical expert, with the experience gained from several previous tours, available to advise those less experienced in the injury patterns, resource constraints and processes of the deployed environment. Their ability to remain one step away from the clinical decision, coupled with extensive experience of similar cases, also made them natural arbitrators when difficult ethical decisions or interpersonal situations arose. The role soon became an essential link to the *chain of command* (CoC) – operating as both liaison and mediator when clinical and military imperatives (or personalities) clashed. As the role developed, so did the experience of this balance and as a group the DMDs developed a deep understanding of the risks taken by leaning further one way or the other.

Initially, DMDs were drawn from a pool of readily identifiable senior clinicians – the defence professors. This small group could not support an enduring operation and so other experienced clinicians were utilised. From ad hoc selection at the beginning, DMD development progressed, until at the height of *Operation Herrick*, there was a clear selection, training and handover process. In recognition of the responsibilities and level of engagement, the post came with acting OF5 (*captain RN, colonel, group captain*) rank during the deployment. It is recognised that this arrangement may well turn out to have been unique to this campaign. The post may not be required to function in the same way with the same training pipeline or selection process in future deployments.[2]

Part of the irony of the DMD role was that they provided the person for the clinical cadre to look to when they felt out of their depth. Research into the way they themselves felt is revealing. The main ethical and non-clinical challenges faced by a cohort of DMDs fell into the following five domains:[3]

- Resource constraints and rationing
- The conflict between military and professional (clinical) obligations
- End-of-life care
- Patient consent for treatment and withdrawal of treatment
- Working in multinational contexts

Each of these areas is discussed in the following subsections. The deployed clinical directors also described the psychological impact of living with the decisions they had made.

Working with limited resources

Issues in this area included the necessity of having to predict and balance the needs of future patients against those of existing patients in the light of present resources, such as blood and beds, and the dilemmas associated with deciding whether and when to prioritise the needs of coalition forces over those of LNs. Evacuation of patients to the United Kingdom inevitably had to balance clinical need with the availability of capacity to manage potential future casualties.

Conflict between military and professional (clinical) obligations

Upholding *medical rules of eligibility* consistently in the light of clinical *mission creep* remained a challenge throughout the campaigns in both Iraq and Afghanistan. Particularly in the former, clear guidance from the medical CoC was not always provided and was, on occasion, frankly unhelpful. Instructions to decide on the eligibility of each individual patient *after* clinical assessment in the emergency department showed a profound a lack of understanding of medical processes and medical professionals. In addition, frequent changes in eligibility for admission occurred and delay of transfer out of the facility of non-UK or Western coalition forces, including local nationals and locally employed civilians, could be complex whilst discussions regarding eligibility for treatment in the United Kingdom and elsewhere were resolved. Transfers to local medical facilities, which invariably offered more restricted capabilities of care, also produced significant ethical and practical dilemmas. On a similar theme, almost inevitably, the post-war treatment of interpreters became a subject of controversy, contrasting perceived legal and moral obligations.

Decisions regarding end-of-life care

As a number of recent high-profile cases have demonstrated, decisions about withholding or withdrawing potentially life-sustaining interventions are invariably associated with ethical challenges, whatever the clinical context. On deployed operations, decisions of this kind are particularly difficult in two contexts: firstly, the levels of injury at which survivability is possible for local casualties unable to access Western levels of support and rehabilitation are almost certain to be very much lower than for Western nationals; secondly, UK (or other Western) casualties with unsurvivable injuries are thousands of miles from their loved ones, but might survive long enough to get home. In the context of Afghanistan particularly, decisions regarding the continuance of treatment in patients with severe spinal injuries, multiple amputations and major burns inevitably involved an assessment of the likely quality of life for each patient in the light of available local resources and medical capability. On the one hand, whereas life in a wheelchair with urinary incontinence is manageable in the United Kingdom, it is not necessarily compatible with long-term survival in rural Helmand Province. Similarly, the years of physiotherapy and multiple surgical episodes likely to be required after catastrophic burns are not generally available in Afghanistan. At the other end of the spectrum, is it ethically appropriate and a justifiable use of resources to keep someone alive long enough to die at home in the presence of their loved ones?

Patient consent

Informed consent for local national casualties was made more difficult by the almost universal need to communicate via an interpreter and the management of children not infrequently involved disagreements with the child's representatives regarding the child's best interests. These representatives might or might not be parents; often they were "uncles," and clarity about whether they actually held *in-loco parentis* responsibility within that cultural and legal framework was lacking.

Working in multinational contexts

The provision of medical support in both campaigns, but especially in Afghanistan, was complicated by the need to work harmoniously across multinational organisations. Inevitably this had organisational consequences, but more surprisingly, it was found that each nation often had their own way of managing a particular condition. Such points of view might be purely clinical, but potentially had a cultural element also.[4] Avoiding or managing potential conflict was a key role of the DMD.

SUPPORTING ETHICAL DECISION-MAKING

The organisational response to the ethical challenges described previously was significant. This section will discuss the key areas of ethical training and development introduced as a consequence of the increased awareness of ethical issues. The first effect was that ethics became a widely discussed topic within the Defence Medical Services (DMS). The *Annual Ethics Symposium* started in 2010 and became a mainstream forum for the discussion of military medical ethics.[5] The first symposium identified the need for enhanced training in medical ethics as part of *pre-deployment training* (PDT) for all personnel. The foundation of that training needed to be the *law of armed conflict*, but it also needed to cover the common issues that were likely to be encountered. A key area discussed in the first symposium was the dual loyalty of the *physician-soldier*. This conflict between the needs of the CoC and the individual patient, both of whom have claims on the clinician, manifests in several ways, including the subordination of the best interests of individual patients in times of resource constraint (triage and rationing), the need to set medical priorities for military purposes (for example anthrax vaccine), the need to breach confidentiality for reasons of operational effectiveness and the imperative to carry out research on soldiers too ill to consent. The British Medical Association has offered useful guidance in the form of the *Armed Forces Ethics Toolkit* to help support DMS personnel in these challenging situations. It is presented as a series of succinct flash-cards highlighting relevant legislation and guidance with clinical examples.[6]

Exactly where the balance point of these dual loyalties sits is hotly debated. The *World Medical Association* makes it clear that it does not feel that this is an issue and that the ethical priorities of the clinician on operations must remain exactly as they should be in civilian practice. Others argue that the deployed clinician does not have the same autonomy as a civilian practitioner and so cannot

be held to the same standards; Kant's argument is that 'ought' implies 'can' – it is only true that you ought to behave in a certain way if your circumstances mean that you can. If your freedom of action is constrained (for example by resources or lawful orders), then so is your ethical behaviour. Thus, our recognised civilian professional codes might not always be applicable.[7] The debate continues, as some would argue that the constraints of working in the *National Health Service* may sometimes be just as severe.[8]

A formal framework to aid ethical decision-making was also developed and, after presentation at the first ethics symposium, was rolled out to the DMS. It now appears in the *Clinical Guidelines for Operations* (CGO). The *four-quadrant approach*

BOX 20.1: Four-quadrant approach to ethical decision making – some detailed areas of discussion under each section

Medical indications
Physiological futility (no hope of fixing)
Quantitative futility (very unlikely to be able to achieve the medical goal)
Qualitative futility (even if successful the intervention results in an outcome so poor as to be undesirable)

Patient preferences
Who else can consent? What do the family want? Has the patient expressed preferences before?

Quality of life
Anticipated cognitive function
Anticipated physical disabilities
Pain and suffering associated with the disease
Burdens of treatment (originally based on neonates, showing how we are having to extrapolate to previously unimagined territories of injury.[9])

Contextual issues
Resources, law, military orders, impact on others (morale, hearts and minds), local context (including beliefs, culture)

(4QA) is intended to provide a structure that ensures that key ethical issues are addressed, allowing the user to come to a considered decision. It does not give answers, but as Sir Isaiah Berlin said, 'Moral risk cannot, at times, be avoided. All we can ask for is that none of the relevant factors be ignored.' The initial step is the recognition that there actually *is* an ethical dilemma, such as deciding whether to treat someone who cannot survive. Once the dilemma is expressed, the user is taken through the four quadrants considering the medical implications of possible choices, the patient's preferences, the probable subsequent quality of life and finally any relevant contextual factors. The user is prompted to recommend a moral action. The process is designed so that the quadrants are weighted by the order in which they appear.

Use of the 4QA has been featured in PDT since 2010, and its use on deployments has now been studied.[10] It would appear to show considerable value, although the way it is used may still require development, and further research into its use in practise is needed. For example, the study population of users was made up only of male doctors. While there are reports of these decisions being multi-disciplinary (even including non-clinicians such as chaplains), decision making still seems mostly to be undertaken by a small 'elite group' (sometimes referred to as a command huddle) and a wider sense of participation is likely to prove beneficial to staff caring for these complex patients.

The tool itself was felt not to change or necessarily improve decision-making, but instead to add structure to discussions. Unsurprisingly it was felt to add less value when the cases were straightforward. A significant limitation was the fact that the tool assumes that the user has all the necessary knowledge (including patient preferences) and indeed it is said that 'good ethics starts with good facts'.[5] Unfortunately, many of these decisions are made on deployment in a state of considerable ignorance in terms of cultural beliefs, expectations and other local context, such as regional health infrastructure capabilities. Where it was felt to be most useful, however, was when discussing patients in whom survivability was uncertain, when the inequalities of local and military facilities were pronounced and when clinicians disagreed.[10] It should be remembered that the 4QA

was designed to allow decisions to be made about the management of a single patient, not to guide decisions about groups of patients, and so while it had considerable value on *Herrick* and *Telic*, it may not translate so well to all contingency operations.

Ethics is thus firmly established within PDT, occurring on an individual basis at courses such as Military Operational Surgical Training and then tested collectively at HOSPEX. Training has tended to be based around demonstration of the 4QA and discussion of the underlying principles and is now supported by an increasing bank of vignettes of ethical dilemmas from recent deployments.

SEVERELY INJURED AND LOCAL NATIONAL PATIENTS

The extreme nature of some of the injuries seen on these operations has been matched by huge advances in medical capability, the result being a shift in the level of injuries which must now be considered survivable. Situations in which treatment used to be clearly futile are now often considered to offer the potential for salvage. This adaptation of the medical system has had two challenging consequences. Firstly, the 'easy' ethical decisions of the past (including cases of clear survivability or futility) are no longer clear cut. Secondly, the inequalities between the parallel healthcare systems (and outcomes) for servicemen and civilians have become even more pronounced.[11]

These conflicting priorities are perhaps most clearly seen on the intensive care unit.[12] At the best of times, the intensive care unit (ICU) is a scarce resource and requires gatekeeping decisions. These are normally based mainly on a patient's need (*triage*) and their likelihood of responding to treatment (*prognosis*). However, with a limited number of beds in a deployed setting, a new pressure is added – *military necessity and responsibility to the CoC*, the need to keep resources available for future troops who are yet to be wounded, for example. The need for resolution of this dual loyalty has been recognised, and the *International Dual Loyalty Working Group*[13] has published guidelines that confirm that the military medical officer is a doctor first, that civilian ethics apply to military clinicians and that military clinicians should triage and treat the sick and wounded according to their need.

While this stance is clear, there are still two considerable problems for the intensivist, who is perhaps at the centre of such dilemmas. First, the CoC may well be ignorant of it, disagree with it or simply choose to overrule it. Second, a deployed field ICU is designed for a pre-screened, fit population of adults destined to be evacuated in a very short timeframe, potentially only hours. It is not scaled to deliver long-term care and is very heavily focused on simply managing the short-term complications of trauma and infectious diseases. It is not equipped to be able to deliver high-level care to civilians with complex, long-term needs. Aside from receiving less than ideal care, these patients denude the unit's resources at a disproportionate rate. These two issues taken together mean that for LNs needing intensive care, there will come a point where the decision to move them into the local healthcare system becomes a compromise between medical and military necessity. Many longer-term strategic arguments might be made to support these decisions, such as the need to keep the local health system challenged and developing in order to prevent dependency and to stimulate growth towards them independently delivering an acceptable level of care, but the decision remains an ethical one. However, there is a risk that many patients will die in the short term, to stimulate the system to save more in the long term. The palatable solutions to these problems in future will be linked to how we engage with and develop LN health services, preparing them to take on this work load early in the campaign.

Even with our own personnel, for whom the ICU is designed, there are difficult ethical questions. Much has been made of whether it is right to keep servicemen alive, even though they are almost certain to die soon, so that they can make it home to be seen by their families.[14] In this situation, we have to consider the British Medical Association guidance[15] regarding prolonging life after unsurvivable injuries. They state that 'when medical treatment ceases to provide a net benefit to the patient...the justification for intervening is gone'. Other factors in this equation include (as discussed earlier) the fact that increasing survivability has made prognostication harder. There is no formal process within the UK military to allow for *advance directives* by which military clinicians could definitely understand patients' wishes before they were severely wounded. Even if there were, it is difficult to accept that views expressed in advance by young men going into battle would necessarily reflect their considered opinion in the event of life-threatening or life-changing injury.

Under the principle of *non-maleficence* (doing no harm), we must, in this context, include risks to aircrew and other personnel as a result of additional missions in a contested environment. The principle of doing no harm to the patient also forces us to consider the risks of remaining in a resource-constrained theatre of war, rather than accessing the comprehensive services available at a UK Major Trauma Centre. Finally, it is difficult to gauge what each patient's *quality of life* will be after these potentially devastating injuries. Rehabilitation medicine has also been moving forwards at a remarkable rate, and quality of life cannot be assessed until after the patient has stabilised and ideally been at least partially rehabilitated; in many cases this may be months after injury. These assessments are certainly far too subjective to be made in a war zone.

MAJOR INCIDENT MANAGEMENT

While *Operations Herrick* and *Telic* forced us to explore further the ethics of treating individuals under operational conditions, they also generated many situations in which multiple casualties occurred. As a result, our understanding of how we manage mass casualty situations has also evolved. Examples have been described in both the land and maritime environments.[16–18] It has been demonstrated that, in general, our processes are broadly fit for purpose. The areas discussed here in which recent deployed experience has led to significant improvements are *command and control, triage* and *mass casualty analgesia*.

Command and control

Command and control of the *front door* of any medical facility has been shown over and over again to be a critical component of the effective management of a multiple casualty incident. In the Role 1 context, this function may be performed by a combat medical technician – the

Battlefield Advanced Trauma Life Support course ensures that all CMTs are taught the principles of the triage sieve.[16] For larger incidents managed at a Role 3 hospital, this *triage* role has traditionally been performed by an experienced clinician[17] as at this stage, the decisions being made are potentially more complex. This was particularly pronounced at sea[18,19] – *RFA Argus* does not allow much flexibility once the patient has started their journey down in the lifts from the receiving flight deck to the *medical treatment facility* (MTF) below. The ability to exert complete control over the movement of personnel was deemed absolutely critical, and it was recommended that the person overseeing triage should have a complete understanding of how triage is done, of the medical treatments that might be ongoing concurrently and, most importantly, of the capability and state of readiness of each part of the MTF. This skill set is not widely available and it was deemed that the most senior emergency department nurse was probably best placed to perform it. Modelling of the impact of patients arriving in small groups ('by the Chinook load') on an MTF would seem to support the need for this level of experience since decisions made prior to the distribution of the patients have critical impacts on the performance of different triage tools.[20]

Triage

One major incident, involving 19 casualties at the Role 3 facility in Camp Bastion, Afghanistan 2010, started a research thread looking into the accuracy of triage systems. The author's experience of this incident (where formal triage was undertaken exactly according to the established protocols in every case, as there was a high level of staffing that day) was that the available systems performed poorly in predicting the sickest casualties. This resulted in an emergency department thoracotomy being performed on a casualty identified as a T2 priority and the first casualty taken to theatre also being categorised as a T2. Retrospective analysis of the *Joint Theatre Trauma Registry* strongly suggested that performance was unacceptably poor with a sensitivity of approximately 55% for patients who needed immediate life-saving intervention.[21] This concept of resource-based analysis of triage

was further developed over prospective studies and also retrospectively using a large civilian trauma data-base.[22] All the results are consistent: namely that our physiological triage systems do not perform as well as we would like, reassuringly perhaps, nor do the systems used elsewhere (for example the *START* system used in the United States).

Research is ongoing to try to both to optimise the physiological parameters of the tools we have in order to improve their performance and also to identify the most accurate mechanistic and anatomical marker that might be combined with the patient's physiology to develop a tool that is more effective. An example is the addition of a level of consciousness assessment to the *Triage Sieve* in the 2011 edition of the *CGOs*. During the evolution of the CGOs across the *Operation Herrick* years, the presence of a tourniquet (an anatomical marker of severity) was successfully added as a T1 defining criterion.

In terms of what we know about physiology, reducing the range of normal for respiratory rate (so that normal is considered to be 12–24 rather than 10–30) seems to have the single biggest impact.[23] Reducing the upper limit of the heart rate as well is also effective but results in much lower sensitivities. An area of promise is the *Shock Index* (*heart rate divided by systolic blood pressure*), which has been shown to be a useful predictor of the need for life-saving intervention in general (sensitivity and specificity around 70%)[24] and also of the need for surgical intervention for life-threatening torso trauma.[25] As a result, the *Shock Index* has been proposed as part of a first-line triage tool once the patient arrives at an MTF.

The use of the patient's triage category as a marker simply of the severity of his* injury has become commonplace, in other words, not to prioritise them against other casualties (they may in fact be the only one) but to warn receiving facilities that they are indeed very unwell (if T1) or relatively stable (if classed as T2 or T3). This equates to what is commonly referred to as *field triage* in

---

* Throughout this book the term his (rather than *his or hers*) has been chosen for ease of reading and because the casualties were very largely male. It is entirely accepted that there were female casualties at all stages of the conflict.

the United Kingdom, a process that can be used to determine whether an individual casualty has to go to a *major trauma centre* or whether they can safely go to a less capable facility such as a *trauma unit*. Although the desire to use the *Triage Sieve* in this way this can be clearly understood, the tools are far too simplistic compared with the processes used in the United Kingdom, and they do not perform well enough to be of significant value in this context.

Major incident analgesia

Inevitably, a major incident is likely to produce large numbers of casualties requiring rapid access to analgesia. Features particular to this environment, including the need to avoid complex and detailed administrative processes and a likely inability to offer detailed and continuous observation, mean that specific solutions are required. Novel methods of battlefield analgesia have been developed and fortunately have been shown to be very effective in major incidents. Perhaps the most obvious is the *fentanyl lozenge*,[16] which would seem ideal as a treatment modality for T2 and T3 casualties. The *Medical Emergency Response Team* also successfully used intranasal fentanyl and ketamine to good effect.

CONSENT AND RECORD KEEPING

Our ability to effectively utilise interpreters has matured through experience, but there are still problems associated with consent and the proper identification of patients, especially in the context of a multiple casualty event. One innovative method that has been explored is the use of pictorial identification and consent, using pictures in the notes, supporting the use of an interpreter, to explain what is proposed and also later as a final patient identity check immediately prior to the start of surgery.[26]

POST-MORTEM IMAGING

Post-mortem imaging has become an important means of establishing a permanent record of injuries sustained, especially in multiple casualty scenarios, or on operations when conventional post-mortem is culturally inappropriate or simply not available. This is critically important for the coroner or equivalent legal process in that country and also allows research to reduce the impact of such incidents in future.[27]

SUPPORT TO HUMANITARIAN OPERATIONS

Long-term exposure to populations in need while the security situation remains unstable has led to a resurgence of interest in the value of military interventions to support humanitarian operations. Local populations may not discriminate between organisations delivering aid based entirely on humanitarian principles and military assistance. Even governments may not truly understand the distinction, with US Secretary Colin Powell stating in 2001 that 'I am serious about making sure we have the best relationship with the NGOs who are such a force multiplier for us, such an important part of our combat team'.[28] This perception that military forces should engage in humanitarian-type operations to improve stability became widely held around the early years of the campaigns in Iraq and Afghanistan, and as a result, *MEDCAPs* (*Medical Civic Action Plans*) became a tool in every commander's arsenal to promote local goodwill and support – winning *hearts and minds*. These were easy to justify, as under the Geneva Conventions, there is a duty of any occupying force 'to ensure sufficient hygiene and public health standards, as well as the provision of food and medical care to the population under occupation…to the fullest extent of the means available to it'.[29]

Hodgetts et al.[30] reviewed the current literature regarding military humanitarianism and found that the term was essentially a misnomer. The motives for military support to the local population are never the same as those of humanitarian organisations whose principles are of *neutrality, impartiality, independence* and *humanity*.

This blurring of the lines between military personnel and humanitarian personnel has recently been more widely recognised as a threat, serving to worsen the security of the humanitarian organisations and to reduce their freedom of movement in the *humanitarian space*. It has been proposed that military humanitarianism be dropped as a term, and if activities are undertaken to facilitate, for example, access to humanitarian supplies, that these be referred to as *Medical Support to Humanitarian Operations*.

Bulstrode noted in 2009 that there was capacity in the DMS to provide some forms of assistance to the local population in all but most kinetic areas and that there was a vacuum from the near or complete collapse of local healthcare infrastructure immediately post fighting that commanders might feel there was a moral pressure to fill.[31] However, he also noted that there had been a change in mindset, from a strong pressure to undertake these activities to a much more hands-off approach. There were several reasons for this, including conflict between the pre-requisites for meaningful interventions and the security risks posed by the kinds of relationships needed to undertake them, and the obvious fact that humanitarian programmes need to be sustainable and integrated and to form part of a longer-term engagement strategy. Successful programmes are typically driven by the needs and wishes of the local community. An example of how this conflicts with the needs of the military operation occurs when the legitimate fear that pattern-setting behaviour would put personnel at risk means that clinics or distribution points are positioned in areas of security (such as forward operating bases), not of need, such as within villages.

Lack of resourcing, in terms of cultural awareness, training, access to interpreters, chaperones and training in tropical and 'third world' medicine, also negatively impacts on such programmes. Now the clinic is not only distant from the need, but the staff cannot communicate effectively with the patients, are likely to make cultural *faux-pas* or underestimate the significance of cultural norms in terms of suitable treatment options and have limited experience of and capability for managing the presenting conditions.

Perceptions of armed forces are also invariably coloured by previous experience of the military amongst those caught up in conflict. Trust is relatively easily lost, but much harder to win back, and people's attitude to those in uniform *must* be understood in the light of earlier interactions with others in uniform, including militias.

These key constraints on the value of the MEDCAPs do not even touch on the impacts on other actors in the area. As has been mentioned, humanitarians are dependent on the local perception of their neutrality and independence to keep them safe. The negative impact of political misinformation programmes on the polio eradication programme in Pakistan demonstrates this perfectly. More than 60 polio workers have been killed since the Taliban banned immunisation in 2012. The ban was in response to allegations that the Central Intelligence Agency had set up a fake hepatitis vaccination programme in the area as part of their attempts to find Osama Bin Laden.[32] In the modern era of 24-hour news and with the prevalence of social media worldwide, it is critical that DMS personnel understand the impact that association (real or perceived) with the military can have on non-governmental organisation personnel.

Another, often forgotten, effect of the MEDCAP is that it physically draws patients to the new facility. These patients are coming from somewhere else, be it a local private healthcare centre or a village traditional healer. In either case, when the facility is open, there is an economic impact on the region, as well as the issue of the effects of withdrawal of a usually more advanced facility when the MTF is withdrawn. The effects on the local health infrastructure may be direct, such as loss of income for the nearby clinic, or indirect, as was seen during *Operation Herrick* with qualified clinicians earning more as interpreters and facilitators.

More recent evidence further emphasises these concerns, suggesting that the *hearts and minds* benefits of MEDCAPs are at best limited and transient – they do not result in meaningful improvements in the health and livelihoods of supported communities.[33] *Medical seminars* have been proposed as an alternative model, concentrating far more on education around proven public health interventions rather than direct delivery of care. Unfortunately, the immediate benefits of this kind of intervention are rarely visible or quantifiable, especially on shorter operations. As such, the inevitable desire of the CoC to be seen to be doing good with under-utilised assets and to consider MEDCAPs is likely to persist.

MEDICAL SUPPORT TO CAPTURED PERSONS[34]

Operations in Iraq and Afghanistan have produced significant changes in the way troops are trained to manage *captured persons*, and medical care has been no exception. Historically, captured persons were clearly identified and managed in accordance with the rules of the *Geneva Conventions*. Recent operations have been conducted against an enemy indistinguishable from the civilian population and who may not follow the established rules of war. On the other hand, in counterinsurgency warfare, the captured person may indeed be a civilian bystander, innocent of any crime, simply unlucky enough to be in the wrong place at the wrong time. Increased media and international scrutiny, and a number of well-publicised incidents in which care of captured persons fell below the standards expected, have driven a much tighter regime for the management of captured persons. The United Kingdom has legal obligations to captured persons, which are monitored by international organisations such as the *International Committee of the Red Cross*.

The medical requirements of captured persons have also evolved, as conflict is increasingly conducted within the civilian population. The chronic medical conditions of the older age group, along with the specific needs of women, adolescents and even children, must be considered. The use of internment in Iraq meant that captured persons were held for extended periods and UK Forces were responsible for their ongoing care during their captivity.

In situations where medical resources are limited, the care of captured persons can be even more challenging. The principle usually adhered to is that captured persons are entitled to the same standard of medical care as would be afforded to UK personnel in theatre. In emergency care, the situation is clear, and captured persons should be managed solely according to medical need. But while complex conditions in deployed UK troops are normally managed with evacuation to the United Kingdom, this may not be an option open to captured persons. Specific consideration needs to be paid to this area during planning. There will undoubtedly be cases where specific judgement calls are required, with command and medical staff in discussion to reach a solution. This will have to balance meeting legal and ethical obligations to the captured persons with the practicalities of theatre capabilities and the legal issues involved in evacuation to a third nation.

For the medical staff, providing care to captured persons has personal challenges. As in previous conflicts, there is a moral tension in providing medical care to the enemy. While the protective emblems of the Geneva Conventions were once almost universally respected, this is no longer the case, and in some instances, medical staff have been specifically targeted. This can lead to clinicians being required to care for individuals who have, until recently, been attempting to kill them. This requires careful management by medical commanders, in order to ensure that the culture of the medical facilities is one that ensures correct treatment, regardless of previous actions.

Interrogation of captured persons may produce information of considerable value to UK forces. Whilst this is a legitimate aim, it is essential that safeguards are in place to ensure the welfare of those being interrogated. The use by US forces of *Behavioural Science Consultation Teams*, which included trained clinicians who used their knowledge to extract information from captured persons, was criticised by the *American Psychological Association*. Clinicians should be free to act solely to provide medical care and must remain separate from the interrogation process. Likewise, they should be encouraged to raise concerns if they feel that an interrogation technique may be harming the health of a captured person.

The *DMS* have introduced specific training to cover this area, and those involved in detention operations have also significantly improved the level of training received. This increased mutual understanding of the standards expected is key to ensuring the correct treatment from both medical and detaining teams. The medical care given to captured persons does produce practical and ethical challenges. That said, the underpinning medical ethics are unchanged, and the core of any decision-making process about detained persons must be that, regardless of any actions they may have committed, they are human beings and are entitled to receive the best attentions that medical staff can provide.

CONCLUSION

The nature and scale of UK military operations in Iraq and Afghanistan have produced many ethical and humanitarian challenges. Most have been effectively and sensitively managed; some have not. The management of captured persons has been reviewed in the glare of media attention and, at least on occasion, has been found wanting. Ethical conundrums that were once managed in private are now subject to the twenty-first century's near universal media attention. Such attention may, on occasion, be ill-informed, prejudicial or unaware of the complexities of the situation. The result is that as well as being potential areas where clinicians are compelled to make difficult decisions, and where there is no *right answer*, commanders and politicians have to be more aware than ever of the moral implications of the actions of those they send into conflict. They also have to recognise that absolute openness is the only sensible course in the event of events occurring, which, for one reason or another, fall short of acceptable standards.

As a result of their recent experience, the UK DMS are probably more aware of, and better prepared for, the ethical challenges they are likely to meet than at any time the recent past. What is equally certain is that every future conflict will present ethical problems that had not been predicted at the start of the campaign.

REFERENCES

1. Mahoney P, Hodgetts TJ, Hicks I. The deployed medical director: Managing the challenges of a complex trauma system. *J R Army Med Corps* 2011;157(3 Suppl 1): S350–S356.
2. Bricknell MCM, Beardmore CE, Williamson RHB. The deployed medical director: Managing the challenges of a complex trauma system. *J R Army Med Corps* 2012;158(1):66.
3. Bernthal EM, Draper HJA, Henning J, Kelly JC. "A band of brothers" – An exploration of the range of medical ethical issues faced by British senior military clinicians on deployment to Afghanistan: A qualitative study. *J R Army Med Corps* 2017;163(3):199–205.
4. Cordell RF. Multinational medical support to operations: Challenges, benefits and recommendations for the future. *J R Army Med Corps* 2012;158(1):22–28.
5. O'Reilly DJ. Proceedings of the DMS ethics symposium. *J R Army Med Corps* 157(4): 405–410.
6. *Ethical Decision Making for Doctors in the Armed Forces. Guidance from the BMA Medical Ethics Committee and Armed Forces Committee.* London: British Medical Association, 2012.
7. Kell J. Following professional codes of practice and military orders in austere environments: A controversial debate on ethical challenges. *J R Army Med Corps* 2015: 161(Suppl 10):i10–i12.
8. Ross DA, Wiliamson RHB Commentary on: Following professional codes of practice and military orders in austere military environments: A controversial debate on ethical challenges. *J R Army Med Corps* 2015;161(Supp 1):i13.
9. Lantos JD, Meadow WL. *Neonatal Bioethics: The Moral Challenges of Medical Innovation.* Baltimore, MD: The Johns Hopkins University Press, 2006.
10. Bernthal EM, Russell RJ, Draper HJA. A qualitative study of the use of the four quadrant approach to assist ethical decision-making during deployment. *J R Army Med Corps* 2014;160(2):196–202.
11. Sokol DK. The medical ethics of the battlefield. *BMJ* 2011;343(3):d3877.
12. Henning J. The ethical dilemma of providing intensive care treatment to local civilians on operations. *J R Army Med Corps* 2009;155(2);84–86.
13. Physicians for Human Rights and the School of Public Health and Primary Health Care University of Cape Town, Health Sciences Faculty. *Dual Loyalty & Human Rights in Health Professional Practice; Proposed Guidelines & Institutional Mechanisms.* 2002. https:// s3.amazonaws.com/PHR_Reports /dualloyalties-2002-report.pdf.
14. Bennett RA. Ethics surrounding the medical evacuation of catastrophically injured

individuals from an operational theatre of war. *J R Army Med Corps* 2016;162(5): 321–323.

15. *End of Life Decisions*. London: British Medical Association, 2009.

16. Reynolds ND, Dalal S. An account of multiple casualties in an austere environment. *J R Army Med Corps* 2012;158(3):181–185.

17. Vassallo DJ. Gerlinger T. Maholtz P et al. Combined UK/US Field Hospital management of a major incident arising from a Chinook helicopter crash in Afghanistan, 28 Jan 2002. *J R Army Med Corps* 2003; 149(1):47–52.

18. Coetzee RH. HMS Ark Royal and the 2003 helicopter crash in the Northern Arabian Gulf. *J R Nav Med Serv* 2010;96(2):96–102.

19. Evans GWL. Receiving mass casualties at sea: The capabilities of the primary casualty receiving facility. *J R Nav Med Serv* 2004;90(2):51–56.

20. Horne ST, Vassallo J. Triage in the Defence Medical Services. *J R Army Med Corps* 2015;161(2):90–93. jramc-2014-000275.

21. Horne S, Vassallo J, Read J et al. UK triage – An improved tool for an evolving threat. *Injury* 2013;44:23–28.

22. Smith JE, Vassallo J. The civilian validation of the Modified Physiological Triage Tool (MPTT): An evidence-based approach to primary major incident triage. *Emerg Med J* 2017;34:810–815.

23. Vassallo SLJ, Horne ST, Ball S, Whitley LJ. UK triage: The validation of a new tool to counter an evolving threat. *Injury* 2014; 45(12):2071–2075.

24. Vassallo J, Horne ST, Ball S, Smith J. Usefulness of the Shock Index as a secondary triage tool. *J R Army Med Corps* 2014;161(1):53–57.

25. Morrison J, Dickson E, Jansen JO, Midwinter M. Utility of admission physiology in the surgical triage of isolated ballistic battlefield torso trauma. *J Emerg Trauma Shock* 2012;5(3):233–237.

26. Matheson AS, Howes RD, Midwinter MJ, Lambert AW. Surgery in an Afghan population: Is pictorial consent and injury pattern recognition identification of patients appropriate? *J R Nav Med Serv* 2010;96(3):158–164.

27. Gibb I, Denton E. Guidelines for the use of computed tomography (CT) in the postmortem – Investigation of deaths in a mass casualty scenario. NHS Improvements. June 2011.

28. Secretary Colin L Powell. Remarks to the National Foreign Policy Conference for Leaders of Nongovernmental Organisations. Washington, DC, 26 October 2001. Avalon.law.yale.edu /spet11/powell_brief31.asp.

29. Convention (IV) respecting the laws and Customs of War on Land and its annex: Regulations concerning the Laws and customs of war on land. The Hague Regulations, 18 October 1907 (arts 27–34, 42–56 and 47–78).

30. Hodgetts T, Mahoney PF, Mozumder A, McLennan J. Care of Civilians during operations *Int J Disaster Med* 2005;3:3–24.

31. Bulstrode C. MEDCAPs – do they work? *J R Army Med Corps* 2009;155(3):182–184.

32. McGirk T. How the bin Laden raid put vaccinators under the gun in Pakistan. *National Geographic*. 2015. http://news.national geographic.com/2015/02/150225-polio -pakistan-vaccination-virus-health/.

33. Cameron E. Do no harm – The limitations of civilian medical outreach and MEDCAP programmes based in Afghanistan. *J R Army Med Corps* 2011;157:3 209–211.

34. Moy RJ. Ethical dilemmas in providing medical care to captured persons on operations. *J R Army Med Corps* 158(1):6–9; with a commentary by RMC McNeil-Love.

21

Deployed experience at sea

INTRODUCTION

The Royal Navy played a key role in the assault on the Al Faw Peninsula conducted by *3 Commando Brigade* on 20–21 March 2003.[1] Secondary objectives were to ensure the safe transit of personnel and equipment by sea and the sustainment of joint forces both afloat and ashore. Royal Navy vessels controlled and maintained defined shipping lanes as well as providing physical protection to vessels in transit. Ships and submarines also served to provide a launch capacity for ordnance and personnel in support of land operations. The size of the deployment, the nature of providing medical care at sea and the variable operational estimates all posed considerable challenges in the planning and implementation of medical care during *Operation Telic* (Figure 21.1).

Following the conflict, at the request of the Iraqi Government, the Royal Navy continued to train the Iraqi Navy to defend her territorial waters and offshore oil infrastructure. British forces working with the US Navy were involved in training and mentoring Iraqi sailors and marines at their main naval base in Umm Qasr until 2011.[2] At the time of writing, Royal Navy vessels and medical personnel continue to maintain a presence in the Persian Gulf. The day-to-day medical work that has continued since 2003 is routine practice for the men and women of the *Royal Navy Medical Services* (RNMS) and will not be further considered in this chapter.

The Royal Navy also contributed to personnel, equipment and expertise in support of operations in Afghanistan. While Afghanistan's geography does not lend itself to maritime operations, Royal Naval medical and support staff have routinely deployed on land alongside the Royal Marines, Army and Royal Air Force (RAF) in support of *Operation Herrick*. On 20 April 2010, *HMS Albion* returned 450 service personnel (including soldiers from *33 Field Hospital*) to the United Kingdom after they were stranded in mainland Europe when volcanic ash from *Eyjafjallajökull* volcano grounded flights for several days.[3] However, this chapter will concentrate on the deployed experience at sea gained during *Operation Telic*, and particularly the first roulement.

DEPLOYED CAPABILITY

A total of 78 vessels, including 16 major Royal Navy and Royal Fleet Auxiliary (RFA) ships, travelled over 5000 miles from the United Kingdom to the Persian Gulf. A great number of the remaining Royal Navy and RFA ships were engaged in escort duties along the route and supported the logistical supply chain, transporting some 9100 ISO containers. The size and nature of the deployment and the distance from home made for a challenging period of medical planning.

In March 2003, the *Operation Telic Naval Task Force*, with standard medical staffing, consisted of the following:

- *HMS Ark Royal* (aircraft carrier), serving as the Flag Ship, operational command and Role 2 Afloat and carrying a general practitioner (GP), chief petty officer medical assistant (CPOMA), petty officer medical assistant (POMA), leading medical assistant (LMA), laboratory technician, three medical assistants (MAs), general duties medical officer (GDMO), dental officer, and leading seaman dental assistant. The R2A

470

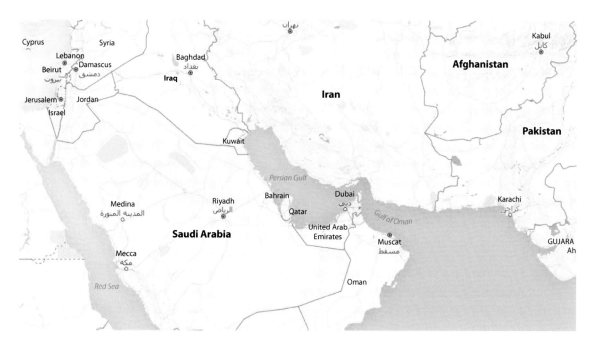

Figure 21.1 Area of operations for *Operation Telic.*

also included an additional POMA, surgeon and anaesthetist.

- *HMS Ocean* (helicopter carrier), carrying a GP, CPOMA, POMA, LMA, and two MAs.
- *HMS Liverpool, HMS Edinburgh* and *HMS York* (Type 42 Destroyers), each with an LMA or POMA and a GDMO.
- *HMS Marlborough* and HMS Richmond (Type 23 Frigates), each with an LMA or POMA and GDMO.
- *HMS Grimsby and HMS Ledbury* (Minehunters), each having a coxswain with additional medical training and access to a limited formulary,
- *RFA Argus* (Aviation Training Ship and Role 3 Afloat), with a GDMO or GP and medical technician (MT), as well as the R3A, which, at full 100-bed capacity, had 24 consultants, 10 registrars, 2 senior house officers, 75 nurses, 32 MAs and 42 Royal Marines Bandsmen.
- *RFA Sir Tristram, RFA Sir Galahad* and *RFA Sir Percivale* (landing ships logistic), each carrying an MT and, if carrying over 100 personnel on board, a GDMO.
- *RFA Fort Austin, RFA Fort Victoria* and *RFA Fort Rosalie* (replenishment ships), each with

an MT and, when carrying over 100 personnel on board, a GDMO.

- *RFA Orangeleaf* (support tanker), carrying an MT and, when carrying over 100 personnel on board, a GDMO
- Fleet submarine with an LMA Submarine [SM], MA (SM) and a GDMO.

Some 14 other Royal Navy and RFA vessels were also involved in the operation to a lesser extent, including *HMS Chatham, HMS Brocklesby* and *HMS Blyth*, which were assigned to the enforcement of United Nations sanctions.

The amphibious force numbered approximately 4000 personnel and included *HQ 3 Commando Brigade, 40 Commando Royal Marines* staff and *42 Commando Royal Marines*, each with embedded RM and Royal Navy medical staff. There were also helicopter air groups aboard *HMS Ark Royal* and *HMS Ocean.*

Operation Telic consisted of 14 roulements (starting March 2003 with *Operation Telic 1* and continuing until *Operation Telic 13*, ending in April 2009). The maritime deployment schedules did not follow the same rotational timelines as land forces, whose subsequent deployments continued until full operational withdrawal in May 2011.

NATURE OF THE CAPABILITY

The sick and wounded are perishable cargo; whether they survive or die is fundamentally affected by the speed with which they are given medical care.... Even those with potentially salvageable wounds may die or, if they survive, may experience serious complicated disabilities if treatment is not correctly timed. In essence, delay in treatment due to evacuation lag is tantamount to denial of care...delayed application of treatment to initially simple wounds can facilitate their conversion into complex, infected, and often life-threatening problems.

–The Triangle of Death, Medical Sustainability in Expeditionary Sea-Based Operations[4]

Role 1 (Primary Care) Afloat (R1A)

The medical manning on board ships and submarines is varied and reflects the embarked population, deployed role and anticipated risks. The basic considerations for all deployments are founded on a strategy of risk identification, assessment and mitigation. By the nature of sea travel, most Royal Naval deployments will result in personnel being far from land and support and having to function, at least for a period, in isolation. In order to reduce the risks of deployment, medical screening is used to identify potential issues and manage them early. The number and skill set of embarked medical staff will again depend on the population, deployed role and anticipated risks. In certain circumstances, operational restrictions may be advised to Command if the appropriate medical capability is not embarked.

Specific anticipated risks for *Operation Telic* included possible enemy use of biological and chemical weapons, use of nuclear and radiological (dirty) weapons, prolonged deployment with a difficult and uncertain supply chain, heat-related illness, infectious gastroenteritis, enemy action using conventional weapons, damage to vessels from floating or submerged mines, contact with local nationals (LNs) or prisoners of war (POWs) and other *disease and nonbattle injury* (DNBI).

There is no central record of all the visits to sickbays during *Operation Telic*, and as such, it is difficult to quantify with any certainty the day-to-day work carried out by MAs and medical officers. No ships were lost and no casualties were sustained from enemy attack at sea. Much of the work is likely to have involved primary care (DNBI), maintaining hygiene standards (public health), promoting primary prevention (occupational health) and ongoing training for both the medical staff and the ship's company. Medical staff aboard ships and deployed with the Royal Marine had access to senior medical advice from within the flotilla (via the Senior Medical Officer (SMO) aboard *HMS Ark Royal* acting as the medical advisor to the UK Maritime Commander or from *UK Fleet Headquarters*.

Role 2 Afloat (R2A)

HMS Ark Royal had a *Role 2 Afloat* (R2A) capability embarked in addition to the ship's regular medical officer (a substantive GP). The embarked R2A facility consisted of a surgeon and anaesthetist (both consultants at OF4 level) and an *operating department practitioner*. The scrub nurse position in the afloat surgical team was filled by the ship's medical department POMA. The latter's primary role on board was to run the stores and pharmacy, ensuring that all embarked equipment remained in date for the duration of the deployment.

The capacity in 2003 was 1/1/1 (one resuscitation bay, one operating theatre table and one Level 3 intensive care unit [ICU] bed) with a further eight ward beds in a 4×2 bunk configuration. The R2A capability would have quickly become overwhelmed dealing with more than two severely injured people at any one time and would have required full support from the ship's medical staff. Blood stocks were held on board and an *emergency donor panel* (EDP) had been organised for use if required. These blood products would not have allowed modern day damage control resuscitation. During *Operation Telic*, no surgical work was performed at the R2A.

At 0430 on 22 March 2003, two Royal Navy Sea King helicopters belonging to *849 Squadron* based on *HMS Ark Royal* collided in mid-air. All seven crewmen on board the two helicopters lost their lives in this incident. The recovery of their bodies and the psychological burden on the crew required the assistance of the medical department.[5]

Role 3 Afloat (R3A)

During *Operation Telic*, all UK maritime surgical work took place aboard *RFA Argus*. *RFA Argus*, the UK's *Primary Casualty Receiving Facility* (PCRF) (Figure 21.2–21.5) was originally requisitioned as *MV Contender Bezant* in 1982 for the Falklands Conflict, when she transported supplies including helicopters and Sea Harriers to the South Atlantic. In 1984, she was purchased for £18 million and converted to an aviation training ship. The PCRF infrastructure was created prior to *Operation Granby* (First Gulf Conflict), with one of the hangars being used as space for a number of interconnecting Portakabins®, which made up the hospital.

Following *Operation Granby*, at the next ship infrastructure upgrade, the Portakabins® were replaced with a steel integral hospital facility, giving the medical capability used for *Operation Telic*.[6] This enhanced capability could, at full capacity, accommodate 100 beds in the format 4/4/10/20/70 layout (four resuscitation bays/four operating theatre tables/10 Level 3 ICU beds/20 Level 2 high dependency unit beds/70 Level 1 ward beds). *RFA Argus* is not marked with a red cross and is colloquially termed a 'grey hull' (Figure 21.3). Her additional roles include acting as a helicopter training vessel and her armament precludes protection or limitation by article two of the *Geneva Convention* outlining the laws of armed conflict. The specialised equipment carried aboard *RFA Argus* included the only computed tomography (CT) scanner in theatre, an image intensifier and laboratory facilities including equipment for an EDP.

RFA Argus sailed with the *Naval Task Force* as an R3A platform from the United Kingdom on 15 January 2003 with a limited number of the R3A medical team already embarked. The full R3A medical team complement embarked in Oman whilst *RFA Argus* was in transit to the Gulf. After several exercises in the southern Gulf, *RFA Argus* was declared operational and ready to receive casualties on 17 February 2003. As the conflict progressed and the frontline moved further inland, *RFA Argus* was withdrawn on 11 April and on 20 May 2003, she returned to Gibraltar.

When fully manned, 43 medical officers, 94 nurses and a number of allied health professionals staffed the R3A. They worked under the maritime operational command of the PCRF's Medical Officer in Charge (MOIC) and the ship's Captain (an RFA officer). While men and women of the R3A were under the clinical operational command of the MOIC and under strategic command of the SMO aboard *HMS Ark Royal*, the position of *RFA Argus* was at all times at the discretion of the ship's Captain, following orders from the Maritime Force Commander.

The PCRF was designed to be environmentally secure with an airtight citadel capable of sealing those working inside the vessel from the external environment. When tested, the pressure produced was not sufficient to form an airtight compartment; instead, a series of filtered air pumps allowed a slightly positive pressure to be created, reducing any potentially contaminated air ingress. Contaminated or potentially contaminated patients were not permitted to be transported to *RFA Argus* until they had undergone full decontamination ashore.

Resupply to *RFA Argus* was by sea from one of the RFA support vessels. Any urgent supplies or equipment requiring dispatch from the United Kingdom were delivered by rotary wing from Kuwait. The standard evacuation chain for injured United Kingdom personnel was via rotary wing to Kuwait and then via fixed wing to the *Royal Centre for Defence Medicine*, then based at Selly Oak Hospital, Birmingham. During the initial and most intense phase of *Operation Telic*, some use was made of the Princess Mary Hospital at *RAF Akrotiri* in Cyprus, prior to definitive repatriation to the United Kingdom.[7]

The Royal Navy and US Navy worked closely at sea, with similarities in working practices and doctrine. *RFA Argus* was linked to a sea-based hospital trauma network known as the *Navy Afloat Trauma*

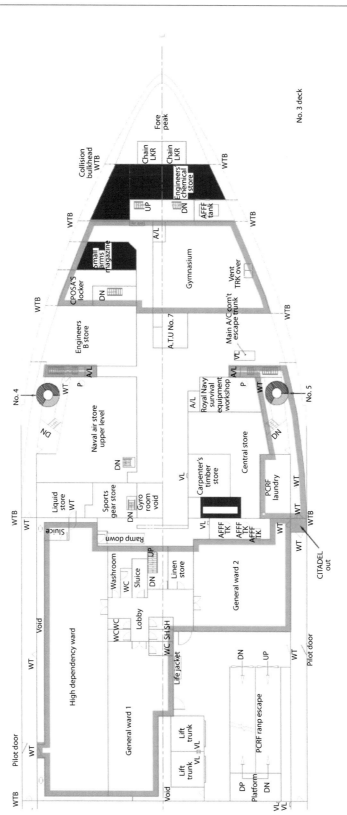

Figure 21.2 (a and b) Layout of Primary Casualty Receiving Facility. The space limitations are evident from these plans. (Continued)

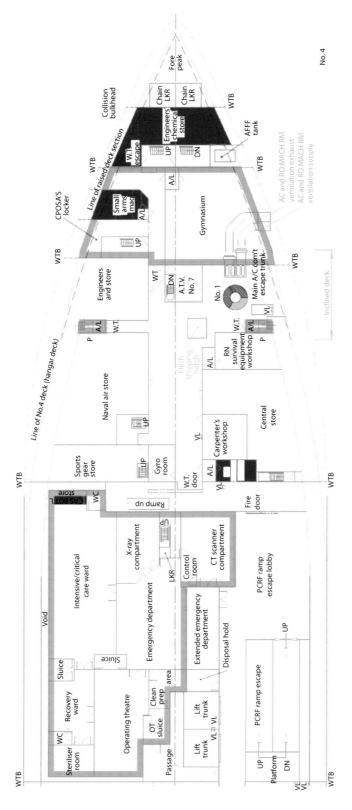

Figure 21.2 (Continued) (a and b) Layout of Primary Casualty Receiving Facility. The space limitations are evident from these plans.

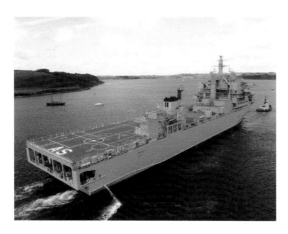

Figure 21.3 *RFA Argus*. Note that the vessel does not bear a red cross.

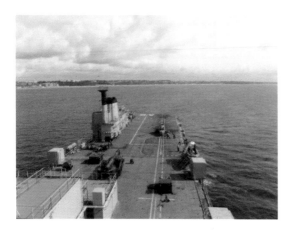

Figure 21.4 Flight deck on *RFA Argus*.

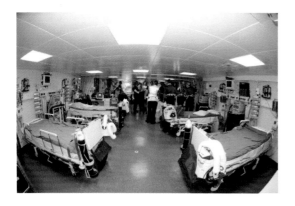

Figure 21.5 ICU on *RFA Argus*.

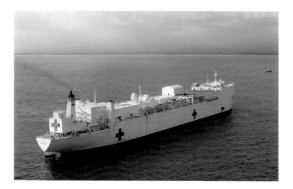

Figure 21.6 *USNS Comfort*.

System (NATS). NATS was designed to maximise efficient use of the total bed capacity afloat and in turn to support military operations up to 100 km inland. The use of the NATS was coordinated by an emergency call system known as RAMPART. Casualties could be triaged centrally and directed to the most appropriate medical care facility. The pooling of allied assets created a total of 12 surgical teams across the fleet, with the ability to continuously receive and manage casualties. In total, there were 120 Level 2 and 3 beds, with a further 1500 Level 1 beds available within the NATS network.[7]

Role 4 Afloat (R4A)

The US Navy deployed the *USNS Comfort* (Figure 21.6) to the Persian Gulf to serve as an afloat trauma centre in support of *Operation Iraqi Freedom*. *USNS Comfort's* staff treated approximately 600 patients, performing 590 surgical procedures and transfusing more than 600 units of blood.[7]

ORGANISATIONAL CHALLENGES

Standardised joint doctrine outlines many of the challenges posed by providing medical operational support in the maritime environment. The current version is very similar to that extant in 2003 and is entitled *Allied Joint Doctrine for Medical Support*.[8] The maritime chapter can be found in Section 1.3.3. A number of important elements of the provision of medical capability in the maritime environment are identified. Ships and, therefore, casualties and medical facilities are mobile and often work within a large area of operation (AO); as a consequence, medical plans must be flexible to allow for this. In the Persian Gulf, this was in part mitigated by the use of NATS to allow maximal coordinated medical coverage to the AO.

Many of the plans and modules designed to work on land will not be suitable for the maritime environment. This was highlighted by the crew of the R3A, who found modular resupply to be unnecessary and cumbersome. When trying to replace individual pieces of equipment, the delivery of a complete replacement module when space is already at premium is unhelpful. External factors such as the weather can alter the risks of injury, hamper the evacuation response and dictate the level of deliverable care. Unlike the land environment, all equipment at sea must be secured to prevent movement in high sea states. Secure stowage may constrain the layout of a medical facility and require bespoke fixings. Compromises may have to be made with the availability and accessibility of ready-to-use items.[9]

It is vital when operating in a maritime environment to ensure that 'the back door' remains open for evacuation. Transport of patients to higher echelons of care or repatriation is essential to ensure capacity for new casualties. Sea states in the Persian Gulf can be variable, and rapid changes in visibility can affect evacuation plans and medical timelines.

A direct attack on a ship is likely to cause a significant number of casualties and hamper the ability of the embarked staff to respond. Coordination between vessels is essential to ensure an appropriate response. During *Operation Telic*, there were no successful ship attacks, but any response would have been coordinated by the UK Maritime commander aboard *HMS Ark Royal*. If additional medical support was required after the primary activity of saving the vessel, this would have been coordinated via the SMO and NATS. It is unrealistic to expect anything more than basic life-saving care to be performed if a vessel is engaged in a contact, as the priority at all times remains the safety and security of the vessel following the order of *Fight – Fire – Flood – Medical*. All those embarked are expected to undertake non-medical tasks in pursuit of this goal, if required, and this must be practised and included in predeployment training.[9]

The medical role of a warship will rarely be its primary one, with command and operational concerns potentially conflicting with best patient care. All the medical teams with the R2A and those providing R1A care were embarked on vessels with a principal war-fighting role. In addition, warships with medical teams embarked are not protected by the Geneva Convention. During *Operation Telic*, *RFA Argus* was primarily deployed to provide medical care but was not designated as a hospital ship, allowing her to get close to the frontline.

Patient access and movement around the PCRF require consideration.[9] In 2003, the transport of patients from the flight deck required the use of an aircraft lift to access the hospital and any boat transfers would have required the use of a man-rated hoist. Level 1 patients were cared for in bunks, with half the available space of a conventional bed, requiring the patient to be sufficiently mobile to climb into an upper bunk space. Caring for patients at height presents risks to both patients and nursing staff. All but routine care within a bunk space is challenging and emergency care is almost impossible.

Whenever patients are moved around a ship, they must be placed in a stretcher and manually carried. This often involves confined lifts, ladders and hatchways. Whole ship coordination is required to open certain external watertight doors and to transit the flight deck.

Storage space for medical staff and equipment is limited by the design of the ship and the operational priorities. While space aboard *RFA Argus* was relatively generous (in naval terms), usable space in and around the purpose-built PCRF was at a premium. Storage space was placed under further pressure by last-minute augmentation and borrowing of equipment. Most embarked medical staff supplemented their modules with personal equipment acquired from local hospitals. On a larger scale, immediately prior to sailing, *RNH Haslar* loaned the PCRF an image intensifier. Careful itemisation and stock accounting were essential to know what equipment was available and where it was stored throughout the vessel. A similar scenario was encountered when embarking R2A onto *HMS Ark Royal*, a situation made all the more challenging as the R2A staff and equipment were effectively a retrofit asset. Resupply was planned either from *RFA Fort George* directly or by *RFA Diligence* retrieving stores that had been flown out from the United Kingdom from shore side in Kuwait. If urgent stores were required, communication and requests could have been made to local allied vessels.

Medical planning is a fluid and evolving process; distances, assets, evacuation and treatment options will depend on the operational situation and Command priorities. On an apparently mundane note, ships normally run at 115 V, and there may be insufficient UK standard three-pin 230 V sockets for the medical equipment. In addition, protected power supplies are essential for laboratory and radiology equipment. Existing 230 V power supplies on protected emergency circuits can be found on certain platforms, but to prevent overload, identification and prioritisation of equipment requiring uninterrupted supply may be required. Management of POWs and LNs needs to be carried out in accordance with guidance from local Command and in accordance with international law.

CLINICAL EXPERIENCE

Primary care perspective

Much of the work out with *RFA Argus* was and remains the core work of the RNMS. This chapter will concentrate on the secondary care work carried out aboard *RFA Argus*.

Role 2 Afloat (R2A)

No surgery was performed by the R2A. However, the helicopter crash on 22 March 2003 highlighted the importance for plans to be in place for care of the dead including the provision of emergency mortuary space and services.

Role 3 Afloat (R3A)

The PCRF pre-deployment training took the form of an annual exercise originally known as *Exercise Strong Resolve*, which later became *Exercise Medical Endeavour*. Pre-deployment training had occurred briefly as an exercise in January 2003 with a partial R3 team. Twenty-five medical personnel sailed from the United Kingdom, their main role being to unpack, set up the equipment and establish standard operating procedures (SOPs). The embarked crew of the PCRF were a mixed compliment of TriService personnel, both regular and reserve. Two of the RAF anaesthetic trainees were nominated to provide the *Critical Care Air Support Team* (CCAST) capability and expected to transfer patients from *RFA Argus*.

The R3A facility aboard *RFA Argus* performed all the UK maritime surgery during *Operation Telic*. As knowledge of, and access to, local care facilities was limited, many of the LN and detainees required more than one operation in order to ensure that the end results were definitive. After the fighting phase was over, these LNs were returned to the Iraqi healthcare facilities. Available records are scarce, serving to emphasise the importance of publishing post-exercise and post-deployment records. It was the belief of the authors Matthews and Mercer[10] that having a wide range of specialties was important in providing care for casualties at R3 and paramount when providing definitive care. Details of the deployed specialities are given in Table 21.1, and operating statistics, in Table 21.2.

Twenty-eight per cent of patients needed more than one operation and one required five procedures. Coalition forces were routinely evacuated

Table 21.1 Clinical specialties on RFA Argus

Specialty	Deployed personnel
General surgeons	3 (+2 trainees)
Trauma and orthopaedic surgeons	2 (+1 trainee)
Urological surgeon	1
Ear nose and throat surgeon	1
Maxillofacial surgeon	1
Plastic surgeon	1
Physicians	2 (+2 trainees)
Paediatrician	1
Ophthalmologist	1
Radiologist	1
Pathologist	1
Neurosurgeons	1
Anaesthetists	4 (+4 trainees)
Intensivists	1 (+2 RAF CCAST trainees)

Source: Matthews JJ, Mercer SJ, *J R Navy Med Serv* 2003;89(3):123–132.

Table 21.2 Operating book statistics from RFA Argus, *Operation Telic*, 23 March–9 April 2003

Type of injury	Number of operations
Total casualties to PCRF	65
Total battle injured patients	36
Total DNBI	29
Casualties brought from point of wounding	15
Total operations	45
Gunshot wound (GSWs)	6
Fragmentation injury	18
Both GSW and fragmentation	7
Extremity injury	28
Laparotomy	2
Thoracotomy	1
Penetrating injury	31
Blunt and penetrating injury	5
Road traffic collision	5
American	1
British	5
Local national	30
Average duration of surgery	132 minutes
Longest duration of surgery	370 minutes

Source: Matthews JJ, Mercer SJ, *J R Navy Med Serv* 2003;89(3):123–132.

from the PCRF within 48 hours, by air to Kuwait. LNs took much longer to evacuate, consuming more resources prior to their repatriation to shore-based field hospitals, holding camps or, if requiring further more complex surgery, to *USNS Comfort*.

PCRF EXPERIENCE OF SOFT TISSUE INJURY

Most penetrating wounds affected soft tissue only, all were explored, longitudinal skin incisions allowed fascial decompression and wound edges were excised. Muscle viability was determined by contractility, bleeding, colour and texture. All non-viable tissue and easily found foreign bodies were removed during surgery. Preoperative Betadine and hydrogen peroxide were used for wash out; postoperatively, washout was performed with 0.9% saline. All open missile wounds were left open for five days prior to delayed closure. Coamoxiclav was administered until 24 hours after closure, with the addition of Metronidazole if the wounds were judged to be

grossly contaminated. To avoid secondary contamination, wound inspection was kept to a minimum after primary debridement and prior to closure. Definitive maritime surgery was usually possible with simple methods; however, complex closures were required on occasion; split skin grafting was common and one pedicle flap was used.

OTHER INJURIES

In total, 21 fractures were managed by the three embarked surgeons. External fixators (both Centrafix® and Hoffman®) were applied to nine limbs (four femurs, two tibias, two wrists and one ulnar). Three patients arrived with Steinman pins and traction via Thomas splint already in situ from R2 land facilities; all injuries were open and contaminated, with extensive soft tissue damage. The operative priorities were to identify salvageable limbs, restore vascular supply and meticulously debride soft tissue with removal of bony splinters; planning involved multidisciplinary discussions between consultants. All fixator pins were placed after discussion with the plastic surgeon to ease subsequent reconstruction. Four patients underwent amputations, one bilateral above knee amputation (having had previous below knee guillotine amputations ashore), one above and one below knee amputation and a shoulder disarticulation following traumatic amputation.[10]

No direct admissions required primary laparotomy, although several required a return to theatre for delayed management and reopening of laparotomies performed ashore at R2 land facilities, for further wound debridement and to manage bleeding. Of note was one paediatric patient who arrived with an open abdomen and 'Bogota bag' with a bullet still in the liver; this was judged too high risk to operate on and left in situ. Pneumothoraces were caused by blast, blunt and penetrating injuries; in total, four patients required a chest drain as their management and one required a thoracotomy.[10]

Only four patients suffered major vessel injury, but none required surgical repair. The image intensifier was utilised on two occasions to perform intraoperative angiography.[10] A US Marine required debridement of an open brain injury. Eight peripheral nerve injuries were identified, and a repair of a transected sciatic nerve was undertaken intraoperatively; the remainder of the injuries in viable limbs were splinted and given physiotherapy. One ophthalmic case was a penetrating eye injury necessitating a microscopic exploration of the globe.

PCRF EXPERIENCE OF PAEDIATRIC SURGERY

Two notable paediatric cases were embarked, one requiring above knee amputation with plastic surgical involvement for skin grafting and the other requiring closure and debridement of a laparotomy wound.

CLINICAL DEVELOPMENTS AND CHALLENGES

The injury pattern seen aboard the PCRF was similar to that of previous conflicts and mirrored that seen on land. Mortality aboard the PCRF was low, as early surgery close to point of wounding proved vital in saving the lives of those seriously injured. Those who were killed or too unstable for transfer were not seen, and a degree of survivor bias can be anticipated to skew the patients and injury patterns seen on the R3A. All but two Iraqi patients had definitive treatment on board *RFA Argus*. Lack of identified evacuation points and the resulting requirement to provide definitive surgery to many of the LNs placed significant additional stress on the R3A. Half of the surgical procedures required more than one operating consultant. This needs to be borne in mind for future deployments of R2A when deploying with a single surgeon. Timelines for operations and resuscitative surgery may need to be relaxed when a surgeon is working alone with unskilled assistance.[10]

Blood was provided from the UK blood transfusion service. Packed cells and fresh frozen plasma were used extensively on the R3A. Meticulous cold chain administration was required to ensure the usability of blood products. There was no ability to obtain platelets except by using whole blood transfusion from the EDP. Point-of-care testing of coagulation was not available.

ISSUES ARISING FROM DEPLOYED EXPERIENCE

Following return from deployment, the PCRF medical staff identified a number of issues that would be addressed in the subsequent maintenance periods. A defects log and record of *issues arising* proved essential for prospective collection of learning points and served as the foundation document for future recommendations, noting the importance of the platform as a whole and of held equipment levels.

Space management on board was a key concern. The PCRF sailed with three operating tables in the main theatre (the fourth operating table was in the minor operating theatre). This resulted in a cramped working environment, and as a result, one table was removed. Future maritime platforms must consider the working medical space required, attempting to take into account the recent changes in trauma management and team working. There was an inadequate single area for scrubbing up, which resulted in delays whilst surgeons prepared to operate and frequent desterilisation requiring rescrubbing and causing further delay. There was also insufficient space for washing equipment between cases. Limited ability to control the theatre temperature and humidity made for an uncomfortable and potentially unsafe working environment. Deck head pendants providing power, suction and piped gas were low and caused several minor injuries to staff working in the operating theatre; temporary foam protection was installed.

There was also a lack of privacy for seeing non-urgent patients. A dedicated consultation area was required in the complex to allow privacy for consultation and examination but was not available. Inadequate storage, small in volume, poorly secured, difficult to access and cumbersome to clean, led to a number of recommendations, including that storage be sealed when not in use and hence be easy to remove and clean.

Experience showed that there were significant equipment issues. Deck head lighting was found to be inflexible and inadequate and the available head torches were of a poor standard. This was particularly apparent when multiple surgical teams were working on the same patient. No theatre table fixings (for example arm boards, leg supports and the equipment required to operate on a prone patient) were provided and local solutions were created – there are now dedicated operating table accessories. The suction provided was insufficient for the large volume of wash required when irrigating contaminated wounds.

Key pieces of equipment, including an image intensifier, were acquired immediately prior to sailing. Other equipment, including the single autoclave, was found to be unreliable and inadequate. Much equipment was appropriated from other sources to augment existing kits, and some expensive equipment was not used. Equipment borrowed from *RNH Haslar* was used in every single orthopaedic case and the military pattern fixator was found to be inadequate for Echelon 3 facilities. A more versatile fixator system was required. No power tools were provided in the module. Two Stryker power systems borrowed from RNH Haslar in the pre-deployment phase allowed application of frames quickly. Battery systems negate the need for air lines in an otherwise crowded environment. Most single specialists brought their own equipment to supplement that provided. The problems of modular resupply in a space-constrained environment have already been mentioned. Proper determination of the required equipment and the establishment of appropriate 'modules' were clearly required.

Communications problems included limited and poor internal communications between departments. Information technology support was also lacking, hampering efforts to control stock and communicate with the UK and local forces ashore. Staffing levels were considered adequate for the casualties received. However, the central sterile services department work was often left until quiet times in the surgical throughput, something that would not be possible in the event of continuous high-level clinical activity. Given the huge investment in specialist equipment in the operating theatres and ICU, it would seem appropriate to have theatres and ICU permanently staffed by a POMA/CPOMA (O) to ensure that they are fully prepared and functional at all times.

FUTURE PLANS AND CAPABILITY

The RNMS will work to support the delivery of the established three Royal Navy key roles and distinctive characteristics as laid out in the strategic document 'The Royal Navy Today, Tomorrow and Towards 2025'. The established three Royal Navy key roles are as follows:

- War fighting – conduct, or be ready to conduct, war fighting at sea and from the sea.
- Maritime security – protect the free, safe and lawful use of the sea where it is vital to UK prosperity and security.
- International engagement – promote UK interests by developing international partnerships.

In order to do this, the Navy and its personnel need to be operationally versatile and capable of contributing to diplomatic, humanitarian and military operations at sea, on land and in the air. Thus, they need to be interoperable and able to operate with the Army, RAF, Government agencies and international allies.

Recently, the T45 destroyers have been introduced and have proved to be a powerful asset. The *Queen Elizabeth Class* aircraft carrier (*CVF – Carrier Vessel Future*) and the *Joint Strike Fighter* will deliver carrier strike capability as part of the *Carrier Enabled Power Projection*. To replace ballistic nuclear Vanguard class submarines, the Royal Navy is preparing the Trident successor programme. Introduction of the Type 26 Global Combat Ship (GCS) in the 2020s will partially replace the T23 frigates. New multi-role mine warfare, hydrography, offshore patrol vessels, fleet tankers and support ships are currently being designed.

Evolved R2A

The R2A team is likely to be a versatile solution for medical support to maritime contingency operations in the future, ranging from a 1/1/1 to a 2/1/2 capability. With the possibility of up to four R2As deploying at any one time, rotas are going to be difficult to maintain, and some specialties may require Tri-Service support. There is also a requirement for ongoing module development. The SOPs, issues arising and lessons identified from each operational deployment of the R2A should be collated as a generic resource. An R2A(Light) is currently being trialled and is likely to form the model for further deployments on the T26 GCS. R2A is currently deployable on the following platforms: *HMS Ocean, RFA Fort Victoria,*

RFA Cardigan Bay, RFA Mounts Bay, RFA Lyme Bay and *RFA Argus.*

Evolved PCRF/R3A

RFA Argus has changed her primary role to that of PCRF. More recent structural upgrades have removed the forward aircraft lift and replaced it with covered housing on the flight deck, allowing triage and sanitisation of the casualties whilst they are protected from the elements. There are now both a ramp and a lift able to take multiple stretchers down to the resuscitation area. Casualty transfer is easier and safer and allows for improved evacuation of the clinical complex in the event of a fire or flood. The PCRF full capability remains 4/4/10/20/70 (see earlier discussion), but the CT scanner has been upgraded to a 64-slice CT scanner and the laboratory facilities have been improved and now include apheresis. PCRF light has a 2/2/5/10/10 configuration. When fully manned, the medical complement is 43 medical officers and 94 nurses.[11] *RFA Argus* deployed most recently in support of the UK's efforts to help the fight against Ebola virus disease in Sierra Leone (*Operation Gritrock*).

While *RFA Argus* has continued to undergo updating with periodic refits and regular maintenance, it is unlikely that a successor vessel will be purchased to replace her when she is decommissioned. The future may well involve smaller-scale support to littoral operations offered by R2A. If larger R3 facilities are required, the RFA Bay Class and the new CVF aircraft carriers have the deck space to accommodate a scalable modular facility similar to that deployed on land. Overall, medical support in the future may well be based on a modular design, perhaps ranging from a Role 2 Afloat (light) supporting a 1/1/1 output to an R2 Enhanced with a range of specialists, a CT scanner and expanded laboratory support.

Provision and resupply of blood and blood products at sea

The provision of blood and its components has become more important with the recognition that they offer the most effective replacement therapy following trauma. In all deployed land environments, provision and resupply of these components present significant challenges, which were effectively overcome on *Operations Herrick* and *Telic*: similar problems apply to the maritime environment. PCRF currently has the capability to hold the following blood products (the numbers quoted are a maximum that could be held on board in terms of space):

- Red cell concentrate (RCC) – Up to 500 units. The shelf life of RCC is 35 days, and they can be resupplied to the ship at sea by air drop.
- Fresh frozen plasma (FFP) – Up to a maximum of 400 units. The shelf life of FFP is two years, and as a result, resupply of this blood product is not usually an issue: FFP cannot currently be resupplied by air drop.
- Cryoprecipitate – Up to a maximum of 20 units. The shelf life of cryoprecipitate is two years; thus, resupply of this blood product is not usually an issue.
- Platelets sourced from the National Health Service Blood and Transplant – Up to a maximum of 16 units. The shelf life of these is between five and seven days, and effective provision is therefore a logistical challenge at sea. In addition, platelets cannot be delivered by air drop. Apheresis platelets taken from pre-screened members (donors) of the personnel on board (EDP) provide an effective source (see Chapter 14).
- Fresh whole blood – From pre-screened members (donors) of the personnel on board (EDP).

Resupply at sea presents a logistical challenge. Frozen blood (favoured by the Dutch) and lyophilised plasma are currently being considered, as they have the potential to negate the need for regular resupply. However, these products would require a prolonged processing step that could be a constraint in an emergency situation and, in the case of lyophilised plasma, do not remove the need for the other blood components. Platelets will always present a challenge, but the effectiveness of apheresis afloat was proved during *Operation Gritrock*. Studies of cold, frozen and lyophilised platelets are ongoing and products are being developed by North Atlantic Treaty Organization partners. Fibrinogen is now available for use in the pre-hospital space.

Plasma options are still primarily based on FFP, but the future may include greater use of *Octaplas®* (lower VCJD [variant Creutzfeldt–Jakob disease] transmission risk) and *Lyoplas®* freeze-fried plasma. Introduction of deployable polymerised chain reaction (PCR) analysers into service raises the possibility of conducting more thorough blood screening on-board, thus facilitating safe apheresis, augmenting EDP management and providing assurance and haemovigilance benefits.

Maritime in transit care

Maritime in transit care (MITC) is a rapidly developing asset. Previously, MITC served to provide advanced first aid[12]; however, recent operations have exercised the deployment of *pre-hospital emergency care*. The MITC is now capable of projecting forward and maintaining in-transit advanced care.[13] It provides the platform for moving casualties to and from maritime medical capabilities in a timely fashion whilst offering appropriate care during transfer. MITC offers both primary and secondary retrieval services. If secondary care is to be offered at sea, an ability to transfer patients without a gap in care provision is essential. A MITC capability is required whenever

- A task group is supporting operations ashore or a unit is dislocated from its medical support.
- There is more than one echelon of medical care within a task group.
- Medical care is being provided out with a task group such as at host nation facilities or during land-based operations with maritime medical support.

CONCLUSION

During recent operations, *RFA Argus* performed well and proved a capable facility, as a consequence it has recently had its service life extended. However, in the current political and financial climate, its replacement is uncertain. In the future, incident reporting and lessons identified for Role 2 or Role 3 medical care on any maritime platform will be owned and acted upon by the new *Deployed Hospital Care (Afloat) Command Team* based at *Naval Command Head Quarters*. Inevitably, there

will a need for close and informed discussion between the DMS and Naval Command regarding the position of Role 3 in the future carrier based fleet. It must not be forgotten that Role 3 Afloat will be a crucial capability not just for Naval operations but also for all three Armed Services in the event of future expeditionary warfare or any major international intervention that involves large numbers of personnel requiring immediate access to advanced care facilities, before these can be established on land, or where the operational situation renders it initially impractical or unsafe to set up such facilities ashore.

The writing of this chapter has demonstrated the difficulties in recording and retention of corporate knowledge and experience. In the future, deployed individuals should be encouraged to keep diaries with the express purpose of recording minor and major learning points. These records post conflict could be security vetted and anonymised. Once compiled, the 'big-data' documents could be searchable and cross-referenced by various categories. If this process were to be adopted, rapid feedback could be relayed to command and a wealth of useful operational information could be conveyed prior to future deployments.

REFERENCES

1. BBC. Peninsula captured; major victory. 2003. http://news.bbc.co.uk/1/hi/uk/2872119.stm (accessed July 28, 2016).
2. MOD. Announcement – Operations in Iraq finish with completion of Royal Navy training mission. 2011. https://www.gov.uk/government/news/operations-in-iraq-finish-with-completion-of-royal-navy-training-mission (accessed 28 July, 2016).
3. BBC. Warship rescues troops and civilians stranded in Spain. 2010. http://news.bbc.co.uk/1/hi/england/devon/8631331.stm (Accessed 28 July, 2016.)
4. Smith AM. The triangle of death: Medical sustainability in expeditionary sea-based operations. *Naval War Coll Rev* 2008;61(2):96.
5. Coetzee RH. *HMS Ark Royal* and the 2003 helicopter crash in the Northern Arabian Gulf. *J R Nav Med Serv* 2010;96(2):96–102.

6. House of Commons Defence Committee. *Medical Care for the Armed Forces, Seventh Report of Session 2007–08.* 7th ed. London: House of Commons, The Stationery Office 2008.

7. Rew D. *Blood, Heat + Dust, Operation Telic and the British Medical Deployment to the Gulf 2003–2009.* Avonworld for: Defence Medical Services, Ministry of Defence, 2005.

8. MOD/NATO. *Allied Joint Doctrine for Medical Support (with UK elements). Edition B Version 1 + UK national elements.* NATO Standardisation Office (NSO) (ed). 2015.

9. Risdall JE, Heames RM, Hill G. Role 2 afloat. *J R Army Med Corps* 2011;157(4):362–364.

10. Matthews JJ, Mercer SJ. 'War surgery at sea': Maritime trauma experience in the Gulf War 2003. *J R Navy Med Serv* 2003; 89(3):123–132.

11. Smith JE, Smith SR, Hill G. The UK maritime Role 3 medical treatment facility: The Primary Casualty Receiving Facility, RFA ARGUS. *J R Nav Med Serv* 2015;101(1):3–5.

12. Whalley L, Smith S. Pre-hospital, maritime in-transit care from a Role 2 Afloat platform. *J R Nav Med Serv* 2013;99(3): 135–136.

13. Bott G, Barnard J, Prior K. Maritime in transit care. *J R Nav Med Serv* 2015;101(2): 104–106.

22

Education, training and human factors

INTRODUCTION

Throughout history, many of the greatest innovations in medicine and surgery have originated during short periods of intense warfare rather than during the longer intervening periods of peace.[1] This chapter will review the subject of human factors in deployed military medicine and the educational and training aspects of *Operations Telic* and *Herrick*. Human factors are considered first because much of the multidisciplinary team training associated with these deployments focussed on this area.

HUMAN FACTORS

As both *Operation Telic* and *Operation Herrick* matured, our clinical results improved significantly.[2] Although some of this success was undoubtedly due to increasing experience and the development of new resuscitation, surgical, anaesthetic and other clinical techniques, it was also the result of exemplary human factors which were refined and rehearsed during pre-deployment training.[3] The field of human factors has been described as:

> 'enhancing clinical performance through an understanding of the effects of teamwork, tasks, equipment, workspace, culture and organisation on human behaviour and abilities and application of that knowledge in clinical settings',[4]

and also as:

> 'the cognitive, social, and personal resource skills that complement technical skills, and contribute to safe and efficient task performance.[5]

Recently, there has been a drive to implement human factors in the *National Health Service* (*NHS*) with the signing of a national concordat by many organisations, including the *General Medical Council*.[6]

The value of human factors was first highlighted in the aviation industry following the investigation of accidents and near misses, where it was thought that approximately 70% of errors occurred as a result of failed communication, poor decision-making or ineffective leadership.[7] Two high-profile medical reports from the US[8] and the UK[9] described how human factors were to blame for morbidity and mortality, and in the medical world, this was echoed by the analysis of two high-profile anaesthetic cases.[1,3,10]

Research, often in conjunction with psychologists and using observational studies, has allowed the development of non-technical skills frameworks for anaesthesia,[11] emergency medicine,[12] surgery[13] and perioperative practitioners.[14] The anaesthetist's non-technical skills framework is reproduced in Table 22.1 and has four separate behaviour categories: task management, team working, situational awareness and decision-making, each category having its own elements. The three published frameworks[4-7,11,14] have much overlap and have been used by the *Defence Medical Services* (UK-DMS) to define the process of the patient journey with rehearsal in pre-deployment training[15] and refinement on operations. Human factors are involved in every stage of the patient pathway depicted in Figure 22.1, with handovers taking place at each stage.[16]

Human factors during *Operation Telic* and *Operation Herrick* will now be discussed with

Table 22.1 Anaesthetists non-technical skills framework

Category	Element
Task Management	Planning and preparing management
	Prioritising
	Providing and maintaining standards
	Identifying and utilising resources
Team Working	Coordinating activities with team members working
	Exchanging information
	Using authority and assertiveness
	Assessing capabilities
	Supporting others
Situational Awareness	Gathering information awareness
	Recognising and understanding
	Anticipating
Decision Making	Identifying options
	Balancing risks and selecting options
	Re-evaluating

Source: Fletcher G, Br J Anaesth 2003;90:580–588.

reference to publications arising from deployed experience.

Pre-hospital phase

The operation of the *Medical Emergency Response Team* (MERT) is described elsewhere (Chapter 3). Operational pre-hospital care is complex and highly dynamic, with exposure to significant risk for all involved. Four discrete levels of care provision have been defined[17] within the Role 1 environment:

- *Care Under Fire* (treatment in a non-permissive environment)
- *Tactical Field Care* (treatment at point of wounding in a permissive or semi-permissive environment)
- *Field Resuscitation* (team-based treatment at a Role 1 facility in a permissive environment)
- *Prolonged Field Care* (additional techniques and management skills that sustain the casualty if there is a delay in medical evacuation)

The management of patients demands careful preparation and planning, maintenance of situational awareness and dynamic risk assessments, re-evaluating and changing patient priorities as the incident threat or patient's pathology

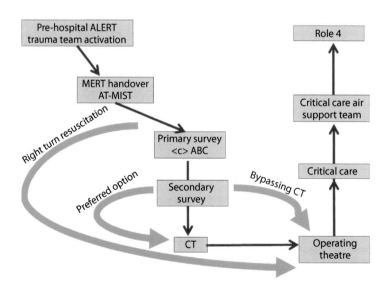

Figure 22.1 Patient pathway for a casualty during *Operation Herrick*.

changes. During *Operations Telic* and *Herrick*, pre-hospital care was required for a diverse population of patients, from injured military personnel (UK, other *International Security Assistance Force* [ISAF] forces and the Afghan National Security Forces) to adult and paediatric local nationals. Transport of suspected enemy combatants raised specific challenges. Mechanisms of injury were diverse, including penetrating and blunt trauma, blast and burns, from battle or non-battle causes, involving individual, multiple or even mass casualties. Battlefield injuries occurred at all times of day, often in remote and austere locations, away from *company aid posts*, and with sometimes dramatic variations in light conditions and weather.

The volume of trauma seen at each Role 1 facility varied widely, often related to the nature and *area of operations* (AO), operational tempo and current missions. AOs continued to evolve, with logistical support and medical resources improving as the infrastructure of each Role 1 facility matured.[18] *Continuous professional development*

whilst deployed is an important tenet of military healthcare governance, and the challenges faced and the solutions generated to facilitate this have been discussed.[19,20] Skill-fade remained a risk throughout each tour and all personnel needed to ensure refresher training remained routine in order to maintain standards.[21]

Figure 22.2 is a simplified schematic diagram of the medical network on *Operation Herrick* showing communication pathways between personnel at different types of medical facility. During *Operation Herrick*, general duties medical officers (GDMOs) were commonly deployed forward to command a company aid post, responsible for pre-hospital emergency care (PHEC), primary healthcare (PHC), medical logistics, medical planning, force protection and personnel management. Distant supervision and support to each GDMO were provided by neighbouring *regimental medical officers* (RMO), deployed secondary care consultants (available by radio-communications form the Role 3 facility) and the *Senior Medical Officer* (SMO) based at Camp Bastion. In the event of a

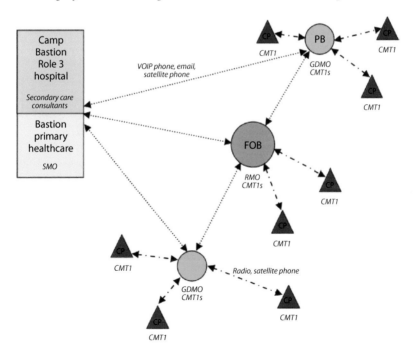

Figure 22.2 Schematic diagram (simplified) of the medical network on *Operation Herrick* showing the communication pathways between the personnel at different types of medical facility. CMT1, Combat Medical Technician class 1; CP, checkpoint; PB, patrol base; VOIP, voice over internet protocol. (From Gumbley AE et al., *J R Army Med Corps* 2013;159:68–72.)

battle incident occurring at a *checkpoint* or during a patrol supported by a combat medical technician (CMT) (or medical assistant [MA]), GDMOs would often provide remote advice and support for medical interventions until patients could be extracted back to the forward operating base (FOB) or patrol base or be picked up directly by the *MERT*.[20] During such an event, excellent communication skills remained the foundation for delivering and executing all other non-technical skills.

Team resource management and human factors (non-technical skills) training are directly transferrable to the Role 1 pre-hospital setting.[22] Unfortunately, training and capability for Role 1 during *Operations Telic* and *Herrick* failed to develop at the same rate as for deployed hospital care.[23] A bespoke Role 1 course with equivalence to the *Military Operational Surgical Training (MOST) course* was never developed, although the MERT course was specifically created and structured to reflect operational challenges and advances and there was a gradual change in the emphasis of *Battlefield Advanced Trauma Life Support* (BATLS) from hospital to pre-hospital care. Systematic

analysis of Role 1 revealed opportunities for developments in training, equipment, personnel, infrastructure, organisation, information and logistics.[24] These deficiencies increase the complexity of any scenario and can impact on a clinician's bandwidth, affecting the delivery of optimum pre-hospital care.

Batham and colleagues completed a qualitative research study to analyse the effect of battlefield conditions on the implementation of frontline pre-hospital trauma interventions (as per BATLS) and the perception of clinical performance.[25] Respondents identified a number of factors that affected their ability to provide a high standard of casualty care (Figure 22.3). Of particular note, respondents' points of reference for acceptable standards were aligned to those provided within the UK NHS. Furthermore, key issues were raised following experiences of dealing with multiple poly-trauma patients and circumstances where personal safety was jeopardised. This article also discussed how numerous environmental, situational, time and clinical pressures resulted in prioritisation of care that was not BATLS protocol compliant; nevertheless, trauma care was

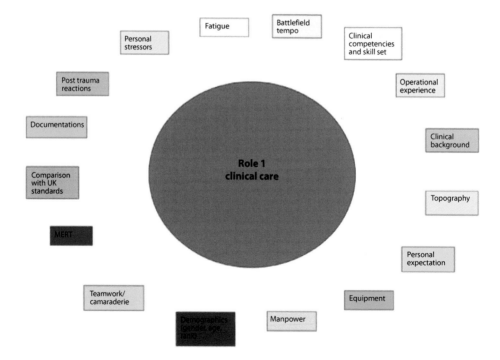

Figure 22.3 Categories of issues identified as affecting clinical care. (From Batham D et al., *J R Army Med Corps* 2012;158:173–180.)

maintained to a high level. Delivery of Role 1 medical care is clearly not comparable to the norms of NHS practice. The BATLS course and *Clinical Guidelines for Operations*[26] were consequently frequently updated and developed to be the overarching doctrine and points of reference for *Operations Telic* and *Herrick*. There is clearly a need for human factors training for all potential Role 1 medical personnel in order to ensure adherence to BATLS protocols despite the complexities of the battle space.

The development of a bespoke Role 1 Course for delivery of human factors and team resource training to address many of the issues raised by Batham and colleagues[25] remains a requirement. Historical stumbling blocks preventing development of this training, including a lack of knowledge regarding the specific challenges, workload, case mix and common non-technical issues involved in working in an FOB[22] have now been addressed. Published Role 1 personal experiences from deployed GDMOs and RMOs now offer good insight into many of the transferable factors and support the development of non-technical training[14] for future contingency operations. Developing educational solutions from a gap analysis of readiness for deploying medical personnel and using simulation tools to enhance decision-making for both individuals and teams constitute two high priorities for *Defence Medical Research and Exploitation*.[27]

Trauma team: Preparing to receive a casualty

The evolved trauma team in Camp Bastion towards the end of operations was a very resource-rich unit. Those involved and their roles are listed in Table 22.2. Salas describes a team as being:

> 'a distinguishable set of two or more people who interact dynamically, interdependently, and adaptively towards a common and valued goal, who have each been assigned specific roles or functions to perform, and who have a limited life-span membership'.[28]

The slight difference between this definition and the complex trauma team in Camp Bastion was that the latter were ready 24 hours a day specifically to deal with a casualty. The ability to provide not only consultant-led care but also consultant-delivered care allowed robust decisions to be made early, based on experience, and ultimately led to this care being described as exemplary.[29] The activation of the trauma team was dependent on pre-determined criteria based on anatomy, physiology and mechanism of injury (Table 22.3), and it was important that this matrix existed so that the team was not activated for every patient arriving at the hospital: this could have led to 'burn out'. Teams were also rotated on a three-to-six-month cycle depending on role, with the clinicians often deploying for two months during very busy periods.

The definition of a leader is 'a person whose ideas and actions influence the thoughts and the behaviour of others'[5]; in other words, they must influence, inspire and direct the actions of the team in order to attain a desired objective. In order to provide consultant-delivered care, the *trauma team leader* (TTL) on operations was a consultant in emergency medicine. The role of rapid assessment and robust decision-making also required an element of management as situations were analysed, goals set, activities co-ordinated and the team directed. Midwinter and colleagues have described some of the difficulties in the decision-making process, with the TTL having a job similar to that of the conductor of an orchestra, with multiple teams all working on a severely injured patient and numerous others supporting the resuscitation.[30] This role has also been described as 'driving the ship', and to allow this to happen, the TTL must be allowed to stand in a position that is completely 'hands off', maintaining a complete overview of what could potentially be a rapidly changing situation.

Once activated, usually by an electronic pager, the trauma team assembled in the emergency department. This period of preparation was vital and commenced with the TTL giving a brief, confirming information from the pre-hospital team and the '9 liner' (the signal sent from the point of wounding, including medical information pertaining to casualty number and injury type as well as important operational constraints such as ongoing hostile activity and helicopter landing site [HLS] details).[31]

Table 22.2 Complex trauma team and designated roles

Team member	Designated role
Emergency Medicine Consultant	Team Leader
Emergency Medicine Registrar	Primary survey doctor
Anaesthetist 1	Airway management
Anaesthetist 2	Large-bore central venous access
Operator Department Practitioner (ODP)	Anaesthetic assistant
Scribe	Trauma nurse co-ordinator responsible for accurate recording of activity in the trauma bay
Emergency Department Nurse 1	Intravenous access and first blood sample
Emergency Department Nurse 2	Drawing up drugs
Emergency Department Nurse 3	Rapid infuser operator and checking blood products
Emergency Department Nurse 3	Rapid infuser operator and checking blood products
Runner	Collect blood products from the laboratory and deliver samples
Orthopaedic Surgeon	Advice to TTL
	Apply pneumatic tourniquet
General Surgeon	Advice to TTL
Plastic Surgeon	Advice to TTL
Radiologist	Perform ultrasound scans
	Prepare for CT scanning
Radiographer	Perform chest and pelvic imaging
Deployed Medical Director	Overall in charge of the clinical aspects of the deployed hospital
Laboratory Manager	Will advise on availability of blood and blood products to activate contingency plans
Theatre Manager	Prepare theatre team for casualty co-ordination of the operating theatre
Ward Master	Provides advice on available beds and planning
Interpreter	To interpret for local nationals
Regimental Sgt Major	Responsible for 'sanitising the patient' – i.e. ensuring that ammunition and weapons do not enter the hospital
Padre	To provide spiritual support to patients and staff

During the briefing, the TTLs also confirmed, based on their experience, the mental model they expected, which was essentially the most likely clinical sequence of events. Specific standard operating procedures were clarified at this time, for example the triggers to move directly into the operating theatre. An immediate move into the operating theatre was termed a 'right turn resuscitation'[32] due to the initial layout of the hospital. The TTL brief not only prepared the team but also encouraged good *followership*, one definition being:

'a process in which subordinates recognise their responsibility to comply with the orders of leaders and take appropriate action consistent with the situation to carry out those orders to the best of their ability. In the absence of orders they estimate the proper action required to contribute to mission performance and take that action'.[33]

Table 22.3 Trauma team activation criteria

1. Mechanism/History
  a. Penetrating trauma
     • Gunshot or shrapnel wound
     • Blast injury (mine/IED/grenade)
     • Stab wound
  b. Blunt trauma
     • Motor vehicle crash with ejection
     • Motorcyclist or pedestrian hit by vehicle >30 km/h
     • Fall >5 m
     • Fatality in the same vehicle
     • Entrapment and/or crush injury
     • Inter-hospital trauma transfer meeting activation criteria
2. Anatomy
     • Injury to two or more body regions
     • Fracture to two or more long bones
     • Spinal cord injury
     • Amputation of a limb
     • Penetrating injury to head, neck, torso, or proximal limb
     • Burns >15% Body Surface Area in adults *or* >10% in children *or* airway burns
     • Airway obstruction
3. Physiology
     • Systolic blood pressure <90 mm Hg or pulse >120 bpm (adults)
     • Respiratory rate <10 or >30 per minute (adults); SpO_2 <90%
     • Depressed level of consciousness or fitting
     • Deterioration in the Emergency Department
     • Age >70 years
     • Pregnancy >24 weeks with torso injury

Source: Ministry of Defence. *Clinical Guidelines for Operations – Joint Service Publication 999.* September 2012. London: MOD.

The most important role of the TTL was to maintain the situational awareness of the team, defined by Endsley as

'the perception of elements in the environment within a volume of time and space, the comprehension of their meaning, and the projection of their status in the near future'.[34]

In complex trauma, the physiological state of the patient could fluctuate, and so decisions regarding transfusion and transfer to the operating theatre had to be made rapidly.

The team was introduced to each other by name, and role and competencies were confirmed. Each member wore a tabard indicating his or her allotted role. Equipment was checked and drugs drawn up in the form of a pre-determined 'wet-pack' of induction drugs, analgesics, antibiotics and tranexamic acid.[35] Contingency planning was also discussed, for example how to deal with a difficult airway and which member of the team would perform a surgical airway. Once the team had assembled, they remained in the trauma bay until dismissed by the TTL. Prior to the arrival of the casualty, a runner was sent to the laboratory to collect blood and blood products, which were delivered in the form of a 'shock pack' supplied in a box with a timer. Products that were not required were returned under the direction of the TTL for use on another patient. In summary, this preparation and planning phase of the trauma team was vital in order to ensure that all members were on 'the same page' and sufficiently briefed to allow a smooth reception and rapid decision making.

Trauma team: Casualty arrival

The critically injured casualty was usually transported from the point of wounding to the Role 3 Hospital in Camp Bastion by the MERT onboard a Chinook CK-47 helicopter. This landed on the HLS outside the hospital and then there was a short transfer by ambulance. The prehospital doctor arrived in the emergency department before the casualty in order to commence the handover. It was important that all team members listened in silence to this handover, which was given the same way every time using the mnemonic AT-MIST (Table 22.4). As the casualty arrived, a five-second check was performed by the team leader. This confirmed that the patient was alive, did not have visible catastrophic haemorrhage and had a patent airway. The primary survey was immediately commenced and conducted following the paradigm <c>ABDCE[36] using a horizontal approach.[37] This process was

Table 22.4 AT-MIST handover

A	Age
T	Time of Injury
M	Mechanism of injury
I	Injuries sustained
S	Signs and symptoms
T	Treatment given

possible as the primary survey was coordinated by the TTL so that in reality, many aspects were performed at the same time; the system has been likened to a 'Formula One pit-stop'.[38] The noise levels were kept to a minimum so that information was conveyed to the TTL and instructions relayed back to individual team members. A typical complex trauma team performing a primary survey using a horizontal approach is shown in Figure 22.4. The initial actions of the trauma team are described in Table 22.5; many of these actions allow the gathering of information towards building a picture for the TTL's situational awareness.[5]

A 'hands-off' TTL who maintains situational awareness allows members of the trauma team to focus on their immediate tasks. This approach seeks to prevent fixation errors from occurring (focusing on a single problem to the detriment of the casualty as a whole).[39] In stressful situations, individuals can very quickly fill their 'bandwidth' (the available mental capacity) and become overloaded, and this too can lead to errors. Should a rapid sequence induction (RSI) be required, this should ideally occur in silence similar to a 'cockpit moment' such as the 'take off' or landing of a plane,[40] with all team members appropriately focused.

Our experience of optimising communication in the *damage control resuscitation* (DCR)–*damage control surgery* (DCS) sequence in major trauma management has been published, suggesting the adoption of a 'Trauma WHO'.[41] The *World Health Organisation* (WHO) introduced a surgical safety checklist with three components: a pre-surgical check, a time out prior to starting surgery and a 'sign out', which has reduced hospital mortality.[42] In time-critical situations such as complex trauma, this checklist may not be appropriate and will hinder the timeliness of interventions.[41] This process

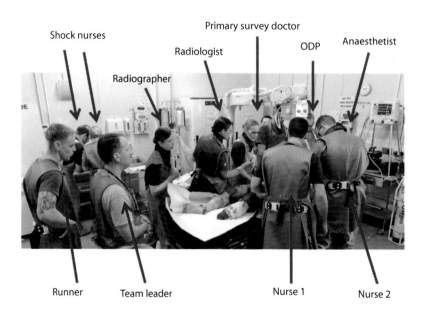

Figure 22.4 Typical complex trauma team undertaking the primary survey.

Table 22.5 Initial management tasks performed by the trauma team in ballistic trauma management

Primary survey <c> ABC

Cervical spine mobilisation (if not already performed)

RSI (if not delivered by MERT)
- Ketamine 1–2 mg/kg
- Suxamethonium 1–2 mg/kg or Rocuronium 1.2 mg/kg

Insertion of a trauma line if indicated (usually in the subclavian vein)

Connection of rapid infusion device and commencement of haemostatic resuscitation

Blood samples for
- Thrombolestomebtry (ROTEM™)
- iSTAT
- Full blood count
- Group and save
- Venous blood gas

Additional intravenous access

Additional drugs administered
- Ketamine (for sedation)
- Fentanyl (up to 500 mcg)
- Neuromuscular blocking drug (Rocuronium)
- Tranexamic acid 1 g
- Tetanus vaccination
- Antiobiotics
- Calcium Chloride (10 mL of 10%)

Focused assessment with sonography for trauma scan (FAST) (by consultant radiologist)

Chest and pelvic digital X-rays (reported by consultant radiologist and viewed by clinicians)

Antibiotics

Swapping C-A-T for pneumatic tourniquets (by orthopaedic surgeons)

Commencement of active warning (using BairHugger™)

was tested and adapted in the field hospital[43] with the four components of the 'Trauma WHO' consisting of

- The Command Huddle
- Snap Brief
- Regular Sit-Reps (Situation Updates)
- Sign out (handover)

COMMAND HUDDLE

The *command huddle* occurred at the end of the secondary survey, when decisions needed to be made regarding the next stage of the patient pathway. Options for onward management included the following:

- An immediate transfer to the operating theatre for DCS. This was typically for a patient who was still actively bleeding and had not responded to early haemostatic resuscitation.
- Transfer to radiology for a computed tomography (CT) scan. *Damage Control Radiology*[44] was the preferred option as much vital information could be gleaned from a 'trauma CT scan'.
- Transfer to critical care. Casualties who had arrived from another facility, who had already had a CT and did not require surgical intervention could be transferred directly to the critical care ward.
- Transfer to the trauma ward for patients who required only Level 3 care.
- Transfer to another facility. Patients who required neurosurgery needed a tactical critical care transfer to the Kandahar Role 3 Hospital (lead by the United States).
- A decision to stop further active treatment and to initiate palliative care. This would require an ethical discussion amongst the team in the command huddle and a method of approaching this has been suggested.[45]

Those personnel involved in the *command huddle* were as follows[41]:

- TTL
- Lead anaesthetist
- Lead trauma surgeon
- Lead orthopaedic surgeon
- Plastic surgeon
- Senior nursing officer
- Deployed medical director

The key decisions that were considered during the *command huddle* were as follows:

- Is treatment futile? This led to termination of active treatment.

- If treatment was to continue, then should the patient be transferred to
  - CT scanner (most favourable option)
  - Operating theatre
  - Critical care
  - Trauma ward
  - Another facility
- If immediate transfer to the operating theatre was required, then which body cavity was to be opened first and which operating table was being used?
- Did the patient require an RSI of anaesthesia? If so, should this be performed in the emergency department or in the operating theatre?
- Were there any ceilings to treatment?

SNAP BRIEF

Once positioned on the operating table and prior to the start of surgery, a snap brief was given. This was led by the TTL prior to handing over to the lead anaesthetist. The key points of information that were communicated included the following[41]:

- The main injuries found on clinical examination and reported radiology. The lead anaesthetist may have been unaware of any additional findings on CT as they were likely to have transferred the patient from CT to theatre and missed the report.
- The current physiological status and degree of physiological stability of the patient.
- The transfusion status including the volume of blood and blood products administered, the estimated ongoing requirements and the current state of the ROTEM™ results.
- The surgical plans and expected timescale of the operation. This might consist of a number of options: these were written out on a white board in theatre, with the trigger points for moving from one plan to another.

SIT REPS

Once surgery was underway a series of SIT REPS (or situation reports)[41] took place. These provided the opportunity to maintain situational awareness by bringing the whole team 'back onto the page'. If too frequent, the SIT REP could be disruptive, so it was conducted only when there was a new piece of

Table 22.6 SIT REP mnemonic

S	Systolic blood pressure
T	Temperature
A	Acidosis
C	Coagulation
K	Kit (Including blood products used)

information or every 30 minutes. The mnemonic STACK can be used to summarise the SIT REP (Table 22.6).

SIGN OUT

At the end of the surgery, there was a formal 'sign out', with a handover to the critical care team who then assumed responsibility for the patient. The lead critical care physician often attended theatre towards the end of the operation for an update and to allow time to prepare to receive the patient.

Critical care air support team

The *Critical Care Air Support Team* (CCAST) evolved throughout the operations, using more sophisticated equipment to push the boundaries of the critical care offered in the air. CCAST also maintained the capability to operate from different air-platforms, unlike many other medical retrieval services, which were tied to a specific airframe. The strategic CCAST was part of *Tactical Medical Wing* (TMW), initially located at *Royal Air Force (RAF) Lyneham* and now at *RAF Brize Norton*. It consisted of two teams, each at high readiness to move 24 hours a day for a period of one month before handing over to a fresh team. At the height of *Operation Herrick*, strategic teams were flying back-to-back missions, with a typical mission length being 24 hours; this was both physically and mentally demanding.

The *tactical CCAST* team was located in the theatre of operations and rotated on a two- or three-month cycle. Teams transferred and retrieved critically ill patients within the theatre of operations in order to deliver them to a higher level of care or for them to receive specialist treatment. Teams flew on a wide variety of air platforms and worked with aircrews from all ISAF nations. Communication within the team and between

CCAST and the individuals involved was vital throughout the patient pathway.

The CCAST team leader was an experienced CCAST nurse. This allowed the consultant anaesthetist/intensivist and second critical care nurse to concentrate on patient care. The team leader concentrated on communication between all the parties involved in a transfer, including the aircrew and the *Aeromedical Liaison Officer* based in the theatre of operations. They also coordinated logistics and communication within the team. Where possible, they were not involved in patient care and stood back to maintain situational awareness. Sometimes, this was not possible, for example if there was more than one patient. The team was encouraged to assist each other within their competency range, maintaining good communication and feeding information to the team leader. As such, communication was vital and once CCAST was activated, the team leader briefed all members on patient information, timelines and aircraft and logistical constraints. An initial medical plan was then briefed to the team by the consultant and mission planning occurred. Simple checklists evolved so that all the 1.5 tonnes of equipment required for a strategic mission as well as any equipment required for each individual patient was checked and packaged in a standardised fashion. This ensured that nothing was forgotten at any point in the patient journey. A series of laminated cards for critical incident management was also developed at the latter end of *Operation Herrick*. This aimed to reduce task fixation by the main operators but also ensured that all team members were empowered to assist within their defined roles.

EDUCATION AND TRAINING

Recently, The *National Institute for Health and Care Excellence* has suggested that healthcare professionals who deliver care to patients with trauma should have up-to-date training in the interventions they are required to provide.[46] The UK-DMS were very much ahead of the curve with this concept and developed and continually adapted training based on current evidence and experience. During the conflict, a number of papers were published on the skill sets and training that were required to become a military

surgeon,[47] a military anaesthetist or other military clinical specialist.[48]

Most of the courses delivered during both *Operation Telic* and *Operation Herrick* were led by those who had recently returned from the conflicts, with input from subject matter experts. The importance of human factors and multidisciplinary training for the teams who were deploying together was recognised and implemented at an early stage. Each individual single service provided their own 'military' pre-deployment training, and this will not be covered in this chapter. However, the remainder of this chapter will review some of the key courses that personnel attended and summarises the publications that resulted from them. In addition, further military training once in the theatre of operations has been documented[49] but will not be covered in this chapter.

Role 1 training

Role 1 care encompasses a variety of key personnel with a diversity of training, experiences, medical knowledge and skills. The aim was to deliver immediate medical care, within the doctrine of the 'platinum 10 minutes' and, thus to minimise morbidity and mortality. The keys to this were effective immediate simple treatment by a 'buddy'. professional medical intervention by Role 1 medical assets and forward projection of specialist care by the MERT. All deployed UK military personnel are trained to deliver basic first aid (as per completion of *Military Annual Training Test* (MATT) 3, *Battlefield Casualty Drills*).[50] In addition to this, the *team medic* role was developed (with a minimum requirement of one in every four soldiers being trained to this level) during *Operation Herrick*.[51] Completion of a three-day course in basic trauma care offered individuals a medical skill set beyond the universal MATT3 level. Commanders quickly recognised the value of this training, and during *Operation Herrick 15*, over four fifths of soldiers on the ground were trained to this standard.[21] The value of basic first aid and *team medic* care has since been recognised as contributing significantly to the number of lives saved.[24]

The medical team construct of the *company aid post* (Role 1 facility) consisted of CMTs or MAs, GDMOs and/or RMOs, all of whom were trained to deliver skilled resuscitation within the 'Golden Hour' following wounding, as laid down in BATLS.[52] BATLS was the minimum training requirement for all Role 1 medical personnel for *Operation Herrick* and *Operation Telic*. Nevertheless, to be better prepared for managing cases at Role 1 and to support CMTs and MAs at remote locations, GDMOs often completed additional non-military pre-deployment courses, sometimes at their own expense, in the following:

- Advanced Paediatric Life Support
- Pre-Hospital Paediatric Life Support
- PHEC
- Major Incident Medical Management and Support

Hodgetts and Findlay published a capability review on Role 1 and stated that

'...delivery of primary health care (PHC) accounts for the majority of Role 1 activity, however as this is less emotive it failed to generate the same leverage for rapid, serial and sustained development of clinical capability and consistent governance [as trauma care]'.[24]

This publication generated 77 recommendations and sub-recommendations intended to enhance the care of patients forward of a field hospital. Following the development of the role of medical regiment healthcare governance warrant officer, *Operation Herrick 15* witnessed a cultural change, with increased event reporting by CMTs. With feedback, risk monitoring and development of clinical standards, a best practice standard for Role 1 healthcare governance was created. It is now intended to address CMT and MA training deficiencies through the development of PHC skills and competencies within the firm base.[21]

In preparation for *Operation Herrick 18*, Parsons and colleagues developed a pre-deployment PHC training course for CMTs in order to improve confidence and capability.[53] Although not validated, the course was successful in achieving its objectives and raised the need to develop a bespoke validated Role 1 course. Wheatley re-analysed the Role 1 Capability

Review and reported through a personal account the issues he considered were still prevalent after completing *Operation Herrick 18*, suggesting solutions for future contingency operations.[54] Two significant training gaps were highlighted during both operational campaigns:

- The management of paediatric patients
- The delivery of optimum analgesia for all injured personnel

Sadly, throughout both campaigns, children continued to be unintended victims of the war fighting. Although paediatric exposure at each FOB was variable and dependent on the nature and phase of operations, paediatric workloads of 11% and 12% were reported. These data have been further supported by studies completed at different times and further along the patients' journey. Walker and colleagues completed a retrospective analysis of all paediatric patients transported by the MERT (May 2006 to December 2007) and reported 7.3% of the clinical workload during this time to be due to paediatrics, most patients having been involved in hostile action.[55] Inwald and colleagues also completed a retrospective review of patients under 16 years of age admitted to intensive therapy unit in Camp Bastion during a period of one year (April 2011 to April 2012),[56] 14% of admissions during this time were paediatric patients (median age, eight years). Clinical experience of managing seriously injured children due to blast and gunshot wounds still cannot be developed in a UK health setting.[57,58]

Although BATLS delivered a 'master class' in paediatric trauma care, Walker and colleagues[55] stated that this should only act as a refresher rather than a primary course and raised the need for the development of a bespoke military paediatric trauma course. As a result, the *Military Advanced Paediatric Life Support* course was developed. This course uses fully immersive simulation training to explore key challenges faced when caring for children in the operational environment.[59] It includes familiarisation with, and use of, the paediatric equipment modules. Difficult cases from previous operational deployments are raised to promote reflection and ethical discussions. Unfortunately, this course has been designed for deployed secondary care personnel, and Role 1 still lacks the equivalent course, thus perpetuating a risk for future contingency operations.

The pathophysiology of pain and benefits of optimum pain relief are known.[60] For *Operations Telic* and *Herrick*, delivering high-quality pain management became an important aspect of military medicine. In 2007, the Surgeon General made delivery of optimum pain relief one of his three main efforts.[60] Inadequate analgesia at Role 1 was reported to be an intolerable capability failing, consistently and objectively identified on *Operations Telic* and *Herrick*.[24] As previously discussed, military pre-hospital care is complex and dynamic. Davey and colleagues commented that:

'a medical officer's actions in terms of analgesia provision may be influenced by a number of factors, in the deployed environment it is often the 'where' that makes their job so challenging. An example would be caring for a traumatic amputee in the back of a vehicle, behind a wall, whilst at risk of persisting enemy fire, following an IED blast, all these factors add complexity to a patients' care before we even begin to consider the human factors involved'.[61]

Compounding the challenges was the reality that many Role 1 locations were manned by a lone inexperienced junior medical practitioner.[62] During pre-deployment training for *Operation Herrick 11* (2010), GDMOs reported a lack of confidence in providing safe and appropriate parenteral analgesia unsupervised. Davey and colleagues then conducted a study to explore experiences and quantify confidence levels of deploying Role 1 medical officers (MOs) regarding their use of parenteral analgesia.[61] Role 1 MOs were often required to achieve optimum analgesic control for rapid casualty extraction, whilst awaiting MERT retrieval and for prolonged field care. Despite the fact that during a BATLS course ketamine was described as the analgesic agent of choice, one MO noted that no formal training was offered and all discussions were anecdotal.[62] In 1972, Austin and Tamlyn commented that 'a new era of pain relief, without central depression, has arrived' in an article in the *Journal of the Royal Army Medical Corps*,[63] as they described the use of ketamine. Addressing the training requirements for the MO was clearly overdue. The training recommendations by Davey and colleagues called for improved analgesic training for all Role 1 clinicians, including simulation training to recreate the circumstances in which pain management is practiced at Role 1.[62] The *specialist interest group* (SIG) for pain subsequently designed a pain management study day and included this in the *Post-Graduate Medical Officers Course*. A significant development introduced by the Pain SIG was the successful trial and introduction of the fentanyl lozenge to augment intramuscular morphine.[64] This deployed analgesic option is now taught on the modern BATLS course.

BATLS COURSE

The concept of DCR was introduced into the UK DMS in 2007.[65] Defence Consultant Advisor Emergency Medicine's directive was towards performing simple interventions well, minimising blood loss and maximising tissue oxygenation and thus optimising patient outcome.[66] Application of knowledge, clinical assessment, resuscitation skills and procedural interventions taught on BATLS represent strong links in the DCR chain of survival. Analysis of data from *Operations Telic* and *Herrick* noted significant numbers of mathematically unexpected survivors. The reasons for this are multifactorial; nevertheless, implementation and revision of the BATLS course have been considered to be a significant contributing factor for many successes.[17] BATLS training provided a dogmatic approach to trauma resuscitation that could be applied to each echelon of care within the conventional military evacuation chain. The course was originally developed from the roots of the *Advanced Trauma Life Support* (ATLS®) course, now in its ninth edition[67] and implemented by the British Army in preparation for mass conflict during a Cold War in Europe.[68] Continued analysis of best practice, clinical doctrine and recent operational experiences has ensured that the BATLS course remains current and credible in mitigating the impact of changing threats. This was evident during *Operations Telic and Herrick* and remains so for future contingency operations. Following analyses of operational experiences, the BATLS manual was periodically updated to account for new generations of resuscitation equipment, clinical protocols, techniques and interventions relevant at point of wounding through to Role 3 care (for example use of topical haemostatic agents).[52] The contents list of the BATLS manual (2008) is given in Table 22.7.

In addition to a medical focus, candidates were taught tactics, techniques and procedures for recognising and responding to improvised explosive device (IED) and mine threats, thereby *preventing* injury.

Prior to attending a three-day course, all candidates were required to revise the previously mentioned subjects. Although the BATLS manual was updated and re-published in 2000, 2005, 2008 and most recently 2014, it must be acknowledged

Table 22.7 Content of the BATLS 2008 edition (current for most of the *Herrick* and *Telic* campaigns)

- Mechanisms and epidemiology of military trauma
- Care under fire
- Tactical field care
- Field resuscitation:
  - Preparation
  - Assessment
  - Critical decisions
- Advanced resuscitation:
  - Emergency department assessment
  - Critical decisions
- Systems trauma management:
  - Chest, abdomen & pelvic trauma
  - Head injury
  - Spinal injury
  - Limb injuries
- Burns
- Paediatric & obstetric trauma
- Pain & analgesia
- Environment
- Forensic and medico-legal
- Intensive care
- BATLS in the CBRN environment
- Prolonged field care
- Treatment of civilians on operations
- Triage
- Helicopter evacuation

that the course has changed significantly more frequently to ensure maximum impact and minimise operational morbidity and mortality. BATLS 2008 teaching used a variety of methodologies, including lectures, case workshops and practical sessions. Candidates from multiple medical disciplines were assessed according to their own expected level of competence, with doctors being taught and assessed on every skill, and nurses, CMTs and MAs assessed on delivering some skills as a provider and some as an assistant. Principal course objectives included confirmation of practical competencies and understanding of a broad range of skills, coupled with an assessment of judgement in a team-based scenario.

For all courses delivered during *Operations Telic* and *Herrick*, a formative assessment and feedback were provided throughout the course. Summative assessment occurred on the last day and included a 10 station *Objective Structured Practical Examination*. Deploying frontline and emergency department medical personnel were required to complete BATLS training for *Operations Herrick* and *Telic*.[25] This standard remains true for future contingency operations.[69] Recent changes have moved the course towards a pre-hospital focus and away from the original more general ATLS©-based concept.

MERT COURSE

Background

The evolution of the MERT capability is described in Chapter 3. Whilst its origins lay in the *Initial Response Team* deployed in Iraq, MERT was the first time critical care capability had been projected from Role 2 or Role 3 forward to the point of wounding. It was born out of necessity and initially resulted in DMS personnel working without role-specific training and with no analysis of training needs. Whilst this process caught up with the capability, it was an enduring theme of MERT training that it was required to respond at very short notice to the changing needs of the service personnel on the ground.

Defining training needs

In the very early days of MERT, 2006–2007, there was no specific competency framework for MERT personnel. RAF paramedics who formed part of the teams had been put through a training pathway designed for the combat search and rescue role. The MERT role was not formally established and the paramedics were augmented by an RAF flight nurse (with aeromedical training), an anaesthetist or emergency physician (consultant or specialist registrar) and an operating department practitioner (ODP). For the last of these, MERT was often their first experience of providing care outside the hospital environment and they deployed without any specific selection, training or validation. Following a training needs analysis, formal team and individual training commenced in 2008 and was provided by *TMW, RAF Lyneham*. Instructional specifications covering a broad range of clinical and administrative learning objectives were produced, as was a clear list of pre-deployment requirements for the various team members. These included

- Helicopter Underwater Escape Training (dunker tank);
- Survival, Evasion, Resistance and Escape Training (SERE); and
- The MERT course.

In addition to the evolving MERT course, the deploying teams were validated during the deploying unit's *mission-specific validation exercises* as part of the hospital exercise (HOSPEX) at Army Medical Services Training Centre (AMSTC).

Challenges of effective MERT training

The key to successful training was being able to accurately recreate the operational MERT environment in order to allow personnel to transfer clinical and non-technical skills to this unique setting and to build confidence in their ability to provide effective care. The course was as much about mental preparation as it was about learning new skills. The MERT environment was unique in its intense workload, kinetic threat and the severity and numbers of casualties seen. Very simply, even for those deploying with previous pre-hospital experience, it was difficult to have absolute confidence that one would be effective in an environment that was so hostile to 'normal' clinical care.

Evolution of the course

Early MERT training took place at *TMW, RAF Lyneham* under the supervision of the training team and the newly created SO2 MERT. Whilst it aimed to identify individuals who did not perform to a required clinical standard or whose non-technical skills were not suitable, there was no formal assessment structure and there was variability of material between courses, in particular in the scenarios the candidates undertook. The course consisted of lectures, skills and equipment workshops, ground-based simulation training and a live flying exercise on either Chinook-CH47 or Merlin aircraft. In 2011, *TMW* moved to *RAF Brize Norton* and for a considerable period did not have sufficient access to training facilities and resources to effectively run the MERT course. Healthcare governance surrounding MERT had considerably evolved, it had become clear that the operational requirements had moved on and the course clearly required restructuring. In line with operational requirements, the course was therefore reviewed and rewritten with a standard set of lectures and scenarios. This provided consistency between courses and a structured assessment matrix for candidates, which provided a framework for the enabling staff to assess individuals. The Tri-Service Lead for pre-hospital emergency medicine (DCA EM) introduced the authority for the course director to decide that a candidate might not be considered to be appropriate or ready for deployment based on aspects of their course performance.

The stated aims of the course given to candidates were as follows:

- Familiarisation with the MERT concept
- Familiarisation with the MERT environment
- Familiarisation with the MERT equipment
- To replicate the challenge of providing emergency care in the MERT environment
- To provide confidence to operate in the MERT environment

Key areas of instruction included patient assessment, resuscitation, pre-hospital anaesthesia, analgesia and sedation, paediatrics, communication and non-technical skills and decision making. The rotary wing environment was covered in detail and an operational update was also provided.

Military Operational Surgical Training course

The *MOST Course* was initially developed by the *Academic Department of Military Surgery* in 2009. This course combined several military surgical courses and its definitive form consisted of a week of whole trauma team training at the Royal College of Surgeons in London. The MOST Course won the *Military and Civilian Health Partnership Award* in November 2010. There was an initial live link with the current team in Camp Bastion for a brief on current injury patterns and case mix and then a series of lectures, workshops, fully immersive simulations and dissection using fresh frozen cadavers. It was intended that teams deploying together would train together as this was considered favourable to excellent practice.[70] Failure to standardise the content of much of the lecture material did, however, remain something of a problem, arising at least in part from a desire to reflect current developments on operations. The highlights for each sub-speciality are summarised.

EMERGENCY MEDICINE

Although not a contributor to the early iterations of MOST, the shift of focus to encompass team working and non-technical skills that coincided with an increase in operational tempo and in team size and complexity drove the inclusion of emergency physicians on the MOST Course as both faculty and delegates from 2010. The opportunity for those individuals who would be deployed as TTLs to practice the role with their deploying colleagues in realistic simulated scenarios with credible formative debriefing was instrumental in improving and standardising how deployed trauma teams were led and operated. Trauma team leadership had previously been a somewhat personality dependent function with marked variation in interpretation of the role, but publishing guidance on how a 'trauma call' should run[37] and then providing a forum in which to practice against this template led to an improvement in standards across the board, particularly driving an increase in awareness and consideration of non-technical skills and human factors. By attending the entire MOST Course, emergency physicians also benefitted from the technical and theoretical training that their anaesthetic and surgical colleagues were undertaking, thus improving the whole team understanding of contemporary trauma lessons as they were brought back from the operational theatre. In addition, other specialists gained from the broader view of their emergency medicine colleagues. This period coincided with the development of major trauma centres and trauma networks, and in many regions, the lessons being learnt on the MOST Course by emergency physicians became the foundations of the trauma team leadership courses that are now a key component in improving trauma care delivery in the NHS and, indeed, the foundations of NHS resuscitation room practice.

TRAUMA SURGERY

During *Operations Telic* and *Herrick*, the MOST Course underwent constant revision to reflect the injuries occurring, so that surgical teams were being trained to treat the most up-to-date injury patterns. For surgeons, it reinforced techniques utilised in trauma and encouraged team interaction. It also allowed assessment of clinicians and formed part of the validation of these individuals prior to deployment. The key operative areas that were addressed were thoracic, neck, abdominal, junctional and vascular trauma. The dissections were undertaken on cadavers and based around case scenarios. Each dissection table was configured with a general and an orthopaedic surgeon and there was anaesthetic, emergency medicine and ODP input depending on scenario.

Thoracic trauma scenarios included the management of lung parenchymal injuries, thoracic vascular injuries and cardiac injuries, emphasising damage control techniques. Similarly, abdominal trauma dissection provided a comprehensive review of solid organ, hollow viscus and vascular trauma, including haemostatic and organ-specific damage control techniques. The course also aided familiarisation and revision of the anatomy and methods of obtaining proximal vascular control. Similarly, the vascular subsection demonstrated vascular damage control techniques, including shunting and relevant limb fasciotomies.

ORTHOPAEDIC SURGERY

Limb trauma has always provided a high surgical workload in war, and the conflicts in Iraq and Afghanistan reflected this. During the early periods of *Operations Telic* and *Herrick*, the surgical team consisted of a single general surgeon and single orthopaedic surgeon. Conflict in the Middle East saw a change in warfare tactics from the predominant use of bullets to blast weapons, which resulted in a well-documented change in wounding patterns and increasing amounts of limb trauma. By the end of the conflict in Afghanistan, the signature injury had become the complex lower limb injury caused by IEDs. There was a marked increase in casualties with severe leg injuries and associated pelvic trauma, and it was recognised that these injuries were very different from the lower limb injuries previously encountered in Iraq. These devastating injuries presented new challenges to the DMS. Consequently, during the latter years of *Operation Herrick*, the surgical team grew massively in size, involving multiple surgeons of varying specialisations, to reflect the challenges of these casualties. The MOST Course adapted in response to both the changing wounding patterns and also the changing make-up of the DCR team. A surgical strategy was developed involving the complete integration of a multidisciplinary team to maximise the outcomes from these complex injuries. Key to the development of this strategy was the opportunity that the MOST Course gave for surgeons of different specialties to train together with a faculty consisting of recently deployed surgeons able to share their experiences. Teamwork across specialties was encouraged, especially in the management of difficult junctional trauma involving scenarios outside set surgical specialties. Vascular, plastic and general surgeons were involved in teaching sessions on limb trauma to reflect the multi-disciplinary team that would be deployed. Simple and complex debridement techniques were taught and the importance of proximal vascular control was emphasised. Cadaveric dissections were used to reflect real-life cases and allowed the opportunity for general, orthopaedic and plastic surgeons to work together, utilising the external fixation techniques and equipment that would be available in the deployed environment. The MOST Course allowed all surgeons, whatever their specialty, to understand the strategy of dealing with limb trauma and also allowed surgeons who generally worked autonomously in their normal practice to gain vital experience of working in a large multi-disciplinary team.

ANAESTHESIA, PAIN AND CRITICAL CARE

The *Department of Military Anaesthesia, Pain and Critical Care* created a *Special Interest Group in Education and Training*, and initial work was published in the *Journal of the Royal Army Medical Corps*.[15] A MOST component was initially developed to cover all the technical and non-technical skills that would be required by a military anaesthetist in the Role 3 Hospital in Camp Bastion and was geared towards them. This was summarised, with a particular emphasis on the management of haemorrhage, by Mercer et al.[35] in the *Journal of Anaesthesia*. Over time, the course was adapted not only to prepare for deployment but also to fulfil the Level 3 Military Anaesthesia Matrix[71] and Higher Military Training Module[48] of the Royal College of Anaesthetists. A summary of the anaesthetic content of the course follows.

A round-robin exercise introduced candidates to all the military specific anaesthetic equipment based in Camp Bastion. There were tutorials complemented by simulation scenarios to ensure competence in the following equipment and techniques (clinical papers used to guide the training are cited):

- Advanced vascular access[72]
- Anaesthetic machines
  - Anaesthetic Machine Light – Triservice Anaesthetic Apparatus[73]
  - Anaesthetic Machine Heavy – Drager Fabius Tiro Anaesthetic Machine
- Critical care ventilator
- Belmont® rapid infuser
- Difficult airway management
- Thromboelastography (ROTEM™)

Several key papers outlining the process and theory of DCR were used as a foundation for the teaching content.[74] There were lectures and small group workshops to ensure that DMS anaesthetists were competent to perform a massive transfusion[75] according to the guidelines of the *Surgeon General's Policy letter*[76] and *Clinical Guidelines for Operations.*[26] This component of training also covered modern concepts, including the acute coagulopathy of shock trauma and the use of near point testing (ROTEM™)[77] to provide the ability to conduct an individually tailored haemostatic resuscitation.

PHEM

The MOST Course provided an introduction to pre-hospital care and outlined how patients would be transported to the hospital and the treatment that they could potentially receive.[78]

SUB-SPECIALITY SPECIFIC WORKSHOPS

The following specialist areas were also covered:

Difficult Airway – This component discussed the issues around the management of the anticipated difficult airway in the deployed environment[79] and the importance of human factors.[80]

Burns – There was a discussion on how to conduct anaesthesia for a casualty with burns in the deployed environment and also a joint lecture with the whole course including ethical considerations.

Paediatrics – A workshop on the management of paediatric casualties was offered, particularly focusing on massive transfusion,[81] equipment and current experience[82] and the management of a child on the critical care at Role 3.[56]

Cardiothoracic Anaesthesia – This was a joint session with the surgeons reviewing the management of cardiothoracic injuries at Role 3,[83] including the management of traumatic cardiac arrest.[84]

Pain Management – An overview of the acute pain guidelines was covered[23,24,85,86] and supplemented by a half-day workshop on regional anaesthesia in the deployed environment.[87]

Critical Care – This workshop provided an overview of critical care at Role 3[16] and covered the deployed critical care Guidelines for Operations. There was also a focus on blast lung injury.[88]

Neuroanaesthesia – There was a focus on the management of patients with traumatic brain injury[89] and how to conduct neuroanaesthesia in the deployed environment.

Imaging – An overview of imaging available in the deployed environment was an important component of the course as there were significant differences between deployed capability and that available in most NHS hospitals.[90]

CCAST – An overview was included of the capabilities of CCAST and how to prepare and package a patient for a CCAST transfer.

OTHER COURSE ELEMENTS

The MOST Course also included focused workshops and discussions. There were discussions on how the Role 4 (Queen Elizabeth Hospital Birmingham) operated,[25,26,91] including specific details of critical care at Role 4[92] and the *Joint Theatre Clinical Case Conference.*[93] An overview of the role of the Deployed Medical Director[94] was provided, including a discussion on difficult decisions including ethics in the deployed environment.[45]

The MOST Course offered the opportunity to use the simulation suite at the Royal College of Surgeons to undertake fully immersive simulation scenarios as a multi-disciplinary trauma team. The simulation suite was 'mocked up' as a trauma bay in Camp Bastion and teams were selected that were deploying together.[95] Scenarios were carefully written and driven to achieve the specific learning objects that are listed in Table 22.8 but essentially cemented the learning from earlier in the course.[15] Following each scenario, usually led by a consultant in emergency medicine, there was an immediate video-assisted debrief focusing on technical and non-technical skills. In order to facilitate the simulation, it was necessary to ensure faculty training and several DMS trainees have undertaken clinical fellowships in simulation.[96]

Defence Anaesthesia Simulation Course

The *Triservice Anaesthetic Apparatus* was originally described by Brigadier Ivan Houghton in 1981,[97] with a subsequent review paper being published by Frazer and Birt.[73] Although not all anaesthetists were in favour of using this equipment,[98] it remained the primary anaesthetic machine for *Operation Telic* and the 'back up' anaesthetic machine for *Operation Herrick.* As a consequence, it was important that DMS

Table 22.8 Examples of learning objectives for fully immersive simulation scenarios

Technical skills	Non-technical skills
Treating trauma patients using clinical guidelines for operations[26]	Practising to receive a casualty as the trauma team and undertaking primary and secondary survey[22,37,95]
Practising administering a massive transfusion according to the Surgeon General's Policy Letter[76]	Conducting a patient assessment using a <C>ABC approach[36] in a horizontal activity[37]
Advanced vascular access (inserting trauma line[72])	Communication • Patient handover (AT-MIST) • Situation updates • Discussion with theatres, critical care and command
Practising using equipment in the trauma bay • Belmont rapid infuser • Difficult airway equipment • Pelvic binders	Command Huddle[41] and decisions to next stage of the patient pathway.
Familiarisation with trauma team paperwork	Team leadership

anaesthetists were familiar with its use prior to deployment.

The *Defence Anaesthesia Simulation Course* is currently a two-day course held at the *Centre for Simulation and Patient Safety* based at Aintree Hospital in Liverpool, a regional high-fidelity simulation centre. The course is for anaesthetists and ODPs with the other roles being played by faculty members. In small teams, the candidates undertake fully immersive simulation scenarios to allow practice with the Tri-Service anaesthetic apparatus and other military anaesthesia equipment with a video-assisted debrief after each scenario. Common problems with the equipment are investigated and military anaesthetic techniques discussed including use in paediatrics.[99] This course is mapped to the higher military module of the Royal College of Anaesthetists.[48]

Surgical Training Denmark

This is a two-day package organised by the Danish Armed Forces, utilising live tissue to demonstrate real-time surgical control of life-threatening traumatic injuries. The course was undertaken by UK personnel every three years, ideally after the MOST Course and just before the team deployed. This course enabled teams to work together in a controlled environment with exposure to high-grade trauma, whilst establishing effective team dynamics. Again like the MOST Course, it replicated time-critical injuries and management. It also enabled the teams to undertake operative management and work in real-time to control the injuries. Like the MOST Course, it encompassed thoracic, abdominal, vascular and junctional trauma. Although this course has attracted a degree of controversy due to its use of live animals, it remains an essential way of learning key lifesaving skills before they are practised on critically injured service personnel.

Critical Care Air Support Team

CCAST (E) COURSE

This was an annual requirement for all nursing and medical members of CCAST and was a one-week course designed to ensure that all team members were up to date with advances in CCAST equipment, competent at basic equipment maintenance and fully informed regarding all equipment capability and constraints. This was vital when working in the extreme and remote conditions of a CCAST retrieval or transfer. The course involved small group tutorials and was assessed with a single best answer question test and practical examination on all the major pieces of equipment.

STRATEGIC CCAST SIMULATION

This 1.5-day course is currently held in the first week of every month in order to give the oncoming strategic CCAST the opportunity to train together in a safe, immersive, simulated environment. Simulations are based on recent missions, allowing dissemination of up-to-date information on case mix, aviation constraints and challenges and logistical issues. Scenarios run as close to real-time as practicable using high-fidelity simulated patients on the ground, the transfer aspect being carried out on either a *Lockheed C-130 Hercules* or a *Boeing C17 Globemaster*. Whilst technical skills are tested in the simulation, the main focus is on the non-technical skills required for a CCAST transfer. This is because CCAST must interact with multiple agencies, carry large amounts of equipment and operate out of multiple air platforms in a variety of environments.

TACTICAL CCAST

This three-day course evolved towards the end of *Operation Herrick* utilising the HOSPEX environment. It allowed the deploying tactical CCAST to train together; not only to rehearse casualty management in scenarios developed following feedback from those recently returning from theatre but also to develop management plans in the event of emergency landings in both permissive and non-permissive environments. The training was assisted by briefings by load master aircrew from the rotary and fixed wing air platforms currently operating in theatre. Live flights on aircraft were

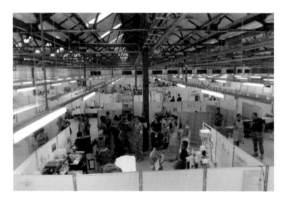

Figure 22.5 HOSPEX. Army Medical Services Training Centre.

included, as many of the team members had not flown on one particular aircraft or other and were therefore unfamiliar with its capability and constraints. In some cases, air sickness was identified as a significant problem.

Scenarios concentrated not only on transfers from a Role 3 hospital but also on retrievals from a Role 2 facility. They emphasised the non-technical skills and operational and logistical issues of transferring patients. These included direct retrieval from the operating theatre on extremely tight time lines and working with ISAF medical colleagues who did not speak English and used different treatment regimens and units of measurement in test results. Lectures were developed using feedback from the most recently deployed team and offered information on non-UK air platforms utilised by CCAST. The issues raised by unfamiliar platforms, especially regarding the airworthiness of equipment and physical constraints that needed to be considered were discussed in detail.

Hospital Exercise

The HOSPEX took place at the AMSTC at Strensall near York (Figure 22.5) and was described as a macrosimulation.[100] HOSPEX evolved dramatically from the time of the end of *Operation Telic* 1.[101] Essentially, a large building was 'mocked up' to replicate the outline of the deployed field hospital with the exact equipment (for example emergency department resuscitation bays, anaesthetic machines, operating tables and paperwork in each department). *HOSPEX* was designed to allow the whole deploying hospital unit the opportunity to practice together in collective training. It allowed personnel not only to rehearse their clinical actions but also to exercise the process of casualty handling from the point of wounding to transfer back to Role 4 by CCAST. Constraints such as limited numbers of radiographers were identified and practice accordingly adjusted. The simulation also included the managerial and logistic aspects of running a deployed hospital.

The exercise lasted from three to five days and matured as both conflicts continued. Towards the end of *Operation Herrick*, teams were mandated to attend two *HOSPEX* exercises. *HOSPEX* also allowed the opportunity to run assurance and validation of the hospital. A description of *HOSPEX* in 2008 has been published.[102]

Scenarios used 'simulated patients' provided by commercial companies who employed live actors who had been injured previously and make-up artists to simulate realistic injury patterns. SimMan 3G® (Laerdal Medical Ltd, Orpington, UK) was also used, and the faculty took advantage of the wireless functions of this mannequin to allow transfer throughout the hospital. The principal advantage of a long exercise was that it allowed clinical conditions to develop over a few days, which was much more realistic than traditional simulation courses that tended to focus on short scenarios. This extended duration allowed patients to arrive via the MERT, undergo a 'trauma call' and be transferred to CT scan and the operating theatre and then to critical care. At the same time, the administration process in the hospital was ongoing. Additional factors which might occur in a deployed environment such as loss of power, indirect fire, captured person reception, oxygen shortage, infectious diseases and even a VIP visit could be inserted into the exercise.

The most significant benefit of *HOSPEX* from the operational point of view was that the deployed hospital team were able to arrive on operations '*ready to hit the ground running*' as they had already met, socialised together and worked through many of the expected scenarios. As has been pointed out by Ramasamy and colleagues when examining surgical logbooks, during busy periods, there is little opportunity for 'in operation' training and so the period of pre-deployment preparation is vital, with instruction needing to take place well in advance of arrival in theatre.[47] Subject matter experts and those who had returned very recently from operations were asked to direct scenarios that were continuously adapted and developed in response to new evidence and experience, ensuring that the training given was as up to date as possible and altered as conditions on the ground and injury patterns changed. Since the end of *Operation Herrick*, the HOSPEX facility has been used to train personnel for the UK Armed Forces response to the Ebola outbreak (*Operation Gritrock*).

CONCLUSIONS

This chapter outlines the importance of human factors along the whole patient pathway during both *Operation Telic* and *Operation Herrick*. The extensive package of pre-deployment clinical training has been described from Role 1 and pre-hospital care to the rest of the hospital team. Of particular significance was the creation of the *Military Operation Surgical Course*, which allowed the whole trauma team to practice together using lectures, workshops, fully immersive simulation scenarios and cadaveric dissection to prepare to receive casualties with very different injury patterns that were not usually encountered in normal NHS practice. Also of significance was the creation of a macrosimulation HOSPEX allowing rehearsal by the whole hospital team at several points in pre-deployment training, with the result that teams arrived in the theatre of operations ready to commence at once. A cautionary note is necessary; maintaining access to training by service medical personnel during times of relatively low operational intensity is always likely to be a challenge, and evidence to date suggests that training budgets *are* seen as areas for cost savings. One can only hope that such measures will not be of a sufficient magnitude to have a negative impact on future care.

REFERENCES

1. Thorson CM, DuBose JJ, Rhee P et al. Military trauma training at civilian centers. *J Trauma Acute Care Surg* 2012;73: S483–S489.
2. Penn-Barwell JG, Roberts SAG, Midwinter MJ et al. Improved survival in UK combat casualties from Iraq and Afghanistan. *J Trauma Acute Care Surg* 2015;78:1014–1020.
3. Mercer SJ, Arul GS, Pugh HEJ et al. Performance improvement through best practice team management – human factors in complex trauma. *J R Army Med Corps* 2014;160:105–108.
4. Catchpole KR, Dale TJ, Hirst DG et al. A multicenter trial of aviation-style training for surgical teams. *J Patient Saf* 2010;6: 180–186.

5. Flin R, O'Connor P, Crichton M. *Safety at the Sharp End: A Guide to Non-Technical Skills*. Farnham: Ashgate, 2008.

6. NHS England. Human factors in healthcare – a concordat from the National Quality Board. 2013. http://www.england.nhs.uk /wp-content/uploads/2013/11/nqb-hum-fact -concord.pdf (accessed 26 April 2016).

7. Helmreich RL, Davies JM. Anaesthetic simulation and lessons to be learned from aviation. *Can J Anaesth* 1997;44:907–912.

8. Kohn LT, Corrigan JM, Donaldson MS. *To Err Is Human: Building a Safer Health System*. Washington, DC: National Academies Press, 2000.

9. Department of Health. *An Organisation with a Memory*. London: The Stationery Office, 2000:VII–XI.

10. Bromiley M. Have you ever made a mistake? *Bull R Coll Anaesth* 2008;48:2442–2445.

11. Fletcher G. Anaesthetists' Non-Technical Skills (ANTS): Evaluation of a behavioural marker system dagger. *Br J Anaesth* 2003;90:580–588.

12. Flowerdew L, Brown R, Vincent C et al. Development and validation of a tool to assess emergency physicians' nontechnical skills. *Ann Emerg Med* 2012;59:376–385.

13. Yule S, Flin R, Paterson-Brown S et al. Development of a rating system for surgeons' non-technical skills. *Med Educ* 2006;40:1098–1104.

14. Mitchell L, Flin R. Non-technical skills of the operating theatre scrub nurse: Literature review. *J Adv Nurs* 2008;63:15–24.

15. Mercer SJ, Whittle C, Siggers B et al. Simulation, human factors and defence anaesthesia. *J R Army Med Corps* 2010;156:365–369.

16. McNicholas J, Henning JD. Major military trauma: Decision making in the ICU. *J R Army Med Corps* 2011;57(S3):S284–S288.

17. Hodgetts TJ, Mahoney PF. Military pre-hospital care: Why is it different? *J R Army Med Corps* 2009;155:4–10.

18. Lyon JD, Stacey M, Simpson R. Preparing for an operational tour as a medical officer in Southern Afghanistan. *J R Army Med Corps* 2010;156:192–196.

19. Defence Medical Services. Healthcare governance and assurance in the defence medical services. *Surgeon General Policy Letter*. 01/09 2009.

20. Randall-Carrick J. Experiences of combat medical technician continuous professional development on operations. *J R Army Med Corps* 2012;158:263–268.

21. Gumbley AE, Claydon MA, Blankenstein TN et al. Medical provision in forward locations in Afghanistan: The experiences of general duties medical officers on Op HERRICK 15. *J R Army Med Corps* 2013;159:68–72.

22. Mercer SJ, Howell M, Simpson R. Simulation training for the frontline – realistic preparation for role 1 doctors. *J R Army Med Corps* 2010;156:87–89.

23. Simpson RG. A Better understanding of deployed Role 1. *J R Army Med Corps* 2012;158:155.

24. Hodgetts TJ, Findlay S. Putting Role 1 first: The Role 1 capability review. *J R Army Med Corps* 2012;158:162–170.

25. Batham D, Finnegan A, Kiernan M et al. Factors affecting front line casualty care in Afghanistan. *J R Army Med Corps* 2012;158:173–180.

26. Ministry of Defence. *Clinical Guidelines for Operations – Joint Service Publication 999*. September 2012. London: MOD.

27. Hodgetts TJ, Mahoney PF. Deconstructing complexity: An innovative strategy for military medical research. *J R Army Med Corps* 2016;162:82–84.

28. Salas E, Rosen MA. Building high reliability teams: Progress and some reflections on teamwork training. *BMJ Qual Saf* 2013;22:369–373.

29. Health Care Commission. Defence Medical Services: A review of the clinical governance of the Defence Medical Services in the UK and Overseas. Commission for Healthcare Audit and Inspection, March 2009. http://www.nhs.uk/Defencemedicine /Documents/Defence_Medical_Services _review%5B1%5D.pdf (accessed 26 February 2010).

30. Midwinter MJ, Mercer S, Lambert AW et al. Making difficult decisions in major military trauma: A crew resource management perspective. *J R Army Med Corps* 2011;157:S299–S304.

31. Bailey CJA, Morrison MJJ, Rasmussen CTE. Military trauma system in Afghanistan: Lessons for civilian systems. *Curr Opin Crit Care* 2013;19:569–577.

32. Tai N, Russell R. Right turn resuscitation: Frequently asked questions. *J R Army Med Corps* 2011;157:S310.

33. Townsend P, Gebhartd JE. For service to work right, skilled leaders need skills in "followership". *Manag Serv Qual* 1997;7:136–140.

34. Endsley MR. Toward a theory of situation awareness in dynamic systems. *Hum Factors* 1995;37:32–64.

35. Mercer SJ, Tarmey NT, Woolley T et al. Haemorrhage and coagulopathy in the Defence Medical Services. *Anaesthesia* 2012;68:49–60.

36. Hodgetts TJ. ABC to ABC: Redefining the military trauma paradigm. *Emerg Med J* 2006;23:745–746.

37. Smith J, Russell R, Horne S. Critical decision-making and timelines in the emergency department. *J R Army Med Corps* 2011;157: 273–276.

38. Mercer S, Park C, Tarmey NT. Human factors in complex trauma. *BJA Educ* 2015;15:231–236.

39. Owen H. Zero harm: A target for error management in anaesthesia. *Bull R Coll Anaesth* 2008;51:2610–2613.

40. Ornato JP, Peberdy MA. Resuscitation. *Resuscitation* 2014;85:173–176.

41. Arul GS, Pugh H, Mercer SJ et al. Optimising communication in the damage control resuscitation–damage control surgery sequence in major trauma management. *J R Army Med Corps* 2012;158:82–84.

42. Van Klei WA, Hoff RG, Van Aarnhem E et al. Effects of the introduction of the WHO "Surgical Safety Checklist" on in-hospital mortality: A cohort study. *Ann Surg* 2012;255:44–49.

43. Arul GS, Pugh H, Mercer SJ et al. Human factors in decision making in major trauma in Camp Bastion, Afghanistan. *Ann Surg* 2015;97:262–268.

44. Chakraverty S, Zealley I, Kessel D. Damage control radiology in the severely injured patient: What the anaesthetist needs to know. *Br J Anaesth* 2014;113:250–257.

45. Bernthal E, Russell RJ, Draper H. A qualitative study of the use of the four quadrant approach to assist ethical decision-making during deployment. *Ann Surg* 2014;160: 196–202.

46. National Institute for Health and Care Excellence. *Major Trauma: Assessment and Initial Management.* London: NICE, 2016.

47. Ramasamy A, Hinsley DE, Edwards DS et al. Skill sets and competencies for the modern military surgeon: Lessons from UK military operations in Southern Afghanistan. *Injury* 2010;41:453–459.

48. Birt DJ, Woolley T. Competencies for the military anaesthetist – a new unit of training. *Bull R Coll Anaesth* 2008;52:2661–2665.

49. Morrison JJ, Forbes K, Woolrich-Burt L. Medium-fidelity medical simulators: Use in a pre-hospital, operational, military environment. *J R Army Med Corps* 2006;152: 132–135.

50. Hodgetts T. *Battlefield Casualty Drills 5th Edition Army Code 71638.* London: MOD. 2007.

51. British Army. *Team Medic Casualty Drills: Aide Memoire, June 2008.* London: MOD, 2008.

52. Defence Medical Services. *Battlefield Advanced Trauma Life Support Course.* London: MOD, 2008.

53. Parsons IT, Rawden MP, Wheatley RJ. Development of pre-deployment primary healthcare training for Combat Medical Technicians. *J R Army Med Corps* 2014;160:241–244.

54. Wheatley RJ. The Role 1 capability review: Mitigation and innovation for Op HERRICK 18 and into contingency. *J R Army Med Corps* 2014;160:211–212.

55. Walker N, Russell R, Hodgetts T. British military experience of pre-hospital paediatric trauma in Afghanistan. *J R Army Med Corps* 2010;156:150–153.

56. Inwald DP, Arul GS, Montgomery M et al. Management of children in the deployed intensive care unit at Camp Bastion, Afghanistan. *J R Army Med Corps* 2013;160:236–240.

57. Pearce P. Preparing to care for paediatric trauma patients. *J R Army Med Corps* 2015;161:i52–i55.

58. Coley E, Roach P, Macmillan AI et al. Penetrating paediatric thoracic injury. *J R Army Med Corps* 2011;157:243–245.

59. Jones CL, Mercer SJ, Mahoney PF. Shaping military training in the era of contingency and revalidation. *Bull R Coll Anaesth* 2016; 97:41–43.

60. Aldington DJ, McQuay HJ, Moore RA. End-to-end military pain management. *Philos Trans R Soc B Biol Sci* 2011;366:268–275.

61. Davey C, Mieville KE, Simpson R et al. A proposed model for improving battlefield analgesia training: Post-graduate medical officer pain management day. *J R Army Med Corps* 2012;158:190–193.

62. Davey C, Mieville KE, Simpson R et al. A survey of experience of parenteral analgesia at Role 1. *J R Army Med Corps* 2012;158:186–189.

63. Austin TR, Tamlyn R. Ketamine: A revolutionary anaesthetic agent for the battle casualty. *J R Army Med Corps* 1972;118:15–23.

64. Aldington D, Jagdish S. The fentanyl "lozenge" story: From books to battlefield. *J R Army Med Corps* 2014;160:102–104.

65. Hodgetts TJ, Mahoney PF, Kirkman E. Damage control resuscitation. *J R Army Med Corps* 2007;153:299–300.

66. Mahoney PF, Hodgetts TJ, Midwinter M et al. The combat casualty care special edition. *J R Army Med Corps* 2007;153:235–236.

67. Advanced Life Support Group. Advanced trauma life support (ATLS®): The ninth edition. *J Trauma Acute Care Surg* 2013;74:1363.

68. Hawley A. Trauma management on the battlefield: A modern approach. *J R Army Med Corps* 1996;142:120–125.

69. Martin-Bates AJ, Jefferys SE. General Duties Medical Officer Role 1 remote supervision in the era of Army Contingency Operations. *J R Army Med Corps* 2016;162:239–241.

70. Tai N, Hill P, Kay A et al. Forward trauma surgery in Afghanistan: Lessons learnt on the modern asymmetric battlefield. *J R Army Med Corps* 2008;154:14–18.

71. Mercer SJ. Training and revalidation in defence anaesthesia. *Bull R Coll Anaesth* 2013;80:16–18.

72. Hulse E, Thomas G. Vascular access on the 21st century military battlefield. *J R Army Med Corps* 2010;156(S1):387–394.

73. Frazer RS, Birt DJ. The Triservice anaesthetic apparatus: A review. *J R Army Med Corps* 2011;156:S380–S384.

74. Dawes R, Thomas GOR. Battlefield resuscitation. *Curr Opin Anaesthesiol* 2009;15:527–535.

75. Doughty H, Woolley T, Thomas G. Massive transfusion. *J R Army Med Corps* 2011; 157:277.

76. Ministry of Defence. *Surgeon Generals Policy Letter – Management of Massive Haemorrhage on Operations*. London: MOD, 2009.

77. Keene DD, Nordmann GR, Woolley T. Rotational thromboelastometry-guided trauma resuscitation. *Curr Opin Crit Care* 2013;19:605–612.

78. Dawes R, Mellor A. Prehospital anaesthesia. *J R Army Med Corps* 2010;156(S4): S289–S294.

79. Mercer S, Lewis S, Wilson S et al. Creating Airway management guidelines for casualties with penetrating airway injuries. *J R Army Med Corps* 2010;156:S355–S360.

80. Mercer SJ, Tarmey NT, Mahoney PF. Military experience of human factors in airway complications. *Anaesthesia* 2013;68: 1080–1081.

81. Bree S, Wood K, Nordmann GR et al. The paediatric transfusion challenge on deployed operations. *J R Army Med Corps* 2010;156:361–364.

82. Nordmann GR. Paediatric anaesthesia in Afghanistan – a review of current experience. *J R Army Med Corps* 2010; 156(S4):325–328.

83. Round JA, Mellor AJ. Anaesthetic and critical care management of thoracic injuries. *J R Army Med Corps* 2010;156:145–149.

84. Smith JE, Rickard A, Wise D. Traumatic cardiac arrest. *J R Soc Med* 2015;108:11–16.

85. Beard DJ, Wood P. Pain in complex trauma: Lessons from Afghanistan. *BJA Educ* 2015;15:207–212.

86. Davenport L, Edwards C, Aldington DJ et al. R4 evolution of the Role 4 UK military pain Service. *J R Army Med Corps* 2010;156(S1):400–404.

87. Connor DJ, Ralph JK, Aldington DJ. Field Hospital Analgesia. *J R Army Med Corps* 2009;159:49–56.

88. Mackenzie IMJ, Tunnicliffe B. Blast injuries to the lung: Epidemiology and management. *Philos Trans R Soc B Biol Sci* 2010;366:295–299.

89. Park C, Moor P, Birch K et al. Operational anaesthesia for traumatic brain injury. *J R Army Med Corps* 2010;156(S1):337–343.

90. Gay D, Miles R. DAT Gay, RM Miles. Use of imaging in trauma decision-making. *J R Army Med Corps* 2011;157:S289–S292.

91. Wood P, Haldane A, Plimmer S. Anaesthesia at Role 4. *J R Army Med Corps* 2010;156: 308–310.

92. Jones C, Chinery J, England K et al. Critical care at Role 4. *J R Army Med Corps* 2010;156:342–348.

93. Willdridge D, Hodgetts T, Mahoney P et al. The Joint Theatre Clinical Case Conference (JTCCC): Clinical governance in action. *J R Army Med Corps* 2010;156:79–83.

94. Mahoney P, Hodgetts T, Hicks I. The deployed medical director: Managing the challenges of a complex trauma system. *J R Army Med Corps* 2011;157:S350–S356.

95. Horne S, Smith JE. Preparation of the resuscitation room and patient reception. *J R Army Med Corps* 2011;157:S267–S272.

96. Mercer S, Jones N, Guha A. A clinical fellowship in simulation in healthcare. *BMJ Careers* 10 February 2010. http://careers .bmj.com/careers/advice/view-article .html?id=20000744.

97. Houghton IT. The Triservice anaesthetic apparatus. *Anaesthesia* 1981;36:1094–1108.

98. Mercer S, Beard DJ. Does the Tri-Service anaesthetic apparatus still have a role in modern conflict? *Bull R Coll Anaesth* 2010;60:18–20.

99. Ralph JK, George R, Thompson J. Paediatric anaesthesia using the Triservice anaesthetic apparatus. *J R Army Med Corps* 2010;156:84–86.

100. Arora S, Sevdalis N. HOSPEX and concepts of simulation. *J R Army Med Corps* 2008; 154:202–205.

101. Cox C, Roberts P. HOSPEX: A historical view and the need for change. *J R Army Med Corps* 2008;154:193–194.

102. Davis TJ, Nader MN, McArthur DJ et al. Hospex 2008. *J R Army Med Corps* 2008; 154:195–197.

23

Developments in equipment and therapeutics

INTRODUCTION

Plato wisely wrote that 'necessity is the mother of invention'[1]; unfortunately, as Louis Foreman remarked much more recently, 'invention is a process; you don't get there overnight'.* Even in times of considerable urgency, where the saving of life is the ultimate end point, a robust, accountable, effective process must be in place to ensure that drug and equipment requirements are met in a timely manner in order to deliver the desired effect. Such a process needs to be rapidly responsive not only to the needs of deployed clinicians and patients but also to developments in the wider clinical world. It is this element of the logistical process that military clinicians must understand and be able to exploit so as to promote care that is responsive to clinical and operational needs and to facilitate the continuous development and deployment of new equipment and therapeutics for deployment.

The opportunity to avoid or mitigate death and injury is an emotive driver of change that demands attention from clinicians on the frontline and in the field hospital, from commanders at all echelons, from the general public and from politicians. Opportunities to manipulate the system by exaggeration of the impact or significance of a change must be balanced against other competing requirements, operational impact and the need for training and maintenance of new equipment. Advice must be scrupulously impartial, expert and coordinated by those in roles

with clinical responsibility for a service or speciality. The pressure to ensure that everything that could be done was being done to reduce death and injury was palpable throughout the conflicts, and with that came a degree of flexibility regarding the processes and additional resources required to support these developments. This allowed very significant advances in equipment, in terms of preventative as well as treatment capabilities, alongside novel uses of new and known therapeutics. Processes were streamlined and military clinical medicine catapulted to the front edge of innovation. The end point of saving lives is evidenced by an unprecedented unexpected survivor rate compared to previous conflicts,[2] a direct result of development based on lessons learned and the enthusiastic embracing of change.

PROCESS OF DEVELOPMENT AND INTRODUCTION OF CLINICAL PRODUCTS INTO THE DEFENCE MEDICAL SERVICES

There has always been innovation within the *Defence Medical Services* (DMS). Porton Down has existed since 1916, investigating the scientific basis of chemical, biological, radiological and nuclear effects and defence strategies. In 2001, it became part of the UK Government's *Defence Evaluation and Research Agency* (DERA), becoming the *Defence Science and Technology Laboratories* (Dstl) when DERA was split and partially privatised. *Dstl* remains a government agency. The stated aim of *Dstl* is to maximise the impact of science and technology for the defence

---

* Louis Foreman – a contemporary American inventor and businessman.

and security of the United Kingdom. At the same time, individual military clinicians and academics have always attempted to identify areas of research and innovation and develop deployable capability in response.

The initiation of projects to feed into the Dstl research programme or into civilian and military academic circles, has several drivers:

- *Clinical necessity* – a capability gap is identified.
- *Clinical interest* – an individual has a specific interest in an area and carries out research to drive this forward.
- *New technology* – exploring how this may be used in a military setting.
- *Obsolescence* – an equipment or drug is no longer produced or support contracts are no longer available and an alternative must be identified.

In the immediate period prior to *Operations Telic* and *Herrick*, there was limited perceived clinical necessity for an effective and rapidly responsive assessment and procurement system. The clinical advances resulting from the recent conflicts in the Falklands and the Baltic states had been embedded and the major capability gaps addressed. The new *Battlefield Ambulance* had been introduced, the limited lifespan of the armoured ambulance had been recognised and a uniform change to Combat 95 had been largely completed. The deployable equipment scalings, however, remained very much based on projected conflicts in temperate climates and predicted warfighting based on recent experience. Each specialty or department serviced its deployed capability using a sequence of *deployable medical modules* each allocated a unique identifying number and designed for use in a particular department, by a particular individual or specialty or for a specific capability. Although subject to review and modification by a responsible senior officer, often but not invariably the *Defence Consultant Advisor* (DCA) for the relevant specialty, these equipment scales would almost inevitably be found not to reflect the requirements of the forthcoming conflicts.

Expertise from individual clinicians has always had a presence in the procurement process. As stated earlier, the DCAs had, and have, a significant role in ensuring that drugs and equipment matched the requirements of deployed capability, but there were also military professorial posts in the major specialties, with departments able to suggest areas of clinical advance and new capability solutions. In addition, overseas fellowships designed to allow trainees to expand their knowledge and experience and the academic journals of the *Royal Army Medical Corps* and *Royal Naval Medical Services* contributed to a culture of *horizon scanning*. All these elements served to drive innovation, but there was a lack of coordination and the process depended very largely on the designated individuals with responsibility for equipment.

Obsolescence management and new technology assessment continued in the background, requiring a continuous process of review and replacement, but the imperative for change was low. However, work did progress in some areas such as the *first field dressing* (FFD), an item that had not changed in decades. The pace of process was slow but considered acceptable; at the time, it didn't seem to need to be any faster.

Figure 23.1 demonstrates the typical process of introducing new equipment and therapeutics. This is a multistage process, and adding in the complexities of military systems (Figure 23.2) and product design (Figure 23.3), as well as issues associated with securing finance to support individual projects, could take many months and in some cases years to come to fruition. The belief that these equipment scales were effectively an insurance policy rather than being required for immediate use inevitably had a deadening effect on the process.

There were avenues in which areas for development could be highlighted beyond obsolescence and personal clinical interest, as already stated. Medical military *lessons learned* were collated from exercises, equipment failure notifications and innovations from the civilian sector. Effective processes were in place and maintained a DMS at a reasonable degree of readiness.

When an item of equipment is required for a specific operation, usually at short notice, the request is usually made by means of an *urgent operational requirement* (UOR). Any product procured using a *UOR* will be available only for that named operation, will be financially supported from the specific operational budget and will not endure in the equipment

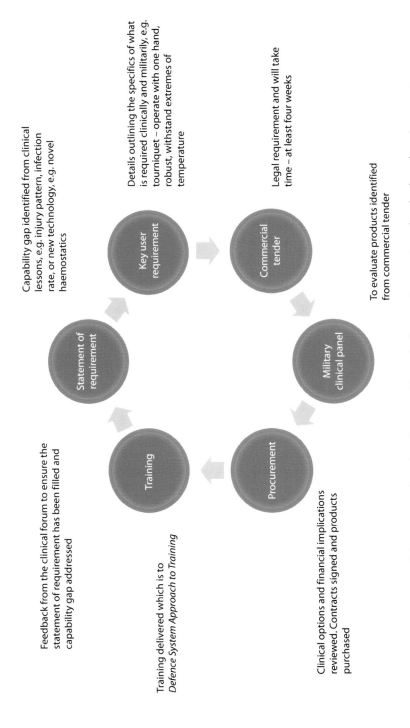

Figure 23.1 Schematic diagram of the process for identifying and introducing equipment into the deployed environment.

Medical capability development process

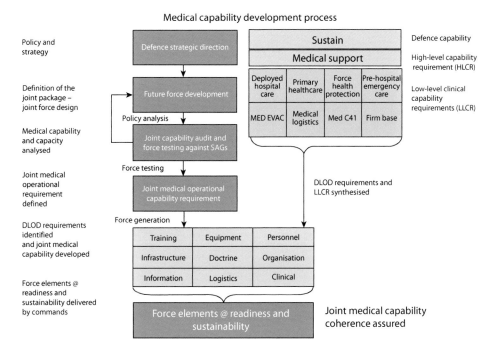

Figure 23.2 Military capability development process.

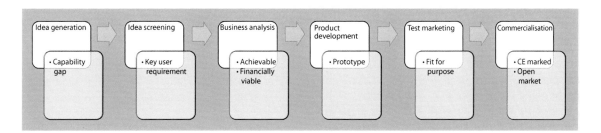

Figure 23.3 Product design.

scales after the end of the operation. Following the end of the operation, therefore, a further, and more complex, procurement process is required, which is discussed in the following sections.

One potential difficulty with the procurement system arose when clinical subject matter experts (SMEs) identified one particular commercially available product as the item of choice for procurement. Although the reasons for this choice might be immediately apparent to the clinicians concerned, these were not always included in the statement of requirement. Because acquisition was (and is) a commercial process carried out by non-clinicians, on occasion, the 'wrong' product was

confirmed for procurement because it was cheaper and fulfilled all the *stated* requirements of the UOR. The obvious way to avoid this was by *very careful* writing of the UOR to ensure that only the item required fulfilled *all* the requirements of the clinicians. However, UORs could not be written to *exclude* a specific product. Inevitably, this was more difficult with very complex items and was a skill that, in general, the DCAs neither had nor had the time to acquire. On occasion, where the only 'evidence' for a particular piece of equipment was expert clinical opinion, it became difficult to override the commercial aspects of the process when a more standard piece of equipment was available and cheaper and no evidence-based case could be made for the preferred alternative. Perhaps, inevitably, these issues led on occasion to clinical frustration with the system. On occasion, the process was halted by clinicians when it became clear that an inappropriate piece of equipment had been endorsed for procurement. Inevitably, this caused delay and wasted money, time and effort.

Further frustration arose when it was perceived that systems designed to prevent wastage in the procurement of "big ticket" items were applied to the acquisition of those costing a few pounds. The legal requirement to go out to tender for such items when clinicians were well aware, for example, of which intravenous cannula they wanted and equally aware that they might have to challenge the process when that item was not selected, was a recurring theme. The small team of staff responsible for medical procurement in *Surgeon General's Department* and the medical logistic chain worked extremely hard throughout the campaigns to ensure that a continuous stream of requests from clinicians was translated into rapid acquisition and deployment. They became expert in facilitating a complex process, and without their efforts in 'translating' the needs of clinicians into achievable procurement goals, many of the advances would either have been significantly delayed or not have happened. The DCAs of the major deployed specialties became adept at ensuring procurement within their areas of responsibility, being fully aware that effective procurement depended on active engagement in the process. In many cases, specialties established equipment committees to filter and assess suggestions for new equipment and therapeutic agents. This largely ensured that time was not wasted processing duplicate or inappropriate requests or requests based on personnel preference that represented little, if any, improvement on the equipment already in service. It was also necessary on occasion to prevent the introduction of items of equipment into theatre by enthusiastic individuals: in the early stage of the campaigns, this was not infrequent (*Medical Emergency Response Team* [MERT] equipment being a notable example) and led to significant amounts of equipment in theatre that was not supported by maintenance contracts or in-house expertise, with which staff were unfamiliar and

untrained and which caused annoyance when it could not be replaced through the normal system.

The ideal system was one that was always alert to potential developments but that rigorously reviewed every item before procurement began. On occasion, problems arose because of a lack of coordination between specialities, although this was not common. Where cooperation was clearly essential, for example in the procurement of expensive items such as the ventilators used in the emergency department (ED), theatres and intensive care unit (ICU), it usually occurred. Where the necessity was less obvious, errors were made, for example acquiring ED trolleys incompatible with the mobile X-ray machines. In order to further refine the system, which had in part been subject to the degree of engagement of the DCAs, towards the later stages of *Operation Herrick*, a *DMS Clinical Materiel Advisory Group* was established to centrally coordinate the process.

Defence procurement, even of relatively small items, is unsurprisingly a complex area from the legal point of view. Over-enthusiastic endorsement of a particular product may raise the risk of an implied contract, and as a consequence, all those involved in acquisition of equipment had to ensure that discussion was focussed on capability gaps rather than particular solutions. Needless to say, this caused some frustration when the process appeared to be taking longer than appeared necessary to procure an item, which, as far as the clinicians were concerned, was obviously the most appropriate solution. However, very large numbers of low priced items such as dressings, tourniquets or needles potentially added up to very considerable sums. It should be no surprise, therefore, that manufacturers and suppliers were extremely keen to retain or acquire contracts. On at least one occasion, ministerial questions were raised as a result of an intervention by an equipment supplier. Such questions inevitably involved a great deal of additional paperwork and time in an already stressed system. On occasion, ill-informed comments by those who should have known better (including accusations of using military personnel as guinea pigs) added unnecessarily to the burden of those engaged in procurement.

The vast majority of medical equipment and drugs were (and are) held in *deployable medical* modules, each module providing the equipment for an individual or team (for example an MERT or *team medic*), department (ED minor injuries or ICU) or capability (surgical or medical). During the campaigns, a thorough review of modules was undertaken to ensure that each was fit for purpose. In most cases, this simply meant regular minor updating of equipment and drugs; on occasion, a radical revision was required, for example of the modules for prehospital care from team medic to pre-hospital doctor, which were realigned with clinical roles.

At all times, the so-called *training tail* had to be considered when introducing equipment to potentially very large numbers of people. Further considerations in the case of replacement kit included the complexity of locating and removing the old equipment from theatre and the potential confusion arising from having two solutions to a given clinical problem. Where there was a significant safety concern regarding the old equipment, or the replacement was *dramatically better*, equipment was generally withdrawn and replaced. Where the change brought only marginal improvement, or the development did not affect the health of patients, stocks of disposables were usually consumed before replacement. When new items offered only marginal improvement over the capability already in service, frequent changes were not endorsed, but a watching brief was kept until the accumulated improvements justified procurement, with its inevitable training requirement and cost.

Appropriate maintenance capabilities also had to be in place for much of the equipment. In some cases, this could be undertaken 'in house', although in the case of complex equipment, it was usually necessary to enter into contracts with the manufacturer. Occasionally, equipment had to be withdrawn not because it failed to function but because it was no longer in production or because maintenance contracts were no longer available. In both cases, a replacement had to be identified and deployed *before* the in-service equipment failed.

PRE-DEPLOYMENT

The advent of the potential conflict of *Operation Telic* can have come as a surprise to very few. Like many conflicts, the period immediately preceding the invasion was suggestive of impending conflict.

Exercise Saif Sareea II was a major military exercise in September and October 2001 involving the UK and Oman military. Over 22,000 UK personnel deployed. Although its main objective was to test the UK's expeditionary warfare strategy, it equally importantly highlighted shortcomings in equipment and practices associated with a deployment to such an austere climate, allowing the military to identify challenges and address these areas.[3] From a medical perspective, the fact that issue combat boots melted in the heat and the SA80 Rifle suffered from stoppages due to sand and heat were worries, but more importantly, the effect of heat on troops and the implications in terms of preventative strategies and treatment options became apparent. At this stage, no one predicted the types, numbers and severity of the casualties that would be seen in the years that followed.

In early 2003, during the preparation for *Operation Telic*, the build-up for deployment and recognition that conflict was likely to occur focused all the elements of the military on the task in hand. The effects of heat had been addressed, with modifications to canvas tents and the establishment of command responsibility to ensure that acclimatisation was carried out, as well as widespread training in the recognition and treatment of heat injury casualties. The lessons learned at this point had been passed from the DMS through the chain of command following the exercise of 2001: the process appeared to work.

EQUIPMENT AND THERAPEUTIC DEVELOPMENT DURING THE CONFLICT

Conflict moves at a rapid place, and the early stages of recognising equipment failures and capability gaps due to the different and austere environment quickly highlighted the need to address these issues in a timely manner. Changes to the process were going to have to occur. Unfortunately, the pace of change and development did not slow during the conflict and the consequences of necessarily short-cutting established processes have had far reaching effects, which are still being addressed today.

As stated previously, equipment procurement by the more rapid *UOR* system lasts only as long as the campaign for which it is acquired. Following the end of the operation, therefore, a further procurement process, using a *statement of requirement (SOR)*, is required for any item required as part of standing capability. Input to generate an SOR for equipment and therapeutics comes from all avenues, as shown in Figure 23.4. SORs are not limited to a single operation and allow items to be taken into the *core (i.e. standing) modules*. As a result, post-conflict, in order to integrate all of the UOR equipment and therapeutics into the core modules and make them available for continued use within the DMS, a large-scale exercise has had to be undertaken and funding streams secured according to clinical priorities.

This has highlighted the importance of data collection and gathering evidence of benefit in sustaining these new capabilities. This process is still ongoing.

Clinical effects were noted and collated. Formal data collected for audit pre-conflict was expanded and data collection systems beginning with the simple *Operational Emergency Department Attendance Register* and moving to the much more complex *Major Trauma Audit for Clinical Effectiveness* were established. This involved the appointment of a

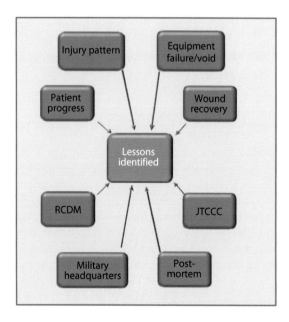

Figure 23.4 Lines of information to identify lessons learned which feed into the statement of requirement and product development.

deployable *trauma nurse coordinator*, a bespoke post that demanded specific pre-deployment training, the production of a new trauma form to capture the data, which was under constant review, and close working relationships with our military allies, allowing sharing of information and audit. Revision of the data collection systems continued throughout both conflicts, and the information was held within the *Joint Theatre Trauma Registry.*[4]

Information from the audits, alongside clinical outcomes at the main receiving hospital for injured service personnel, the *Queen Elizabeth Hospital Birmingham (Royal Centre for Defence Medicine [RCDM])*, post-mortem findings, injury patterns, current ballistic and war threat information from command headquarters, as well as intelligence gathering, was collated and informed by discussion at the weekly *Joint Theatre Clinical Case Conference* (JTCCC). By these means, critical medical intelligence was passed to those best placed to address the issues raised. This facilitated rapid policy change and the authority to develop, procure and deliver new equipment and therapies. Examples included the development of clothing offering protection to the perineum, eye protection, the acquisition of blood warming capability for MERT and effective systems for vascular access during resuscitation.

DEVELOPMENT OF EQUIPMENT AND THERAPEUTICS ALREADY IN USE

Change is not easy, especially in the context of operating in an alien environment with the ongoing threat of war fighting. Even small changes that had begun to take shape prior to the conflict, but with which personnel were not yet completely familiar, caused concern. The following sections discuss only a very small sample of the many changes and additions made to medical devices and drugs over the two campaigns.

First field dressing

The FFD, an absorbent dressing bandage that had remained the mainstay of initial treatment for decades, had recently been replaced by the

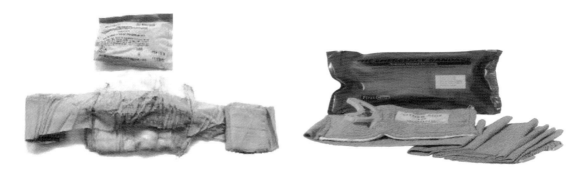

Figure 23.5 Field dressings. The old *FFD* (a) and the new *emergency care bandage* (b).

emergency care bandage, after assessment by emergency medicine specialists under the supervision of the DCA (Figure 23.5). A pragmatic decision was made that existing stock piles would be used up (at the time this was largely for training purposes), and as a consequence, the new bandage was only just reaching frontline troops in 2003.

The initial tendency, in some cases, was to utilise both systems, placing the FFD on a wound and then wrapping the emergency care bandage around to hold it in place, a 'belts and braces' approach to medicine, which was a common theme throughout the conflicts. This specific practice was recognised and with targeted training the correct use was quickly implemented.[5]

The *emergency care bandage* was reviewed several times during the conflict. The need for larger versions for abdominal injuries and extensive soft tissue wounds became evident as injury patterns evolved and the *abdominal bandage* and *blast bandage* were procured. This procurement was very much targeted to deliver effect, with the need to limit any training burden and exploit the ease of familiarity influencing the key user requirements. This addition occurred without any major problems and the new bandages became an additional element in the armoury of front line troops.

A specific concern in relation to the emergency bandage was pressure from commercial suppliers to procure the bandage with an integral pressure bar. This bar would allow the dressing to be used as a tourniquet and was commonly used by other armed forces to good effect. Given that all UK troops were issued with a separate tourniquet of known effectiveness, the issue was carefully

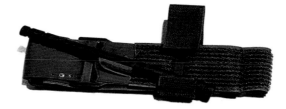

Figure 23.6 CAT™.

considered. It was concluded by UK SMEs that a tourniquet effect was not always required and might be used inappropriately if it formed part of the routine dressing. It was further felt that on those occasions when a tourniquet was genuinely needed, the Combat Application Tourniquet™ (CAT) was more likely to be effective than using the tourniquet element of the emergency bandage (Figure 23.6). To that end, the DMS continued to use the simple emergency care bandage in conjunction with a tourniquet, with good outcomes, testament to understanding the potential complications of over-engineering a product.

Combat tourniquet

The tourniquet had gone out of favour in civilian practice and no longer formed part of routine haemorrhage control. The medical tourniquet held in the military modules was tired and impractical; made from rubber that perished in storage, it was far from intuitive to use. It very quickly became apparent from early in the conflicts that with an increasing frequency of amputated limbs, a robust, effective, easily applicable tourniquet was needed.

Tourniquets improvised from cable ties and belts had been used but were unacceptable given the delay associated with their application and their variability in effectiveness. There was a clinical imperative to address this issue and a high priority was assigned to finding a solution. A UOR was produced detailing the basic requirements to be fulfilled and the procurement process accelerated, with the timely arrival of the CAT™ in theatre shortly thereafter.

The first iteration of the tourniquet did not have a name and time label on it; this was added later as it was understood that capturing the time of application was important and that pre-hospital documentation was difficult to achieve. Other modifications have included strengthening the windlass and, most recently, a single-loop buckle. The effectiveness of the tourniquet is now almost universally accepted and some armed forces have adopted clothing with tourniquets built in. This approach has not been adopted by the UK Military.

The development of the tourniquet continued throughout the conflicts. Its clinical effects and potential complications were monitored, and alternative products were reviewed several times, but the CAT™ continued to be fit for purpose.[6–10] In 2016, a formal SOR was raised to bring the tourniquet into core equipment schedules.

The surgical tourniquet used within the field hospital was due for an upgrade, but this came late on in the conflict as the available model was fit for purpose. This change came about in line with changes to the resuscitation process of the seriously injured casualty undergoing resuscitation, transfer to the computed tomography (CT) scanner and then to theatre. A more easily mobile tourniquet was needed with audible and visual alarms if the inflatable cuff failed, a new element to a product that was previously acceptable.

Recombinant factor VIIa

Despite immense pressure to save lives and reduce morbidity, this did not mean that the regulatory framework stipulated by the UK *Medical and Health Products Regulatory Agency* could be ignored. However, if a drug was to be used 'off license', a specific military process was available. This involved a detailed review of any proposed change in practice by the *UK Advisory Group on*

Military Medicine, a committee of senior civilian and military subject matter experts who would review the information, assess any risk and advise the Surgeon General accordingly. The Surgeon General would then be able to issue a *policy letter* endorsing use under specific conditions.

At the start of the conflicts, recombinant factor VIIa (rFVIIa), a product that aided coagulation and therefore stopped bleeding, was recognised as an adjunct to standard methods of haemorrhage control in European trauma guidelines. Its initial use in trauma was documented in 1999 by the Israeli Defence Force and it had been used subsequently for this indication but was only licensed in the United Kingdom for the treatment of haemophilia. It was also very expensive and most effective when the patient was not in extremis with deranged coagulation and acidosis. Evidence suggested, therefore, that it should not be seen as a 'last ditch' intervention, when futility was likely in the face of standard treatments. These factors were taken into consideration and clinicians were given clear guidelines regarding how and when this product should be used with its inclusion into the *Clinical Guidelines for Operations* and a Surgeon General's policy letter adding weight to this.[11] Given the controversy around this drug, its use was closely monitored throughout the conflict, with frequent reviews, and found to be in line with the parameters set.[12,13] In general, the impressions gained by deployed clinicians suggested little, if any, effect.[14] As the conflict continued and resuscitation management developed with the advent in 2009 of point-of-care testing utilising *Rotational Thromboelastometry* (ROTEM) to target the management of coagulopathy using component blood products, the use of rFVIIa dropped considerably. By 2012, evidence concerning clinical outcomes following use of the drug underwent an international review, and it was deemed no longer appropriate for use outside the treatment of haemophilia.[15] Accordingly, the military adhered to the civilian guidance and it was withdrawn.

Tranexamic acid

This drug was discovered in 1962 and is an antifibrinolytic drug, which has been shown to reduce bleeding. It was generally used in gynaecology for the treatment of heavy menstrual periods but also commonly in surgical specialities such as urology and orthopaedics. In 2010, a large randomised controlled trial involving 274 hospitals in 40 countries was undertaken looking at the effects of early administration of a short course of tranexamic acid (TXA) on death, vascular occlusive events and the receipt of blood transfusion in trauma patients. This trial, CRASH-2 (Clinical Randomisation of an Antifibrinolytic in Trauma), demonstrated that TXA safely reduced the risk of death in bleeding trauma patients.[16] A further review of the data in 2011 refined the details of dosage and timing of delivery.[17] Immediately following from this, the North Atlantic Treaty Organization (NATO) Blood Panel directed that NATO forces should include TXA in the treatment of trauma patients with uncontrolled bleeding, and it was introduced into clinical practice by the DMS and deployed accordingly.[18] Its use was subsequently pushed forward to the pre-hospital clinicians and incorporated into their clinical protocols to ensure timely delivery as part of forward resuscitation. Further work was undertaken to understand and assess the effect of its administration on total blood product use, thromboembolic complications and mortality and how it works in conjunction with the targeted ROTEM directed treatment of coagulopathy. The studies[19,20] showed favourable outcomes.

The potential of TXA does not end there in that there is a school of thought that consideration should be given to issuing TXA to all frontline troops in future conflicts in order to ensure that it is delivered within the beneficial window, especially if the timelines in future operations are likely to be prolonged.[21] In effect, this drug, which was seldom used outside of specialist practice, has become a high-profile, lifesaving, forward delivered medicine during the conflicts and the available data augmented the evidence for its effectiveness.

DEVELOPMENT OF EQUIPMENT AND THERAPEUTICS NEW TO THE DEFENCE MEDICAL SERVICES

The nature of the conflicts, in terms of the patterns of wounding and mobility of medical assets around the battle space, in conjunction with close clinical governance feedback loops shaping clinical practice, led to two major changes in clinical approach:

- The defining of damage control resuscitation – which included optimising the patient pathway, reducing timelines, establishing damage control surgery and 'right turn resuscitation' and targeting specific clinical therapies.
- The formation of the MERT, a modification of the existing *Incident Response Team* (Figure 23.7)

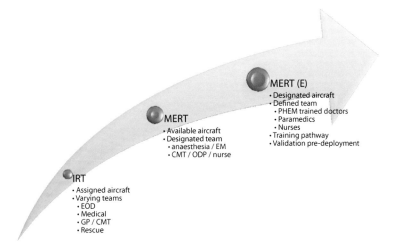

Figure 23.7 The development of the enhanced MERT capability. Brief descriptions of the clinical enhancements offered by each level of capability are given. EM, emergency medicine; CMT, combat medical Technician; ODP, operating department practitioner; PHEM, pre-hospital emergency medicine.

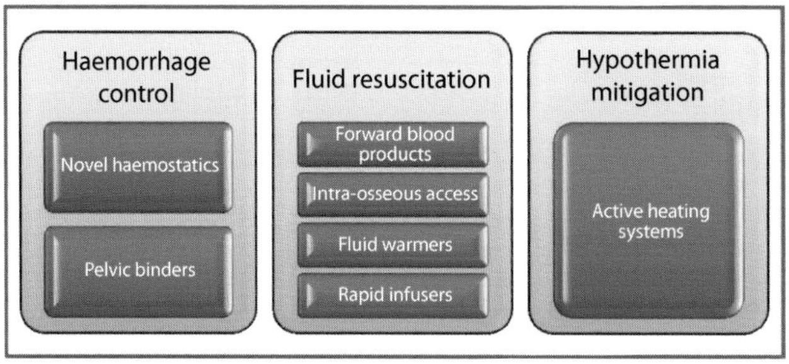

Figure 23.8 Lines of development for MERT clinical practice.

The changes in injury patterns and advances in the forward projection of medical capability meant that the equipment to facilitate this and the training to operate in a potentially very hostile environment were required. The main areas affected are discussed in the following subsections (and shown in Figure 23.8).

Haemorrhage control

It was recognised prior to the conflict that haemorrhage was a major cause of preventable death and an academic review was ongoing.[22] As the conflict began, this area became an operational imperative that demanded the rapid development of a strategy for a novel haemostatic. The tourniquet and emergency care bandage had addressed limb haemorrhage, but junctional wounds were still problematic. Solutions were sought and the procurement and implementation of these were undertaken as a UOR and delivered in a timely manner with constant horizon scanning for improved products and the ability to implement changes as appropriate.

Novel haemostatics

The first iteration of the novel haemostatic was *QuikClot*™. In the timeframe available, it was commercially ready and deemed the product with the best clinical performance available at the time. *QuikClot*™ (granular zeolite, derived from volcanic rock) was proven in swine models to be effective at controlling devastating haemorrhage from large vessels, but generated tissue temperatures up to 57°C raising concern over associated tissue necrosis. The distribution of this product was therefore limited to the professional medic and it was only deployed for use on *Operations Telic* and *Herrick* with clear guidance regarding how and when it was to be used. Training consisted of a video and practical hands-on training, which was delivered in the pre-deployment phase and repeated once the medic was in theatre. This method of training amongst the UK medics was evaluated and found to be effective.[23] To monitor its use and potential complications, an audit form was completed post use by the receiving hospital practitioner, which was returned to RCDM for review. The product was utilised by multiple nations within the area of operations as it was one of the few products available for junctional massive tissue loss casualties. It was not uncommon for the product to be used outside its directed use, by personnel not trained to use it, and although no formal data are available to quantify this, it was recognised that the product was far from ideal. This drove a need to find alternatives in a timely manner, including modifications to QuikClot™ delivery itself. To try and contain the QuikClot™ powder, the company delivered the granules in a teabag-like mesh bag, which assisted with targeted therapy but did not reduce the heat generation and potential complications from it to any great degree.[24]

HemCon™ (chitosan, derived from crushed shellfish) was the next available product that had performed comparably in animal models to QuikClot™ but did not produce exothermia. It also allowed for more easily targeted and anatomically wider use, proving useful in some surgical fields to good effect.[25] QuikClot™ and HemCon™ were used simultaneously for a period, with both being used by medics and the latter more widely. At the time, Quikclot™ was believed to be more effective if more

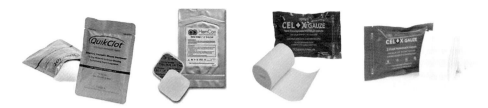

Figure 23.9 Development of topical haemostatic provision.

difficult to use, hence its distribution only to qualified medics. Both were phased out when Celox™ was introduced. There had been a commercial race to produce a haemostatic that would address the military need, and although still under an UOR, the process to determine which was the most suitable for UK DMS was thorough and academically driven under the responsibility of successive DCAs in emergency medicine. Celox™ (chitosan impregnated gauze) was found to be the best product, providing a chemical haemostasis with very few limitations on its use (including use internally).[26] This continues to be the case in 2017 following a recent review with only the presentation, from a roll (which was found to have excess wastage of the product) to the Z-fold version, being altered (Figure 23.9).

The use of haemostatic dressings and agents is one of the main advances of recent decades. However, it can be claimed that the ideal haemostatic has not yet been recognised; therefore this area needs to remain in the focus of the DMS.

Pelvic binders

The predominantly improvised explosive device-related blast injuries caused significant pelvic damage, and a solution for stabilisation of the pelvis and control of potentially life-threatening haemorrhage pre-hospital was clearly required (Figure 23.10). Under a UOR, an 'off-the-shelf' immediate solution was selected as, like the tourniquet, an effective improvised alternative was not available. Few products were on the market at the time, and the *SAM™ Pelvic binder* was procured. The initial iteration was blue and orange, but the company manufactured a version in more military colours (Figure 23.11). Appropriate training was delivered, emphasising that it is the mechanism of injury that is the most important indicator in the need for

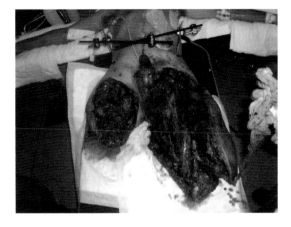

Figure 23.10 Bilateral above knee amputations with pelvic disruption.

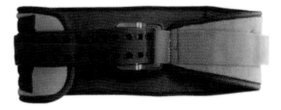

Figure 23.11 Military pelvic binder.

application. It was noted that the position of the binder could move during transit, and this was investigated and found to be a common finding.[27] Further training was targeted to address this issue, and it was highlighted on pre-deployment courses such as *Battlefield Advanced Trauma Life Support*. The pelvic binder has been reviewed since the end of the conflicts, with the SAM™ pelvic being considered still to be fit for purpose.

An area that started to be explored, within the realm of haemorrhage control, was the use of an abdominal tourniquet. This is not a new concept, as the *Military Anti Shock Trousers* delivered an element of this capability, but it was established that rapid proximal control of a bleeding vessel was sometimes required. As part of damage control surgery, it was not uncommon for the chest or abdomen to be opened in order to compress the aorta to allow for recognition and treatment of a distal bleeding point. It was postulated that if there could be external compression of the abdominal aorta, a similar effect could be achieved whilst the patient was rapidly transferred to a surgical facility. Initial low-level research demonstrated that the abdominal aorta could be compressed using an abdominal tourniquet, but the full consequences of this remain unknown.[28] The device has not been sanctioned for use by UK service personnel, but the research and evidence concerning its use is being monitored.

Fluid resuscitation

Pre-hospital fluid resuscitation prior to the conflict consisted of a crystalloid being delivered at room temperature via an intravenous cannula, hastened if necessary by the use of a pressure bag. Given the degree of blood loss and resuscitation that was required by the casualties in these conflicts, this strategy was inadequate. Each area of the process was investigated, problems were identified and solutions were sought for early resolution. Medically perhaps the most important systemic changes of the conflicts, the new resuscitation regimes, were the result of clinical, academic and scientific efforts coordinated across a broad range of specialties.

Intravenous access

The patterns of injury predominantly involving the limbs meant that the conventional sites for venous cannulation were often unavailable for use. In addition, frontline medics were not always confident about inserting intravenous cannulas due to limited practical exposure and difficult conditions. This meant that an alternative method of delivering fluid to the hypovolaemic casualty was required – a capability gap was highlighted. The intraosseous (IO) route was well established in the paediatric population, and there were products that assisted

in the placement of IO cannula in an adult. A rapid review of available products was undertaken and a military choice made. Two products were procured – EZIO™ and FAST™.

EZ IO™

The EZ-IO (Figure 23.12) was introduced in 2006 and was initially delivered with both the power driver and the manual driver depending on the setting, as space and weight within the dismounted medic's bergen were at a premium. The manual driver was later withdrawn. The first needles to be available were the paediatric (pink) and the adult size (blue), but the longer (yellow) needle was added later as it was noted that the humeral site was being utilised more often and the larger build of some service personnel necessitated the use of a longer needle to penetrate their large muscle bulk. The product designers worked with the military to overcome this problem. A minor flaw was reported and subsequently addressed – it was noted that on CT scan, it appeared that the EZ-IO needle had bent. This was thought to be due to the movement of the casualties' arm after insertion into the humerus. Instant feedback was given that this was a clinical effect rather than a design fault and this was incorporated into the training package, with post-insertion care highlighted as an area of risk.

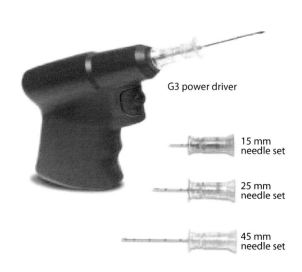

G3 power driver

15 mm needle set

25 mm needle set

45 mm needle set

Figure 23.12 EZ-IO battery driver.

FAST™

The FAST (Figure 23.13) was identified for IO access into the sternum. At the same time a specific decision was made not to procure the EZ-IO™ sternal needle. It was felt that a clear difference between the sites and needle choices was required to ensure that there was no confusion and that the wrong (peripheral) EZ-IO™ needle was not used on the sternum. Such an error risked the possibility of insertion through the sternum with potentially devastating consequences.

The FAST™ device was not without its early problems. The initial model had a separate device that was required in order to remove the cannula from the sternum; simply pulling at the cannula risked separation of the metal tip of the cannula from its plastic tube, leaving a metallic foreign body within the sternum.[29] The product designers overcame this problem by improving the metal and plastic joint with the result that the specific remover was no longer required. This latter design was used for the rest of the conflict, although a new product has recently been released that is lighter and consists of a single piece with no requirement for a sighting template.

Comprehensive training packages were delivered and altered as required, with any necessary changes being identified. Reviews of both devices were undertaken during and after the conflict, which confirmed that IO access, utilising these devices, was very effective.[30–32]

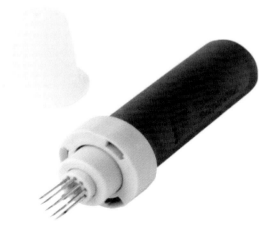

Figure 23.13 FAST device™.

Fluid warmers

It is well recognised that infusing cold fluid into a trauma casualty has negative effects, and therefore, a method of warming intravenous fluid is required. In civilian hospitals, fluid warmers are commonly used and often combine fluid warming with a rapid infusion capability. This is no different in the military, although during the conflict, there was a change from the *Level One™* device to the *Belmont Rapid Infuser™*, as it was deemed the more appropriate product after a thorough review. However, in the pre-hospital setting, blood warming is a relatively new concept, and therefore, few products were available.

In the early stages of *Operation Herrick*, crystalloid infusion fluids were warmed in a microwave before use on the MERT. The need for an effective practical fluid warmer became significantly greater when blood products were pushed forward onto the helicopter. The helicopter started to carry packed red cells and plasma, which were stored at the required temperature range of <5°C, necessitating the need for warming as part of the administration process. Once the capability gap was recognised, and in line with established processes, a rapid review was undertaken and a product was identified. As this was to be used in aircraft, it needed to undergo airworthiness testing, which can take as long as nine months to complete due to the complexities of the test and the potential risks of interference with the aircraft electronics or fire aboard the airframe. There was no shortcut. In addition, international airworthiness certificates did not have UK recognition, so irrespective of clearance having been achieved in, for example, the United States, the full process had to be repeated in the United Kingdom. Even expedited, this element held back the delivery of this product, which was then further delayed by the initial selection failing the tests. As a result, an alternative product was selected, and after successful airworthiness testing, the EnFlow™ was procured by the DMS.

The EnFlow™ device was utilised to good effect. Although it was one of the best products on the market, the device was unable to achieve the optimal temperature at the flow rates needed for the level of aggressive resuscitation that the casualties demanded. This was recognised, and the training delivered was targeted at managing the flow rates in a pragmatic manner, balancing the urgency of requirement against the effects of cold fluid on the casualty. Recently, the manufacturers of EnFlow™ have stopped production, and after a recent investigation of available products, the DMS has opted for the BuddyLite™, which is a device used extensively by allied forces.

To date, no pre-hospital fluid warmer exists that fits the criteria of being light, compact, robust and battery operated but is able to deliver the heating of cold fluids to body temperature at high flow rates. Although there are multiple companies exploring this and new devices using novel techniques, the DMS will continue to horizon scan for the product that will deliver to its needs.

Forward blood products

The cold chain requirements needed to maintain the low temperatures at which blood is stored are problematic, especially in an environment in which temperatures can be as high as 50°C. It was not practical to put a blood fridge on board the aircraft, and even then, a power supply would have been required. An alternative solution was sought, and the 'Golden Hour Boxes' were developed. These look like simple cardboard boxes and hold thermal plates that keep the products at the correct

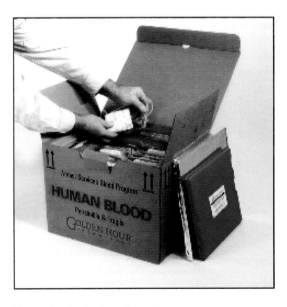

Figure 23.14 Golden hour box.

temperature for up to 72 hours without the need for external power (Figure 23.14). This technology remains extant and has not only facilitated blood on the MERT but also has the potential to allow the use of blood products in supporting small-scale forward operations.[33]

The transport and storage of blood create a large logistical burden, but this capability is now inherent in DMS clinical practice and expected to be available in contingency operations in the future, especially for isolated teams.

Further research is required to optimise the cold chain as it currently remains a potential weak link within the delivery of care in forward operations of the DMS.

Hypothermia mitigation

The final area for discussion of new products is that of *hypothermia mitigation systems*. Even in the high temperatures of Iraq and Afghanistan, a casualty who has been stripped in order to gain clinical access will lose body heat rapidly, especially when he or she is transported in a helicopter. This was well evidenced, and targeted strategies were required to address this as hypothermia increases the mortality and morbidity of injured casualties.

Passive warming, by placing a casualty in a sleeping bag or wrapping him or her in the already available silver ambulance sheet, whilst better than nothing, was not effective, so an active system was required. Active systems provide heat to the casualty. Two main systems were identified, the *Hypothermia Mitigation Prevention Kit* (HPMK™) and the *Blizzard Blanket*™ (Figure 23.15). An element of confusion with regard to procurement occurred in that both delivered the required capability. Frontline commanders had the ability to purchase medical equipment they deemed necessary within a limited budget, and so, both of these products appeared in theatre at the same time. This did not give any clinical concern as both have similar effects and deliver a comparable result, but in terms of procurement and establishing a contract, a single product was required. DMS practice requires that a single product is purchased so as not to cause confusion or add to any training, maintenance or logistical burden. Economies of scale are also more likely to be possible with a single supplier. Advice was sought from the clinical end-users not only to gauge their preference but also to gain a set of *key user requirements*. Other available products were invited into the trial, and eventually, the Blizzard™ was chosen by the DMS. There was a delay in this decision as there was some objection from the HPMK™ manufacturer as their product had performed better in terms of robustness when dragged with a casualty in situ. Given that this was not a main function of the product, it was given little weighting. The Blizzard™ remained the device of choice and its procurement was easily justifiable.

The active heating system is a chemical pack that produces an exothermic reaction, delivering temperatures of up to 42°C, and as such, there were several reported incidents of accidental thermal burns to skin. These were highlighted quickly via the feedback chain of the JTCCC, and training was immediately reviewed with re-enforcement of the message that packs were not to be placed directly against the skin. Further work with the Blizzard™ progressed, and smaller heat packs more amenable to dismounted troops were developed; these are now held within the appropriate modules.

CHALLENGES FOR THE FUTURE

A significant number of new innovations, updates on old themes and changes to practice occurred during the last conflict. As with any research or exploration into new areas, many more questions arise than answers. Iraq and Afghanistan offered short casualty timelines with a secure logistic trail and funding to support the requirements.

The future is uncertain, but some elements are predictable and projects are already in place to find solutions. These areas can be grouped around prolonged timelines, limited resupply and far forward medical teams. Simple questions such as how far forward can we take oxygen? How can we self-sustain oxygen production at high flow rates? How do we optimise the cold chain with limited power and minimal space? How do we heat fluid rapidly in the pre-hospital area? remain to be addressed. Solutions to these questions do not currently exist within the commercial sector but are the subjects of ongoing research. There can be no doubt that future conflicts will produce challenges that are as

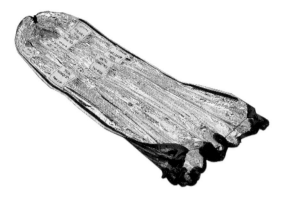

Figure 23.15 Blizzard® heating system.

yet unforeseen. The DMS can now say with confidence that it has the structures to address these issues as they arise.

CONCLUSION

The Iraq and Afghanistan conflicts provided drive and innovation to implement new technologies and changes to clinical treatment pathways designed to deliver high-quality clinical care. The process of development remained robust throughout although flexible enough to deliver what was required within the timeframe demanded. Frustrating as the system was, there was no example of a significant clinical development that was prevented by failure to procure the relevant equipment. The war-fighting imperative was paramount. The consequences of expediting certain steps in the procurement process were understood and the risks mitigated on a case-by-case basis. It was recognised that good equipment, although expensive, is ultimately cost-effective in preventing morbidity and mortality, whether it be short-term or lifelong. Review of DMS equipment and therapeutics is an ongoing process with necessary emphasis on innovation and research led from the highest level and supported fully at all levels. It is expected that future operations will bring with them new challenges and that the systems currently in place and lessons learnt from the past will continue to ensure that the DMS is capable of reacting rapidly and effectively so that it remains able to deliver clinical effect as it has done in the recent campaigns.

REFERENCES

1. Plato. *The Republic, Book II.* 369c.
2. Penn-Barwell J, Roberts S, Midwinter M et al. Improved survival in UK combat casualties from Iraq and Afghanistan: 2003–2012. *J Trauma Acute Care Surg* 2015;78(5): 1014–1020.
3. Ministry of Defence. *Exercise Saif Sareea II. Report by the Comptroller and Auditor General HC 1097. Session 2001–2002.* 1 August 2002. London: MOD.
4. Smith J, Hodgetts T, Mahoney P et al. Trauma governance in the UK Defence Medical Services. *J R Army Med Corps* 2007;153(4):239–242.
5. Hodgetts T, Russell R, Russell M, Mahoney P, Kenward G. Evaluation of clinician attitudes to the implementation of novel haemostatics. *J R Army Med Corps* 2005;151:176–178.
6. Mahoney P, Hodgetts T, Russell R, Russell M. Novel haemostatic techniques in military medicine. *J R Army Med Corps* 2005;151(3): 139–141.
7. Brodie S, Hodgetts TJ, Lambert P et al. Tourniquet use in combat trauma: UK military experience. *J R Army Med Corps* 2007;153(4):310–313. Reproduced in *J Spec Operations Med* 9(1):74–77.
8. Mawhinney AC, Kirk SJ. A systematic review of the use of tourniquets and topical Haemostatic agents in conflicts in Afghanistan and Iraq. *J R Navy Med Serv* 2015;101(2):147–154.
9. Clasper JC, Brown KV, Hill PF. Limb complications following pre-hospital tourniquet use. *J R Army Med Corps* 2009;155(3): 200–202.
10. Taylor DM, Vater GM, Parker PJ. An evaluation of two tourniquet systems for the control of prehospital lower limb haemorrhage. *J Trauma* 2011;71(3):591–595.
11. Hodgetts T, Mahoney P, Kirkman E, Russell R, Thomas R. UK Defence Medical Services guidance for use of recombinant factor VIIa in the deployed military setting. *J R Army Med Corps* 2007;153(4): 307–309.
12. Davies E, Smith A, Mahoney P, Midwinter M. Activated recombinant factor VIIa in British military trauma: An audit of use against SGPL guidelines. 2010 Military Surgery Meeting (abstract). *J R Army Med Corps* 2010;156(3):178.
13. Smith JE, Fawcett R. The use of recombinant activated factor VII in a patient with penetrating chest trauma and ongoing pulmonary haemorrhage. *Mil Med* 2012;177(5):614–616.
14. Smith JE. The use of recombinant activated factor VII (rFVIIa) in the management of patients with major haemorrhage in military hospitals over the last 5 years. *Emerg Med J* 2013;30:316–319.
15. Simpson E, Lin Y, Stanworth S et al. Recombinant factor VIIa for the prevention and treatment of bleeding in patients without haemophilia. *Cochrane Database Syst Rev* 2012;(3):CD005011.
16. The CRASH-2 Collaborators. Effects of tranexamic acid on death, vascular occlusive events, and blood transfusion in trauma patients with significant haemorrhage (CRASH-2): A randomised, placebo-controlled trial. *Lancet* 2010;376:23–32.
17. The CRASH-2 Collaborators. The importance of early treatment with tranexamic acid in bleeding trauma patients: An exploratory analysis of the CRASH-2 randomised controlled trial. *Lancet* 2011;377(9771):1096–1101, 1101.e1–1101.e2.
18. Heier HE, Badloe J, Bohonek M et al. The use of tranexamic acid in bleeding combat casualties. *Mil Med* 2015;180(80): 844–846.
19. Morrison JJ, Dubose JJ, Rasmussen TE, Midwinter MJ. Military Application of Tranexamic Acid in Trauma Emergency Resuscitation (MATTERs) study. *Arch Surg* 2012;147(2):113–119.
20. Morrison JJ, Ross JD, Dubose JJ, Jansen JO, Midwinter MJ, Rasmussen TE. Association of cryoprecipitate and tranexamic acid with improved survival following wartime injury: Findings from the MATTERs II Study. *JAMA Surg* 2013;148(3):218–225.

21. Wright C. Battlefield administration of tranexamic acid by combat troops: A feasibility analysis. *J R Army Med Corps* 2014;160(4):271–272.

22. Mahoney P, Hodgetts T, Russell R, Russell M. Novel haemostatic techniques in military medicine. *J R Army Med Corps* 2005;151(3):139–141.

23. Hodgetts T, Russell R, Russell M, Mahoney P, Kenward G. Evaluation of clinician attitudes to the implementation of novel haemostatics. *J R Army Med Corps* 2005;151:176–178.

24. Lawton G, Granville-Chapman J, Parker PJ. Novel haemostatic dressings. *J R Army Med Corps.* 2009;155(4):309–314.

25. Morrison JJ, Mountain AJ, Galbraith KA, Clasper JC. Penetrating pelvic battlefield trauma: Internal use of chitosan-based haemostatic dressings. *Injury* 2010;41(2): 239–241.

26. Arul GS, Bowley DM, DiRusso S. The use of Celox gauze as an adjunct to pelvic packing in otherwise uncontrollable pelvic haemorrhage secondary to penetrating trauma. *J R Army Med Corps.* 2012;158(4):331–333; discussion 333–334.

27. Bonner TJ, Eardley WG, Newell N et al. Accurate placement of a pelvic binder improves reduction of unstable fractures of the pelvic ring. *J Bone Joint Surg Br* 2011;93(11):1524–1528.

28. Taylor DM, Coleman M, Parker PJ. The evaluation of an abdominal aortic tourniquet for the control of pelvic and lower limb hemorrhage. *Mil Med* 2013; 178(11):1196–1201.

29. Fenton P, Bali N, Sargeant I, Jeffrey SLA. A complication of the use of an intra-osseous needle. *J R Army Med Corps* 2009;155(2):110–111.

30. Cooper BR, Mahoney PF, Hodgetts TJ, Mellor A. Intra-osseous access (EZ-IO®) for resuscitation: UK military combat experience. *J R Army Med Corps* 2007; 153(4):314–316.

31. Lewis P, Wright C. Saving the critically injured trauma patient: A retrospective analysis of 1000 uses of intraosseous access. *Emerg Med J* 2015;32(6):463–467.

32. Vassallo J, Horne S, Smith SE. Intra-osseous access in the military operational setting. *J R Navy Med Serv* 2014;100(1):34–37.

33. Maung N, Doughty H, MacDonald S, Parker P. Transfusion support by UK Role 1 medical team: A 2 year experience from Afghanistan. *J R Army Med Corps* 2015;162(6):440–444.

24

The research dimension

INTRODUCTION

Military medicine, and in particular the management of military trauma, has a number of distinct differences when compared to civilian practice. The mechanism of injury in the military context often involves higher whole body energy transfer, either as a result of blast from an explosive device or from high-velocity gunshot wounds (GSWs). The injuries often occur in remote, hostile environments, with the result that access to professional medical care can occur only when the patient is evacuated to a more permissive environment, increasing the time from point of injury to definitive medical treatment. On the other hand, the deployed medical system, including the level of medical training that individual service personnel undergo, is often far more capable and immediately available than that which would be expected in a civilian environment. It is therefore not always possible to take the findings from civilian research and apply them directly to the military setting. *Defence Science and Technology Laboratories* (Dstl) are configured to address these issues by providing research from bench-side modelling to clinical translational studies, which will influence patient care in the field. This chapter aims to highlight some of the lessons learnt at *Dstl* and how the findings of research studies undertaken have been translated into clinical practice. It will also review the impact that this research has had on military patient care and consider how some of these findings have been adopted (and adapted) within civilian practice in the United Kingdom.

OVERVIEW AND CLINICAL CONTEXT

The paramount importance of controlling haemorrhage is embodied in the <C>ABC principle of casualty management,[1] the introduction of the <C> component, control of major external haemorrhage, being a significant change in the trauma paradigm and reflecting the importance of bleeding as a cause of avoidable death on the battlefield. An important tool in this approach is the *Combat Application Tourniquet*™ (CAT).[2] However, in a significant proportion of casualties, the site of blood loss is not amenable to control using CAT™, and other strategies have had to be developed. During *Operation Telic* and the early stages of *Operation Herrick*, recombinant activated factor VII (rFVIIa) was being proposed as an adjunct to haemorrhage control, following clinical reports of success by the Israeli Defence Forces.[3,4] *Dstl* was asked to conduct a series of studies to examine the efficacy of rFVIIa in controlling haemorrhage in a series of models representative of battlefield injuries and resuscitation. These studies are detailed in this chapter. The output of the rFVIIa studies formed part of the evidence base underpinning the case for consultant-led use of rFVIIa in selected cases. rFVIIa was credited with a number of lives saved[5,6] before its use was discontinued as a consequence of changes in casualty management and guidance from the manufacturers (in part because of the risk of thromboembolic complications[7]) as well as the development of other treatment strategies. This chapter details the models used to assess the limitations of pre-hospital resuscitation strategies extant at the beginning of *Operation Herrick*, which had an impact on developing amended resuscitation strategies for prolonged field care of blast casualties. Studies making the case for pre-hospital oxygen availability for these casualties are also described. These models evolved further to provide scientific evidence supporting pre-hospital administration of blood products, which was being pioneered by the *Defence Medical Services* (*DMS*) in the latter stages of *Operation Herrick*.

The second half of the chapter describes translational research into the detection and underpinning mechanisms of acute trauma coagulopathy (ATC) in battlefield casualties, with deployed research at the Role 3 medical facility in Camp Bastion. This part of the research established the role of *Rotational Thromboelastometry* (ROTEM™) as a near patient test for guiding haemostatic resuscitation. At the same time, *Dstl* was conducting studies into a potential pharmacological treatment of blast lung, focusing on the use of rFVIIa, which had been the subject of a number of case studies of its successful use in treating alveolar bleeding of medical origin. The outcome of this latter research was the demonstration that rFVIIa did not help in blast lung. Although negative results are less 'exciting' than positive results, they are nonetheless important clinically in ruling out treatments that are unlikely to be effective and may be harmful.

The chapter also considers research into the treatment of limb injury, examining the impact of different wound dressings in a model of high energy limb wounds and the effects of blast on the vascular endothelium. The chapter concludes with studies into the development of future treatments such as the use of a haemoglobin-based oxygen carrier, which does not require refrigeration for early resuscitation, better use of patient physiology to assess the efficacy of resuscitation (microvascular flow in addition to macrovascular pressure) and the impact of analgesic drugs on the response to resuscitation. Such issues will be particularly important in future conflicts where there may be prolonged field care.

COMBAT CASUALTY CARE RESEARCH PROGRAMME

The *Combat Casualty Care Research Programme* is an integrated suite of projects designed to address DMS' research needs for casualty care. The programme covers a broad spectrum of topics ranging from the pathophysiological and immunological impact of militarily relevant injuries to the effects of these disturbances on the response to early treatment. However, some injury types (particularly blast injuries) and treatment constraints (such as delayed or protracted evacuation), whilst not unique to the military environment, are much more common amongst military casualties. These aspects are therefore usually under-researched by the civilian scientific community. The *Combat Casualty Care Research Programme* at *Dstl* aims to address these gaps and form a bridge between the published literature and some of the research needs of the DMS.

Dstl Porton Down has a long history of studying military injuries and developing in vivo, in vitro and computational models (simulations) in order to address the military's research needs. The work is conducted in close collaboration with clinical colleagues at the Royal Centre for Defence Medicine (RCDM), who have direct experience of the clinical issues faced by combat casualties and insights into the potential clinical implications of emerging strategies. Coupling this clinical insight with the scientific rigour, and in many respects unique capabilities, of *Dstl* produces a very powerful basis for integrative research. A further capability, allowing systematic observation and scientific monitoring of the impact of treatment at the Camp Bastion hospital, led to unique translational research. All of the experimental studies involving living animals at *Dstl* Porton Down reported in this chapter were conducted in accordance with the Animals (Scientific Procedures) Act, 1986.

NATURE OF BATTLEFIELD INJURIES AND THE RESULTING PATHOPHYSIOLOGICAL CHALLENGE

Injuries from explosions are complex and are usually classified according to the component of the explosion that caused them.[8] To understand these injuries, we must therefore consider the component parts of an explosion and how they interact with the body.

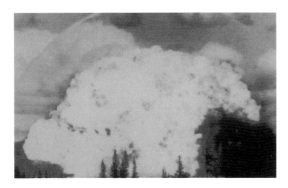

Figure 24.1 Open air blast. This photograph clearly shows the expanding ball of combustion products (the blast wind) as well as the expanding shock front (shock wave), top left.

Injuries due to the shock wave are defined as *primary blast injuries* and are almost (but not completely) unique to injuries caused by explosions (Figure 24.1). Gas-containing organs are particularly susceptible, and 'blast lung', characterised by pulmonary contusion and the rapid development of pulmonary oedema with a consequent reduction in pulmonary gas transfer is an example of this type of injury[9,10] On *Operation Herrick*, this was seen in approximately 11% of severely injured casualties who also suffered other (particularly penetrating) injuries.[11,12] Secondary and tertiary blast injuries are caused, respectively, by fragments or debris (usually penetrating injuries) and translation of the victim against solid objects (usually blunt injuries).

The common features from all of the studies of severely injured military casualties on *Operations Telic* and *Herrick* are extensive tissue damage and severe blood loss and, in a variable but clinically significant minority, blast lung resulting in hypoxaemia. This sets the scene for the research into haemorrhage control and resuscitation strategies that was initiated at the beginning of *Operation Telic* in 2002 and evolved through *Operation Herrick* to the present day.

HAEMOSTATIC EFFECTS OF rFVIIa

Haemorrhage was the leading cause of battlefield deaths throughout *Operations Telic* and *Herrick*[13-15] and is the second leading cause of civilian trauma deaths. In recent years, the majority of those who succumb to blood loss have done so before arriving in a hospital.[13] A major advance in the immediate treatment of severely injured battlefield casualties was the evolution of the *Airway/Breathing/Circulation* (ABCDE) paradigm into the <C>ABCDE approach with the addition of treatment of catastrophic haemorrhage (<C>) before moving on to ABC.[1] Consequently, considerable efforts were expended to improve haemostatic strategies and to devise new approaches to controlling bleeding, including improvements in tourniquet design, haemostatic dressings and topical adjuncts. All of these were reported as having utility in the appropriate setting.[16-19] However, in some circumstances where there is incompressible haemorrhage, the anatomical site of bleeding precludes the effective use of these adjuncts. rFVIIa is an agent administered intravenously that, in theory, preferentially targets the site of bleeding by interacting with locally exposed tissue factor and activated platelets to promote haemostasis.[20]

rFVIIa was developed to treat patients with haemophilia types A and B[20] and is licensed for this specific use. The first anecdotal reports of the successful use of rFVIIa to promote haemostasis in a coagulopathic trauma patient (with a military GSW) who did not have a pre-existing coagulopathy were in 1999.[21] There followed several anecdotal short case reports of successful and unsuccessful use of rFVIIa after trauma, which were reviewed by Martinowitz.[3] In a number of clinical reports where rFVIIa was deemed effective, it was in the context of reducing the haemorrhage or the need for blood products, rather than increasing survival.[22-24] However, there was a paucity of prospective randomised controlled trial evidence supporting the use of rFVIIa in trauma casualties or models of trauma. *Dstl* was therefore asked to assess the potential efficacy of rFVIIa in a model of battlefield haemorrhage. Two series of experimental studies addressed this issue.

The aim of the first study was to determine whether a single dose of rFVIIa, as the only haemostatic intervention, could improve survival and reduce blood loss in a model of severe incompressible haemorrhage (abdominal aortotomy in terminally anaesthetised pigs). A subsidiary aim was to compare the consequences of two resuscitation strategies (hypotensive and normotensive resuscitation with 0.9% saline) on the efficacy of rFVIIa. The model used in the first study involved substantial haemorrhage from a discrete longitudinal lesion in the abdominal aorta, but relatively little other tissue damage beyond the surgery itself. Since a large volume of injured tissue could act as an effective 'sink' for any administered rFVIIa, the aim of the second study was to determine whether the tissue damage resulting from a ballistic injury to the muscle of the hind limb, causing extensive muscle damage, reduced the efficacy of rFVIIa.

The first study was conducted on four groups of terminally anaesthetised pigs. All of the animals were subjected to a controlled haemorrhage of 40% of the initial blood volume, followed by the administration of either rFVIIa (180 µg/kg, designed to be the equivalent of a human haemostatic dose given a reduced responsiveness of pigs to human rFVIIa) or placebo. One minute after drug/placebo administration, a longitudinal aortotomy was created in the infra-renal aorta and resuscitation commenced to either a hypotensive target corresponding to the *Battlefield Advanced Trauma Life Support* (BATLS) guidance or a normotensive target corresponding to the Advanced Trauma Life Support (ATLS®) guidance that was extant at the time. The animals were then maintained according to the relevant resuscitation protocol for the following six hours, or until death, whichever came sooner.

This study showed clearly that the administration of rFVIIa significantly prolonged survival time and reduced the volume of blood loss. The increase in survival time was clinically meaningful since it fell within the anticipated timescale for evacuation of military battlefield casualties to a surgical facility.[25] The fluid resuscitation strategy also influenced outcome and the efficacy of rFVIIa, with a statistically significant increase in survival time being seen only in animals with hypotensive targets (as advocated by *Battlefield Advanced Trauma Life Support* doctrine) rather than those with normotensive targets. Perhaps not surprisingly, the resuscitation strategy also influenced the degree of uncontrolled haemorrhage and amount of intravenous fluid required, with a smaller volume of uncontrolled haemorrhage and a lower intravenous fluid requirement being associated with hypotensive targets.[25] There was no evidence of microthrombi associated with the use of rFVIIa.[25]

In the second study, three groups of terminally anaesthetised pigs were investigated. Two of the groups were subjected to a ballistic injury to the hamstring muscle, which caused extensive soft tissue damage, while the third group was not given a ballistic injury. All groups had a controlled haemorrhage of 30% blood volume followed by an infrarenal aortotomy. Five minutes after the aortotomy, one ballistic injury group and the non-ballistic injury group were given rFVIIa (180 µg/kg) (in contrast to the first study where rFVIIa was given immediately before aortotomy), while the remaining ballistic injury group received placebo (saline). All groups were then given hypotensive resuscitation and maintained for up to six hours or until death, whichever came sooner.

rFVIIa, compared to placebo, significantly increased survival time after combined ballistic injury and uncontrolled haemorrhage. However, there was no difference in survival time between the groups given rFVIIa in the presence and absence of ballistic injury, indicating that the presence of tissue damage had not reduced the efficacy of the dose of rFVIIa used in this study (Figure 24.2). Again, there was no evidence of microthrombi associated with the use of rFVIIa.

Clinical impact of the rFVIIa haemostatic research

Evidence of the efficacy of rFVIIa in two related models of severe uncompressible haemorrhage, without evidence of microthrombotic complications, was presented to the Surgeon General at the time when decisions were being made about the off-label use of rFVIIa for battlefield injury. These experimental studies addressed the gaps in knowledge based on the current clinical and other available experimental evidence. rFVIIa was used extensively before the advent of haemostatic resuscitation and has been credited with saving a number of lives.[5,6] rFVIIa eventually fell out of use, due to concerns regarding thromboembolic complications as its use became more extensive,[7] a widespread impression amongst clinicians of little if any benefit from its use and most importantly the advent of ROTEM guided resuscitation with targeted blood components. Since then, there have been further developments in mechanical methods of addressing previously incompressible haemorrhage using devices such as abdominal tourniquets; haemostatic

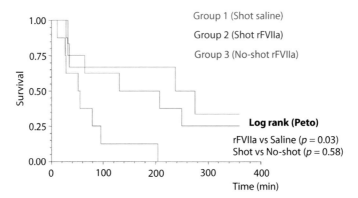

Figure 24.2 Kaplan-Meier survival curve for three groups of anaesthetised pigs following ballistic hind-limb injury (groups 1 and 2) or no ballistic injury (group 3), haemorrhage, infra-renal aortotomy and hypotensive resuscitation (all groups) and treated with either rFVIIa (groups 2 and 3) or placebo (group 1).

foam, which can be injected into body cavities; and endovascular techniques such as resuscitative endovascular balloon occlusion of the aorta. These latter developments represent areas of active research by a number of groups, but none have yet been accepted into routine clinical use. Since these techniques also have clinical penalties associated with their use, there is always a possibility that the use of intravenous agents, such as rFVIIa, may be revisited in future austere environments, with the benefit of an extensive evidence base from *Operations Telic* and *Herrick* as a means of identifying indications and contraindications for their use.

DEVELOPMENT OF MODELS OF BATTLEFIELD INJURY AT PORTON DOWN TO ASSESS THE IMPACT OF RESUSCITATION STRATEGIES

Wherever possible, models requiring the use of living animals are avoided. However, investigations of the pathophysiology of blast injuries rely on complex interactions between a variety of body systems, such as the pulmonary, cardiovascular and inflammatory systems, that could not be modelled without recourse to living animals. Detailed accounts of the consideration and development underpinning the series of models used are given elsewhere[26–28] and are briefly summarised here.

The model has to be representative of battlefield injuries that are potentially survivable given the level of care available to battlefield casualties

and must also reflect realistic timescales, including extended evacuation times such as those seen in the early phases of *Operations Telic* and *Herrick*. The key features of the original model are summarised in Table 24.1.

Several established models of uncontrolled and incompressible haemorrhage were in use by various research groups when this work was initiated. These were critically evaluated to determine if any were suitable for the programme's needs before a model[27] was finally developed to assess the physiological limitations of the BATLS protocols extant at the time[29] and the model was developed to assess the new (novel) hybrid resuscitation strategy.[30]

Finally, as clinical resuscitation practice evolved during *Operation Herrick*, and the importance of

Table 24.1 Key features of the original large animal model for blast-resuscitation studies

- An injury severe enough to require resuscitation to maintain life for up to eight hours
- An assumption of no surgical intervention for up to eight hours
- Capability to provide data on survival and physiological state from the onset of resuscitation up to a maximum of eight hours
- Able to deliver reproducible and quantifiable without introducing bias due to sensitivity to confounding factors.

the recently recognised TIC became apparent, the model was further refined to reflect a clinically relevant (shock-driven) coagulopathy, reduced pre-hospital timelines and pre-hospital use of blood products.[28]

FLUID RESUSCITATION

Hypotensive resuscitation: Identifying the problem

At the beginning of *Operation Telic*, British military doctrine for resuscitation advocated a hypotensive strategy until evacuation to surgical care.[29] This was in accordance with the National Institute for Health and Care Excellence guidelines and US military practice.[31] However, there were serious concerns regarding this approach when delayed evacuation was likely to be imposed because of operational issues such as intense local hostile action, remote terrain or adverse weather conditions, and the concerns were amplified when blast injuries were considered. The consequences of blast lung include hypoxaemia[32] and a range of cardiovascular[33-35] and microcirculatory[36] disturbances that may further compromise nutritive tissue blood flow. There was therefore concern that the low tissue blood flow state inherent in hypotensive resuscitation might be compounded by poor arterial oxygenation, leading to an overwhelmingly inadequate tissue oxygen delivery. Conversely, it was also known that blast injury could lead to a degree of myocardial compromise,[35] which could limit the response to a more aggressive resuscitation strategy. There was therefore no evidence to promote either a hypotensive or a normotensive resuscitation strategy after blast injury. The first step to resolving the problem was to investigate the physiological response to resuscitation after combined blast injury and haemorrhage.

The aim of the initial study was to compare normotensive and hypotensive strategies and their implications for survival over an eight-hour period of resuscitation. Controlled haemorrhage was used in this study to avoid systematic bias that would be introduced in an uncontrolled haemorrhage model as a result of an anticipated difference in amounts of blood loss in blast and non-blast groups.[26] This study was not intended to address the issue of

re-bleeding, as this is likely to be highly dependent on the nature of the model (or clinical injury) and would have confounded the interpretation of the physiological data.

The study was conducted in terminally anaesthetised pigs. Two injury patterns were included: haemorrhage (loss of 30% estimated total blood volume, consistent across all groups) either alone or preceded by a survivable primary blast injury. The study compared the consequences of prolonged hypotensive and normotensive resuscitation after each injury type. The target for the hypotensive group was a systolic arterial pressure (SBP) of 80 mm Hg, corresponding to a palpable radial pulse, that for the normotensive group, an SBP of 110 mm Hg, was attained using the ATLS® strategy of infusing 2 L/70 kg 0.9% saline followed by further aliquots as necessary to attain and maintain the target SBP. All resuscitation was conducted with 0.9% saline at an infusion rate of 3 mL/kg/min, as this was the most commonly available fluid and likely infusion rate in a military pre-hospital setting.

The most important finding of this study[37,38] was a clear, statistically and clinically significant difference in survival times between groups. When the data were stratified into those subjected to blast and sham (no) blast before haemorrhage, those in the blast group given normotensive resuscitation had a significantly longer survival time than did those given hypotensive resuscitation: none of the animals given hypotensive resuscitation survived beyond 209 minutes after the onset of resuscitation, while approximately two thirds of those given normotensive resuscitation survived for the full 480 minutes of the study. In the sham blast strand, survival was equally good with both hypotensive and normotensive resuscitation, but those given hypotensive resuscitation had a much greater physiological compromise.

A detailed assessment of oxygen transport suggested that the problem with hypotensive resuscitation after combined blast injury and haemorrhage was related to oxygen delivery.[38] Despite maximal oxygen extraction, it was clear that oxygen delivery was grossly inadequate during hypotensive resuscitation after combined blast and haemorrhage, and whole body oxygen consumption was found to be reduced in this group.[38] The implication of these data was that normotensive resuscitation restored organ perfusion sufficiently to satisfy demand for oxygen, even in those where blood oxygenation was impaired after blast.

This physiological study therefore demonstrated that prolonged hypotensive resuscitation is incompatible with survival after primary blast injury and haemorrhage. However, over shorter timescales of up to one hour, it was possible to sustain life using a hypotensive strategy. Even in the absence of blast injury, hypotensive resuscitation after haemorrhage allows significant physiological deterioration likely to cause later clinical problems, including coagulopathy[39] and the development of inflammatory complications.[40]

Although the model used in this study did not allow us to comment on the likelihood of normotensive resuscitation re-initiating haemorrhage, which may itself affect survival,[41] the study did demonstrate that aggressive resuscitation did not overwhelm the functional capacity of the blast injured myocardium. Normotensive resuscitation could be incorporated into resuscitation protocols following blast, or suspected blast injury, dependent on clinical judgement regarding the risk of rebleeding.

SOLUTION TO THE LIMITATIONS OF HYPOTENSIVE RESUSCITATION: (NOVEL) HYBRID RESUSCITATION

To address the limitations of prolonged hypotensive resuscitation, particularly when blast lung was also present, a new approach, termed 'novel hybrid' was designed at Porton Down in consultation with RCDM and the then Defence Consultant Advisor in Emergency Medicine. Although 'novel hybrid' was the original term used to reference this resuscitation strategy, since it has been in use for 11 years, the consensus is that the term 'novel' should now be omitted and the strategy referred to simply as 'hybrid'.

This approach combined initial hypotensive resuscitation for the first hour, to allow a degree of clot stabilisation, with a revised target arterial blood pressure thereafter in an attempt to improve tissue perfusion and, hence, oxygen delivery. The likelihood of causing re-bleeding during the normotensive phase was a serious concern, so the model was changed to include an uncompressed Grade IV liver injury that, in consultation with clinical colleagues, was viewed as a survivable but serious battlefield injury at risk of re-bleeding. During the pilot phase of model development, it was shown that aggressive fluid resuscitation (to a normotensive target) initiated within 5 minutes of a Grade IV liver injury caused exsanguination.

The new hybrid resuscitation strategy reversed the metabolic acidosis caused by shock during the haemorrhagic and hypotensive phases in both blast and non-blast injury strands and significantly increased survival time in the blast strand (Figure 24.3). There was no evidence of enhanced bleeding from the Grade IV liver injury.[27,42]

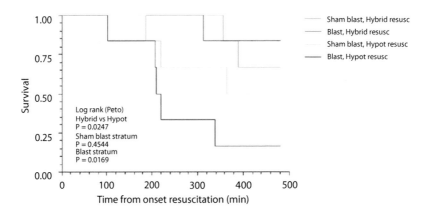

Figure 24.3 Kaplan-Meier survival plots for four groups of animals subjected to either sham blast (Sham blast) or blast (Blast), haemorrhagic shock and hybrid (Hybrid) or hypotensive (Hypot) resuscitation with 0.9% saline. (From Doran CM et al., *J Trauma Acute Care Surg [Internet]* 2012;72(4):835–843.)

Furthermore, the improved perfusion associated with hybrid resuscitation also attenuated the coagulopathy that developed during hypotensive resuscitation, despite a slightly larger volume of crystalloid being used with hybrid resuscitation.[30,43] Finally, the reduction in shock with hybrid resuscitation led to a reduced inflammatory response in both blast and non-blast strands.[42]

HYPOTENSIVE VS. HYBRID RESUSCITATION RESEARCH: CLINICAL IMPACT

This formed part of the evidence base evaluated by the DMS in modifying BATLS, which now advocates consideration of revising the hypotensive blood pressure target in suitable casualties after the first hour during protracted evacuation.[44]

Investigating the potential to reduce logistical burden using hypertonic solutions to reduce volume required for resuscitation: Hypertonic saline dextran

The initial demonstration of the novel hybrid resuscitation strategy utilised 0.9% saline as the only resuscitation fluid. It was possible that further advantage could be gained by initiating resuscitation with a hypertonic solution, for example *hypertonic saline dextran* (HSD). Hypertonic solutions have been advocated for far-forward military resuscitation[45] since they possess a significant logistical benefit in terms of reduced weight burden; 250 mL of HSD is reputed to be equivalent to 3 L of 0.9% saline with respect to early plasma volume expansion. Hypertonic solutions are also known to dampen the systemic inflammatory response that develops after trauma and which is thought to be part of the aetiology underlying later complications.[46–48] This benefit of HSD has been shown in a number of clinical studies.[48–50] In addition, hypertonic solutions have been shown to confer microcirculatory benefit, possibly improving the distribution of blood flow in tissue.[51] Consistent with this, in an early study, we found that HSD reduced the metabolic acidosis during hypotensive resuscitation after haemorrhage alone.[52] Unfortunately, this beneficial effect was not apparent after combined blast injury and haemorrhage.

A possible explanation for this at the time was that the microcirculatory effect of HSD was simply not sufficient to overcome the very poor tissue oxygen delivery due to combined low arterial oxygen content (due to blast lung) and low flow (due to the hypotension).[52] However, a resuscitation strategy that promotes better tissue perfusion might allow the beneficial effects of HSD to become apparent after combined blast injury and haemorrhage.

An extension of the hybrid study therefore evaluated whether HSD, as part of a resuscitation strategy employing the hybrid blood pressure profile, was at least as effective as 0.9% saline in relation to survival. Furthermore, we sought to determine whether HSD was superior to 0.9% saline with respect to physiological changes by limiting the initial deterioration in acid base status during the hypotensive phase of resuscitation and enhancing the acid base improvement during the normotensive phase. This study therefore compared the effectiveness of hybrid resuscitation when the resuscitation was commenced with HSD versus normal saline. The maximum amount of HSD was limited to 500 mL/70 kg and the fluid was given in controlled aliquots to avoid over-shooting the target blood pressure and increasing the risk of re-bleeding from an uncompressed haemorrhage model.

Surprisingly, HSD was associated with a significantly reduced survival time in the blast/haemorrhage groups.[27] Poor survival in the group subjected to combined blast injury and haemorrhage and subsequently resuscitation with HSD was due to poor responsiveness to HSD.[27]

HSD (for initial resuscitation) was therefore inferior to 0.9% saline when haemorrhage was complicated with primary blast injury. By contrast, HSD did show a significant physiological benefit when used after haemorrhage in the absence of primary blast injury. However, this benefit may not outweigh the risk of overshooting the target blood pressure during resuscitation, especially in austere circumstances where accurate, continuous measurement of arterial blood pressure is impossible.

HSD STUDIES: CLINICAL IMPACT

The output from the experimental study of HSD use resulted in a recommendation not to deploy HSD to Afghanistan. This avoided a potentially dangerous strategy in a situation where the majority of casualties were injured in explosions and where it would be impossible to form a clear clinical opinion (in the early phase of their treatment, when HSD would be given) of whether the casualty had suffered blast lung.

Nonetheless, HSD may have a role (in circumstances where the logistical benefit of weight reduction is very important) for resuscitating casualties where primary blast injury can definitely be excluded. Should HSD be used in these circumstances, very careful titration of HSD to target blood pressures would be necessary, imposing its own burden on those responsible for resuscitating the casualty under difficult circumstances.

When the risk of re-bleeding is too great to implement hybrid resuscitation: The role of supplementary oxygen

The strategies described hitherto focused on improving tissue perfusion. These were investigated first because forward deployment of oxygen in a military setting is especially problematic: pressurised cylinders represent a substantial additional hazard in an environment where there is a ballistic threat, although newer technologies to generate oxygen in situ may provide a solution in the future. Unfortunately, there will always be a cohort of casualties in whom the injuries pose an unacceptably high risk of re-bleeding. In theory, oxygen administration should make a significant impact when initial arterial saturation is low (for example in blast lung), but less so when initial saturation is approaching 100%. A further study was therefore undertaken to assess the effects of elevated FiO_2 in combination with hypotensive resuscitation on survival after combined blast injury and haemorrhage. The primary outcome variable was again survival, and secondary outcomes included the animal's physiological state.

The study was conducted on two groups of terminally anaesthetised Large White pigs. Both groups were subjected to primary blast injury followed by the model of controlled/uncontrolled haemorrhage (Grade IV liver injury). A hypotensive resuscitation strategy using normal saline was used throughout. Thirty minutes after the onset of resuscitation, one group of animals were given elevated inspired oxygen, titrated to increase oxygen saturation to 95%. The second (control) group continued to breathe air throughout. Administration of supplementary oxygen successfully increased PaO_2 and SaO_2, and there were no difficulties in titrating SaO_2 to a target value of 95%. In a field situation, this could be achieved using pulse oximetry.

Survival times were significantly longer in the oxygen-treated group compared to animals breathing air. The improved survival was associated with an arrest of the development of metabolic acidosis in the oxygen-treated group. Supplementary oxygen can therefore be used to 'buy time' in blast-injured hypovolaemic casualties, but its impact is likely to be limited by the poor tissue perfusion associated with hypotensive resuscitation. However, in casualties in whom there is a high risk of re-bleeding and an elevation in arterial blood pressure later in the resuscitation process (hybrid resuscitation) poses an unacceptable risk, supplemental oxygen has a clear role to increase survival times during protracted evacuation to surgical care. This provides a potential alternative to hybrid resuscitation for DMS clinicians during prolonged evacuation of blast casualties.[27,53] This use of supplementary oxygen to a pre-defined arterial saturation level is in accordance with published guidelines relating to the use of emergency oxygen in adults.[54]

SUPPLEMENTARY OXYGEN STUDIES: CLINICAL IMPACT

These findings were reported to RCDM, who in turn presented them to the Advisory Group on Military Medicine to make the case for deploying oxygen forward, for example on *Medical Emergency Response Teams* (MERTs).

ATC: The rationale for early use of packed red blood cell:fresh frozen plasma

The next major change impacting on resuscitation was a re-evaluation of the impact of *trauma-induced coagulopathy* (TIC) on outcome after severe injury.[55-57] This resulted in a drive to identify techniques aimed at early detection and proactive treatment of TIC. A joint research effort by *Dstl* and RCDM in the United Kingdom and at Bastion evaluated methods of near-patient testing to target early detection and treatment of TIC in severely injured casualties. The culmination of this aspect of research[58] was the deployment of ROTEM for near patient testing in Bastion.

TIC has an evolving pathology in the patient, often starting with the consequences of tissue hypoperfusion and developing through phases that can include the consequences of shock-driven acidosis, hypothermia, iatrogenic (and auto-genic) haemodilution and clotting factor consumption.[55,57] The initial phase of trauma-related coagulopathy is referred to as *acute trauma coagulopathy*, which includes both anticoagulation and fibrinolysis.

The evolving understanding of the mechanism(s) of ATC has, to some extent, driven therapy. Current therapy focuses on early and aggressive use of blood products such as plasma and fibrinogen,[55,57] as well as red cells, with an emphasis on a high ratio of plasma to red cells, while the use of colloids and crystalloids is limited.[59] An empirical approach of administering blood products as early as possible was adopted clinically on *Operation Herrick*. Initially, this involved early and aggressive in-hospital use of blood products. However, the MERT was able to project fresh frozen plasma (FFP) and packed red blood cells (pRBC) in the pre-hospital arena.[60] By contrast, at the time if blood products were used at all, civilian helicopter ambulance services in the United Kingdom projected pRBC without plasma into the pre-hospital arena. Since pre-hospital projection of pRBC and FFP does have significant logistical implications (including ensuring appropriate storage conditions and traceability) and some clinical hazards (such as possible transfusion reactions and infection), especially in austere circumstances, it was important to determine whether earlier (pre-hospital) administration confers advantage compared to immediate in-hospital administration. Furthermore, to aid in the translation of military 'lessons learned' into the civilian setting, it was important to compare the military (pre-hospital pRBC and FFP) and civilian (pre-hospital pRBC alone) putative 'best practices' to the original (often current) standard

of care (limited use of crystalloid fluid). These considerations formed the basis of a prospective study at *Dstl*, which involved the development of a novel model of battlefield injury that incorporated a relevant (shock-driven) coagulopathy and the establishment of a porcine blood bank to provide the blood products for the study.

The aim of the study was to compare three treatments (pRBC and FFP, pRBC alone and 0.9% saline alone) for simulated pre-hospital hypotensive resuscitation in a model of complex trauma involving both tissue injury and hemorrhagic shock, with and without concomitant blast injury in terminally anaesthetised pigs. The simulated 'pre-hospital' phase was followed by a simulated 'in-hospital' phase, which involved normotensive resuscitation in all cases with pRBC:FFP (1:1) ratio. The principal outcome variable was coagulopathy 30 minutes into the in-hospital phase, corresponding to the time when surgical decisions are made, often based on the patient's physiological and coagulopathic state. The secondary outcomes included physiological changes and volumes of the various fluids needed for resuscitation, using current standard clinical endpoints based on pressure-driven targets.[31,44]

The principal finding was that use of blood products for 'pre-hospital' resuscitation attenuated the coagulopathy that developed in the control group, which was given 0.9% saline only in the 'pre-hospital' phase (representing the clinical standard of care for all except MERT at the time) (Figure 24.4). A superficially surprising finding was that the use of pRBC alone in the pre-hospital phase was as effective as pRBC and FFP (1:1 ratio) in avoiding ATC in this model (Figure 24.4). This finding is consistent with the concept that it is tissue hypoperfusion and possibly reduced oxygen delivery that are the early drivers of ATC.[39,61] In this model, therefore, 'pre-hospital' use of blood products did confer benefit extending into relevant 'in-hospital' phases, even when aggressive resuscitation strategies are employed from the outset in the in-hospital phase.

Secondary findings related to changes in physiological state and volumes of fluid used for resuscitation. All groups developed a significant degree of shock during the pre-hospital phases, seen as a marked fall in base excess and elevated lactate levels. In the non-blast injury strand only, pre-hospital

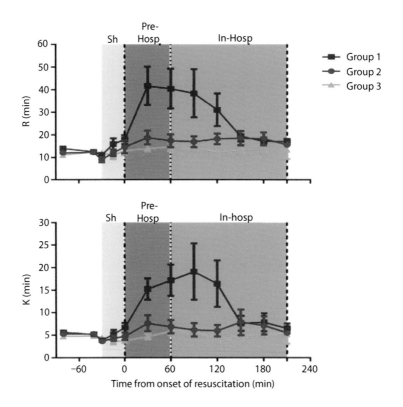

Figure 24.4 Effects of tissue injury and haemorrhage, followed by a shock phase (Sh), pre-hospital hypotensive resuscitation phase (Pre-Hosp) and in-hospital normotensive resuscitation phase (In-Hosp) on TEG R time (clot initiation), K time (clot dynamics). Note that increased R time indicates delayed clotting and increased K time represents reduced clot dynamics (i.e. coagulopathy). Treatment groups differed in the fluid used for resuscitation during pre-Hosp; group 1 (n = 9) received 0.9% saline, group 2 (n = 9) received 1:1 PRBCs and FFP and group 3 (n = 6) received PRBCs without FFP. All groups received PRBC:FFP (1:1) during the in-hospital phase. The first three data points represent, respectively, baseline value, followed immediately before and immediately after tissue injury and haemorrhage. Mean ± SEM. (From Watts S et al., *Shock [Internet]* 2015;44(Suppl 1):138–148.)

pRBC and FFP appeared to afford the greatest protection against shock, which is counterintuitive since, predictably, arterial oxygen content was highest in the group given pre-hospital PRBC alone. Unfortunately, it was not possible to compare statistically the cumulative burden of shock between pRBC with FFP and pRBC alone due to the different distributions in the two groups, but the overall levels of both base excess and lactate in the pRBC alone group was nearer the saline group than the group given pRBC and FFP. It is clear that oxygen extraction was maximal in all of the groups during the pre-hospital phase (equally high oxygen extraction ratio and low mixed venous oxygen content in all groups[28]), suggesting that the low blood flow state

inherent in hypotensive resuscitation was the limiting factor. It is possible that the better performance of pRBC with FFP may reflect a beneficial effect of the plasma on the microvasculature, possibly via an action on the endothelium and/or glycocalyx,[62–64] which optimised local control and oxygen delivery. Additionally, the buffering capacity of FFP may also have played a part in reducing the acidosis.

However, it is of clinical significance that the shock-reducing effect of pRBC and FFP was not apparent in the blast injury strand of the study. It is possible that any benefit of pRBC and FFP was lost in the blast injured strand because the concomitant presence of lung injury and the subsequent hypoxaemia, when combined with the effects of reduced tissue perfusion during hypotensive resuscitation, could not be overcome by any microvascular effect of the plasma. There remains, therefore, a capability gap in this aspect of resuscitation, which may be addressed by the use of a *haemoglobin-based oxygen carrier* (HBOC; see section 'Lessons Learned and Examples of Future Directions').

The overall volume of fluid needed for resuscitation was considerably less in the groups given pre-hospital blood products. This difference was due to a much greater volume of saline being needed in the groups given pre-hospital saline, and the magnitude is likely to be of clinical significance especially given the emerging concerns regarding the deleterious effect of crystalloid on the vascular endothelium and inflammatory responses.[65] In a military context, the reduction in volume of pre-hospital fluid requirement is likely to have a logistical benefit, although the cooling required for blood products to some degree negates this.

Haemostatic resuscitation studies: Clinical impact

In conclusion, this study provides evidence that use of pre-hospital blood products confers advantage compared to the old standard of care (limited crystalloid administration) and supports a treatment strategy that was started pragmatically by clinicians on the MERT in Afghanistan. If FFP is not available, then pRBC alone has a clear benefit over saline.[28]

DEPLOYED RESEARCH: AETIOLOGY OF TRAUMA COAGULOPATHY

Research conducted at Role 3 in Camp Bastion evolved and matured as the facility developed. Initial studies focused on immediate clinical applications such as methods for allowing early detection of TIC. Later studies had longer-term goals and focused on developing an understanding of TIC in battlefield casualties, which required specialised laboratory facilities and staffing, which are detailed elsewhere.[60] Many of these studies were conducted as collaborations between *Dstl*, RCDM, international colleagues and university departments,[60,66] particularly *St Thomas' Hospital, London* and *Birmingham University*. The support of all of the clinical staff

and the clinical biomedical laboratory at the Role 3 Medical Treatment Facility (Field Hospital) in Camp Bastion (R3 Bastion) is gratefully acknowledged.

As we have already considered, the initial deployed research at R3 Bastion was conducted against a background of renewed recognition of the problems caused by trauma coagulopathy in the seriously injured and in view of the need for rapid diagnosis of this condition and timely monitoring of the patient's response to treatment. The first study focused on the early detection of trauma coagulopathy in severely injured battlefield casualties using near patient tests that provided feedback to the attending clinicians. ROTEM™ was found to be a robust technique that could be applied in a busy Role 3 hospital.[67] A subsequent study identified a means, using interim values reported by ROTEM™, to reduce the time required to identify the presence of coagulopathy.[58] A further study showed, for the first time, that coagulopathic blood, unlike normal blood, was not stable with respect to ROTEM™ analysis for a period of hours after collection. The apparent degree of coagulopathy attenuated over time,[68] which has important implications for interpretation of ROTEM™ analysis of such samples: for example collection of blood in a pre-hospital setting for later analysis in-hospital could underestimate the presence of coagulopathy.

The ROTEM™ studies described earlier were conducted by deployed clinicians, who were also responsible for the clinical management of patients at R3 Bastion. As the research questions became more detailed, it was apparent that a deployed research laboratory was needed (Figures 24.5 and 24.6). In addition, conducting time-consuming and time-critical analyses concurrently with clinical duties was not feasible, hence the need for experienced scientific staff, with the capacity to evaluate ongoing results and to conduct some of the analyses. The focus of this work was the aetiology of trauma coagulopathy, and the deployed research was designed to integrate with experimental studies conducted at *Dstl Porton Down* and university-based research in the United Kingdom.[60]

The effect of military trauma, and in particular blast injuries, on haemostasis had not been previously studied. Understanding the effect would help to tailor resuscitation protocols and provide

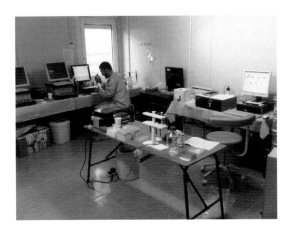

Figure 24.5 Deployed research laboratory at Role 3 Bastion.

clearer insight in applying civilian studies to military trauma.

Fifty-three sequential patients sustaining injuries from explosions (blast) or gunshot with major blood loss presenting to Role 3 Bastion, and who survived into their first surgery, were assessed and blood was taken on admission for haemostatic studies. After routine coagulation tests were performed, the waste plasma was frozen locally, then shipped back via a cold chain to the United Kingdom, where the samples were stored at −80°C and analysed at *St. Thomas' Hospital, London.* The results of these analyses were presented as an abstract and oral presentation at the *Military Health Systems Research Symposium* in 2016.[69] All 53 patients were male, with a median (range) age of 25 (19–35). The patients had a range of injury severities (*Injury Severity Score* [ISS] 21 [1–75]). Overall, there was clear evidence of clinically significant

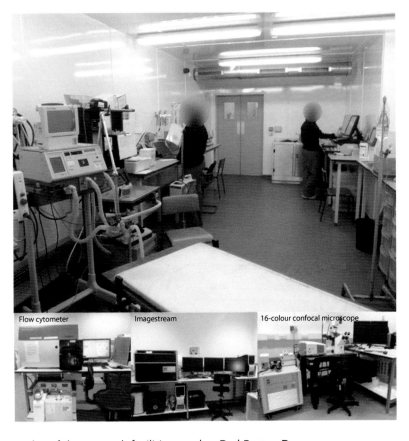

Figure 24.6 Examples of the research facilities used at *Dstl Porton Down.*

shock in this cohort of patients (admission pulse rate, 110 [36–183] bpm, pH 7.25 [6.67–7.47]; base deficit [BD], 6 mM [27 mM deficit to 4 mM excess]). Forty two percent (22/53) had received tranexamic acid prior to admission.

Admission haemostatic values are shown in Table 24.2. There was clear evidence of coagulopathy, with clinically significant elevations in prothrombin times. There was also clear evidence of clot formation and thrombin generation (elevations in prothrombin fragment [PF] 1 + 2) and very active fibrinolysis, with D-dimer and plasmin–antiplasmin complex levels uniformly (and in some patients massively) above normal levels. There was intense activity in the control mechanisms of fibrinolysis. The median values of both tissue plasminogen activator and its inhibitor were at, or just above, the upper end of the normal range, but the range of values extended far above the upper end of normal. Platelet counts were within the normal range, although it must be appreciated that this gives no indication of platelet function, which is key for haemostasis. Clotting substrates were broadly within normal levels, although the range for many of the factors (including fibrinogen) did extend below the normal range. In interpreting these data, it should be acknowledged that the impact of reduced clotting factor levels on coagulation has generally been assessed in the context of a single factor reduction, and the possible synergistic effects of depressing several factors simultaneously are yet to be thoroughly investigated. In addition, it has been argued that 'normal levels' of key substrates such as fibrinogen are based on an uninjured population in whom, at the time, there is no massive demand for clotting. Consequently, 'normal' levels for the uninjured state may be below optimal for a casualty with multiple injuries with a widespread demand for clotting activity to achieve haemostasis,[70] and parallels have been drawn with the physiological elevations in fibrinogen seen in pregnancy as the body presumably prepares for potential haemorrhage during childbirth.[70]

Forty-five patients had complete datasets for BD, ISS, PAP and D-dimers. There were differences between blast and GSW mechanisms in median ISS (25 vs. 16) and BD (7.5 vs. 4.0 mM), but these did not attain statistical significance ($P = 0.094$ and $P = 0.184$, respectively). The data were stratified into three shock bands (BE <6, 6–12 and >12 mM) and three ISS bands (<15, 15–40 and >40). A three-way analysis of variance (for mechanism, shock and injury severity) indicated that a significantly higher fibrinolysis (PAP, $P < 0.0001$; D-dimers, $P = 0.0008$)

Table 24.2 Admission values of haemostatic variables in 53 patients on admission to Role 3 Bastion

	Cohort median values	Cohort range	Published normal range
PT sec	18.68	13.8–30.9	12–15.9
Prothrombin fragment 1 + 2, pmol/L	1,600	24–2,566	200–1200
D-dimer, ng/mL	3,222	256–8648	<145
Plasmin–antiplasmin complexes (PAP), µg/L	5138	930–37,000	150–800
t-PA antigen, ng/mL	17	3–108	1–15
PAI-1 activity, ng/mL	31	11–119	0–33
Platelet count, × 10⁹/L	249	60–483	150–450
Clauss fibrinogen, g/L	1.91	0.57–3.19	1.5–4
Prothrombin, iu/mL	0.75	0.39–1.16	0.5–1.5
Factor V, iu/mL	0.54	0.13–1.06	0.5–1.5
Factor VII, iu/mL	0.70	0.36–1.43	0.5–1.5
Factor X, iu/mL	0.79	0.02–1.18	0.5–1.5

was associated with blast vs. GSW. The additional effect of injury severity was only significant for PAP (the lower ISS band was different to the other two, $P = 0.001$), but not for D-Dimer ($P = 0.8238$). The effect of shock level was not significant for either PAP ($P = 0.5106$) or D-dimer ($P = 0.9982$).

The patients were coagulopathic on admission to hospital, with markedly reduced fibrinogen and factor V levels and a lesser reduction in other coagulation factors. Markers of fibrinolysis (t-PA, PAP and D-dimers) were greatly increased with evidence of good thrombin generation (elevated PF 1 + 2). Importantly, there appears to be a difference in fibrinolysis between blast and GSW that is related to mechanism of injury, in addition to any effect of injury severity. Further analysis is yet to be completed on these data.

USE OF rFVIIa IN THE TREATMENT OF BLAST LUNG

Blast lung is a primary blast injury (caused by the shock wave from the explosion) that is characterised by contusions of the lungs and, in some casualties, further pulmonary compromise that evolves over approximately 24–48 hours and requires intensive care therapy. In addition, the hypoxaemia caused by the lung damage can immediately limit the efficacy of hypotensive resuscitation in casualties who have also suffered significant haemorrhage as a consequence of secondary blast injury.[38]

Incidence of blast lung

Because of the clinical implications of blast lung, its incidence was monitored carefully by RCDM throughout *Operations Telic* and *Herrick*. An analysis of military casualties from terrorist bombings in Northern Ireland[71] found that blast lung was frequently identified at post-mortem examination, but in the majority of cases, death could also be attributed to other causes such as penetrating wounds, head injuries or traumatic amputations. In general, the incidence of blast lung in survivors admitted to hospitals was low (approximately 1–2%),[71] but higher percentages were reported for explosions in confined spaces (for example figures ranging from 63% to 94% of critically injured civilian survivors in the Madrid train bombings[72,73]). With regard to

Operation Telic, Ramasamy et al.[74] provided evidence that the incidence of primary blast injury was very small (approximately 3.8% of casualties sustained in explosive events). However, extreme caution should be exercised in general application of this headline data since Ramasamy et al.[74] focused almost exclusively (91.3% of cases reported in the paper) on a 'special' type of 'explosive device', the *explosively formed projectile improvised explosive device* (EFP-IED). This device is very focused in its action and produces a directional projectile threat. Ramasamy et al. themselves state very explicitly, '*We report a different pattern of injury caused by the EFP-IED compared with conventional explosive devices*',[74] A very recent review of military casualties[75] concluded that 71% of combat casualties admitted to medical treatment facilities during 2003–2006 were the result of explosions, and the proportion of these suffering blast lung injury was very small (3.6%). However, the definition of blast lung (a *primary* blast injury) used in this study could have significantly underestimated the true incidence since '*Patients found to have rib-fractures, scapula fractures, or open wounds to the chest were included in the study but were considered to have injuries caused by secondary or tertiary explosive mechanisms*',[75] Whilst this is a very 'safe' definition of blast lung for circumstances where it is essential to exclude all other possibilities, it will exclude blast lung injury when it co-exists with other injury types (which is common with conventional munitions and terrorist bombs) and hence may underestimate the occurrence of blast lung in current in military casualties. More recent assessments of casualties from *Operation Herrick* reported the incidence of blast lung to be approximately 11% in casualties who also suffered other (particularly penetrating) injuries.[11,12]

The differences in the reported incidence of blast lung in various conflicts therefore do not represent errors or shortcomings in the individual analyses but rather emphasise the importance of the context of the explosion, which has a profound effect on the nature, type and frequency of the injuries. The common element in all of these studies is a group of casualties who have extensive tissue damage and severe blood loss and, in a variable but clinically significant minority, also have blast lung resulting in hypoxaemia.

Pathophysiology of blast lung

Coupling of the shock wave into the thorax leads to widespread rupture of blood vessels (particularly small vessels) in the lung, causing blood contamination of the alveoli and small airways (usually without parenchymal laceration). The contusions may range from scattered petechiae to confluent haemorrhages involving the whole lung and may continue to spread over the ensuing hours and days.[76] A physiological shunt may be established and the lung compliance will decrease, resulting in stiffer lungs and hypoxia.[77] The injury may progress to *acute respiratory distress syndrome*,[78] often within 24–48 hours,[79,80] with the worst of the respiratory distress and hypoxemia being seen within the first 72 hours.[77,79–82] Blast lung is therefore a condition that evolves (and can worsen) over a period of hours following blast exposure, and a casualty who may not appear too severe initially may become critically ill later. Fortunately, if the casualty survives, then the lung damage resolves over ensuing months and lung function returns to normal within approximately one year,[83] although it must be stressed that this finding is based on a small case series.

Recently, a large amount of research has been directed towards understanding the pathology of blast lung, which in time will underpin new treatment strategies. This has been reviewed in detail elsewhere.[10] Of particular relevance to this chapter is the observation that free haemoglobin and extravasated blood have been shown to induce free radical reactions, which cause oxidative damage[84] and initiate or augment a pro-inflammatory response.[85] Free haemoglobin also causes an accumulation of inflammatory mediators and chemotactic attractants,[86] thereby amplifying the initial pulmonary problem. It is therefore possible that strategies to limit the intrapulmonary bleeding may attenuate the acute pulmonary impairment that evolves over the first 24–48 hours after blast exposure and hence reduce the demands made on intensive care facilities.

rFVIIa offered a potential treatment to limit intrapulmonary bleeding in blast lung and was being used off label in both *Operations Telic* and *Herrick* to limit 'conventional' traumatic haemorrhage in casualties. In addition, there were isolated reports of rFVIIa being successful in limiting intrapulmonary haemorrhage (from large vessels) as a consequence of a GSW to the thorax[87] and diffuse alveolar haemorrhage due to a range of medical conditions. Two case reports[88–90] were of particular interest because the rFVIIa was instilled via the airway (or on one occasion given by nebulisation) rather than the conventional intravenous route. In the case series by Heslet et al.[89] intrapulmonary rFVIIa resolved the bleeding in all six patients studied, including the first case in which previous intravenous administration had been ineffective. A later study from a separate group[88] elected to administer rFVIIa by the intrapulmonary rather than intravenous route. In both cases, the intrapulmonary bleeding was controlled after intrapulmonary rFVIIa.[88]

As a consequence of the need to develop an effective treatment for blast lung, and the potential for rFVIIa to provide this solution, two sequential studies were conducted at *Dstl*, the first to examine the efficacy of intravenous rFVIIa in a model of combined blast lung and haemorrhagic shock and the second to assess the potential of inhaled (nebulised) rFVIIa to limit the development of blast lung.

INTRAVENOUS rFVIIa IN A MODEL OF COMBINED BLAST LUNG AND HAEMORRHAGIC SHOCK

The aim of the study was to assess the effects of a single intravenous dose of human rFVIIa in combination with hypotensive resuscitation on survival after combined blast injury and haemorrhage. The effects of rFVIIa were compared to the effects of elevated FiO_2 (which was reported previously[91,92]). The primary outcome variable was survival and secondary outcomes included physiological state.

The study was conducted in terminally anaesthetised Large White pigs subjected to a primary blast injury, haemorrhage and an uncompressed Grade IV liver injury, followed by hypotensive resuscitation with 0.9% saline. Thirty minutes after the onset of resuscitation, one group of animals were given rFVIIa (180 µg/kg). The control group was given placebo and both groups continued to breathe air throughout the study.

Survival times in the group treated with rFVIIa were not significantly different from those seen in the placebo-treated animals ($P = 0.649$). Arterial oxygen saturation in the rFVIIa group was higher than that seen in the placebo group and achieved statistical significance at 45 minutes after onset of resuscitation, suggesting that rFVIIa did have some beneficial effects, although clearly, this was not sufficient to overcome the penalties of tissue hypoperfusion associated with hypotensive resuscitation. Reassuringly, there was no evidence of microthrombi formation associated with the use of rFVIIa.

However, an unexpected penalty was found to be associated with the administration of rFVIIa when a detailed analysis of clotting was performed on blood samples from the pigs used in this study.[93] As expected, there was an enhancement of clotting (assessed using thromboelastography) immediately after the administration of rFVIIa, but this was followed by an exaggerated deterioration in coagulation. A second, or delayed, dose of rFVIIa was simulated in an in vitro study where blood from these animals was 'spiked' with rFVIIa prior to thromboelastography. In the animals treated with intravenous rFVIIa, the effect of the second (in vitro) dose of rFVIIa was attenuated. These findings have implications for austere, resource-constrained military settings since a boost in clotting might reduce immediate blood loss. However, this needs to be balanced against the loss of responsiveness over time should additional doses be necessary.[93]

It was therefore concluded that a single, early intravenous dose of rFVIIa was not, by itself, sufficient to modify blast lung.[53] However, there remained the potential that targeted application of the rFVIIa into the lungs might improve its efficacy, as had already been reported in medical causes of diffuse alveolar haemorrhage.[88,89]

INHALED rFVIIa IN A MODEL OF ISOLATED BLAST LUNG

The aim of this study was to determine whether nebulised rFVIIa, administered by inhalation, could attenuate the development of blast lung by limiting bleeding into lung tissue and attenuating any secondary inflammatory responses. A secondary outcome of the study was to assess whether rFVIIa, administered by inhalation would enter into the circulation since a local action within the lungs without penetration into the circulation would obviate the risk of thromboembolic events that were a concern with pro-coagulant drugs such as rFVIIa.

The assessment of rFVIIa in isolated blast lung did not require the use of a large animal model. The initial part of this body of work therefore involved developing a small animal model of blast lung and characterising the deposition of active rFVIIa in the lung (Figure 24.7).[94]

There was evidence of systemic absorption of rFVIIa administered by inhalation since there

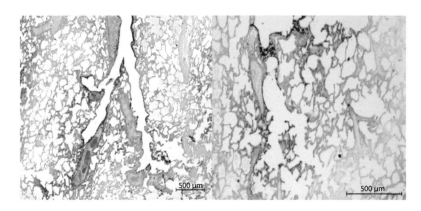

Figure 24.7 Photomicrograph showing deposition of nebulised rFVIIa in rabbit lung (DAB, brown stain) throughout the respiratory tree from main primary bronchioles (left) down to individual alveolar air spaces (right). (From Smith JE. Inhaled recombinant activated factor VII [rFVIIa] in the management of blast lung injury. MD Thesis, University of Newcastle.)

was an elevation in plasma rFVIIa above baseline 2 hours after blast exposure in animals given rFVIIa, but not in those given placebo. This difference did not reach statistical significance, but the trend was clear.[94]

The degree of blast lung was determined by measuring the amount of blood-borne iron bound transferrin by electron paramagnetic resonance: this technique has previously been used to quantify blast lung, and a fall in iron-bound transferrin has been shown to correlate with the degree of blast lung.[95] Blast exposure resulted in a significant fall in circulating iron-bound transferrin, which is an established measure of blast lung. However, no significant difference was seen between rFVIIa- and placebo-treated groups in the pattern of change in iron bound transferrin.[94] Furthermore, there was no significant difference between treatment groups in the circulating levels of inflammatory cytokines (interleukin [IL]-6) or chemokines (macrophage inflammatory protein [MIP-2]). These data suggest that although rFVIIa was successfully deposited in the lungs, it did not attenuate blast lung or the inflammatory response associated with blast lung.[96]

Clinical implications: rFVIIa in the treatment of blast lung

The overall clinical implications of the studies evaluating the impact of rFVIIa on blast lung were that a single dose of rFVIIa had little potential to attenuate blast lung regardless of whether it was administered intravenously or by inhalation. Furthermore, although there was no evidence of microembolic complications associated with rFVIIa in these studies, there was evidence that a single, early dose might attenuate the efficacy of later doses. The overall conclusion was that rFVIIa should not be recommended as a treatment for blast lung and that other avenues such as modified ventilation strategies might provide a more immediate method of supporting casualties whilst research into novel methods of haemostasis in lung tissue were being explored.

TREATMENT OF LIMB INJURIES

Data from conflicts in Iraq and Afghanistan have shown that extremity injury occurs in approximately 50% of combat casualties.[97] The majority of these casualties were injured by IEDs.[98,99] In addition, although the majority of extremity wounds are penetrating soft tissue wounds, around a quarter involve a fracture, of which the vast majority are open fractures.[98] Studies of high-energy, complex and heavily contaminated wounds have identified high rates of infectious complications[100,101] and eventual osteomyelitis.[102] It has also been demonstrated that the rate of vascular injury is higher than in previous conflicts, with about 12% of combat wounded from Iraq and Afghanistan having a vascular injury.[103]

The long-term impact of military extremity trauma is currently under investigation. Recent reports suggest that some functional outcomes after lower limb amputation are better than after lower limb salvage[104] and that more than half of 214 casualties with extremity vascular injury had unfavourable outcomes.[105]

There was a clear need for extremity trauma research to support the DMS during *Operations Telic* and *Herrick*, and as a consequence, two programmes of work were initiated to address the following clinical questions: what dressing should be applied at Role 2E/Role 3 to reduce infection and what are the central physiological consequences of restoring blood flow to a blast injured ischaemic limb? This led to the development of two separate studies; one study investigated the anti-microbial effects of wound dressings, and the other, the impact of blast exposure on vascular endothelium.

Anti-microbial effects of wound dressings used post-initial debridement

The complications that occur after military trauma place a significant burden on the casualty and medical systems alike and can result in poor functional recovery. One such complication is wound infection, and *Staphylococcus aureus* is the most common pathogen identified in delayed infection. Prevention of extremity war wound infection remains a clinical challenge, and due to the heterogeneity of traumatic injuries on the battlefield, interpreting the results of any randomised controlled trial can be problematic. As a result, pre-clinical evaluation of strategies to reduce wound infection are necessary.

A model of a contaminated soft tissue injury was needed as existing models of wound contamination were restricted to superficial injury. A rabbit model of a high-energy soft tissue muscle injury contaminated with *S. aureus* was developed and is described in detail elsewhere.[106] This model was used in two separate experimental studies. The first study evaluated the anti-microbial activity of gauze soaked in either saline, povidine–iodine or chlorhexidine or the commercial dressing *Acticoat®* over a 48-hour post-injury period, and the second, a seven-day study, evaluated the anti-microbial activity of a saline-soaked gauze dressing and three commercially available dressings, *Inadine®*, *Acticoat®* and *Activon®* Tulle. A group treated with saline soaked gauze with systemic antibiotic administration was also included. The primary outcome was a statistically significant reduction ($P < 0.05$) in tissue *S. aureus* at two or seven days post-injury respectively.

There was no statistical or clinically significant difference in bacterial counts at 48 hours between the dressings evaluated in the two-day study.[107] However, the antibiotic, *Inadine®* and *Acticoat®* groups had statistically significantly lower bacterial counts (mean, 7.13 [95% confidence interval, 0.00–96.31] $\times$ 10^2; 1.66 [0.94–2.58] $\times$ 10^5; 8.86 [0.00–53.35] $\times$ 10^4 cfu/g, respectively) and the *Activon®* Tulle group had significantly higher counts (2.82 [0.98–5.61] $\times$ 10^6 cfu/g) than the saline-soaked gauze control (7.58 [1.65–17.83] $\times$ 10^5 cfu/g) in the seven-day study.[108]

The secondary outcome measurements in both studies included bacteraemias, observational data, whole blood determination and lymph node histopathology. Due to the longer duration of the second study, additional analysis was undertaken including enzyme-linked immunosorbent assay for plasma biomarkers and polymerase chain reaction (PCR) array analysis of muscle tissue wound healing gene expression and muscle histopathology. There were no bacteraemias or significant differences in observational data or whole blood determination. Neither were there any significant differences in lymph node cross-sectional area or morphology for the dressings in both studies. There was some significant but potentially

counter-intuitive variation in the plasma cytokines IL-4, tumour necrosis factor α and MCP-1 in comparison to the control saline group.

PCR array data demonstrated more general changes in gene expression in the *Activon®* Tulle group than the *Inadine®* or *Acticoat®* dressings, with a limited number of genes showing significantly altered expression compared to control. There were no significant differences in muscle loss or pathology, nor were there any statistically significant differences in lymph node cross-sectional area or morphology.

In summary, a recovery model of contaminated deep soft tissue injury was developed that can be used to assess anti-microbial dressings. The wound model demonstrated statistically significant changes in *S. aureus* counts over a seven-day protocol but not over a two-day study, indicating that any anti-microbial effects potentially augment the host's natural defence mechanisms but that the potency of the anti-microbial effects are small when the bacterial burden is high.

Impact of blast exposure on vascular endothelium

Revascularisation after a critical period of ischaemia leads to reperfusion injury. Two issues are of immediate clinical concern: the effect of reperfusion of a limb on the body as a whole and the functionality of the reperfused limb. There was evidence that muscle can tolerate warm ischaemia for six hours,[109] but the influence of concurrent injuries such as hypovolaemia can reduce this tolerance,[110] and the effects of blast in this context had not been evaluated. Blast may adversely affect the limb's ability to extract oxygen and recover function after reperfusion, as an alteration of endothelial function post-blast could lead to gross disturbances in regional haemodynamics and, hence, in the immediate response of the limb to revascularisation. An assessment of the blast effects on the endothelium was necessary.

A model of blast exposure to the hind limbs of rabbits has been described elsewhere.[111] Briefly, terminally anaesthetised rabbits were subjected to one of four blast exposures (*high*, *medium*, *low* or *no blast*) to the gastrocnemius muscle. Blood samples were analysed for circulating endothelial cells pre-injury and at 1, 6 and 11 hours post-injury together with analysis for endothelial activation pre-injury and at 1, 6 and 12 hours post-injury. Post-mortem tissue (12 hours post-injury) was analysed for both protein and mRNA expression and also for histopathology.

The study demonstrated that blast injury to the hind limbs of anaesthetised rabbits causes activation of and damage to the endothelium. The magnitude of the effect is related to the level of blast loading, with low blast exposures resulting in endothelial activation and with endothelial damage (evidenced by circulating endothelial cells) evident only after high blast exposure. Changes to the endothelium ultimately resulted in changes in the histological appearance of muscle tissue at and around the site of injury with oedema, cell infiltrate and also necrosis. It is not known whether the changes observed in this study correspond to a functional change that would either impact on functional outcomes or significantly influence casualty management, but results may be suggestive of an exacerbated damaging effect of blast injury on haemorrhage and resulting shock.

LESSONS LEARNED AND EXAMPLES OF FUTURE DIRECTIONS

Resuscitation

The experimental studies of haemostatic resuscitation showed that early (simulated pre-hospital) use of blood products attenuated the development of ATC after haemorrhagic shock in models of trauma with and without blast injury. As we move beyond *Operation Herrick* into an era when prolonged care in relatively austere environments may be the issue, the advantages of fluids that do not require frozen storage (and careful thawing), or even use of fridges, become increasingly important. Part of the solution may be increased use of products such as fibrinogen or dried plasma, but this does not address the issue of oxygen transport, which is an important physiological consideration for managing not only shock but also early coagulopathy. *Dstl* has already made significant headway in addressing the oxygen transport element and has completed a study using an HBOC

(MP4, Sangart),[112] which had already been in Phase 2 clinical trials. One formulation of MP4 does not require refrigerated storage. In the presence of blast injury, MP4 was found to be significantly better than saline for reversal of shock associated with haemorrhage and hypotensive resuscitation, while PRBC with FFP was intermediate. By contrast, in the absence of blast injury PRBC with FFP was significantly better than saline, while MP4 and PRBC alone were intermediate.[112] This leads to the suggestion that plasma may aid resuscitation, possibly by improving the microcirculation. However, in the presence of blast injury, loading of oxygen into the blood in the lungs becomes a significant issue. The resulting reduction in arterial oxygen content after blast, coupled with a reduction in tissue blood flow during haemorrhagic shock and hypotensive resuscitation, may depress oxygen delivery to the point where the beneficial effects of plasma cannot be seen. Under these circumstances, the altered oxygen carrying properties (oxygen association/disassociation curves) of MP4 may provide significant benefit in the lungs and in the tissues when combined with the patient's own haemoglobin. Future studies may therefore be able to combine HBOC with a dried plasma solution to obtain a physiological and logistical 'best of both worlds'. Other studies, with an immediate clinical impact, will address the use of fresh whole blood and platelets, which represent current emerging clinical practice.

Endpoints of resuscitation and the microcirculation

Current resuscitation strategies use blood pressure, or a proxy measure of blood pressure such as the presence or absence of a palpable peripheral or central pulse, as primary targets. This approach results in casualties arriving in hospital in a wide range of physiological states. Similarly, individual animals in a defined model of trauma may develop marked variation in their degree of shock despite being resuscitated to identical clinical endpoints.[113] To some degree, the worst of the shock states may be attenuated by the use of better resuscitation fluids, such as blood products, but unfortunately, even with these superior fluids, the problem still persists. This effect is likely to be exaggerated and of greater clinical importance with prolonged evacuation. The underpinning reason for this variation rests with differences in individual haemodynamic responses to trauma, haemorrhage and resuscitation. The development of shock, and possibly of early coagulopathy, has a greater relation to tissue blood flow than to arterial blood pressure. Consequently, some individuals who have initiated a lesser vasoconstrictor response to haemorrhage will tolerate lower blood pressures or demand more fluid based on pressure-driven targets and hence be better resuscitated. By contrast, those who generate a profound vasoconstrictor response sacrifice tissue flow to maintain pressure and may become grossly under-resuscitated because they do not cross the pressure threshold to trigger fluid resuscitation. *Dstl* has been assessing tissue perfusion and oxygenation in experimental studies, which utilised current pressure-driven targets for resuscitation. There was a correlation between the vascular response in skeletal muscle (assessed using *near-infrared spectroscopy*, to determine tissue oxygenation) during the early shock and resuscitation phase and the degree of shock (assessed using base excess) 60 minutes later at the end of a simulated 'pre-hospital' resuscitation phase. Furthermore, microcirculatory assessment using *Sidestream Dark Field* revealed wide variation between individual animals in the degree of sublingual microvascular perfusion during shock and resuscitation. Interestingly, when microvascular perfusion was assessed in the haemostatic resuscitation study, the coagulopathy was found to develop only in the sub-group of saline-treated animals that had poor microvascular perfusion. Coagulopathy did not seem to develop in animals treated with saline if microvascular perfusion was good, nor in animals treated with blood products, even when microvascular perfusion was poor (Hutchings, Watts, Kirkman, unpublished data). This emphasises the important interplay between fluids used for resuscitation, resuscitation targets and individual physiological responses. It is far too early to form any firm conclusions based on these findings, but they do raise the interesting possibility that with more intelligent resuscitation targets, we may be able to individualise resuscitation in casualties more effectively. Whilst it is not anticipated that the use of these flow-related targets will ever replace pressure safeguards (to avoid re-bleeding), supplementary flow assessment targets may help to reduce physiological deterioration and make better use of limited resources in an austere environment. A number of studies to address this issue are already underway or being planned.

Battlefield pain management: Secondary cardiovascular effects of analgesic agents

Pain management is an important aspect of the treatment of battlefield casualties. Clearly, analgesic agents must provide effective pain control for severely injured casualties, but in choosing the optimal agent, secondary pharmacological effects must also be considered in the context of the specific constraints of casualty management. Of particular relevance to this chapter are the cardiovascular effects of analgesic agents in the context of trauma. These cardiovascular effects cannot be extrapolated from a simple knowledge of the effects of the agents in the uninjured, since the effects are probably the result of interactions with complex central nervous pathways engaged as part of the response to injury. A number of groups have demonstrated profound effects of mu (μ) opioid analgesic agents on the cardiovascular response to blood loss. In rats and rabbits, mu (μ) opioid agonists such as morphine delay the point of decompensation during simple haemorrhage[114-117]; by contrast, in sheep, the point of decompensation is hastened.[118]

A deleterious effect of morphine?

The delay in decompensation induced by morphine during haemorrhage does not provide protection to the casualty, indeed it maybe deleterious. At least three independent groups have shown in models of haemorrhage in the rat that mortality is increased, despite the apparent better (higher) blood pressure during severe haemorrhage.[119-121] This effect becomes relevant when there are long delays before full cardiovascular resuscitation. The effects on survival in sheep are unknown but clearly may be different from those in rats given the fundamental difference in the effects of morphine on the response to haemorrhage in these two species. Since battlefield casualties, especially in austere contingency operations, may be subject to a long evacuation chains, the topic is of importance to the DMS. A programme to investigate the effects of morphine on the cardiovascular response to simulated haemorrhage in volunteers has been conducted in collaboration with *James Cook University Hospital, Middlesbrough, UK*. The part of the trial investigating the effects of morphine in simple haemorrhage has shown a clear difference between morphine and placebo, with the direction of effect in humans being similar to that previously reported for rats. This raises the possibility that morphine, and perhaps other mu (μ) opioid agonists, may have deleterious cardiovascular effects after haemorrhage when there are long delays before full resuscitation. Further studies, in models relevant to battlefield injury, are now needed to determine whether other mu (μ) opioid agents such as fentanyl also have these limitations.

CONCLUSION

The combat casualty care research programme is an integrated suite of translational research work-streams that successfully addressed a range of questions for *DMS* during *Operations Telic* and *Herrick*. The same programme continues to address issues relevant to military, as well as civilian, trauma casualties into the future. It is a close collaboration between senior clinicians at RCDM and elsewhere and scientists at *Dstl*. Much of the research has been conducted at Porton Down, benefiting from a unique collection of facilities, resources and capabilities that together allow the development of models of battlefield injury relevant to current battlefield casualties. In addition, important components of the research have been conducted at other sites, including deployed research at Role 3 Bastion. The research links into civilian centres established through Dstl and the importance of its role in coordinating combined initiatives under National direction led by the DMS should not be underestimated.

The main focus has been resuscitation strategies for seriously injured battlefield casualties, including those with blast injuries, together with the impact of delayed evacuation. These studies evolved into investigations into haemostatic resuscitation and ATC. Other studies examined aspects of wound management, and the pathophysiological and immunological consequences of high energy trauma. The output of this work provided underpinning evidence for changes in clinical practice by the DMS. Future work is building on this experience and established capabilities and collaborations to examine issues such as resuscitation during prolonged field care, physiological targets to individualise resuscitation, novel fluids for resuscitation and the impact of concurrent pharmacological therapy.

REFERENCES

1. Hodgetts TJ, Mahoney PF, Russell MQ, Byers M. ABC to ABC: Redefining the military trauma paradigm. *Emerg Med J* 2006;23(10):745–746.
2. Brodie S, Hodgetts TJ, Ollerton J, McLeod J, Lambert P, Mahoney P. Tourniquet use in combat trauma: UK military experience. *J R Army Med Corps* 2007;153(4):310–313.
3. Martinowitz U, Michaelson M, Israeli Multidisciplinary rFVIIa Task Force. Guidelines for the use of recombinant activated factor VII (rFVIIa) in uncontrolled bleeding: A report by the Israeli Multidisciplinary rFVIIa Task Force. *J Thromb Haemost* 2005;3:640–648.
4. Martinowitz U, Kenet G, Lubetski A, Luboshitz J, Segal E. Possible role of recombinant activated factor VII (rFVIIa) in the control of hemorrhage associated with massive trauma. *Can J Anaesth* 2002;49(10):S15–S20.
5. Spinella PC, Perkins JG, McLaughlin DF et al. The effect of recombinant activated factor VII on mortality in combat-related casualties with severe trauma and massive transfusion. *J Trauma* 2008;64(2):286–293; discussion 293–294.
6. Mitra B, Cameron PA, Parr MJ, Phillips L. Recombinant factor VIIa in trauma patients with the 'triad of death'. *Injury* 2012;43(9): 1409–1414.
7. Smith JE. The use of recombinant activated factor VII (rFVIIa) in the management of

patients with major haemorrhage in military hospitals over the last 5 years. *Emerg Med J* 2013;30(4):316–369.

8. Belanger HG, Scott SG, Scholten J, Curtiss G, Vanderploeg RD. Utility of mechanism-of-injury-based assessment and treatment: Blast Injury Program case illustration. *J Rehabil Res Dev* 2005;42(4):403–412.

9. Elsayed NM. Toxicology of blast overpressure. *Toxicology* 1997;121(1):1–15.

10. Kirkman E, Watts S. Characterization of the response to primary blast injury. *Philos Trans R Soc Lond B Biol Sci* 2011; 366(1562):286–290.

11. Smith JE. The epidemiology of blast lung injury during recent military conflicts: A retrospective database review of cases presenting to deployed military hospitals, 2003–2009. *Philos Trans R Soc Lond B Biol Sci* 2011;366(1562):291–294.

12. Aboudara M, Mahoney PF, Hicks B, Cuadrado D. Primary blast lung injury at a NATO Role 3 hospital. *J R Army Med Corps* 2014;160(2):161–166.

13. Eastridge BJ, Mabry RL, Seguin P et al. Death on the battlefield (2001-2011): Implications for the future of combat casualty care. *J Trauma Acute Care Surg* 2012;73(6 Suppl 5):S431–S437.

14. Pannell D, Brisebois R, Talbot M et al. Causes of death in Canadian Forces members deployed to Afghanistan and implications on tactical combat casualty care provision. *J Trauma* 2011;71(5 Suppl 1): S401–S407.

15. Edwards S, Smith J. Advances in military resuscitation. *Emerg Nurse* 2016;24(6): 25–29.

16. Pusateri AE, Holcomb JB, Kheirabadi BS, Alam HB, Wade CE, Ryan KL. Making sense of the preclinical literature on advanced hemostatic products. *J Trauma Inj Infect Crit Care* 2006;60(3):674–682.

17. King RB, Filips D, Blitz S, Logsetty S. Evaluation of possible tourniquet systems for use in the Canadian Forces. *J Trauma Inj Infect Crit Care* 2006;60(5):1061–1071.

18. Wedmore I, McManus JG, Pusateri AE, Holcomb JB. A special report on

the chitosan-based hemostatic dressing: Experience in current combat operations. *J Trauma Inj Infect Crit Care* 2006;60(3):655–658.

19. Alam HB, Burris D, DaCorta JA, Rhee P. Hemorrhage control in the battlefield: Role of new hemostatic agents. *Mil Med* 2005;170(1):63–69.

20. Hedner U. Mechanism of action, development and clinical experience of recombinant FVIIa. *J Biotechnol* 2006;124(4): 747–757.

21. Kenet G, Walden R, Eldad A, Martinowitz U. Treatment of traumatic bleeding with recombinant factor VIIa. *Lancet* 1999;354(9193):1879.

22. Dutton RP, McCunn M, Hyder M et al. Factor VIIa for correction of traumatic coagulopathy. *J Trauma Inj Infect Crit Care* 2004;57(4):709–719.

23. Biss TT, Hanley JP. Recombinant activated factor VII (rFVIIa/NovoSeven) in intractable haemorrhage: Use of a clinical scoring system to predict outcome. *Vox Sang* 2006;90(1):45–52.

24. Harrison TD, Laskosky J, Jazaeri O, Pasquale MD, Cipolle M. "Low-dose" recombinant activated factor VII results in less blood and blood product use in traumatic hemorrhage. *J Trauma Inj Infect Crit Care* 2005;59(1):150–154.

25. Sapsford W, Watts S, Cooper G, Kirkman E. Recombinant activated factor VII increases survival time in a model of incompressible arterial hemorrhage in the anesthetized pig. *J Trauma Inj Infect Crit Care* 2007;62(4):868–879.

26. Garner JP, Watts S, Parry C, Bird J, Kirkman E. Development of a large animal model for investigating resuscitation after blast and hemorrhage. *World J Surg [Internet]* 2009;33(10):2194–2202.

27. Kirkman E, Watts S, Cooper G. Blast injury research models. *Philos Trans R Soc Lond B Biol Sci* 2011;366(1562):144–159.

28. Watts S, Nordmann G, Brohi K et al. Evaluation of prehospital blood products to attenuate acute coagulopathy of trauma in a model of severe injury and shock

in anesthetized pigs. *Shock [Internet]* 2015;44(Suppl 1):138–148.

29. Battlefield Advanced Trauma Life Support (BATLS). *J R Army Med Corps* 2001;147(3):314–321.

30. Doran CM, Doran CA, Woolley T et al. Targeted resuscitation improves coagulation and outcome. *J Trauma Acute Care Surg [Internet]* 2012;72(4):835–843.

31. NICE. Pre-hospital initiation of fluid replacement therapy in trauma. National Institute for Health and Care Excellence. NICE; 2004:1–32.

32. Damon EG, Yelverton JT, Luft UC, Mitchell K, Jones RK. Acute effects of air blast on pulmonary function in dogs and sheep. *Aerosp Med* 1971;42(1):1–9.

33. Guy RJ, Kirkman E, Watkins PE, Cooper GJ. Physiologic responses to primary blast. *J Trauma* 1998;45(6):983–987.

34. Ohnishi M, Kirkman E, Guy RJ, Watkins PE. Reflex nature of the cardiorespiratory response to primary thoracic blast injury in the anaesthetised rat. *Exp Physiol* 2001;86(3):357–364.

35. Harban F, Kirkman E, Kenward CE, Watkins PE. Primary thoracic blast injury causes acute reduction in cardiac function in the anaesthetised pig. *J Physiol (Lond)* 2001;533:81P.

36. Žunić G, Romić P, Vueljić M, Jovanikić O. Very early increase in nitric oxide formation and oxidative cell damage associated with the reduction of tissue oxygenation is a trait of blast casualties. *Vojnosanit Pregl* 2005;62(4):273–280.

37. Garner JP. Resuscitation after blast and haemorrhage. MD Thesis, Newcastle University.

38. Garner J, Watts S, Parry C, Bird J, Cooper G, Kirkman E. Prolonged permissive hypotensive resuscitation is associated with poor outcome in primary blast injury with controlled hemorrhage. *Ann Surg [Internet]* 2010;251(6):1131–1139.

39. Brohi K, Cohen MJ, Ganter MT et al. Acute traumatic coagulopathy: Initiated by hypoperfusion: Modulated through the protein C pathway? *Ann Surg* 2007;245(5):812–818.

40. Lee CC, Marill KA, Carter WA, Crupi RS. A current concept of trauma-induced multiorgan failure. *Ann Emerg Med* 2001;38(2):170–176.

41. Bickell WH, Wall MJ, Pepe PE et al. Immediate versus delayed fluid resuscitation for hypotensive patients with penetrating torso injuries. *N Engl J Med* 1994;331(17):1105–1109.

42. Jacobs N. Novel resuscitation strategies for casualties of blast and haemorrhage. MD Thesis, Newcastle University.

43. Doran CM. Effect of resuscitation strategies on coagulation following haemorrhage and blast exposure. MD Thesis, Newcastle University.

44. UK Defence Medical Education Training Agency. Battlefield Advanced Life Support. 2006.

45. Dubick MA, Atkins JL. Small-volume fluid resuscitation for the far-forward combat environment: Current concepts. *J Trauma Inj Infect Crit Care* 2003;54(5 Suppl):S43–S45.

46. Alam HB, Sun L, Ruff P, Austin B, Burris D, Rhee P. E- and P-selectin expression depends on the resuscitation fluid used in hemorrhaged rats. *J Surg Res* 2000;94(2):145–152.

47. Bahrami S, Zimmermann K, Szelényi Z et al. Small-volume fluid resuscitation with hypertonic saline prevents inflammation but not mortality in a rat model of hemorrhagic shock. *Shock* 2006;25(3):283–289.

48. Bulger EM, Cuschieri J, Warner K, Maier RV. Hypertonic resuscitation modulates the inflammatory response in patients with traumatic hemorrhagic shock. *Ann Surg* 2007;245(4):635–641.

49. Rizoli SB, Rhind SG, Shek PN et al. The immunomodulatory effects of hypertonic saline resuscitation in patients sustaining traumatic hemorrhagic shock: A randomized, controlled, double-blinded trial. *Ann Surg [Internet]* 2006;243(1):47–57.

50. White H, Cook D, Venkatesh B. The role of hypertonic saline in neurotrauma. *Eur J Anaesthesiol Suppl* 2008;42(Suppl 42):104–109.

51. Zakaria ER, Tsakadze NL, Garrison RN. Hypertonic saline resuscitation improves intestinal microcirculation in a rat model of hemorrhagic shock. *Surgery* 2006;140(4):579–587; discussion 587–588.

52. Kirkman E, Watts S, Garner JP, Parry C, Bird J, Hesketh A. *Strategies for the Resuscitation of Combined Blast and Haemorrhage Casualties.* Dstl, 2006. Report No.: Dstl/TR19030.

53. Granville-Chapman J. Adjuncts to pre-hospital resuscitation strategies for haemorrhagic shock and blast injury: Supplemental oxygen and recombinant activated factor VII. MD Thesis, Newcastle University.

54. Leach RM, Davidson AC. Use of emergency oxygen in adults. *BMJ* 2009;338(1):a2790.

55. Asehnoune K, Faraoni D, Brohi K. What's new in management of traumatic coagulopathy? *Intensive Care Med* 2014;40(11):1727–1130.

56. Maegele M, Schöchl H, Cohen MJ. An update on the coagulopathy of trauma. *Shock* 2014;41(Suppl 1):21–25.

57. Cap A, Hunt BJ. The pathogenesis of traumatic coagulopathy. *Anaesthesia* 2014;70(Suppl 1):96–101, e32–e34.

58. Woolley T, Midwinter M, Spencer P, Watts S, Doran C, Kirkman E. Utility of interim ROTEM(®) values of clot strength, A5 and A10, in predicting final assessment of coagulation status in severely injured battle patients. *Injury* 2013;44(5):593–599.

59. Pidcoke HF, Aden JK, Mora AG et al. Ten-year analysis of transfusion in Operation Iraqi Freedom and Operation Enduring Freedom: Increased plasma and platelet use correlates with improved survival. *J Trauma Acute Care Surg* 2012;73(6 Suppl 5):S445–S452.

60. Nordmann G, Woolley T, Doughty H, Dalle Lucca J, Hutchings S, Kirkman E. Deployed research. *J R Army Med Corps* 2014;160(2):92–98.

61. Brohi K, Cohen MJ, Ganter MT et al. Acute coagulopathy of trauma: Hypoperfusion induces systemic anticoagulation and hyperfibrinolysis. *J Trauma* 2008;64(5):1211–1217; discussion 1217.

62. Pati S, Matijevic N, Doursout M-F et al. Protective effects of fresh frozen plasma on vascular endothelial permeability, coagulation, and resuscitation after hemorrhagic shock are time dependent and diminish between days 0 and 5 after thaw. *J Trauma Inj Infect Crit Care* 2010;69(Suppl 1):S55–S63.

63. Torres LN, Sondeen JL, Ji L, Dubick MA, Torres Filho I. Evaluation of resuscitation fluids on endothelial glycocalyx, venular blood flow, and coagulation function after hemorrhagic shock in rats. *J Trauma Acute Care Surg* 2013;75(5):759–766.

64. Torres LN, Sondeen JL, Dubick MA, Filho IT. Systemic and microvascular effects of resuscitation with blood products after severe hemorrhage in rats. *J Trauma Acute Care Surg* 2014;77(5):716–723.

65. Peng Z, Pati S, Potter D et al. Fresh frozen plasma lessens pulmonary endothelial inflammation and hyperpermeability after hemorrhagic shock and is associated with loss of syndecan 1. *Shock* 2013;40(3):195–202.

66. Kirkman E, Watts S. Combat Casualty Care research programme. *J R Army Med Corps* 2014;160(2):109–116.

67. Doran CM, Woolley T, Midwinter MJ. Feasibility of using rotational thromboelastometry to assess coagulation status of combat casualties in a deployed setting. *J Trauma* 2010;69(Suppl 1):S40–S48.

68. Jansen JO, Luke D, Davies E, Spencer P, Kirkman E, Midwinter MJ. Temporal changes in ROTEM®-measured coagulability of citrated blood samples from coagulopathic trauma patients. *Injury* 2013;44(1):36–39.

69. Woolley T, Gwyther R, Parmar K et al. Haemostatic changes in military casualties in Afghanistan. *Military Health System Research Symposium.* 2016.

70. Fries D, Martini WZ. Role of fibrinogen in trauma-induced coagulopathy. *Br J Anaesth* 2010;105(2):116–121.

71. Mellor SG, Cooper GJ. Analysis of 828 servicemen killed or injured by explosion in Northern Ireland 1970–84: The

Hostile Action Casualty System. *Br J Surg* 1989;76(10):1006–1110.

72. de Ceballos JPG, Turégano-Fuentes F, Pérez-Díaz D, Sanz-Sánchez M, Martin-Llorente C, Guerrero-Sanz JE. 11 March 2004: The terrorist bomb explosions in Madrid, Spain – an analysis of the logistics, injuries sustained and clinical management of casualties treated at the closest hospital. *Crit Care* 2005;9(1):104–111.

73. Martí M, Parrón M, Baudraxler F, Royo A, Gómez León N, Alvarez-Sala R. Blast injuries from Madrid terrorist bombing attacks on March 11, 2004. *Emerg Radiol* 2006;13(3):113–122.

74. Ramasamy A, Harrisson SE, Clasper JC, Stewart MPM. Injuries from roadside improvised explosive devices. *J Trauma* 2008;65(4):910–914.

75. Ritenour AE, Blackbourne LH, Kelly JF et al. Incidence of primary blast injury in US military overseas contingency operations: A retrospective study. *Ann Surg* 2010;251(6):1140–1144.

76. Cooper GJ. Protection of the lung from blast overpressure by thoracic stress wave decouplers. *J Trauma* 1996;40(3 Suppl):S105–S110.

77. Cohn SM. Pulmonary contusion: Review of the clinical entity. *J Trauma Inj Infect Crit Care* 1997;42(5):973–979.

78. Cooper GJ, Townend DJ, Cater SR, Pearce BP. The role of stress waves in thoracic visceral injury from blast loading: Modification of stress transmission by foams and high-density materials. *J Biomech* 1991;24(5):273–285.

79. Gans L, Kennedy T. Management of unique clinical entities in disaster medicine. *Emerg Med Clin North Am* 1996;14(2):301–326.

80. Mellor SG. The pathogenesis of blast injury and its management. *Br J Hosp Med* 1988;39(6):536–539.

81. Katz E, Ofek B, Adler J, Abramowitz HB, Krausz MM. Primary blast injury after a bomb explosion in a civilian bus. *Ann Surg* 1989;209(4):484–488.

82. Leibovici D, Gofrit ON, Stein M et al. Blast injuries: Bus versus open-air bombings – a comparative study of injuries in survivors of open-air versus confined-space explosions. *J Trauma Inj Infect Crit Care* 1996;41(6):1030–1035.

83. Hirshberg B, Oppenheim-Eden A, Pizov R et al. Recovery from blast lung injury: One-year follow-up. *Chest* 1999;116(6):1683–1688.

84. Gorbunov NV, Asher LV, Ayyagari V, Atkins JL. Inflammatory leukocytes and iron turnover in experimental hemorrhagic lung trauma. *Exp Mol Pathol* 2006;80(1):11–25.

85. Gorbunov NV, Elsayed NM, Kisin ER, Kozlov AV, Kagan VE. Air blast-induced pulmonary oxidative stress: Interplay among hemoglobin, antioxidants, and lipid peroxidation. *Am J Physiol* 1997;272(2 Pt 1):L320–L334.

86. Gorbunov NV, McFaul SJ, Januszkiewicz A, Atkins JL. Pro-inflammatory alterations and status of blood plasma iron in a model of blast-induced lung trauma. *Int J Immunopathol Pharmacol* 2005;18(3):547–556.

87. Tien HCN, Gough MRC, Farrell R, Macdonald J. Successful use of recombinant activated coagulation factor VII in a patient with massive hemoptysis from a penetrating thoracic injury. *Ann Thorac Surg* 2007;84(4):1373–1374.

88. Estella A, Jareño A, Perez-Bello Fontaiña L. Intrapulmonary administration of recombinant activated factor VII in diffuse alveolar haemorrhage: A report of two case stories. *Cases J* 2008;1(1):150.

89. Heslet L, Nielsen JD, Levi M, Sengeløv H, Johansson PI. Successful pulmonary administration of activated recombinant factor VII in diffuse alveolar hemorrhage. *Crit Care* 2006;10(6):R177.

90. Heslet L, Nielsen JD, Nepper-Christensen S. Local pulmonary administration of factor VIIa (rFVIIa) in diffuse alveolar hemorrhage (DAH) – a review of a new treatment paradigm. *Biologics [Internet]* 2012;6:37–46.

91. Granville-Chapman J, Kirkman E, Mahoney P, Midwinter M, Watts S. Supplementary oxygen improves survival time during prolonged hypotensive resuscitation after blast injury and haemorrhage. *Br J Surg* 2010;97(S2):190.

92. Watts S, Granville-Chapman J, Mahoney P, Midwinter M, Hodgetts T, Kirkman E. *Effects of Increased Inspired Oxygen (FiO₂) on Survival after Combined Blast Injury and Haemorrhage.* Dstl CR v., 2009.

93. Woolley T. Effects of recombinant activated Factor VII and supplementary oxygen on coagulopathy after trauma. MD Thesis, University of Newcastle, 2013.

94. Smith JE. Inhaled recombinant activated factor VII (rFVIIa) in the management of blast lung injury. MD Thesis, University of Newcastle.

95. Gorbunov NV, McFaul SJ, Van Albert S, Morrissette C, Zaucha GM, Nath J. Assessment of inflammatory response and sequestration of blood iron transferrin complexes in a rat model of lung injury resulting from exposure to low-frequency shock waves. *Crit Care Med* 2004;32(4):1028–1034.

96. Watts S, Spear A, Smith JE, Doran C, Taylor C, Kirkman E. *Inhaled Recombinant Factor VII (rFVIIa) in the Treatment of Blast Lung.* Dstl CR, 2012.

97. Owens BD, Kragh JFJ, Wenke JC, Macaitis J, Wade CE, Holcomb JB. Combat wounds in operation Iraqi Freedom and operation Enduring Freedom. *J Trauma Inj Infect Crit Care* 2008;64(2):295–299.

98. Owens BD, Kragh JF, Macaitis J, Svoboda SJ, Wenke JC. Characterization of extremity wounds in Operation Iraqi Freedom and Operation Enduring Freedom. *J Orthop Trauma* 2007;21(4):254–257.

99. Ramasamy A, Harrisson S, Lasrado I, Stewart MPM. A review of casualties during the Iraqi insurgency 2006 – a British field hospital experience. *Injury* 2009;40(5): 493–497.

100. Murray CK, Wilkins K, Molter NC et al. Infections in combat casualties during Operations Iraqi and Enduring Freedom. *J Trauma* 2009;66(4 Suppl):S138–S144.

101. Petersen K, Riddle MS, Danko JR et al. Trauma-related infections in battlefield casualties from Iraq. *Ann Surg* 2007;245(5): 803–811.

102. Brown KV, Murray CK, Clasper JC. Infectious complications of combat-related mangled extremity injuries in the British military. *J Trauma* 2010;69(Suppl 1): S109–S115.

103. White JM, Stannard A, Burkhardt GE, Eastridge BJ, Blackbourne LH, Rasmussen TE. The epidemiology of vascular injury in the wars in Iraq and Afghanistan. *Ann Surg* 2011;253(6):1184–1189.

104. Doukas WC, Hayda RA, Frisch HM et al. The Military Extremity Trauma Amputation/ Limb Salvage (METALS) study: Outcomes of amputation versus limb salvage following major lower-extremity trauma. *J Bone Joint Surg Am* 2013;95(2):138–145.

105. Scott DJ, Arthurs ZM, Stannard A, Monroe HM, Clouse WD, Rasmussen TE. Patient-based outcomes and quality of life after salvageable wartime extremity vascular injury. *J Vasc Surg* 2014;59(1):173–179.e1.

106. Eardley WGP, Martin KR, Taylor C, Kirkman E, Clasper JC, Watts SA. The development of an experimental model of contaminated muscle injury in rabbits. *Int J Low Extrem Wounds* 2012;11(4):254–263.

107. Eardley WGP, Martin KR, Kirkman E, Clasper JC, Watts SA. The efficacy of antimicrobial wound dressings used in the management of military complex extremity injury: A pre-clinical ramdomised controlled trial. *Br J Surg* 2011;98(S2):21.

108. Guthrie HC, Martin KR, Taylor C et al. A pre-clinical evaluation of silver, iodine and Manuka honey based dressings in a model of traumatic extremity wounds contaminated with *Staphylococcus aureus. Injury* 2014;45(8):1171–1178.

109. Burkhardt GE, Gifford SM, Propper B, Spencer JR, Williams K, Jones L et al. The impact of ischemic intervals on neuromuscular recovery in a porcine (*Sus scrofa*) survival model of extremity vascular injury. *J Vasc Surg* 2011;53(1):165–173.

110. Hancock HM, Stannard A, Burkhardt GE et al. Hemorrhagic shock worsens neuromuscular recovery in a porcine model

of hind limb vascular injury and ischemia-reperfusion. *J Vasc Surg* 2011;53(4):1052–1062; discussion 1062.

111. Spear AM, Davies EM, Taylor C et al. Blast wave exposure to the extremities causes endothelial activation and damage. *Shock* 2015;44(5):470–478.

112. Kirkman E, Burhop K, Hutchings S et al. Physiological effects of "pre-hospital" resuscitation with HBOC compared to saline and packed red cells: Plasma in two models of severe injury. 2016.

113. Kirkman E, Watts S. Haemodynamic changes in trauma. *Br J Anaesth* 2014;113(2):266–275.

114. Ohnishi M, Kirkman E, Marshall HW, Little RA. Morphine blocks the bradycardia associated with severe hemorrhage in the anesthetized rat. *Brain Res* 1997;763(1):39–46.

115. Ohnishi M, Kirkman E, Hiraide A, Little RA. Bradycardia and hypotension associated with severe hemorrhage are reversed by morphine given centrally or peripherally in anesthetized rats. *J Trauma* 1998;45(6):1024–1030.

116. Evans RG, Ludbrook J. Effects of mu-opioid receptor agonists on circulatory responses to simulated haemorrhage in conscious rabbits. *Br J Pharmacol* 1990;100(3):421–426.

117. Evans RG, Ludbrook J, Van Leeuwen AF. Role of central opiate receptor subtypes in the circulatory responses of awake rabbits to graded caval occlusions. *J Physiol (Lond)* 1989;419:15–31.

118. Frithiof R, Rundgren M. Activation of central opioid receptors determines the timing of hypotension during acute hemorrhage-induced hypovolemia in conscious sheep. *Am J Physiol Regul Integr Comp Physiol* 2006;291(4):R987–R996.

119. Molina PE, Zambell KL, Zhang P, Vande Stouwe C, Carnal J. Hemodynamic and immune consequences of opiate analgesia after trauma/hemorrhage. *Shock* 2004;21(6):526–534.

120. Feuerstein G, Siren AL. Effect of naloxone and morphine on survival of conscious rats after hemorrhage. *Circ Shock* 1986;19(3):293–300.

121. Little RA, Kirkman E, Ohnishi M. Opioids and the cardiovascular responses to haemorrhage and injury. *Intensive Care Med* 1998;24(5):405–414.

Appendix A: Forces deployed on *Operation Telic*

This list is kept short for clarity and includes official abbreviations for ease of reference. Apart from *Royal Artillery*, it does not include Combat Support Arms (*Royal Engineers*, *Royal Corps of Signals* and *Intelligence Corps*) or Combat Service Support (e.g. *Royal Logistic Corps* and *Army Medical Services*), which are essential components of any major deployed force and were present throughout the campaigns.

The main sources of this information are Historical Branch (Army) and Tim Ripley's *Operation TELIC – The British Campaign in Iraq 2003–2009* (Telic–Herrick Publications, 2016), www.operationtelic.co.uk. Some units changed their role during a tour or straddled two *Operation Telic* deployments. For instance, QRH commenced *Operation Telic 3* as a Ground Holding battlegroup but were later shifted to a Security Sector Reform role; the *1st Battalion, Argyll* and *Sutherland Highlanders* were in theatre during both *Telic 3* and *Telic 4*.

Main combat forces deployed on *Operation Telic*

Telic 1 **(Feb–Jun 2003):** 1st (UK) Armoured Division Commander: Major General Robin Brims (Jan–May 2003), Major General Peter Wall (May–July 2003)

- 7 Armoured Brigade (commanded by Brigadier Graham Binns). Four battlegroups:
  - *The Royal Scots Dragoon Guards (SCOTS DG)*
  - *2nd Royal Tank Regiment (2 RTR)*
  - *1st Battalion, The Royal Regiment of Fusiliers (1 RRF)*
  - *1st Battalion, The Black Watch (1 BW)*
  - *Also: 3rd Regiment, Royal Horse Artillery*
- 16 Air Assault Brigade (Brigadier Jacko Page). Four battlegroups:
  - *1st Battalion, The Parachute Regiment (1 PARA)*
  - *3rd Battalion, The Parachute Regiment (3 PARA)*
  - *1st Battalion, The Royal Irish Regiment (1 R IRISH)*
  - *3rd Regiment Army Air Corps*
  - *Also: 7 Parachute Regiment, Royal Horse Artillery*
- 3 Commando Brigade RM (Brigadier Jim Dutton RM). Three battlegroups:
  - *40 Commando, Royal Marines*
  - *42 Commando, Royal Marines*
  - *15th Marine Expeditionary Unit (US Marine Corps)*

(Continued)

(Continued) Main combat forces deployed on *Operation Telic*

	Also: *29 Commando Regiment, Royal Artillery*
	• 102 Logistics Brigade (Brigadier Shaun Cowlam)
	• Other Divisional assets:
	• *1st The Queen's Dragoon Guards*
	• *Other units as listed in the MOD's The Fight for Iraq January–June 2003, p. 152*

Telic 2 (Jul–Oct 2003):
Headquarters Multi-National Division (South East)
(Maj Gen Graeme Lamb)

19 Mechanised Brigade (Brigadier Bill Moore)

National Support Component HQ (tri-service HQ providing logistic support from July 2003–May 2009, based at Shaibah Logistic Base/Umm Qasr/Basra Airport)

• Ground holding (framework) battlegroups:
  • *1st Battalion, The King's Own Scottish Borders (1 KOSB) (Task Force Maysan)*
  • *1st Battalion, The King's Regiment (1 KINGS)*
  • *1st Battalion, The Queen's Lancashire Regiment (1 QLR)*
  • *40 Regiment, Royal Artillery*
• Surge/reinforcement battlegroups:
  • *1st Battalion, The Royal Green Jackets (1 RGJ) (Divisional asset)*
  • *2nd Battalion, The Light Infantry (2 LI)*

Telic 3 (Nov 2003–Apr 2004):
HQ MND(SE)
(Maj Gen Andrew Stewart)

20 Armoured Brigade (Brigadiers David Rutherford-Jones/Nick Carter)

• Ground Holding Battlegroups:
  • *1st Battalion, The Light Infantry (1 LI) (TF Maysan)*
  • *1st Battalion, The Royal Regiment of Wales (1 RRW)*
  • *The Queen's Royal Hussars (QRH)*
  • *26 Regiment Royal Artillery*
• Surge/reinforcement battlegroups:
  • *1st Battalion, The Royal Scots (The Royal Regiment) (1 RS) (reinforcing other units)*
  • *2nd Battalion, The Parachute Regiment (2 PARA)*
  • *1st Battalion, The Argyll and Sutherland Highlanders (1 A&SH)*

Telic 4 (May–Oct 2004):
HQ MND(SE)
(Maj Gen William Rollo)

1 Mechanised Brigade
(Brig Andrew Kennett)

• Ground holding battlegroups:
  • *1st Battalion, The Princess of Wales's Royal Regiment (1 PWRR) (TF Maysan)*
  • *1st Battalion, The Cheshire Regiment (1 CHESHIRE)*
  • *1st Battalion, The Royal Welch Fusiliers (1 RWF)*
  • *1st Royal Horse Artillery*
• Surge/reinforcement battlegroups:
  • *40 Commando, Royal Marines/1st Battalion, The Royal Highland Fusiliers (1 RHF)*
  • *1st Battalion, The Black Watch (1 BW)*

(Continued)

(Continued) Main combat forces deployed on *Operation Telic*

Telic 5 (Nov 2004–Apr 2005):
HQ MND(SE)
(Maj Gen Jonathan Riley)

4 Armoured Brigade
(Brigadiers Paul Gibson/Chris Deverell)

- Ground holding battlegroups:
  - *1st Battalion, Welsh Guards (1 WG) (TF Maysan)*
  - *1st Battalion, The Duke of Wellington's Regiment (1 DWR)*
  - *Royal Dragoon Guards (RDG)*
  - *4 Regiment Royal Artillery*

- Surge/reinforcement battlegroups:
  - *1st Battalion, Scots Guards (1 SG)*
  - *2nd Battalion, The Princess of Wales's Royal Regiment (2 PWRR)*
  - *1st Battalion, The Royal Highland Fusiliers (1 RHF)*
  - *1st The Queen's Dragoon Guards (QDG)*

Telic 6 (May–Oct 2005):
HQ MND(SE)
(Maj Gen Jim Dutton RM)

12 Mechanised Brigade
(Brigadiers Chris Hughes/John Lorimer)

- Ground holding battlegroups:
  - *1st Battalion, The Royal Anglian Regiment (1 R ANGLIAN)*
  - *1st Battalion, The Royal Irish Regiment (1 R IRISH)*
  - *1st Battalion, The Staffordshire Regiment (1 STAFFORDS) (TF Maysan)*
  - *1st Battalion, Coldstream Guards (1 COLDM GDS)*
  - *19 Regiment, Royal Artillery*
- Surge/reinforcement/reserve/rear ops battlegroups:
  - *1st Battalion, The Royal Regiment of Wales (1 RRW)*
  - *The Light Dragoons (LD)*
  - *The King's Royal Hussars (KRH)*

Telic 7 (Nov 2005–Apr 2006):
HQ MND(SE)
(Maj Gen John Cooper)

7 Armoured Brigade
(Brig Patrick Marriott)

- Ground holding battlegroups:
  - *1st Battalion, The Highlanders (1 HIGHLANDERS)*
  - *The Royal Scots Dragoon Guards (SCOTS DG) (TF Maysan)*
  - *3rd Royal Horse Artillery*
- Reserve/rear ops battlegroups:
  - *1st Battalion, The King's Own Royal Border Regiment (I KORBR)*
  - *1st Battalion, The Royal Regiment of Fusiliers (1 RRF)*
  - *9/12th Royal Lancers (9/12 L)*
  - *2nd Battalion, The Parachute Regiment (2 PARA)*

(Continued)

(Continued) Main combat forces deployed on *Operation Telic*

Telic 8 **(May–Oct 2006):**
HQ MND(SE)

(Maj Gen Richard Shirreff)
20 Armoured Brigade
(Brig James Everard)

- Ground holding battlegroups:
  - *1st Battalion, The Light Infantry (1 LI)*
  - *2nd Battalion, The Royal Anglian Regiment (2 R ANGLIAN)*
  - *1st Battalion, The Devonshire and Dorset Light Infantry (1 DDLI)*
  - *1st Battalion, The Princess of Wales's Royal Regiment (1 PWRR)*
  - *The Queen's Royal Hussars (QRH) (TF Maysan)*
- Surge/reinforcement/reserve/rear ops battlegroups:
  - *1st The Queen's Dragoon Guards (QDG)*
  - *2nd Battalion, The Royal Regiment of Fusiliers (2 RRF)*
  - *1st Battalion, Grenadier Guards (1 GREN GDS)*

Telic 9 **(Nov 2006–Apr 2007):**
HQ MND(SE)
(Maj Gen Jonathan Shaw)

19 Light Brigade
(Brig Tim Evans)

- Ground holding battlegroups:
  - *2nd Battalion, The Duke of Lancaster's Regiment (2 LANCS)*
  - *1st Battalion, The Staffordshire Regiment (1 STAFFORDS)*
  - *1st Battalion, The Royal Green Jackets (1 RGJ)/renamed 2nd Battalion, The Rifles (2 RIFLES) on 1 Feb 2007*
  - *1st Battalion, The Yorkshire Regiment (1 YORKS)*
- Reserve/rear ops battlegroups:
  - *Queen's Royal Lancers (QRL) (TF Maysan)*
  - *40 Regiment Royal Artillery*

Telic 10 **(May–Oct 2007):**
HQ MND(SE)
(Maj Gen Graham Binns)

1 Mechanised Brigade
(Brig James Bashall)

- Ground holding battlegroups:
  - *4th Battalion, The Rifles (4 RIFLES)*
- Reserve/rear ops battlegroups:
  - *1st Battalion, Irish Guards (1 IG)*
  - *2nd Battalion, The Royal Welsh Regiment (2 R WELSH)*
  - *1st Royal Horse Artillery*
  - *King's Royal Hussars (KRH) (TF Maysan)*

Telic 11 **(Nov 2007–May 2008):**
HQ MND(SE)
(Maj Gen Barney White-Spunner)

4 Mechanised Brigade
(Brig Julian Free)

- Strike/manoeuvre battlegroups:
  - *1st Battalion, Scots Guards (1 SG)*
  - *1st Battalion, The Duke of Lancaster's Regiment (2 LANCS)*
- Reserve/rear ops battlegroups:
  - *1st Battalion, The Royal Regiment of Scotland (1 SCOTS)*
  - *1st Battalion, The Mercian Regiment (1 MERCIAN)*

(Continued)

(Continued) Main combat forces deployed on *Operation Telic*

Telic 12 **(May–Nov 2008):**
HQ MND(SE)
(Maj Gen Andy Salmon)

7 Armoured Brigade
(Brig Sandy Storrie)

- Military Transition Team (MiTT) operations:
  - *The Royal Scots Dragoon Guards (SCOTS DG)*
  - *2nd Battalion, The Royal Anglian Regiment (2 R ANGLIAN)*
  - *4th Battalion, The Royal Regiment of Scotland (4 SCOTS)*
  - *1st Battalion, The Royal Regiment of Fusiliers (1 RRF)*
  - *3rd Royal Horse Artillery*

Telic 13 **(Nov 2008–May 2009):**
HQ MND(SE)
(Maj Gen Andy Salmon)

20 Armoured Brigade
(Brig Tom Beckett)

- Military Transition Team (MiTT) operations:
  - *1st Royal Tank Regiment (1 RTR)*
  - *1st Battalion, The Yorkshire Regiment (1 YORKS)*
  - *1st Battalion, The Princess of Wales's Royal Regiment (1 PWRR)*
  - *5th Battalion, The Rifles (5 RIFLES)*
  - *26 Regiment Royal Artillery*

Appendix B: Forces deployed on *Operation Herrick*

This list is kept short for clarity and includes official abbreviations for ease of reference. It does not include Combat Support Arms (*Royal Artillery, Royal Engineers, Royal Corps of Signals* and *Intelligence Corps*) or Combat Service Support (e.g. *Royal Logistic Corps* and *Army Medical Services*), which are essential components of any major deployed force and were present throughout the campaigns.

Detached units or elements reinforcing the principal battlegroups are included only if manning the Warrior, Mastiff, Viking and Warthog groups, in which case parent regiments are generally mentioned. In addition, a Danish mechanised reconnaissance squadron and an Estonian mechanised infantry platoon were attached to *Task Force Helmand* from *Herrick 4* onward. The Danish contingent increased to 750 personnel and took charge of Battle Group Centre around Lashkar Gah from *Herrick 7*, also deploying a troop of three Leopard 2 tanks from November 2007, before leaving Afghanistan in May 2014. The Army Air Corps provided up to eight Apache attack helicopters and four Lynx battlefield utility helicopters each tour from *Herrick 4* onwards. The Royal Air Force provided six Chinook helicopters, one of which was always on standby for casualty evacuation with the *Medical Emergency Response Team*, accompanied by two Apache gunships.

The main sources for this information include Historical Branch (Army), Leigh Neville's *The British Army in Afghanistan 2006–14: Task Force Helmand* (Osprey Publishing, 2015) and David Reynolds' *AFGHANISTAN Britain's War in Helmand – An Historical Account* (DRA Publishing, 2017)

Main combat forces deployed on *Operation Herrick*

Herrick 1 (1 Oct 2004–30 Apr 2005)
1st Battalion, The Worcestershire and Sherwood Foresters Regiment (1 WFR)

Herrick 2 (29 Mar–2 Oct 2005)
2nd Battalion, The Royal Gurkha Rifles (2 RGR)

Herrick 3 (3 Oct 2005–3 Apr 2006)
1st Battalion, The Royal Gloucestershire, Berkshire and Wiltshire Light Infantry (1 RGBW)

Herrick 4 (16 Air Assault Brigade) (Apr–Oct 2006)
3 PARA Battle Group, in keeping with its envisioned peace support role, deployed with mainly unarmoured vehicles (Land Rover Snatch vehicles and Pinzgauer trucks, together with machine-gun mounted Land Rover Wolf Weapon Mount Installation Kits (WMIKs). There was no armoured mobility protection for infantry. The Battle Group had a tracked armoured squadron in the reconnaissance role, known as the *Brigade Reconnaissance Force*, equipped with Combat Vehicles Reconnaissance Tracked (CVRTs), particularly Scimitars (armed with 30 mm cannon), which served Task Force Helmand well throughout *Op Herrick*.

(Continued)

(Continued) Main combat forces deployed on *Operation Herrick*

Principal manoeuvre units:
- 3rd Battalion, The Parachute Regiment (3 PARA)
- 1st Battalion, The Royal Irish Regiment (1 R IRISH)

Brigade Reconnaissance Force:
- D Squadron, The Household Cavalry Regiment (HCR)

Afghan National Army/Police (ANA/ANP) Mentoring:
- 7th Parachute Regiment Royal Horse Artillery

Theatre Reserve Battalion (from Cyprus):
- 2nd Battalion, The Royal Regiment of Fusiliers (2 RRF)

Herrick 5 (*3 Commando Brigade*) (Oct 2006–Apr 2007)

The Royal Marines had Viking Armoured All-Terrain Vehicles (an amphibious, two-cabin tracked personnel carrier, which provided better protection against mines and improvised explosive device). They also began to receive Enhanced WMIKS (E-WMIK) with increased armour protection.

Principal manoeuvre unit:
- 42 Commando, Royal Marines

Theatre Reserve and ANA/ANP Mentoring:
- 45 Commando, Royal Marines

Brigade Reconnaissance Force: *C Squadron, The Light Dragoons (LD)*

Herrick 6 (*12 Mechanised Brigade*) (Apr–Oct 2007)

New capabilities on this tour included the Mastiff and the Warrior. The Mastiff 1 Protected Patrol Vehicle (a six-wheeled, heavily armoured and machine gun-equipped vehicle capable of carrying eight infantrymen) provided the protected mobility that had previously been lacking. The Mastiffs were initially crewed by *2 Royal Tank Regiment*, as the theatre 'Mastiff Group'. The Warrior Infantry Fighting Vehicle was first deployed to Helmand in September 2007 and was operated by the *Armoured Infantry Company*, known as the 'Warrior Group', initially provided by the Scots Guards. *39 Regiment Royal Artillery* also deployed a battery equipped with the Guided Multiple Launch Rocket System (GMLRS).

Principal manoeuvre units:
- *1st Battalion, Grenadier Guards (1 GREN GDS)* (also ANA/ANP Mentoring)
- 1st Battalion, The Royal Anglian Regiment (1 R ANGLIAN)
- *1st Battalion, The Worcestershire and Sherwood Foresters Regiment (1 WFR)* (renamed the *2nd Battalion, The Mercian Regiment (Worcesters and Foresters) (2 MERCIAN)* in August 2007)

Theatre Reserve:
- 1st Battalion, The Royal Welsh Regiment (Royal Welch Fusiliers) (1 R WELSH)

Brigade Reconnaissance Force: *B Squadron, The Light Dragoons (LD)*

Mastiff Group: *2nd Royal Tank Regiment (2 RTR)*

Warrior Group: *Right Flank Company, 1st Battalion, Scots Guards (1 SG)*

Herrick 7 (*52 Infantry Brigade*) (Oct 2007–Apr 2008)

ANA/ANP mentoring:
- 2nd Battalion, The Yorkshire Regiment (Green Howards) (2 YORKS)

Principal manoeuvre units:
- 40 Commando, Royal Marines
- 1st Battalion, Coldstream Guards (1 COLDM GDS)
- 1st Battalion, The Royal Gurkha Rifles (1 RGR)
- 4th Regiment, Royal Artillery
- Danish Battle Group (as Battle Group Centre)

(Continued)

(Continued) Main combat forces deployed on *Operation Herrick*

Brigade Reconnaissance Force: *C Squadron, The Household Cavalry Regiment (HCR)*
Mastiff Group: *B Squadron, The King's Royal Hussars (KRH)*
Warrior Group: drawn from the *Scots Guards*

Herrick 8 (16 Air Assault Brigade) (Apr–Oct 2008)
Principal manoeuvre units:
- 2nd Battalion, The Parachute Regiment (2 PARA)
- 3rd Battalion, The Parachute Regiment (3 PARA)
- 1st Battalion, The Royal Irish Regiment (1 R IRISH) (also ANA Mentoring)
- The Argyll & Sutherland Highlanders, 5th Battalion The Royal Regiment of Scotland (5 SCOTS)
- Danish Battle Group (as Battle Group Centre)

Theatre Reserve: *2nd Battalion, The Princess of Wales's Royal Regiment (2 PWRR)*
Brigade Reconnaissance Force: *1 Squadron, The Household Cavalry Regiment (HCR)*
Warrior Group: *The Highlanders, 4th Battalion The Royal Regiment of Scotland (4 SCOTS)*
Mastiff Group: *The Royal Highland Fusiliers, 2nd Battalion The Royal Regiment of Scotland (2 SCOTS)*
Viking Group: *The Queen's Royal Lancers (QRL)*

Herrick 9 (3 Commando Brigade) (Oct 2008–Apr 2009)
ANA/ANP mentoring:
- 1st Battalion, The Rifles (1 RIFLES)

Principal manoeuvre units:
- 45 Commando, Royal Marines (as Battle Group North)
- 2nd Battalion, The Royal Gurkha Rifles (2 RGR) (as Battle Group North-West)
- Danish Battle Group (as Battle Group Centre)
- 1st The Queen's Dragoon Guards (QDG) (as Battle Group South)

Theatre Reserve: *42 Commando, Royal Marines*
Warrior Group: *1st Battalion, The Princess of Wales's Royal Regiment (1 PWRR)*
Mastiff Group: *3rd Battalion, The Yorkshire Regiment (3 YORKS)*
Viking Group: *Armoured Support Company (45 Commando, Royal Marines)*

Herrick 10 (19 Light Brigade) (Apr–Oct 2009)
ANA/ANP Mentoring:
- (ANA): 2nd Battalion, The Mercian Regiment (Worcesters and Foresters) (2 MERCIAN)
- (ANP): 2nd Battalion, The Royal Gurkha Rifles (2 RGR)

Principal manoeuvre units:
- The Black Watch, 3rd Battalion The Royal Regiment of Scotland (3 SCOTS)
- 2nd Battalion, The Rifles (2 RIFLES)
- 4th Battalion, The Rifles (4 RIFLES)
- Danish Battle Group (as Battle Group Centre)

Brigade Reconnaissance Force: *The Light Dragoons (LD)*
Warrior Group: *2nd Battalion, Welsh Guards (2 WG)*
Mastiff Group: *206 Pioneer Squadron, Royal Logistic Corps*
Viking Group: *2nd Royal Tank Regiment (2 RTR)*

Herrick 11 (11 Light Brigade) (Oct 2009–Apr 2010)
ANA/ANP Mentoring:
- (ANA): *2nd Battalion, The Yorkshire Regiment (Green Howards) (2 YORKS)*
- (ANP): *1st Battalion, The Royal Anglian Regiment (1 R ANGLIAN)*

(Continued)

(Continued) Main combat forces deployed on *Operation Herrick*

Principal manoeuvre units:

- 1st Battalion, Grenadier Guards (1 GREN GDS)
- 1st Battalion, Coldstream Guards (1 COLDM GDS)
- 3rd Battalion, The Rifles (3 RIFLES)
- 1st Battalion, The Royal Welsh (Royal Welch Fusiliers) (1 R WELSH)
- Danish Battle Group (as Battle Group Centre)

Reinforced by:

- The Royal Scots Borderers, 1st Battalion The Royal Regiment of Scotland (1 SCOTS)
- *4th Battalion, The Duke of Lancaster's Regiment (4 LANCS) (as Theatre Reserve Battalion)*

Brigade Reconnaissance Force: *B Squadron, The Household Cavalry (HCR)*

Warrior Group: *Right Flank Company, 1st Battalion, The Scots Guards (1 SG)*

Herrick 12 (4 Mechanised Brigade) **(Apr–Oct 2010)**

ANA/ANP Mentoring:

- (ANA): *The Royal Scots Borderers, 1st Battalion The Royal Regiment of Scotland (1 SCOTS)*
- (ANP): *C Squadron, Royal Dragoon Guards (RDG), and 1st Battalion, The Mercian Regiment (Cheshire) (1 MERCIAN)*

Principal manoeuvre units:

- 1st Battalion, Scots Guards (1 SG)
- 40 Commando, Royal Marines
- *1st Battalion, The Duke of Lancaster's Regiment (1 LANCS) (as Theatre Reserve Battalion)*
- *1st Battalion, The Royal Gurkha Rifles (1 RGR)*
- Danish Battle Group (as Battle Group Centre)

Mastiff Group: *B Squadron, Royal Dragoon Guards (RDG)*

Viking Group: *D Squadron, Royal Dragoon Guards (RDG)*

Herrick 13 (16 Air Assault Brigade) **(Oct 2010–Apr 2011)**

The Viking vehicle was superseded by the better armoured Warthog Amphibious and all-terrain vehicle from the end of *Herrick 12*, with the Viking Group being renamed the Warthog Group.

ANA/ANP Mentoring:

- (ANA): *1st Battalion, Irish Guards (1 IG)*
- (ANP): *The Argyll & Sutherland Highlanders, 5th Battalion The Royal Regiment of Scotland (5 SCOTS)*

Principal manoeuvre units:

- 2nd Battalion, The Parachute Regiment (2 PARA)
- 3rd Battalion, The Parachute Regiment (3 PARA)
- 1st Battalion, The Royal Irish Regiment (1 R IRISH)
- The Royal Highland Fusiliers, 2nd Regiment The Royal Regiment of Scotland (2 SCOTS)
- Danish Battle Group (as Battle Group Centre)

Brigade Reconnaissance Force: *The Household Cavalry Regiment (HCR)*

Mastiff Group: *2nd Royal Tank Regiment (2 RTR)*

Warthog Group: *2nd Royal Tank Regiment (2 RTR)*

Herrick 14 (3 Commando Brigade) **(Apr–Oct 2011)**

ANA/ANP Mentoring:

- (ANA): *3rd Battalion, The Mercian Regiment (Staffords) (3 MERCIAN)*
- (ANP): *2nd Battalion, The Royal Gurkha Rifles (2 RGR)*

(Continued)

(Continued) Main combat forces deployed on *Operation Herrick*

Principal manoeuvre units:
- 1st Battalion, The Rifles (1 RIFLES)
- 42 Commando, Royal Marines
- 45 Commando, Royal Marines
- The Highlanders, 4th Battalion The Royal Regiment of Scotland (4 SCOTS)
- Danish Battle Group (as Battle Group Centre)(handing over Lashkar Gah in July)

Brigade Reconnaissance Force: *9th/12th Royal Lancers (9/12 L)*
Warthog Group: *Royal Scots Dragoon Guards (SCOTS DG)*

Herrick 15 (*20 Armoured Brigade*) (Oct 2011–May 2012)
ANA/ANP Mentoring:
- (ANA): *2nd Battalion, The Rifles (2 RIFLES)*
- (ANP): *1st Battalion, The Princess of Wales's Royal Regiment (1 PWRR)*

Principal manoeuvre units:
- *The Queen's Royal Hussars (QRH)* (in infantry role)
- The Black Watch, 3rd Battalion The Royal Regiment of Scotland (3 SCOTS)
- 1st Battalion, The Yorkshire Regiment (Prince of Wales's Own) (1 YORKS)
- 5th Battalion, The Rifles (5 RIFLES)
- 2nd Battalion, The Mercian Regiment (Worcesters and Foresters) (2 MERCIAN)
- Danish Battle Group

Warrior Group: *3rd Battalion, The Yorkshire Regiment (Duke of Wellington's) (3 YORKS)*
Warthog Group: *1st The Queen's Dragoon Guards (QDG)*

Herrick 16 (*12 Mechanised Brigade*) (May–Oct 2012)
ANA/ANP Mentoring:
- (ANA): *3rd Battalion, The Rifles (3 RIFLES)*
- (ANP): *1st Battalion, The Royal Welsh (Royal Welch Fusiliers) (1 R WELSH)*

Principal manoeuvre units:
- *The King's Royal Hussars (KRH)* (in infantry role)
- 1st Battalion, Grenadier Guards (1 GREN GDS)
- 1st Battalion, Welsh Guards (1 WG)
- 1st Battalion, The Royal Anglian Regiment (1 R ANGLIAN)
- 3rd Battalion, The Yorkshire Regiment (Duke of Wellington's) (3 YORKS)
- Danish Battle Group

Brigade Reconnaissance Force: *The Light Dragoons (LD)*

Herrick 17 (*4 Mechanised Brigade*) (Oct 2012–Apr 2013)
ANA/ANP Mentoring:
- (ANA): *The Royal Scots Borderers, 1st Battalion The Royal Regiment of Scotland (1 SCOTS)*
- (ANP): *Royal Dragoon Guards (RDG)*

Principal manoeuvre units:
- 40 Commando Royal Marines
- 1st Battalion, Scots Guards (1 SG)
- 1st Battalion, The Mercian Regiment (Cheshire) (1 MERCIAN)
- 1st Battalion, The Duke of Lancaster's Regiment (1 LANCS)
- 1st Battalion, The Royal Gurkha Rifles (1 RGR)
- Danish Battle Group

Brigade Recce Force: *B Squadron, The Queen's Royal Lancers (QRL)*

(Continued)

(Continued) Main combat forces deployed on *Operation Herrick*

Herrick 18 (1 Mechanised Brigade) (Apr–Oct 2013)

ANA/ANP Mentoring:
- (ANA): *4th Battalion, The Rifles (4 RIFLES)*
- (ANP): *The Royal Highland Fusiliers, 2nd Battalion The Royal Regiment of Scotland (2 SCOTS)*

Principal manoeuvre units:
- 1st Battalion, Irish Guards (1 IG)
- 2nd Battalion, The Duke of Lancaster's Regiment (2 LANCS)
- *1st Battalion, The Royal Regiment of Fusiliers* (1 RRF) (also providing Warrior Group)
- Danish Battle Group

Brigade Reconnaissance Force: *The Household Cavalry Regiment (HCR)*

Warthog Group: *2nd Royal Tank Regiment* (2 RTR) (also ANA Mentoring)

Herrick 19 (7 Armoured Brigade) (Oct 2013–Jun 2014)

Principal manoeuvre units (supporting the Afghan National Security Forces):
- The Highlanders, 4th Battalion The Royal Regiment of Scotland (4 SCOTS)
- 2nd Battalion, The Royal Anglian Regiment (2 R ANGLIAN)
- 3rd Battalion, The Mercian Regiment (Staffords) (3 MERCIAN)
- *Danish Battle Group* (withdrawn May 2014)

Brigade Reconnaissance Force: *9th/12th Royal Lancers (Prince of Wales's)*

Kabul Support Unit:
- August 2013–February 2014: *Royal Scots Dragoon Guards (SCOTS DG)*
- February–August 2014: *1st Battalion, Coldstream Guards (1 COLDM GDS)*

HERRICK 20 (20 Armoured Brigade) (Jun–Nov 2014)

Principal units (covering the withdrawal):
- 1st Battalion, The Princess of Wales's Royal Regiment (1 PWRR)
- 2nd Battalion, The Rifles (2 RIFLES)
- 5th Battalion, The Rifles (5 RIFLES) (with elements from 7th Battalion)

Brigade Reconnaissance Force: *1st The Queen's Dragoon Guards (QDG)*

Warthog Group: *C Squadron, The Queen's Royal Hussars (QRH)*

Kabul Support Unit (February–August 2014): *1st Battalion, Coldstream Guards (1 COLDM GDS)*

Brigade deployments to *Operation Herrick*

Herrick

4 (Mar–Oct 06): *16 Air Assault Brigade*

5 (Oct 06–Apr 07): *3 Commando Brigade*

6 (Apr–Oct 07): *12 Mechanised Brigade*

7 (Sep 07–Apr 08): *52 Infantry Brigade*

8 (Apr–Oct 08): *16 Air Assault Brigade*

9 (Oct 08–Apr 09): *3 Commando Brigade*

10 (Apr–Oct 09): *19 Light Brigade*

11 (Oct 09–Apr 10): *11 Light Brigade*

12 (Apr–Oct 10): *4 Mechanised Brigade* (formation of RC(SW) with new command structure, with a CO for CS Med Regt as well as for BSN R3(UK))

13 (Nov 10–Apr 11): *16 Air Assault Brigade*

14 (Mar–Oct 11): *3 Commando Brigade*

15 (Sep 11–Apr 12) 20 Armoured Brigade

16 (Apr–Oct 12) 12 Mechanised Brigade

17 (Nov 12–Apr 13) 4 Mechanised Brigade

18 (Apr–Oct 13) 1 Mechanised Brigade

19 (Nov 13–Apr 14) 7 Armoured Brigade

20 (Apr–Sep 14) 20 Armoured Brigade

Appendix C: Medical units deployed on *Operations Telic* and *Herrick*

Table C.1 *Operation Telic 1* Medical units

Maritime component	Lines of communication component	Air component	Joint force logistics component (JFLogC)	British Forces Cyprus
PCRF (RFA *ARGUS*)	1 CS Med Regt 5 GS Med Regt 16 CS Med Regt 3 Cdo Bde Med Sqn 3 Casevac Sqn	Medical centres (in all Deployed Operational Bases) 1 Air Evac Sqn 2 Air Evac Sqn	4 GS Med Regt 33 Fd Hosp (relief in place by 202 Fd Hosp on 17 March 2003) 34 Fd Hosp (relief in place by 202 Fd Hosp on 15 May 2003) Aeromed facility at Kuwait City International Airport	TPMH, Aeromed Facility at RAF Akrotiri

Abbreviations: PCRF, Primary Casualty Receiving Facility; RFA, Royal Fleet Auxiliary; CS, close support; GS, general support; Med Regt, Medical Regiment; Cdo Bde, Commando Brigade; Sqn, squadron; Fd Hosp, field hospital; TPMH, The Princess Mary's Hospital, Akrotiri, Cyprus.

Table C.2 Medical Regiment Deployments on Operations Telic and Herrick

Iraq – Operation Telic 1–13		Afghanistan – Operation Herrick 4–20	
Telic 1 (Mar–Jun 03)	1 CS Med Regt, 16 CS Med Regt, 4 GS Med Regt, 5 GS Med Regt		
Telic 2 (Jul–Nov 03)	3 CS Med Regt (returned to UK on formation of UK Med Gp)		
Telic 3 (Nov 03–May 04)	CS Sqn: 22 Med Sqn (from 4 GS Med Regt)		
Telic 4 (May–Nov 04)	CS Sqn: A Sqn (5 GS Med Regt)		
Telic 5 (Nov 04–Apr 05)	CS Sqn: B(30) CS Sqn (1 CS Med Regt)		
Telic 6 (May–Nov 05)	RHQ: 5 GS Med Regt		
	CS Sqn: 16 CS Med Sqn (3 CS Med Regt)		
	RHQ: 3 CS Med Regt		
	CS Sqn: 12 CS Sqn (3 CS Med Regt)		
Telic 7 (Nov 05–Apr 06)	RHQ: 1 CS Med Regt		
	CS Sqn: 29 CS Med Sqn (1 CS Med Regt)	H 4 (Apr–Sep 06)	16 CS Med Regt
Telic 8 (May–Oct 06)	CS Sqn: D Sqn (5 GS Med Regt)	H 5 (Oct 06–Apr 07)	Med Sqn, Commando Logistic Regt
Telic 9 (Nov 06–May 07)	CS Sqn: 24 (Lt) Med Sqn (3 CS Med Regt)	H 6 (May–Oct 07)	4 GS Med Regt
Telic 10 (May–Nov 07)	CS Sqn: 16 CS Med Sqn (3 CS Med Regt)	H 7 (Nov 07–Apr 08)	5 GS Med Regt
Telic 11 (Dec 07–Apr 08)	RHQ, CS Sqn and (for the 1st time) Hosp Sqn: 1 CS Med Regt	H 8 (May–Oct 08)	16 CS Med Regt
Telic 12 (May–Nov 08)	RHQ, CS Sqn and Hosp Sqn: 3 CS Med Regt	H 9 (Nov 08–Apr 09)	Med Sqn, Commando Logistic Regt
Telic 13 (Dec 08–Apr 09)	CS Sqn: 30 Sqn (1 Med Regt)	H 10 (Apr–Nov 09)	2 Med Regt
		H 11 (Oct 09–Apr 10)	33 Fd Hosp (RHQ, Spt Sqn & Med Regt role)
		H 12 (Apr–Oct 10)	3 Med Regt
		H 13 (Oct 10–Apr 11)	16 Med Regt
		H 14 (Apr–Oct 11)	Med Sqn, Commando Logistic Regt
		H 15 (Oct 11–Apr 12)	1 Med Regt
		H 16 (Apr–Oct 12)	4 Med Regt
		H 17 (Oct 12–Apr 13)	3 Med Regt
		H 18 (Apr–Oct 13)	5 Med Regt
		H 19 (Oct 13–Apr 14)	2 Med Regt
		H 20 (Apr–Sep 14)	1 Armoured Med Regt

Abbreviations: CS, close support; GS, general support; Hosp Sqn, Hospital Squadron; Lt, light; Med Regt, Medical Regiment; RHQ, Regimental Headquarters; Sqn, squadron.

Table C.3 Field hospital deployments on *Operations Telic* and *Herrick*

Iraq – *Op Telic* 1–13 (2003–2009)		Afghanistan – *Op Fingal* (2001–2002, Bagram) and *Op HERRICK 4–20* (Camp Bastion Hospital) (2001–2014)	
		Op Fingal (Dec 01–May 02) (Bagram, North Afghanistan)	34 Fd Hosp
Telic 1 (Feb–Jun 03)	22 Fd Hosp, 33 Fd Hosp, 34 Fd Hosp, 202 Fd Hosp		
Telic 2 (Jul–Nov 03)	33 Fd Hosp		
Telic 3 (Nov 03–May 04)	22 Fd Hosp		
Telic 4A (May–Aug 04)	207 Fd Hosp		
Telic 4B (Aug–Nov 04)	256 Fd Hosp		
Telic 5 (Nov 04–Apr 05)	33 Fd Hosp		
Telic 6 (May–Nov 05)	205 Fd Hosp		
Telic 7 (Nov 05–Apr 06)	34 Fd Hosp		
Telic 8 (May–Oct 06)	22 Fd Hosp (RHQ & Sp Sqn only); RAF Hosp Sqn	*H 4* (Apr–Sep 06)	22 Fd Hosp (Hospital Squadron)
Telic 9 (Nov 06–May 07)	33 Fd Hosp	*H 5* (Oct 06–Apr 07)	RN Hosp Sqn
Telic 10 (May–Nov 07)	34 Fd Hosp	*H 6A* (May–Jul 07)	212 Fd Hosp
		H 6B (Jul–Oct 07)	208 Fd Hosp
Telic 11 (Dec 07–Apr 08)	1 CS Med Regt (providing RHQ, Sp, CS & Hosp Sqns)	*H 7A* (Nov 07–Jan 08)	201 Fd Hosp
		H 7B (Jan–Apr 08)	243 Fd Hosp
Telic 12 (May–Nov 08)	3 CS Med Regt (providing RHQ, Sp, CS & Hosp Sqns)	*H 8A* (May–Jul 08)	203 Fd Hosp
		H 8B (Jul–Oct 08)	204 Fd Hosp
Telic 13 (Dec 08–Apr 09)	22 Fd Hosp	*H 9* (Nov 08–Apr 09)	RN Hosp Sqn
		H 10A (Apr–Jul 09)	202 Fd Hosp
		H 10B (Jul–Nov 09)	Danish Fd Hosp
		H 11 (Oct 09–Apr 10)	33 Fd Hosp (RHQ, Spt Sqn & Med Regt role)
		H 11A (Oct 09–Jan 10)	
		H 11B (Jan–Apr 10)	256 Fd Hosp
			205 Fd Hosp
		H 12 (Apr–Oct 10)	34 Fd Hosp
		H 13A (Oct 10–Jan 11)	207 Fd Hosp
		H 13B (Jan–Apr 11)	212 Fd Hosp
		H 14 (Apr–Oct 11)	RN Hosp Sqn
		H 15A (Oct 11–Jan 12)	208 Fd Hosp
		H 15B (Jan–Apr 12)	201 Fd Hosp
		H 16 (Apr–Oct 12)	22 Fd Hosp
		H 17A (Oct 12–Jan 13)	243 Fd Hosp
		H 17B (Jan–Apr 13)	204 Fd Hosp
		H 18 (Apr–Oct 13)	33 Fd Hosp
		H 19A (Oct 13–Jan 14)	203 Fd Hosp
		H 19B (Jan–Apr 14)	202 Fd Hosp
		H 20 (Apr–Sep 14)	34 Fd Hosp

Abbreviations: CS Med Regt, Close Support Medical Regiment; Fd Hosp, field hospital; RAF, Royal Air Force; RHQ, Regimental Headquarters; RN, Royal Navy; Sp Sqn, Support Squadron.

Table C.4 *Operation Herrick* medical commanders

H 4–5:	Comd UK JF Med Gp, OC BSN Role 2E
H 6–9:	Comd UK JF Med Gp, OC BSN Role 3(UK)
H 10–11:	Comd Med JFSP(A), Comd UK JF Med Gp, CO BSN Role 3(UK)
H 12–19:	Comd Med JFSP(A), CO CS Med Regt, CO BSN Role 3(UK)
H 20:	Reversion to preH 10 construct: Comd UK JF Med Gp, CO BSN Role 3(UK)

Appendix D: Publications by subject

This appendix lists DMS and associated academic publications by subject matter. Many of the articles in this list appear more than once. For example:

Davey CMT, Mieville KE, Simpson R, Aldington D. A survey of experience of parenteral analgesia at Role 1. *J R Army Med Corps* 2012 Sep;158(3):186–189.

will be found under both *Pain Management* and under *Primary care and Medicine at Role 1*. Inevitably, decisions regarding the placing of papers will be, to some extent, subjective, but I hope I have achieved a degree of consistency and uniformity. In general, I have only included *personal experiences* when they have been published in academic journals. Interested readers are referred in particular to *The Medic—The Royal Army Medical Corps Magazine*, which contains a great deal of unit information, and the magazines of the other Corps of the DMS for a wide range of other personal reports.

ABDOMINAL TRAUMA

Arul GS, Sonka BJ, Lundy JB et al. Management of complex abdominal wall defects associated with penetrating abdominal trauma. *J R Army Med Corps* 2015 Mar;161(1):46–52.

Arul GS, Sonka BJ, Lundy JB et al. Managing combat laparostomy: Author's reply. *J R Army Med Corps* 2015 Dec;161(4):352.

Bowley DM, Gross K. Blunt abdominal trauma. In: Nessen SC, Lounsbury DE, Hetz SP (eds.). *War Surgery in Afghanistan and Iraq: A Series of Cases 2003–2007*. Washington, DC: Office of the Surgeon General, 2008, 441 p. ISBN: 0981822800.

Bowley DM, Jansen JO, Nott D et al. Difficult decisions in the surgical care of military casualties with major torso trauma. *J R Army Med Corps* 2011 Sep;157(3 Suppl 1):S324–S333.

Bowley DM, Tai N, Parker P, Mahoney P. Military Surgery. In: Boffard K (ed.). *Manual of Definitive Surgical Trauma Care*. 3rd ed. London: CRC Press, 2011, 304 p.. ISBN: 9781444102826.

Bowley DM, Gillingham S, Mercer S et al. Pneumoperitoneum without visceral trauma: An under recognised phenomenon after blast injury? *J R Army Med Corps* 2013 Dec;159(4):312–313.

Brogden TG, Garner JP. Anorectal injury in pelvic blast. *J R Army Med Corps* 2013 Mar;159(Suppl 1):i26–i31.

Brooks A, Price V, Simms M. FAST on operational military deployment. *Emerg Med J* 2005 Apr;22(4):263–265.

Edgar IA, Hadjipavlou G, Terry M. Penetrating abdominal trauma: Prevalence from a UK Field hospital during contemporary operations *J R Army Med Corps* 2015;161:73–75.

Findlay IG, Edwards T, Lambert AW. Damage control laparotomy. *Br J Surg* 2004 Jan;91:83–85.

Fries CA, Penn-Barwell J, Tai NR et al. Management of intestinal injury in deployed UK hospitals. *J R Army Med Corps* 2011 Dec;157(4):370–373.

Janson JO (on behalf of the Torso Trauma Working Group of the Academic Department of Surgery and Trauma, Royal Centre for Defence Medicine). Selective non-operative management of abdominal injury in the military setting (consensus statement). *J R Army Med Corps* 2011 Sep;157(3):237–242.

Lamb CM, Berry JE, DeMello WF, Cox C. Secondary abdominal compartment syndrome after military wounding. *J R Army Med Corps* 2010 Jun;156(2):102–103.

Lamb CM, Garner JP. Managing combat laparotomy (letter with original authors' reply). *J R Army Med Corps* 2015 Dec;161(4):351–352.

Leong MJ, Edgar I, Terry M. Penetrating abdominal injury: UK military experience from the Afghanistan conflict. *J R Nav Med Serv* 2016;102(2):8–12.

Lundy JB, Oh JS, Chung KK et al. Frequency and relevance of acute peri-traumatic pulmonary thrombus diagnosed by computed tomographic imaging in combat casualties. *J Trauma Acute Care Surg* 2013 Aug;75(2 Suppl 2):S215–S220.

Morrison JJ, Midwinter M, Jansen J. Management of ballistic thoraco-abdominal injuries: Analysis of recent operational experience. 2010 Military Surgery Meeting (abstract). *J R Army Med Corps* 2010 Sep;156(3):184.

Morrison JJ, Clasper JC, Gibb I, Midwinter M. Management of penetrating abdominal trauma in the conflict environment: The role of computed tomography scanning. *World J Surg* 2011 Jan;35(1):27–33.

Morrison JJ, Midwinter MJ, Jansen JO. Ballistic thoracoabdominal injury: Analysis of recent military experience in Afghanistan. *World J Surg* 2011 Mar;35:1396–1401.

Morrison JJ, Dickson EJ, Jansen JO, Midwinter MJ. Utility of admission physiology in the surgical triage of isolated ballistic battlefield torso trauma. *J Emerg Trauma Shock* 2012 Jul;5(3):233–237.

Morrison JJ, Poon H, Garner J et al. Non-therapeutic laparotomy in combat casualties. *J Trauma Acute Care Surg* 2012 Dec;73(6 Suppl 5):S479–S482.

Morrison JJ, Rasmussen TE. Non-compressible torso haemorrhage: A review with contemporary definitions and management strategies. *Surg Clin North Am* 2012 Aug;92(4):843–858.

Morrison JJ, Stannard A, Rasmussen TE et al. Injury pattern and mortality of noncompressible torso hemorrhage in UK combat casualties. *J Trauma Acute Care Surg* 2013 Aug;75(2 Suppl 2):S263–S268.

Morrison JJ, Ross JD, Rasmussen T et al. Resuscitative endovascular balloon occlusion of the aorta (REBOA): A gap analysis of severely injured UK combat casualties. *Shock* 2014 May;41(5):388–393.

Mossadegh S, Tai N, Midwinter M, Parker P. Improvised explosive device related pelvi-perineal trauma: Anatomic injuries and surgical management. *J Trauma Acute Care Surg* 2012 Aug;73(2 Suppl 1):S24–S31.

Mossadegh S, Midwinter M, Sapsford W, Tai N. Military treatment of splenic injury in the era of non-operative management. *J R Army Med Corps* 2013 Jun;159(2):110–113.

Pengelly S, Matheson A, Howes D et al. Military torso trauma: Which, or how many, surgeons deploy (abstract)? *World J Surg* 2009;33:144.

Read JA, Ingram M. Massive haemorrhage following penetrating abdominal trauma. *J R Nav Med Serv* 2008;94(2):68–70.

Sharrock AE, Barker T, Yuen HM et al. Management and closure of the open abdomen after damage control laparotomy for trauma. A systematic review and meta-analysis. *Injury* 2016 Feb;47(2):296–306.

Smith IM, Beech ZKM, Lundy JB, Bowley DM. A prospective observational study of abdominal injury management in contemporary military operations: Damage control laparotomy is associated with high survivability and low rates of fecal diversion. *Ann Surg* 2015;261(4):765–773.

Smith IM, Naumann DN, Marsden ME et al. Scanning and war: Utility of FAST and CT in the assessment of battlefield abdominal trauma. *Ann Surg* 2015 Aug;262(2):389–396.

Smith JE, Midwinter M, Lambert AW. Avoiding cavity surgery in penetrating torso trauma: The role of the computed topography scan. *Ann Surg* 2010;92:486–488.

Stannard A, Benson C, Bowley DM et al. Central vascular injuries in deployed military personnel: A contemporary experience. *J R Army Med Corps* 2008;154(3):188.

Stannard A, Morrison JJ, Scott DJ et al. The epidemiology of non-compressible torso hemorrhage in the wars in Iraq and Afghanistan. *J Trauma Acute Care Surg* 2013;74:830–834.

Tai, NR, Mossadegh S, Sapsford W. Military treatment of splenic injury in the era of non-operative management. *J R Army Med Corps* 2013 Jun;159(2):110–113.

Wood AM, Trimble K, Louden MA et al. Selective non-operative management of ballistic solid organ injury in the deployed military setting. *J R Army Med Corps* 2010 Mar;156(1):21–24.

ANAESTHESIA

Barnard EB, Moy RJ, Kehoe AD et al. Rapid sequence induction of anaesthesia via the intraosseous route: A prospective observational study. *Emerg Med J* 2015 Jun;32(6):449–452.

Bateman R, Wedgewood J, Henning J. Case report: Use of remifentanil infusion with the tri-service anaesthetic apparatus. *J R Nav Med Serv* 2005;91(1):48–49.

Bateman RM, McNicholas JJ. Overview of 12 months anaesthetic activity in a UK field hospital on enduring operations in Iraq. *J R Nav Med Serv* 2006;92(2):51–56.

Birt DJ, Woolley T. Competencies for the military anaesthetist – A new unit of training. *Bull R Coll Anaesth* 2008 Nov;52:2661–2666.

Brogden TG, Bunin J, Kwon H. Strategies for ventilation in acute, severe lung injury after combat trauma. *J R Army Med Corps* 2015 Mar;161(1):14–21.

Clasper JC, Aldington D. Regional anaesthesia, ballistic limb trauma and acute compartment syndrome (editorial). *J R Army Med Corps* 2010 Jun;156(2):77–78.

Davenport L, Edwards D, Edwards C et al. Evolution of the Role 4 U.K. military pain service. *J R Army Med Corps* 2010 Dec;156(4 Suppl 1):398–401.

Henning JD, Bateman R. Excess delivery of isoflurane liquid from a syringe driver. *Anaesthesia* 2004 Dec;59(12):1251.

Henning JD. The Tri-service anaesthetic apparatus – An alternative configuration. *Anaesthesia* 2006 Nov;61(11):1123.

Hughes S, Birt D. Continuous peripheral nerve blockade on OP HERRICK 9. *J R Army Med Corps* 2009 Mar;155(1):57–58.

Lewis S, Jagdish S. Total intravenous anaesthesia for war surgery. *J R Army Med Corps* 2010 Dec;156(4 Suppl 1):S301–S307.

Ley S, Bell G. Draw-over or push over during manual ventilation with the Tri-Service Anaesthetics Apparatus? *Anaesthesia* 2016 Apr;71(4):474–475.

Mercer S, Beard DJ. Does the Tri-Service anaesthetic apparatus still have a role in modern conflict? *Bull R Coll Anaesth* 2010 Jan;60:18–20.

Mercer SJ, Lewis SE, Wilson SJ et al. Creating airway management guidelines for casualties with penetrating airway injuries. *J R Army Med Corps* 2010 Dec;156(4 Suppl 1):S355–S360.

Mercer SJ, Tarmey N, Mahoney PF. Military experience of human factors in airway complications. *Anaesthesia* 2013 Oct;68:1081–1082.

Moy RJ, Sharpe D, Russell R. Ketamine in military pre-hospital practice for anaesthesia and analgesia (abstract). *J R Army Med Corps* 2015;161(1):73–75.

Nordmann GR. Paediatric anaesthesia in Afghanistan: A review of the current experience. *J R Army Med Corps* 2010;156(4):S323–S326.

Park CL, Moor P, Birch K, Shirley PJ. Operational anaesthesia for the management of traumatic brain injury. *J R Army Med Corps* 2010;156(4):S335–S341.

Parkhouse DA. Anaesthetics. *J R Army Med Corps* 2004;150(2):124–133.

Parkhouse DA. The future for military anaesthesia after operations in Afghanistan. *J R Army Med Corps* 2010;156(4):S285–S286.

Ralph JK, George R, Thompson J. Paediatric anaesthesia using the Triservice anaesthetic apparatus. *J R Army Med Corps* 2010 Jun;156(2):84–86.

Round J, Mellor A. Anaesthetic and critical care management of thoracic injury. *J R Army Med Corps* 2010 Sep;156(3):145–149.

Stansfield T, Hay H. Spinal anaesthetic with patient wearing enhanced combat body armour (image). *J R Army Med Corps* 2008;154:85.

Tarmey NT, Park CL, Fox M et al. Anaesthesia for overseas operations: UK Military guidelines. *Med Corps Int Forum* 2013;(3):4–7.

Tarmey NT, Easby D, Park CL. Paediatric anaesthesia for overseas operations: UK Military guidelines. *Med Corps Int Forum* 2014;(1):32–35.

Thomas D, Wee M, Clyburn P et al. Blood transfusion and the anaesthetist: Management of massive haemorrhage. *Anaesthesia* 2010 Nov;65(11):1153–1161.

Wood P, Gill M, Edwards D et al. Clinical and microbiological evaluation of epidural and regional anaesthesia catheters in injured UK military personnel. *J R Army Med Corps* 2016 Aug;162(4):261–265.

Wood PR, Haldane AG, Plimmer SE. Anaesthesia at Role 4. *J R Army Med Corps* 2010;156 (4 Suppl 1):308–310.

Woods KL, Aldington D. Current epidural practice – Results of a survey of military anaesthetists. *J R Army Med Corps* 2010 Dec;156(4 Suppl 1):393–397.

Wyldbore M, Aldington DJ. Effective pain management in the armed forces. *Pain Europe [Internet]* 2013 Jun;(2):8–9. http://www .paineurope.com/healthcare-professional /paineurope/features/details/article/effec tive-pain-management-in-the-armed-forces .html

ATTITUDES TO THE CONFLICTS

Berndtsson J, Dandeker C, Yden K. Swedish and British public opinion of the Armed Forces after a decade of war. *Armed Forces Soc* 2015 Apr;41(2):307–328.

Gribble R, Wessely S, Klein S et al. The UK's Armed Forces: Public support for the troops but not their missions? In: Park A, Clery E, Curtice J et al. (eds.). *British Social Attitudes: The 29th Report*. Natcen Social Research. London, 2012, pp. 138–154.

Gribble R, Wessley S, Klein S et al. British public opinion after a decade of war: Attitudes to Iraq and Afghanistan. *Politics* 2015 Jun;35(2):128–150.

Hines LA, Gribble R, Wessely S et al. Are the armed forces understood and supported by the public? A view from the United Kingdom. *Armed Forces Soc* 2015 Oct;41(4):688–713.

Pinder RJ, Murphy D, Hatch SL et al. A mixed methods analysis of the perceptions of the media by members of the British Armed Forces during the Iraq War. *Armed Forces Soc* 2009;36(1):131–152.

BALLISTIC AND BLAST INJURY

Abbotts R, Harrison SE, Cooper GL. Primary blast injuries to the eye: A review of the evidence. *J R Army Med Corps* 2007 Jun;153(2):119–123.

Aboudara M, Mahoney PF, Hicks B, Cuadrado D. Primary blast lung injury at a NATO Role 3 hospital. *J R Army Med Corps* 2014 Jun;160(2):161–166.

Aboudara M, Hicks B, Cuadrado D et al. Impact of primary blast lung injury during combat operations in Afghanistan (letter). *J R Army Med Corps* 2016 Feb;162(1):75.

Barnard EB, Johnston A. Images in clinical medicine. Blast lung. *N Eng J Med* 2013 Mar;14;368(11):1045.

Barnard EB, Rimmer J, Johnston A. Pulmonary puzzle: A precordial crunch. *Thorax* 2013 Jan;68(8):794–795.

Barton SJ, Kaleel S, Rayatt S, Peart F. Healing Hands: Management of a shrapnel wound injury in the dominant hand of a serviceman, sustained in the Iraq conflict (abstract). *J R Army Med Corps* 2005 Mar;151(2):108.

Baxter D, Sharp DJ, Feeney C et al. Pituitary dysfunction after blast traumatic brain injury: The UK BIOSAP Study. *Ann Neurol* 2013 Oct;74(4):527–536.

Blanch RJ, Scott RA. Primary blast injury of the eye. *J R Army Med Corps* 2008 Mar;154(1):76.

Bowley DM, Gillingham S, Mercer S et al. Pneumoperitoneum without visceral trauma: An under recognised phenomenon after blast injury? *J R Army Med Corps* 2013 Dec;159(4):312–313.

Boyd MC, Mountain AJ, Clasper JC. Improvised skeletal traction in the management of ballistic femoral fractures. *J R Army Med Corps* 2009 Sep;155(3):194–196.

Breeze J. Obtaining multi-national consensus on future combat face and neck protection – Proceedings of the Revision Military Protection Workshop (letter). *J R Army Med Corps* 2012 Jun;158(2):141–142.

Breeze J, Opie N, Monaghan A, Gibbons AJ. Isolated orbital wall blowout fractures due to primary blast injury (letter). *J R Army Med Corps* 2009 Mar;155(1):70.

Breeze J, Cooper H, Pearson CR et al. Ear injuries sustained by British service personnel subjected to blast trauma. *J Laryngol Otol* 2011 Jan;125(1):13–17.

Breeze J, Gibbons AJ, Hunt NC et al. Mandibular fractures in British military personnel secondary to blast trauma sustained in Iraq and Afghanistan. *Br J Oral Maxillofac Surg* 2011 Dec;49(8):607–611.

Breeze J, Horsfall I, Hepper A, Clasper J. Face, neck, and eye protection: Adapting body armour to counter the changing patterns of injuries on the battlefield. *Br J Oral Maxillofac Surg* 2011 Dec;49(8):602–606.

Breeze J, Masterson L, Banfield G. Outcomes from penetrating ballistic cervical injury. *J R Army Med Corps* 2012 Jun;158(2):96–100.

Breeze J, Leason J, Gibb I et al. Characterisation of explosive fragments injuring the neck. *Br J Oral Maxillofac Surg* 2013 Dec;51(8):e263–e266.

Breeze J, Carr DJ. Energised fragments, bullets and fragment simulating projectiles. In: Bull AMJ, Clasper J, Mahoney PF (eds.). *Blast Injury Science and Engineering.* Springer, Cham, Switzerland: Springer International Publishing, 2016, pp. 219–226.

Breeze J, Tong DC. Damage control surgery and combat-related maxillofacial and cervical injuries: A systematic review. *Br J Oral Maxillofac Surg* 2016 Jan;54(1):8–12.

Calderbank P, Porter K, Anderson P et al. Urethral injury due to blast: A new pattern (abstract)? *J R Army Med Corps* 2010 Sep;156(3):183.

Carr DJ, Horsfall I, Malbon C. Is behind armour blunt trauma a real threat to users of body armour? A systematic review. *J R Army Med Corps* 2016 Feb;162(1):8–11.

Chalioulias K, Sim KT, Scott R. Retinal sequelae of primary ocular blast injuries. *J R Army Med Corps* 2007 Jun;153(2):124–125.

Clasper JC, Aldington D. Regional anaesthesia, ballistic limb trauma and acute compartment syndrome (editorial). *J R Army Med Corps* 2010 Jun;156(2):77–78.

Coley E, Roach P, Macmillan AI et al. Penetrating paediatric thoracic injury. *J R Army Med Corps* 2011 Sep;157(3):243–245.

Cooper B, Mellor A, Bruce A et al. Paediatric thoracic damage control resuscitation for ballistic injury: A case report. *J R Army Med Corps* 2007 Dec;153(4):317–318.

Cross AM, Davis C, Penn-Barwell J et al. The incidence of pelvic fractures with traumatic lower limb amputation in modern warfare due to improvised explosive devices. *J R Nav Med Serv* 2014;100(2):152–156.

Davies E, Boylan M, Hawker JJ, Banerjee B. Don't forget the fragment! An unusual case of occult fragment embolization following penetrating neck injury. *J R Army Med Corps* 2011 Dec;157(4):396–398.

Eardley WG, Stewart MP. Early management of ballistic hand trauma. *J Am Acad Orthop Surg* 2010 Feb;18(2):118–126.

Eardley W, Stitson D, Miles R, Clasper J. Exploring the role of whole body computed tomography (WBCT) in the early management of combat casualties from explosive devices (abstract). *J R Army Med Corps* 2010 Sep;156(3):181.

Eardley WG, Beaven A, Sargeant I. Endoscopic evaluation of a complex ballistic injury. *J R Army Med Corps* 2011 Dec;157(4):399–401.

Eardley WG, Brown KV, Bonner TJ et al. Infection in conflict wounded. *Philos Trans R Soc Lond B Biol Sci* 2011 Jan;366(1562):204–218.

Eardley WG, Watts SA, Clasper JC. Modelling for conflict: The legacy of ballistic research and current extremity in vivo modelling. *J R Army Med Corps* 2013 Jun;159(2):73–83.

Edwards MJ, Lustik M, Eichelberger MR et al. Blast injury in children: An analysis from Afghanistan and Iraq, 2002–2010. *J Trauma Acute Care Surg* 2012 Nov;73(5):1278–1283.

Edwards MJ, Lustik M, Carlson T et al. Surgical interventions for pediatric blast injury: An analysis from Afghanistan and Iraq 2002 to 2010. *J Trauma Acute Care Surg* 2014 Mar;76(3):854–858.

Gibb IE. Computed tomography of projectile injuries. *Clin Radiol* 2008 Oct;63(10):1167–1168.

Gibbons AJ, Breeze J. The face of war: The initial management of modern battlefield ballistic facial injuries. *J Mil Veterans Health* 2011 Apr;19(2):15–18.

Gibbons AJ, Mackenzie N, Breederveld RS. Use of a custom designed external fixator system to treat ballistic injuries to the mandible. *Int J Oral Maxillofac Surg* 2011 Jan;40(1):103–105.

Goonewardene SS, Mangat KS, Sargeant ID et al. Tetraplegia following cervical spine cord contusion from indirect gunshot injury effects. *J R Army Med Corps* 2007 Mar;153(1):52–53.

Haldane AG. Traumatic pneumorrhachis. *J R Army Med Corps* 2010 Dec;156(4 Suppl 1):S318–S320.

Harrison SE, Kirkman E, Mahoney P. Lessons learnt from explosive attacks. *J R Army Med Corps* 2007 Dec;153(4):278–282.

Hinsley DE, Phillips SL, Clasper JS. Ballistic fractures during the 2003 Gulf Conflict – Early prognosis and high complication rate. *J R Army Med Corps* 2006 Jun;152(2):96–101.

Jacobs N, Rourke K, Hicks A et al. Lower limb injuries caused by improvised explosive devices: Proposed "Bastion" classification and prospective validation. *Injury* 2014 Sep;45(9):1422–1428.

Johnston AM, West AT, Kendrew JM et al. Delayed haemoptysis from explosive device fragments. *Lancet* 2013 Sep;382(9898):1152.

Johnston AM, Ballard M. Primary blast lung injury. *Am J Respir Crit Care Med* 2015 Jun;191(12):1462–1463.

Jones N, Thandi G, Fear NT et al. The psychological effects of improvised explosive devices (IEDs) on UK military personnel in Afghanistan. *Occup Environ Med* 2014 Jul;71(7):466–471.

Kirkman E, Watts S. Characterization of the response to primary blast injury. *Philos Trans R Soc Lond B Biol Sci* 2011 Jan;366(1562)286–290.

Mackenzie IMJ, Tunnicliffe B. Blast injuries to the lung: Epidemiology and management. *Phil Trans R Soc Lond B Biol Sci* 2011 Jan;366(1562)295–299.

Mackenzie I, Tunnicliffe B, Clasper J et al. What the intensive care doctor needs to know about blast-related lung injury. *J Intensive Care Soc* 2013 Oct;14(4):303–312.

Macmillan AIM. Teamwork and ballistic trauma. *Surgeons' News* 2011 Jan:52–53.

Masouros SD, Newell N, Ramasamy A et al. Design of a traumatic injury simulator for assessing lower limb response to high loading rates. *Ann Biomed Eng* 2013 Sep;41(9):1957–1967.

McKinlay J, Smith JE. Penetrating brain injury: A case of survival following blast fragmentation injuries to the head. *J R Nav Med Serv* 2013;99(2):55–56.

Mellor AJ, Woods D. Serum neutrophil gelatinase-associated lipocalin in ballistic injuries: A comparison between blast injuries and gunshot wounds. *J Crit Care* 2012 Aug;27(4):419.

Morrison JJ, Mahoney PF, Hodgetts T. Shaped charges and explosively formed penetrators: Background for clinicians. *J R Army Med Corps* 2007 Sep;153(3):184–187.

Morrison JJ, Midwinter M, Jansen J. Management of ballistic thoraco-abdominal injuries: Analysis of recent operational experience. 2010 Military Surgery Meeting (abstract). *J R Army Med Corps* 2010 Sep;156(3):184.

Morrison JJ, Clasper JC, Gibb I, Midwinter M. Management of penetrating abdominal trauma in the conflict environment: The role of computed tomography scanning. *World J Surg* 2011 Jan;35(1):27–33.

Morrison JJ, Midwinter MJ, Jansen JO. Ballistic thoracoabdominal injury: Analysis of recent military experience in Afghanistan. *World J Surg* 2011 Mar;35:1396–1401.

Mossadegh S, Tai N, Midwinter M, Parker P. Improvised explosive device related pelvi-perineal trauma: Anatomic injuries and surgical management. *J Trauma Acute Care Surg* 2012 Aug;73(2 Suppl 1):S24–S31.

Mossadegh S, Midwinter M, Parker P, Improvised explosive device-related pelvi-perineal trauma: UK Military experience, literature review and lessons for civilian trauma teams (editorial). *Bull R Coll Surg Engl* 2013 Oct;95(9):1–5.

Mossadegh S, He S, Parker P. Bayesian scoring systems for military pelvic and perineal blast injuries: Is it time to take a new approach? *Mil Med* 2016 May;181(5 Suppl):127–131.

Nordmann G, Galbraith K, Mellor A. Raised creatine kinase as an indicator of inadequate muscle debridement in ballistic injuries. *J Intensive Care Soc* 2009;10(2):122–124.

Pengelly S, Moore N, Burgess D. Home-made explosive found inside injured Afghan. *J R Army Med Corps* 2015 Jun;161(2):150–152.

Penn-Barwell JG, Sargeant ID et al. Gun-shot injuries in UK military casualties – Features associated with wound severity. *Injury* 2016 May;47(5):1067–1071.

Poon H, Morrison JJ, Clasper JC et al. Use and complications of operative control of arterial inflow in combat casualties with traumatic lower-extremity amputations caused by improvised explosive devices. *J Trauma Acute Care Surg* 2013 Aug;75(2 Suppl 2):S233–S237.

Ramasamy A, Harrisson SE, Clasper JC et al. Injuries from roadside improvised explosive devices. *J Trauma* 2008:65:910–914.

Ramasamy A, Harrisson SE, Stewart MPM, Midwinter M. Penetrating missile injuries during the Iraqi insurgency. *Ann R Coll Surg Engl* 2009;91:551–558.

Ramasamy A, Hill A, Clasper JC. Improvised explosive devices: Pathophysiology, injury profiles and current medical management. *J R Army Med Corps* 2009;155(4):265–272.

Ramasamy A, Hill AM, Hepper AE et al. Blast mines: Physics, injury mechanisms and vehicle protection. *J R Army Med Corps* 2009;155(4):258–264.

Ramasamy D, Hinsley DE, Brooks AJ. The use of three-dimensional computed tomography reconstruction in the assessment of penetrating ballistic trauma. *Emerg Med J* 2009;26:228.

Ramasamy A, Hill AM, Masouros S, Gibb I et al. Blast-related fracture patterns: A forensic biomechanical approach. *J R Soc Interface* 2011 May;8(58):689–698.

Ramasamy A, Hill AM, Phillip R. The modern "deck-slap" injury – Calcaneal blast fractures from vehicle explosions. *J Trauma* 2011 Dec; 71(6):1694–1698.

Ramasamy A, Hill AM, Spyridon D et al. Evaluating the effect of vehicle modification in reducing injuries from landmine blasts. An analysis of 2212 incidents and its application for humanitarian purposes. *Accid Anal Prev* 2011 Sep;43(5):1878–1886.

Ramasamy A, Masouros SD, Newell N et al. In-vehicle extremity injuries from improvised explosive devices: Current and future foci. *Phil Trans R Soc* 2011;366:160–170.

Ramasamy A, Hill AM, Masouros S et al. Outcomes of IED foot and ankle blast injuries. *J Bone Joint Surg Am* 2013 Mar;95(5):e25.

Ramasamy MA, Hill AM, Phillip R et al. FASS is a better predictor of poor outcome in lower limb blast injury than AIS: Implications for blast research. *J Orthop Trauma* 2013 Jan;27(1):49–55.

Scott TE, Kirkman E, Haque M, Gibb IE et al. Primary blast lung injury – A review. *Br J Anaesth* 2017 Mar;118(3):311–316.

Singleton JA, Gibb IE, Bull AM et al. Primary blast lung injury prevalence and fatal injuries from explosions: Insights from postmortem computed tomographic analysis of 121 improvised explosive device fatalities. *J Trauma Acute Care Surg* 2013 75(2 Suppl 2):S269–S274.

Singleton JA, Gibb IE, Bull AM, Clasper JC. Blast-mediated traumatic amputation: Evidence for a revised, multiple injury mechanism theory. *J R Army Med Corps* 2014;160(2):175–179.

Singleton JA, Walker NM, Gibb IE et al. Case suitability for definitive through knee amputation following lower extremity blast trauma: Analysis of 146 combat casualties, 2008–2010. *J R Army Med Corps* 2014;160:187–190.

Smith JE. Blast lung injury. *J R Nav Med Serv* 2011;97(3):99–105.

Smith JE. The epidemiology of blast lung injury during recent military conflicts: A retrospective database – Review of cases presenting to deployed military hospitals 2003–2009. *Phil Trans R Soc B* 2011;366:291–294.

Spurrier E, Singleton JA, Masouros S et al. Blast injury in the spine: Dynamic response index is not an appropriate model for predicting injury. *Clin Orthop Relat Res* 2015 Sep;473(9):2929–2935.

Spurrier E, Gibb I, Masouros S, Clasper J. Identifying spinal injury patterns in underbody blast to develop mechanistic hypotheses. *Spine (Phila Pa 1976)* 2016 Mar;41(5):E268–E275.

Stapley SA, Cannon LB. An overview of the pathophysiology of gunshot and blast injury with resuscitation guidelines. *Curr Orthop* 2006;20(5):322–332.

Woods DR, Phillip R, Quinton R. Managing endocrine dysfunction following blast injury to the male external genitalia. *J R Army Med Corps* 2013 Mar;159(Suppl 1):45–48.

BALLISTIC PROTECTION

Breeze J. Editorial: The problems of protecting the neck from combat wounds. *J R Army Med Corps* 2010 Sep;156(3):137–138.

Breeze J. Editorial: Saving faces: The UK future facial protection programme. *J R Army Med Corps* 2012 Dec;158(4):284–287.

Breeze J. Obtaining multi-national consensus on future combat face and neck protection – Proceedings of the Revision Military Protection Workshop (letter). *J R Army Med Corps* 2012 Jun;158(2):141–142.

Breeze J, Horsfall I, Hepper A, Clasper J. Face, neck, and eye protection: Adapting body armour to counter the changing patterns of injuries on the battlefield. *Br J Oral Maxillofac Surg* 2011 Dec;49(8):602–606.

Breeze J, Watson CH, Horsfall I, Clasper J. Comparing the comfort and potential military performance restriction of neck collars from the body armor of six different countries. *Mil Med* 2011 Nov;176(11):1274–1277.

Breeze J, Allanson-Bailey LS, Hunt NC et al. Surface wound mapping of battlefield occulo-facial injury. *Injury* 2012 Nov;43(11):1856–1860.

Breeze J, Midwinter MJ. Editorial: Prospective computerised surface wound mapping will optimise future body armour design. *J R Army Med Corps* 2012 Jun;158(2):79–81.

Breeze J, Clasper JC. Ergonomic assessment of future methods of ballistic neck protection. *Mil Med* 2013 Aug;178(8):899–903.

Breeze J, Helliker M, Carr DJ. An integrated approach towards future ballistic neck protection materials selection. *Proc Inst Mech Eng H* 2013 May;227(5):581–587.

Breeze J, James GR, Hepper AE. Perforation of fragment simulating projectiles into goat skin and muscle. *J R Army Med Corps* 2013 Jun;159(2):84–89.

Breeze J, Leason J, Gibb I et al. Computed tomography can improve the selection of fragment simulating projectiles from which to test future body armour materials. *Mil Med* 2013 Jun;178(6):690–695.

Breeze J, Midwinter MJ, Pope D et al. Developmental framework to validate future designs of ballistic neck protection. *Br J Oral Maxillofac Surg* 2013 Jan;51(1):47–51.

Breeze J, West A, Clasper J. Anthropometric assessment of cervical neurovascular structures using CTA to determine zone-specific vulnerability to penetrating fragmentation injuries. *Clin Radiol* 2013 Jan;68(1):34–38.

Breeze J, Granger CJ, Pearkes TD, Clasper JC. Ergonomic assessment of enhanced protection under body armour combat shirt neck collars. *J R Army Med Corps* 2014 Mar;160(1):32–37.

Breeze J, Newbery T, Pope D, Midwinter MJ. The challenges in developing a finite element injury model of the neck to predict penetration of explosively propelled projectiles. *J R Army Med Corps* 2014 Sep;160(3):220–225.

Breeze J, Allanson-Bailey LS, Hepper AE, Lewis E. Novel method for comparing coverage by future methods of ballistic facial protection. *Br J Oral Maxillofac Surg* 2015 Jan;53(1):3–7.

Breeze J, Allanson-Bailey LS, Hepper AE, Midwinter MJ. Demonstrating the effectiveness of body armour: A pilot prospective computerised surface wound mapping trial performed at the Role 3 hospital in Afghanistan. *J R Army Med Corps* 2015 Mar;161(1):36–41.

Breeze J, Allanson-Bailey LS, Hunt NC et al. Using computerised surface wound mapping to compare the potential medical effectiveness of enhanced protection under body armour combat shirt collar designs. *J R Army Med Corps* 2015 Mar;161(1):22–26.

Breeze J, Baxter D, Carr D, Midwinter MJ. Defining combat helmet coverage for protection against explosively Propelled Fragments. *J R Army Med Corps* 2015 Mar;161(1):9–13.

Breeze J, Carr DJ, Mabbott A et al. Refrigeration and freezing of porcine tissue does not affect the retardation of fragment simulating projectiles. *J Forensic Leg Med* 2015 May;32:77–83.

Breeze J, Fryer R, Hare J et al. Clinical and post mortem analysis of combat neck injury used to inform a novel coverage of armour tool. *Injury* 2015 Apr;46(4):629–633.

Breeze J, Fryer R, Lewis EA, Clasper J. Defining the minimum anatomical coverage required to protect the axilla and arm against penetrating ballistic projectiles. *J R Army Med Corps* 2016 Aug;162(4):270–275.

Breeze J, Lewis EA, Fryer R. Optimising the anatomical coverage provided by military body armour systems. In: Bull AMJ, Clasper J, Mahoney PF, *Blast Injury Science and Engineering*. Springer International Publishing 2016, pp. 291–299.

Breeze J, Lewis EA, Fryer R et al. Defining the essential anatomical coverage provided by military body armour against high energy projectiles. *J R Army Med Corps* 2016 Aug;162(4):284–290.

Breeze J, Tong DC, Powers D et al. Optimising ballistic facial coverage from military fragmenting munitions: A consensus statement. *Br J Oral Maxillofac Surg* 2017 Feb;55(2):173–178.

Lewis E, Pigott MA, Randall A, Hepper AE. The development and introduction of ballistic protection of the external genitalia and peritoneum. *J R Army Med Corps* 2013 Mar;159(Suppl 1):i15–i17.

Mahoney PF, Carr DJ, Delaney RJ et al. Does preliminary optimisation of an anatomically correct skull-brain model using simple stimulants produce clinically realistic ballistic injury fracture patterns? *Int J Legal Med* 2017 Jul;131(4):1043–1053.

Ramasamy A, Hill AM, Hepper AE et al. Blast mines: Physics, injury mechanisms and vehicle protection. *J R Army Med Corps* 2009;155(4):258–264.

CHEMICAL, BIOLOGICAL RADIATION AND NUCLEAR

Bland DJ, Rona RJ, Coggon D et al. Urinary isotopic analysis in the UK Armed Forces: No evidence of depleted uranium absorption in combat and other personnel in Iraq. *Occup Environ Med* 2007 Jul;64(12):834–838.

Henning JD, Lockey DJ. The protection of critically ill patients in a military chemical warfare environment. *Resuscitation* 2005 Feb;64(2):237–239.

Nordmann GR, Woolley T. Unusual critical incident: Chemical gas alert. *Anaesthesia* 2003;58:926.

CHEST TRAUMA

Barnard EB, Rimmer J, Johnston A. Pulmonary puzzle: A precordial crunch. *Thorax* 2013 Jan;68(8):794–795.

Blenkinsop G, Mossadegh S, Ballard M, Parker P. What is the optimal device length and insertion site for needle thoracostomy in UK Military casualties? A computed tomography study. *J Spec Oper Med* 2015 Fall;15(3):60–65.

Calderbank P, Bowley D, Tai N. Mediastinal great vessel injury. In: Doll D, Degiannis E (eds.). *Penetrating Trauma: A Practical Guide on Operative Technique and Peri-Operative Management*. Springer-Verlag Berlin Heidelberg: Springer, 2011. ISBN: 978-3642435225.

Coley E, Roach P, Macmillan AI et al. Penetrating paediatric thoracic injury. *J R Army Med Corps* 2011 Sep;157(3):243–245.

Cooper B, Mellor A, Bruce A et al. Paediatric thoracic damage control resuscitation for ballistic injury: A case report. *J R Army Med Corps* 2007 Dec;153(4):317–318.

Haldane AG. Traumatic pneumorrhachis. *J R Army Med Corps* 2010 Dec;156(4 Suppl 1):S318–S320.

Johnston AM, West AT, Kendrew JM et al. Delayed haemoptysis from explosive device fragments. *Lancet* 2013 Sep;382(9898):1152.

Johnston AM, Ballard M. Primary blast lung injury. *Am J Respir Crit Care Med* 2015 Jun;191(12):1462–1463.

Jugg BJ, Smith AJ, Rudall SJ, Rice P. The injured lung: Clinical issues and experimental models. *Philos Trans R Soc Lond B Biol Sci* 2011 Jan;366(1562):306–309.

Keneally R, Szpisjak D. Thoracic trauma in Iraq and Afghanistan. *J Trauma Acute Care Surg* 2013 May;74(5):1292–1297.

Lundy JB, Oh JS, Chung KK et al. Frequency and relevance of acute peri-traumatic pulmonary thrombus diagnosed by computed tomographic imaging in combat casualties. *J Trauma Acute Care Surg* 2013 Aug;75 (2 Suppl 2):S215–S220.

Morrison JJ, Midwinter M, Jansen J. Management of ballistic thoraco-abdominal injuries: Analysis of recent operational experience. 2010 Military Surgery Meeting (abstract). *J R Army Med Corps* 2010 Sep;156(3):184.

Morrison JJ, Mellor A, Midwinter M et al. Is pre-hospital thoracotomy necessary in the military environment? *Injury* 2011 May;42(5):469–473.

Morrison JJ, Midwinter MJ, Jansen JO. Ballistic thoracoabdominal injury: Analysis of recent military experience in Afghanistan. *World J Surg* 2011 Mar;35:1396–1401.

Morrison JJ, Midwinter MJ, Jansen JO. Survivorship bias following military thoracic injuries: Reply (letter). *World J Surg* 2011 Dec;35(12):2828.

Morrison JJ, Dickson EJ, Jansen JO, Midwinter MJ. Utility of admission physiology in the surgical triage of isolated ballistic battlefield torso trauma. *J Emerg Trauma Shock* 2012 Jul;5(3):233–237.

Morrison JJ, Poon H, Rasmussen TE et al. Resuscitative thoracotomy following wartime injury. *J Trauma Acute Care Surg* 2013 Mar;74(3):825–829.

Morrison JJ, Ross JD, Rasmussen T et al. Resuscitative endovascular balloon occlusion of the aorta (REBOA): A gap analysis of severely injured UK combat casualties. *Shock* 2014 May;41(5):388–393.

Pengelly S, Matheson A, Howes D et al. Military torso trauma: Which, or how many, surgeons deploy (abstract)? *World J Surg* 2009;33:144.

Singleton JA, Gibb IE, Bull AM et al. Primary blast lung injury prevalence and fatal injuries from explosions: Insights from postmortem computed tomographic analysis of 121 improvised explosive device fatalities. *J Trauma Acute Care Surg* 2013 75(2 Suppl 2): S269–S274.

Smith JE, Midwinter M, Lambert AW. Avoiding cavity surgery in penetrating torso trauma: The role of the computed topography scan. *Ann Surg* 2010;92:486–488.

Round J, Mellor A. Anaesthetic and critical care management of thoracic injury. *J R Army Med Corps* 2010 Sep;156(3):145–149.

Scott TE, Kirkman E, Haque M, Gibb IE et al. Primary blast lung injury – A review. *Br J Anaesth* 2017 Mar;118(3):311–316.

Senanayake EL, Poon H, Graham TR, Midwinter MJ. UK specialist cardiothoracic management of thoracic injuries in military casualties sustained in the wars in Iraq and Afghanistan. *Eur J Cardiothorac Surg* 2014 Jun;45(6):e202–e3207.

Smith JE, Midwinter M, Lambert AW. Avoiding cavity surgery in penetrating torso trauma: The role of the computed topography scan. *Ann Surg* 2010;92:486–488.

Stannard A, Benson C, Bowley DM et al. Central vascular injuries in deployed military personnel: A contemporary experience. *J R Army Med Corps* 2008;154(3):188.

Stannard A, Morrison JJ, Scott DJ et al. The epidemiology of non-compressible torso hemorrhage in the wars in Iraq and Afghanistan. *J Trauma Acute Care Surg* 2013;74:830–834.

COMMUNICABLE AND INFECTIOUS DISEASES

Bailey MS, Boos CJ, Vautier G et al. Gastroenteritis outbreak in British troops, Iraq. *Emerg Infect Dis* 2005 Oct;11(10):1626–1628.

Bailey MS, Green AD, Ellis CJ et al. Clinical guidelines for the management of cutaneous Leishmaniasis in British military personnel. *J R Army Med Corps* 2005 Jun;151(2):73–80.

Bailey M, Gallimore CI, Lines LD et al. Viral gastroenteritis outbreaks in deployed British troops during 2002–7. *J R Army Med Corps* 2008 Sep;154(3):156–159.

Bailey MS, Trinick TR, Dunbar JA et al. Undifferentiated febrile illnesses amongst British troops in Helmand, Afghanistan. *J R Army Med Corps* 2011 Jun;157(2):150–155.

Bailey MS, Caddy AJ, McKinnon KA et al. Outbreak of zoonotic cutaneous Leishmaniasis with local dissemination in Balkh, Afghanistan. *J R Army Med Corps* 2012 Sep;158(3):225–228.

Brown D, Gray J, MacDonald P et al. Outbreak of acute gastroenteritis associated with Norwalk-like viruses among British military personnel – Afghanistan, May 2002. *MMWR* 2002 Jun;51(22):477–479.

Connor P, Hutley E, Mulcahy HE, Riddle MS. Enteric disease on Operation HERRICK. *J R Army Med Corps* 2013 Sep;159(3):229–236.

Cooper NK, Bricknell MC, Holden GR, McWilliam C. Pertussis – A case finding study amongst returnees from OP Herrick. *J R Army Med Corps* 2007 Jun;153(2):114–116.

Dunbar J, Cooper B, Hodgetts T et al. An outbreak of human external ophthalmomyiasis due to *Oestrus ovis* in Southern Afghanistan. *Clin Infect Dis* 2008 Jun;46(11):e124–e126.

Gallimore CI, Pipkin C, Shrimpton H et al. Detection of multiple enteric virus strains within a foodborne outbreak of gastroenteritis: An indication of the source of contamination. *Epidemiol Infect* 2005 Feb;133(1):141–147.

Green AD, Terrell A. Cutaneous leishmaniasis in the UK Armed Forces. *CDR Weekly* 2005;15:42.

Hennessy EP, Green AD, Connor MP et al. Norwalk virus infection and disease is associated with ABO histo-blood group type. *J Infect Dis* 2003 Jul;188(1):176–177.

Keene DD, Tong JL, Roughton S, Fadden SJ. A force protection audit: Antimalarial chemoprophylaxis following evacuation from Afghanistan (abstract). *J R Army Med Corps* 2010 Mar;156(1):60.

Keene DD, Tong JL, Roughton S, Fadden SJ. Anti-malarial chemoprophylaxis following evacuation from Afghanistan. *J R Army Med Corps* 2012 Mar;158(1):38–40.

Lonsdale N, Green N, Penn-Barwell JG. Malaria chemoprophylaxis in British casualties returning from Afghanistan. *J R Nav Med Serv* 2013;99(3):166–168.

Matheson A, Williams R, Bailey MS. Cutaneous Leishmaniasis in Royal Marines from Oruzgan, Afghanistan. *J R Army Med Corps* 2012 Sep;158(3):221–224.

Meynard J-B, Summers RH, Faulde MK et al. Epidemie de dengue en Afghanistan: Une fausse alerte. *Medecine Tropicale* 2006 Mar;66:98–99.

Murphy D, Dandeker C, Horn O et al. UK Armed Forces response to an informed consent policy for anthrax vaccination: A paradoxical effect? *Vaccine* 2006 Apr;24(16):3109–3114.

Murphy D, Hull L, Horn O et al. Anthrax vaccination in a military population before the war in Iraq: Acceptance, side effects and choice. *Vaccine* 2007 Nov;25(44):7641–7648.

Murphy D, Hotopf M, Marteau T, Wessely S. Multiple vaccinations, health and recall bias in UK Armed Forces deployed to Iraq. *BMJ* 2008 Jun;337:a22.

Murphy D, Marteau T, Hotopf M et al. Why do UK military personnel refuse the anthrax vaccination? *Biosecur Bioterror* 2008 Sep;6(3):237–342.

Murphy D, Strong A. Investigating factors associated with reporting concerns towards malaria prophylaxis, and the contents of concerns amongst UK Service Personnel deployed to the Iraq conflict between 2003–2006: A mixed methods study. *J R Army Med Corps* 2010 Mar;156(1):28–31.

Murphy D, Marteau TM, Wessely S. A longitudinal study of UK military personnel offered anthrax vaccination: informed choice, symptom reporting, uptake and pre-vaccination health. *Vaccine* 2012 Feb;30(6):1094–1100.

Musa F, Tailor R, Gao A et al. Contact lens-related microbial keratitis in deployed British military personnel. *Br J Ophthalmol* 2010 Aug;94(8):988–993.

Naumann DN, Baird-Clarke CD, Ross DA. Fleas on operations in Afghanistan – Environmental health measures on the front line. *J R Army Med Corps* 2011;157(3):226–228.

Naumann DN, Lundy J, Burns et al. Routine deworming of children at deployed military healthcare facilities. *Pediatr Infect Dis J* 2013;32(9):931–932.

Newman E, Johnstone P, Bridge H et al. Seroconversion for infectious pathogens among UK military personnel deployed to Afghanistan, 2008–2011. *Emerg Infect Dis* 2014;20(12):2015–2022.

Penn-Barwell J, Finnikin S, Sargeant I, Porter K. *Staphylococcus aureus* osteomyelitis complicating septic arthritis in a UK soldier serving in Iraq. *J R Army Med Corps* 2009;155:208–209.

Ross A, Holden G, Tuck JJH. Mitigating the risk against operationally acquired pertussis. *Int Review Armed Forces Med Serv* 2006;79(3):172–177.

Sellers E, Ross DA, Green AD. Improvements in compliance with medical force protection measures by simplification of the anti-malarial chemoprophylaxis regime. *J R Army Med Corps* 2011;157:156–159.

Stacey M, Blanch RJ. A case of external ophthalmomyiasis in a deployed UK soldier. *J R Army Med Corps* 2008;154:60–62.

Tuck J, Green AD, Roberts KI. Falciparum malaria: An outbreak in a military population on an operational deployment. *Mil Med* 2003 Aug;168(8):639–642.

Wood P, Gill M, Edwards D et al. Clinical and microbiological evaluation of epidural and regional anaesthesia catheters in injured UK military personnel. *J R Army Med Corps* 2016 Aug;162(4):261–265.

CRITICAL CARE AIR SUPPORT TEAMS (CCAST)

Barnard EB, Mora AG, Bebarta VS. Preflight variables are associated with increased ventilator days and 30-day mortality in trauma casualties evacuated by critical care air transport teams: An exploratory retrospective study. *Mil Med* 2016 May;181(5Suppl):132–137.

Bennett RA. Ethics surrounding the medical evacuation of catastrophically injured individuals from an operational theatre of war. *J R Army Med Corps* 2016 Oct;162(5):321–323.

Flutter C, Ruth M, Aldington D. Pain management during Royal Air Force Strategic Aeromedical evacuations. *J R Army Med Corps* 2009 Mar;155(1):61–63.

Haites EM, Turner S. Are CCAST patients developing a metabolic acidosis in-flight and if so is lactate monitoring necessary (abstract)? *J R Army Med Corps* 2010 Dec;156(4 Suppl 1):S402.

Lamb D. The introduction of new critical care equipment into the aeromedical evacuation service of the Royal Air Force. *Intensive Crit Care Nurs* 2003 Apr;19(2):92–102.

Lamb D. Collaboration in practice – Assessment of an RAF CCAST. *Br J Nurs* 2006 May;15:552–556.

Nicholson-Roberts TC, Berry R. Prehospital trauma and aeromedical transfer. A military perspective. *Contin Educ Anaesth Crit Care Pain* 2012;12:186–189.

Patterson CM, Woodcock T, Mollan IA et al. United Kingdom military aeromedical evacuation in the Post 9/11 era. *Aviat Space Environ Med* 2014;85(10):1005–1012.

Turner S, Ruth MJ, Bruce DL. "In flight catering": Feeding critical care patients during aeromedical evacuation. *J R Army Med Corps* 2008;154(4):282–283.

Turner S, Ruth M, Tipping R. Critical care air support teams and deployed intensive care. *J R Army Med Corps* 2009 Jun;155(2):171–174.

DAMAGE CONTROL RESUSCITATION AND SURGERY

Blenkinsop G, Mossadegh S, Ballard M, Parker P. What is the optimal device length and insertion site for needle thoracostomy in UK military casualties? A computed tomography study. *J Spec Oper Med* 2015 Fall;15(3):60–65.

Boutefnouchet T, Gregg R, Tidman J et al. Emergency red cells first: Rapid response or speed bump? The evolution of a massive transfusion protocol for trauma in a single UK centre. *Injury* 2015 Sep;46(9):1772–1778.

Bowles F, Hawksley OJ. Blood product use during role 3 trauma calls: Are products used appropriately and wastage minimised? *J R Army Med Corps* 2014;160(3):258.

Bree S, Wood K, Nordmann GR, McNicholas J. The paediatric transfusion challenge on deployed operations. *J R Army Med Corps* 2010 Dec;156(4 Suppl 1):361–364.

Breeze J, Tong DC. Damage control surgery and combat-related maxillofacial and cervical injuries: A systematic review. *Br J Oral Maxillofac Surg* 2016 Jan;54(1):8–12.

Doran CM, Doran CA, Woolley T et al. Targeted resuscitation improves coagulation and outcome. *J Trauma Acute Care Surg* 2012 Apr;72(4):835–843.

Doughty H, Tidman J. Implementation and revision of a massive transfusion protocol. *Transfus Med* 2010;20(Suppl 1):40, PO30.

Doughty HA, Woolley T, Thomas GOR. Massive transfusion. *J R Army Med Corps* 2011 Sep;157(3 Suppl 1):S277–S283.

Doughty H. Military management of massive haemorrhage. In: Thomas D, Thompson J, Ridler BMF (eds.). *All Blood Counts – A Manual for Blood Conservation and Patient Blood Management.* 2nd ed. tfm Publishing Ltd., 2016.

Eardley W, Stitson D, Miles R, Clasper J. Exploring the role of whole body computed tomography (WBCT) in the early management of combat casualties from explosive devices (abstract). *J R Army Med Corps* 2010 Sep;156(3):181.

Gay DAT, Miles RM. Damage control radiology: An evolution in trauma imaging (Use of imaging in trauma decision making). *J R Army Med Corps* 2011 Sep;157(3 Suppl 1):s289–s292.

Hodgetts T, Mahoney P, Russell MQ, Byers M. ABC to <C>ABC: Redefining the military trauma paradigm. *Emerg Med J* 2006 Oct;23(10):745–746.

Hodgetts TJ, Mahoney PF, Kirkman E. Damage control resuscitation. *J R Army Med Corps* 2007;153(4):299–300.

Holcomb JB, Jenkins D, Rhee P et al. damage control resuscitation: Directly addressing the early coagulopathy of trauma. *J Trauma Acute Care Surg* 2007 Feb;62(2):307–310.

Hunt BJ, Woolley T, Parmar K et al. Haemostatic changes following military trauma and major blood loss. *J Thromb Haemost* 2013:11(Suppl 2):672.

Kirkman E, Watts S, Hodgetts T et al. A Proactive approach to the coagulopathy of trauma: The rationale and guidelines for treatment. *J R Army Med Corps* 2007 Dec;153(4):302–306.

Lamb CM, MacGoey P, Navarro AP, Brooks AJ. Damage control surgery in the era of damage control resuscitation. *Br J Anaesth* 2014 Aug;113(2):242–249.

Middleton SWF, Nott DM, Midwinter MJ, Lambert AW. Is damage control surgery appropriate in vascular trauma in the field? *J R Nav Med Serv* 2010;96:76–82.

Midwinter MJ. Damage Control Surgery in the era of damage control resuscitation. *J R Army Med Corps* 2009 Dec;155(4):323–326.

Midwinter MJ, Woolley T. Resuscitation and coagulopathy in the severely injured trauma patient. *Phil Trans R Soc Lond B Biol Sci* 2011 Jan;366(1562):192–203.

Moor P, Rew D, Midwinter MJ, Doughty H. Editorial. Transfusion for trauma: Civilian lessons from the battlefield? *Anaesthesia* 2009;64(5):469–472.

Morrison JJ, Ross JD, Poon H et al. Intra-operative correction of acidosis, coagulopathy and hypothermia in combat casualties with severe haemorrhagic shock. *Anaesthesia* 2013 Aug;68(8):846–850.

Nordmann GR, McNicholas JJ, Templeton PA et al. Paediatric trauma management on deployment. *J R Army Med Corps* 2011;157 (3 Suppl 1):S334–S343.

Penn-Barwell JG, Fries CA, Bennett PM et al. The injury burden of recent combat operations: Mortality, morbidity, and return to service of U.K. naval service personnel following combat trauma. *Mil Med* 2013;178(11):1222–1226.

Rees PSC, Inwald D P, Hutchings S. Echocardiography, performed during damage control resuscitation can be used to monitor the haemodynamic response to volume infusion in the deployed military critical care unit. *Heart* 2013;99(Suppl 2):A71.

Sharpe D, Barneby E, Russell R. New approaches to the management of traumatic external haemorrhage. *Trauma* 2011;13:47–55.

Stansfield T, Hill G, Louden M et al. Right turn or pause at the crossroads? 2010 Military Surgery Meeting (abstract). *J R Army Med Corps* 2010;156(3):183.

Tai NRM, Russell R. Right turn resuscitation: Frequently asked questions. *J R Army Med Corps* 2011;157(3 Suppl 1):S310–S314.

Tai N, Parker P The damage control surgery set: Rethinking for contingency. *J R Army Med Corps* 2013 Dec;159(4):314–315.

Tarmey N, Woolley T, Jansen JO et al. Evolution of coagulopathy monitoring in military damage-control resuscitation. *J Trauma Acute Care Surg* 2012;73:S417–S422.

Thomas D, Wee M, Clyburn P et al. Blood transfusion and the anaesthetist: Management of massive haemorrhage. *Anaesthesia* 2010 Nov;65(11):1153–1161.

Wright C, Mahoney P, Hodgetts T et al. fluid resuscitation: A defence medical services Delphi study into current practice. *J R Army Med Corps* 2009;155(2):99–104.

DEPLOYED EXPERIENCE AT SEA

Ablett D, Herbert LJ, Brogden T. The role played by Royal Navy Medical Assistants on Operation Herrick 9. Can we do more to prepare them for future operations in Afghanistan? *J R Nav Med Serv* 2010;96(1):17–22.

Bott G, Barnard J, Prior K. Maritime in transit care. *J R Nav Med Serv* 2015;101(2):104–106.

Coetzee RH. HMS Ark Royal and the 2003 helicopter crash in the Northern Arabian Gulf. *J R Nav Med Serv* 2010;96(2):96–102.

Evans GW. Receiving mass casualties at sea: The capabilities of the Primary Casualty receiving facility. *J R Nav Med Serv* 2004;90(2):51–56.

Matthews JJ, Mercer SJ. 'War Surgery at Sea': Maritime trauma experience in the Gulf War 2003. *J R Nav Med Serv* 2003;89(3):123–132.

Mercer SJ, Heames RM. Anaesthesia and critical care aspects of Role 2 Afloat. *J R Nav Med Serv* 2013;99(3):140–143.

Risdall JE, Heames RM, Hill G. Role 2 Afloat. *J R Army Med Corps* 2011;157(4):362–364.

Smith JE, Smith SR, Hill G. The UK maritime Role 3 medical treatment facility: The Primary Casualty Receiving Facility, RFA ARGUS. *J R Nav Med Serv* 2015;101(1):3–5.

Whalley L, Smith S. Pre-hospital, maritime in-transit care from a Role 2 Afloat platform. *J R Nav Med Serv* 2013;99(3):135–136.

Whybrow D, Jones N, Evans C et al. The mental health of deployed UK maritime forces. *Occup Environ Med* 2016 Feb;73(2):75–82.

DIET AND LIFESTYLE

Azari J, Dandeker C, Greenberg N. Cultural stress: How interactions with and among foreign populations affect Military personnel. *Armed Forces Soc* 2010 Jan;36(4):585–603.

Boos CJ, Croft AM. Smoking rates in the staff of a military field hospital before and after wartime deployment. *J R Soc Med* 2004 Jan;97(1):20–22.

Boos CJ, Wheble GA, Campbell MJ et al. Self-administration of exercise and dietary supplements in deployed British Military personnel during Operation TELIC 13. *J R Army Med Corps* 2010 Mar;156(1):32–36.

Boos CJ, White SH, Bland SA, McAllister PD. Dietary supplements and military operations: Caution is advised. *J R Army Med Corps* 2010 Mar;156(1):41–43.

Boos CJ, Simms P, Morris FR, Fertout M. The use of exercise and dietary supplements among British soldiers in Afghanistan. *J R Army Med Corps* 2011 Sep;157(3):229–232.

Browne T, Iversen A, Hull L et al. How do experiences in Iraq affect alcohol use amongst male UK Armed Forces personnel? *Occup Environ Med* 2008 Sep;65(9):628–633.

Debell F, Fear NT, Head M, Batt-Rawden S et al. A systematic review of the comorbidity between PTSD and alcohol misuse. *Soc Psychiatry Psychiatr Epidemiol* 2014 Sep;49(9):1401–1425.

Fear N, Iversen A, Chatterjee A et al. Risky driving among regular Armed Forces personnel from the United Kingdom. *Am J Prev Med* 2008 Aug;35:230–236.

Greene T, Buckman J, Dandeker C, Greenberg N. The influence of culture clash on deployed troops. *Mil Med* 2010 Dec;175(12):958–963.

Henderson A, Langston V, Greenberg N. Alcohol misuse in the Royal Navy. *Occup Med* 2009;59:25–31.

Hooper R, Rona, R, Jones M et al. Cigarette and alcohol use in the UK Armed Forces, and their association with combat exposure: A prospective study. *Addict Behav* 2008 Aug;33(8):1067–1071.

Jones E, Fear NT. Alcohol use and misuse within the military: A review. *Int Rev Psychiatry* 2011 Apr;23(2):166–172.

Okpala NCE, Ward NJ, Bhullar A. Seatbelt use among military personnel during operational deployment. *Mil Med* 2007;172(12):1231–1233.

Parsloe L, Jones N, Fertout M et al. Rest and recuperation in the UK Armed Forces. *Occup Med (Lond)* 2014 Dec;64(8):616–621.

Rona R, Jones M, Fear N et al. Alcohol misuse and functional impairment in the UK Armed Forces. *Drug Alcohol Depend* 2010 Apr;108(1–2):37–42.

Sherriff R, Forbes H, Greenberg N et al. Risky driving among UK regular forces: Changes over time. *BMJ Open* 2015;5:e008434 doi 10.1136/bmjopen_2015.008431

Stansfield T, Winkworth K, Wilkinson D. Recreational opioid use in Afghan patients admitted to Camp Bastion Role 3 Hospital (abstract). *J R Army Med Corps* 2010;156(3):182.

Thandi G, Sundin J, Dandeker C et al. Risk-taking behaviours among reserves: A UK perspective. *Occup Med (Lond)* 2015 Jul;65(5):413–416.

Thandi G, Sundin J, Knight T et al. Alcohol misuse in the United Kingdom Armed Forces: A longitudinal study. *Drug Alcohol Depend* 2015 Nov;156:78–83.

EAR, NOSE AND THROAT (ENT)

Breeze J, Cooper H, Pearson CR et al. Ear injuries sustained by British service personnel subjected to blast trauma. *J Laryngol Otol* 2011 Jan;125(1):13–17.

Jones GH, Pearson CR. The use of personal hearing protection in hostile territory and the effect of health promotion activity: Advice falling upon deaf ears. *J R Army Med Corps* 2016 Aug;162(4):280–283.

Patil M, Breeze J. Use of hearing protection on military operations *J R Army Med Corps* 2011;157:381–384.

Pearson C. The characteristics of pure tone audiograms in a sample of Royal Marines after Operation Herrick 9. *J R Nav Med Serv* 2011;97(3):123–126.

EDUCATION AND TRAINING

Arora S, Sevdalis N. HOSPEX and concepts of simulation. *J R Army Med Corps* 2008 Sep;154(3):202–205.

Benavides LC, Smith IM, Benavides JM et al. Deployed skills training for whole blood collection by a special operations expeditionary surgical team. *J Trauma Acute Care Surg* 2017 Jun;82(6S Suppl 1):S96–S102.

Birt DJ, Woolley T. Competencies for the military anaesthetist – A new unit of training. *Bull R Coll Anaesth* 2008 Nov;52:2661–2666.

Budd, ME, Hitchinson M, Doughty H. Development of a training programme for a deployed military transfusion nurse. *Transfus Med* 2013;23(Suppl 2):48–49.

Cooper D, Troth T, Chin EJ, Hughes J. Graduate medical education in combat support hospitals: An enlightening experience in a British-led combat support hospital. *Mil Med* 2014;179(7):697–701.

Cox CW, Roberts P. HOSPEX: A historical view and the need for change. *J R Army Med Corps* 2008 Sep;154(3):193–194.

Davey CM, Mieville KE, Simpson R, Aldington D. A proposed model for improving battlefield analgesia training: Post-graduate medical officer pain management day. *J R Army Med Corps* 2012 Sep;158(3):190–193.

Davies TJ, Nadin MN, McArthur DJ et al. Hospex 2008. *J R Army Med Corps* 2008 Sep;154(3):195–197.

Davis M, Driscoll P, Hanson J, Wieteska S. The Advanced Life Support Group's view of HOSPEX. *J R Army Med Corps* 2008 Sep;154(3):206–208.

Dow WA. Operational pre-deployment training and its usefulness to medical personnel deploying as individual replacements to areas of operations *J R Nav Med Serv* 2006;92(3):136–139.

DuBose J, Rodriguez C, Martin M et al. The Eastern Association for the Surgery of Trauma Military Ad Hoc Committee: Preparing the surgeon for war: Present practices of US, UK, and Canadian militaries and future directions for the US military. *J Trauma Acute Care Surg* 2012 Dec;73(6):S423–S430.

Eardley WG, Taylor DM, Parker PJ. Training tomorrow's military surgeons: Lessons from the past and challenges for the future. *J R Army Med Corps* 2009 Dec;155(4):249–252.

Eardley WG, Taylor DM, Parker PJ. Training in the practical application of damage control and early total care operative philosophy – Perceptions of UK orthopaedic specialist trainees. *Ann R Coll Surg Engl* 2010 Mar;92(2):154–158.

Fries CA, Rickard RF. Surgical training in Camp Bastion, Afghanistan. *J R Nav Med Serv* 2012;98(2):23–26.

Gould M, Meeks D, Gibbs T et al. What are the psychological effects of delivering and receiving 'high-risk' survival resistance training? *Mil Med* 2015 Feb;180(2):168–177.

Greenberg N, Langston V, Fear NT et al. An evaluation of stress education in the Royal Navy. *Occup Med (Lond)* 2009 Jan;59(1):20–24.

Jones CL, Mercer SJ, Mahoney PF. Shaping military training in the era of contingency and revalidation. *Bull R Coll Anaesth* 2016 Jan;97:41–43.

Keogh B, Willett K. Lessons from war must be remembered. *J R Nav Med Serv* 2012;98(1):3–4.

Mercer SJ. Training and revalidation in defence anaesthesia. *Bull R Coll Anaesth* 2013 Jul;80:14–16.

Mercer SJ, Howell M, Simpson R. Simulation training for the frontline – Realistic preparation for Role 1 doctors. *J R Army Med Corps* 2010 Jun;156(2):87–89.

Mercer SJ, Whittle C, Siggers B et al. Simulation, human factors and defence anaesthesia. *J R Army Med Corps* 2010 Dec;156(Suppl 4):365–369.

Mercer SJ. Training and revalidation in defence anaesthesia. *Bull R Coll Anaesth* 2013 Jul;80:14–16.

Morrison JJ, Forbes K, Woolrich-Burt L et al. Medium-Fidelity Medical Simulators: Use in a pre-hospital, operational, military environment. *J R Army Med Corps* 2006 Sep;152(3):132–135.

Parker PJ. Training for war: Teaching and skill-retention for the deployed surgical team. *J R Army Med Corps* 2008 Mar;154(1):3–4.

Parsons IT, Rawdon MP, Wheatley RJ. Development of pre-deployment primary healthcare training for combat medical technicians. *J R Army Med Corps* 2014;160(3):241–244.

Ramasamy A, Hinsley DE, Edwards DS et al. Skill sets and competencies for the modern military surgeon: Lessons from UK military operations in Southern Afghanistan. *Injury* 2010 May;41(5):453–459.

Randall-Carrick JV. Experiences of combat medical technician continuous professional development on operations. *J R Army Med Corps* 2012 Sep;158(3):263–267.

Shastri-Hurst N, Naumann DN, Bowley DM, Whitbread T. Military surgery in the new curriculum: Whither general surgery training in uniform? *J R Army Med Corps* 2015;161(2):100–105.

Smith JE, Charlton KW, Piper N. Immediate life support training in an operational environment. *J R Nav Med Serv* 2003;89(3):133–135.

Wesson M. Lessons learnt from America – Reflections from a fellowship examining the prevention, recognition and treatment of operational stress injuries in US Army serving personnel. *J R Nav Med Serv* 2010;96(3):175–184.

EMERGENCY MEDICINE (EXCLUDING TRAUMA RESUSCITATION)

Hodgetts T. Personal view: A day in the life of an emergency physician at war. *Emerg Med J* 2004;21(2):129–130.

Horne S, Smith JE. Preparation of the Resuscitation Room and Patient Reception. *J R Army Med Corps* 2011 Sep;157(3 Suppl 1):S267–S272.

Milligan C, Higginson I, Smith JE. Emergency department staff knowledge of massive transfusion for trauma: The need for an evidence based protocol. *Emerg Med J* 2011 Oct;28(10):870–872.

Reavley PDA, Black JJM. Attendances at a Field Hospital emergency department during operations in Iraq November 2003 to March 2004 (Operation Telic III). *J R Army Med Corps* 2006;152:231–235.

Russell R, Hodgetts T, Ollerton J et al. The Operational Emergency Department Attendance Register: A new epidemiological tool. *J R Army Medical Corps* 2007;153(4):244–250.

Smith JE, Russell RJ. Critical decision making and timelines in the emergency department. *J R Army Med Corps* 2011;157(3 Suppl 1):S273–S276.

Stalker A, Ollerton J, Everington S et al. Three year review of emergency department admissions – Op HERRICK 4 to 9. *J R Army Med Corps* 2011;157(3):213–217.

EQUIPMENT INCLUDING NOVEL HAEMOSTATICS

Arul GS, Bowley DM, DiRusso S. The use of Celox gauze as an adjunct to pelvic packing in otherwise uncontrollable pelvic haemorrhage secondary to penetrating trauma. *J R Army Med Corps* 2012 Dec;158(4):331–333; discussion 333–334.

Dharm-Datta S, Hill G. Improvised equipment for skeletal traction on operations. *J R Army Med Corps* 2007 Jun;153(2):144.

Eardley WG. The combination tool: A significant cause of morbidity in deployed personnel. *J R Army Med Corps* 2005 Mar;151(1):59.

Hewitt-Smith A, Laird C, Porter K, Bloch M. Haemostatic dressings in prehospital care. *Emerg Med J* 2013 Oct;30(10):784–789.

Hodgetts T, Russell R, Mahoney PF et al. Evaluation of clinician attitudes to the implementation of novel haemostatic techniques. *J R Army Med Corps* 2005 Sep;151(3):176–178.

Jeyanathan J, Webster BB, Hawksley OJ, Mellor AJ. A comparison of performance between Teflon and polyurethane safety cannulae at extremes of operating temperatures. *J R Army Med Corps* 2012 Jun;158(2):120–122.

Johnston AM, Batchelor NK, Wilson D. Evaluation of a disposable sheath bronchoscope system for use in the deployed field hospital. *J R Army Med Corps* 2014 Sep;160(3):217–219.

Kyle T, Le Clerc S, Thomas A et al. The success of battlefield surgical airway insertion in severely injured military patients: A UK perspective. *J R Army Med Corps* 2016 Dec;162(6):460–464.

Lamb D. The introduction of new critical care equipment into the aeromedical evacuation service of the Royal Air Force. *Intensive Crit Care Nurs* 2003 Apr;19(2):92–102.

Lawton G, Granville-Chapman J, Parker PJ. Novel haemostatic dressings. *J R Army Med Corps* 2009 Dec;155(4):309–314.

Mahoney PF, Russell R, Russell MQ, Hodgetts TJ. Novel haemostatic techniques in military medicine. *J R Army Med Corps* 2005 Sep;151(3):139–142.

Morrison JJ, Mountain AJ, Galbraith KA, Clasper JC. Penetrating pelvic battlefield trauma: Internal use of chitosan-based haemostatic dressings. *Injury* 2010 Feb;41(2):239–241.

Morrison JJ, Ross JD, Rasmussen T et al. Resuscitative endovascular balloon occlusion of the aorta (REBOA): A gap analysis of severely injured UK combat casualties. *Shock* 2014 May;41(5):388–393.

Rowlands TK, Clasper J. The Thomas splint – A necessary tool in the management of battlefield injuries. *J R Army Med Corps* 2003;149(4):291–293.

Rutherford J, Adams S. The Afghanistan Fracture Pan. *J R Army Med Corps* 2011;157:3.

Sharpe D, Barneby E, Russell R. New approaches to the management of traumatic external haemorrhage. *Trauma* 2011;13:47–55.

Technical tip: Removal of tungsten carbide rings. *J R Army Medical Corps* 2013;159(1):64–64.

ETHICS, LEGAL, AND HUMANITARIAN ISSUES

Bennett RA. Ethics surrounding the medical evacuation of catastrophically injured individuals from an operational theatre of war. *J R Army Med Corps* 2016 Oct;162(5):321–323.

Bernthal EM, Russell RJ, Draper HJ. A qualitative study of the use of the four-quadrant approach to assist ethical decision-making during deployment. *J R Army Med Corps* 2014 Jun;160(2):196–202.

Bernthal EM, Draper HJA, Henning J, Kelly JC. "A band of brothers" – An exploration of the range of medical ethical issues faced by British senior military clinicians on deployment to Afghanistan: A qualitative study. *J R Army Med Corps* 2016 Oct;163(3):199–205.

Henning J. The ethical dilemma of providing intensive care treatment to local civilians on operations. *J R Army Med Corps* 2009 Jun;155(2):84–86.

Hodgetts T, Mahoney PF, Mozumder A, McLennan J. Care of civilians during operations. *Int J Disast Med* 2005;3(1–4):3–24.

Kelly J. Following professional codes of practice and military orders in austere military environments: A controversial debate on ethical challenges. *J R Army Med Corps* 2015 Dec;161(Suppl 1):i10–i12.

Matheson AS, Howes RD, Midwinter MJ, Lambert AW. Surgery in an Afghan population: Is pictorial consent and injury pattern recognition identification of patients appropriate? *J R Nav Med Serv* 2010;96(3):158–163.

Moy RJ. Ethical dilemmas in providing medical care to captured persons on operations. *J R Army Med Corps* 2012 Mar;158(1):6–9.

O'Reilly DJ. Proceedings of the DMS ethics symposium. *J R Army Med Corps* 2011 Dec;157(4):405–410.

Ross DA, Wiliamson RHB. Commentary on: Following professional codes of practice and military orders in austere military environments: A controversial debate on ethical challenges. *J R Army Med Corps* 2015;161(Supp 1):i13.

FACE AND NECK TRAUMA AND MAXILLOFACIAL SURGERY

Banfield G. Penetrating neck injury in Iraq and Afghanistan. 2010 Military Surgery Meeting (abstract). *J R Army Med Corps* 2010;156(3):180.

Breeze J. Head, face and neck injuries sustained by British Servicemen in Iraq and Afghanistan (abstract) *J R Army Med Corps* 2010 Sep;156(3):179.

Breeze J. Editorial: Saving faces: The UK future facial protection programme. *J R Army Med Corps* 2012 Dec;158(4):284–287.

Breeze J, Gibbons AJ. Are soldiers at increased risk of third molar symptoms when on operational tour in Iraq? A prospective cohort study. *J R Army Med Corps* 2007 Jun;153(2):102–104.

Breeze J, Bryant D. Current concepts in the epidemiology and management of battlefield head, face and neck trauma. *J R Army med Corps* 2009 Dec;155(4):274–278.

Breeze J, Opie N, Monaghan A, Gibbons AJ. Isolated orbital wall blowout fractures due to primary blast injury (letter). *J R Army Med Corps* 2009 Mar;155(1):70.

Breeze J, Gibbons A, Opie N, Monaghan A. Maxillofacial injuries in military personnel treated at the Royal Centre for Defence Medicine June 2001 to December 2007. *Br J Oral Maxillofac Surg* 2010 Dec;48(8):613–616.

Breeze J, Monaghan A, Williams M et al. Five months surgery in the multinational field hospital in Afghanistan with an emphasis on oral and maxillofacial injuries. *J R Army Med Corps* 2010 Jun;156(2):125–128.

Breeze J, Gibbons AJ, Combes JG, Monaghan AM. Oral and maxillofacial surgical contribution to 21 months of operating theatre activity in Kandahar Field Hospital: 1 February 2007–31 October 2008. *Br J Oral Maxillofac Surg* 2011 Sep;49(6):464–468.

Breeze J, Gibbons AJ, Hunt NC et al. Mandibular fractures in British military personnel secondary to blast trauma sustained in Iraq and Afghanistan. *Br J Oral Maxillofac Surg* 2011 Dec;49(8):607–611.

Breeze J, McVeigh K, Lee JJ et al. Management of Maxillofacial wounds sustained by British Service Personnel in Afghanistan. *Int J Oral Maxillofac Surg* 2011 May;40(5):483–486.

Breeze J, Allanson-Bailey LS, Hunt NC et al. Mortality and morbidity from combat neck injury. *J Trauma Acute Care Surg* 2012 Apr;72(4):969–974.

Breeze J. Obtaining multi-national consensus on future combat face and neck protection – Proceedings of the Revision Military Protection Workshop (letter). *J R Army Med Corps* 2012 Jun;158(2):141–142.

Breeze J, Allanson-Bailey LS, Hunt NC et al. Surface wound mapping of battlefield occulo-facial injury. *Injury* 2012 Nov;43(11):1856–1860.

Breeze J, Brazier W, Monaghan AM. Intra-oral injury assessment and recording in evacuated military personnel. *Int J Oral Maxillofac Surg* 2013 Mar;42(3):419.

Breeze J, Leason J, Gibb I et al. Characterisation of explosive fragments injuring the neck. *Br J Oral Maxillofac Surg* 2013 Dec;51(8):e263–e266.

Carr DJ, Lewis E, Horsfall I. A systematic review of military head injuries. *J R Army Med Corps* 2017 Feb;163(1):13–19.

Davies E, Boylan M, Hawker JJ, Banerjee B. Don't forget the fragment! An unusual case of occult fragment embolization following penetrating neck injury. *J R Army Med Corps* 2011 Dec;157(4):396–398.

Feldt BA, Salinas NL, Rasmussen TE, Brennan J. The Joint Facial and Invasive Neck Trauma (J-FAINT) project, Iraq and Afghanistan 2003–2011. *Otolaryngol Head Neck Surg* 2013 Mar;148(3):403–408.

Gibbons AJ, Mackenzie N. Lessons learned in oral and maxillofacial surgery from British Military deployments in Afghanistan. *J R Army Med Corps* 2010 Jun;156(2):113–116.

Gibbons AJ, Breeze J. The face of war: The initial management of modern battlefield ballistic facial injuries. *J Mil Veterans Health* 2011 Apr;19(2):15–18.

Gibbons AJ, Mackenzie N, Breederveld RS. Use of a custom designed external fixator system to treat ballistic injuries to the mandible. *Int J Oral Maxillofac Surg* 2011 Jan;40(1):103–105.

Hale RG, Lew T, Wenke JC. Craniomaxillofacial battle injuries: Injury patterns, conventional treatment limitations and direction of future research. *Singapore Dent J* 2010 Jun;31(1):1–8.

McVeigh K, Breeze J, Jeynes P et al. Clinical strategies in management of complex maxillofacial injuries sustained in British military personnel. *J R Army Med Corps* 2010 Jun;156(2):110–113.

Petersen K, Colyer MD, Hayes DK et al. Prevention of infections associated with combat-related eye, maxillofacial, and neck injuries. *J Trauma* 2011;71:S264–S269.

Richardson PS Dental Morbidity in United Kingdom Armed Forces, Iraq 2003. *Mil Med* 2005;170(6):536–541.

Richardson PS. Dental risk assessment for military personnel. Mil Med 2005;170(6):542–545.

Tong DC, Breeze J. Damage control surgery and combat-related maxillofacial and cervical injuries: A systematic review. *Br J Oral Maxillofac Surg* 2016;54(1):8–12.

Wordsworth M, Thomas R, Breeze J et al. The surgical management of facial trauma in British soldiers during combat operations in Afghanistan. *Injury* 2017;48(1):70–74.

HISTORY

Cox CW, Roberts P. HOSPEX: A historical view and the need for change. *J R Army Med Corps* 2008 Sep;154(3):193–194.

Gaunt C, Gill J, Aldington D. British military use of morphine: A historical review. *J R Army Med Corps* 2009 Mar;155(1):46–49.

Jones E, Fear NT, Wessely S. Shell shock and mild traumatic brain injury: A historical review. *Am J Psychiatry* 2007 Nov;164(11):1641–1645.

Kinch KJ, Clasper JC. A brief history of war amputation. *J R Army Med Corps* 2011 Dec;157(4):374–380.

Mahan JK. Closure of the Bastion Role 3 on 22 Sep 2014. *J R Nav Med Serv* 2014;100(3):231.

Mahan JK. Final address: Closure of the Bastion Role 3 on 22 Sep 2014. *The Medic (The Royal Army Medical Corps Magazine)* 2014;4(2):15–16.

Olson CM Jr, Bailey J, Mabry R et al. Forward aeromedical evacuation: A brief history, lessons learned from the Global War on Terror, and the way forward for US policy. *J Trauma Acute Care Surg* 2013;75:S130–S136.

Vassallo D. A short history of Camp Bastion Hospital: The two hospitals and unit deployments. *J R Army Med Corps* 2015 Mar;161(1):79–83.

Vassallo D. A short history of Camp Bastion Hospital: Bastion's catalytic role in advancing casualty care. *J R Army Med Corps* 2015 Jun;161(2):160–166.

Vassallo D. A short history of Camp Bastion Hospital: Preparing for war, national recognition and Bastion's legacy. *J R Army Med Corps* 2015 Dec;161(4):355–360.

HUMAN FACTORS

Arul GS, Pugh HEJ, Mercer SJ, Midwinter MJ. optimising communication in the damage control resuscitation – Damage control surgery sequence in major trauma management. *J R Army Med Corps* 2012 Jun;158(2):82–84.

Arul GS, Pugh HE, Mercer SJ, Midwinter MJ. Human factors in decision making in Major Trauma in Camp Bastion, Afghanistan. *Ann R Coll Surg Engl* 2015 May;97(4):262–268.

Bowley DM, Jansen JO, Nott D et al. Difficult decisions in the surgical care of military casualties with major torso trauma. *J R Army Med Corps* 2011 Sep;157(3 Suppl 1):S324–S333.

Bricknell MCM, Beardmore CE, Williamson RH. The deployed medical director: Managing the challenges of a complex trauma system (letter). *J R Army Med Corps* 2012 Mar;158(1):66.

Bricknell MCM, Beardmore C, Williamson RHB. Letter. *J R Army Med Corps* 2012;158(1):64–67.

Macmillan AIM. Teamwork and ballistic trauma. *Surgeons' News* 2011 Jan:52–53.

Mahoney PF, Hodgetts TJ, Hicks I. The deployed medical director: Managing the challenges of a complex trauma system. *J R Army Med Corps* 2011 Sep;157(3 Suppl 1):S350–S356.

McNicholas JJ, Henning JD. Major military trauma: Decision making in the ICU. *J R Army Med Corps* 2011 Sep;157(3 Suppl 1):S284–S288.

Mercer SJ, Whittle CL, Mahoney PF. Lessons from the battlefield: Human factors in defence anaesthesia. *Br J Anaesth* 2010 Jul;105(1):9–20.

Mercer SJ, Tarmey N, Mahoney PF. Military experience of human factors in airway complications. *Anaesthesia* 2013 Oct;68:1081–1082.

Mercer S, Arul GS, Pugh HE. Performance improvement through best practice team management: Human factors in complex trauma. *J R Army Med Corps* 2014 Jun;160(2):105–108.

Mercer S, Park C, Tarmey NT. Human factors in complex trauma. *BJA Educ* 2015 Oct;15(5):231–236.

Midwinter MJ, Mercer S, Lambert AW, De Rond MJ. Making difficult decisions in major military trauma: A crew resource management perspective. *J R Army Med Corps* 2011 Sep;157(Suppl 3):S299–S304.

INFECTION AND INFECTION CONTROL

Brown KV, Murray KC, Clasper JC Infectious complications of combat-related mangled extremity injuries in the British Military. *J Trauma* 2010 Jul;69(1):S109–S115.

D'Avignon LC, Chung KK, Saffle JR et al. Prevention of infections associated with combat-related burn injuries. *J Trauma* 2011 Aug;71(2 Suppl 2):S282–S289.

Eardley WG, Brown KV, Bonner TJ et al. Infection in conflict wounded. *Philos Trans R Soc Lond B Biol Sci* 2011 Jan;366(1562):204–218.

Eardley WG, Watts SA, Clasper JC. Limb wounding and antisepsis: Iodine and chlorhexidine in the early management of extremity injury. *Int J Low Extrem Wounds* 2012 Sep;11(3):213–223.

Forgione MA, Moores LE, Wortmann GW; Prevention of Combat-related Infections Guidelines Panel. Prevention of infections associated with combat-related central nervous system injuries. *J Trauma* 2011 Aug;71(2 Suppl 2):S258–S263.

Hospenthal DR, Green AD, Crouch HK. Prevention of Combat-related Infections Guidelines Panel. Infection prevention and control in deployed military medical treatment facilities. *J Trauma* 2011 Aug;71(2 Suppl 2): S290–S298.

Hospenthal DR, Murray CK, Andersen, RC et al. Guidelines for the prevention of infections associated with combat-related injuries: 2011 update: Endorsed by the Infectious Diseases Society of America and the Surgical Infection. *J Trauma Acute Care Surg* 2011 Aug;71(2):S210–S234.

Hutley EJ, Green AD. Infection in wounds of conflict – Old lessons and new challenges. *J R Army Med Corps* 2010 Dec;155(4):315–319.

Johnston AM. Focus on sepsis and intensive care. *J R Army Med Corps* 2009 Jun;155(2):129–132.

Johnston AM, Easby D, Ewington I. Sepsis management in the deployed field hospital. *J R Army Med Corps* 2013 159(3):175–180.

Jones A, Morgan D, Walsh A et al. Importation of multidrug-resistant *Acinetobacter* spp infections with casualties from Iraq. *Lancet Infect Dis* 2006 Jun;6(6):317–318.

Martin GJ, Dunne JR, Cho JM, Solomkin JS. Prevention of Combat-related Infections Guidelines Panel. Prevention of infections associated with combat-related thoracic and abdominal cavity injuries. *J Trauma* 2011 Aug;71(2 Suppl 2):S270–S281.

Matheson A, Hutley E, Green AD. The evolving challenge of war wounds *Microbiologist* 2011;12(4):26–29.

Murray CK, Wilkins K, Molter NC et al. Infections complicating the care of combat casualties during operations Iraqi Freedom and Enduring Freedom. *J Trauma* 2011;71(1 Suppl):S62–S73.

Murray CK, Obremskey WT, Hsu JR et al. Prevention of infections associated with combat-related extremity injuries. *J Trauma* 2011;71:S235–S257.

Parker PJ. Pre-hospital antibiotic administration. *J R Army Med Corps* 2008 Mar;154(1):5–6.

Penn-Barwell JG, Fries CA, Sargeant ID et al. Aggressive soft tissue infections and amputation in military trauma patients. *J R Nav Med Serv* 2012;98(2):14–18.

Petersen K, Colyer MD, Hayes DK et al. Prevention of infections associated with combat-related eye, maxillofacial, and neck injuries. *J Trauma* 2011;71:S264–S269.

INTENSIVE CARE

Barnard EB, Mora AG, Bebarta VS. Preflight variables are associated with increased ventilator days and 30-day mortality in trauma casualties evacuated by critical care air transport teams: An exploratory retrospective study. *Mil Med* 2016 May;181(5Suppl):132–137.

Birch K. Who benefits from intensive care in the field? *J R Army Med Corps* 2009 Jun;155(2):122–124.

Brogden TG, Bunin J, Kwon H. Strategies for ventilation in acute, severe lung injury after combat trauma. *J R Army Med Corps* 2015 Mar;161(1):14–21.

Harris CC, McNicholas JJ. Paediatric intensive care in the field hospital. *J R Army Med Corps* 2009 Jun;155(2):157–159.

Henning DC, Smith JE, Patch D, Lambert AW. A comparison of civilian (National Confidential Enquiry into Patient Outcome and Death) trauma standards with current practice in a deployed field hospital in Afghanistan. *Emerg Med J* 2011 Apr;28(4):310–312.

Henning JD, Lockey DJ. The protection of critically ill patients in a military chemical warfare environment. *Resuscitation* 2005 Feb;64(2):237–239.

Henning J, Mellor A, Hoffman A, Mahoney P. Military intensive care part 3: Future directions. *J R Army Med Corps* 2007 Dec;153(4):288–290.

Henning J, Scott T, Price S. Nutrition of the critically ill patient in field hospitals on operations. *J R Army med Corps* 2008 Dec;154(4):279–281.

Henning J. The ethical dilemma of providing intensive care treatment to local civilians on operations. *J R Army Med Corps* 2009 Jun;155(2):84–86.

Hoffman A, Henning J, Mellor A, Mahoney PF. Military intensive care part 2: Current practice. *J R Army Med Corps* 2007 Dec;15(4):286–287.

Hutchings SD, Rees PSC. Trauma resuscitation using echocardiography in a deployed military intensive care unit. *J Intensive Care Soc* 2013 Apr;14(2):120–125.

Hutchings S, Howarth G, Rees P, Midwinter M. Conducting clinical research in the deployed intensive care unit: Challenges and solutions. *J R Nav Med Serv* 2013;99(3):151–315.

Hutchings S, Risdall J, Lowes T. Intensive care in the Defence Medical Services. *J Intensive Care Soc* 2014 Jan;15(1):24–27.

Inwald DP, Arul GS, Montgomery M et al. Management of children in the deployed intensive care unit at Camp Bastion, Afghanistan. *J R Army Med Corps* 2014 Sep;160(3):236–240.

Janson JO, Turner S, Johnston AM. Nutritional management of critically ill trauma patients in the deployed military setting. *J R Army Med Corps* 2011 Sep;157(3 Suppl 1):S344–S349.

Johnston AM. Focus on sepsis and intensive Care. *J R Army Med Corps* 2009 Jun;155(2):129–132.

Johnston AM, Henning JD. Outcomes of patients treated at Bastion Hospital Intensive Care Unit in 2009. *J R Army Med Corps* 2014 Dec;160(4):323.

Jones CPL, Chinery JP, England K, Mahoney P. Critical Care at Role 4. *J R Army Med Corps* 2010 Dec;156(Suppl 4):S342–S348.

Lockey DJ, Nordman GR, Field JM et al. The deployment of an intensive care facility with a military field hospital to the 2003 conflict in Iran. *Resuscitation* 2004 Sep;62(3):261–265.

Mackenzie I, Tunnicliffe B, Clasper J et al. What the intensive care doctor needs to know about blast-related lung injury. *J Intensive Care Soc* 2013 Oct;14(4):303–312.

McNicholas JJ, Henning JD. Major military trauma: Decision making in the ICU. *J R Army Med Corps* 2011 Sep;157(3 Suppl 1):S284–S288.

Morrison JJ, Ross JD, Poon H et al. Intraoperative correction of acidosis, coagulopathy and hypothermia in combat casualties with severe haemorrhagic shock. *Anaesthesia* 2013 Aug;68(8):846–850.

Nesbitt I, Almond M, Freshwater D. Renal Replacement in the Deployed Setting. *J R Army Med Corps* 2011;157:2 179–181.

Parent P, Trottier VJF, Bennet DR et al. Are IVC filters required in combat support hospitals? *J R Army Med Corps* 2009;155:210–212.

Ralph JK, Lowes T. Neurointensive care. *J R Army Med Corps* 2009 Jun;155(2):147–151.

Roberts MJ, Fox MA, Hamilton-Davies C. The experience of the intensive care unit in a British Army field hospital during the 2003 Gulf Conflict. *J R Army Med Corps* 2003;149:284–290.

Round J, Mellor A. Anaesthetic and critical care management of thoracic injury. *J R Army Med Corps* 2010 Sep;156(3):145–149.

Scott T, Davies M, Dutton C et al. Intensive care follow-up in UK military casualties: A one-year pilot. *J Intensive Care Soc* 2014;15(2):113–116.

Shah K, Pirie S, Compton L et al. Utilization profile of the trauma intensive care unit at the Role 3 Multinational Medical Unit at Kandahar Airfield between May 1 and Oct. 15, 2009. *Can J Surg* 2011 Dec;54(6):S130–S134.

Shirley P. Operational critical care, intensive care and trauma. *J R Army Med Corps* 2009;155(2):133–140.

Thornhill R, Tong JL, Birch K, Chauhan R. Field intensive care – Weaning and extubation. *JR Army Med Corps* 2010;156(4):S311–S317.

Turner S, Ruth M, Tipping R. Critical Care Air Support Teams and deployed intensive care. *J R Army Med Corps* 2009 Jun;155(2):171–174.

INTERNAL MEDICINE

Bailey MS. Medical and DNBI admissions to the Role 3 field hospital at Camp Bastion during Operation Herrick (letter). *J R Army Med Corps* 2016 Feb;162(1):76–77.

Bailey MS, Trinick TR, Dunbar JA et al. Undifferentiated febrile illnesses amongst British troops in Helmand, Afghanistan. *J R Army Med Corps* 2011 Jun;157(2):150–155.

Bailey MS, Davies GW, Freshwater DA, Timperley AC. Medical and DNBI admissions to the UK Role 3 field hospital in Iraq during Op TELIC (letter). *J R Army Med Corps* 2016 Aug;162(4):309.

Barnard EB, Baladurai S, Badh T, Nicol E. Challenges of managing toxic alcohol poisoning in a resource-limited setting. *J R Army Med Corps* 2014 Sep;160(3):245–250.

Bland DJ, Rona RJ, Coggon D et al. Urinary isotopic analysis in the UK Armed Forces: No evidence of depleted uranium absorption in combat and other personnel in Iraq. *Occup Environ Med* 2007 Jul;64(12):834–838.

Bolton JPG, Gilbert PH, Tamayo BCC. Heat illness on Operation Telic in summer 2003: The experience of the heat illness treatment unit in Northern Kuwait *J R Army Med Corps* 2006 Sep;152(3):148–155.

Bruce AS, Tunstall C, Boulter MJ, Coneybeare A. A treatment algorithm for mass heat casualties. *J R Army Med Corps* 2008 Mar;154(1):19–20.

Bullock C, Johnston AM. Upper extremity deep vein thrombosis in a military patient *J R Army Med Corps* 2016 Aug;162(4):299–301.

Connor P, DeLegge M. Ward based enteral and supplemental nutrition on operations. *J R Army Med Corps* 2008 Dec;154(4):276–278.

Cox AT, Lentaigne J, White S et al. A 2-year review of the general internal medicine admissions to the British Role 3 Hospital in Camp Bastion, Afghanistan. *J R Army Med Corps* 2016 Feb;162(1):56–62.

Cox AT, Linton TD, Bailey K et al. An evaluation of the burden placed on the general internal medicine team at the Role 3 Hospital In Camp Bastion by UK Armed Forces personnel presenting with symptoms resulting from previously identified disease. *J R Army Med Corps* 2016 Feb;162(1):18–22.

Craig DG, Adam MG, Proffitt A et al. Venous thromboembolism: Reducing the risk in a Role 3 setting. *J R Army Med Corps* 2014 Dec;160(4):304–309.

Grainge C, Heber M. The Role of The physician in modern military operations: 12 Months experience in Southern Iraq. *J R Army Med Corps* 2005 Jun;151(2):101–104.

Gutierrez RL, Goldberg M, Young P et al. Management of service members presenting with persistent and chronic diarrhea, during or upon returning from deployment. *Mil Med* 2012 Jun;177(6):627–634.

Hamilton S, Dickson SJ, Smith JE. Hyponatraemia on an operational deployment in southern Iraq-a case series. *J R Nav Med Serv* 2006;92(3):114–117.

Hill NE, Fallowfield JL, Delves SK et al. Changes in gut hormones and leptin in military personnel during operational deployment in Afghanistan. *Obesity* 2015 Mar;23(3):608–614.

Lamb L, Ross D, Lalloo D et al. Management of venomous bites and stings in British Military personnel deployed in Iraq, Afghanistan and Cyprus. *J R Army Med Corps* 2008 Dec:154 (4 Suppl):2–40.

Mitchell J, Simpson R, Whitaker J. Cold injuries in contemporary conflict. *J R Army Med Corps* 2012 Sep;158(3):248–251.

Nesbitt I, Almond M, Freshwater D. Renal replacement in the deployed setting. *J R Army Med Corps* 2011;157:179–181.

Newman ENC, Johnstone P, Hatch R et al. Undifferentiated febrile illnesses amongst British troops in Helmand, Afghanistan (letter with original authors' reply). *J R Army Med Corps* 2012;158(2):143–144.

Parent P, Trottier VJF, Bennet DR et al. Are IVC Filters Required in Combat Support Hospitals? *J R Army Med Corps* 2009;155:210–212.

Stacey M, Woods D, Ross D, Wilson D. Heat illness in military populations: Asking the right questions for research. *J R Army Med Corps* 2014;160(2):121–124.

Woods DR, Phillip R, Quinton R. Managing endocrine dysfunction following blast injury to the male external genitalia. *J R Army Med Corps* 2013 Mar;159(Suppl 1):45–48.

INTRAOSSEOUS ACCESS

Barnard EB, Moy RJ, Kehoe AD et al. Rapid sequence induction of anaesthesia via the intraosseous route: A prospective observational study. *Emerg Med J* 2015 Jun;32(6):449–452.

Barratt J, Re: Reasons for not using intraosseous access in critical illness (letter). *Emerg Med J* 2013 Jun;30(6):516–517.

Cooper BR, Mahoney PF, Hodgetts TJ, Mellor A. Intra-osseous access (EZ-IO®) for resuscitation: UK military combat experience. *J R Army Med Corps* 2007 Dec;153(4):314–316.

Fenton P, Bali N, Sargeant I, Jeffrey SL. A Complication of the use of an intra-osseous needle. *J R Army Med Corps* 2009 Jun;155(2):110–111.

Lewis P, Wright C. Saving the critically injured trauma patient: A retrospective analysis of 1000 uses of intraosseous access (abstract). *Emerg Med J* 2015 Jun;32(6):463–467.

Taylor DM, Bailey MS. A complication of the use of an intra-osseous needle (letter). *J R Army Med Corps* 2010;156(2):132.

Vassallo J, Horne S, Smith JE. Intra-osseous access in the military operational setting. *J R Nav Med Serv* 2014;100(1):34–37.

JUNCTIONAL TRAUMA

Parker P. Consensus statement on decision making in junctional trauma care; Limb Trauma Working Group. *J R Army Med Corps* 2011 Sep;157(3 Suppl 1):S293–S295.

Tai N, Dickson EJ. Military junctional trauma. *J R Army Med Corps* 2009;155(4):285–292.

Walker NM, Eardley W, Clasper JC. UK combat-related pelvic junctional vascular injuries 2008–2011: Implications for future intervention. *Injury* 2014 Oct;45(10):1585–1589.

LIMB (PERIPHERAL) TRAUMA

Barton SJ, Kaleel S, Rayatt S, Peart F. Healing hands: Management of a shrapnel wound injury in the dominant hand of a serviceman, sustained in the Iraq conflict (abstract). *J R Army Med Corps* 2005 Mar;151(2):108.

Beech Z, Parker P. Internal fixation on deployment: Never, ever, clever? *J R Army Med Corps* 2012 Mar;158(1):4–5.

Belmont PJ, McCriskin BJ, Hsiao MS et al. The nature and incidence of Musculoskeletal combat wounds in Iraq and Afghanistan (2005–2009). *J Orthop Trauma* 2013 May;27(5):e107–e113.

Birch R, Misra P, Stewart MP et al. Nerve injuries sustained during warfare: Part I: Epidemiology. *J Bone Joint Surg Br* 2012 Apr;94(4):523–528.

Birch R, Misra P, Stewart MP et al. Nerve injuries sustained during warfare: Part II: Outcomes. *J Bone Joint Surg Br* 2012 Apr;94(4):529–535.

Boyd MC, Mountain AJ, Clasper JC. Improvised skeletal traction in the management of ballistic femoral fractures. *J R Army Med Corps* 2009 Sep;155(3):194–196.

Brown KV, Tai N, Midwinter M, Clasper JC. Ballistic extremity vascular injuries. Abstract – Military surgery 2008. *J R Army Med Corps* 2008 Sep;154(3):188.

Brown KV, Ramasamy, A, Tai N, Clasper J. Complications of Extremity Vascular Injuries in Conflict. *J Trauma* 2009 Apr;66(4):S145–S149.

Brown KV, Dharm-Datta S, Potter BK et al. Comparison of development of heterotopic ossification in injured US and UK Armed Services personnel with combat-related amputations: Preliminary findings and hypotheses regarding causality. *J Trauma* 2010 Jul;69(1):S116–S122.

Brown KV, Murray KC, Clasper JC Infectious complications of combat-related mangled extremity injuries in the British Military. *J Trauma* 2010 Jul;69(1):S109–S115.

Brown KV, Henman P, Stapley S, Clasper JC. Limb salvage of severely injured extremities after military wounds. *J R Army Med Corps* 2011 Sep;157(3 Suppl 1):S315–S323.

Clasper JC, Phillips SL. Early failure of external fixation in the management of war injuries. *J R Army Med Corps* 2005 Jun;151(2):81–86.

Clasper JC, Standley D, Heppell S et al. Limb compartment syndrome and fasciotomy. *J R Army Med Corps* 2009 Dec;155(4):298–301.

Clasper JC, Aldington D. Regional anaesthesia, ballistic limb trauma and acute compartment syndrome (editorial). *J R Army Med Corps* 2010 Jun;156(2):77–78.

Clasper J, Standley D, Heppell D et al. The use of compression bandaging in fasciotomy wounds. *Wounds* 2012 Apr;8(1):89–94.

Cross AM, Davis C, Penn-Barwell J et al. The incidence of pelvic fractures with traumatic lower limb amputation in modern warfare due to improvised explosive devices. *J R Nav Med Serv* 2014;100(2):152–156.

Dharm-Datta S, Hill G. Improvised equipment for skeletal traction on operations. *J R Army Med Corps* 2007 Jun;153(2):144.

Eardley WG. The combination tool: A significant cause of morbidity in deployed personnel. *J R Army Med Corps* 2005 Mar;151(1):59.

Eardley WG, Stewart MP. Early management of ballistic hand trauma. *J Am Acad Orthop Surg* 2010 Feb;18(2):118–126.

Eardley WG, Taylor DM, Parker PJ. Amputation and the assessment of limb viability: Perceptions of two hundred and thirty two orthopaedic trainees. *Ann R Coll Surg Engl* 2010 Jul;92(5):411–416.

Eardley WG, Watts SA, Clasper JC. Limb wounding and antisepsis: Iodine and chlorhexidine in the early management of extremity injury. *Int J Low Extrem Wounds* 2012 Sep;11(3):213–223.

Foong DPS, Jose RM, Jeffery S, Titley OG. Fasciotomy: A call for proper placement. *The Surgeon* 2011 Oct;9(5):249–254.

Foong DP, Evriviades D, Jeffery SL. Integra™ permits early durable coverage of improvised explosive device (IED) amputation stumps. *J Plast Reconstr Aesthet Surg* 2013 Dec;66(12):1717–1724.

Guthrie HC, Clasper JC, Kay AR, Parker PJ; Limb trauma and wounds working groups. Initial extremity war wound debridement: A multidisciplinary consensus. *J R Army Med Corps* 2011 Jun;157(2):170–175.

Guyver PM, Baden JM, Standley DM, Stewart M. The management of hand injuries in a Role 2 enhanced or Role 3 facility: Part 2. *J R Nav Med Serv* 2012;98(1):29–33.

Guyver PM, Mountain AJC, Jeffery SLA. Application of topical negative pressure for traumatic amputations. *Ann R Coll Surg Engl* 2013 Apr;95(3):226–227.

Hanna K, Jeffery S. Radial forearm flaps as durable soft tissue coverage for local nationals being treated in the field hospital setting. *J R Army Med Corps* 2013 Mar;159(1):21–23.

Hinsley DE, Phillips SL, Clasper JS. Ballistic fractures during the 2003 Gulf Conflict – Early prognosis and high complication rate. *J R Army Med Corps* 2006 Jun;152(2):96–101.

Jacobs N, Rourke K, Hicks A et al. Lower limb injuries caused by improvised explosive devices: Proposed "Bastion" classification and prospective validation. *Injury* 2014 Sep;45(9):1422–1428.

Jansen JO, Thomas GOR, Adams SA et al. Early management of proximal traumatic lower extremity amputation and pelvic injury caused by improvised explosive devices (IEDs). *Injury* 2012 Jul;43(7):976–979.

Jeffery SLA. Advanced wound therapies in the management of severe military lower limb trauma: A new perspective. *Eplast* 2009 Jul;9(28):266–277.

Jeffrey S, Fries A. Hand fasciotomies in military trauma (abstract). *J R Army Med Corps* 2010 Sep;156(3):182.

Ladlow P, Phillip R, Etherington J et al. Functional and Mental Health Status of United Kingdom Military Amputees Post Rehabilitation. *Arch Phys Med Rehabil* 2015 Nov;96(11):2048–2054.

Middleton S, Clasper J, Compartment syndrome of the foot – Implications for military surgeons. *J R Army Med Corps* 2010 Dec;156(4):241–244.

Mitchell J, Simpson R, Whitaker J. Cold injuries in contemporary conflict. *J R Army Med Corps* 2012 Sep;158(3):248–251.

Morrison JJ, Hunt N, Midwinter M, Jansen J. Associated injuries in casualties with traumatic lower extremity amputations caused by improvised explosive devices. *Br J Surg* 2012 Mar;99(3):362–366.

Morrison JJ, Rasmussen TE, Midwinter MJ, Jansen JO. Authors' reply: Associated injuries in casualties with traumatic lower extremity amputations caused by improvised explosive devices (letter). *Br J Surg* 2012 Jul;99:1021.

Neal PK. An exploration of the experiences of wound healing in military traumatic amputees and its impact on their rehabilitation. *J R Army Med Corps* 2015;161(Suppl):i64–i68.

Penn-Barwell JG, Bennett PM, Powers D Standley D. Isolated hand injuries on operational deployment: An examination of epidemiology and treatment strategy. *Mil Med* 2011;176(12):1404–1407.

Penn-Barwell JG, Fries CA, Sargeant ID et al. Aggressive Soft Tissue Infections and Amputation in Military Trauma Patients. *J R Nav Med Serv* 2012;98(2):14–18.

Penn-Barwell JG, Bennett PM, Fries CA et al. Severe open tibial fractures in combat trauma: Management and preliminary outcomes. *Bone Joint J* 2013;95-B:101–105.

Penn-Barwell JG, Myatt RW, Bennett PM et al. Medium-term outcomes following limb salvage for severe open tibia fracture are similar to trans-tibial amputation. *Injury* 2015 Feb;46(2):288–291.

Poon H, Morrison JJ, Clasper JC et al. Use and complications of operative control of arterial inflow in combat casualties with traumatic lower-extremity amputations caused by improvised explosive devices. *J Trauma Acute Care Surg* 2013 Aug;75(2 Suppl 2):S233–S237.

Ramalingam T. Extremity injuries remain a high surgical workload in a conflict zone: Experiences of a British Field hospital In Iraq, 2003. *J R Army Med Corps* 2004;150:187–190.

Ramasamy A, Hill AM, Phillip R. The modern "deck-slap" injury – Calcaneal blast fractures from vehicle explosions. *J Trauma* 2011 Dec;71(6):1694–1698.

Ramasamy A, Hill AM, Phillip R et al. FASS is a better predictor of poor outcome in lower limb blast injury than AIS: Implications for blast research. *J Orthop Trauma* 2013 Jan;27(1):49–55.

Rowlands TK, Clasper J. The Thomas splint– a necessary tool in the management of battlefield injuries. *J R Army Med Corps* 2003;149(4):291–293.

Stannard A Burkhardt G, Keltz et al. Quality of limb salvage following wartime extremity vascular injury: Results of a novel patient-based outcomes study (abstract). *J R Army Med Corps* 2010;156(3):178.

Staruch RM, Jackson PC, Hodson J et al. Comparing the surgical timelines of military and civilians traumatic lower limb amputations. *Ann Med Surg (Lond)* 2016 Feb;6:81–86.

Taylor CJ, Hettiaratchy S, Jeffery SL et al. Contemporary approaches to definitive extremity reconstruction of military wounds. *J R Army Med Corps* 2009 Dec;155(4):302–307.

Taylor CJ, Chester DL, Jeffery SL. Functional splinting of upper limb injuries with gauze-based topical negative pressure wound therapy. *J Hand Surg Am* 2011 Nov;36(11):1848–1851.

Trull B, Hearn M, Jeffery S. Residual limb hyperhidrosis: Use of botulinum-A toxin to improve prosthesis fit and function. *Wounds UK* 2011;7:92–97.

Wesson M. Lessons learnt from America – Reflections from a fellowship examining the prevention, recognition and treatment of operational stress injuries in US Army serving personnel. *J R Nav Med Serv* 2010;96(3):175–184.

MAJOR INCIDENTS, MASS GATHERINGS AND TRIAGE

Clarke JE, Davis PR. Medical evacuation and triage of combat casualties in Helmand Province, Afghanistan: October 2010–April 2011. *Mil Med* 2012 Nov;177(11):1261–1266.

Cross JD, Wenke JC, Ficke JR, Johnson AE. Data-driven disaster management requires data: Implementation of a military orthopaedic trauma registry. *J Surg Orthop Adv* 2011 Spring;20(1):56–61.

Doughty, HA, Frith, L. and Harris, C. The demand for group O blood in a mass casualty situation. *Transfus Med* 2005;15(Suppl 1):4. SI07.

Doughty H, Glasgow S, Kristoffersen E. Mass casualty events: Blood transfusion emergency preparedness across the continuum of care. *Transfusion* 2016 Apr;56(Suppl 2):S208–S216.

Evans GW. Receiving mass casualties at sea: The capabilities of the Primary Casualty receiving facility. *J R Nav Med Serv* 2004;90(2):51–56.

Gibb I, Denton E. Guidelines for the use of computed tomography (CT) in the postmortem – Investigation of deaths in a mass casualty scenario. *NHS Improvements June 2011*.

Gibb I, Denton E. Guidelines for imaging the injured blast/ballistic patient in a mass casualty scenario. *NHS Improvements 2011*.

Glasgow SM, Allard S, Rackham R, Doughty H. Going for gold: Blood planning for the London 2012 Olympic Games. *Transfus Med* 2014 Jun;24(3):145–153.

Horne S, Vassallo J, Read J, Ball S. UK triage – An improved tool for an evolving threat. *Injury* 2013 Jan;44(1):23–28.

Horne ST, Vassallo J. Triage in the Defence Medical Services. *J R Army Med Corps* 2015 Jun;161(2):90–93.

Morrison JJ, Dickson EJ, Jansen JO, Midwinter MJ. Utility of admission physiology in the surgical triage of isolated ballistic battlefield torso trauma. *J Emerg Trauma Shock* 2012 Jul;5(3):233–237.

Nordmann GR, Woolley T. Unusual critical incident: Chemical gas alert. *Anaesthesia* 2003;58:926.

Potter D, Kehoe A, Smith JE. The sensitivity of pre-hospital and in-hospital tools for the identification of major trauma patients presenting to a major trauma centre. *J R Nav Med Serv* 2013;99(1):16–19.

Reynolds ND, Dalal S. An account of multiple casualties in an austere environment. *J R Army Med Corps* 2012;158:181–185.

Ross RA, Selwood P. Multiple casualties in the Bastion UK role 3 hospital: Personal reflections on the positive evolution of deployed military hospital care. *J R Nav Med Serv* 2014;100(2):210–214.

Russell R, Hodgetts TJ, Mahoney PF, Russell M. An international approach to disaster preparedness and response for both military and civilian environment. *Int Rev Armed Forces Med Serv* 2007:80(3);161–165.

Smith JE, Vassallo J. Major incident triage: The civilian validation of the modified physiological triage tool. *Emerg Med J* 2016;33(12):908.

Thomas R, Woolley T, Doughty H. Guidelines on massive transfusion. Emergency guidelines for ACDS(H) on behalf of DoH. Preparation for 2012 Olympics. 2012.

Vassallo DJ, Gerlinger T, Maholtz P et al. Combined UK/US Field Hospital management of a major incident arising from a Chinook helicopter crash In Afghanistan, 28 Jan 2002 *J R Army Med Corps* 2003;149:47–52.

Vassallo J, Horne ST, Ball S et al. Usefulness of the Shock Index as a secondary triage tool. *J R Army Med Corps* 2014 May;161(1):53–57.

Vassallo J, Horne S, Ball S, Whiteley J UK Triage – The validation of a new tool for an evolving threat *Injury* 2014;45(12):2071–2075.

MENTAL HEALTH

Azari J, Dandeker C, Greenberg N. Cultural stress: How interactions with and among foreign populations affect military personnel. *Armed Forces Soc* 2010 Jan;36(4):585–603.

Banwell E, Greenberg N, Smith P et al. What happens to the mental health of UK service personnel after they return home from Afghanistan? *J R Army Med Corps* 2016 Apr;162(2):115–119.

Boos CJ, Croft AM. Smoking rates in the staff of a military field hospital before and after wartime deployment. *J R Soc Med* 2004 Jan;97(1):20–22.

Brunger H, Ogden J, Malia K et al. Adjusting to persistent post-concussive symptoms following mild traumatic brain injury and subsequent psycho-educational intervention: A qualitative analysis in military personnel. *Brain Inj* 2014;28(1):71–80.

Browne T, Iversen A, Hull L et al. How do experiences in Iraq affect alcohol use amongst male UK Armed Forces personnel? *Occup Environ Med* 2008 Sep;65(9):628–633.

Buckman JEJ, Sundin J, Greene T et al. The impact of deployment length on the health and well-being of military personnel: A systematic review of the literature. *Occup Environ Med* 2011 Jan;68(1):69–76.

Buckman J, Forbes H, Clayton T et al. Early service leavers: A study of the factors associated with premature separation from the UK Armed Forces and the mental health of those that leave early. *Eur J Public Health* 2013 Jun;23(3):410–415.

Bull S, Thandi G, Keeling M et al. Medical and Welfare Officers beliefs about post-deployment screening for mental health disorders in the UK Armed Forces: A qualitative study. *BMC Public Health* 2015 Apr;15:338.

Burdett H, Jones N, Fear NT et al. Early psychosocial intervention following operational deployment: Analysis of a free text questionnaire response. *Mil Med* 2011 Jun;176(6):620–625.

Burdett H, Fear NT, Jones N et al. Use of a two-phase process to identify possible cases of mental ill health in the UK military. *Int J Methods Psychiatr Res* 2016 Sep;25(3):168–177.

Campion BH, Hacker-Hughes JG, Devon M et al. Psychological morbidity during the 2002 deployment to Afghanistan. *J R Army Med Corps* 2006 Jun;152(2):91–93.

Campion B, Jones N, Keeling M et al. Cohesion, Leadership, Mental Health Stigmatisation and Perceived Barriers to Care in UK Military Personnel. *J Ment Health* 2016 Jun;20:1–9.

Campion, BH Jones, N, Wessely, S. Greenberg, N. Mental health and psychological support in UK armed forces personnel deployed to Afghanistan and Iraq 2009–2014. *J Ment Health* In press.

Cawkill P, Jones M, Fear NT et al. Mental health of UK Armed Forces medical personnel post-deployment. *Occup Med (Lond)* 2015 Mar;65(2):157–164.

Coetzee RH, Simpson RG, Greenberg N. Detecting post-deployment mental health problems in primary care. *J R Army Med Corps* 2010 Sep;156(3):196–199.

Cohn S, Dyson C, Wessely S. Early accounts of Gulf War illness and the construction of narratives in UK service personnel. *Soc Sci Med* 2008 Dec;67(11):1641–1649.

Dandeker C, Wessely S, Iversen A et al. What's in a Name? Defining and caring for 'veterans': The United Kingdom in International Perspective. *Armed Forces Soc* 2006 Jan;32(2):161–177.

Dandeker C. from victory to success: The changing mission of western armed forces. In Angstrom J, Duyvesteyn I (eds.). *Modern War and the Utility of Force*. Oxon: Routledge, 2010, pp. 16–38. ISBN: 978-0415622349.

Dandeker, C. What "success" means in Afghanistan Iraq and Libya. In Burk J. (ed.). *How 911 Changed Our Ways of War*. Stanfrod, CA: Stanford University Press, 2015, pp. 116–148.

Debell F, Fear NT, Head M, Batt-Rawden S et al. A Systematic review of the comorbidity between PTSD and alcohol misuse. *Soc Psychiatry Psychiatr Epidemiol* 2014 Sep;49(9):1401–1425.

De Burgh HT, White CJ, Fear NT, Iversen AC. The impact of deployment to Iraq or Afghanistan on partners and wives of military personnel. *Int Rev Psychiatry* 2011 Apr;23(2):192–200.

Du Preez J, Sundin J, Wessely S, Fear NT. Unit cohesion and mental health in the UK Armed Forces. *Occup Med (Lond)* 2012 Jan;62(1):47–53.

Fear N, Iversen A, Chatterjee A et al. Risky driving among regular Armed Forces personnel from the United Kingdom. *Am J Prev Med* 2008 Aug;35:230–236.

Fear NT, Jones M, Murphy D et al. What are the consequences of deployment to Iraq and Afghanistan on the mental health of the UK Armed Forces? A cohort study. *Lancet* 2010 May;375(9728):1783–1797.

Fear NT, Sundin J, Wessely S. What is the impact on mental health and wellbeing of military service in general and deployment in particular? A UK perspective. In: Venables KM (ed.). *Current Topics in Occupational Epidemiology*. Oxford University Press, 2013.

Fertout M, Jones N, Greenberg N et al. A review of United Kingdom Armed Forces' approaches to prevent post-deployment mental health problems. *Int Rev Psychiatry* 2011 Apr;23(2):135–143.

Fertout M, Jones N, Greenberg N. Third location decompression for individual augmentees after a military deployment. *Occup Med (Lond)* 2012 Apr;62(3):188–195.

Fertout M, Jones N, Keeling M, Greenberg N. Mental health stigmatisation in deployed UK Armed Forces: A principal components analysis. *J R Army Med Corps* 2015 Dec;161(Suppl 1): i69–i76.

Foran HM, Garber BG, Zamorski MA et al. Post-deployment military mental health training: Cross-national evaluations. *Psychol Serv* 2013 May;10(2):152–160.

Forbes HJ, Fear NT, Iversen A, Dandeker C. The mental health of UK Armed Forces personnel: The impact of Iraq and Afghanistan. *RUSI J* 2011 May;156(2):14–20.

Forbes HJ, Jones N, Woodhead C et al. What are the effects of having an illness or injury whilst deployed on post deployment mental health? A population based record linkage study of UK Army personnel who have served in Iraq or Afghanistan. *BMC Psychiatry* 2012 Oct;12:178.

Forbes HJ, Boyd CF, Jones N et al. Attitudes to mental illness in the U.K. Military: A comparison with the general population. *Mil Med* 2013 Sep;178(9):957–965.

Frappell-Cooke W, Gulina M, Green K et al. Does trauma risk management reduce psychological distress in deployed troops? *Occup Med (Lond)* 2010 Dec;60(8):645–665.

Frappell-Cooke W, Wink P, Wood A. The psychological challenge of genital injury. *J R Army Med Corps* 2013 Mar;159(Suppl 1):i52–i56.

Goodwin L, Jones M, Rona RJ et al. Prevalence of delayed-onset posttraumatic stress disorder in military personnel: Is there evidence for this disorder? Results of a prospective UK cohort study. *J Nerv Ment Dis* 2012 May;200(5):430–437.

Goodwin L, Ben-Zion I, Fear NT et al. Are reports of psychological stress higher in occupational studies? A systematic review across occupational and population based studies. *PLoS One* 2013 Nov;8(11):e78693.

Goodwin L, Bourke JH, Forbes H et al. Irritable bowel syndrome in the UK military after deployment to Iraq: What are the risk factors? *Soc Psychiatry Psychiatr Epidemiol* 2013 Nov;48(11):1755–1765.

Goodwin L, Rona RJ. PTSD in the armed forces: What have we learned from the recent cohort studies of Iraq/Afghanistan? *J Ment Health* 2013 Oct;22(5):397–401.

Goodwin L, Wessely S, Fear NT. The future of "big data" in suicide behaviors research: Can we compare the experiences of the U.S. and U.K. Armed Forces. *Psychiatry* 2015;78(1):25–28.

Goodwin L, Wessely S, Hotopf M et al. Are common mental disorders more prevalent in the UK serving military compared to the general population? *Psychol Med* 2015 Jul;45(9):1881–1891.

Gould M, Greenberg N and Hetherton J. Stigma and the military: Evaluation of a PTSD Psychoeducational Program. *J Trauma Stress* 2007 Aug;20(4):505–515.

Gould M, Sharpley J, Greenberg N. Patient characteristics and clinical activities at a British military department of community mental health. *Br J Psych Bull* 2008;32:99–102.

Gould M, Adler A, Zamorski M et al. Do stigma and other perceived barriers to mental health care differ across Armed Forces? *J R Soc Med* 2010 Apr;103(4):148–156.

Gould M, Meeks D, Gibbs T et al. What are the psychological effects of delivering and receiving 'high-risk' survival resistance training? *Mil Med* 2015 Feb;180(2):168–177.

Greenberg N, Cawkill P, Sharpley J. How to TRiM away at post traumatic stress reactions: Traumatic risk management-now and the future. *J R Nav Med Serv* 2005;91(1):26–31.

Greenberg N, Browne T, Langston V, McAllister P. Operational mental health: A user's guide for medical staff. *J R Nav Med Serv* 2007;93(1):5–11.

Greenberg N, Henderson A, Langston V et al. Peer responses to perceived stress in the Royal Navy. *Occup Med (Lond)* 2007 Sep;57(6):424–429.

Greenberg N, Langston V, Gould M. Culture – What is its effect on stress in the military? *Mil Med* 2007;172:931–935.

Greenberg N, Thomas, S, Murphy D, Dandeker C. Occupational stress and job satisfaction in media personnel assigned to the Iraq War (2003): A qualitative study. *Journalism Pract* 2007 Sep;1(3):356–371.

Greenberg N, Langston V, Jones N. Trauma risk management (TRiM) in the UK Armed Forces. *J R Army Med Corps* 2008 Jul;154(2):124–127.

Greenberg N, Fear N, Jones E. Medically unexplained symptoms in military personnel. *Psychiatry* 2009 May;8(5):170–173.

Greenberg N, Langston V, Fear NT et al. An evaluation of stress education in the Royal Navy. *Occup Med (Lond)* 2009 Jan;59(1):20–24.

Greenberg N, Wessely S. The dangers of inflation: Memories of trauma and post-traumatic stress disorder. *Br J Psychiatry* 2009 Jun;194(6):479–480.

Greenberg N, Langston V, Everitt B et al. A cluster randomised controlled trial to determine the efficacy of Trauma Risk Management (TRiM) in a military population. *J Trauma Stress* 2010 Aug;23(4):430–436.

Greenberg N, Jones E, Jones N et al. The injured mind in the UK Armed Forces. *Philos Trans R Soc Lond B Biol Sci* 2011 Jan;366(1562):261–267.

Greenberg N, Langston V, Iversen A and Wessely. S. The acceptability of "Trauma Risk Management (TRiM)" within the UK Armed Forces. *Occup Med (Lond)* 2011 May;61(3):184–189.

Greenberg N. What's so special about military veterans? *Int Psych* 2014;11(2):79–80.

Greene T, Buckman J, Dandeker C, Greenberg N. The influence of culture clash on deployed troops. *Mil Med* 2010 Dec;175(12):958–963.

Greene T, Greenberg N, Buckman J, Dandeker C. How communication with families can both help and hinder service members' mental health and occupational effectiveness on deployment. *Mil Med* 2010 Oct;175(10):745–749.

Gribble R, Wessely S, Klein S et al. Public awareness of UK veterans' charities. *RUSI J* 2014 Feb;159(1):50–57.

Hacker-Hughes J, Cameron F, Eldridge R et al. Going to war does not have to hurt: Preliminary findings from the British deployment to Iraq. *Br J Psych* 2005;186:536–537.

Hacker-Hughes J, Abdul-Hamid WK, Fossey MJ. Flash to bang: Psychological trauma, veterans and military families: Can services cope? *J R Army Med Corps* 2015 Dec;161(4):298–299.

Harrison J, Sharpley J, Greenberg N. The management of post-traumatic stress reactions in the military. *J R Army Med Corps* 2008 Jun;154(2):110–114.

Harvey SB, Hatch SL, Jones M et al. The long-term consequences of military deployment: A 5-year cohort study of United Kingdom reservists deployed to Iraq in 2003. *Am J Epidemiol* 2012 Dec;176(12):1177–1184.

Hatch S, Harvey S, Dandeker C et al. Life in and after the Armed Forces: Social networks and the mental health in the UK military. *Sociol Health Illn* 2013 Sep;35(7):1045–1064.

Head M, Goodwin L, Debell, F et al. Posttraumatic stress disorder and alcohol misuse: Comorbidity in UK military personnel. *Soc Psychiatry Psychiatr Epidemiol* 2016 Feb;51(8):1171–1180.

Henderson A, Greenberg N, Langston V et al. Peer responses to perceived stress in the Royal Navy. *Occup Med (Lond)* 2007 Sep;57(6):424–429.

Henderson A, Langston V, Greenberg N. Alcohol misuse in the Royal Navy. *Occup Med* 2009;59:25–31.

Hibberd J, Greenberg N. Coping with the impact of working in a conflict zone: A comparative study of diplomatic staff. *J Occup Environ Med* 2011 Apr;53(4):352–357.

Hicks T, Banks R, Fear NT, Greenberg N. Acceptability of anxiety management within UK armed forces. *Occup Med (Lond)* 2013 Sep;63(6):439–441.

Hines LA, Goodwin L, Jones M et al. Factors affecting help seeking for mental health problems after deployment to Iraq and Afghanistan. *Psychiatr Serv* 2014 Jan;65(1):98–105.

Hines LA, Sundin J, Rona RJ et al. Posttraumatic stress disorder post Iraq and Afghanistan: Prevalence among military subgroups. *Can J Psychiatry* 2014 Sep;59(9):468–479.

Hooper R, Rona, R, Jones M et al. Cigarette and alcohol use in the UK Armed Forces, and their association with combat exposure: A prospective study. *Addict Behav* 2008 Aug;33(8):1067–1071.

Horn O, Hull L, Jones, M et al. Is there an Iraq War Syndrome? Comparison of the health of UK service personnel after the Gulf and Iraq Wars. *Lancet* 2006 May;367(9524):1742–1746.

Hotopf M. Hull L, Fear N et al. The health of UK military personnel who deployed to the 2003 Iraq War: A cohort study. *Lancet* 2006 May;367(9524):1731–1741.

Hotopf M, Wessely S. Neuropsychological changes following military service in Iraq: Case proven, but what is the significance? *JAMA* 2006 Aug;296(5):574–575.

Hughes JG, Earnshaw M, Greenberg N et al. The use of psychological decompression in military operational environments. *Mil Med* 2008 Jun;173(6):534–538.

Hunt EJF, Wessely S, Jones N et al. The mental health of the UK Armed Forces: Where facts meet fiction. *Eur J Psychotraumatol* 2014 Aug;5:23617.

Iversen A, Nicolaou V, Greenberg N et al. What happens to British veterans when they leave the Armed Forces? *Eur J Public Health* 2005 Apr;15(2):175–184.

Iversen A, Dyson C, Smith N et al. "Goodbye and good luck": The mental health needs and treatment experiences of British ex Service personnel. *Br J Psychiatry* 2005 Jun;186:480–486.

Iversen A, Liddell K, Fear N et al. Consent, Confidentiality and the Data Protection Act: Epidemiological research and hard-to-engage cohorts. *Br Med J* 2006 Jan;332(7534):165–169.

Iversen A, Fear N, Simonoff E et al. Pre-enlistment vulnerability factors and their influence on health outcomes in UK Military personnel. *Br J Psychiatr* 2007;191:506–511.

Iversen AC, Fear NT, Ehlers A et al. Risk factors for post-traumatic stress disorder amongst UK Armed Forces Personnel. *Psychol Med* 2008 Apr;38(4):511–522.

Iversen A, Greenberg N. Mental health of regular and reserve military veterans. *Adv Psychiatr Treat* 2009;15:100–106.

Iversen AC, Van Staden L, Hacker-Hughes J et al. The prevalence of common mental disorders and PTSD in the UK military: Using data from a clinical interview based study. *BMC Psychiatry* 2009 Oct;9:68–79.

Iversen A, Van Staden L, Hughes JH et al. Help seeking and receipt of treatment among United Kingdom Service Personnel. *Br J Psychiatry* 2010 Aug;197(2):149–155.

Iversen AC, Van Staden L, Hacker Hughes J et al. The stigma of mental health problems and other barriers to care in the UK Armed Forces. *BMC Health Serv Res* 2011;11:31.

Jones E, Fear NT. Alcohol use and misuse within the military: A review. *Int Rev Psychiatry* 2011 Apr;23(2):166–172.

Jones E, Fear NT, Wessely S. Shell shock and mild traumatic brain injury: A historical review. *Am J Psychiatr* 2007 Nov;164(11):1641–1645.

Jones M, Fear N, Greenberg N et al. Do medical services personnel who deployed to the Iraq War have worse mental health than other deployed personnel? *Eur J Public Health* 2008 Aug;18(4):422–427.

Jones M, Rona R, Hooper R, Wessely S. The burden of psychological symptoms in UK Armed Forces. *Occup Environ Med* 2006 Aug;56(5):322–328.

Jones M, Sundin J, Goodwin L et al. What explains post-traumatic stress disorder (PTSD) in UK service personnel: Deployment or something else? *Psychol Med* 2013 Aug;43(8):1703–1712.

Jones N, Greenberg N, Fear, NT et al. The operational mental health consequences of deployment to Iraq for UK Forces. *J R Army Med Corps* 2008 Jun;154(2):102–106.

Jones N, Fear N, Greenberg N et al. Occupational outcomes in soldiers hospitalized with mental health problems. *Occup Med (Lond)* 2009 Oct;59(7):459–465.

Jones N, Fear NT, Jones M et al. Long-term military work outcomes in soldiers who become mental health casualties when deployed on operations. *Psychiatry* 2010 Winter;73(4):352–364.

Jones N, Burdett H, Wessely S, Greenberg N. The subjective utility of early psychosocial interventions following combat deployment. *Occup Med (Lond)* 2011 Mar;61(2):102–107.

Jones N, Seddon R Fera NT et al. Leadership, cohesion, morale and the mental health of UK Armed Forces in Afghanistan. *Psychiatry* 2012 Spring;75(1):49–59.

Jones N, Fertout M, Parsloe L, Greenberg N. An evaluation of the psychological impact of operational rest and recuperation in United Kingdom Armed Forces personnel: A post-intervention survey. *J R Soc Med* 2013 Nov;106(11):447–455.

Jones N, Jones M, Fear NT et al. Can mental health and readjustment be improved in UK military personnel by a brief period of structured post-deployment rest (third location decompression)? *Occup Environ Med* 2013 Jul;70(7):439–445.

Jones N, Twardzicki M, Fertout M et al. Mental Health, Stigmatising beliefs, barriers to care and help-seeking in a non-deployed sample of UK army personnel. *Psychol Psychother* 2013 Jan;3:129.

Jones N, Fear NT, Rona R et al. Mild traumatic brain injury (mTBI) among UK military personnel whilst deployed in Afghanistan in 2011. *Brain Inj* 2014;28(7):896–899.

Jones N, Mitchell P, Clack J et al. Mental health and psychological support in UK armed forces personnel deployed to Afghanistan in 2010 and 2011. *Br J Psychiatry* 2014 Feb;204(2):157–162.

Jones N, Thandi G, Fear NT et al. The psychological effects of improvised explosive devices (IEDs) on UK military personnel in Afghanistan. *Occup Environ Med* 2014 Jul;71(7):466–471.

Jones N, Twardzicki M, Ryan J et al. Modifying attitudes to mental health using comedy as a delivery medium. *Soc Psychiatry Psychiatr Epidemiol* 2014 Oct;49(10):1667–1676.

Jones N, Greenberg N. The use of Threshold Assessment Grid triage (TAG-triage) in mental health assessment. *J R Army Med Corps* 2015 Dec;161(Suppl 1):i46-i51.

Jones N, Keeling M, Thandi G, Greenberg N. Stigmatisation, perceived barriers to care, help seeking and the mental health of British Military personnel. *Soc Psychiatry Psychiatr Epidemiol* 2015 Dec;50(12):1873–1883.

Jones N, Campion B, Keeling M, Greenberg N. Cohesion, leadership, mental health stigmatisation and perceived barriers to care in UK military personnel. *J Ment Health* 2016 Jun;27:1–9.

Keeling M, Knight T, Sharp D et al. Contrasting beliefs about screening for mental disorders among UK military personnel returning from deployment to Afghanistan. *J Med Screen* 2012 Dec;19(4):206–211.

Keeling M, Wessely S, Dandeker C et al. Relationship difficulties among UK Military personnel: The impact of socio-demographic, military and deployment-related factors. *Marriage Fam Rev* 2015 Apr;51(3):275–303.

Keeling M, Woodhead C, Fear N. Interpretative phenomenological analysis of soldier's experience of being married and serving in the British Army. *Marriage Fam Rev* 2016 Jan;52(6):511–534.

Keller RT, Greenberg N, Bobo WV et al. Soldier peer mentoring care and support: Bringing psychological awareness to the front. *Mil Med* 2005 May;170(5):355–361.

Kennedy I, Whybrow D, Jones N et al. A service evaluation of self-referral to military mental health teams. *Occup Med (Lond)* 2016 Jul;66(5):394–398.

Kramer J, Green AD. Thinking outside of the box. *Health Protection Matters: The Magazine of the Health Protection Agency* 2005;3:8–9.

Langston V, Greenberg N, Fear N et al. Stigma and mental health in the Royal Navy: A mixed methods paper. *J Ment Health* 2010 Feb;19(1):8–16.

Lucas PA, Page PR, Phillip RD, Bennett AN. The impact of genital trauma on wounded servicemen: Qualitative study. *Injury* 2014 May;45(5):825–829.

MacManus D, Wessely S. Why do some ex-armed forces personnel end up in prison? *BMJ* 2011 Jun;342:d3898.

MacManus D, Dean K, Al Bakir M et al. Violent behaviour in UK military personnel returning home after deployment. *Psychol Med* 2012 Aug;42(8):1663–1673.

MacManus D, Dean K, Iversen A et al. Influence of pre-enlistment antisocial behaviour on behavioural outcomes among UK military personnel. *Soc Psychiatry Psychiatr Epidemiol* 2012;47:1353–1358.

MacManus D, Dean K, Jones M et al. Violent offending by UK military personnel deployed to Iraq and Afghanistan: A data linkage cohort study. *Lancet* 2013 Mar;381(9870):907–917.

MacManus D, Wessely S. Veteran mental health services in the UK: Are we headed in the right direction? *J Ment Health* 2013 Aug;22(4):301–305.

MacManus D, Fossey M, Watson S, Wessely S. Former Armed Forces personnel in the criminal justice system. *Lancet Psychiatry* 2014 Dec;2(2):121–122.

MacManus D, Jones N, Wessely S et al. The mental health of the UK Armed Forces in the 21st century: Resilience in the face of adversity. *J R Army Med Corps* 2014 Jun;160(2):125–130.

MacManus D, Rona RJ, Dickson H et al. Aggressive and violent behaviour among military personnel deployed to Iraq and Afghanistan: Prevalence and link with deployment and combat exposure. *Epidemiol Rev* 2015;37:196–212.

McAllister PD, Blair SPR, Philpott S. A field mental health team in the general support medical setting. *J R Army Med Corps* 2004 Jun;150(2):107–112.

McAllister P, Greenberg N, Henderson M. Occupational psychiatry in the armed forces: Should depressed soldiers carry guns? *Advances in Psychiatric Treatment* 2011;17(5):350–356.

Messenger K, Farquharson L, Stallworthy P et al. The experiences of security industry contractors working in Iraq: An interpretative phenomenological analysis. *J Occup Environ Med* 2012 Jul;54(7):859–867.

Mulligan K, Jones N, Woodhead C et al. Mental health of UK personnel while on deployment in Iraq. *Br J Psychiatry* 2010 Nov;197(5):405–410.

Mulligan K, Fear NT, Jones N et al. Psycho-educational interventions designed to prevent deployment-related psychological ill-health in Armed Forces personnel: A review. *Psychol Med* 2011 Apr;41(4):673–686.

Mulligan K, Fear NT, Jones N et al. Post-deployment battlemind training for the U.K. Armed Forces: A cluster randomized controlled trial. *J Consult Clin Psychol* 2012 Jun;80(3):331–341.

Mulligan K, Jones N, Davies M et al. Effects of home on the mental health of British forces serving in Iraq and Afghanistan. *Br J Psychiatry* 2012 Sep;201(3):193–198.

Murphy D, Hooper R, French C et al. Is increased reporting of symptomatic ill health in Gulf War veterans related to how one asks the question? *J Psychosom Res* 2006 Aug;61(2): 181–186.

Murphy D, Iversen A, Greenberg N. The Mental Health of Veterans. *J R Army Med Corps* 2008 Jun;154(2):136–139.

Murphy D, Greenberg N, Bland D. Health concerns in UK Armed Forces personnel. *J R Soc Med*, 2009:102:143–147.

Murphy D, Sharp D. Exploring pre-enlistment and military factors associated with the morale of members of the UK Armed Forces. *Mil Med* 2011 Jan;176(1):13–18.

Murphy D, Hunt E, Luzon O, Greenberg N. Exploring pathways to care for members of the UK Armed Forces receiving treatment for PTSD: A qualitative study. *Eur J Psychotraumatol* 2014 Feb;5. doi: 10.3402/ejpt.v5.21759

Murphy D, Hodgman G, Carson C et al. Mental health and functional impairment outcomes following a 6-week intensive treatment programme for UK military veterans with post-traumatic stress disorder (PTSD): A naturalistic study to explore dropout and health outcomes at follow-up. *BMJ Open* 2015 Mar;5(3):e007051.

Murphy D, Palmer E, Wessely S et al. Prevalence and associations between traumatic brain injury and mental health difficulties within UK veterans accessing support for mental health difficulties. *Psychol Res* 2015 Nov;5(11):613–623.

Murphy D, Weijers B, Palmer E, Busuttil W. Exploring Patterns in Referrals toCombat Stress for UK Veterans with Mental Health Difficulties between 1994 and 2014. *Int J Emerg Mental Health Hum Resilience* 2015;17(3):652–658.

Murphy D. Detailing the clinical pathways at Combat Stress for UK veterans experiencing symptoms of complex post traumatic stress disorder. *Healthcare Couns Psychother J* 2016;14(1):24–27.

Osorio C, Greenberg N, Jones N et al. Combat exposure and post-traumatic stress disorder among Portuguese special operation forces deployed in Afghanistan. *Mil Psychol* 2013;25(1):70–81.

Osorio C, Jones N, Fertout, Greenberg. Perceptions of stigma and barriers to care among UK military personnel deployed to Afghanistan and Iraq. *Anxiety Stress Coping* 2013 Sep;26(5):539–557.

Osorio C, Jones N, Fertout M, Greenberg N. Changes in stigma and barriers to care over time in U.K. Armed Forces deployed to Afghanistan and Iraq between 2008 and 201. *Mil Med* 2013 Aug;178(8):846–853.

Osorio C, Jones N, Jones E et al. Combat Experiences and their relationship to post-traumatic stress disorder symptom clusters in UK military personnel deployed to Afghanistan. *Behav Med* 2017 Mar 10:1–10.

Pinder RJ, Murphy D, Hatch SL et al. A mixed methods analysis of the perceptions of the media by members of the British Armed Forces during the Iraq War. *Armed Forces Soc* 2009;36(1):131–152.

Pinder RJ, Fear, NT, Wessely S et al. Mental Health Care Provision in the U.K. Armed Forces *Mil Med* 2010 Oct;175(10):805–810.

Pinder R, Iversen A, Kapur N et al. Self harm and attempted suicide in UK Armed Forces Personnel: Results of a cross sectional survey. *Int J Soc Psychiatry* 2012 Jul;58(4):433–439.

Rona RJ. Long-term consequences of mild traumatic brain injury. *Br J Psychiatry* 2012 Sep;201(3):172–174.

Rona RJ, Hooper R, Jones M et al. Screening for physical and psychological illness in the British Armed Forces: III The value of a questionnaire to assist a Medical Officer to decide who needs help. *J Medical Screening* 2004;11:158–161.

Rona RJ, Jones M, French C et al. Screening for physical and psychological illness in the British Armed Forces: I The acceptability of the pro-gramme. *J Med Screen* 2004;11(3):148–152.

Rona R, Hyams C, Wessely S. Screening for psy-chological illness in military personnel. *JAMA* 2005;293:1257–1260.

Rona R, Hooper R, French C et al. The meaning of self-perception of health in the UK Armed Forces. *Br J Health Psychol* 2006;11:703–715.

Rona R, Hooper R, Greenberg N et al. Medical downgrading, self-perception of health and psychological symptoms in the British Armed Forces. *Occup Environ Med* 2006 Apr;63(4):250–254.

Rona R, Jones M, Hooper R et al. Mental health screening in armed forces before the Iraq War and prevention of subsequent psychologi-cal morbidity: Follow up study. *BMJ* 2006 Nov;333(7576):991.

Rona R, Fear N, Hull L, Wessely S. Women in novel occupational roles: Mental health trends in the UK Armed Forces. *Int J Epidemiol* 2007 Apr;36(2):319–326.

Rona RJ, Fear NT, Hull L. Mental health con-sequences of overstretch in the UK Armed Forces: First phase of a cohort study. *BMJ* 2007 Sep;335(7620):603.

Rona R, Hooper R, Jones M et al. The contribu-tion of prior psychological symptoms and combat exposure to post Iraq deployment mental health in the UK military. *J Trauma Stress* 2009 Feb;22(1):11–19.

Rona RJ, Jones M, Iversen A et al. The impact of post-traumatic stress disorder on impairment in the UK military at the time of the Iraq War. *J Psychiatr Res* 2009 Mar;43(6):649–655.

Rona R, Jones M, Fear N et al. Alcohol mis-use and functional impairment in the UK Armed Forces. *Drug Alcohol Depend* 2010 Apr;108(1–2):37–42.

Rona RJ, Jones M, Fear NT et al. Mild traumatic brain injury in UK military personnel returning from Afghanistan and Iraq: Cohort and cross-sectional analyses. *J Head Trauma Rehabil* 2012 Jan–Feb;27(1):33–44.

Rona RJ, Jones M, Fear NT et al. Frequency of mild traumatic brain injury in Iraq and Afghanistan: Are we measuring incidence or prevalence? *J Head Trauma Rehabil* 2012;27(1):75–82.

Rona R, Jones M, Sundin J et al. Predicting persistent posttraumatic stress disorder (PTSD) in UK military personnel who served in Iraq: A longitudinal study. *J Psychiatric Res* 2012;46:1191–1198.

Rona RJ, Jones M, Goodwin L et al. Risk fac-tors for headache in the UK military: Cross-sectional and longitudinal analyses. *Headache* 2013 May;53(5):787–798.

Rona RJ, Jones M, Keeling M, Hull L et al. Mental Health Consequences of Overstretch in the UK Armed Forces 2007–2009. *Lancet Psychiatry* 2014;1:531–538.

Rona R, Jones M, Hull L et al. Anger in the UK Armed Forces: Strong association with mental health, childhood antisocial behavior and combat role. *J Nerv Ment Dis* 2015;203:15–22.

Rowe M, Murphy D, Wessely S, Fear NT. Exploring the impact of deployment to Iraq on relation-ships. *Mil Behav Health* 2015;1:10–18.

Rowe S, Keeling M, Fear N, Wessely S. Perceptions of the impact of a military career has on children. *Occup Med (Lond)* 2014 Oct;64(7): 490–496.

Scott JN. Diagnosis and outcome of psychiatric referrals to the field mental health team, 202 Field Hospital, Op Telic. *J R Army Med Corps* 2005;151:95–100.

Seddon RL, Jones E, Greenberg N. The role of chaplains in maintaining the psychological health of military personnel: An historical and contemporary perspective. *Mil Med* 2011 Dec;176(12):1357–1361.

Sharp ML, Fear NT, Rona R et al. Stigma as a barrier to seeking healthcare among military personnel with mental health problems. *Epidemiol Rev* 2015;37:144–162.

Sharpley JG, Fear NT, Greenberg N et al. Pre-deployment stress briefing: Does it have an effect? *Occup Med (Lond)* 2008 Jan;58(1):30–34.

Sheriff R, Forbes H, Greenberg N et al. Risky driving among UK regular forces: Changes over time. *BMJ Open* 2015 Sep;5(9): e008434.

Stevelink SA, Malcolm EM, Mason C et al. The prevalence of mental health disorders in (ex-) military personnel with a physical impairment: A systematic review. *Occup Environ Med* 2014;72(4):243–251.

Stevelink SA, Malcolm EM, Fear NT. Visual impairment, coping strategies and impact on daily life: A qualitative study among working-age UK ex-service personnel. *BMC Public Health* 2015 Nov;15:1118.

Stevelink SA, Malcolm EM, Gill PC et al. The mental health of UK ex-servicemen with a combat-related or a non-combat-related visual impairment: Does the cause of visual impairment matter? *Br J Ophthalmol* 2015 Aug;99(8):1103–1108.

Stevelink SA, Fear NT. Psychosocial impact of visual impairment and coping strategies in female ex-Service personnel. *J R Army Med Corps* 2016 Apr;162(2):129–133.

Sundin J, Fear NT, Hull L. Rewarding and unrewarding aspects of deployment to Iraq and its association with psychological health in UK military personnel. *Int Arch Occup Environ Health* 2010 Aug;83(6):653–663.

Sundin J, Fear NT, Iversen A et al. PTSD after deployment to Iraq: Conflicting rates, conflicting claims. *Psychol Med* 2010 Mar;40(3):367–382.

Sundin J, Jones N, Greenberg N et al. Mental health among commando, airborne and other UK infantry personnel. *Occup Med (Lond)* 2010 Oct;60(7):552–559.

Sundin J, Forbes H. Fear NT et al. The impact of the conflicts of Iraq and Afghanistan: A UK perspective. *Int Rev Psychiatry* 2011 Apr;23(2):153–159.

Sundin J, Mulligan K, Henry S. Impact on mental health of deploying as an individual augmentee in the U.K. Armed Forces. *Mil Med* 2012 May;177(5):511–516.

Sundin J, Herrell RK, Hoge CW et al. Mental health outcomes in US and UK military personnel returning from Iraq. *Br J Psychiatry* 2014 Mar;204(3):20.

Tate R, Jones M, Fear N et al. How many mailouts? Could attempts to increase the response rate in the Iraq war cohort study be counterproductive? *BMC Med Res Methodol* 2007;7:51.

Thandi G, Sundin J, Knight T et al. Alcohol misuse in the United Kingdom Armed Forces: A longitudinal study. *Drug Alcohol Depend* 2015 Nov;156:78–83.

Trevillion, Kylee, Williamson E, Thandi G et al. A systematic review of mental disorders and perpetration of domestic violence among military populations. *Soc Psychiatry Psychiatr Epidemiol* 2015 Sep;50(9):1329–1346.

Turner MA, Kiernan MD, McKechanie AG et al. Acute military psychiatric casualties from the war in Iraq. *Br J Psychiatry* 2005 Jun;186:476–479.

Van Hoorn LA, Jones N, Busuttil W et al. Iraq and Afghanistan veteran presentations to Combat Stress, since 2003. *Occup Med (Lond)* 2013 Apr;63(3):238–241.

Van Staden L, Fear NT, Iversen A et al. Transition back into civilian life: A study of personnel leaving the UK Armed Forces via "military prison". *Mil Med* 2007 Sep;172(9):925–930.

Van Staden LN, Fear N, Iversen A et al. Young military veterans show similar help seeking behaviour. *Br Med J* 2007;334(7590):382.

Vermetten E, Greenberg N, Boeschoten MA et al. Deployment-related mental health support: Comparative analysis of NATO and allied ISAF partners. *Eur J Psychotraumatol* 2014 Aug;5. doi: 10.3402/ejpt.v5.23732

Wessely S. When being upset is not a mental health problem. *Psychiatry* 2004;67:153–157.

Wessely S. Risk, psychiatry and the military. *Br J Psychiatry* 2005 Jun;186:459–466.

Wessely S. War stories. *Br J Psychiatry* 2005 Jun;186:473–475.

Wessely S. The London attacks – Aftermath: Victimhood and resilience. *N Engl J Med* 2005 Aug;353(6):548–550.

Wessely S. Twentieth century theories on combat motivation and breakdown. *J Contemp Hist* 2006;41:268–286.

Wessely S, Bryant R, Greenberg N et al. Does psychoeducation help prevent post traumatic distress? *Psychiatry* 2008;71:287–302.

Wesson M, Whybrow D, Gould M et al. An Initial evaluation of the clinical and fitness for work outcomes of a military group behavioural activation programme. *Behav Cogn Psychother* 2014 Mar;42(2):243–247.

White CJ, de Burgh HT, Fear NT et al. The impact of deployment to Iraq or Afghanistan on military children: A review of the literature. *Int Rev Psychiatry* 2011 Apr;23(2):210–217.

Whybrow, D. Behavioural activation for the treatment of depression in military personnel. *J R Army Med Corps* 2013 Mar;159(1):15–20.

Whybrow D, Jones N, Greenberg N. Corporate knowledge of psychiatric services available in a combat zone. *Mil Med* 2013 Feb;178(2):e241–e247.

Whybrow D, Jones N Greenberg N. Promoting organizational well-being: A comprehensive review of Trauma Risk Management. *Occup Med (Lond)* 2015 Jun;65(4):331–336.

Whybrow D, Jones N, Evans C et al. The mental health of deployed UK maritime forces. *Occup Environ Med* 2016 Feb;73(2):75–82.

Wilson J, Jones M, Hull L et al. Does prior psychological health influence recall of military experiences? A prospective study. *J Trauma Stress* 2008 Aug;21(4):385–393.

Wilson J, Jones M, Fear NT et al. Is previous psychological health associated with the likelihood of Iraq War deployment? An investigation of the "healthy warrior effect". *Am J Epidemiol* 2009 Jun;169(11):1362–1369.

Wilson MM, McAllister PD, Hacker Hughes JG et al. Do military uniform and rank impact on the therapeutic relationship between military mental health clients and clinicians? *J R Army Med Corps* 2007 Sep;153(3):170–171.

Woodhead C, Wessely S, Jones N et al. Impact of exposure to combat during deployment to Iraq and Afghanistan on mental health by gender. *Psychol Med* 2012 Sep;42(9):1985–1996.

NEUROTRAUMA AND NEUROSURGERY (INCLUDING MTBI)

Baxter D, Sharp DJ, Feeney C et al. Pituitary dysfunction after blast traumatic brain injury: The UK BIOSAP Study. *Ann Neurol* 2013 Oct;74(4):527–536.

Breeze J, Gibbons A, Shief C et al. Combat-related craniofacial and cervical injuries: A five-year review from the British Military. *J Trauma* 2011 Jul;71(1):108–113.

Breeze J, West A, Clasper J. Anthropometric assessment of cervical neurovascular structures using CTA to determine zone-specific vulnerability to penetrating fragmentation injuries. *Clin Radiol* 2013 Jan;68(1):34–83.

Brunger H, Ogden J, Malia K et al. Adjusting to persistent post-concussive symptoms following mild traumatic brain injury and subsequent psycho-educational intervention: A qualitative analysis in military personnel. *Brain Inj* 2014;28(1):71–80.

Carr DJ, Lewis E, Horsfall I. A systematic review of military head injuries. *J R Army Med Corps* 2017 Feb;163(1):13–19.

Dharm-Datta S, Gough MR, Porter PJ et al. Successful outcomes following neurorehabilitation in military traumatic brain injury patients in the United Kingdom. *J Trauma Acute Care Surg* 2015 Oct;79(4 Suppl 2):S197–S203.

DuBose JJ, Barmparas G, Inaba K et al. Isolated severe traumatic brain injuries sustained during combat operations: Demographics, mortality outcomes, and lessons to be learned from contrasts to civilian counterparts. *J Trauma* 2011 Jan;70(1):11–16; discussion 16–18.

Eardley WG, Bonner TJ, Gibb IE, Clasper JC. Spinal fractures in current military deployments. *J R Army Med Corps* 2012 Jun;158(2):101–105.

Fear NT, Jones E, Groom M et al. Symptoms of post-concussional syndrome are non-specifically related to mild traumatic brain injury in UK Armed Forces personnel on return from deployment in Iraq: An analysis of self-reported data. *Psychol Med* 2009 Aug;39(8):1379–1387.

French DD, Bair MJ, Bass E et al. Central nervous system and musculoskeletal medication profile of a veteran cohort with blast-related injuries. *J Rehabil Res Dev* 2009;46(4):463–468.

Hawley CA, de Burgh HT, Russell RJ, Mead A. Traumatic brain injury recorded in the UK joint theatre trauma registry among the UK Armed Forces. *J Head Trauma Rehabil* 2015 Jan–Feb;30(1):E47–E56.

Jones E, Fear NT, Wessely S. Shell shock and mild traumatic brain injury: A historical review. *Am J Psychiatry* 2007 Nov;164(11):1641–1645.

Jones N, Fear NT, Rona R et al. Mild traumatic brain injury (mTBI) among UK military personnel whilst deployed in Afghanistan in 2011. *Brain Inj* 2014;28(7):896–899.

McKinlay J, Smith JE. Penetrating brain injury: A case of survival following blast fragmentation injuries to the head. *J R Nav Med Serv* 2013;99(2):55–56.

Mellor A, Ralph JK, Harrisson SE. Neurosurgery in Helmand: What could we do, what should we do? *J R Nav Med Serv* 2009;95(3):136–141.

Murphy D, Palmer E, Wessely S et al. Prevalence and associations between traumatic brain injury and mental health difficulties within UK veterans accessing support for mental health difficulties. *Psychol Res* 2015 Nov;5(11):613–623.

Park CL, Moor P, Birch K, Shirley PJ. Operational anaesthesia for the management of traumatic brain injury. *J R Army Med Corps* 2010;156(4):S335–S341.

Park CL, Garner JP. Massive subcutaneous emphysema after cervical gunshot wound. *Trauma* 2016;18(3):241–242.

Possley DR, Petfield JL, Schoenfeld AJ et al. Complications associated with military spine injuries. *Spine J* 2012;12(9):762–768.

Ralph JK, Lowes T. Neurointensive care. *J R Army Med Corps* 2009 Jun;155(2):147–151.

Risdall JE, Menon DK. Traumatic Brain Injury. *Phil Trans R Soc B* 2011;366:241–250.

Roberts SA, Toman E, Belli A, Midwinter MJ. Decompressive craniectomy and cranioplasty: Experience and outcomes in deployed UK military personnel. *Br J NeuroSurg* 2016; 30(5):529–535.

Rona RJ. Long-term consequences of mild traumatic brain injury. *Br J Psychiatry* 2012;Sep;201(3):172–174.

Rona RJ, Jones M, Fear NT et al. Mild traumatic brain injury in UK military personnel returning from Afghanistan and Iraq: Cohort and cross-sectional analyses. *J Head Trauma Rehabil* 2012 Jan–Feb;27(1):33–44.

Rona RJ, Jones M, Fear NT et al. Frequency of mild traumatic brain injury in Iraq and Afghanistan: Are we measuring incidence or prevalence? *J Head Trauma Rehabil* 2012;27(1):75–82.

Smith JE, Kehoe A, Harrison SE et al. Outcome of penetrating intracranial injuries in a military setting. *Injury* 2014 45(5):874–878.

NUTRITION

Connor P, DeLegge M. Ward based enteral and supplemental nutrition on operations. *J R Army Med Corps* 2008 Dec;154(4):276–278.

Duff S, Price S, Gray J. The role of nutrition in injured military personnel at Role 4: Current practice. *J R Army Med Corps* 2008 Dec;154(4):284–291.

Fallowfield JL, Delves SK, Hill NE et al. Energy expenditure, nutritional status, body composition and physical fitness of Royal Marines during a 6-month operational deployment in Afghanistan. *Br J Nutr* 2014 Sep;112(5):821–829.

Henning J, Scott T, Price S. Nutrition of the critically ill patient in field hospitals on operations. *J R Army Med Corps* 2008 Dec;154(4):279–281.

Hill N, Fallowfield J, Price S, Wilson D. Military nutrition: Maintaining health and rebuilding injured tissue. *Philos Trans R Soc Lond B Biol Sci* 2011 Jan;366(1562)231–240.

Janson JO, Turner S, Johnston AM. Nutritional management of critically ill trauma patients in the deployed military setting. *J R Army Med Corps* 2011 Sep;157(3 Suppl 1):S344–S349.

Turner S, Ruth MJ, Bruce DL. "In flight catering": Feeding critical care patients during aeromedical evacuation. *J R Army Med Corps* 2008;154(4):282–283.

OBSTETRICS AND GYNAECOLOGY

Faulconer ER, Irani S, Dufty N, Bowley D. Obstetric complications on deployed operations: A guide for the military surgeon. *J R Army Med Corps* 2016 Oct;162(5):326–329.

OPHTHALMOLOGY

Abbotts R, Harrison SE, Cooper GL. Primary blast injuries to the eye: A review of the evidence. *J R Army Med Corps* 2007 Jun;153(2):119–123.

Ansell M, Breeze J, McAlister V et al. Management of devastating ocular trauma – Experience of maxillofacial surgeons deployed to a forward field hospital. *J R Army Med Corps* 2010 Jun;156(2):106–109.

Aslam S, Griffiths MF. Eye casualties during Operation Telic. *J R Army Med Corps* 2005 Mar;151(1):34–36.

Banerjee PJ, Xing W, Bunce C et al. Triamcinolone during pars plana vitrectomy for open globe trauma: A pilot randomised controlled clinical trial. *Br J Ophthalmol* 2016 Jul;100(7):949–955.

Barnard EB, Baxter D, Blanch R. Anterior chamber gas bubbles in open globe injury. *J R Nav Med Serv* 2013;99(2):53–54.

Blanch RJ, Scott RA. Primary blast injury of the eye. *J R Army Med Corps* 2008 Mar;154(1):76.

Blanch RJ, Scott RAH. Military ocular injury: Presentation, assessment and management. *J R Army Med Corps* 2009 Dec;155(4):279–284.

Blanch RJ, Bindra MS, Jacks AS, Scott RAH. Ophthalmic Injuries in British Armed Forces in Iraq and Afghanistan. *Eye (Lond)* 2011 Feb;25(2):218–223.

Blanch RJ, Ahmed Z, Berry M, Scott RA et al. Animal models of retinal injury. *Invest Ophthalmol Vis Sci* 2012 May;53(6):2913–2920.

Blanch RJ, Good PA, Shah P et al. Visual outcomes after blunt ocular trauma. *Ophthalmol* 2013 Aug;120(8):1588–1591.

Blanch RJ, Ahmed Z, Thompson AR et al. Caspase-9 mediates photoreceptor death after blunt ocular trauma. *Invest Ophthalmol Vis Sci* 2014 Sep;55(10):6350–6357.

Chalioulias K, Sim KT, Scott R. Retinal sequelae of primary ocular blast injuries. *J R Army Med Corps* 2007 Jun;153(2):124–125.

Chaudhary R, Upendran M, Campion N et al. The role of computerised tomography in predicting visual outcome in ocular trauma patients. *Eye (Lond)* 2015 Jul;29(7):867–871.

Dunbar J, Cooper B, Hodgetts T et al. An outbreak of human external ophthalmomyiasis due to *Oestrus ovis* in Southern Afghanistan. *Clin Infect Dis* 2008 Jun;46(11):e124–e126.

Malcolm E, Stevelink SAM, Fear NT. Care pathways for UK and US service personnel who are visually impaired. *J R Army Med Corps* 2014 Sep;160(3):1–5.

Musa F, Tailor R, Gao A et al. Contact lens-related microbial keratitis in deployed British military personnel. *Br J Ophthalmol* 2010 Aug;94(8):988–993.

Ollerton JE, Hodgetts TJ. Operational morbidity analysis: Ophthalmic presentations during Operation Telic. *J R Army Med Corps* 2010;156(1):37–40.

Parker P, Mossadegh S, McCrory C. A comparison of the IED-related eye injury rate in ANSF and ISAF forces at the UK R3 Hospital, Camp Bastion, 2013. *J R Army Med Corps* 2014 Mar;160(1):73–74.

Petersen K, Colyer MD, Hayes DK et al. Prevention of infections associated with combat-related eye, maxillofacial, and neck injuries. *J Trauma* 2011;71:S264–S269.

Ritchie JV, Horne ST, Perry J et al. Ultrasound triage of ocular blast injury in the military emergency department. *Mil Med* 2012 Feb;177(2):174–178.

Scott RAH. The injured eye. *Phil Trans R Soc B* 2011;366:251–260.

Scott RAH. Management of ocular trauma by maxillo-facial surgeons at the Role 3, ISAF Hospital Kandahar over a 21 month period. *J R Army Med Corps* 2012;158(2):142.

Scott RAH. Letter and authors' reply. *J R Army Med Corps* 2012 Sep;158(3):142–143.

Scott RAH. The science from ocular war injuries. *Acta Ophthalmol* 2014 Sep;92:S253.

Scott RAH, Blanch RJ, Morgan-Warren PJ. Aspects of ocular war injuries. *Trauma* 2014;17(2):83–92.

Stacey M Blanch RJ. A Case of external ophthalmomyiasis in a deployed UK soldier. *J R Army Med Corps* 2008;154:60–62.

Stevelink SA, Malcolm EM, Fear NT. Visual impairment, coping strategies and impact on daily life: A qualitative study among working-age UK ex-service personnel. *BMC Public Health* 2015 Nov;15:1118.

Stevelink SA, Malcolm EM, Gill PC et al. The mental health of UK ex-servicemen with a combat-related or a non-combat-related visual impairment: Does the cause of visual impairment matter? *Br J Ophthalmol* 2015 Aug;99(8):1103–1108.

Stevelink SA, Fear NT. Psychosocial impact of visual impairment and coping strategies in female ex-Service personnel. *J R Army Med Corps* 2016 Apr;162(2):129–133.

ORGANISATION OF MEDICAL SERVICES

Ablett D, Herbert LJ, Brogden T. The role played by Royal Navy Medical Assistants on Operation Herrick 9. Can we do more to prepare them for future operations in Afghanistan? *J R Nav Med Serv* 2010;96(1):17–22.

Bailey JA, Morrison JJ, Rasmussen TE. Military trauma systems in Afghanistan: Lessons for civil systems? *Curr Opin Crit Care* 2013 Dec;19(6):569–577.

Bricknell MCM. Reporting clinical activity on military operations – Time for some standardisation. *J R Army Med Corps* 2005 Sep;151(3):142–144.

Bricknell MCM. Reflections on medical aspects of ISAF IX in Afghanistan. *J R Army Med Corps* 2007 Mar;153(1):44–51.

Bricknell MCM, Beardmore CE, Williamson RH. The deployed medical director: Managing the challenges of a complex trauma system (letter). *J R Army Med Corps* 2012 Mar;158(1):66.

Bricknell MCM, Nadin M. Lessons from the organisation of the UK medical services deployed in support of Operation TELIC (Iraq) and Operation HERRICK (Afghanistan). *J R Army Med Corps* 2017 Aug;163(4):273–279.

Bulstrode C. MEDCAPS – Do they work? *J R Army Med Corps* 2009 Sep;155(3):182–183.

Childers R, Parker P. The cost of deploying a Role 2 medical asset to Afghanistan. *Mil Med* 2015 Nov;180(11):1132–1134.

Cordell RF, Cooney MS, Beijer D. Audit of the effectiveness of command and control arrangements for medical evacuation of seriously ill or injured casualties in Southern Afghanistan 2007. *J R Army Med Corps* 2008 Dec;154(4):227–230.

Cordell RF. Multinational medical support to operations: Challenges, benefits and recommendations for the future. *J R Army Med Corps* 2012 Mar;158(1):22–28.

Davis PR, Rickards AC, Ollerton JE. Determining the composition and benefit of the Pre-Hospital Medical Response Team in the conflict setting. *J R Army Med Corps* 2007 Dec;153(4):269–273.

Diehle J, Greenberg N; (King's Centre). Counting the Costs (the healthcare burden associated with service in the British Armed Forces between 1991 and 2014) King's College London, King's Centre for Military Health Research and Help for Heroes Report: Nov 2015.

Grant S, Wheatley RJ. A system for the management, display and integration of pre-hospital healthcare activity in the deployed environment. *J R Army Med Corps* 2014 Dec;160(4):298–303.

Hettiaratchy S, Tai N, Mahoney P, Hodgetts T. UK's NHS trauma systems: Lessons from military experience. *Lancet* 2010 Jul;376(9736):149–151.

Jackson PC, Foster M, Fries A et al. Military trauma care in Birmingham: Observational study of care requirements and resource utilisation. *Injury* 2014;45(1):44–49.

Naumann DN, Baird-Clarke CD, Ross DA. Restoring the equilibrium – Medical force protection and training for Role 1 staff. *J R Army Med Corps* 2010;156:3–4.

Rew DA. Strategic clinical manpower planning in the defence medical services beyond Op Herrick. *J R Army Med Corps* 2011;157:207–208.

Tai N. Civilian trauma care and the Defence Medical Services a prospectus for partnership? *J R Army Med Corps* 2009;155(4):246–247.

Tai NR, Brooks A, Midwinter M et al. Optimal clinical timelines a consensus from the academic department of military surgery and trauma. *J R Army Med Corps* 2009 Dec;155(4):253–256.

Tai N, Parker P The damage control surgery set: Rethinking for contingency. *J R Army Med Corps* 2013 Dec;159(4):314–315.

Verey A, Keeling M, Thandi G et al. UK support services for families of wounded, injured or sick Service personnel: The need for evaluation. *J R Army Med Corps* 2016 Oct;162(5):324–325.

Withnall RDJ, Smith M, Graham DJ et al. Telemedicine in the UK Defence Medical Services: Time for an upgrade? *J R Army Med Corps* 2016 Oct;162(5):318–320.

PAEDIATRICS AND PAEDIATRIC TRAUMA

Arul GS, Reynolds J, DiRusso S et al. Paediatric admissions to the British military hospital at Camp Bastion, Afghanistan. *Ann R Coll Surg Engl* 2012 Jan;94(1):52–57.

Bree S, Wood K, Nordmann GR, McNicholas J. The paediatric transfusion challenge on deployed operations. *J R Army Med Corps* 2010 Dec;156(4 Suppl 1):361–364.

Coley E, Roach P, Macmillan AI et al. Penetrating paediatric thoracic injury. *J R Army Med Corps* 2011 Sep;157(3):243–245.

Cooper B, Mellor A, Bruce A et al. paediatric thoracic damage control resuscitation for ballistic injury: A case report. *J R Army Med Corps* 2007 Dec;153(4):317–318.

Dua A, Via KC, Kreishman P et al. Early management of pediatric vascular injuries through humanitarian surgical care during U.S. military operations. *J Vasc Surg* 2013;58(3):695–700.

Edwards MJ, Lustik M, Eichelberger MR et al. Blast injury in children: An analysis from Afghanistan and Iraq, 2002–2010. *J Trauma Acute Care Surg* 2012 Nov;73(5):1278–1283.

Edwards MJ, Lustik M, Carlson T et al. Surgical interventions for pediatric blast injury: An analysis from Afghanistan and Iraq 2002 to 2010. *J Trauma Acute Care Surg* 2014 Mar;76(3):854–858.

Gurney I. Paediatric Casualties During Op TELIC. *J R Army Med Corps* 2004 Dec;150(4):270–272.

Harris CC, McNicholas JJ. Paediatric intensive care in the field hospital. *J R Army Med Corps* 2009 Jun;155(2):157–159.

Heller D. Child patients in a field hospital; during the 2003 Gulf War. *J R Army Med Corps* 2005 Mar;151(1):41–43.

Hillman CM, Rickard A, Rawlins M, Smith JE. Paediatric traumatic cardiac arrest: Data from the Joint Theatre Trauma Registry. *Emerg Med J* 2014;31(9):790.

Hillman CM, Rickard A, Rawlins M, Smith JE. Paediatric traumatic cardiac arrest: Data from the Joint Theatre Trauma Registry. *J R Army Med Corps* 2016 Aug;162(4)276–279.

Inwald DP, Arul GS, Montgomery M et al. Management of children in the deployed intensive care unit at Camp Bastion, Afghanistan. *J R Army Med Corps* 2014 Sep;160(3):236–240.

Mckechnie PS, Wertin T, Parker P, Eckert M. Pediatric surgery skill sets in Role 3: The Afghanistan experience. *Mil Med* 2014 Jul;179(7):762–765.

Naumann DN, Lundy J, Burns et al. Routine Deworming of Children at Deployed Military Healthcare Facilities. *Pediatr Infect Dis J* 2013;32(9):931–932.

Neff LP, Cannon JW, Morrison JJ et al. Clearly defining pediatric massive transfusion: Cutting through the fog and friction with combat data. *J Trauma Acute Care Surg* 2015 Jan;78(1):22–28.

Nordmann GR. Paediatric anaesthesia in Afghanistan: A review of the current experience. *J R Army Med Corps* 2010;156(4):S323–S326.

Nordmann GR, McNicholas JJ, Templeton PA et al. Paediatric trauma management on deployment. *J R Army Med Corps* 2011;157 (3 Suppl 1):S334–S343.

Pearce P. Preparing to care for paediatric trauma patients. *J R Army Med Corps* 2015;161:i52–i55.

Ralph JK, George R, Thompson J. Paediatric anaesthesia using the Triservice anaesthetic apparatus. *J R Army Med Corps* 2010 Jun;156(2):84–86.

Tarmey NT, Easby D, Park CL. Paediatric anaesthesia for overseas operations: UK Military guidelines. *Med Corps Int Forum* 2014;(1):32–35.

Villamaria CY, Morrison JJ, Fitzpatrick CM et al. Wartime vascular injuries in the pediatric population of Iraq and Afghanistan: 2002–2011. *J Pediatr Surg* 2014 Mar;49(3):428–432.

Walker N, Russell RJ, Hodgetts TJ. British military experience of pre-hospital paediatric trauma in Afghanistan. *J R Army Med Corps* 2010 Sep;156(3):150–153.

White CJ, de Burgh HT, Fear NT et al. The impact of deployment to Iraq or Afghanistan on military children: A review of the literature. *Int Rev Psychiatry* 2011 Apr;23(2):210–217.

Woods KL, Russell RJ, Bree S et al. The pattern of paediatric trauma on operations. *J R Army Med Corps* 2013;158(1):34–37.

PAIN MANAGEMENT

Aldington D. Pain – How to avoid it. *Trans Med Soc Lond* 2009;126:187–191.

Aldington DJ, Mcquay HJ, Moore RA. End-to-end military pain management. *Philos Trans R Soc Lond B Biol Sci* 2011 Jan;27;366(1562):268–275.

Aldington D, Kerns R. Battlefield to Bedside to Recovery. *IASP Clin Update* 2011 Sep;19(5):1–6.

Aldington D. Pain management in victims of conflict. *Curr Opin Support Palliat Care* 2012 Jun;6(2):172–176.

Aldington D, Jagdish S. The fentanyl 'lozenge' story: From books to battlefield. *J R Army Med Corps* 2014 Jun;160(2):102–104.

Aldington D, Small C, Edwards D et al. A survey of post-amputation pains in serving military personnel. *J R Army Med Corps* 2014 Mar;160(1):38–41.

Beard DJ, Wood P. Pain in complex trauma: Lessons from Afghanistan. *BJA Educ* 2015 Aug;15(4):207–212.

Connor DJ, Ralph JK, Aldington DJ. Field hospital analgesia. *J R Army Med Corps* 2009 Mar;155(1):49–56.

Davey CM, Mieville KE, Simpson R, Aldington D. A survey of experience of parenteral analgesia at Role 1. *J R Army Med Corps* 2012 Sep;158(3):186–189.

Davey CM, Mieville KE, Simpson R, Aldington D. A proposed model for improving battlefield analgesia training: Post-graduate medical officer pain management day. *J R Army Med Corps* 2012 Sep;158(3):190–193.

Edwards D, Bowden M, Aldington DJ. Pain management at role 4. *J R Army Med Corps* 2009 Mar;155(1):58–61.

Flutter C, Ruth M, Aldington D. Pain management during Royal Air Force strategic aeromedical evacuations. *J R Army Med Corps* 2009 Mar;155(1):61–63.

Flutter C, Aldington D. Pain priorities in pre-hospital care. *Anaesth Int Care Med* 2011 Sep;12(9):380–382.

Fowler M, Slater TM, Garza TH et al. Relationships between early acute pain scores, autonomic nervous system function, and injury severity in wounded soldiers. *J Trauma* 2011 Jul;71(1 Suppl):S87–S90.

French DD, Bair MJ, Bass E et al. Central nervous system and musculoskeletal medication profile of a veteran cohort with blast-related injuries. *J Rehabil Res Dev* 2009;46(4):463–468.

Gaunt C, Gill J, Aldington D. British military use of morphine: A historical review. *J R Army Med Corps* 2009 Mar;155(1):46–49.

Jagdish S, Aldington D. The use of opioids during rehabilitation after combat-related trauma. *J R Army Med Corps* 2009 Mar;155(1):64–66.

Jones CP, Chauhan R, Aldington D. Use of Intramuscular Morphine in Trauma Patients. *Anaesthesia* 2014 Jul;69(7):796–797.

Keene D, Rea W, Aldington D. Acute pain management in trauma. *Trauma* 2011 May;13(3):167–179.

Le Feuvre P, Aldington D. Know Pain Know Gain: Proposing a treatment approach for phantom limb pain. *J R Army Med Corps* 2014 Mar;160(1):16–21.

Looker J, Aldington D. Pain scores – As easy as counting to three. *J R Army Med Corps* 2009 Mar;155(1):42–43.

Mercer SJ, Chavan S, Tong JL et al. The early detection and management of neuropathic pain following combat injury. *J R Army Med Corps* 2009 Jun;155(2):94–98.

Mercer SJ, Whittle CL, Mahoney PF. Lessons from the battlefield: Human factors in defence anaesthesia. *Br J Anaesth* 2010 Jul;105(1):9–20.

Park CL, Roberts DE, Aldington DJ, Moore RA. Prehospital analgesia: Systematic review of evidence. *J R Army Med Corps* 2010 Dec;156(4 Suppl 1):295–300.

Tarmey NT, Park CL, Aldington D et al. Acute Pain Management on Overseas Operations: UK Military Guidelines. *Medical Corps Int Forum* 2014;3:40–43.

Wyldbore M, Aldington D. Trauma pain – A military perspective. *Br J Pain* 2013;7(2):74–78.

PELVIC TRAUMA

Adams SA. Pelvic ring injuries in the military environment. *J R Army Med Corps* 2009 Dec;155(4):293–296.

Arul GS, Bowley DM, DiRusso S. The use of Celox gauze as an adjunct to pelvic packing in otherwise uncontrollable pelvic haemorrhage secondary to penetrating trauma. *J R Army Med Corps* 2012 Dec;158(4):331–333; discussion 333–334.

Bonner TJ, Eardley WG, Newell N et al. Accurate placement of a pelvic binder improves reduction of unstable fractures of the pelvic ring. *J Bone Joint Surg Br* 2011 Nov;93(11):1524–1528.

Cross AM, Davis C, Penn-Barwell J et al. The incidence of pelvic fractures with traumatic lower limb amputation in modern warfare due to improvised explosive devices. *J R Nav Med Serv* 2014;100(2):152–156.

Durrant JJ, Ramasamy A, Salmon MS et al. Pelvic fracture-related urethral and bladder injury. *J R Army Med Corps* 2013 Mar;159(Suppl 1):i132–i139.

Eardley W, Bonner T, Gibb I, Clasper J. Pelvic fractures in current military deployments (abstract). *J R Army Med Corps* 2010 Sep;156(3):181.

Matheson A, Howes D, Standley D et al. Transpelvic gunshot wounds: Potential multidisciplinary mayhem! *World J Surg* 2009;33:144.

Morrison JJ, Mountain AJ, Galbraith KA, Clasper JC. Penetrating pelvic battlefield trauma: Internal use of chitosan-based haemostatic dressings. *Injury* 2010 Feb;41(2):239–241.

Jansen JO, Thomas GOR, Adams SA et al. Early management of proximal traumatic lower extremity amputation and pelvic injury caused by improvised explosive devices (IEDs). *Injury* 2012 Jul;43(7):976–979.

Mossadegh S, Tai N, Midwinter M, Parker P. Improvised explosive device related pelvi-perineal trauma: Anatomic injuries and surgical management. *J Trauma Acute Care Surg* 2012 Aug;73(2 Suppl 1):S24–S31.

Poon H, Morrison JJ, Apodaca AN et al. The UK military experience of thoracic injury in the wars in Iraq and Afghanistan. *Injury* 2013 44(9):1165–1170.

Ramasamy A, Bhullar TPS. Posterior fracture dislocation of the hip from a warrior Turret injury. *J R Army Med Corps* 2006;152:236–238.

Richardson JJ, Bowley DM, Karandikar SS. Sacral nerve stimulation for the treatment of faecal incontinence secondary to a pelvic war injury: A case report. *J R Army Med Corps* 2014;160(1):58–60.

Walker NM, Eardley W, Clasper JC. UK combat-related pelvic junctional vascular injuries 2008–2011: Implications for future intervention. *Injury* 2014 Oct;45(10):1585–1589.

Webster C, Masouros S, Gibb et al. Fracture patterns in pelvic blast injury: A retrospective analysis and implications for future preventative strategies. *Bone Joint J Orthopaedic Proc Supplement* 2015;97(Suppl 8):14.

PERSONAL EXPERIENCES

Arul GS, Bree S, Sonka B et al. The secret lives of the Bastion Bakers. *BMJ* 2014 Dec;349:g7448.

Chinery J, Lane C, Faulconer E, Round J. Operation Telic 8 & 9: Battle casualties in Basra City (abstract). *J R Army Med Corps* 2008 Sep;154(3):191–192.

Cooper DJ. A personal view – 6 Months in a FOB. *J R Army Med Corps* 2010 Mar;156(1):57–59.

Edgar S. The personal experiences of the regimental aid post. 1st Bn the Royal Regiment of Fusiliers. Op TELIC, Iraq. *J R Army Med Corps* 2004 Mar;150(1):27–31.

Grainge C, Heber M. The Role Of The physician in modern military operations: 12 Months experience In Southern Iraq. *J R Army Med Corps* 2005 Jun;151(2):101–104.

Gumbley AE, Claydon MA, Blankenstein TN, Fell TH. Medical provision in forward locations in Afghanistan: The experiences of general duties medical officers on Op HERRICK 15. *J R Army Med Corps* 2013 Jun;159(2):68–72.

Hodgetts T. Personal view: A day in the life of an emergency physician at war. *Emerg Med J* 2004;21(2):129–130.

Lim F. A day in Helmand – A personal view. *J R Nav Med Serv* 2009;95(3):142–144.

Lyon JD, Stacey M, Simpson R. Preparing for an operational tour as a medical officer in southern Afghanistan. *J R Army Med Corps* 2010 Sep;156(3):192–196.

Parker PJ. Experiences of medical care with the 250th Forward Surgical Team (Airborne) during a military operation into Northern Iraq in 2003. *Mil Med* 2007 Feb;172(2):127.

Wilkinson G. Nursing in Afghanistan. *J R Nav Med Serv* 2009;95(1):28–29.

PHARMACOLOGY AND THERAPEUTICS

Davies E, Smith A, Mahoney P, Midwinter M. Activated recombinant factor VIIa in British military trauma: An audit of use against SGPL guidelines (abstract). *J R Army Med Corps* 2010 Sep;156(3):178.

Gokhale SG, Scorer T, Doughty H. Freedom from frozen: The first British Military use of lyophilised plasma in forward resuscitation. *J R Army Med Corps* 2016 Feb;162(1):63–65.

Heier HE, Badloe J, Bohonek M et al. Use of tranexamic acid in bleeding combat casualties. *Mil Med* 2015 Aug;180(8):844–846.

Hodgetts TJ, Mahoney PF, Kirkman E et al. UK Defence Medical Services guidance for use of recombinant factor VIIa (rFVIIa) in the deployed military setting. *J R Army Med Corps* 2007 Dec;153(4):307–309.

Morrison JJ, Dubose JJ, Rasmussen TE, Midwinter MJ. Military Application of Tranexamic Acid in Trauma Emergency Resuscitation (MATTERs) Study. *Arch Surg* 2012 Feb;147(2):113–119.

Smith JE, Fawcett R, Randalls B. The use of recombinant activated factor VII in a patient with penetrating chest trauma and ongoing pulmonary hemorrhage. *Mil Med* 2012;177(5):614–616.

Smith JE. The use of recombinant activated factor VII (rFVIIa) in the management of patients with major haemorrhage in military hospitals over the last 5 years. *Emerg Med J* 2013;30:316–319.

Trull B, Hearn M, Jeffery S. Residual limb hyperhidrosis: Use of botulinum-A toxin to improve prosthesis fit and function. *Wounds UK* 2011;7:92–97.

Wright C. Battlefield administration of tranexamic acid by combat troops: A feasibility analysis. *J R Army Med Corps* 2014;160:271–272.

PLASTIC SURGERY AND BURNS

D'Avignon LC, Chung KK, Saffle JR et al. Prevention of infections associated with combat-related burn injuries. *J Trauma* 2011 Aug;71(2 Suppl 2):S282–S289.

Evriviades D, Jeffery S, Cubison T, Lawton G, Gill M, Mortiboy D. Shaping the military wound: Issues surrounding the reconstruction of injured servicemen at the Royal Centre for Defence Medicine. *Trans R Soc Lond B Biol Sci* 2011 Jan;366(1562):219–230.

Foster MA, Moledina J, Jeffery SL. Epidemiology of U.K. military burns. *J Burn Care Res* 2011 May–Jun;32(3):415–420.

Jeevaratnam JA, Pandya AN. One year of burns at a Role 3 medical treatment facility in Afghanistan. *J R Army Med Corps* 2014 Mar;160(1):22–26.

Jeffery SLA. Current Burn Wound Management. *Trauma* 2009 Dec;11:241–248.

Jeffery SLA. Exudate monitoring in traumatic wounds. *Wounds UK* 2013;9(2):40–44.

Jeffery SLA. The Management of combat wounds: The British Military experience. *Adv Wound Care* 2016 Oct;5(10):464–473.

Maitland L, Lawton G, Baden J et al. The role of military plastic surgeons in the management of modern combat trauma: An analysis of 645 cases. *Plast Reconstr Surg* 2016 Apr;137(4):717e–724e.

Martin NAJ, Macleod BMG, Pandya AN et al. Pyrotechnic signal flare (miniflare) injuries. *J R Army Med Corps* 2009 Sep;155(3):197–199.

Martin NA, Lundy JB, Rickard RF. Lack of precision of burn surface area calculation by UK Armed Forces medical personnel. *Burns* 2014 Mar;40(2):246–250.

Rickard RF, Martin NA, Lundy JB. Imprecision in TBSA calculation (letter). *Burns* 2014 Feb;40(1):172–173.

PRE-HOSPITAL CARE

Apodaca AN, Morrison JJ, Spott MA et al. Improvements in the hemodynamic stability of combat casualties during en route care. *Shock* 2013 Jul;40(1):5–10.

Barnard EB, Moy RJ, Kehoe AD et al. Rapid Sequence Induction of Anaesthesia via the Intraosseous route: A prospective observational study. *Emerg Med J* 2015 Jun;32(6):449–452.

Barnard EB, Mora AG, Bebarta VS. Preflight variables are associated with increased ventilator days and 30-day mortality in trauma casualties evacuated by critical care air transport teams: An exploratory retrospective study. *Mil Med* 2016 May;181(5Suppl):132–137.

Blackbourne LH, Baer DG, Eastridge BJ et al. Military medical revolution: Prehospital combat casualty care. *J Trauma Acute Care Surg* 2012 Dec;73(6 Suppl 5):S372–S377.

Blackbourne LH, Baer DG, Eastridge BJ et al. Military medical revolution: Deployed hospital and en route care. *J Trauma Acute Care Surg* 2012 Dec;73(6 Suppl 5):S378–S387.

Calderbank P, Woolley T, Mercer S et al. Doctor on board? What is the optimal skill-mix in military pre-hospital care? *Emerg Med J* 2011 Oct;28(10):882–883.

Clasper JC, Brown KV, Hill P. Limb complications following pre-hospital tourniquet use. *J R Army Med Corps* 2009 Sep;155(3):200–202.

Davis PR, Rickards AC, Ollerton JE. Determining the composition and benefit of the pre-hospital medical response team in the conflict setting. *J R Army Med Corps* 2007 Dec;153(4):269–273.

Dawes R. Does placing two pre-hospital fluid warmers in series increase output temperature significantly? National Institute of Academic Anaesthesia Showcase 2009 *J R Army Med Corps* 2010;156(1):61.

Dawes R, Thomas GO. Battlefield resuscitation. *Curr Opin Crit Care* 2009 Dec;15(6):527–535.

Edgar IA, Thompson CJ, Hunter S et al. Does the method of aeromedical evacuation from the point of wounding to a field hospital have an effect on subsequent blood product usage and patient physiology? *J R Nav Med Serv* 2014;100(1):12–17.

Fenton P, Bali N, Sargeant I, Jeffrey SL. A complication of the use of an intra-osseous needle. *J R Army Med Corps* 2009 Jun;155(2):110–111.

Flutter C, Aldington D. Pain priorities in pre-hospital care. *Anaesth Int Care Med* 2011 Sep;12(9):380–382.

Guyver PM, Lambert AW. Vascular access on the front line. *J Vasc Access* 2004;9:142–144.

Haldane AG. Advanced airway management – A medical emergency response team perspective. *J R Army Med Corps* 2010 Sep;156(3):159–161.

Hervig T, Doughty H, Ness P et al. Prehospital use of plasma: The blood bankers' perspective. *Shock* 2014 May;41(Suppl 1):39–43.

Hewitt-Smith A, Laird C, Porter K, Bloch M. Haemostatic dressings in prehospital care. *Emerg Med J* 2013 Oct;30(10):784–789.

Hodgetts T, Mahoney P, Evans G, Brooks A. Battlefield Advanced Trauma Life Support (part one). *J R Army Med Corps* 2006;152 (4 Suppl 1).

Hodgetts T, Mahoney P, Evans G, Brooks A. Battlefield Advanced Trauma Life Support (part two). *J R Army Med Corps* 2006;152(4 Suppl 1).

Hodgetts T, Mahoney P, Evans G, Brooks A. Battlefield Advanced Trauma Life Support (part three). *J R Army Med Corps* 2006;152(4 Suppl 1).

Hodgetts T, Mahoney P, Russell MQ, Byers M. ABC to <C>ABC: Redefining the military trauma paradigm. *Emerg Med J* 2006 Oct;23(10):745–746.

Hodgetts TJ, Mahoney PF. Military pre-hospital care: Why is it different? *J R Army Med Corps* 2009 Mar;155(1):4–8.

Hulse EJ, Thomas GO. Vascular access on the 21st century military battlefield. *J R Army Med Corps* 2010 Dec;156(4 Suppl 1):385–390.

Kehoe A, Jones A, Marcus S et al. Current controversies in military pre-hospital critical care. *J R Army Med Corps* 2011 Sep;157(3 Suppl 1): S305–S309.

Kyle T, Le Clerc S, Thomas A et al. The success of battlefield surgical airway insertion in severely injured military patients: A UK perspective. *J R Army Med Corps* 2016 Dec;162(6):460–464.

Kyle T, Greaves I, Beynon A et al. Ionised calcium levels in major trauma patients who received blood en route to a military medical treatment facility. *J Emerg Med* In press.

Le Clerc S, McLennan J, Kyle A et al. Predicting when to administer blood products during tactical aeromedical evacuation: Evaluation of a US model. *J Spec Operations Med* 2014 Jan;14(4):48–52.

Mercer SJ, Lewis SE, Wilson SJ et al. Creating airway management guidelines for casualties with penetrating airway injuries. *J R Army Med Corps* 2010 Dec;156(4 Suppl 1): S355–S360.

Morrison JJ, Oh J, DeBose JJ et al. En-route care capability from point of injury impacts mortality after severe wartime injury. *Ann Surg* 2013 Feb;257(2):330–334.

Nicholson-Roberts TC, Berry R. Prehospital trauma and aeromedical transfer. A military perspective. *Contin Educ Anaesth Crit Care Pain* 2012;12:186–189.

Olson CM Jr, Bailey J, Mabry R et al. Forward aeromedical evacuation: A brief history, lessons learned from the Global War on Terror, and the way forward for US policy. *J Trauma Acute Care Surg* 2013;75:S130–S136.

O'Reilly D, König T, Tai N. Field trauma care in the 21st century. *J R Army Med Corps* 2008;154(4):257–264.

O'Reilly DJ, Morrison JJ, Jansen JO et al. Initial UK Experience of Prehospital Blood Transfusion in Combat Casualties. *J Trauma Acute Care Surg* 2014 Sep;77(3 Suppl 2):S66–S70.

O'Reilly DJ, Morrison JJ, Jansen JO et al. Prehospital blood transfusion in the en route management of severe combat trauma: A matched cohort study. *J Trauma Acute Care Surg* 2014:77;(3 Suppl 2):S114–S120.

Park CL, Roberts DE, Aldington DJ, Moore RA. Prehospital analgesia: Systematic review of evidence. *J R Army Med Corps* 2010 Dec;156(4 Suppl 1):295–300.

Pugh HEJ, Le Clerc S, Mclennan J. A review of pre-admission advanced airway management in combat casualties, Helmand Province 2013. *J R Army Med Corps* June 2015;161:121–126.

Quayle JM, Thomas GOR. A Pre-hospital Technique for Controlling Haemorrhage from Traumatic Perineal and High Amputation Injuries. *J R Army Med Corps* 2011;157:419–420.

Sharpe D, Barneby E, Russell R. New approaches to the management of traumatic external haemorrhage. *Trauma* 2011;13:47–55.

Smith IM, James RH, Dretzke J, Midwinter MJ. Pre-hospital blood product resuscitation for trauma: A systematic review. *Shock* 2016;46(1):3–16.

Stannard A, Rasmussen TE, Midwinter M et al. Outcomes of non-compressible haemorrhage on the battlefield. 2010 Military Surgery Meeting (abstract). *J R Army Med Corps* 2010;156(3):179.

Tarmey NT, Park CL, Bartells OJM. Prehospital cardiopulmonary resuscitation time in traumatic arrest. *J Trauma Acute Care Surg* 2012 March;72(6 Suppl 5):800–801.

Therien SP, Nesbitt ME, Duran-Stanton AM, Gerhardt RT. Prehospital medical documentation in the Joint Theater Trauma Registry: A retrospective study. *J Trauma* 2011 Jul;71(1 Suppl):S103–S108.

Thomas A. An overview of the Medical Emergency Response Team (MERT) in Afghanistan: A paramedic's perspective. *J Paramed Pract* 2014;6(6):296–302.

Walker N, Russell RJ, Hodgetts TJ. British military experience of pre-hospital paediatric trauma in Afghanistan. *J R Army Med Corps* 2010 Sep;156(3):150–153.

Watts S, Nordmann G, Brohi K et al. Evaluation of prehospital blood products to attenuate acute coagulopathy of trauma in a model of severe injury and shock in anesthetized pigs *Shock* 2015 Aug;44:138–148.

Whalley L, Smith S. Pre-hospital, maritime in-transit care from a Role 2 Afloat platform. *J R Nav Med Serv* 2013;99(3):135–136.

Wheatley RJ. The Role 1 capability review: Mitigation and innovation for Op HERRICK 18 and into contingency. *J R Army Med Corps* 2014;160:211–212.

Wood RJ, Jeevaratnam JA, Clasper JC. Aspects of military pre-hospital care. *J Paramed Pract* 2011;3(2):64–69.

Wright C. Battlefield administration of tranexamic acid by combat troops: A feasibility analysis. *J R Army Med Corps* 2014;160:271–272.

PRIMARY CARE AND MEDICINE AT ROLE 1

Aye Maung N, Doughty H, MacDonald S, Parker P. Transfusion support by a UK Role 1 medical team: A two-year experience from Afghanistan. *J R Army Med Corps* 2016 Dec;162(6):440–444.

Batham D, Fiinnegan A, Kiernan M et al. Factors affecting front line casualty care in Afghanistan. *J R Army Med Corps* 2012 Sep;158(3):173–180.

Batham DR, Wall CM. An audit of the quality of deployed DMICP records on Operation HERRICK 14. *J R Army Med Corps* 2012 Sep;158(3):213–216.

Benavides LC, Smith IM, Benavides JM et al. Deployed skills training for whole blood collection by a special operations expeditionary surgical team. *J Trauma Acute Care Surg* 2017 Jun;82(6S Suppl 1):S96–S102.

Chinery J, Lane C, Faulconer E, Round J. Operation Telic 8 & 9: Battle casualties in Basra City (abstract). *J R Army Med Corps* 2008 Sep;154(3):191–192.

Coetzee RH, Simpson RG, Greenberg N. Detecting post-deployment mental health problems in primary care. *J R Army Med Corps* 2010 Sep;156(3):196–199.

Cooper DJ. A personal view – 6 Months in a FOB. *J R Army Med Corps* 2010 Mar;156(1):57–59.

Davey CM, Mieville KE, Simpson R, Aldington D. A survey of experience of parenteral analgesia at Role 1. *J R Army Med Corps* 2012 Sep;158(3):186–189.

Dawes R, Thomas GO. Battlefield resuscitation. *Curr Opin Crit Care* 2009 Dec;15(6):527–535.

Driver J, Nelson TG, Simpson R, Wall C. To refer or not to refer: A qualitative study of reasons for referral from Role 1. *J R Army Med Corps* 2012 Sep;158(3):208–212.

Driver J, Simpson R, Wall C, Nelson TG. Dermatology on Operation HERRICK. *J R Army Med Corps* 2012 Sep;158(3):232–237.

Edgar S. The personal experiences of the regimental aid post. 1st Bn the Royal Regiment of Fusiliers. Op TELIC, Iraq. *J R Army Med Corps* 2004 Mar;150(1):27–31.

Gumbley AE, Claydon MA, Blankenstein TN, Fell TH. Medical provision in forward locations in Afghanistan: The experiences of general duties medical officers on Op HERRICK 15. *J R Army Med Corps* 2013 Jun;159(2):68–72.

Guyver PM, Lambert AW. Vascular access on the front line. *J Vasc Access* 2004;9:142–144.

Hawksley OJ, Jeyanathan J, Mears K, Simpson R. A survey of primary health care provision at a forward operating base in Afghanistan during operation HERRICK 10. *J R Army Med Corps* 2011 Jun;157(2):145–149.

Hodgetts T, Greasley LA. Impact of deployment of personnel with chronic conditions to forward areas. *J R Army Med Corps* 2003 Dec;149(4):277–283.

Hodgetts T, Mahoney P, Russell MQ, Byers M. ABC to <C>ABC: Redefining the military trauma paradigm. *Emerg Med J* 2006 Oct;23(10):745–746.

Hodgetts TJ, Findlay S. Putting Role 1 first: The Role 1 Capability review. *J R Army Med Corps* 2012 Sep;158(3):162–170.

Hulse EJ, Thomas GO. Vascular access on the 21st century military battlefield. *J R Army Med Corps* 2010 Dec;156(4 Suppl 1):385–390.

McAllister PD, Blair SPR, Philpott S. A field mental health team in the general support medical setting. *J R Army Med Corps* 2004 Jun;150(2):107–112.

Mercer SJ, Howell M, Simpson R. Simulation training for the frontline – Realistic preparation for Role 1 doctors. *J R Army Med Corps* 2010 Jun;156(2):87–89

Naumann DN, Baird-Clarke CD, Ross DA. Restoring the equilibrium – Medical force protection and training for Role 1 staff. *J R Army Med Corps* 2010;156:3–4.

Nelson TG, Wall C, Driver J, Simpson R. Op Herrick primary care casualties: The forgotten many. *J R Army Med Corps* 2012 Sep;158(3):252–255.

Parker PJ. Casualty evacuation timelines: An evidence based review. *J R Army Med Corps* 2007;153(4):274–277.

Parsons IT. The health of the Role 1 doctor. *J R Army Med Corps* 2015;161(4):300–303.

Simpson RG. A Better understanding of Deployed Role 1. *J R Army Med Corps* 2012 Sep;158(3):155.

RADIOLOGY AND IMAGING

Breeze J, Leason J, Gibb I et al. Characterisation of explosive fragments injuring the neck. *Br J Oral Maxillofac Surg* 2013 Dec;51(8): e263–e266.

Chaudhary R, Upendran M, Campion N et al. The role of computerised tomography in predicting visual outcome in ocular trauma patients. *Eye (Lond)* 2015 Jul;29(7):867–871.

Eardley W, Stitson D, Miles R, Clasper J. Exploring the role of whole body computed tomography (WBCT) in the early management of combat casualties from explosive devices (abstract). *J R Army Med Corps* 2010 Sep;156(3):181.

Gay DAT, Miles RM. Damage control radiology: An evolution in trauma imaging (Use of imaging in trauma decision making). *J R Army Med Corps* 2011 Sep;157(3 Suppl 1):s289–s292.

Gibb IE. Computed tomography of projectile injuries. *Clin Radiol* 2008 Oct;63(10):1167–1168.

Gibb I, Denton E. Guidelines for the use of computed tomography (CT) in the postmortem – Investigation of deaths in a mass casualty scenario. *NHS Improvements June 2011.*

Gibb I, Denton E. Guidelines for imaging the injured blast/ballistic patient in a mass casualty scenario. *NHS Improvements 2011.*

Graham RNJ. Battlefield radiology. *Br J Radiol* 2012 Dec;85(1020):1556–1565.

Hutchings SD, Rees PSC. Trauma resuscitation using echocardiography in a deployed military intensive care unit. *J Intensive Care Soc* 2013 Apr;14(2):120–125.

Jeffery S. Wound imaging: From Waterloo to tomorrow. *Br J Nurs* 2014 Aug;23(15):S3.

Kinnear-Mellor R, Newton K, Woolley T, Rickard R. Predictive utility of cardiac ultrasound in traumatic cardiac arrest in a combat casualty. *J R Army Med Corps* 2016 Feb;162(1):68–70.

Lundy JB, Oh JS, Chung KK et al. Frequency and relevance of acute peri-traumatic pulmonary thrombus diagnosed by computed tomographic imaging in combat casualties. *J Trauma Acute Care Surg* 2013 Aug;75 (2 Suppl 2):S215–S220.

O'Reilly D Kilbey J. Analysis of the Initial 100 Scans from the First CT Scanner deployed by the British Armed Forces in a land environment. *J R Army Med Corps* 2007;153:165–167.

Ramasamy A, Hensley DE, Brooks AJ. The Use of improvised bullet markers with 3D CT reconstruction in the evaluation of penetrating trauma. *J R Army Med Corps* 2008;154:239–241.

Ramasamy D, Hinsley DE, Brooks AJ. The use of three-dimensional computed tomography reconstruction in the assessment of penetrating ballistic trauma. *Emerg Med J* 2009;26:228.

Rees PSC, Inwald D P, Hutchings S. Echocardiography, performed during damage control resuscitation can be used to monitor the haemodynamic response to volume infusion in the deployed military critical care unit. *Heart* 2013;99(Suppl 2):A71.

Ritchie JV, Horne ST, Perry J et al. Ultrasound triage of ocular blast injury in the military emergency department. *Mil Med* 2012 Feb;177(2):174–178.

Rushambuza, R. The role of diagnostic CT imaging in the acute assessment of battlefield external genital injuries. *J R Army Med Corps* 2013;159(Suppl 1):i21–i25.

Singleton JA, Gibb IE, Bull AM et al. Primary blast lung injury prevalence and fatal injuries from explosions: Insights from postmortem computed tomographic analysis of 121 improvised explosive device fatalities. *J Trauma Acute Care Surg* 2013;75(2 Suppl 2):S269–S274.

Smith IM, Naumann DN, Marsden ME et al. Scanning and war: Utility of FAST and CT in the assessment of battlefield abdominal trauma, *Ann Surg* 2015 Aug;262(2):389–396.

Smith JE, Midwinter M, Lambert AW. Avoiding cavity surgery in penetrating torso trauma: The role of the computed topography scan. *Ann Surg* 2010;92:486–488.

Watchorn J, Miles R, Moore N. The role of CT angiography in military trauma. *Clin Radiol* 2013 Jan;68(1):39–46.

REHABILITATION

Aldington D, Small C, Edwards D et al. A survey of post-amputation pains in serving military personnel. *J R Army Med Corps* 2014 Mar; 160(1):38–41.

Bahadur S, McGilloway E, Etherington J. Injury severity at presentation is not associated with long-term vocational outcome in British Military brain injury. *J R Army Med Corps* 2016 Apr;162(2):120–124.

Brown KV, Dharm-Datta S, Potter BK et al. Comparison of development of heterotopic ossification in injured US and UK armed services personnel with combat-related amputations: Preliminary findings and hypotheses regarding causality. *J Trauma* 2010 Jul;69(1):S116–S122.

Brunger H, Ogden J, Malia K et al. Adjusting to persistent post-concussive symptoms following mild traumatic brain injury and subsequent psycho-educational intervention: A qualitative analysis in military personnel. *Brain Inj* 2014;28(1):71–80.

Dharm-Datta S, Gough MR, Porter PJ et al. Successful outcomes following neurorehabilitation in military traumatic brain injury patients in the United Kingdom. *JTrauma Acute Care Surg* 2015 Oct;79(4 Suppl 2):S197–S203.

Edwards DS, Phillip RD, Bosanquet N et al. What is the magnitude and long-term economic cost of care of the British Military Afghanistan amputee cohort? *Clin Orthop Relat Res* 2015 Sep;473(9):2848–2855.

French DD, Bair MJ, Bass E et al. Central nervous system and musculoskeletal medication profile of a veteran cohort with blast-related injuries. *J Rehabil Res Dev* 2009;46(4):463–468.

Jones N, Fear NT, Jones M et al. Long-term military work outcomes in soldiers who become mental health casualties when deployed on operations. *Psychiatry* 2010 Winter;73(4):352–364.

Kent J, Sherman KE. Intrinsic variability in the early unaided gait of bilateral C-leg® users. *Gait Posture* 2014 Jun;39(S1):S82.

Kinch KJ, Clasper JC. A brief history of war amputation. *J R Army Med Corps* 2011 Dec;157(4):374–380.

Ladlow P, Phillip R, Etherington J et al. Functional and mental health status of United Kingdom Military amputees post rehabilitation. *Arch Phys Med Rehabil* 2015 Nov;96(11):2048–2054.

Ladlow P, Phillip R, Coppack R et al. Influence of immediate and delayed lower-limb amputation compared with lower-limb salvage on functional and mental health outcomes post-rehabilitation UK military. *J Bone Joint Surgery Am* 2016;98:1996–2005.

Malcolm E, Stevelink SAM, Fear NT. Care pathways for UK and US service personnel who are visually impaired. *J R Army Med Corps* 2014 Sep;160(3):1–5.

McGilloway E, Mitchell J, Dharm-Datta S et al. The Mayo Portland Adaptability Inventory-4 outcome measure is superior to UK FIM+FAM in a British military population. *Brain Inj* 2016 Jul;28:1–5.

Penn-Barwell JG, Myatt RW, Bennett PM et al. Medium-term outcomes following limb salvage for severe open tibia fracture are similar to trans-tibial amputation. *Injury* 2015 Feb;46(2):288–291.

Pope S, Vickerstaff AL, Wareham AP. Lessons Learned From Early Rehabilitation of Complex Trauma at the Royal Centre for Defence Medicine. *J R Army Med Corps* 2017;163:124–131.

Trull B, Hearn M, Jeffery S. Residual limb hyperhidrosis: Use of botulinum-A toxin to improve prosthesis fit and function. *Wounds UK* 2011;7:92–97.

RESEARCH

Dretzke J, Smith IM, James RH, Midwinter MJ. Protocol for a systematic review of the clinical effectiveness of pre-hospital blood components compared to other resuscitative fluids in patients with major traumatic haemorrhage. *Syst Rev* 2014 Oct;3:123.

Fries CA, Ayalew Y, Penn-Barwell JG et al. Prospective randomised controlled trial of nanocrystalline silver dressing versus plain gauze as the initial post-debridement management of military wounds on wound microbiology and healing. *Injury* 2014 Jul;45(7):1111–1116.

Harvey DJR, Hardman JG. Computational modelling of lung injury: Is there potential for benefit? *Phil Trans R Soc Lond B Biol Sci* 2011 Jan;366(1562)300–305.

Hutchings S, Howarth G, Rees P, Midwinter M. Conducting clinical research in the deployed intensive care unit: Challenges and solutions. *J R Nav Med Serv* 2013;99(3):151–155.

Jugg BJ, Smith AJ, Rudall SJ, Rice P. The injured lung: Clinical issues and experimental models. *Philos Trans R Soc Lond B Biol Sci* 2011 Jan;366(1562):306–309.

Kirkman E, Watts S, Cooper G. Blast injury research models. *Philos Trans R Soc Lond B Biol Sci* 2011 Jan;366(1562)144–159.

Kirkman E, Watts S. Combat Casualty Care research programme. *J R Army Med Corps* 2014 Jun;160(2):109–116.

Mahoney PF, Carr DJ, Delaney RJ et al. Does preliminary optimisation of an anatomically correct skull-brain model using simple simulants produce clinically realistic ballistic injury fracture patterns? *Int J Legal Med* 2017 Jul;131(4):1043–1053.

Masouros SD, Newell N, Ramasamy A et al. Design of a traumatic injury simulator for assessing lower limb response to high loading rates. *Ann Biomed Eng* 2013 Sep;41(9):1957–1967.

Mellor AJ, Woods D. Serum neutrophil gelatinase-associated lipocalin in ballistic injuries: A comparison between blast injuries and gunshot wounds. *J Crit Care* 2012 Aug;27(4):419.

Mossadegh S, Midwinter M, Parker P. Developing a cumulative anatomic scoring system for military perineal and pelvic blast injuries. *J R Army Med Corps* 2013 Mar;159 (Suppl 1):i40–i44.

Mossadegh S, He S, Parker P. Bayesian scoring systems for military pelvic and perineal blast injuries: Is it time to take a new approach? *Mil Med* 2016 May;181(5 Suppl):127–131.

Nordmann G, Woolley T, Doughty H. Deployed research. *J R Army Med Corps* 2014;160:92–98.

Perel O, Prieto-Merino D, Shakur H et al. Predicted early death in patients with traumatic bleeding: Development and validation of prognostic model. *BMJ* 2012;345:e5166.

Ramasamy A, Newell N, Masouros S. From the battlefield to the laboratory; the use of clinical data analysis in developing models of lower limb blast injury. *J R Army Med Corps* 2014;160(2):117–120.

Stannard A, Scott DJ, Ivatury RA et al. A collaborative research system for functional outcomes following wartime extremity vascular injury. *J Trauma Acute Care Surg* 2012;73(2):S7–S12.

RESERVE FORCES' MENTAL HEALTH

Browne T, Hull L, Horn O et al. Explanations for the increase in mental health problems in UK reserve forces who have served in Iraq. *B J Psych* 2007 Jun;190:484–489.

Dandeker C, Greenberg N, Orme G. The UK's Reserve Forces: Retrospect and prospect. *Armed Forces Soc* 2011 Apr;37(2):341–360.

Harvey SB, Hatch SL, Jones M et al. Coming home: Social functioning and the mental health of UK reservists on return from deployment to Iraq or Afghanistan. *Ann Epidemiol* 2011 Sep;21(9):666–672.

Iversen A, Greenberg N. Mental health of regular and reserve military veterans. *Adv Psychiatr Treat* 2009;15:100–106.

Jones N, Wink P, Brown RA et al. A clinical follow-up study of reserve forces personnel treated for mental health problems following demobilisation. *J Ment Health* 2011 Apr;20(2):136–145.

Thandi G, Sundin J, Dandeker C et al. Risk-taking behaviours among reserves: A UK perspective. *Occup Med (Lond)* 2015 Jul;65(5):413–416.

ROLE 4

Breeze J, Gibbons A, Opie N, Monaghan A. Maxillofacial injuries in military personnel treated at the Royal Centre for Defence Medicine June 2001 to December 2007. *Br J Oral Maxillofac Surg* 2010 Dec;48(8):613–616.

Davenport L, Edwards D, Edwards C et al. Evolution of the Role 4 U.K. military pain service. *J R Army Med Corps* 2010 Dec;156 (4 Suppl 1):398–401.

Duff S, Price S, Gray J. The role of nutrition in injured military personnel at Role 4: Current practice. *J R Army Med Corps* 2008 Dec;154(4):284–291.

Edwards D, Bowden M, Aldington DJ. Pain management at role 4. *J R Army Med Corps* 2009 Mar;155(1):58–61.

Evriviades D, Jeffery S, Cubison T, Lawton G, Gill M, Mortiboy D. Shaping the military wound: Issues surrounding the reconstruction of injured servicemen at the Royal Centre for Defence Medicine. *Trans R Soc Lond B Biol Sci* 2011 Jan;366(1562):219–230.

Glennie JS, Bailey MS. UK Role 4 Military infectious diseases at Birmingham Heartlands Hospital in 2005–9. *J R Army Med Corps* 2010 Sep;156(3):162–164.

Jackson PC, Foster M, Fries A et al. Military trauma care in Birmingham: Observational study of care requirements and resource utilisation. *Injury* 2014;45(1):44–49.

Jones CPL, Chinery JP, England K, Mahoney P. Critical Care at Role 4. *J R Army Med Corps* 2010 Dec;156(Suppl 4):S342–S348.

Pope S, Vickerstaff AL, Wareham AP. Lessons learned from early rehabilitation of complex trauma at the Royal Centre for Defence Medicine. *J R Army Med Corps* 2017;163:124–131.

SPINE AND NERVE TRAUMA

Birch R, Misra P, Stewart MP et al. Nerve injuries sustained during warfare: Part I: Epidemiology. *J Bone Joint Surg Br* 2012 Apr;94(4):523–528.

Birch R, Misra P, Stewart MP et al. Nerve injuries sustained during warfare: Part II: Outcomes. *J Bone Joint Surg Br* 2012 Apr;94(4):529–535.

Bird JH, Luke DP, Ward NJ et al. Management of unstable cervical spine injuries in Southern Iraq during Op TELIC. *J R Army Med Corps* 2005 Sep;151(3):179–185.

Blair JA, Patzkowski JC, Schoenfeld AJ et al. Skeletal Trauma Research Consortium (STReC). Are spine injuries sustained in battle truly different? *Spine J* 2012 Sep;12(9):824–829.

Breeze J, Gibbons A, Shief C, et al. Combat-related craniofacial and cervical injuries: A five-year review from the British Military. *J Trauma* 2011 Jul;71(1):108–113.

Breeze J, Masterson L, Banfield G. Outcomes from penetrating ballistic cervical injury. *J R Army Med Corps* 2012 Jun;158(2):96–100.

Goonewardene SS, Mangat KS, Sargeant ID et al. Tetraplegia following cervical spine cord contusion from indirect gunshot injury effects. *J R Army Med Corps* 2007 Mar;153(1):52–53.

Patzkowski JC, Blair JA, Schoenfeld AJ et al. Multiple associated injuries are common with spine fractures during war. *Spine J* 2012;12(9):791–797.

Spurrier E, Singleton JA, Masouros S et al. blast injury in the spine: Dynamic response index is not an appropriate model for predicting injury. *Clin Orthop Relat Res* 2015 Sep;473(9):2929–2935.

Spurrier E, Gibb I, Masouros S, Clasper J. Identifying spinal injury patterns in underbody blast to develop mechanistic hypotheses. *Spine (Phila Pa 1976)* 2016 Mar;41(5):E268–E275.

White SH, Dickson S, Colman T et al. Back pain in a Bangladeshi worker in Iraq. *J R Army Med Corps* 2010;156(1):44–46.

SURGERY IN GENERAL

Clasper JC, Midwinter MJ. Forward Surgery. *J R Army Med Corps* 2007 Sep;153(3):149–151.

Dharm-Datta S, McLenaghan J. Medical lessons learnt from the US and Canadian experience of treating combat casualties from Afghanistan and Iraq. *J R Army Med Corps* 2013 Jun;159(2):102–109.

Granville-Chapman J, Stewart MPM, Kay A. A review of field hospital surgical discharge letters in Summer 2007, Iraq: Burden by surgical specialty and NHS standards (abstract). *J R Army Med Corps* 2008 Sep;154(3):188–189.

Howes R, Webster C, Garner J. Appendicitis in a deployed military setting: Diagnosis, management and impact on the fighting force. *J R Army Med Corps* 2017 Apr;163(2):111–114.

Jacobs N, Taylor DM, Parker PJ. Changes in surgical workload at the JF Med Gp Role 3 Hospital, Camp Bastion, Afghanistan, November 2008-November 2010. *Injury* 2012 Jul;43(7):1037–1040.

Parker PJ, Adams SA, Williams D, Shepherd A. Forward surgery on Operation Telic – Iraq 2003. *J R Army Med Corps* 2005 Sep;151(3):186–191.

Parker PJ, Stapley SA, Porter K. Editorial: Lessons of war. *Bone Joint J* 2015 Dec.

Proffitt A, Faulconer R, Kreishman P et al. An unusual cause of peritonitis in a deployed environment. *J R Army Med Corps* 2015 Mar;161(1):69–70.

Ramasamy A, Brooks A, Midwinter MK et al. Surgical workload during Operation Herrick (abstract). *J R Army Med Corps* 2008;154(3):189.

Rew DA, Clasper J, Kerr G. Surgical workload from an integrated UK field hospital during the 2003 Gulf conflict. *J R Army Med Corps* 2004;150:99–106.

Tai N, Hill P, Kay A, Parker P. Forward trauma surgery in Afghanistan: Lessons learnt on the modern asymmetric battlefield. *J R Army Med Corps* 2008 Mar;154(1):14–18.

THROMBOELASTOMETRY (ROTEM®)

Doran CM, Woolley T, Midwinter MJ. Feasibility of using rotational thromboelastometry to assess coagulation status of combat casualties in a deployed setting. *J Trauma* 2010 Jul;69(Suppl 1):S40–S48.

Hunt H, Stanworth S, Curry N et al. Thromboelastography (TEG) and rotational thromboelastometry (ROTEM) for trauma induced coagulopathy in adult trauma patients with bleeding. *Cochrane Database Syst Rev* 2015 Feb;(2):CD010438.

Jansen JO, Luke D, Davies E et al. Temporal changes in ROTEM®-measured coagulability of citrated blood samples from coagulopathic trauma patients. *Injury* 2013 Jan;44(1):36–39.

Keene DD, Nordmann GR, Woolley T. Rotational Thromboelastometry (ROTEM®) guided trauma resuscitation. *Curr Opin Crit Care* 2013 Dec;19(6):605–612.

Walker C, Ingram M, Edwards D et al. Use of thromboelastometry in the assessment of coagulation before epidural insertion after massive transfusion. *Anaesthesia* 2011 Jan;66(1):52–55.

Woolley T, Midwinter M, Spencer P et al. Utility of interim ROTEM® values of clot strength, A5 and A10, in predicting final assessment of coagulation status in severely injured battle patients. *Injury* 2013 May;44(5):593–599.

TOURNIQUETS

Brodie S, Hodgetts TJ, Lambert P et al. Tourniquet use in combat trauma: UK military experience. *J R Army Med Corps* 2007 Dec;153(4):310–313. Reproduced in *J Spec Operations Med* 2009;9(1):74–77.

Clasper JC, Brown KV, Hill P. Limb complications following pre-hospital tourniquet use. *J R Army Med Corps* 2009 Sep;155(3):200–202.

Mawhinney AC, Kirk SJ. A systematic review of the use of tourniquets and topical Haemostatic agents in conflicts in Afghanistan and Iraq. *J R Nav Med Serv* 2015,101(2):147–154.

Parker PJ, Clasper J. The military tourniquet. *J R Army Med Corps* 2007 Mar;153(1):10–12.

Stewart SK, Duchesne JC, Khan MA. Improvised tourniquets: Obsolete or obligatory? *J Trauma Acute Care Surg* 2015 Jan;78(1):178–183.

Taylor DM, Vater GM, Parker PJ An evaluation of two tourniquet systems for the control of prehospital lower limb hemorrhage. *J Trauma* 2011 Sep;71(3):591–595.

Taylor DM, Coleman M, Parker PJ. The evaluation of an abdominal aortic tourniquet for the control of pelvic and lower limb hemorrhage. *Mil Med* 2013;178(11):1196–1201.

TRANSFUSION MEDICINE AND HAEMATOLOGY

Allcock, EC, Woolley T, Doughty H et al. The clinical outcome of UK Military personnel who received a massive transfusion in Afghanistan during 2009. *J R Army Med Corps* 2011 Dec;157(4):365–369.

Aye Maung N, Doughty H, MacDonald S, Parker P. Transfusion support by a UK Role 1 medical team: A two-year experience from Afghanistan. *J R Army Med Corps* 2016 Dec;162(6):440–444.

Benavides LC, Smith IM, Benavides JM et al. Deployed skills training for whole blood collection by a special operations expeditionary surgical team. *J Trauma Acute Care Surg* 2017 Jun;82(6S Suppl 1):S96–S102.

Bhangu A, Nepogodiev D, Doughty H, Bowley DM. Intraoperative cell salvage in a combat support hospital: A prospective proof of concept study. *Transfusion* 2013 Apr;53(4):805–810.

Bhangu A, Nepogodiev D, Doughty H, Bowley DM. Meta-analysis of plasma to red blood cell ratios and mortality in massive blood transfusions for trauma. *Injury* 2013 Dec;44(12):1693–1699.

Boutefnouchet T, Gregg R, Tidman J et al. Emergency red cells first: Rapid response or speed bump? The evolution of a massive transfusion protocol for trauma in a single UK centre. *Injury* 2015 Sep;46(9):1772–1778.

Bowles F, Hawksley OJ. Blood product use during role 3 trauma calls: Are products used appropriately and wastage minimised? *J R Army Med Corps* 2014;160(3):258.

Bree S, Wood K, Nordmann GR, McNicholas J. The paediatric transfusion challenge on deployed operations. *J R Army Med Corps* 2010 Dec;156(4 Suppl 1):361–364.

Budd ME, Hitchinson M, Doughty H. Development of a training programme for a Deployed Military Transfusion Nurse'. *Transfus Med* 2013;23(Suppl 2):48–49.

Curry N, Rourke C, Davenport R et al. Early cryoprecipitate for major haemorrhage in trauma: A randomised controlled feasibility trial. *Br J Anaesth* 2015 Jul;115(1):76–83.

Davies E, Smith A, Mahoney P, Midwinter M. Activated recombinant factor VIIa in British military trauma: An audit of use against SGPL guidelines (abstract). *J R Army Med Corps* 2010 Sep;156(3):178.

Davies RL. Should whole blood replace the shock pack? *J R Army Med Corps* 2016 Feb;162(1):5–7.

Doughty HA. Why did soldiers donate blood in Afghanistan? *Transfus Med* 2002;12 (Suppl 1):52.

Doughty HA. Transfusion support for trauma. *Blood Matters* 2009;28,(Summer Issue):10–12.

Doughty, H. Recent developments in military transfusion and the impact on civilian practice. *Blood Transplant Matters* 2014 May;42:4–5.

Doughty, H. Military management of massive haemorrhage. In: Thomas D, Thompson J, Ridler BMF (eds.). *All Blood Counts – A Manual for Blood Conservation and Patient Blood Management*. 2nd ed. Shrewsbury: tfm Publishing Ltd., 2016.

Doughty, HA, Frith, L. and Harris, C. The demand for group O blood in a mass casualty situation. *Transfus Med* 2005;15(Suppl 1):4. SI07.

Doughty H, Tidman J. Implementation and revision of a massive transfusion protocol. *Transfus Med* 2010;20(Suppl 1):40. PO30.

Doughty H, Tidman J, Fleetwood P. Polytrauma answers. *CPD News (May)* 2011;36:3–4.

Doughty HA, Woolley T, Thomas GOR. Massive transfusion. *J R Army Med Corps* 2011 Sep;157(3 Suppl 1):S277–S283.

Doughty H, Glasgow S, Kristoffersen E. Mass casualty events: Blood transfusion emergency preparedness across the continuum of care. *Transfusion* 2016 Apr;56(Suppl 2): S208–S216.

Doughty H, Thompson P, Cap AP et al. A Proposed field emergency donor panel questionnaire and triage tool. *Transfusion* 2016 Apr;56(Suppl 2):S119–S127.

Doughty H, Scorer T. Transfusion support for deployed surgical operations. In *The British Deployed Surgical Manual*. Ministry of Defence. London, in press.

Dretzke J, Smith IM, James RH, Midwinter MJ. Protocol for a systematic review of the clinical effectiveness of pre-hospital blood components compared to other resuscitative fluids in patients with major traumatic haemorrhage. *Syst Rev* 2014 Oct;3:123.

Edgar IA, Thompson CJ, Hunter S et al. Does the method of aeromedical evacuation from the point of wounding to a field hospital have an effect on subsequent blood product usage and patient physiology? *J R Nav Med Serv* 2014;100(1):12–17.

Glasgow SM, Allard S, Rackham R, Doughty H. Going for gold: Blood planning for the London 2012 Olympic Games. *Transfus Med* 2014 Jun;24(3):145–153.

Gokhale SG, Scorer T, Doughty H. Freedom from frozen: The first British military use of lyophilised plasma in forward resuscitation. *J R Army Med Corps* 2016 Feb;162(1):63–65.

Gregg, R, Boutefnouchet, T, Steadman, J et al. An evaluation of predictive scores for massive transfusion in a trauma cohort clinically judged to be at high risk of major haemorrhage. *Haematologica* 2013;98(Suppl 1):189.

Gregg R, Boutefnouchet T, Tidman J et al. An evaluation of Predictive Scores for Massive Transfusion in a trauma cohort clinically judged to be at high risk of major haemorrhage. *Transfus Med* 2013;23(Suppl 2):S137.

Gregg R, Boutefnouchet T, Tidman J Dought H. An evaluation of the influence of major transfusion protocol design on the ability of trauma teams to predict massive transfusion. *Vox Sanguinis* 2013 Jun;105(Suppl 1):25–26.

Heier HE, Badloe J, Bohonek M et al. Use of tranexamic acid in bleeding combat casualties. *Mil Med* 2015 Aug;180(8):844–846.

Hennessy EP, Green AD, Connor MP et al. Norwalk virus infection and disease is associated with ABO histo-blood group type. *J Infect Dis* 2003 Jul;188(1):176–177.

Hervig T, Doughty H, Ness P et al. Prehospital use of plasma: The blood bankers' perspective. *Shock* 2014 May;41(Suppl 1):39–43.

Hodgetts TJ, Mahoney PF, Kirkman E et al. UK Defence Medical Services guidance for use of recombinant factor VIIa (rFVIIa) in the deployed military setting. *J R Army Med Corps* 2007 Dec;153(4):307–309.

Holcomb JB, Jenkins D, Rhee P et al. Damage control resuscitation: Directly addressing the early coagulopathy of trauma. *J Trauma Acute Care Surg* 2007 Feb;62(2):307–310.

Hunt BJ, Woolley T, Parmar K, et al. Haemostatic changes following military trauma and major blood loss. *J Thromb Haemost* 2013:11 (Suppl 2):672.

Jansen JO, Morrison JJ, Midwinter MJ, Doughty H. Changes in blood transfusion practices in the UK role 3 medical treatment facility in Afghanistan, 2008–2011. *Transfus Med* 2014 Jun;24(3):154–161.

Jenkins DH, Rappold JF, Badloe JF et al. Trauma hemostasis and oxygenation research position paper on remote damage control resuscitation: Definitions, current practice and knowledge gaps. *Shock* 2014 May;41 (Suppl 1):3–12.

Kirkman E, Watts S, Hodgetts T et al. A Proactive approach to the coagulopathy of trauma: The rationale and guidelines for treatment. *J R Army Med Corps* 2007 Dec;153(4):302–306.

Mercer SJ, Tarmey NT, Woolley T et al. Haemorrhage and coagulopathy in the Defence Medical Services. *Anaesthesia* 2013 Jan;68(Suppl 1):49–60.

Modgil K, Doughty H. Blood brothers at TEDxBrum. *Bull R Coll Pathol* 2015 Jan;169:10.

Moor P, Rew D, Midwinter MJ, Doughty H. Editorial. Transfusion for trauma: Civilian lessons from the battlefield? *Anaesthesia* 2009;64(5):469–472.

Morrison JJ, Ross JD, Dubose JJ et al. Association of cryoprecipitate and tranexamic acid with improved survival following wartime injury: Findings from the MATTERs II Study. *JAMA Surg* 2013 Mar;148 74(3):218–225.

Neff LP, Cannon JW, Morrison JJ et al. Clearly defining pediatric massive transfusion: Cutting through the fog and friction with combat data. *J Trauma Acute Care Surg* 2015 Jan;78(1):22–28.

O'Reilly DJ, Morrison JJ, Jansen JO et al. Initial UK Experience of Prehospital Blood Transfusion in Combat Casualties. *J Trauma Acute Care Surg* 2014 Sep;77(3 Suppl 2):S66–S70.

O'Reilly DJ, Morrison JJ, Jansen JO et al. Prehospital blood transfusion in the en route management of severe combat trauma: A matched cohort study. *J Trauma Acute Care Surg* 2014:77;(3 Suppl 2):S114–S20.

Parker P, Nordmann G, Doughty H. Taking transfusion forward. *J R Army Med Corps* 2015;161(1):2–4.

Scorer T, Doughty H. Acute transfusion reactions: An update. *J R Nav Med Serv* 2014;100(3):316–320.

Smith JE, Fawcett R, Randalls B. The Use of recombinant activated factor VII in a patient with penetrating chest trauma and ongoing pulmonary hemorrhage. *Mil Med* 2012;177(5):614–616.

Smith JE. The use of recombinant activated factor VII (rFVIIa) in the management of patients with major haemorrhage in military hospitals over the last 5 years. *Emerg Med J* 2013;30:316–319.

Starkey K, Keene,D, Morrison JJ et al. Impact of high ratios of plasma-to-red-cell-concentrate on the incidence of acute respiratory distress syndrome in UK transfused combat casualties. *Shock* 2013;40(1):15–20.

Strandenes G, Berséus O, Cap AP et al. Low titer group O whole blood in emergency situations. *Shock* 41(Suppl 1):70–75.

Tappenden J. Artificial blood substitutes. *J R Army Med Corps* 2007;153(1):3–9.

Tarmey N, Woolley T, Jansen JO et al Evolution of coagulopathy monitoring in military damage-control resuscitation. *J Trauma Acute Care Surg* 2012;73:S417–S422.

Thomas D, Wee M, Clyburn P et al. Blood transfusion and the anaesthetist: Management of massive haemorrhage. *Anaesthesia* 2010 Nov;65(11):1153–1161.

Thomas R, Woolley T, Doughty H. Guidelines on massive transfusion. Emergency guidelines for ACDS(H) on behalf of DoH. Preparation for 2012 Olympics. 2012.

Tidman J, Doughty H. Implementation and revision of a massive transfusion protocol. *Transfus Med* 2010;20(Suppl s1):15–16.

Watts S, Nordmann G, Brohi K et al. Evaluation of prehospital blood products to attenuate acute coagulopathy of trauma in a model of severe injury and shock in anesthetized pigs. *Shock* 2015 Aug;44:138–148.

Wild G, Anderson D Lund P. Round Afghanistan with a fridge. *J R Army Med Corps* 2013;159(1):24–29.

Williams DJ, Thomas GO, Pambakian S et al. First military use of activated Factor VII in an APC-III pelvic fracture. *Injury* 2005 Mar;36(3):395–399.

Woolley T, Hunt BJ, Parmar K et al. Haemostatic changes following military trauma and major blood loss, *J Thromb Haemost* 2013;11(S2):290–1019.

Woolley T, Badloe J, Bohonek M et al. NATO Blood Panel Perspectives on changes to military pre-hospital resuscitation policies: Current and future practice. *Transfusion* 2016 Apr;56(Suppl 2):S217–S223.

TRAUMA SCORING, GOVERNANCE, DATA ANALYSIS AND MODELLING

Batham DR. Clinical governance on Operation Herrick 9 – A personal perspective. *J R Nav Med Serv* 2011;97(2):50–55.

Batham DR, Wall CM. An audit of the quality of deployed DMICP records on Operation HERRICK 14. *J R Army Med Corps* 2012 Sep;158(3):213–216.

Breeze J, Fryer R, Hare J et al. Clinical and post mortem analysis of combat neck injury used to inform a novel coverage of armour tool. *Injury* 2015 Apr;46(4):629–633.

Bricknell MCM. Reporting Clinical activity on military operations – Time for some standardisation. *J R Army Med Corps* 2005 Sep;151(3):142–144.

O'Connell KM, Littleton-Kearney MT, Bridges E, Bibb SC. Evaluating the Joint Theater Trauma Registry as a data source to benchmark casualty care. *Mil Med* 2012 May;177(5):546–552.

Cross JD, Wenke JC, Ficke JR, Johnson AE. Data-driven disaster management requires data: Implementation of a military orthopaedic trauma registry. *J Surg Orthop Adv* 2011 Spring;20(1):56–61.

Fowler M, Slater TM, Garza TH et al. Relationships between early acute pain scores, autonomic nervous system function, and injury severity in wounded soldiers. *J Trauma* 2011 Jul;71(1 Suppl):S87–S90.

Gross KR, Rickard RF, Eastridge BJ et al. Review of the Fifth Annual Joint Theater Trauma System Trauma Conference. *J Trauma Acute Care Surg* 2015 Jun;79 (4 Suppl 2):S70–S74.

Hawley CA, de Burgh HT, Russell RJ, Mead A. Traumatic brain injury recorded in the UK joint theatre trauma registry among the UK Armed Forces. *J Head Trauma Rehabil* 2015 Jan–Feb;30(1):E47–E56.

Hewitt-Smith A. The use of clinical audit during a successful medical engagement in Afghanistan. *J R Army Med Corps* 2012 Sep 158(3):259–262.

Hodgets TJ, Davies S, Midwinter M et al. Operational Mortality of UK service personnel in Iraq and Afghanistan: A one year analysis 2006–7. *J R Army Med Corps* 2007 Dec;153(4):252–254.

Hodgetts TJ, Davies S, Russell R, McLeod J. Benchmarking the UK military deployed trauma system. *J R Army Med Corps* 2007 Dec;153(4):237–238.

Horn O, Sloggett A, Ploubidis GB et al. Upward trends in symptom reporting in the UK Armed Forces. *Eur J Epidemiol* 2010 Feb;25(2):87–94.

Keene DD, Penn-Barwell JG, Wood P et al. Died of Wounds: A mortality review. *J R Army Med Corps* 2016 Oct;162(5):355–360.

Lewin IJS. Contingency: The likely spectrum of injuries based upon a review of three recent undeveloped theatres of operations – Corporate, Telic 1 and Herrick 4. *J R Nav Med Serv* 2014;100(1):40–43.

Mann-Salinas EA, Le TD, Shackelford SA et al. Evaluation of Role 2 (R2) medical resources in the Afghanistan combat theater: Initial review of the Joint Trauma System R2 Registry. *J Trauma Acute Care Surg* 2016 Nov;8(5 Suppl 2; Proceedings of the 2015 Military Health System Research Symposium):S121–S127.

Marsden ME, Sharrock AE, Hansen CL et al. British Military surgical key performance indicators: Time for an update? *J R Army Med Corps* 2016 Oct:162(5):373–378.

Martin M, Oh J, Currier H et al. An analysis of in-hospital deaths at a modern combat support hospital. *Trauma Acute Care Surg* 2009 Apr;66(4):S51–S61.

McLeod J, Hodgetts T, Mahoney P. Combat "Category A" calls: Evaluating the pre-hospital timelines in a military trauma system. *J R Army Med Corps* 2007 Dec;153(4):266–268.

Mossadegh S, Midwinter M, Parker P. Developing a cumulative anatomic scoring system for military perineal and pelvic blast injuries. *J R Army Med Corps* 2013 Mar;159(Suppl 1):i40–i44.

Ollerton J, Hodgetts T, Russell R. Operational morbidity analysis of soft tissue injuries during Operation Telic. *J R Army Med Corps* 2007;153(4):263–265.

Ollerton JE, Hodgetts TJ. Operational morbidity analysis: Ophthalmic presentations during Operation Telic. *J R Army Med Corps* 2010;156(1):37–40.

Penn-Barwell JG, Fries CA, Bennett PM et al. Mortality, survival and residual injury burden of Royal Navy and Royal Marine combat casualties sustained in 11-years of operations in Iraq and Afghanistan. *J R Nav Med Serv* 2014;100(2):161–165.

Penn-Barwell JG, Roberts SAG. Midwinter M. Improved survival in UK combat casualties from Iraq and Afghanistan: 2003–2012 *J Trauma Acute Care Surg* 2015 May;78(5):1014–1020.

Pinder R, Boyko E, Gackstetter G et al. Profile of two cohorts: UK and US prospective studies of military health. *Int J Epidemiol* 2012;41(5):1272–1282.

Ramasamy A, Harrisson S, Lasrado I, Stewart MPM. A review of casualties during the Iraqi insurgency 2006 – A British field hospital experience. *Injury* 2009 May;40(5):493–497.

Russell R, Hodgetts T, Ollerton J et al. The Operational Emergency Department Attendance Register: A new epidemiological tool. *J R Army Medical Corps* 2007;153(4):244–250.

Russell R, Hodgetts T, Macleod J et al. The role of trauma scoring in developing trauma clinical governance in the Defence Medical Services. *Philos Trans R Soc* 2011;366:171–191.

Russell R, Hunt N, Delaney R. The Mortality Peer Review Panel: A report on the deaths on operations of UK Service personnel 2002–2013. *J R Army Med Corps* 2014;160(2):150–154.

Singleton JA, Gibb IE, Bull AM et al. Primary blast lung injury prevalence and fatal injuries from explosions: Insights from postmortem computed tomographic analysis of 121 improvised explosive device fatalities. *J Trauma Acute Care Surg* 2013 75(2 Suppl 2):S269–S274.

Singleton JA, Gibb IE, Hunt NC et al. Identifying future 'unexpected' survivors: A retrospective cohort study of fatal injury patterns in victims of improvised explosive devices. *BMJ Open* 2013;3:e003130 doi 10.1136/bmjopen_2013-003130

Smith JE, Hodgetts T, Mahoney P et al. Trauma governance in the UK Defence Medical Services. *J R Army Med Corps* 2007;153(4):239–242.

Smith IM, Naumann DN, Guyver P et al. Inter-observer variability in injury severity scoring after combat trauma: Different perspectives, different values? *J Spec Oper Med* 2015 Summer;15(2):86–93.

Stannard A, Bowley DM, Tai NR et al. Mechanism and profile of fatal injury in modern counter insurgency warfare. *Br J Surg* 2007;94(S2):73.

Stannard A, Tai NR, Bowley DM et al. Key performance indicators in British Military trauma. *World J Surg* 2008 Aug;32(8):1870–1873.

Starkey KJ, Hodgetts TJ, Russell R, Mahoney PF. Combat trauma survival: Where is the proof of good outcome? *J R Army Med Corps* 155(3):226–232.

Therien SP, Nesbitt ME, Duran-Stanton AM, Gerhardt RT. Prehospital medical documentation in the Joint Theater Trauma Registry: A retrospective study. *J Trauma* 2011 Jul;71(1 Suppl):S103–S108.

Tubb CC, Oh JS, Do NV et al. Trauma care at a multinational United Kingdom-led role 3 combat hospital: Resuscitation outcomes from a multidisciplinary approach. *Mil Med* 2014;179(11):1258–1262.

Ward NJ, Okpala E. Analysis of 47 road traffic accident admissions to BMH Shaibah. *J R Army Med Corps* 2005 Mar;151(1):37–40.

Willdridge DJ. Hodgetts TJ, Mahoney PF et al. The Joint Theatre Clinical Case Conference (JTCCC): Clinical governance in action. *J R Army Med Corps* 2010 Jun;156(2):79–83.

TRAUMATIC AMPUTATION

Brown KV, Ramasamy A, McLeod J et al. Predicting the need for early amputation in ballistic mangled extremity injuries. *J Trauma* 2009 Apr;66(4 Suppl):S93–S98.

Brown KV, Dharm-Datta S, Potter BK et al. Comparison of development of heterotopic ossification in injured US and UK armed services personnel with combat-related amputations: Preliminary findings and hypotheses regarding causality. *J Trauma* 2010 Jul;69(1):S116–S122.

Brown KV, Clasper JC. The changing pattern of amputations. *J R Army Med Corps* 2013 Dec;159(4):300–303.

Clasper J, Amputations of the lower limb: A multidisciplinary consensus. *J R Army Med Corps* 2007 Sep;153(3):172–174.

Cross AM, Davis C, Penn-Barwell J et al. The incidence of pelvic fractures with traumatic lower limb amputation in modern warfare due to improvised explosive devices. *J R Nav Med Serv* 2014;100(2):152–615.

Eardley WG, Taylor DM, Parker PJ. Amputation and the assessment of limb viability: Perceptions of two hundred and thirty two orthopaedic trainees. *Ann R Coll Surg Engl* 2010 Jul;92(5):411–416.

Guyver PM, Mountain AJC, Jeffery SLA. Application of topical negative pressure for traumatic amputations. *Ann R Coll Surg Engl* 2013 Apr;95(3):226–227.

Jacobs N, Rourke K, Hicks A et al. Lower limb injuries caused by improvised explosive devices: Proposed "Bastion" classification and prospective validation. *Injury* 2014 Sep;45(9):1422–1428.

Jansen JO, Thomas GOR, Adams SA et al. Early management of proximal traumatic lower extremity amputation and pelvic injury caused by improvised explosive devices (IEDs). *Injury* 2012 Jul;43(7):976–979.

Kinch KJ, Clasper JC. A brief history of war amputation. *J R Army Med Corps* 2011 Dec;157(4):374–380.

Ladlow P, Phillip R, Etherington J et al. Functional and mental health status of United Kingdom military amputees post rehabilitation. *Arch Phys Med Rehabil* 2015 Nov;96(11):2048–2054.

Ladlow P, Phillip R, Coppack R et al. Influence of immediate and delayed lower-limb amputation compared with lower-limb salvage on functional and mental health outcomes post-rehabilitation UK military. *J Bone Joint Surgery Am* 2016;98:1996–2005.

Morrison JJ, Hunt N, Midwinter M, Jansen J. Associated injuries in casualties with traumatic lower extremity amputations caused by improvised explosive devices. *Br J Surg* 2012 Mar;99(3):362–366.

Morrison JJ, Rasmussen TE, Midwinter MJ, Jansen JO. Authors' reply: Associated injuries in casualties with traumatic lower extremity amputations caused by improvised explosive devices (letter). *Br J Surg* 2012 Jul;99:1021.

Penn-Barwell JG, Bennett PM, Kay A et al. Acute bilateral leg amputation following combat injury in UK servicemen. *Injury* 2014 Jul;45(7):1105–1110.

Penn-Barwell JG, Myatt RW, Bennett PM et al. Medium-term outcomes following limb salvage for severe open tibia fracture are similar to trans-tibial amputation. *Injury* 2015 Feb;46(2):288–291.

Singleton JA, Gibb IE, Bull AM, Clasper JC. Blast-mediated traumatic amputation: Evidence for a revised, multiple injury mechanism theory. *J R Army Med Corps* 2014;160(2):175–179.

Singleton JA, Walker NM, Gibb IE et al. Case suitability for definitive through knee amputation following lower extremity blast trauma: Analysis of 146 combat casualties, 2008–2010. *J R Army Med Corps* 2014;160:187–190.

TRAUMATIC CARDIAC ARREST

Bhangu A, Nepogodiev D, Bowley D. Outcomes following military traumatic cardiorespiratory arrest: The role of surgery in resuscitation. *Resuscitation* 2013 Jan;84(1):e23–e24.

Hillman CM, Rickard A, Rawlins M, Smith JE. Paediatric traumatic cardiac arrest: Data from the Joint Theatre Trauma Registry. *Emerg Med J* 2014;31(9):790.

Hillman CM, Rickard A, Rawlins M, Smith JE. Paediatric traumatic cardiac arrest: Data from the Joint Theatre Trauma Registry. *J R Army Med Corps* 2016 Aug;162(4)276–279.

Kinnear-Mellor R, Newton K, Woolley T, Rickard R. Predictive utility of cardiac ultrasound in traumatic cardiac arrest in a combat casualty. *J R Army Med Corps* 2016 Feb;162(1):68–70.

Morrison JJ, Poon H, Rasmussen TE. Re: Traumatic cardio-respiratory arrest on the battlefield (letter). *J Trauma Acute Care Surg* 2013 Aug;75(2):343–345.

Smith JE, Hunt PAF, Le Clerc S. Challenging the dogma of traumatic cardiac arrest management: A military perspective. *Emerg Med J* 2015;32:955–960.

Stansfield T, Hill G, Louden M et al. Right turn or pause at the crossroads? 2010 Military Surgery Meeting (abstract). *J R Army Med Corps* 2010;156(3):183.

Tai NRM, Russell R. Right Turn Resuscitation: Frequently asked questions. *J R Army Med Corps* 2011;157(3 Suppl 1):S310–S314.

Tarmey N, Park C, Bartels O et al. Outcomes following military traumatic cardiorespiratory arrest; a prospective observational study. *Resuscitation* 2011;82(9):1194–1197.

UROLOGY AND ANDROLOGY

Calderbank P, Porter K, Anderson P et al. Urethral injury due to blast: A new pattern (abstract)? *J R Army Med Corps* 2010 Sep;156(3):183.

Davendra MS, Webster CE, Kirkman-Brown J et al. Genitouirnary Working group (Trauma). Blast injury to the perineum. *J R Army Med Corps* 2013 Mar;159(Suppl 1):i1–i3.

Durrant JJ, Ramasamy A, Salmon MS et al. Pelvic fracture-related urethral and bladder injury. *J R Army Med Corps* 2013 Mar;159(Suppl 1): i132–i139.

Frappell-Cooke W, Wink P, Wood A. The psychological challenge of genital injury. *J R Army Med Corps* 2013 Mar;159(Suppl 1):i52–i56.

Hill NE, Woods DR, Delves SK et al. The gonadotrophic response of Royal Marines during an operational deployment in Afghanistan. *Andrology* 2015 Mar;3(2):293–297.

Jones GH, Bowley D. Traumatic andropause after combat injury: A rare phenomenon. 2010 Military Surgery Meeting (abstract). *J R Army Med Corps* 2010 Sep;156(3):183.

Jones GH, Kirkman-Brown J, Sharma DM, Bowley D. Traumatic andropause after combat injury. *BMJ Case Rep* 2015 Aug;2015. doi: 10.1136 /bcr-2014-207924

Lewis E, Pigott MA, Randall A, Hepper AE. The development and introduction of ballistic protection of the external genitalia and peritoneum. *J R Army Med Corps* 2013 Mar;159(Suppl 1):i15–i17.

Lucas PA, Page PR, Phillip RD, Bennett AN. The impact of genital trauma on wounded servicemen: Qualitative study. *Injury* 2014 May;45(5):825–829.

Mossadegh S, Midwinter M, Parker P. Developing a cumulative anatomic scoring system for military perineal and pelvic blast injuries. *J R Army Med Corps* 2013 Mar;159(Suppl 1):i40–i44.

Mossadegh S, Midwinter M, Parker P, Improvised explosive device-related pelvi-perineal trauma: UK military experience, literature review and lessons for civilian trauma teams (editorial). *Bull R Coll Surg Engl* 2013 Oct;95(9):1–5.

Mossadegh S, He S, Parker P. Bayesian scoring systems for military pelvic and perineal blast injuries: Is it time to take a new approach? *Mil Med* 2016 May;181(5 Suppl):127–131.

Rushambuza, R. The role of diagnostic CT imaging in the acute assessment of battlefield external genital injuries. *J R Army Med Corps* 2013;159:(Suppl 1):i21–i25.

Sharma DM, Genitourinary Working Group (Trauma). The management of genito-urinary war injuries: A multidisciplinary consensus. *J R Army Med Corps* 2013;(Suppl 1):57–59.

Sharma DM, Bowley DM. Immediate surgical management of combat-related injury to the external genitalia. *J R Army Med Corps* 2013 Mar;159(Suppl 1):i18–i20.

Sharma DM, Webster CE, Kirkman-Brown et al. Blast injury to the perineum. *J R Army Med Corps* 2013 159 (Suppl):i1–i13.

Uppal L, Anderson P, Evriviades D. Complex lower genitourinary reconstruction following combat related injury. *J R Army Med Corps* 2013 Mar;159(Suppl 1):i49–i51.

Watchorn JC, Standley DM, Smith JE et al. The initial management of complete urethral disruption in a deployed military field hospital. *Injury Extra* 2012:43:65–67.

Williams RJ, Fries CA, Midwinter M et al. Battlefield scrotal trauma: How should it be managed in a deployed military hospital? *Injury* 2013 Sep;44(9):1246–1249.

Woods DR, Phillip R, Quinton R. Managing endocrine dysfunction following blast injury to the male external genitalia. *J R Army Med Corps* 2013 Mar;159(Suppl 1):45–48.

VASCULAR

Brown KV, Tai N, Midwinter M, Clasper JC. Ballistic extremity vascular injuries. Abstract – Military surgery 2008. *J R Army Med Corps* 2008 Sep;154(3):188.

Brown KV, Ramasamy, A, Tai N, Clasper J. Complications of extremity vascular injuries in conflict. *J Trauma* 2009 Apr;66(4):S145–S149.

Dua A, Via KC, Kreishman P et al. Early management of pediatric vascular injuries through humanitarian surgical care during U.S. military operations. *J Vasc Surg* 2013;58(3):695–700.

Jeevaratnam JA, Exton R, Cubison TC. The vascular supply of muscles in war injuries: A century on. *Eur J Plast Surg* 2014;37(7):409–410.

Markov NP, DuBose JJ, Scott D et al. Anatomic distribution and mortality of arterial injury in the wars in Afghanistan and Iraq with comparison to a civilian benchmark. *J Vasc Surg* 2012 Sep;56(3):728–736.

Poon H, Morrison JJ, Clasper JC et al. Use and complications of operative control of arterial inflow in combat casualties with traumatic lower-extremity amputations caused by improvised explosive devices. *J Trauma Acute Care Surg* 2013 Aug;75(2 Suppl 2):S233–S237.

Stannard A, Benson C, Bowley DM et al. Central vascular injuries in deployed military personnel: A contemporary experience. *J R Army Med Corps* 2008;154(3):188.

Stannard A Burkhardt G, Keltz et al. Quality of limb salvage following wartime extremity vascular injury: Results of a novel patient-based outcomes study (abstract). *J R Army Med Corps* 2010;156(3):178.

Stannard A, Brown K, Benson C et al. Outcome after vascular trauma in a deployed military trauma system. *Br J Surg* 2011 Feb;98(2):228–234.

Stannard A, Scott DJ, Ivatury RA et al. A collaborative research system for functional outcomes following wartime extremity vascular injury. *J Trauma Acute Care Surg* 2012;73(2):S7–S12.

Stannard JJ, Brown K, Benson C et al. Vascular trauma: Survivability and surgical outcome in a deployed military trauma system. *Br J Surg* 2009;96(S1):6–6(1).

Villamaria CY, Morrison JJ, Fitzpatrick CM et al. Wartime vascular injuries in the pediatric population of Iraq and Afghanistan: 2002–2011. *J Pediatr Surg* 2014 Mar;49(3):428–432.

Walker NM, Eardley W, Clasper JC. UK combat-related pelvic junctional vascular injuries 2008–2011: Implications for future intervention. *Injury* 2014 Oct;45(10):1585–1589.

Watson JDB, Houston R, Morrison JJ et al. A retrospective cohort comparison of expanded polytetrafluoroethylene to autologous vein for vascular reconstruction in modern combat casualty care. *Ann Vasc Surg* 2015;29:822–829.

White JM, Rasmussen TE, Clouse WD et al. Vascular injury rates from the wars in Iraq and Afghanistan (abstract). *J R Army Med Corps* 2010;156(3):179.

White JM, Stannard A, Burkhardt GE et al. The epidemiology of vascular injury in the wars in Iraq and Afghanistan. *Ann Surg* 2011;253(6):1184–1189.

VETERANS' AFFAIRS

Buckman J, Forbes H, Clayton T et al. early service leavers: A study of the factors associated with premature separation from the UK Armed Forces and the mental health of those that leave early. *Eur J Public Health* 2013 Jun;23(3):410–415.

Burdett H, Greenberg N, Fear NT and Jones N. The mental health of military veterans in the UK. *International Psychiatry* 2014;11(4):86–87.

Cross JD, Johnson AE, Wenke JC et al. Mortality in female war veterans of operations enduring freedom and Iraqi freedom. *Clin Orthop Relat Res* 2011 Jul;469(7):1956–1961.

Dandeker C, Wessely S, Iversen A et al. What's in a name? Defining and caring for 'veterans': The United Kingdom in International Perspective. *Armed Forces Soc* 2006 Jan;32(2):161–177.

Doll D, Bowley DM. Veterans' health-surviving acute injuries is not enough. *Lancet* 2008 Mar;371(9618):1053–1055.

French DD, Bair MJ, Bass E et al. Central nervous system and musculoskeletal medication profile of a veteran cohort with blast-related injuries. *J Rehabil Res Dev* 2009;46(4):463–468.

Greenberg N. What's so special about military veterans? *Int Psych* 2014;11(2):79–80.

Gribble R, Wessely S, Klein S et al. Public awareness of UK veterans' charities. *RUSI J* 2014 Feb;159(1):50–57.

Hacker-Hughes J, Abdul-Hamid WK, Fossey MJ. Flash to bang: Psychological trauma, veterans and military families: Can services cope? *J R Army Med Corps* 2015 Dec;161(4):298–299.

Iversen A, Dyson C, Smith N et al. "Goodbye and Good Luck": The mental health needs and treatment experiences of British ex Service personnel. *Br J Psychiatry* 2005 Jun;186:480–486.

Iversen A, Nicolaou V, Greenberg N et al. What happens to British veterans when they leave the Armed Forces? *Eur J Public Health* 2005 Apr;15(2):175–184.

Iversen A, Greenberg N. Mental health of regular and reserve military veterans. *Adv Psychiatr Treat* 2009;15:100–106.

MacManus D, Wessely S. Why do some ex-armed forces personnel end up in prison? *BMJ* 2011 Jun;342:d3898.

MacManus D, Wessely S. Veteran mental health services in the UK: Are we headed in the right direction? *J Ment Health* 2013 Aug;22(4):301–305.

MacManus D, Fossey M, Watson S, Wessely S. Former Armed Forces personnel in the Criminal Justice System. *Lancet Psychiatry* 2014 Dec;2(2):121–122.

Murphy D, Iversen A, Greenberg N. The mental health of veterans. *J R Army Med Corps* 2008 Jun;154(2):136–139.

Murphy D, Hodgman G, Carson C et al. Mental health and functional impairment outcomes following a 6-week intensive treatment programme for UK military veterans with post-traumatic stress disorder (PTSD): A naturalistic study to explore dropout and health outcomes at follow-up. *BMJ Open* 2015 Mar;5(3). doi: 10.1136/bmjopen-2014-007051

Murphy D, Weijers B, Palmer E, Busuttil W. Exploring patterns in referrals to combat stress for UK veterans with mental health difficulties between 1994 and 2014. *Int J Emerg Mental Health Hum Resilience* 2015;17(3):652–658.

Murphy D. Detailing the clinical pathways at Combat Stress for UK veterans experiencing symptoms of complex post traumatic stress disorder. *Healthcare Couns Psychother J* 2016;14(1):24–27.

Stevelink SA, Malcolm EM, Mason C et al. The prevalence of mental health disorders in (ex-) military personnel with a physical impairment: A systematic review. *Occup Environ Med* 2014;72(4):243–251.

Stevelink SA, Malcolm EM, Fear NT. Visual impairment, coping strategies and impact on daily life: A qualitative study among working-age UK ex-service personnel. *BMC Public Health* 2015 Nov;15:1118.

Stevelink SA, Malcolm EM, Gill PC et al. The mental health of UK ex-servicemen with a combat-related or a non-combat-related visual impairment: Does the cause of visual impairment matter? *Br J Ophthalmol* 2015 Aug;99(8):1103–1108.

Stevelink SA, Fear NT. Psychosocial impact of visual impairment and coping strategies in female ex-Service personnel. *J R Army Med Corps* 2016 Apr;162(2):129–133.

Woodhead C. An estimate of the veteran population in England: Based on data from the 2007 Adult Psychiatric Morbidity Survey. *Population Trends* 2009;138(1):50–54.

WOUNDS AND WOUND MANAGEMENT

Barton SJ, Kaleel S, Rayatt S, Peart F. Healing Hands: Management of a shrapnel wound injury in the dominant hand of a serviceman, sustained in the Iraq conflict (abstract). *J R Army Med Corps* 2005 Mar;151(2):108.

D'Avignon LC, Chung KK, Saffle JR et al. Prevention of infections associated with combat-related burn injuries. *J Trauma* 2011 Aug;71(2 Suppl 2):S282–S289.

Eardley WG, Watts SA, Clasper JC. Limb wounding and antisepsis: Iodine and chlorhexidine in the early management of extremity injury. *Int J Low Extrem Wounds* 2012 Sep;11(3):213–223.

Evriviades D, Jeffery S, Cubison T, Lawton G, Gill M, Mortiboy D. Shaping the military wound: Issues surrounding the reconstruction of injured servicemen at the Royal Centre for Defence Medicine. *Trans R Soc Lond B Biol Sci* 2011 Jan;366(1562):219–230.

Foong DP, Evriviades D, Jeffery SL. Integra™ permits early durable coverage of improvised explosive device (IED) amputation stumps. *J Plast Reconstr Aesthet Surg* 2013 Dec;66(12):1717–1724.

Forgione MA, Moores LE, Wortmann GW; Prevention of Combat-related Infections Guidelines Panel. Prevention of infections associated with combat-related central nervous system injuries. *J Trauma* 2011 Aug;71 (2 Suppl 2):S258–S263.

Fries CA, Jeffery SL, Kay AR. Topical negative pressure and military wounds – A review of the evidence. *Injury* 2011 May;42(5):436–440.

Fries CA, Ayalew Y, Penn-Barwell JG et al. Prospective randomised controlled trial of nanocrystalline silver dressing versus plain gauze as the initial post-debridement management of military wounds on wound microbiology and healing. *Injury* 2014 Jul;45(7):1111–1116.

Guthrie HC, Clasper JC, Kay AR, Parker PJ; Limb trauma and wounds working groups. Initial extremity war wound debridement: A multidisciplinary consensus. *J R Army Med Corps* 2011 Jun;157(2):170–175.

Guyver PM, Mountain AJC, Jeffery SLA. Application of topical negative pressure for traumatic amputations. *Ann R Coll Surg Engl* 2013 Apr;95(3):226–227.

Hankin E, Jeffery S. Challenges of treating modern military trauma wounds. *Wounds Int* 2011;2(2):7–12.

Hospenthal DR, Green AD, Crouch HK. Prevention of Combat-Related Infections Guidelines Panel. Infection prevention and control in deployed military medical treatment facilities. *J Trauma* 2011 Aug;71(2 Suppl 2):S290–S298.

Hospenthal DR, Murray CK, Andersen, RC et al. guidelines for the prevention of infections associated with combat-related injuries: 2011 Update: Endorsed by the Infectious Diseases Society of America and the Surgical Infection. *J Trauma Acute Care Surg* 2011 Aug;71(2):S210–S234.

Hutley EJ, Green AD. Infection in wounds of conflict – Old lessons and new challenges. *J R Army Med Corps* 2010 Dec;155(4):315–319.

Jeffery SLA. Advanced wound therapies in the management of severe military lower limb trauma: A new perspective. *Eplasty* 2009 Jul;9(28):266–277.

Jeffery SLA. Current burn wound management. *Trauma* 2009 Dec;11:241–248.

Jeffery SLA. Exudate monitoring in traumatic wounds. *Wounds UK* 2013;9(2):40–44.

Jeffery SLA. The Management of combat wounds: The British Military experience. *Adv Wound Care* 2016 Oct;5(10):464–473.

Jones A, Morgan D, Walsh A et al. Importation of multidrug-resistant *Acinetobacter* spp infections with casualties from Iraq. *Lancet Infect Dis* 2006 Jun;6(6):317–318.

Long VS. Jeffery SLA. Using topical negative pressure in a military field hospital. *Wounds UK* 2012;22(8):244–245.

Martin GJ, Dunne JR, Cho JM, Solomkin JS: Prevention of Combat-related Infections Guidelines Panel. Prevention of infections associated with combat-related thoracic and abdominal cavity injuries. *J Trauma* 2011 Aug;71(2 Suppl 2):S270–S281.

Matheson A, Hutley E, Green AD. The evolving challenge of war wounds *Microbiologist* 2011;12(4):26–29.

Murray CK, Obremskey WT, Hsu JR et al. Prevention of infections associated with combat-related extremity injuries. *J Trauma* 2011;71:S235–S257.

Neal PK. An exploration of the experiences of wound healing in military traumatic amputees and its impact on their rehabilitation. *J R Army Med Corps* 2015;161(Suppl):i64–i68.

Penn-Barwell J, Fries C, Street C et al. Use of topical negative pressure therapy in patients with high energy combat wounds – A case series. *JBJS* 2011;93:51–52.

Penn-Barwell JG, Fries CA, Street L, Jeffery S. Use of topical negative pressure in British servicemen with combat wounds. *ePlasty* 2011;11:e35.

Penn-Barwell JG, Fries CA, Sargeant ID et al. Aggressive soft tissue infections and amputation in military trauma patients. *J R Nav Med Serv* 2012;98(2):14–18.

Poon H, Le Cocq H, Mountain A, Sargeant I. 'Dermal fenestration' with negative pressure wound therapy: A new technique for managing the soft tissue injury associated with high-energy complex foot fractures. *J Foot Ankle Surg* 2015 Oct;55(1):161–165

Russell F, Jeffery S. Use of Renasys™ gauze and port to simplify negative pressure dressing techniques. *Wounds UK* 2010;6:125–130.

Savage JM Jeffery SLA. Use of 3D photography in complex-wound assessment. *J Wound Care* 2013 Mar;22(3):156, 158–160.

Staruch R, Jeffery S. Variable topical negative pressure therapy for wound care. *Wounds UK* 2011:7;26–33.

St Mart JP, Jeffery S, Clark J. Using negative pressure wound therapy to manage severe military trauma wounds. *Wounds UK* 2009:5:56–64.

Taylor C, Jeffery SLA. Management of military wounds in the modern era. *Wounds UK* 2009:5:50–58.

Taylor CJ, Hettiaratchy S, Jeffery SL et al. Contemporary approaches to definitive extremity reconstruction of military wounds. *J R Army Med Corps* 2009 Dec;155(4):302–307.

Appendix E: Extracts from the key findings of the CQC Report *Defence Medical Services: A Review of Compliance with the Essential Standards of Quality and Safety*

PRIMARY HEALTHCARE MEDICAL SERVICES DEPLOYED OPERATIONS (AFGHANISTAN)

Outcome 4: Care and welfare of people who use services

The primary healthcare medical services in Afghanistan were fully compliant with this standard. There were no minor concerns. The services were judged compliant as we found that military personnel and entitled civilians had efficient and quick access to a range of excellent primary healthcare and medical emergency services delivered by well trained, committed and competent staff.

The range of primary healthcare services included health needs assessment, screening and treatment, occupational health, dental services, rehabilitation, community mental health services and health promotion and emergency services. Patients were involved in their plan of care and treatment options, and risks and benefits were fully explained. Patients reported that they received clear information from the medical centre staff and were confident in the teams providing care and treatment.

Outcome 6: Cooperating with other providers

The primary healthcare medical services in Afghanistan were fully compliant with this standard. There were no minor concerns. The services were judged compliant as we found that patients who either had accidents, were injured or became ill whilst on military operations, received effective and well coordinated primary healthcare services. This included health promotion and education as well as treatment, delivered by teams of specialist staff working effectively together. Relevant information was shared in a confidential way and services providing medical transfer and transport worked and trained together to provide effective and well coordinated services.

Outcome 9: Management of medicines

The primary healthcare medical services in Afghanistan were compliant with this standard. However, there were, some minor concerns relating to communication difficulties, which did at times impact on the timely prescribing of medication. Medication storage in some of the forward operating bases did not always fully meet policy requirements. Risk assessments and actions to mitigate against risk were in place. We judged the service to be compliant as we found that medicines were handled safely, securely and appropriately. Patients were given clear information about medicines. The use, effect and possible side-effects of all medication was well explained to patients. Staff had access to relevant policies and clinical guidance and support.

Outcome 16: Assessing and monitoring the quality of service provision

The services in Afghanistan were compliant with this standard. However, there were some minor concerns about keeping medical records up to date when treatment was provided outside the main primary healthcare medical centre, and with the connectivity with IT recording systems for medical records in the UK. At times, operational issues caused communication delays between the primary healthcare medical centre and the forward operating bases. Nevertheless, services were judged compliant as we found that there was a culture of continuous improvement, which was promoted and supported. There was an audit lead and committee that oversaw audit and ongoing evaluation of services. The outcomes from these activities were used to change and improve services and to advise and educate Service personnel. Patients using the primary healthcare services provided regular feedback about the services they used, which was used to make improvements to services. Staff were supported through a network of clinical supervision. Services identified the risks of working in hostile and remote conditions and took action to mitigate or remove risks as far as possible.

HOSPITAL HEALTHCARE DEPLOYED OPERATIONS (AFGHANISTAN)

Outcome 4: Care and welfare of people who use services

The hospital services in Afghanistan were fully compliant with this standard. There were no

minor concerns. The services were judged compliant as we found that patients experienced exemplary hospital treatment, care and support. Fundamental to this was the multi-disciplinary approach to effective team working from all the staff we encountered. The hospital provided intensive care and high-dependency facilities, as well as surgical, medical and accident and services. The hospital had an extensive range of diagnostic testing facilities, including access to a well-equipped, X-ray department with computerised tomography (CT) scanners and laboratory facilities. The hospital was designed primarily to manage and provide acute resuscitation and damage control surgery for battle injury casualties. Non-battle injuries resulting from accidents or illness were also treated. We considered the provision of trauma care to be exemplary. The hospital was UK-led, but multinational in its staffing complement. This included clinicians from the USA and Denmark working alongside the predominantly territorial army field hospital unit, who were staffing and managing the hospital at the time of the inspection visit. Patients told us that they were impressed with the care they had received and by the instruction and information that was shared with them about their care and treatment.

Outcome 5: Meeting nutritional needs

The hospital services in Afghanistan were fully compliant with this standard. There were no minor concerns. The service was judged compliant as we found that patients were supported to have adequate nutrition and hydration. The hospital provided choices of food and drink for patients to meet their diverse needs, ensuring that the food they provided was nutritionally balanced and supported their health. The hospital could cater for special diets.

Outcome 6: Cooperating with other providers

The hospital services in Afghanistan were fully compliant with this standard. There were no minor concerns. We found that patients received safe and coordinated care, treatment and support where more than one provider was involved or where patients were moved between services. The care and treatment provided within the field hospital involved a range of clinical and clinical support staff at every stage of the patient pathway. These staff worked very closely together and developed systems so that the care provided was both seamless and integrated. Regular clinical meetings were held to review and monitor patients within the hospital and those transferred to the UK for further treatment.

Outcome 8: Cleanliness and infection control

The hospital services in Afghanistan were fully compliant with this standard. There were no minor concerns. The hospital was clean, well-lit and well maintained. There were appropriate arrangements in place to safely manage infection prevention and control. These included regular monitoring and auditing, clear cleaning schedules, protective clothing for staff and training for staff. Patients were protected against the risk of exposure to infections through the systems and processes in place.

Outcome 9: Management of medicines

The hospital services in Afghanistan were fully compliant with this standard. There were no minor concerns. The hospital was keeping patients and staff safe by having systems in place to ensure that medicines were managed and handled safely and securely. Systems were in place for auditing and monitoring medicines and staff had access to relevant policies and guidance, training and clinical support.

DEFENCE MEDICAL REHABILITATION CENTRE

Outcome 1: Respecting and involving people who use services

The Defence Medical Rehabilitation Centre was fully compliant with this standard. There were no minor concerns. Patients benefited from a working ethos that promoted their right to be treated with dignity and consideration, and that promoted privacy, understanding and confidentiality. Patients understood the care, treatment and the support available to them. They were able to express their views, which were taken into account in the way the services were provided. The patients we spoke with in the centre were very positive in relation to patient respect and involvement, services meeting their needs and making informed choices about their healthcare.

Outcome 4: Care and welfare of people who use services

The Defence Medical Rehabilitation Centre was compliant with this standard. However, there were some minor concerns that some patients were distressed at having to relocate from their accommodation from one ward to another at weekends. Other patients said that they felt there was a need for medical boards to receive more direction to assist with grading and continued treatment. The centre was judged as compliant because patients experienced effective and appropriate care tailored to meet their individual needs. The use of the social model of disability, with its emphasis on ability and independence, allowed patients to take risks, to build confidence and to attain their full rehabilitation potential. Patients felt they received a high standard and quality of care from a committed and competent team of staff.

Outcome 6: Co-operating with other providers

The Defence Medical Rehabilitation Centre was fully compliant with this standard with no minor concerns. Patients received coordinated care, treatment and support where more than one provider was involved, or when they were moved between services. Staff had developed very effective relationships with a number of healthcare providers, government departments and charitable organisations to work in cooperation with others. This provided coordinated care, treatment and support when patients received services from other organisations.

Outcome 14: Supporting workers

The Defence Medical Rehabilitation Centre was fully compliant with this standard with no minor concerns. Staff had access to training, support and supervision, and guidance for the care and treatment of patients. We found that well-planned induction programmes were in place for all military and civilian staff. Safe recruitment processes for the employment of locum staff were in place. Training needs were identified, staff attended the required mandatory training and they received regular supervision and appraisals. We found well-led and well-managed teams of staff, and staff felt supported and confident in their roles. The patients we spoke with in the centre were very positive about the competence of staff providing the services and the help and support they received.

Outcome 16: Assessing and monitoring the quality of service provision

The Defence Medical Rehabilitation Centre was fully compliant with this standard. There were no minor concerns. Processes and systems were in place to manage risks and influence decision-making so that patients benefited from safe, quality, care, treatment and support. These included programmed audits, risk assessment and risk registers, research programmes, implementing relevant clinical guidelines and patient feedback systems. Clear governance arrangements were in place. Staff in the centre were involved in training to develop treatment and rehabilitation services, not just at the centre, but throughout the rehabilitation services. Staff were aware of their roles and responsibilities for the safety and continuous improvement of services. The defence medical rehabilitation centre had strong and effective clinical and managerial leadership.

REGIONAL REHABILITATION UNITS

Outcome 1: Respecting and involving people who use services

All the regional rehabilitation units inspected were judged as compliant with this standard. There was

a minor concern in one of the units, which related to the age and layout of the building and the inadequate accommodation for patients attending rehabilitation treatment programmes. A further minor concern related to the lack of immediate accessibility of all patient information on the electronic patient record system. In the regional rehabilitation units inspected, we found that patients were fully involved in their rehabilitation programme. Patients were given sufficient information to understand the care, treatment and support choices available to them and to manage their illnesses or injuries. Their privacy and dignity was respected and systems were in place to take account of their views and experiences to influence the way services were provided. The patients interviewed in the regional rehabilitation units were very positive about services meeting their needs and in providing information about their current and future healthcare needs.

Outcome 4: Care and welfare of people who use services

All of the regional rehabilitation units we inspected were judged as fully compliant with this standard. We found that patients were fully involved in the planning and monitoring of their treatment plans. Their needs were thoroughly assessed by a multidisciplinary team of staff to ensure that there was clear diagnosis of their needs and a tailored treatment plan implemented. We found that patients experienced effective and appropriate individual care and treatment programmes. The patients interviewed in the regional rehabilitation units were very positive about the level of individual support they received and the quality of treatment provided.

Outcome 6: Cooperating with other providers

All the regional rehabilitation units inspected were judged as fully compliant with this standard. We found that patients received coordinated care, treatment and support where more than one provider was involved, or where patients were moved between services. Regional rehabilitation units had developed effective working relationships with a number of other service providers across the NHS for investigations and specialist healthcare treatment.

Outcome 14: Supporting workers

All the regional rehabilitation units inspected were judged as fully compliant with this standard. Staff working in these units had access to a range of training and development opportunities to develop and maintain their knowledge and practice. Staff felt well-supported, and received regular supervision and appraisals. Patients attending the regional units for treatment were confident that care was delivered by competent teams of staff.

Outcome 16: Assessing and monitoring the quality of service provision

All the regional rehabilitation units we inspected were judged as fully compliant with this standard. We found that patients benefitted from treatment and support as there were effective processes in place to manage risks and monitor hoe services were delivered. Planned programmes of audit activity were in place, risk registers were used to effectively manage risks, and feedback from patients was used to inform and develop practice. Staff were aware of their responsibilities for the safety and quality of care and treatment. We found these units to be very well-led and managed.

Appendix F: Summary of the report *Treating Injury and Illness arising on Military Operations* National Audit Office 2010

SUMMARY

1. A total of 522 personnel have been seriously injured on operations in Iraq and Afghanistan between October 2001 and the end of October 2009.1 On operations, personnel have attended medical facilities some 125,000 times for minor injury and illness2 since 2006, and a further 1,700 for mental health conditions. Some 6,900 people have been evacuated back to the UK from Iraq and Afghanistan since 2003 for serious injuries and a range of other medical conditions. The nature of the very serious injuries suffered by some personnel necessitates long and complex treatment and rehabilitation; they and their families may face considerable life-long challenges. We have estimated that the cost of medical care as a result of military operations was £71 million in 2008-09.

2. Medical support is key to the psychological and physical well-being of military personnel on operations and underpins morale and physical capability. The Ministry of Defence (the Department) aims, as part of its duty of care, to deliver the highest possible standards of treatment to those deployed on operations. Not all injuries occur as a direct result of battle. A significant number of personnel need treatment for illnesses such as gastrointestinal disorders and non-battlefield injuries, including those incurred during accidents or physical training.

3. This report assesses the Department's provision of medical care to Service personnel who were injured or suffered health problems, mental or physical, resulting from operations in Iraq and Afghanistan. We focused on the level of medical care provided, whether it is timely, sufficient and is available on an appropriate scale. We assessed the impact of minor injuries and illness in terms of "manpower days lost", a simple measure of the impact on operational capability. We have not examined clinical judgements or the management of individual patients' care.

4. In examining the Department's treatment of those seriously injured on operations we focused on the effectiveness of medical support, in particular:

   - Measures of the success of treatment in saving lives
   - Speed of evacuation from the battlefield, and back to the UK
   - Capability of the field hospital to stabilise major trauma casualties
   - Capacity of medical care and rehabilitation back in the UK.

5. For minor injury, illness and mental healthcare we examined:
   - Trends in overall rates on operations and, for mental health, following deployment;
   - The balance of healthcare delivered at forward bases, in the field hospital and in the UK
   - Mental health support in place for personnel on operations.

We have not examined services for veterans. The majority of personnel seriously injured on operations in Iraq and Afghanistan have not, to date, completed their treatment within the Department's rehabilitation services. We attempted to compare medical treatment with that of coalition forces but a lack of published data seriously limited our analysis.

SERIOUS INJURY

5. *The quality of trauma care on operations is demonstrated by the numbers of "unexpected survivors", who would usually be expected to die given the severe nature of their injuries.* Through mathematical modelling and clinical peer review, the Department has identified 75 unexpected UK, coalition and local survivors from Iraq and Afghanistan between April 2006 and July 2008. We calculate the rate of unexpected survivors as a proportion of all seriously injured survivors to be up to 25 per cent. The Department's and the NHS' methodology for calculating unexpected survivors differs and so a direct comparison is not easy, but ostensibly its unexpected survivor rate compares favourably with that achieved by the best NHS hospitals. Over the same period, the number of deaths identified among UK personnel that could be avoided, given the operational circumstances, is very low.

6. *The strength of the Department's clinical care on operations has been underpinned by a clear focus on trauma care for the seriously wounded and a number of other factors, in particular:*
   - The field hospital being designed specifically to deal with trauma casualties
   - Trauma teams being consultant-led and multi-disciplinary
   - Strong performance in rapidly evacuating casualties from the battlefield to the field hospital
   - Numerous developments in first-aid practices and technologies, and in the protocols for treating major trauma
   - Strong clinical governance

7. *The field hospital in Afghanistan is close to capacity but has been able to manage casualty levels.* The Department determines the levels of staff and facilities required using several factors including the size of population served, casualty estimates, the availability of coalition medical facilities, the distribution of deployed forces and predicted rates of minor injury and illness. The Department formally reviews capacity at the field hospital every six months as part of operational planning and, to meet demand, increased medical staff numbers from 2006 and facilities in 2009. The Department's August 2009 review concluded that, following the latest increases, resources are sufficient but the hospital continued to be close to capacity. The field hospital has increased capacity further for short periods of high casualty levels by using contingent equipment, such as ventilators, and calling off-duty medical staff to assist.

8. *The Department will need to manage the potential impact of the future Regional Trauma Networks on the clinical experience of military medical personnel deploying in future.* Regional Trauma Networks are to be introduced in the NHS, where a hospital in each region will be an identified major trauma centre. When not on operations, military medical staff maintain their clinical skills working in the NHS, the majority in six Trusts hosting military hospital units. Some of these Trusts may not become major trauma centres and therefore will receive fewer complex trauma patients.

9. Seriously injured personnel evacuated to the UK are treated in the NHS, the majority at Selly Oak hospital, under a contract between the Department and University Hospital Birmingham Foundation Trust. The vast majority of patients then move to the Department's rehabilitation facility, Headley Court, Surrey. The medical care and rehabilitation of personnel who have been seriously injured on military operations is a long, complex process. *Military commanders and the patients to whom we spoke have confidence in*

the clinical treatment at Selly Oak and Headley Court.

10. *Casualty numbers from military operations are placing increasing demands on Selly Oak and Headley Court but have been managed to date by taking measures to increase capacity for these patients.* To manage increased levels of military casualties, some civilian care at Selly Oak has been outsourced to private providers and other NHS facilities, and agency staff and bed numbers have increased at Headley Court. Military casualties peaked in July 2009, and consequently took one-third of Selly Oak's 90 trauma and orthopaedic ward beds and the military-managed ward reached 80 per cent of capacity. Throughout 2009, the number of operational patients at Headley Court exceeded the 28 beds originally set aside for complex trauma but not overall bed numbers.

11. *Current contingency plans for providing further capacity have recently improved but there is scope for further development.* The Department has a joint plan with the Department of Health outlining how capacity to deal with high and sustained levels of military casualties could be enhanced. Contingency planning for increased casualty levels has recently been strengthened through the development of a voluntary regional agreement to continue to treat military patients at Selly Oak by diverting some civilian trauma patients to other hospitals in the region. The Department is currently reviewing its contingency plan with the Department of Health. There is scope for improvement, for example by modelling the capacity required under different casualty scenarios and defining clear indicators for when each level of contingency would be required. The Department has developed contingency plans to expand the provision of rehabilitation for seriously injured patients by providing Headley Court-led services in other existing rehabilitation centres and constructing more ward space.

MINOR INJURY AND ILLNESS

12. *A certain level of disease and minor injury is expected on military operations. However, rates in Afghanistan have almost doubled from 4 to 7 per cent of deployed personnel per week between 2006 and 2009, although they remain within the Department's planning assumption of up to 10 per cent.* The rate of digestive disorders has also more than doubled in Afghanistan over the same period. There are particular spikes around the six-monthly rotations of deployed units. The increase in minor injury and illness in-theatre between October 2006 and September 2009 represents a financial cost of some £0.7 million and a small reduction in operational capability of 6,700 days lost. However, there is a risk that operational capability will be reduced further if rates continue to rise.

13. *Rising rates of disease and minor injury demonstrate that the Department needs to do more to assess which prevention measures should be improved to halt the increase.* There are likely to be several contributing factors to the increase, including the basic living conditions at some forward operating bases, the intensity of operations and improved reporting. However, the Department's data do not allow it to quantify the significance of any individual factor. The Department seeks to control levels of disease and minor illness in several ways.

14. *Some evacuated personnel have completed treatment within a short period on return to the UK.* For example, our analysis shows 13 per cent of treatment for musculoskeletal injuries is completed within two weeks of evacuation. This illustrates the need for the Department to assess whether it could be more cost-effective to provide more treatment and rehabilitation on operations where it is possible to deliver equivalent treatment.

MENTAL HEALTH

15. *The Department has taken several steps to provide support on operations to personnel at risk of developing mental health conditions but there are weaknesses in follow-up for those who deploy individually.* The Department deploys mental health specialists and a small proportion of personnel are referred to this specialist psychiatric support while on operations (0.2 per cent in Afghanistan; 0.8 per cent in Iraq in 2008-09). The Department does not routinely

screen personnel on return from operations, and relies on personnel seeking help and the non-medical stress management processes it has introduced for personnel on, and following, deployment. There is inconsistent access to non-medical stress management processes on return to the UK for personnel who deploy individually rather than as part of a unit or who move units following deployment. The Department is currently developing its stress management processes to address this problem.

DATA

16. *The clinical governance and audit of major trauma on operations is good but the Department does not collect or analyse all required medical data relating to operations.* The Department holds regular conference calls discussing patient cases, collects data to identify unexpected survivors and avoidable deaths, and military medical research has supported developments in trauma care. The Department generally has the data it needs for day-to-day management of individual patients; however, it is unable to assess fully the impact of operations on the health of Service personnel. The Department could do more analysis with the data it collects on outcomes, treatment timelines and on injury and illness rates, including benchmarking with coalition partners. To support this, data collection needs to be improved further and some steps are being taken to do so. The Department does not seek to identify or analyse the full costs of treating operational casualties.

VALUE FOR MONEY CONCLUSION

17. The Department's clinical treatment and rehabilitation of the seriously injured is highly effective. The Department has a clear focus on providing a high level of care and rehabilitation to seriously injured personnel on operations and in the UK, and outcomes achieved are good relative to the seriousness of injuries sustained.

18. The Department's attention has understandably focused on treating seriously injured personnel. The Department takes steps to minimise the level of minor injury and illness on operations.

However, preventive measures currently in place have not been sufficient to halt the rising trend – from four to seven per cent in Afghanistan between 2006 and 2009. This trend represents a small reduction in operational capability. To date, the rate has remained within the Department's planning assumption but it is the rise which is of concern as, should it persist, it presents a risk to value for money through the continued reduction in operational capability. Preventing illness is intuitively more cost-effective than the associated costs of evacuation and treatment, and would minimise the impact on capability, but the Department has not assessed the relative costs and benefits of improving specific prevention measures.

19. The Department has improved its patient data and now generally has the data it needs for day-to-day management. However, the Department has not done enough analysis to understand fully whether its healthcare system is optimised to provide effective medical care that is value for money and to manage future risks to delivery. In particular:

The Department has not modelled potential demand for secondary care and rehabilitation, and there is scope to improve contingency planning further to ensure that future capacity could deal effectively with high and sustained numbers of casualties.

The Department has not analysed treatment timelines or collected adequate information on the costs of delivering care, which would enable it to make better decisions on the most cost-effective models of care.

RECOMMENDATIONS

20. Against this background we make the following recommendations:

a. *The numbers of serious battlefield casualties have increased since 2006, and contingency plans to extend capacity at Selly Oak and Headley Court have been strengthened.* As part of its ongoing work to improve further its contingency planning, the Department should model the capacity required under different casualty scenarios. Specifically for secondary care, the Department should build on the clear decision-making structures in place by:

– Establishing clear indicators of when each level of contingency should be enacted

– Determining which categories of patient should remain at Selly Oak

– Defining the most appropriate destination for categories of military patients if treated nationally

– Assessing how experience in treating military trauma would be transferred in those cases.

For rehabilitation, the Department should assess the feasibility of its contingency plans for increasing the capacity of Regional Rehabilitation Units to take more operational patients.

b. *The rate of minor injury and illness has almost doubled in three years although it remains within the Department's planning assumption.* The Department needs to take further steps to halt the rising trend through:

– Researching systematically why the rate of minor injury and illness has increased

– Improving prevention, identifying the most cost-effective prevention measures and developing alternative means for delivering environmental health at forward positions

– Strengthening governance for minor injuries and illness, for example through introducing weekly conference calls to discuss performance.

The Department should also assess the benefit of treating more minor injuries on operations, including through enhancing rehabilitation services at the field hospital, rather than evacuating personnel to the UK, although this would need to be balanced against the cost and impact on UK care.

c. *The Services have non-medical stress management processes to oversee personnel at risk of developing mental health problems during and following deployment, and encourage them to seek treatment. These processes are more difficult to deliver to personnel who do not deploy as part of a regular formed unit or who move to a new unit after deployment.* The Department should

implement stress management processes for these personnel.

d. The Department is currently unable to assess fully the impact of operations on the health of Service personnel because it does not centrally collate accurate and complete medical data. There is also scope for the Department to make greater use of its existing data to support decisions on further developments in care. The Department should:

– Improve further its medical data, including consistently recording where military operations are the primary cause of an injury or illness, and addressing the variability of data entry, including on operations (recognising this is most feasible in the field hospital)

– Analyse available data to identify and understand the cause of long-term trends in disease and minor injury, and benchmark performance and practices against coalition partners

– Collate the costs of medical support required as a result of operations

– Identify research and benchmarking required to support further improvements in medical care and rehabilitation, including making better use of the varied existing information sources to monitor the efficiency of treatment and rehabilitation for specific conditions, and benchmarking performance on unexpected survivors.

e. *The future introduction of Regional Trauma Networks in the NHS may impact on the clinical experience military medical staff obtain because some of the Trusts where the majority work may not become a major trauma centre.* Given that its current contracts end in 2011, the Department now needs to assess the impact of Regional Trauma Networks on the clinical experience and professional development of its medical staff and consider options for alternative locations for maintaining the clinical experience of military medical staff, if necessary. This assessment should also take into account the potential benefits to the NHS of sharing military trauma experience.

Appendix G: Campaigns in Iraq and Afghanistan reading list

The lists here represent only a small selection of the books written about the campaigns in Iraq and Afghanistan. With the exception of the official reports, they tend to fall into the categories of analysis (both political and military) and memoir. Both groups should be approached with circumspection. It is inevitable that the analysis of such controversial events risks authorial bias and memoirs are inevitably personal. No single book offers a rounded perspective, but taken together, they offer a nuanced picture of the conflicts: why they were fought, how they were fought and what it was like to fight them.

OFFICIAL REPORTS

Chilcot, Sir John. *The Iraq Inquiry*. 6 July 2016. http://www.iraqinquiry.org.uk/. Known as the Chilcot Report, this definitive report examines in detail the decisions that led to the UK invading Iraq in 2003.

Forbes, Sir Thayne. *The Report of Al Sweady Inquiry*. December 2014. https://www.gov.uk/government/uploads/system/uploads/attachment_data/file/388292/Volume_1_Al_Sweady_Inquiry.pdf

Gage, Sir William. *The Report of the Baha Mousa Inquiry*. 2011. https://www.gov.uk/government/uploads/system/uploads/attachment_data/file/279190/1452_i.pdf

Lessons Exploitation Centre. *Operation HERRICK Campaign Study* (British Army: Directorate Land Warfare, 2015) Redacted version available at https://www.gov.uk/government /uploads/system/uploads/attachment_data /file/492757/20160107115638.pdf

Ministry of Defence. *Operations In Iraq – First Reflections*. 7 July 2003. http://www.globalsecurity.org/military/library/report/2003/iraq2003operations_ukmod_july03.pdf

Ministry of Defence. *Operation Telic – United Kingdom Military Operations In Iraq*. National Audit Office, 11 December 2003. https://www.nao.org.uk/wp-content /uploads/2003/12/030460.pdf

Ministry of Defence. *The Fight for Iraq (January–June 2003) – The British Army's Role in Liberating a Nation: A Pictorial Account*. London: Ministry of Defence, 2004.

Ministry of Defence. *Operations in Iraq, January 2005–May 2009 (Op TELIC 5-13) An Analysis from a Land Perspective*. London: MOD 29 November 2010, released to the public September 2016.

GENERAL

Bailey J, Iron R, Strachan H (Eds). *British Generals in Blair's Wars*. Farnham: Ashgate, 2013.

Barry, B. *Harsh Lessons – Iraq, Afghanistan and the Changing Character of War* Abingdon: Routledge, for International Institute for Strategic Studies, 2017.

Collins D. *In Foreign Fields – Heroes of Iraq and Afghanistan in Their Own Words*. Reading: Monday Books, 2007.

Dannatt R. *Leading from the Front*. Bantam, 2010.

Dannatt R. *Boots on the Ground: Britain and Her Army since 1945*. London: Profile Books, 2017.

Elliott, C. *High Command – British Military Leadership in the Iraq and Afghanistan Wars*. London: Hurst & Company, 2015.

Jackson M. *Soldier: The Autobiography*. London: Corgi, 2008.

Ledwidge F. *Losing Small Wars. British Military Failure in Iraq and Afghanistan*. New Haven, CT: Yale University Press, 2011; new edition 2017.

Richards D. *Taking Command*. London: Headline, 2014.

IRAQ

Beharry, J (with Nick Cook). *Barefoot Soldier – A Story of Extreme Valour*. London: Sphere, 2006.

Cockburn P. *The Occupation: War and Resistance in Iraq*. London: Verso, 2007.

Cockburn P. *Muqtada al Sadr and the Fall of Iraq*. Faber and Faber, 2008.

Docherty L. *Desert of Death*. London: Faber and Faber, 2007.

Fairweather J. *A War of Choice: Honour, Hubris and Sacrifice: The British in Iraq*. London: Jonathan Cape, 2011.

Fox R. *Iraq Campaign 2003 – Royal Navy and Royal Marines*. London: Agenda Publishing, 2003.

Greenstock J. *Iraq – The Cost of War*. London: William Heinemann, 2016.

Holmes R. *Dusty Warriors*. London: Harper Perennial, 2007 (1 PWRR).

Ivison K. *Red One – A Bomb Disposal Expert on the Front Line*. London: Weidenfeld & Nicolson, 2010.

Keegan J. *The Iraq War*. London: Hutchinson, 2004.

Mills D. *Sniper One*. London: Michael Joseph, 2007 (1 PWRR).

Mockaitis TR. *Iraq and the Challenge of Counterinsurgency*. Westport, CT: Praeger, 2008.

Newsinger J. *British Counterinsurgency*. 2nd ed. Basingstoke: Palgrave Macmillan, 2015.

Nicol M. *Last Round*. London: Weidenfeld & Nicolson, 2005.

Nicol M. *Iraq – A Tribute to Britain's Fallen Heroes*. Edinburgh: Mainstream Publishing, 2008.

Nicol M. *Condor Blues – British Soldiers at War*. Edinburgh: Mainstream Publishing, 2007.

North R. *Ministry of Defeat – The British War in Iraq 2003–2009*. London: Continuum, 2009.

Ricks TE. *Fiasco: The American Military Adventure in Iraq*. London: Penguin, 2007.

Ripley T. *Operation TELIC – The British Campaign in Iraq 2003–2009*. Lancaster, UK: Telic-Herrick Publications, 2016. www.operationtelic.co.uk

Stewart R. *Occupational Hazards: My Time Governing in Iraq*. London: Picador, 2007.

Synnott H. *Bad Days in Basra: My Turbulent Time as Britain's Man in Southern Iraq*. London: I B Tauris, 2008.

Ucko DH, Egnell R. *Counterinsurgency in Crisis – Britain and the Challenges of Modern Warfare*. New York: Columbia University Press, 2015.

Williams AT. *A Very British Killing – The Death of Baha Mousa*. London: Jonathan Cape, 2012.

AFGHANISTAN

Allen C. *With the Paras in Helmand – A Photographic Diary*. Barnsley: Pen & Sword, 2010.

Annet R. *Lifeline in Helmand. RAF Battlefield Mobility in Afghanistan*. Barnsley: Pen & Sword, 2010.

Barry B. *Harsh Lessons – Iraq, Afghanistan and the Changing Character of War*. Abingdon: Routledge, for International Institute for Strategic Studies, 2017.

Beattie DMC. *An Ordinary Soldier*. London: Simon and Schuster, 2009.

Benitz M. *Six Months without Sundays: The Scots Guards in Afghanistan*. Edinburgh: Birlinn, 2011.

Bishop P. *3 Para*. London: Harper Perennial, 2007.

Bishop P. *Ground Truth*. London: Harper Perennial, 2009 (3 Para).

Black Watch. *Aviation Assault Battle Group*. Barnsley: Pen & Sword Military, 2011.

Bury P. *Callsign Hades*. London: Simon & Schuster, 2010 (Royal Irish Regiment).

Cartwright J. *Sniper in Helmand*. Barnsley: Pen & Sword, 2011 (Royal Anglian Regt).

Cowper-Coles S. *Cables from Kabul: The Inside Story of the West's Afghanistan Campaign.* London: Harper Press, 2012.

Dannatt R. *Leading from the Front.* London: Bantam, 2010.

Doherty R. *Helmand Mission – With the Royal Irish Battlegroup in Afghanistan 2008.* Barnsley: Pen & Sword, 2009.

Dorney R. *The Killing Zone.* London: Ebury, 2012 (Grenadier Guards).

Evans M. *Code Black: Cut off and Facing Overwhelming Odds: The Siege of Nad Ali.* London: Coronet, 2015 (Coldstream Guards).

Evans M (with Sharples A). *Under the Bearskin: A Junior Officer's Story of War and Madness.* London: Coronet, 2017 (Coldstream Guards).

Fairweather J. *The Good War – Why We Couldn't Win The War or the Peace in Afghanistan.* London: Jonathan Cape, 2014.

Farrell T, Osinga F, Russell JA (Eds.). *Military Adaptation in Afghanistan.* Stanford, CA: Stanford University Press, 2013.

Farrell T. *Unwinnable – Britain's War in Afghanistan 2001–2014.* London: Bodley Head, 2017.

Fergusson J. *A Million Bullets: The Real Story of the British Army in Afghanistan.* London: Bantam, 2008.

Grey S. *Operation Snakebite: The Explosive True Story of an Afghan Desert Siege.* London: Penguin Books, 2010 (2 Yorks).

Hammond MDFC. *Immediate Response.* London: Penguin, 2010.

Harnden T. *Dead Men Risen: The Welsh Guards and the Real Story of Britain's War in Afghanistan.* London: Quercus, 2011.

Hennessy P. *The Junior Officers' Reading Club.* London: Allen Lane, 2009; Penguin, 2010 (Grenadier Guards).

Hennessy P. *Kandak: Fighting with Afghans.* London: Allen Lane, 2012.

Jakobsen PV, Thruelsen PD. *Clear, Hold, Train: Denmark's Military Operations in Helmand 2006–2010.* Copenhagen: Danish Foreign Policy Yearbook, 2011.

Kemp R, Hughes C. *Attack State Red.* London: Michael Joseph, 2009 (Royal Anglian Regt).

Kiley S. *Desperate Glory: At War in Helmand with Britain's Air Assault Brigade.* London: Bloomsbury, 2009.

Lewis R. *Company Commander.* London: Virgin, 2012 (2 Para).

Lothian G. *An Artist in Afghanistan.* Helensburgh: Cranston Fine Arts, 2015.

Mayhew E. *A Heavy Reckoning: War, Medicine and Survival in Afghanistan and Beyond.* London: Wellcome Collection, 2017.

Mercer J. *We Were Warriors: One Soldier's Story of Brutal Combat.* London: Sidgwick & Jackson, 2017 (29 Commando Regiment Royal Artillery).

Monty B. *A Sniper's Conflict.* Barnsley: Pen & Sword, 2014.

Neville L. *The British Army in Afghanistan 2006–14. Task Force Helmand.* Oxford: Osprey Publishing, 2015.

Nicol J. *Medic.* London: Penguin 2009.

Ormrod M. *Man Down.* London: Bantam Press, 2009 (40 Cdo Royal Marines).

Parker H. *Anatomy of a Soldier.* London: Faber & Faber, 2016.

Reynolds D. *Afghanistan Britain's War in Helmand – An Historical Account.* Plymouth, UK: DRA Publishing, 2017.

Southeby-Tailyour E. *3 Commando Brigade: Helmand Assault.* London: Ebury, 2010.

Streatfeild R. *Honourable Warriors – Fighting the Taliban in Afghanistan.* Barnsley: Pen & Sword, 2015 (The Rifles).

Tootal S. *Danger Close: Commanding 3 PARA in Afghanistan.* London: John Murray, 2009.

Index

Page numbers followed by f and t indicate figures and tables, respectively.

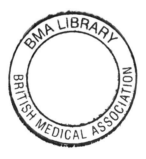

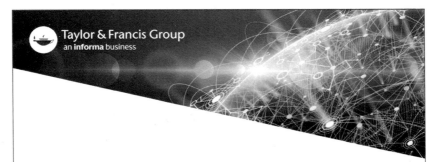